THE LYMPHOMAS

THE LYMPHOMAS

GEORGE P. CANELLOS,
MD, FRCP
William Rosenberg Professor
  of Medicine
Harvard Medical School
Dana-Farber Cancer Institute
Boston, Massachusetts

T. ANDREW LISTER,
MD, FRCP, FRCPath
Professor of Medical Oncology
  and Director
ICRF Medical Oncology Unit
Department of Medical
  Oncology
St. Bartholomew's Hospital
West Smithfield
London, England

JEFFREY L. SKLAR,
MD, PhD
Professor of Pathology
Harvard Medical School

Director, Divisions of
  Molecular Oncology and
  Diagnostic Molecular
  Biology
Brigham and Women's Hospital
Boston, Massachusetts

W.B. SAUNDERS COMPANY
A Division of Harcourt Brace & Company
Philadelphia   London   Toronto   Montreal   Sydney   Tokyo

W.B. SAUNDERS COMPANY
A Division of Harcourt Brace & Company

The Curtis Center
Independence Square West
Philadelphia, Pennsylvania 19106

Library of Congress Cataloging-in-Publication Data

The lymphomas / [edited by] George P. Canellos, T. Andrew Lister,
Jeffrey L. Sklar. — 1st ed.

    p.   cm.

    ISBN 0–7216–5030–9

    1. Lymphomas.   I. Canellos, George P. (George Peter)
II. Lister, T. A. (Thomas Andrew)   III. Sklar, Jeffrey L.
    [DNLM: 1. Lymphoma.   WH 525 L9852 1998]
    RC280.L9L953   1998   616.99′446—dc21

DNLM/DLC   97–22034

THE LYMPHOMAS

ISBN 0–7216–5030–9

Printed in the United States of America.

Last digit is the print number: 9   8   7   6   5   4   3   2   1

Contributors

James O. Armitage, MD
Professor and Chair, Department of Internal Medicine, University of Nebraska Medical Center
Omaha, Nebraska
Bone Marrow Transplantation for Malignant Lymphoma; Peripheral T-Cell Lymphoma

Clara D. Bloomfield, MD
William G. Pace III Professor of Cancer Research; Director, Comprehensive Cancer Center; Deputy Director, Arthur G. James Cancer Hospital and Research Institute; and Director, Division of Hematology and Oncology, Ohio State University Medical Center, Columbus, Ohio
Major Cytogenetic Findings in Non-Hodgkin's Lymphoma

Beverly Buck, BS
Instructor in Radiation Therapy, Harvard Medical School; Education and Development Coordinator, Joint Center for Radiation Therapy, Boston, Massachusetts
Principles of Radiation Therapy for Lymphomas

George P. Canellos, MD, FRCP
William Rosenberg Professor of Medicine, Harvard Medical School, Dana-Farber Cancer Institute, Boston, Massachusetts
Hodgkin's Disease

Ronald A. Castellino, MD
Chairman Department of Radiology, Memorial Sloan Kettering Cancer Center, New York, New York; Professor of Radiology, Cornell University Medical College, New York
Diagnostic Radiology

Bruce A. Chabner, MD
Professor of Medicine, Harvard Medical School; Chief, Department of Medical Hematology and Oncology, Massachusetts General Hospital, Boston, Massachusetts
Principles of Chemotherapy for Lymphomas

Bertrand Coiffier, MD
Professor of Hematology, Université Claude Bernard; Head, Department of Hematology, Centre Hospitalier Lyon Sud, Lyon, France
Non-Hodgkin's Lymphoma in Elderly Patients; Lymphoma and Pregnancy

Derek Crowther, PhD, MB B Chir, MSe, FRCP, FRCR
Professor and Director, Department of Medical Oncology, Manchester University; Director of Medical Oncology, Christie Hospital, Manchester, England
Biologic Therapy for Lymphomas

Riccardo Dalla-Favera, MD
Professor of Pathology and Genetics and Development, Columbia University College of Physicians and Surgeons, New York, New York
The Biology of High-Grade Non-Hodgkin's Lymphoma

N. Dhedin, MD
Physician, Centre Hospitalier Lyon Sud, Lyon, France
Lymphoma and Pregnancy

Horst Dürkop, MD
Klinikum Benjamin Franklin (Universitätsklinikum Benjamin Franklin), Berlin, Germany
Biology of Hodgkin's Disease

Howard A. Fine, MD
Assistant Professor of Medicine, Harvard Medical School, Dana-Farber Cancer Institute, Boston, Massachusetts
Primary Central Nervous System Lymphoma

Richard I. Fisher, MD
Professor of Medicine, Loyola University Medical Center, Stritch School of Medicine; Director, Oncology Institute, and Director, Hematology/Oncology, Loyola University Medical Center, Maywood, Illinois
Diffuse Large Cell and Immunoblastic Lymphomas

Hans-Dieter Foss, MD
Klinikum Benjamin Franklin (Universitätsklinikum Benjamin Franklin), Berlin, Germany
Biology of Hodgkin's Disease

Gianluca Gaidano, MD, PhD
Assistant Professor, Division of Internal Medicine, Department of Medical Sciences, University of Torino at Novara, Novara, Italy
The Biology of High-Grade Non-Hodgkin's Lymphoma

Ellen R. Gaynor, MD
Associate Professor of Medicine, Loyola University Stritch School of Medicine, Maywood, Illinois
Diffuse Large Cell and Immunoblastic Lymphomas

Mary K. Gospodarowicz, MD, FRCPC
Professor, Department of Radiation Oncology, University of Toronto School of Medicine; Ontario Cancer Institute/Princess Margaret Hospital, Toronto, Ontario, Canada
Primary Extranodal Lymphomas

Henrik Griesser, MD
Professor, Department of Pathology, Julius-Maximilians
University; Chief, Division of Applied Cytology,
Institute of Pathology, University Medical Center,
Würzburg, Germany
*Developmental and Functional Biology of B and T
Lymphocytes*

Thomas M. Grogan, MD
Professor of Pathology and Head of Hematopathology,
University of Arizona Medical Center, Tucson, Arizona
Immunohistochemistry of Lymphomas

Hermann Herbst, MD
University Hospital Eppendorf Institute of Pathology,
Hamburg, Germany
Biology of Hodgkin's Disease

Richard T. Hoppe, MD
Henry S. Kaplan–Harry Lebeson Professor of Cancer
Biology and Chairman, Department of Radiation
Oncology, Stanford University, Stanford, California
*Mycosis Fungoides and Other Cutaneous
Lymphomas*

Michael Hummel, PhD
Klinikum Benjamin Franklin (Universitätsklinikum
Benjamin Franklin), Berlin, Germany
Biology of Hodgkin's Disease

Elaine S. Jaffe, MD
Chief, Hematopathology Section, and Deputy Chief,
Laboratory of Pathology, National Cancer Institute,
National Institutes of Health, Bethesda, Maryland
*Histopathology of the Non-Hodgkin's Lymphomas
and Hodgkin's Disease*

Eva Klein, MD
Professor, Research Group Leader, Microbiology and
Tumor Biology Center, Karolinska Institute, Stockholm,
Sweden
Epstein-Barr Virus and Human Lymphomas

George Klein, MD, DSc
Professor, Research Group Leader, Microbiology and
Tumor Biology Center, Karolinska Institute, Stockholm,
Sweden
Epstein-Barr Virus and Human Lymphomas

Stanley J. Korsmeyer, MD
Professor of Medicine and Pathology and Investigator,
Howard Hughes Medical Institute, Washington
University School of Medicine, St. Louis, Missouri
The Biology of Low-Grade Malignant Lymphoma

Alexandra M. Levine, MD
Professor of Medicine and Chief, Division of Hematology,
University of Southern California School of Medicine;
Deputy Clinical Director, USC/Norris Cancer Center,
Los Angeles, California
*Lymphoma in the Setting of Human
Immunodeficiency Virus Infection*

Albert Y. Lin, MD, MPH
Medical Officer, U.S. Food and Drug Administration,
Rockville, Maryland
*Epidemiology of Hodgkin's Disease and Non-
Hodgkin's Lymphoma*

T. Andrew Lister, MD, FRCP, FRCPath
Professor of Medical Oncology and Director, ICRF
Medical Oncology Unit, Department of Medical
Oncology, St. Bartholomew's Hospital, West Smithfield,
London, England
*Follicular Lymphoma; "Diffuse" Low-Grade
B-Cell Lymphomas*

Jay S. Loeffler, MD
Associate Professor of Radiation Oncology, Harvard
Medical School, and Director of the Proton Beam
Center, Massachusetts General Hospital, Boston,
Massachusetts
Primary Central Nervous System Lymphoma

Ian T. Magrath, MB, BS, FRCP, FRCPath
Professor of Pediatrics, University of the Uniformed
Services in the Health Sciences; Chief, Lymphoma
Biology Section, Pediatric Branch, National Cancer
Institute, Bethesda, Maryland
*Burkitt's Lymphoma: The Small Noncleaved Cell
Lymphomas*

Tak W. Mak, PhD
Full Professor, Departments of Medical Biophysics and
Immunology, University of Toronto; Senior Staff
Scientist, Princess Margaret Hospital/Ontario Cancer
Institute, Toronto, Ontario, Canada
*Developmental and Functional Biology of B and T
Lymphocytes*

Karen C. Marcus, MD
Assistant Professor, Department of Radiation Oncology/
Joint Center for Radiation Therapy, Harvard Medical
School, Boston, Massachusetts
Principles of Radiation Therapy for Lymphomas

Peter M. Mauch, MD
Associate Professor, Department of Radiation Oncology,
Harvard Medical School, Boston, Massachusetts
Principles of Radiation Therapy for Lymphomas

Krzysztof Mrózek, MD, PhD
Senior Research Associate, Cytogenetics Research
    Laboratory, Division of Medicine, Roswell Park Cancer
    Institute, Buffalo, New York
    Major Cytogenetic Findings in Non-Hodgkin's
        Lymphoma

Ama Rohatiner, MD, FRCP
Reader in Medical Oncology, ICRF Medical Oncology
    Unit; Consultant Physician, Department of Oncology,
    St. Bartholomew's Hospital, West Smithfield, London,
    England
    Follicular Lymphoma; "Diffuse" Low-Grade
        B-Cell Lymphomas

Saul A. Rosenberg, MD
Maureen Lyles D'Ambrogio Professor of Medicine and
    Radiation Oncology, Emeritus, Stanford University,
    Stanford, California
    Hodgkin's Disease

Arthur T. Skarin, MD, FACP, FCCP
Associate Professor of Medicine, Harvard Medical School;
    Associate Physician, Department of Medicine, Dana-
    Farber Cancer Institute, Boston, Massachusetts
    Approach to the Patient with Suspected
        Lymphoma; Paraneoplastic Syndromes;
        Disorders that Mimic Lymphomas or May
        Predate Lymphoma

Jeffrey L. Sklar, MD, PhD
Professor of Pathology, Harvard Medical School; Director,
    Divisions of Molecular Oncology and Diagnostic
    Molecular Biology, Brigham and Women's Hospital,
    Boston, Massachusetts
    Introduction to Molecular Biology; Molecular
        Diagnosis of Lymphoma and Related Disorders

Harald Stein, MD
Professor of Pathology, Free University (Freie Universität
    Berlin); Director, Institute of Pathology, Klinikum
    Benjamin Franklin (Universitätsklinikum Benjamin
    Franklin), Berlin, Germany
    Biology of Hodgkin's Disease

Simon B. Sutcliffe, BSc, MD, FRCP, FRCPC
Vice-President, British Columbia Cancer Agency, and
    Director, Vancouver Cancer Centre, Vancouver Cancer
    Centre, Vancouver, British Columbia, Canada
    Primary Extranodal Lymphomas

Tak Takvorian, MD
Assistant Professor of Medicine, Harvard Medical School,
    Dana-Farber Cancer Institute, Boston, Massachusetts
    Lymphoblastic Lymphoma

Margaret A. Tucker
Chief, Genetic Epidemiology Branch, National Cancer
    Institute, National Institutes of Health, Bethesda,
    Maryland
    Epidemiology of Hodgkin's Disease and Non-
        Hodgkin's Lymphoma

Julie M. Vose, MD
Associate Professor, University of Nebraska Medical
    Center, Omaha, Nebraska
    Bone Marrow Transplantation for Malignant
        Lymphoma

Wyndham H. Wilson, MD, PhD
Senior Investigator, Medicine Branch, Division of Clinical
    Science, National Cancer Institute, National Institutes
    of Health, Bethesda, Maryland
    Principles of Chemotherapy for Lymphomas

Mary M. Zutter, MD
Associate Professor of Pathology, Washington University
    School of Medicine, St. Louis, Missouri
    The Biology of Low-Grade Malignant Lymphoma

Preface

In the field of cancer medicine the malignant lymphomas have been the subject of remarkable progress in basic and clinical investigation. The product of this effort has been an accumulation of knowledge that, until now, has never been assembled in one volume. This book attempts to fill this void by bringing together chapters written by noted experts covering the full range of clinical and basic topics relevant to these cancers.

In the early years, information gained by the empirical approach to malignant lymphoma generally outpaced understanding of the fundamental biologic or immunologic principles underlying the pathogenesis of these disorders. The relative rate of advancement in these two areas of knowledge may now be reversed. As described in the first portion of this book, increasing information on normal and abnormal lymphopoiesis has provided a much fuller picture of the processes leading to malignant lymphoma, along with important clinical implications for the management of the various disorders that evolve from neoplastic lymphopoiesis. Molecular biologic and genetic discoveries have improved the primary diagnosis of lymphoproliferative processes, have permitted better assessment of prognosis, and have provided means for the detection of minimal neoplastic disease within various histologic groups. Categorization of major subgroups of non-Hodgkin's lymphomas and Hodgkin's disease, which historically has relied on histopathology, is under continuing revision, especially with respect to non-Hodgkin's lymphoma. Aided by new biologic markers, a delineation of newly defined subcategories, such as mantle cell lymphoma, lymphoma of mucosa-associated lymphoid tissue, and anaplastic large cell lymphoma, has been possible. These categories reflect a better appreciation for the natural history of lymphoma subtypes and differences in response to conventional therapies.

The clinical and therapeutic challenges of the malignant lymphomas are presented with a review of current treatment modalities of chemotherapy and radiation therapy, including a chapter on the management of lymphoma during pregnancy and in older age groups. We have also included chapters that deal with diseases that resemble lymphoma and require specific, organized approaches to therapy. These discussions on disease management take into account the view that initial therapeutic advances, based on the empirical use of conventional-dose combination chemotherapy, may have reached a plateau of efficiency limited to certain subgroups and patients with favorable prognostic features. Antiproliferative agents that work by inhibiting DNA synthesis or by damaging DNA probably have a defined and limited role in achieving cures in these diseases. Emerging knowledge of the mechanisms of drug resistance as outlined in this book will likely have relevance to patients who become refractory to conventional doses of drugs. However, new targets, which may be antigenic in nature, related in some way to cytokine action, or involved in certain aspects of cell cycle regulation, will be required to treat indolent lymphomas containing populations of cells with low proliferative indices. In any event, we are surely in the midst of a biologic revolution that is yielding a quantity and depth of new knowledge that cannot help but contribute to our understanding of and better therapy for the malignant lymphomas.

The editors are pleased to thank all of those who have helped prepare this volume, whether as authors, secretaries, or friendly advisors. They gratefully acknowledge the inspiration of their mentors as colleagues in the field, some who are no longer alive, particularly the late Gordon Hamilton-Fairley, first Professor of Medical Oncology at St. Bartholomew's Hospital, and the late Henry Kaplan of Stanford University, a visionary giant in the field of lymphoma biology as treatment. At the same time, it is testimony to the rapidity with which the field of lymphoma oncology has developed that most of the major contributors to the field are still alive, and we are pleased that many of these individuals are authors of this volume.

GEORGE P. CANELLOS
T. ANDREW LISTER
JEFFREY L. SKLAR

Contents

Section **ONE**

BASIC CONSIDERATIONS

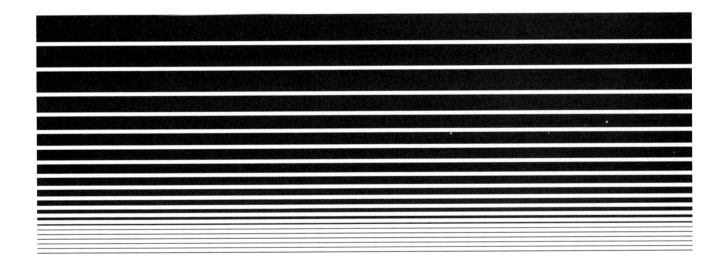

▬ Introduction to Molecular Biology ▬

Jeffrey L. Sklar

The future will likely look back on the last two decades of the twentieth century as the era that ushered in the first real insights into the fundamental biologic mechanisms that cause human cancers. Results obtained from the study of lymphomas have often been in the forefront of this revolution. The knowledge gained from these studies is already having significant impact on the diagnosis of lymphomas and in due course will undoubtedly affect approaches to the therapy of these diseases. The discoveries that account for this new understanding of the biology of cancer, including lymphoma, are based in turn on rapid advances in the fields of molecular biology. Today, more so than ever, oncologists, hematologists, pathologists, and other physicians who care for patients with lymphoma must have a grounding in the basic principles of molecular biology and the methods of this field relevant to lymphoma. Toward this end, this chapter briefly reviews the essential elements of molecular biology as it pertains to malignant lymphoma and related disorders.

CHROMOSOMES, GENES, AND DNA

All features and properties of individual cells, and ultimately the organisms composed of them, are a function of the genes expressed by those cells.[1, 2] The genes of human somatic (nongermline) cells reside in DNA distributed among 46 chromosomes (22 pairs of autosomes and 2 sex chromosomes, with one member of each autosomal pair plus a sex chromosome derived from one or the other parent). The chromosome pairs are numbered in order roughly according to descending size and DNA content, except for the two sex chromosomes X and Y.

An individual chromosome contains one very long, continuous double helix of DNA composed of two intertwined strands (Fig. 1–1). A large amount of DNA is accommodated within a chromosome by wrapping the double helix around beads of histone proteins, coiling of this string of beads, and looping out of the coil from a central proteinaceous chromosome scaffold.[3] Individual strands of DNA have polarity, with one end of each strand designated 5′ and the other 3′. The two strands in the double helix have opposite polarity and are consequently said to be antiparallel.[4] Each DNA strand consists of polymers of nucleotides–

deoxyribose sugars bearing a nitrogenous purine or pyrimidine base on one end and a phosphate group at the other. Adjacent nucleotides in a strand of DNA are linked through these phosphate groups. There are four types of nucleotides in DNA, distinguished by the base they bear: adenosine (A), thymidine (T), guanosine (G), and cytosine (C). The sequences of nucleotides within the two strands of the DNA are such that A always appears opposite to T, and G opposite C. Through their bases, A in one strand forms two hydrogen bonds with T in the opposite strand, and G forms three hydrogen bonds with C. Under most physiologic conditions, the two strands are held together mostly by these hydrogen bonds between complementary sequences of the nucleotides. Heat, high pH, or exposure to certain chemical denaturants disrupts the hydrogen bonds between complementary sequences, leading to strand separation.[5] Strands containing complementary sequences spontaneously reassemble into double helices when incubated together at appropriate temperatures, pH, and ionic strength. This propensity for the reassembly, or annealing, of complementary sequences into double-stranded DNA is the basis for many techniques in molecular biology, including most molecular methods used to diagnose and detect lymphomas.

Genes consist of stretches of DNA that generally encode the synthetic information for the chains of amino acids representing the polypeptide products of most genes. For a few genes, the final product is an RNA, a polymer of nucleotides consisting of the same four basic types as in DNA, except that the sugar ribose moiety of the nucleotides has a hydroxy group at one position where it is lacking in the nucleotides of DNA, and uridine (U) replaces T. Additionally, all genes include some noncoding, regulatory sequences at either end. Within the coding sequence of the gene, each successive three nucleotides in the coding strand dictates the incorporation into the eventual polypeptide product of a different one of the 20 amino acids that are the basic components of proteins. Nucleotide triplets encoding the signal for incorporation of a specific amino acid are termed "codons." Certain other codons provide the signal for initiation or termination of polypeptide synthesis. The sequences of codons within the DNA and of amino acids within the polypeptide products of genes are colinear; that is, the order of codons in the gene is preserved in the order of amino acids within the polypeptide. However, in most eukaryotic genes, the coding sequences are not continuous

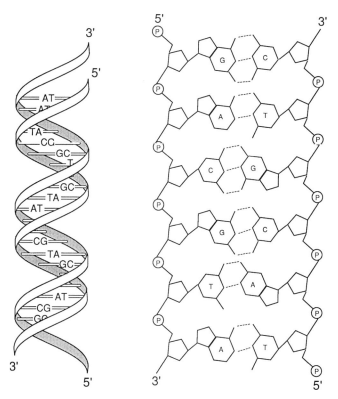

Figure 1–1. The structure of DNA. On the left is shown a schematic representation of the double helix illustrating the two intertwined sugar phosphate backbones held together by purine-pyrimidine base pairs. The double helix has been unwound on the right to demonstrate greater detail of the molecule in two dimensions. P indicates phosphate groups linking adjacent ribose units, to which are joined purine (A, adenine; G, guanine) or pyrimidine (T, thymine; C, cytosine) bases. G forms three hydrogen bonds with C, and A forms two hydrogen bonds with T. The sequences shown are arbitrary.

because of the gaps made up of noncoding nucleotide sequences of varying size that interrupt the coding sequences.[6] These gaps, which generally have no known function and may be mere evolutionary remnants of gene development,

are called "introns," and the remaining portions of the gene are called "exons."

Altogether, each haploid set of 23 human chromosomes contains about 3.3×10^9 nucleotide pairs (often called "base pairs," in reference to the nitrogenous bases that make up the nonsugar portion of the nucleotide), or about 7 billion base pairs per normal diploid cell. The total nuclear DNA content of the cell is referred to as the "genome." There are estimated to be about 75,000 to 100,000 different genes scattered throughout the human genome. Except for those genes on sex chromosomes in males, every gene is present in two copies, or alleles—one on each homologue of the 22 autosome chromosome pairs. Collectively, the base pairs within all genes comprise only about 5% or less of the DNA within cells; the remainder of the DNA may have some structural role or may be functionless (so-called junk DNA), as appears to be the case for most intronic DNA. An international effort is under way to determine the complete nucleotide sequence of all human DNA. As part of this larger project, the nucleotide sequence of all human genes is being determined, a goal that is expected to be achieved by the year 2000 and one that certainly has many implications for the diagnosis and treatment of lymphoma and all other cancers.

GENE EXPRESSION

As mentioned earlier, the sequence of codons within genes specifies the sequence of amino acids in polypeptides. Proteins are sometimes made up of a single polypeptide and hence may be the products of only one gene. Quite often proteins consist of aggregates of several specific polypeptide subunits encoded at different sites within the genome and therefore are the products of several genes.[7] The synthesis of an individual polypeptide from the sequence of codons within a gene begins by the transcription of the nucleotide sequence in the coding strand (or antisense strand) of the DNA into a strand of RNA composed of a sequence of ribonucleotides complementary to that of the DNA template

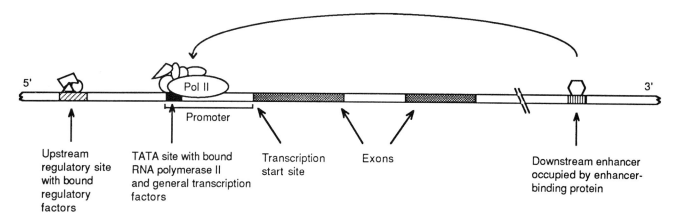

Figure 1–2. Gene structure and transcription. A prototypic eukaryotic gene is illustrated along with the control sites and regulatory proteins responsible for transcription of the DNA within that gene. The relative positions of the critical control sites are indicated, although not to scale. The gene is transcribed from the 5′ to the 3′ end (left to right in the figure) beginning from the transcriptional start site at the end of the promoter sequence. Regulatory factors, here shown bound to an upstream control site (the position of such sites is variable among different genes), accelerate or inhibit assembly of the transcription complex at the TATA site (named for a widely conserved tetrameric nucleotide sequence within promoters) by mechanisms that may involve bending of DNA and direct interaction with transcription factors. An enhancer-binding protein located at the enhancer, here shown far downstream of the coding sequence of the gene, presumably accelerates transcription complex formation by interacting with transcription factors at the TATA site after bending of the DNA brings these two sites close together.

from which it is derived. Transcription starts near a site in the DNA termed the "promoter," at which a complex of proteins controlling the initiation of transcription assembles (Fig. 1–2).[8, 9] These proteins include one of three different types of RNA polymerases, the enzymes directly responsible for RNA synthesis (RNA polymerase II being the one that transcribes most genes affecting differentiated properties of individual tissues), and various accessory proteins called "transcription factors," which facilitate recognition of the promoter.[10, 11] Assembly of this complex may be assisted or inhibited by proteins referred to as "activators" and "repressors." There are also sequences in the DNA, termed "enhancers," which may lie at considerable distances from the promoter, on either side of the gene or even within introns, that somehow stimulate assembly of the transcription complex, probably after looping out of the DNA between the two sites and participation in formation of the initiation complex by proteins that bind to the enhancer sequence.[12]

After formation of the initiation complex, RNA polymerase moves along the coding strand of the gene in a 3′-to-5′ direction, building the RNA molecule from the 5′-to-3′ end by successively adding nucleotides to the growing strand of RNA according to the DNA sequence encountered as the polymerase proceeds through the gene. Transcription continues beyond the gene, sometimes for long distances, before the polymerase falls off the DNA. The immediate product of transcription is rapidly processed first by cleavage near AAUAAA sequences following the coding sequence and the attachment of a string of A nucleotides (polyA) to the cleaved 3′-end of the RNA.[13, 14] The intronic sequences are spliced out of the RNA by a specialized structure called the "spliceosome," and the 5′ of the RNA is modified by addition of 7-methyl Gppp (the cap, in which "p" stands for phosphate).[15] Once it has been polyadenylated, spliced, and capped, the mature messenger RNA (mRNA) is transported through pores in nuclear membrane to the cytoplasm, where it serves as the template for translation into polypeptide sequences.

Most gene activity is controlled at the level of transcription. The programmed turning on and off of sets of genes under various signals external or internal to the cell during embryogenesis accounts for the development of the organism and the eventual establishment of a continuously active set of genes in terminally differentiated tissues. Lymphomas, as well as cancer as a whole, arise from the dysregulation of genes or sets of genes. Transcription factors play a major role in the control of gene transcription, and increasingly aberrations of the genes for transcription factors or for the genes that control expression or the activity of transcription factors are being found to be involved in the transformation of normal cells to malignancy.[16, 17]

Once in the cytoplasm, the mRNA is bound by ribosomes, the organelles that function as the platform on which the polypeptide is constructed.[18] Individual ribosomes recognize the 5′-cap and then scan the adjacent RNA until it finds a nearby AUG nucleotide triplet, which is the initiator codon (as well as the codon for the amino acid methionine; in polypeptides that do not begin with methionine, this amino acid is eventual cleaved away). Starting at the initiator codon, the ribosome ratchets along the RNA, codon by codon, adding an amino acid for each codon to the growing end of the polypeptide. Construction

of the polypeptide begins at the amino, or N, terminus and concludes at the carboxy, or C, terminus. The codon sequence is actually read by small transfer RNA (tRNA) molecules, of which there are more than 20 varieties bearing different amino acids attached to their 3′ ends. As the ribosome moves to a new codon, a tRNA enters a pocket in the ribosome and anneals to the codon by a complementary anticodon sequence that distinguishes each type of tRNA and determines the amino acid with which the tRNA is charged. The ribosome then transfers the amino acid from the tRNA to the growing polypeptide and advances to the next codon. The ribosome continues down the mRNA until it encounters a UAG, UAA, or UGA codon (terminator or nonsense codons), which signals the ribosome to release the mRNA and the completed polypeptide. Besides the requirement for ribosomes and tRNA, each step in polypeptide synthesis—initiation, elongation, and termination—depends on the participation of a set of catalytic protein factors, which successively associate and disassociate from the ribosome as it moves through the coding sequence of the mRNA template.

Newly synthesized polypeptides can have a number of destinations.[19] Some polypeptides synthesized on free ribosomes in the cytoplasm remain in the cytoplasm, where they assume a particular conformation owing to interactions of the various amino acids (a process that actually starts as the polypeptide first begins to emerge from the ribosome) and may aggregate with other polypeptides. Folding of polypeptide chains into the proper conformation is aided by a group of proteins, termed "chaperones," that bind to and stabilize the nascent polypeptide as it emerges from the ribosome.[20] After folding in the cytoplasm, another category of polypeptides containing short runs of certain basic amino acids (nuclear localization sequences) pass through pores in the nuclear into the nucleus.[21] Still other polypeptides are secreted by the cell or become embedded in the cytoplasmic membrane. Both of these latter types of polypeptides contain so-called signal sequences of amino acids that thread the nascent polypeptide through the membrane of the endoplasmic reticulum, an extensive network of membrane-lined channels within the cytoplasm.[22] Membrane-associated polypeptides, which are often receptors or ligands for receptors on other cells, remain attached to the membrane of the endoplasmic reticulum through one or more domains of hydrophobic amino acids that span the membrane. Secreted polypeptides collect in the endoplasmic reticulum, where they may aggregate with other polypeptides and are usually glycosylated by various enzymes that add carbohydrates to particular amino acids. Glycosylated proteins move to the Golgi apparatus and then are transported by secretory vesicles that fuse with the cytoplasmic membrane, dumping their contents into the extracellular space. A similar process delivers cell surface proteins to the cytoplasmic membrane, but as the vesicle fuses at this site, the proteins remain tethered to the membrane.

Proteins synthesized by the cell account for all aspects of cellular biology and behavior, whether normal or neoplastic. In addition, proteins, and sometimes the carbohydrates borne by them, have served as important antigenic markers for the immunohistochemical characterization of tumors. Among lymphomas, membrane-bound proteins have been especially useful as markers for the diagnosis and classification of the many subtypes of these neoplasms.

THE CELL CYCLE AND ITS CONTROL

Ultimately, the changes in cells that render them malignant are manifest by the final common characteristic of unrestricted or dysfunctional cellular proliferation. This essential phenotypic feature of all cancers reflects disturbances in the cell cycle—the stereotypic pattern of events that control the division of somatic cells (Fig. 1–3).[23, 24] The life of a dividing cell is usually diagrammed as having four distinct phases: M, G_1, S, and G_2. M (for mitosis) phase involves the process by which the chromosomes, duplicated earlier in the cell cycle, are distributed to the two daughter cells that result from the binary fission of the original parental cell. The duplication of the chromosomes occurs during S (for synthesis) phase, when the DNA is replicated. G_1 (for gap) phase represents the interval between M and the next S phase, and G_2 phase intervenes between S and the following M. Nondividing cells that have withdrawn from the cell cycle, invariably at a point early in G_1, are sometimes said to be in G_0. All cells that are not in mitosis, and are histologically indistinguishable from one another, are said to be in interphase.

Great progress has been made over recent years in discovering the molecules that control the phases of the cell cycle.[23, 25] The critical factors appear to be a set of proteins in which one subunit, termed a "cyclin-dependent kinase" (cdk), is catalytic and the other subunit, the cyclin, regulates the activity of the cdk. So far, four major cdks—1, 2, 4, and 6—have been discovered (cdk1 is usually referred to as "cdc2" after the homologous protein from yeast, in which genes controlling the cell cycle were first described). There are at least six cyclins—A, B, D1 through D3, and E. The relative levels of the three types of cyclin D vary among tissues; their functional differences are unclear, and they are usually assumed to have similar roles. Consequently, they are often collectively referred to as "cyclin D." Passage through the early part of G_1 appears to be promoted by cdk4 and 6, each bound to cyclin D. Preceding entry into S phase, levels of cdk2-cyclin E rise as the cdk2 and 6 fall.[26] Acting in combination just prior to S phase, these cdk-cyclin complexes seem to power the cell past a so-called restriction point, beyond which the cell becomes committed to completing mitosis, irrespective of the effects of external growth factors. Cyclin A, which binds to cdk2, appears before S phase begins and is required for continued DNA synthesis. Toward the end of S phase, cdc2–cyclin B and cdc2–cyclin A appear and continue to increase in concentration through G_2. These cdk-cyclin complexes govern the events that accompany mitosis, such as condensation of chromatin (the extended state of chromosomes during interphase) into the tightly packed chromosomes of mitosis, the dissolution of the nuclear membrane, and the reorganization of microtubular proteins into the mitotic spindle apparatus that draws the chromosomes apart toward opposite poles in the dividing cell.

The precise substrates for cdk proteins during the cell cycle are not fully known. Presumably, cdks, when activated by binding to cyclins and through interactions with other proteins (which in turn may be kinases or phosphorylases), add phosphates to certain protein targets, thereby altering their activities. For example, a family of transcription factors collectively termed "E2F" induces transcription of genes necessary for nucleotide and DNA synthesis preceding the entry of the cell into S phase. During G_1, E2F is sequestered and inactivated by the rb protein, which was discovered because the gene encoding this protein is deleted and/or mutated in the cells of retinoblastoma. Cdk-cyclin complexes in G_1 and cdk2–cyclin A in S phase phosphorylate rb, releasing active E2F.

A feature of the cell cycle directly relevant to lymphoma and other cancers is checkpoint control.[27] In normal cells, damage to DNA in G_1 or incomplete DNA synthesis in S halts further progression in the cell cycle. Abnormalities in the proteins that sense these deficiencies occur in cancers and may contribute to genetic instability—the tendency to accumulate mutations and aberrations in chromosome number that characterize many cancers in advanced stages and may drive these cancers to more aggressive behavior.

GENES AND CANCER

One of the key concepts that have shaped current understanding of the fundamental biology of cancer is that tumors initially arise from single cells that acquire a sufficient number of mutations in critical genes, permitting these cells to escape the normal inhibitory controls preventing continued proliferation.[16, 17] In general, these mutations affect two broad categories of genes: oncogenes and tumor suppressor genes.[28–30] Mutations involving oncogenes are activating, usually leading to increased expression of the gene, to constitutive activity of the gene product at inappropriate times in the cell cycle, or to hyperactivity of the product. These genes often have normal functions during

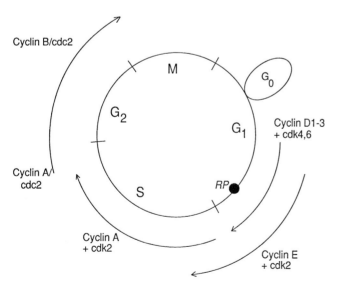

Figure 1–3. Diagram of the cell cycle showing the principal proteins involved in its regulation. As conventionally depicted, the cycle operates in a clockwise manner. Cells may withdraw from the cycle by entering a replicatively quiescent state, represented by the tangential pathway G_0, for variable periods. RP indicates the restriction point, beyond which the cycle becomes impervious to exogenous influences, such as those exerted by growth factors. The roles of the different cyclins and cyclin-dependent kinases are described in the text.

embryogenesis or at times of rapid cellular proliferation. The ability of many oncogenic retroviruses to transform cells that they infect derives from the fact that the genomes of these viruses have incorporated portions of cellular oncogenes that have become activated as a result of the insertion process or through subsequent evolution within the virus.[31] In contrast, mutations involving tumor suppressor genes are inactivating. In normal cells, these genes usually suppress or negatively regulate cell division, and mutations that decrease their activity remove these inhibitory controls. Since one copy of a tumor suppressor gene is usually sufficient for proper control over cellular division, both alleles must be inactivated to produce a phenotypic effect. Overall, hematopoietic neoplasms, including lymphomas, display more mutation of oncogenes than of tumor suppressor genes, the latter being more prevalent in solid tumors. Mutant genes associated with inherited predispositions to cancer usually fall into the class of tumor suppressors.

Several kinds of mutations lead to activation of oncogenes and inactivation of tumor suppressor genes. Missense mutations are usually single-base substitutions in which one codon is changed to another. Such changes can be activating or inactivating, depending on the gene and the replacement of amino acids that occurs in the polypeptide product. Substitutions of single bases can also create nonsense codons that cause premature termination of polypeptide synthesis. Similar results may arise from insertions or deletions of one or a few base pairs, which shift the codon-reading frame out of phase so that a nonsense codon appears downstream. Frame shift and nonsense mutations seem to be particularly common as mechanisms for inactivating certain tumor suppressor genes. Another frequent mechanism for destroying tumor suppresser gene function is the deletion of large segments of DNA, removing the entire gene along with considerable stretches of flanking sequence on either side. In fact, deletion of one tumor suppressor allele and missense or nonsense mutation in the second allele represent the standard scenario for inactivation of tumor suppressor genes found in human tumors.[32] Some of these deletions involving tumor suppressor genes are detectable under the microscope as losses of whole regions in metaphase chromosomes. More often, such deletions are detected only molecularly through the disappearance from tumor cells of polymorphic sequence markers closely linked to a tumor suppressor gene. These polymorphic markers occur in the form of numerous scattered, genetically neutral variations in sequence, frequently consisting of varying numbers of tandemly repeated dinucleotides or trinucleotides, many of which have been mapped throughout the genome. Recurrent deletion of one or the other allele for a polymorphism at a particular site in tumor cells compared with normal cells, a finding referred to as "loss of heterozygosity" (LOH), is often the first clue to the existence of a nearby tumor suppressor gene for that type of tumor.[33]

A final category of mutation that happens to be especially common in hematopoietic neoplasms, including lymphoma, is chromosome translocation.[34] Such mutations are usually detectable as exchanges of segments between chromosomes in spreads of metaphase nuclei under the microscope, and they have several possible consequences for the genes at the breakpoints in the participating chromosomes. Most commonly, the domains from genes on the two chromosomes are fused to produce a chimeric polypeptide with novel properties. Occasionally, translocations lead to overexpression of a gene near the breakpoint, sometimes owing to stabilization of a transcript having altered structure outside the coding region, or to increased promoter activity due to distant effects of enhancers or other regulatory elements brought into range of the promoter by the translocation. Truncation of a polypeptide as a result of breakage within a gene is also sometimes found. In general, all of these changes activate the genes associated with them, indicating that the affected genes act as oncogenes.

MOLECULAR BIOLOGIC METHODS RELEVANT TO CANCER

METHODS FOR THE CLONING AND MANIPULATION OF GENES

The rapid pace of progress in molecular biology and in applications of this field to oncology has been fueled in large part by the development of methods to study the structure and function of nucleotide sequences within DNA and RNA. The most important of these methods is molecular cloning of DNA.[35] This technique permits the production of large amounts of homogeneous DNA fragments, which can then be easily analyzed and manipulated in a variety of ways. In its most common form, molecular cloning involves the insertion of DNA fragments in vitro into the genome of a bacteriophage or the DNA of a plasmid using restriction enzymes and polynucleotide ligase. Restriction enzymes are purified from bacteria, where they protect the organism from invading foreign DNA by cleaving DNA that has not been appropriately modified, usually by methylation of bases, at sites specific to the particular species. These sites consist of short sequences of nucleotides four to eight base pairs in length. More than 100 such enzymes with many different site specificities are known. Cleavage frequently occurs by nicking the two strands of the DNA at the restriction sites several base pairs apart, so that short single-stranded overhangs created at the ends of the resulting fragments are complementary. Annealing of these overhangs facilitates the joining of fragments from disparate sources, provided the fragments to be joined were generated by digestion with the same restriction enzyme. Once the overhangs have annealed, the nicks remaining between the ends of the fragments in both strands can be sealed by the ligase enzyme purified from *Escherichia coli*. Alternatively, fragments can be joined by adding complementary homopolymers (such as polyG and polyC) to the 3′ ends of fragments using the enzyme terminal transferase, then annealing the two fragments and sealing the joint with ligase. This method permits the joining of fragments produced by methods other than restriction cleavage, but it leaves a run of G:C base pairs at the junctions between fragments. Still a third method for joining fragments of DNA is to ligate short pieces of DNA containing complementary, overhanging sequences (so-called linkers or adapters) to the ends of fragments before annealing the fragments together and sealing the joints with ligase.

The bacteriophages and plasmids into which DNA fragments are inserted act as vectors to carry these fragments along with that of the vector. Each type of vector has different advantages: bacteriophages accommodate larger inserts (up to approximately 25 kilobases [kb], or thousands of base pairs) and offer ease of screening the recombinant genomes for the cloned DNA of interest, whereas the plasmids, being stably maintained as freely replicating, small DNA circles in the bacterial host, are simpler to propagate and can be stored conveniently as frozen pure DNA. A special type of composite vector, called a "cosmid," has an insert capacity of approximately 50 kb but is much more difficult to manipulate than standard plasmids or bacteriophage.

The DNA of both bacteriophages and plasmids vectors have been engineered to have restriction sites that can be readily opened to accept insertion of DNA fragments for cloning. To introduce the recombinant bacteriophage genomes into the bacterial host, the DNA must be packaged into virions by incubating with extracts of infected cells containing unassembled virion proteins. The packaged DNA can then be used to infect bacteria in culture, or on the surface of agar plates to produce plaques, each one of which represents the offspring of an individual recombinant virus. Recombinant plasmids can be directly transfected into bacteria by heat-shocking bacteria in the presence of plasmid DNA coprecipitated with calcium phosphate. Transfected bacteria can be grown in liquid culture or spread on agar plates to produce individual colonies containing the recombinant plasmid (growth of untransfected cells is suppressed by adding an antibiotic to the medium or agar and using plasmids containing genes conferring resistance to the drug). Individual plaques and colonies can be checked quickly for the insert of interest by transferring material directly from the plate to a nylon membrane briefly applied to the surface of the plate and then removed. This membrane may be incubated with a specific, radiolabeled fragment of DNA to test for sequences in the plaques of colonies to which this fragment anneals (such fragments are often referred to as "probes"; see later). Occasionally, the contents of plaques or colonies transferred to membranes are screened for the production of polypeptide sequences from the recombinant vector DNA by using antibodies directed against these polypeptides. Plaques and colonies are not destroyed by the transfer procedure, and once the positive spot on the membrane is matched to a plaque or colony on the plate, the bacteriophage or bacteria containing the DNA of interest can be selected for expansion. Abundant amounts of recombinant vector can be generated in bacteria grown in liquid culture or on plates, the vector DNA extracted from the bacteriophage or bacteria, and cloned insert released by digestion with appropriate restriction enzyme.

Besides fragments of genomic DNA, molecular cloning is often used to amplify cDNAs, or double-stranded DNA versions of the RNA sequences containing the transcribed portions of genes. These cDNAs are synthesized by using the enzyme reverse transcriptase, originally isolated from the virions of retroviruses, to copy the RNA into a single strand of DNA, followed by synthesis of a second, complementary strand of DNA. The cDNA is inserted into vector DNA after adding linkers to the ends or tailing with G or C.

New vectors with the capacity to carry very large fragments of genomic DNA have been critical for rapid progress over the last few years in the molecular cloning of specific regions of the human genome, including many regions relevant to cancer and lymphoma. Foremost among these vectors have been yeast and bacterial artificial chromosomes (YACs and BACs, respectively).[36] YACs, which must be propagated in yeast hosts, have been constructed from centromeres (the elements to which the spindle fibers attach, ensuring segregation of daughter chromosomes during mitosis), replication centers (sequences at which DNA replication starts), and telomeres (chromosome ends) derived from yeast chromosomes.[37] The remainder of the DNA sequence in these vectors may be derived from any source and can be larger than 1000 kb. BACs, which are grown in *E. coli*, just as a true bacterial chromosome, are circular, contain merely a replication origin to permit extrachromosome DNA synthesis, and will accept up to approximately 300 kb of foreign DNA.[38]

Several libraries of human DNA in YACs have been produced, and the individual members of these libraries have been mapped to many parts of the human genome, permitting investigators attempting to clone sites defined by genetic or cytogenetic data to focus quickly on small groups of YACs, or contigs, that cover the regions spanning those sites. Similar but less complete mapping has been accomplished with BACs. Additionally, information about DNA sequences surrounding polymorphisms allows efficient identification of a YAC or BAC containing that polymorphism and any closely linked region of DNA. These YACs and BACs can be used to select cDNAs for genes contained within the DNA carried in the vector. Since the locations of many DNA polymorphisms have been mapped within the human genome, it is therefore possible to move from the chromosome position of a cytogenetic aberration or site of LOH determined by deletion of a specific polymorphism to genes within the vicinity of those abnormalities. These genes can then be checked for mutations or sequence rearrangements in human cancers. This procedure for gene isolation has been extensively employed to find oncogenes and tumor suppressor genes in recent years.

The ability to insert DNA into eukaryotic cells has been a major breakthrough that greatly advanced the molecular analysis of cancer. Many methods are now available to achieve this objective. DNA coprecipitated with calcium phosphate may be directly taken up by cells in culture. Experiments performed in this manner were instrumental in first demonstrating that activated oncogenes were present in the genomes of transformed cells and could transmit the transformed phenotype to cells in culture.[39] Uptake can be increased by packaging DNA in small vesicles of artificial lipid membranes called "liposomes" (a process called "lipofection") or by subjecting the cells to brief electrical shock in the presence of the DNA (a method called "electroporation"). Even higher percentages of cells may acquire exogenous DNA introduced by means of eukaryotic viral vectors, particularly those constructed from retroviruses.[40] In experimental mouse systems, tumor cells infected by retroviral vectors carrying constitutively active genes for cytokines have been given to animals bearing various types of tumors to stimulate systemic immune responses against the tumors.[41] The oncogenic properties of a number of genes have been tested by infection of bone marrow stem cells, which have then been used to repopulate the marrow of lethally irradiated recipient mice.[42] Viral vectors have also been tried as vehicles to transduce genes into cells of intact animals, including humans.[43] Such efforts at gene therapy in human patients have attempted to supply functional alleles to cells and tissues in which mutations have destroyed gene function.[44]

Another method used in certain situations for introducing DNA into eukaryotic cells is direct injection with extremely fine needles. So-called transgenic mice are now routinely constructed by injecting genes into fertilized oocytes, which are then implanted in the uteri of surrogate mothers.[45] All cells in the resulting transgenic animals contain the transgene, expression of which can be targeted to a particular tissue by placing the coding sequence of the transgene behind a promoter known to be active only in that tissue. Induction of tumors by such transgenes has been considered important evidence for the oncogenic potential of a gene. That only a few tumors arise over the lifetime of such transgenic animals despite the widespread expression of the transgene within a tissue has been taken as evidence of genetic changes in multiple genes being required for malignant transformation of cells—a central tenet of modern cancer biology.[46]

A special type of transgenic mouse that has provided a valuable form of genetic analysis is the knockout mouse.[47, 48] Construction of these animals begins by injecting a recombinant, defective version of a gene into ES tissue culture cells. These cells, derived from a murine embryonic carcinoma, support a particularly high rate of homologous recombination between the injected transgene and the corresponding endogenous gene, such that insertion of the transgene into the genomic DNA of the ES cell disrupts and inactivates the endogenous gene under analysis. The injected ES cells are manipulated into early embryos, which are then inserted into uteri of surrogate mothers. The offspring of this procedure are chimeras in which the ES cells have contributed to the development of various tissues within the mouse, hopefully including the germline tissues, thereby enabling further breeding of animals with altered genomes. After testing for disruption of the target gene, and nonchimeric animals are bred and homozygous mice produced from those animals in which one copy has been found to be destroyed. Alternatively, it is now often possible to convert heterozygous ES knockout cells to homozygosity in vitro to significantly reduce the breeding time required to generate homozygous animals. Knockout mice prepared in this manner have helped elucidate the role of genes in tissue differentiation and sometimes in tumor suppression, although the interpretation of these experiments is often complicated by the essential tendency of many genes toward early embryo development (leading to blighting of the embryo early on) and the apparent redundancy of the genome for genes controlling many developmental and cancer-related functions (leading to no or only subtle effects).

TECHNIQUES FOR THE ANALYSIS OF MACROMOLECULES

Understanding of the advances in the molecular biology of lymphoma, including an increasing number of clinical applications of molecular biology to these disorders, calls for a familiarity with a core set of basic techniques commonly used to detect and analyze three macromolecules of the cell: DNA, RNA, and proteins.

Gel Electrophoresis

Most of the common techniques of molecular biology rely fundamentally on gel electrophoresis as an essential separatory procedure. In this procedure, an electric field drives charged macromolecules through a matrix composed of polyacrylamide or agarose.[49] In most situations, the criterion of separation is primarily the size of the macromolecule, with the matrix acting as a sieve to retard larger molecules, such that after sufficient time in the electric field, different-sized molecules within a mixture applied to the top of the gel will form a series of discrete bands within the gel, each band appearing at a distance from the origin inversely proportional to the size of the molecules in that band. The ability to distinguish small differences in the size of macromolecules by this simple procedure can be extraordinary. For example, single base pair differences in DNA fragments several hundred base pairs in length are routinely detected by polyacrylamide gel electrophoresis. In general, agarose gels are used to separate larger fragments (≥1 kb) of DNA and RNA, whereas polyacrylamide gels are used for smaller fragments.[50] Proteins are usually analyzed in polyacrylamide gels containing the detergent sodium dodecyl sulfate (SDS), which denatures the polypeptides by disrupting hydrogen bonds, as well as hydrostatic and other forces between amino acid side chains, thereby permitting separation based primarily on the number of amino acids in the polypeptide.[51, 52]

Probes and the Detection of Macromolecules

Detection of macromolecules whether in gels or elsewhere is a constant issue in molecular biology. DNA is usually detected with radioactivity, either by labeling the DNA directly with radioactive phosphorus, or indirectly, by annealing radiolabeled DNA or RNA probes having complementary sequences to the target DNA. RNA is almost always detected by the annealing of radiolabeled probes. Radiolabeling is done in basically two ways: (1) DNA is copied in vitro by the enzyme DNA polymerase from *E. coli* (to produce a DNA probe) or RNA polymerase (to produce an RNA probe) using nucleotides containing radioactive phosphorus atoms[53, 54] or (2) a single phosphate group containing radioactive phosphorus is added to the 5′ end of a DNA probe by the enzyme polynucleotide kinase.[55] DNA and RNA probes can also be labeled in vitro by incorporating into the probe nucleotides that have had biotin or digoxigenin covalently attached to them.[56, 57] Antibodies conjugated with peroxidase or alkaline phosphatase are used to recognize the derivitized bases, and the binding of antibody is detected in turn by incubating the complexes with a substrate that is converted by the conjugated enzyme to an insoluble colored product.[58] In certain situations, antibody conjugated to a fluorescent tag is used to identify the location of an annealed probe. However, in general, such chromogenic or fluorescent methods fail to achieve the sensitivity offered by radioactivity.

The use of probes to detect complementary sequences within target DNA or RNA has been pivotal in basic and applied molecular biology.[59] An important operational principle governing the use of probes is that the affinity of a probe for a target sequence depends on the size of the probe and the degree of complementarity between the sequences in the probe and the target. This affinity can be measured by comparing the conditions under which the duplexes of probe and target strands (usually referred to as hybrids) form. Low salt, high temperature, and the presence of chemical denaturants such as urea and formamide favor single strands over hybrids and are said to constitute conditions of high stringency. Increasing numbers of mismatched bases between probe and target require reduced stringency for hybridization to occur and also raise the likelihood that nonspecific binding will take place. By precisely manipulating the factors that affect hybridization, sequence differences as small as a single nucleotide between

the probe and the target, using very short probes, can be distinguished.

Southern and Northern Blots

A long-standing mainstay technique that makes use of both gel electrophoresis and hybridization between probes and DNA targets is Southern blot analysis (named for its inventor, E. M. Southern) (Fig. 1–4).[60] This technique is used to identify the presence of a particular sequence within DNA (e.g., the presence of viral genomes in the DNA extracted from cells) or to detect alterations in DNA sequences (e.g., those occurring as a consequence of chromosome translocations). The technique is usually performed on total

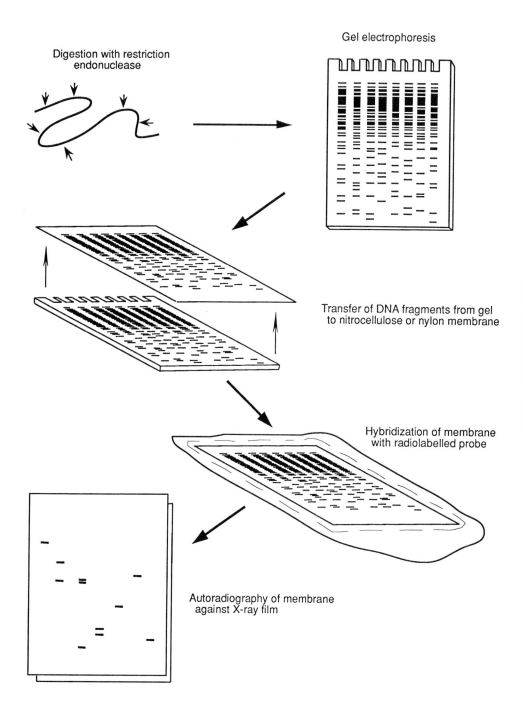

Digestion with restriction endonuclease

Gel electrophoresis

Transfer of DNA fragments from gel to nitrocellulose or nylon membrane

Hybridization of membrane with radiolabelled probe

Autoradiography of membrane against X-ray film

Figure 1–4. Schematic representation of the Southern blot hybridization procedure. The steps involved in the procedure are described in the text. The various lanes in the gel depict digests of total cellular DNA by different restriction enzymes. Bands formed by DNA fragments of varying sizes are illustrated in both the gel and the membrane, although these bands are actually invisible.

DNA extracted from a tissue or cells. Each analysis requires about 5 μg of DNA—the equivalent of approximately 0.5 mg of wet tissue, or 5 million cells. The DNA is digested with one or sometimes two bacterial restriction enzymes, and the resulting mixture of DNA fragments is separated by electrophoresis in an agarose gel. The result is an invisible ladder of thousands of bands, each containing DNA fragments of identical size. The DNA fragments making up these bands are denatured by briefly soaking the gel in alkali and then transferring to a nylon membrane by laying the membrane against the surface of the gel and drawing buffer from a reservoir through the gel and membrane, either by putting an absorbent material against the membrane or by applying a low vacuum to the membrane surface.

On drying of the membrane, the single strands of DNA transferred to the membrane become immobilized where they contact the nylon, preserving the relative positions of the bands as they were in the agarose gel. The membrane is then incubated with a radiolabeled probe (sometimes consisting of RNA, in which case it is sometimes referred to as a "riboprobe," but more commonly a heat-denatured double-stranded DNA fragment) containing sequence complementary to a particular region of DNA under analysis. After sufficient time (usually overnight) to allow for hybridization between complementary sequences in the probe and target fragments on the membrane, the membrane is rinsed, dried, and placed against a sheet of x-ray film in the dark for autoradiography. The autoradiogram produced when the x-ray film is developed hours to days later displays dark bands at positions corresponding to the size of the DNA fragments containing the sequence complementary to the probe.

A variation of the Southern blot technique is used to analyze RNA. In this procedure, waggishly termed Northern blot analysis, RNA extracted from the cell is first subjected to agarose gel electrophoresis and then transferred to a nylon membrane, in a manner quite similar to that used in Southern blot analysis.[61, 62] The membrane is incubated with a radiolabeled probe, rinsed, dried, and autoradiographed. Bands appear in the resulting autoradiogram at positions reflecting the size of the RNA containing sequence complementary to the probe.

There are several obvious differences between Southern and Northern blot techniques. First, RNA generally requires much more care in preparation than does DNA. RNA is relatively unstable compared with DNA (the relative stabilities being consistent with the roles of these molecules in the cell—the mediation by RNA of levels of gene expression that vary over time and under different conditions versus the transmission by DNA of hereditary potential from cell to cell). Additionally, since RNA is rapidly degraded by ribonucleases released from lysosomes in devitalized cells, RNA must be quickly extracted from cells to separate the RNA from the ribonucleases. Alternatively, the cells must be stored frozen until the RNA is extracted promptly after thawing. Sometimes total RNA extracted from cells is analyzed, but the large amount of ribosome RNA (a non-polyadenylated structural component of all ribosomes) may obscure smaller amounts of similarly sized polyadenylated RNA in Northern blots. Therefore, polyadenylated RNA is purified before electrophoresis by hybridization and elution form columns or agarose beads bearing polyT complementary to the polyA tails at the 3′ ends of the RNA. Another

major difference between Southern and Northern blot analyses is that digestion with restriction enzymes is not performed on RNA (indeed, no degradative enzymes with specificity for short sequences comparable to restriction enzymes are available for RNA). The sizes of most mature RNA species, however, fall conveniently within the range of size of polynucleotides well resolved by agarose gels. Furthermore, because RNA, which is primarily single-stranded, may form short regions of intramolecular hybrids, accurate sizing of the molecules requires conditions of electrophoresis in which the interstrand and intrastrand hybrid formation is reduced, usually by using gels containing the chemicals urea, formaldehyde, or formamide. Finally, for reasons that are unclear, Northern blots are less sensitive than Southern blots, so that more cellular equivalents of RNA are required for Northern blot analysis, despite the fact that the complexity of the RNA is far lower than DNA and RNA molecules for most expressed genes are present in many copies within the cell.

Polymerase Chain Reaction

Hybridization between complementary nucleotide sequences is also critical in what is currently the most widely used technique in molecular biology—the polymerase chain reaction (PCR).[63–66] PCR permits the in vitro amplification of defined regions of DNA provided that sequences surrounding the region to be amplified are known (Fig. 1–5). Four key reagents used in the PCR procedure are (1) template DNA (such as whole cellular DNA extracted from a tissue biopsy specimen); (2) heat-resistant DNA polymerase purified from the thermophilic bacterium *Thermus aquaticus* (Taq polymerase); (3) two oligonucleotide primers consisting of single-stranded pieces of DNA 15 to 40 nucleotides long; and (4) the four deoxynucleoside triphosphates. The oligonucleotide primers are constructed to complement the sequences in the opposite strands of the template on either side of the region intended for amplification. These primers determine entirely the specificity of the amplification.

PCR amplification is carried out in repeated cycles of DNA synthesis in which the DNA polymerase copies the template sequences by extending the 3′ end of the primers hybridized to the two strands of the template (like most DNA polymerases, Taq polymerase cannot initiate DNA synthesis de novo but only can add nucleotides to preexisting 3′ ends). Each cycle of synthesis involves rapid shifts in temperature, accomplished by special incubators (termed "thermal cyclers") designed for this purpose, to allow template denaturation, annealing of the two primers, and primer extension. DNA synthesized in each earlier cycle of primer extension becomes template for each subsequent cycle. Typically, 20 to 60 cycles are performed over several hours. The product of amplification is a homogeneous set of fragments having a size corresponding precisely to the distance between the sequences in the template complementary to the primers, which themselves become embedded at the 5′ ends of the two product strands. Theoretically, the number of product fragments accumulated per template after n cycles of synthesis is 2^n, or about 10^6 fragments following 20 cycles. The whole process is extremely efficient, and amplification products can frequently be detected from

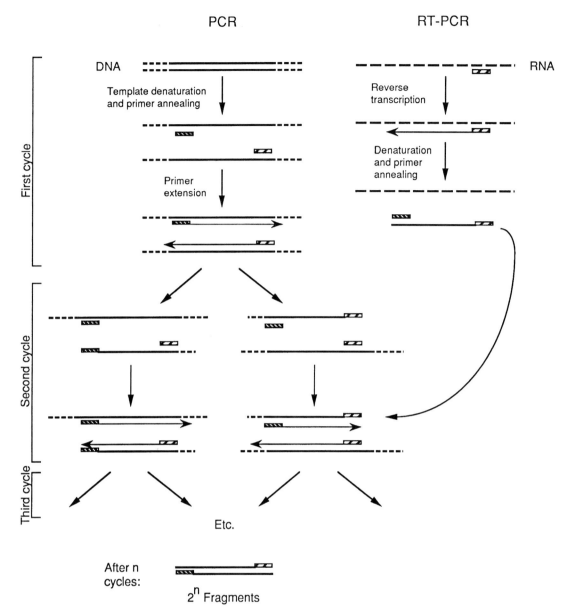

Figure 1–5. Schematic representation of amplification of DNA sequences by polymerase chain reaction (PCR) and of RNA sequences by RT-PCR (see text).

a single template molecule in a reaction of 30 to 40 cycles. With adequate numbers of cycles (sometimes aided by replenishing primer and polymerase at some point during the reaction), sufficient amplification from a few micrograms of total DNA is achieved to directly visualize the product in an agarose or polyacrylamide gel illuminated by ultraviolet light after staining of the DNA with ethidium bromide.

Several modifications of the original PCR protocol have been introduced to expand the usefulness of the technique. For example, RNA sequences can be amplified by first synthesizing a cDNA from the RNA using the enzyme reverse transcriptase (reverse transcription of RNA followed by PCR is often referred to as "RT-PCR").[67] Furthermore, standard PCR is limited to amplification of a few kilobases of sequence. Amplification of longer products up to 20 or more kilobases in length (so-called long-range PCR) has been achieved by altering the reaction conditions and switching to another heat-resistant polymerase.[68, 69] The requirement for sequence information on both sides of a target sequence also has been overcome by ligating a defined sequence to one end of a DNA fragment or by adding a homopolymer with terminal transferase, so that PCR is possible when sequence on only one side of the region to be amplified is known (a procedure sometimes called "anchored PCR").[70] Finally, PCR with oligonucleotide primers containing a mismatched base can be used to create site-specific mutations in DNA, which can then be assayed for function in vivo by insertion of mutant DNA fragments into genes of expression vectors.[71]

In Situ Hybridization Methods

Two other different hybridization techniques, with unfortunately similar names, have figured prominently in the molecular biologic studies of cancer and lymphoma. "In situ hybridization" refers to the direct hybridization of probes to RNA within cells and tissues on microscope slides.[72] These probes may be labeled with radioactivity (usually with ^{35}S in place of phosphorus) or nonradioactive chemical tags. Hybridization of a radioactive probe is detected by overlaying the slide with a thin, translucent film of photographic emulsion, which is developed while still on the slide after sufficient time of exposure. Hybridization of chemically tagged probes is detected using antibodies conjugated to enzymes capable of catalyzing a chromogenic reaction. In either case, the results are viewed through the light of the microscope to determine the distribution and extent of expression by a specific gene identified by the probe used in the hybridization.

In contrast, "in situ fluorescent hybridization" (universally referred to as FISH) is directed against DNA within either metaphase or interphase chromosomes.[73–76] The probes used in FISH usually consist of YACs, BACs, recombinant bacteriophage genomes, cosmids, or sometimes whole libraries of DNA from individual chromosomes (so-called chromosome painting probes), each containing chemically labeled nucleotides detectable with antibodies tagged with various fluorochromes. The location of the hybridized probe is visualized through a standard fluorescent microscope or one equipped with a digital camera connected to a computer having the capacity for imaging processing. FISH can be used to map genes and DNA to specific sites in the genome and to detect abnormalities in chromosome structure (such as chromosome translocations, deletions, and duplications).

Nucleotide Sequence Analysis and Methods of Mutation Detection

With the characterization of so many genes implicated in cancer and other human diseases over the the last few years, a topic of growing interest has been the efficient identification of point mutations within these genes. Mutation detection can involve either the screening of entire genes for mutations anywhere within the DNA of that gene or the evaluation of specific sites within genes for mutations that commonly occur at that site or were previously found in the genes of a separate specimen from the patient (for instance, a tumor-specific mutation detected at a primary site later sought in followup tissue samples). Ultimately, definitive mutation detection can always be accomplished by complete nucleotide sequence analysis (Fig. 1–6).[77, 78] This is a rather complicated, labor-intensive procedure in which (as most commonly done) a single-stranded DNA (or cDNA) to be sequenced is used as a template for in vitro DNA synthesis directed by DNA polymerase. Four separate reactions are carried out, each beginning at the same primer flanking the DNA to be sequenced. (Recall from the discussion of PCR that most DNA polymerases require primers to initiate DNA synthesis.) The reactions are performed in the presence of the four nucleotides, one of which is labeled with ^{35}S to permit detection of the products. The difference between the four reactions is the inclusion of a chain-terminating nucleotide analog (2′,3′-dideoxynucleoside triphosphate) for one or the other of the four bases in DNA, so that some portion of the primer-extension reaction will stop whenever the nucleotide complementary to the dideoxy analogue

added to the reaction appears in the template. The result of each reaction is a series of radioactive, single-stranded products, all having the same 5′ end and varying in length by the distance between the positions of the nucleotides complementary to the analogue in the template. The products of the four reactions are analyzed by electrophoresis in adjacent lanes of a polyacrylamide gel, followed by autoradiography of the gel. The sequence for the template is assembled by reading up the autoradiogram, moving back and forth from lane to lane, noting which lane contains the next band nearest the bottom. A nucleotide corresponding to the nucleotide analogue used in the reaction to generate the lane is added to the deduced sequence for each band that appears in that lane.

Because of the significant work involved in the manual sequence analysis of DNA, efforts have been made to automate sequence analysis as much as possible. So far, these efforts have amounted to developing a set of fluorescent tags to label the separate primer extension products.[79] This permits running all four reactions in the same lane of the electrophoretic gel and assembly of the sequence by computerized readers that scan the gel at different wavelengths.[80] Such automated sequence analysis has been crucial in the ongoing mission to sequence all human DNA.

The laboriousness of complete sequence analysis has also prompted development of simpler, although less definitive, methods to detect mutations at specific sites and over some region within DNA.[81] For mutation detection at specific sites, the most extensively used technique has been allele-specific oligonucleotide (ASO) hybridization.[82] In this procedure, a labeled oligonucleotide probe about 15 to 20 nucleotides long is prepared to match the sequence spanning the position of the mutation. DNA to be tested for the mutation is amplified from cells or tissues by PCR. The products of amplification are usually denatured and applied directly to a nylon membrane, which is then hybridized with the oligonucleotide probe. Under the proper conditions of stringency, a single nucleotide mismatch between the oligonucleotide probe and normal target DNA is sufficient to detect substantially greater hybridization of the oligonucleotide to the normal DNA (or, in the commonly encountered situation, to homozygous normal DNA versus heterozygous mutant). In testing for a particular base substitution, an oligonucleotide matching the mutant sequence can be used. This probe hybridizes more efficiently to the mutant PCR product than does an oligonucleotide containing normal sequence.

The effectiveness of ASO hybridization has led to widely heralded efforts now under way to create technology whereby whole genes can be interrogated for mutations by placing arrays of oligonucleotides that cover the entire gene sequence on small chips and hybridizing labeled PCR products to these chips.[83, 84] Currently, however, scanning of genes for mutations at numerous positions is usually attempted using either of two electrophoretic techniques based on the altered conformation of DNA fragments containing mutations. The more popular of these relies on the principle of single-strand conformational polymorphism (SSCP).[85–87] Radiolabeled, double-stranded PCR products are denatured and quickly reannealed to allow intrastrand bonds to form. After reannealing, the DNA strands are separated by polyacrylamide electrophoresis under non-

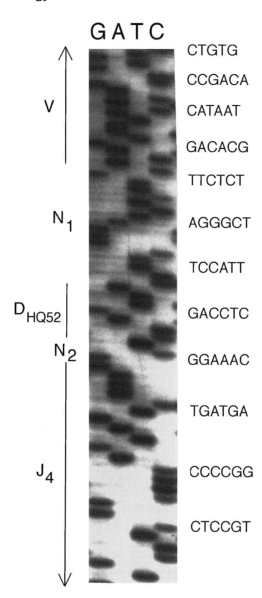

Figure 1–6. Autoradiogram of a DNA sequencing gel. Analysis was performed on a fragment of DNA amplified by polymerase chain reaction (PCR) from a rearranged immunoglobulin heavy chain gene of B-cell lymphoma. The nucleotide sequence in the antisense strand across the VDJ junction is shown (see Chapter 7). The four sequencing reactions carried out with chain-terminating dideoxynucleotides were loaded in the order indicated at the top, with the letter standing for the dideoxynucleotide used in that reaction. The sequence determined from the pattern of bands is shown at the right, with the first base in each group aligned opposite the corresponding band and the following bases reading downward from that point.

denaturing conditions, followed by autoradiography. The three-dimensional structures assumed by each strand, and the consequent electrophoretic mobility of those structures in the gels, can be affected by single nucleotide differences within the nucleotide sequence of that strand.

The second conformationally based technique used for gene scanning is denaturing gradient gel electrophoresis (DGGE).[88, 89] This technique uses an increasing gradient of chemical denaturants incorporated into a polyacrylamide gel to induce local separation of strands in double-stranded PCR products as they move through the gel. The concentration of denaturant within the gradient at which strand separation first occurs is strongly dependent on the precise sequence of nucleotides in that region of the DNA. Any single-strandedness greatly reduces mobility of the fragment in the gel, resulting in bands at the position in the gel where the

concentration of denaturant has begun to open the double helix. In both DGGE and SSCP, the appearance of bands at positions other than that generated from normal DNA denotes the presence of a mutation. Each technique is limited to analysis of fragments about 200 to 500 base pairs long. Although DGGE is more cumbersome than SSCP, principally because the pouring of gradient gels demands extra care, DGGE has the advantage that it can be performed with unlabeled DNA that is rendered fluorescent by staining the gel with ethidium bromide. Unfortunately, neither technique detects all mutations within DNA.

Methods of Protein Analysis

Besides straightforward SDS–polyacrylamide gel electrophoresis to size polypeptides, as mentioned earlier, there are two additional basic techniques commonly applied directly to the analysis of proteins: Western blot analysis and immunohistochemistry. An essential reagent for both techniques is antibody directed against the protein under analysis.[58] These antibodies may be produced by immunized animals. The antibodies raised by such immunizations are polyclonal and directed against several epitopes on the protein. Alternatively, monoclonal antibodies with specificity for only one epitope may be produced by the fusion in vitro of single lymphocytes obtained from an immunized mouse with immortalized myeloma cells and the propagation of the resulting hybridomas in the ascitic fluid of mice or in culture. In generating either polyclonal or monoclonal antibodies, the protein immunogen used these days is likely to be a polypeptide expressed from a cDNA inserted into *E. coli* by way of a plasmid vector that supplies the bacterial promoter and ribosome binding site for synthesis of the human protein in the bacterial host.[90] To facilitate the purification of the protein from bacteria, the coding sequence is frequently linked to a sequence dictating the synthesis of some short, distinctive polypeptide tag for which an antibody is available or which greatly increases the affinity of the protein to some chromatographic matrix.

In Western blot analysis (another twist on the term "Southern blot" because of the procedural similarities of the two techniques), or immunoblotting, mixtures of proteins are separated into bands by polyacrylamide gel electrophoresis, followed by transfer of the proteins from the gel to a nitrocellulose membrane by an electric field applied to the surface of gel, perpendicular to the original direction of electrophoresis.[58, 91, 92] The membrane is then incubated with the antibody to the protein of choice. The binding of antibody to a particular band in the membrane is detected by a second-stage antibody that recognizes the constant region of the first antibody and is conjugated to some type of detector, such as an enzyme that deposits an insoluble reaction product at the site of binding or generates a chemiluminescent signal that can be captured on x-ray film in the dark.

Immunohistochemistry, although developed before in situ hybridization, is analogous to the latter technique in that it detects gene products in cells and tissue sections and permits direct correlation with the microscopic anatomy of tissues.[93] The success of immunohistochemistry is dependent on the individual antibody preparation and, most important, on the preserved antigenicity of the proteins within the cells under examination. Antigen preservation is best achieved in frozen sections; however, the morphology in most of these sections is inferior to that in the standard formalin-fixed, paraffin-embedded tissues used for routine histologic examination. Recently, it has been found that heating of paraffin-embedded sections in dilute urea solutions (the so-called antigen rescue procedure) somehow restores the antigenicity of certain epitopes, expanding the potential usefulness of immunohistochemistry.[94] Binding of antibody to antigen within cells and tissues on the microscope slide is detected by using antibodies conjugated to enzymes that catalyze a chromogenic reaction, the product of which can be seen under the microscope at the location of the antigen.

Techniques for investigating the physical interactions of proteins along pathways that control cell metabolism and growth have also contributed significantly in recent years to advancing understanding of the biology of cancer. One such technique is the coimmunoprecipitation of proteins from extracts of cells by antibodies against one or the other protein within a complex.[58] Following precipitation, the proteins within the complex can be separated by SDS–polyacrylamide gel electrophoresis to determine the other protein constituents associated with the antigen in the complex.

A second, widely applied technique to assess or discover protein interactions is the so-called yeast two-hybrid system or interaction trap.[95] This is a genetic technique based on the principle that the DNA-binding domain and the activation domain of a transcription factor need not be linked in the same polypeptide but only held together by noncovalent forces to activate transcription of a cognate promoter. In fact, one DNA-binding domain may substitute for another in this combination. Building on this principle, coding sequence for a test polypeptide (the bait) in the two-hybrid system is fused to coding sequence of a DNA-binding domain within an expression vector. This vector is used to search for protein sequences that interact with the bait by inserting the vector into a culture of yeast carrying an expression library of cDNAs fused to the sequence for the activation domain of a transcription factor. These yeast also harbor a reporter gene that can be activated by the activation domain expressed by the library and is located behind the DNA-binding site recognized by the binding domain encoded by the vector containing the sequences of the bait. The yeast are spread on the surface of an agar plate and the transcription of the reporter gene monitored by either growth of colonies under selective conditions or the production of a distinct color within the colony. Transcription of the reporter gene within the colony indicates that the cDNA in the cells of that colony directed the synthesis of polypeptide or region of a polypeptide that interacted with the bait, bringing together the activation domain with the DNA-binding domain of the transcription factor. The cDNA within the yeast can be removed, amplified, and sequenced to determine the identity of the interacting protein.

The need to sequence directly the amino acids of polypeptides is rather limited these days. Most amino acid sequence is analyzed indirectly by sequencing nucleotides within DNA, which is a far more efficient process than is amino acid sequence analysis. In those situations where direct analysis of amino acid sequence is indicated (such as in coimmunoprecipitation studies to identify unknown proteins brought down by the antibody), small fragments of the polypeptide for analysis are usually prepared by cleavage of the protein with a specific endopeptidase. The amino acids of a peptide fragment are released sequentially from the N-terminus by chemical modification followed by treatment with acid,[96] and each amino acid released is identified by chromatography on paper or through columns. Alternatively, and with increasing frequency, amino acid sequence is being deduced by mass spectroscopy of small polypeptide fragments. Even relatively short stretches of amino acid sequence are sufficient to permit construction of oligonucleotides (or sets of oligonucleotides because of the redundancy of codons for most amino acids) that can be used to probe cDNA libraries for nucleotide sequences encoding the protein under examination.[97] Once the cDNA is obtained, the full amino acid sequence can be determined from the codon contents of this molecule. The relationship of the

the protein can be confirmed by expressing the cDNA within *E. coli* and demonstrating similar physical and functional properties to the protein originally isolated, including the ability to raise cross-reacting antibodies within immunized animals.

By itself, knowledge of the amino acid sequence of a protein is often sufficient these days to infer key functional features about that protein. As amino acid sequences information on proteins has expanded dramatically in recent years, a variety of sequence motifs shared proteins have become apparent, although these homologies are frequently subtle and are identified only by the computer programs that compare newly acquired sequences with data bases of known protein sequences. In many instances, understanding of the function of a protein or a domain within a protein the sequence of which is stored in the data base provides a valuable clue to the role of a recently discovered protein or gene within the cell.

REFERENCES

1. Alberts B, Bray D, Lewis J, et al: Molecular Biology of the Cell, 3rd ed. New York, Garland, 1994.
2. Lodish H, Baltimore D, Berk A, et al: Molecular Cell Biology, 3rd ed. New York, Freeman, 1995.
3. Adolph KW (ed): Chromosomes and Chromatin, vols 1–3. Boca Raton, FL, CRC Press, 1988.
4. Dickerson RE, Drew HR, Conner BN, et al: The anatomy of A-, B-, and Z-DNA. Science 1982; 216:475.
5. Cantor CR, Schimmel PR: Biophysical Chemistry, vol 3. San Francisco, Freeman, 1980.
6. Sharp PA: RNA splicing and genes. JAMA 1988; 260:3035.
7. Branden C, Tooze J: Introduction to Protein Structure. New York, Garland, 1991.
8. McKinney JD, Heintz N: Transcriptional regulation in the eukaryotic cell cycle. Trends Biochem Sci 1991; 16:430.
9. Mitchell PJ, Tjian R: Transcriptional regulation in mammalian cells by sequence-specific DNA binding proteins. Science 1989; 245:371.
10. Pabo CO, Sauer RT: Transcription factors: Structural families and principles of DNA recognition. Ann Rev Biochem 1992; 61:1053.
11. Greenblatt J: RNA polymerase–associated transcription factors. Trends Biochem Sci 1991; 16:408.
12. Schleif R: DNA looping. Ann Rev Biochem 1992; 61:199.
13. Richardson JP: Transcriptional termination. Crit Rev Biochem Molec Biol 1993; 28:1.
14. Sachs A, Wahle E: Poly(A) tail metabolism and function in eucaryotes. J Biol Chem 1993; 268:22955.
15. Nevins J: The pathway of eukaryotic mRNA formation. Ann Rev Biochem 1983; 52:441.
16. Cooper GM: Oncogenes, 2nd ed. Boston, Jones and Bartlett, 1995.
17. Bishop JM, Weinberg RA (eds): Molecular Oncology. New York, Scientific American, 1996.
18. Merrick WC: Mechanism and regulation of eukaryotic protein synthesis. Microbiol Rev 1992; 56:291.
19. Rothman JE: Mechanisms of intracellular protein transport. Nature 1994; 372:59.
20. Gething MJ, Sambrook J: Protein folding in the cell. Nature 1992; 355:33.
21. Silver PA: How proteins enter the nucleus. Cell 1991; 64:489.
22. Nunnari J, Walter P: Protein targeting to and translocation across the membrane of the endoplasmic reticulum. Curr Opin Cell Biol 1992; 4:573.
23. Nasmyth K: Viewpoint: Putting the cell cycle in order. Science 1996; 274:1643.
24. Sherr CJ: Cancer cell cycles. Science 1996; 274:1672.
25. King RW, Deshaies RJ, Peters J-M, Kirschner MW: How proteolysis drives the cell cycle. Science 1996; 274:1652.
26. Stillman B: Cell cycle control of DNA replication. Science 1996; 274:1659.
27. Elledge SJ: Cell cycle checkpoints: Preventing an identity crisis. Science 1996; 274:1664.
28. Bishop JM: Molecular themes in oncogenesis. Cell 1991; 64:235.
29. Weinberg RA: Tumor suppressor genes. Science 1991; 254:1138.
30. Perkins AS, Stern DF: Molecular biology of cancer: Oncogenes. *In* DeVita VT, Hellman S, Rosenberg SA (eds): Cancer: Principles and Practice of Oncology, 5th ed. Philadelphia, JB Lippincott, 1997, p 79.
31. Zur Hausen H: Viruses in human cancers. Science 1991; 254:1167.
32. Cavenee W, Hansen M, Nordenskjold M, et al: Genetic origin of mutations predisposing to retinoblastoma. Science 1985; 228.
33. Lasko D, Cavenee WK, Nordenskjold M: Loss of constitutional heterozygosity in human cancer. Ann Rev Genet 1991; 25:281.
34. Rabbitts TH: Chromosomal translocations in human cancer. Nature 1994; 372:143.
35. Watson JD, Gilman M, Witkowski J, Zoller M: Recombinant DNA, 2nd ed. New York, Scientific American, 1992.
36. Monaco AP, Larin Z: YACs, BACs, PACs, and MACs: Artificial chromosomes as research tools. Trends Biotechnol 1994; 12:280.
37. Ramsey M: Yeast artificial chromosome cloning. Mol Biotechnol 1994; 1:181.
38. Shizuya H, Birren B, Kim U-J, et al: Cloning and stable maintenance of 300-kilobase-pair fragments of human DNA in *Escherichia coli* using an F-factor-based vector. Proc Natl Acad Sci U S A 1992; 89:8794.
39. Shih C, Shilo B-Z, Goldfarb MP, et al: Passage of phenotypes of chemically transformed cells via transfection of DNA and chromatin. Proc Natl Acad Sci U S A 1981; 76:5714.
40. Danos O, Mulligan RC: Safe and efficient generation of recombinant retroviruses with amphotropic and ecotropic host ranges. Proc Natl Acad Sci U S A 1988; 85:6460.
41. Dranoff G, Jaffee E, Lazenby A, et al: Vaccination with irradiated tumor cells engineered to secrete murine granulocyte-macrophage colony-stimulating factor stimulates potent, specific, and long-lasting antitumor immunity. Proc Natl Acad Sci U S A 1993; 90:3539.
42. Daley GQ, Van Etten RA, Baltimore D: Induction of chronic myelogenous leukemia in mice by the P210*bcr/able* gene of the Philadelphia chromosome. Science 1990; 247:824.
43. Crystal RG: Transfer of genes to humans: Early lessons and obstacles to success. Science 1995; 270:404.
44. Anderson WF: Human gene therapy. Science 1992; 256:808.
45. Grosveld F, Kollias G (eds): Transgenic Animals. New York, Academic Press, 1992.
46. Stewart TA, Pattengale PK, Leder P: Spontaneous mammary adeno-carcinomas in transgenic mice that carry and express MTV/*myc* fusion genes. Cell 1984; 38:627.
47. Capecchi MR: Altering the genome by homologous recombination. Science 1989; 244:1288.
48. Gossen J, Vijg J: Transgenic mice as model systems for studying gene mutations in vivo. Trends Genet 1993; 9:27.
49. Andrews AT: Electrophoresis. Oxford, UK, Clarendon Press, 1986.
50. Southern EM: Gel electrophoresis of restriction fragments. Methods Enzymol 1979; 68:152.
51. Weber K, Osborn M: Proteins and sodium dodecyl sulfate: Molecular weight determination on polyacrylamide gels and related procedures. *In* Neurath H, Hill RL (eds): The Proteins, 3rd ed, vol 1. New York, Academic Press, 1975, p 179.
52. Hames BD, Rickwood D (eds): Gel Electrophoresis of Proteins: A Practical Approach. New York, Oxford University Press, 1990.
53. Rigby PWJ, Dieckmann M, Rhodes C, Berg P: Labeling deoxyribonucleic acid to high specific activity in vitro by nick translation with DNA polymerase I. J Mol Biol 1977; 113:237.
54. Feinberg AP, Vogelstein B: A technique for radiolabeling DNA restriction endonuclease fragments to high specific activity. Anal Biochem 1983; 132:6.
55. Richardson CC: Polynucleotide kinase from *Escherichia coli* infected with bacteriophage T4. Nucleic Acids Res 1971; 2:815.
56. Chan VT, Fleming KA, McGee JO: Detection of sub-picogram quantities of specific DNA sequences on blot hybridization with biotinylated probes. Nucleic Acids Res 1985; 13:8083.
57. Leary JJ, Brigati DJ, Ward DC: Rapid and sensitive colorimetric method for visualizing biotin-labeled DNA probes hybridized to DNA or RNA immobilized on nitrocellulose: Bio-blots. Proc Natl Acad Sci U S A 1983; 80:4045.
58. Harlow E, Lane D: Antibodies: A Laboratory Manual. Cold Spring Harbor, NY, Cold Spring Harbor Laboratory, 1988.

59. Wetmur JG: DNA probes: Applications of the principles of nucleic acid hybridization. Crit Rev Biochem Mol Biol 1991; 26:227.
60. Southern E: Detection of specific sequences among DNA fragments separated by gel electrophoresis. J Mol Biol 1975; 98:503.
61. Alwine JC, Kemp DJ, Stark GR: Method for detection of specific RNAs in agarose gels by transfer to diabenzyloxymethyl paper and hybridization with DNA probes. Proc Natl Acad Sci U S A 1977; 74:5350.
62. Thomas PS: Hybridization of denatured RNA and small DNA fragments transferred to nitrocellulose. Proc Natl Acad Sci U S A 1980; 77:5201.
63. Saiki RK, Scharf S, Faloona F, et al: Enzymatic amplification of β-globin genomic sequences and restriction site analysis for diagnosis of sickle cell anemia. Science 1985; 230:1350.
64. Saiki R, Bugawan T, Horn G, et al: Analysis of enzymatically amplified beta-globin and HLA-DQ DNA with allele-specific oligonucleotide probes. Nature (London) 1986; 324:163.
65. Mullis KB, Faloona FAS: Specific synthesis of DNA in vitro via a polymerase-catalyzed chain reaction. Methods Enzymol 1987; 155:335.
66. Saiki RK, Gelfand DH, Stoffel S, et al: Primer-directed enzymatic amplification of DNA with a thermostable DNA polymerase. Science 1988; 239:487.
67. Kawasaki ES, Clark SS, Coyne MY, et al: Diagnosis of chronic myelogenous leukemia and acute leukemia by detection of leukemia-specific mRNA sequences amplified in vitro. Proc Natl Acad Sci U S A 1988; 85:5689.
68. Cheng S, Fockler C, Barnes WM, Higuchi R: Effective amplification of long targets from cloned inserts and human genomic DNA. Proc Natl Acad Sci U S A 1994; 91:5695.
69. Barnes WM: PCR amplification of up to 35-kb DNA with high fidelity and high yield from λ templates. Proc Natl Acad Sci U S A 1994; 91:2216.
70. Loh EY, Elliott JF, Cwirla S, et al: Polymerase chain reaction with single-sided specificity: Analysis of T-cell receptor delta chain. Science 1989; 243:217.
71. Higuchi R: Using PCR to engineer DNA. In Ehrlich HA (ed): PCR Technology. New York, Freeman, 1992, pp 61–70.
72. Angerer LM, Angerer RC: Localization of mRNAs by in situ hybridization. Methods Cell Biol 1991:35.
73. Langer-Safer P, Levine M, Ward D: Immunological method for mapping genes on *Drosophila* polytene chromosomes. Proc Natl Acad Sci U S A 1982; 79:4381.
74. Lichter P, Cremer T, Tang CJ, et al: Rapid detection of human chromosome 21 aberrations by in situ hybridization. Proc Natl Acad Sci U S A 1988; 85:9664.
75. Pinkel D, Landegent J, Collins C, et al: Fluorescent in situ hybridization with human chromosome–specific libraries: Detection of trisomy 21 and translocations of chromosome 4. Proc Natl Acad Sci U S A 1988; 87:9138.
76. Joos S, Fink TM, Ratsch A, Lichter P: Mapping and chromosome analysis: The potential of fluorescence in situ hybridization. J Biotechnol 1994; 35:135.
77. Maxam AM, Gilbert W: A new method for sequencing DNA. Proc Natl Acad Sci U S A 1977; 74:560.
78. Sanger F, Nicklen S, Coulson AR: DNA sequencing with chain-terminating inhibitors. Proc Natl Acad Sci U S A 1977; 74:5463.
79. Smith L, Sanders J, Kaiser R, et al: Fluorescence detection in automated DNA sequence analysis. Nature 1986; 321:674.
80. Adams MD, Kerlavage AR, Kelley JM, et al: A model for high-throughput automated DNA sequencing and analysis core facilities. Nature 1994; 368(6470):474.
81. Mashal RD, Sklar J: Practical methods of mutation detection. Curr Opin Genet Develop 1996; 6:275.
82. Studencki AB, Wallace RB: Allele-specific hybridization using oligonucleotide probes of very high specific activity: Discrimination of the human beta A- and beta S-globin genes. DNA 1984; 3(1):7.
83. Lennon GG, Lehrach H: Hybridization analyses of arrayed cDNA libraries. Trends Genet 1991; 7:314.
84. Kozal MJ, Shah N, Shen N, et al: Extensive polymorphisms observed in HIV-1 grade B protease gene using high-density oligonucleotide arrays. Nature Med 1996; 2:753.
85. Orita M, Iwahana H, Kanazawa H, et al: Detection of polymorphisms of human DNA by gel electrophoresis as single-strand conformation polymorphisms. Proc Natl Acad Sci U S A 1989; 86:2766.
86. Orita M, Suzuki Y, Sekiya T, Hayashi K: Rapid and sensitive detection of point mutations and DNA polymorphisms using the polymerase chain reaction. Genomics 1989; 5(4):874.
87. Sheffield VC, Beck JS, Kwitek AE, et al: The sensitivity of single-strand conformation polymorphism analysis for the detection of single base substitutions. Genomics 1993; 16(2):325.
88. Myers RM, Lumelsky N, Lerman LS, Morley AA: Detection of single-base substitutions in total genomic DNA. Nature 1985; 313:495.
89. Myers RM, Maniatis T, Lerman LS: Detection and localization of single base changes by denaturing gradient gel electrophoresis. Method Enzymol 1987; 155:501.
90. Yarranton GT: Mammalian recombinant proteins: Vectors and expression systems. Curr Opin Biotechnol 1990; 1:133.
91. Burnette WN: Western blotting: Electrophoretic transfer of proteins from sodium dodecyl sulfate-polyacrylamide gels to unmodified nitrocellulose and radiographic detection with antibody and radioiodinated protein A. Anal Biochem 1981; 125:195.
92. Renart J, Sandoval IV: Western blots. Methods Enzymol 1984; 104:455.
93. Larsson L: Tissue preparation methods for light microscopic immunohistochemistry. Appl Immunohistochem 1993; 1:2.
94. Gown A, de Weber N, Battifora H: Microwave antigenic unmasking: A revolutionary new technique for routine immunohistochemistry. Appl Immunohistochem 1993; 1:256.
95. Fields S, Sternglanz R: The two-hybrid system: An assay for protein-protein interactions. Trends Genet 1994; 10:286.
96. Walsh KA, Ericsson LH, Parmelee DC, Titani K: Advances in protein sequencing. Ann Rev Biochem 1981; 50:261.
97. Yang J, Ye J, Wallace DC: Computer selection of oligonucleotide probes from amino acid sequences for use in gene library screening. Nucleic Acids Res 1984; 12:837.

Chapter Two

——Developmental and Functional —— Biology of B and T Lymphocytes

Henrik Griesser
Tak W. Mak

Prior to their delineation as B or T cells, lymphocytic precursors emerge from pluripotential stem cells originating at sites of general hematopoiesis such as fetal liver and adult bone marrow. Stem cells presumably produce more committed, incompletely differentiated cell types. Indirect evidence for the existence of a common lymphoid progenitor for B, T, and natural killer (NK) cells may have come from mice with targeted germline mutation of the Ikaros gene.[1] This gene encodes a zinc finger DNA-binding protein that is highly expressed in lymphoid cells. Ikaros gene knockout mice lack T, B, and NK cells, but no defect is seen in the maturation of myeloid and erythroid lineages. From the 7th gestational week onward the lymphoid precursors, committed to T or B lineage, migrate into the primary lymphoid organs where they enter a highly regulated program of differentiation. T cells in the thymus and B cells in the bone marrow pass through stages of negative and positive selection that removes lymphocytes with useless, defective, or self-reactive antigen receptors. Mainly, those lymphocytes survive that are properly equipped for recognition of foreign antigen.

This chapter reviews different events that influence B and T lymphocyte maturation and shape the antigen receptor repertoires. T and B cells have structurally similar antigen receptors, the T-cell receptor (TCR) and immunoglobulin (Ig) molecules. They use common mechanisms for their immune receptor gene assembly, and they activate similar, but not identical, signal transduction pathways on antigen receptor and coreceptor stimulation. In the periphery, T and B cells serve different purposes. T cells are involved mainly in cellular immunity, and B cells are major players in the humoral immune response. This is accounted for by differences in the differentiation events of the two lymphoid lineages in secondary lymphoid organs such as spleen, lymph nodes, and extranodal lymphoid tissues. The first part of the chapter concentrates on the biologic aspects of T lymphocytes that play a central role in immune regulation. The second part outlines B-cell development. Interactions between T and B cells are emphasized in the discussion of antigen-dependent B-cell maturation and activation.

T LYMPHOCYTES

T cells undergo a radical selection process in the thymus. Their antigen-recognition molecules, the TCRs for antigen, allow them to react specifically against exogenous or endogenous antigens. Unlike Ig molecules, TCRs do not recognize soluble antigens and rather interact with antigens bound to special-presentation molecules encoded by the major histocompatibility complex (MHC).[2] TCR molecules are physically associated with a variety of other surface molecules, including CD3, CD4 or CD8, CD2, integrin receptors, CD45, or CD28 molecules. Engagement of these coreceptors is necessary for a complete response of a T cell that specifically recognizes an antigen. The specific antigen binding leads to T-lymphocyte transformation into blast cells and initiates their clonal expansion.

Different T-lymphocyte subpopulations have different effector functions: They mediate destruction of virus-infected cells by cytotoxic T cells, or they secrete hormone-like lymphokines as T-helper cells and support antigen-dependent B-cell differentiation or expansion of cytotoxic T cells. CD4-expressing cells typically interact with cells displaying MHC class II (MCH II) and function as helper cells to regulate other cellular responses. CD8 lymphocytes recognize MHC I molecules and are primarily cytotoxic.

THE T-CELL RECEPTOR, ITS CORECEPTORS AND LIGANDS
The T-Cell Receptor for Antigen

TCRs are disulfide-linked heterodimeric polypeptide molecules consisting mainly of α-β chains. In 5% to 10% of mature T lymphocytes an alternative TCR is found composed of γ-δ chains.[3–5] Depending on glycosylation patterns and individual allelic variations, TCR α chains are 40 to 50 kilodaltons (kD) and TCR β chains are 40- to 45-kD glycoproteins. Human TCRγ1 and γ2 encoded proteins are 35 to 55 kD and δ chains are 40 to 60 kD. The TCR chains attain great diversity by the random rearrangement of multiple variable (V), diversity (D), and joining (J) genes. Together these gene segments encode the extracellular TCR

V domain that binds antigens and MHC molecules. TCR constant (C) regions contain four functional domains. The first distal extracellular domain of all four TCR polypeptides is likely to have a similar folding structure as Ig C1 regions. A cysteine residue encoded by a separate exon sits between the transmembrane spanning region and the C1 domain. The cysteine residue is covalently bound through a sulfhydryl linkage to the equivalent cysteine on the corresponding partner chain (α-β, γ-δ). This region is designated as a "connecting peptide" or "hinge region." Human Cγ2-encoded proteins lack a cysteine residue at the hinge region and interact with the δ chain noncovalently.[6] The third C region is hydrophobic, appears to span the membrane, and comprises positively charged amino acids at conserved sites. All TCR polypeptides have a fourth, very short intracellular cytoplasmic region of unknown function.

TCRs are noncovalently associated with the CD3 complex (Fig. 2–1) that is responsible for the signal transduction on antigenic stimulation.[7] CD3 peptides have long cytoplasmic domains containing conserved amino acid motifs (Y-L). These motifs are important for the communication with other molecules involved in signal transduction, such as ZAP-70 and its associated kinases.[8, 9] The CD3 multimer consists of the invariant CD3γ, δ, ε, and the homodimeric ζ-ζ or, in mice, heterodimeric ζ-η chains. The η chain represents an alternatively spliced protein product of the ζ chain.[10] Structural and functional data implicate different roles for CD3γ, δ, ε molecules on the one hand and the ζ-ζ and ζ-η dimers on the other. ζ chains are not members of the Ig superfamily, and they have important roles in the signal transduction of NK cells. Both chain compositions form two parallel signal transduction units, both being capable of eliciting interleukin-2 (IL-2) production.[8]

Coreceptors

Mature T cells express either the CD4 or the CD8 receptor on the surface that binds to nonpolymorphic regions of the MHC II or MHC I molecules, respectively. These coreceptors stabilize the binding of the TCR complex to antigen and participate in the signal transduction.[11, 12] Data obtained from CD4- and CD8-deficient mice confirm that CD4 molecules are mainly responsible for helper activity. Mice without CD8 cells are severely impaired in MHC I–dependent responses against viruses.[13, 14]

CD4 molecules are expressed as monomers on the cell surface of T cells, some monocytes and macrophages, follicular dendritic reticulum cells (FDCs), Langerhans cells of the skin, thymic dendritic cells, some B cells, and microglial cells in the brain.[15] As mentioned earlier, CD4 molecules probably interact with nonpolymorphic sites within MHC II domains.[16, 17] CD4 contacts MHC II along a surface including one side of the complementarity-determining region 1 (CDR1)-like and CDR3-like loops of the N-terminal domain and a part of the second Ig-like domain.[18] After CD3 stimulation, CD4 molecules move in close association with the TCR/CD3 complex. CD4-TCR/CD3 association and, consequently, antigen-specific signal transduction, is dependent on the physical interaction between CD4 molecules and the protein tyrosine kinase (PTK) p56lck.

CD8 molecules are transmembrane glycoproteins that form disulfide-linked heterodimers consisting of an α chain and a β chain. Sometimes homodimers of CD8α occur. Human T cells can alter the relative number of CD8αα and CD8αβ dimers on the cell surface on stimulation. A subset of human intestinal CD8+ intraepithelial lymphocytes (IELs) expresses CD8αα homodimers rather than the more usual CD8αβ heterodimers.[19] CD8 molecules interact with a nonpolymorphic region on MHC I molecules.[20] The short cytoplasmic portion of only the α chain of CD8 contains conserved cysteine motifs at basic amino acid residues for physical association with p56lck,[21, 22] but only 10% to 25% of p56lck is associated with CD8α. Cross-linking of CD8 and p56lck does not substantially increase TCR-mediated signals, which differs from the functional findings for CD4-p56lck.

CD2, a glycoprotein and member of the Ig superfamily, is expressed at early stages of thymic T-cell differentiation and maintained on almost all peripheral T cells.[23] The major role of CD2 molecules is the enhancement of the TCR/CD3–mediated response, particularly in resting and naive T cells.[24] CD2 binds with very high affinity to its ligand lymphocyte functional antigen-3 (LFA-3), which is expressed on the surface of nearly all nucleated cells. This is a major factor in stabilizing initial cell-cell interactions and adhesion before specific TCR activation. TCR activation leads to increased CD2 surface expression. This interaction may be important for initial functional binding of T-helper cells to antigen-presenting cells (APCs), of cytotoxic T cells to their targets, and of immature thymocytes to epithelial or bone marrow–derived stromal cells.

CD45 phosphatase activity is essential for CD2-mediated

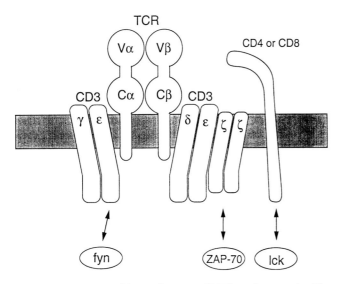

Figure 2–1. Structure of the T-cell receptor (TCR) signaling complex. The membrane-bound αβ TCR has extracellular variable (V) domains, invariable extracellular constant (C) domains, and transmembrane domains. The TCR chains are associated with different CD3 molecules (γ, δ, ε) and the ζ chain dimer. Furthermore, CD8 or CD4 receptors are required for corecognition of MHC I or II molecules, respectively. *Arrows* indicate the association of cytoplasmic domains of the TCR coreceptors with their signaling molecules, the protein tyrosine kinases p56lck, p59fyn, and ZAP-70.

tyrosine kinase activation, phospholipase C-γ1 (PLC-γ1) phosphorylation, and IL-2 production.[25] CD45 is a major transmembrane glycoprotein forming about 10% of all surface molecules on leukocytes and hematopoietic progenitor cells.[26] The intracellular CD45 region comprises two subdomains, repeated in tandem, that contain protein tyrosine phosphatase activity. T and B cells express different isoforms of CD45 with a molecular weight ranging from 180 to 235 kD because of differential splicing of the four variable exons 4, 5, 6, and 7 in the NH_2-terminal domain of the molecule. Expression of different isoforms depends on the cellular differentiation and activation stage. B cells express the highest molecular weight form of 220 kD. Macrophages, CD34+ precursor cells, immature CD4+/CD8+ thymocytes, and memory T cells mainly express the low-molecular-weight (LMW) CD45 isoform of 180 kD. Other peripheral T cells and mature CD4+ or CD8+ thymocytes express multiple isoforms.[27, 28] Activated T cells express LMW, and resting T cells express high-molecular-weight (HMW) forms. Antibodies detecting the expression of variable exons or restricted epitopes of CD45 are available. The CD45 isoforms identified by antiexon 4, antiexon 5, and antiexon 6 specific monoclonal antibodies are also known as CD45RA, CD45RB, and CD45RC, respectively. The antibody CD45RO recognizes the 180-kD LMW form of CD45. Different isoforms of CD45 display major differences in glycosylation patterns and therefore differences in negatively charged sugar residues on the cell surface. HMW forms interfere with physical contacts of specific ligand/receptor pairs. LMW CD45 isoforms, which carry less sialic acids and a negative charge, may allow increased cell-cell interactions such as is found in activated and memory T cells. Exon switching of CD45 molecules on T-cell activation may also influence the interaction of CD45 with intercellular receptors on other cells and/or lateral ligands expressed on the same cell.[26] The lowest-molecular-weight CD45 isoform (CD45RO) may be the ligand for CD22 molecules found on B cells.[29] Activated and memory T cells thus might be involved in T-cell-dependent B-cell activation by production of cytokines and directly by physical association between CD45RO and CD22. CD45 associates not only with the TCR/CD3 complex but also preferentially interacts with T-cell accessory molecules.[30] The integrin receptor LFA-1 preferentially associates with the HMW CD45 isoforms, whereas CD2 aggregates with LMW isoforms. CD4 and CD8 accessory molecules presumably interact with CD45RC. HMW CD45 isoforms thus may hamper and LMW isoforms promote lateral movement of surface proteins to contact sites between two cells, which, for example, could partly account for rapid responses typical of memory T cells.

Major Histocompatibility Complexes

The TCRαβ receptors physiologically recognize antigen when presented on the cell surface in the context with a self-MHC molecule. This phenomenon is termed "MHC restriction."[2] MHC molecules are subdivided into class I and class II molecules. Class I molecules are expressed on cells of almost all somatic tissues. Class II molecules are restricted to certain cell types such as macrophages, dendritic cells, B cells, and activated T cells. Regulation of MHC expression specifically occurs at the transcriptional level and can be influenced by cytokines (e.g., interferon-γ[IFN-γ]). Peptides destined for presentation on MHC I molecules are generated from proteins degraded in the cytosol ("endogenous antigens") and transported into the endoplasmic reticulum (ER) where they are complexed to MHC I.[31, 32] They then move to the plasma membrane via the Golgi's complex and post-Golgi's vesicles. MHC II molecules present peptides derived from proteins entering the cell from an outside milieu ("exogenous antigens") via phagocytosis, endocytosis, or internalization of membrane molecules.

MHC I molecules contain an MHC-encoded α or heavy chain of 44 kD and a non-MHC encoded, noncovalently associated 12-kD β or light chain known as "$β_2$-microglobulin." Class II molecules comprise a 32- to 34-kD α chain and a smaller 29- to 32-kD β chain. Class II α and β heterodimers complex with an invariant chain in the ER and are routed to an acidic endosomal-endolysosomal compartment. Class II heterodimers are loaded with peptides in phagolysosomes after degradation of the invariant chain. Peptide-MHC II complexes are shuttled to the cell surface and corecognized by CD4+ T lymphocytes. The number of naturally processed peptides bound to MHC I after infection of cells with live influenza virus has been estimated to be between 220 and 540 copies.[33] It has been suggested that MHC peptides are constitutively occupied with peptides and that different MHC alleles "select" for different motifs out of the supply from cellular proteins. Thus, MHC molecules themselves may govern the selection of specific peptides out of crude cellular protein lysates.[33]

TCRγδ cells can function as cytotoxic T cells without the need to recognize classic MHC I or II molecules.[3] The physiologic role and the potential ligands of γδ T lymphocytes, however, are still unclear.

V REGION DIVERSITY OF THE T-CELL RECEPTORS

TCR molecules are structurally similar to Ig chains and therefore belong to the Ig gene superfamily.[34] TCR molecules have a large extracellular portion consisting of a C and a V domain. The V region is assembled from two or three gene segments: a V segment, a short J gene segment, and (in TCRβ or TCRδ genes) a D segment, which lies between the V and J segments in the assembled gene. An estimated 10^{19} different combinations occur for the TCRαβ molecules.[5] However, actual numbers might differ. Genomic deletions of long stretches of V gene segments[35–37] can greatly shape the TCR V region repertoire. Positive or negative selection of T cells expressing certain TCR V(D)J combinations during thymic maturation or postthymic circulation also adds to the variety. The momentary activation of lymphocyte subsets by environmental antigens, such as bacterial or retroviral superantigens, influences the variety of V domains.[38–42] The combinatorial diversity of the TCRγδ molecules is calculated to be lower (approximately 10^{13} combinations) considering that at most 8 functional Vγ, 5 Jγ, 10 Vδ, 3 Dδ, and 3 Jδ segments can be rearranged to form functional TCRγ and δ-chain genes.[43] However, the actual V region diversity of both TCRαβ and TCRγδ molecules is likely to be larger than that calculated from simple combinatorial diversity due to the extensive junctional variation at joining sites of V-D, D-D, and J-D gene segments.

Distinct regions of the TCR may interact separately with peptide antigens or with polymorphic epitopes of the surrounding MHC molecules.[5] TCR molecules, very similar to Ig receptor molecules, contain three hypervariable regions or CDRs in the V domain. These hypervariable loops cluster together to form the antigen/MHC binding site. The CDR1 and/or CDR2 regions of TCRα chains, encoded by V region genes, seem to play a role critical to the fine specificity of MHC recognition. The most variable portions of TCR (CDR3), encoded by β V-D-J and α V-J joints, may mainly contribute to T-cell antigen specificity.[44, 45]

Germline V, D, and J gene segments are flanked by a set of conserved nucleotides, heptamers, and nonamers. They function as recombination signal sequences for V-D, D-J, or V-J joining and are recognized by a recombinase enzyme system.[46] These signal sequences are separated by a nonconserved spacer (Fig. 2–2). The spacer situated 3′ of the V or D gene segment is 21 to 23 base pairs (bp) long (about two turns of the DNA helix). It is 11 or 12 bp long (about one turn of the double helix) when located 5′ of the D or J gene segment. Flanking sequences with a one-turn spacer signal can rearrange only to a two-turn signal. This probably ensures joining of appropriate gene segments. Thus, one V and one J can recombine, but more than one D segment can join. This has frequently been described for Dδ1-Dδ2, Dδ1-Dδ3, and Dδ1-Dδ2-Dδ3 joinings.[47] Intervening DNA stretches are either deleted or retained if the two segments are joined in an opposite transcriptional orientation. At the coding ends, the joining is commonly imprecise through differential trimming of recombining gene termini by exonucleases. Among coding ends that do not show nucleotide loss, there is a unique type of nucleotide addition. These seem to be inverted repeats of the last one or two nucleotides (termed "P nucleotides").[48] Introduction of sometimes more than 10 nucleotides in random sequence between V-D, D-D, D-J, or V-J junctions generates N diversity. The addition of these nontemplate-directed N-nucleotides is probably mediated by the enzyme terminal desoxynucleotidyl transferase (TdT).[49] This process contributes significantly to the potential diversity of the immune receptor, but it may also result in the generation of stop codons at the coding junctions.[50] Somatic hypermutation, a major mechanism for increased Ig V region diversity, does not seem to occur among TCR genes.[5, 43]

The V(D)J recombination is probably initiated by duplex DNA cleavage and is dependent on the machinery for general duplex DNA repair as well as on two lymphocyte-specific proteins termed "RAG1" and "RAG2."[51] The involvement of double-strand DNA breakage in rearrangement processes then has to be restricted to particular cell cycle intervals because the persistence of double-strand breaks in the S phase would be deleterious to the cell. Posttranslational modification of RAG1 and RAG2 may influence the fine control of these recombinations. In B progenitor cell lines and normal murine thymocytes RAG2 protein accumulates preferentially in the G_0/G_1 phase of the cell cycle, declines sharply before cell entry into the S phase, and remains low throughout the remainder of the cell cycle. This may indicate that V(D)J recombination occurs preferentially within G_0/G_1.[52] Expression of the *RAG1* and *RAG2* genes strictly correlates with V(D)J recombinase activity. Their transcripts occur in pre-B and pre-T cells but not in later stages of lymphocyte development.[53] During T-cell development, *RAG1* gene expression does not seem to occur in prothymocytes or mature thymocytes either.[54] *RAG1*-deficient mice have small lymphoid organs because of a lack of mature B and T cells. The maturational arrest occurs at an early developmental stage in these animals. Development and function of NK cells (in which TCR homologues are postulated for antigen recognition) and development of macrophages or granulocytes is not impaired.[55, 56]

Genomic Organization of the T-Cell Receptors

TCR polypeptides generally form mutually exclusive pairs of TCRαβ or TCRγδ heterodimers.[5] TCRδ chains can rarely

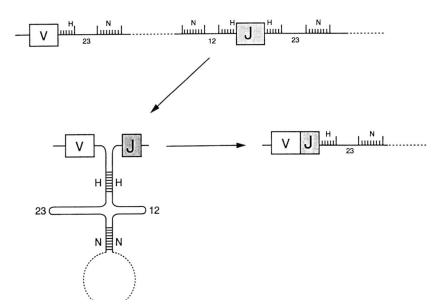

Figure 2–2. Signals involved in the joining of variable (V) and joining (J) region genes during rearrangement. Hypothetical V and J segments are illustrated with associated heptamer (H) and nonamer (N) sequences separated by spacers of 12 or 23 base pairs in length. Consensus H and N sequences align during the rearrangement. A loop is formed containing intervening sequences. After excision of the loop the V and J sequences join, forming the V domain.

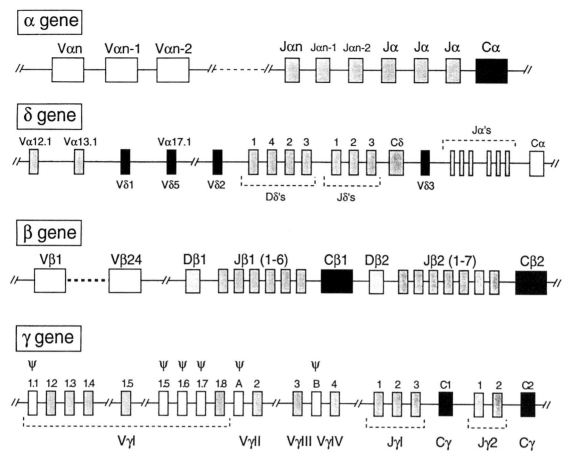

Figure 2–3. Organization of the human T-cell receptor (TCR) genes. All four TCR gene loci contain multiple V region and several J region segments 5′ to either one (TCRα, δ) or two (TCRβ, γ) C region genes. Diversity (D) gene segments are present in the TCR β and δ chains. Multiple V pseudogenes (ψ) occur in the TCRγ locus. The TCRδ genes are nested between the Vα and Jα segments. The Vδ3 segment maps 3′ to the Cδ locus in an inverse orientation.

bind to a β chain instead of an α chain.[57] Because of allelic exclusion, each T cell usually expresses only one TCR product.[58]

TCRα chain genes map to the long arm of chromosome 14 (14q11-12)[59] and harbor the TCRδ genes between its V and J region gene sequences (Fig. 2–3). Approximately 50 Vα gene segments are spread out over more than 750 kilobases (kb).[60, 61] More than 80 Jα gene segments are dispersed over an area of at least 50 kb of DNA.[62–65] D region coding sequences have not been identified, but N region diversification exists in the V-J junctional regions. The α-chain locus contains only one C region gene composed of four exons.[62]

TCR δ-chain gene sequences occupy the space between the Vα and the Jα gene cluster (see Fig. 2–3). Only one Cδ region gene exists. Three joining gene segments (Jδ 1 to 3) localize 3.4, 5.7, and 12 kb upstream of the first Cδ exon.[66] Most early fetal δ rearrangements involve C-proximal Jδ segments (Jδ3), whereas most δ chains at a later developmental stage and in peripheral T cells use C-distal Jδ segments (Jδ1). Until now, 10 different Vδ gene segments have been characterized, with 6 Vδ gene segments being functional. Vδ3 maps 3′ to Cδ and upstream to Jα genes in an inverse orientation. Most of the γδ T cells use Vδ1 or Vδ2 segments, and T cells of early ontogenic origin use predominantly Vδ2 segments.[67, 68] V region segments can be shared between the TCRα and δ locus.[3, 69] Four D gene segments have been

characterized.[70, 71] Since joining of several D segments can occur during recombination, variability of γ-δ heterodimers might be considerably higher than one would expect from their limited number of functional V genes.[47] TCR-αβ-bearing cells usually delete both alleles of the δ locus.

The TCR β-chain locus spans about 600 kb on chromosome 7q35.[72] More than 60 different V region gene segments belong to 20 subfamilies.[73] They are mapped to the 5′ end of the two D-J-C clusters.[74] All Vβ gene segments rearrange to both Jβ clusters with similar frequency.[5, 75] The two C region genes of the β chain are approximately 8 kb apart. Their amino acid sequences are highly homologous.[76] Two J gene clusters, Jβ1 and Jβ2, are each located 2 to 5 kb 5′ to the C region genes (see Fig. 2–3). They contain six and seven J gene segments, respectively. Rearrangements in the TCRβ locus more frequently involve D-Jβ2 than D-Jβ1 joining; consequently, postrearrangement deletion of the DJCβ1 gene segments is common.[77]

The TCRγ chain gene maps to the short arm of chromosome 7 (7p15), where it spans a distance of approximately 160 kb.[78] Only 10 of the 15 known Vγ segments undergo rearrangement, and only 8 are functional (V1.2 to 1.5, 1.8, and 2 to 4).[79, 80] The other V gene segments are pseudogenes that are not expressed at the protein level due to transcriptional or translational defects. The TCRγ locus contains five known J segments (see Fig. 2–3). They can be divided in two groups comprising (1) Jγ1.1, Jγ1.2, and

Jγ1.3 located upstream of Cγ1 and (2) Jγ2.1 and Jγ2.3 located upstream of Cγ2.[81] Both Cγ segments are structurally similar to the Cα and Cβ genes but have three instead of four exons.[82] Exon 2 sequences are different between Cγ1 and Cγ2. Cγ2 has two or three copies of the second exon, but none of these code for the cysteine residue believed to be important for interchain disulfide linkage.[83] Thus, it depends on the Cγ gene usage whether (Cγ1) or not (Cγ2) the TCRγ chain can form a disulfide bond with the TCRδ chain.[84]

Regulatory Genes for T-Cell Receptor Gene Rearrangements

Rearrangement processes in both Ig and TCR genes are tightly regulated despite the use of a common recombinase and expression of RAG genes in early B and T cells. TCR genes are efficiently rearranged only in T and not B cells, and vice versa for the Ig genes.

After V(D)J rearrangement, a promoter 5′ to the recombined V segment initiates transcription resulting in a primary RNA message. Remaining sequences between V-D-J and C exons are excised by splicing. The final processed mRNA is translated to the immune receptor polypeptide. TCR promoters are active in cells of both TCRαβ and TCRγδ lineage.[85] The promoter regions contain a binding site for leucine zipper transcription factors belonging to the cAMP response element binding protein/activating transcription factor (CREB/ATF) family.[86] Although the promoter itself is not T-cell specific, it may potentiate the activity of the 3′ enhancer. Multiple additional upstream regulatory sequences control the promoter genes. These sequences comprise regulatory binding sites for tissue-specific and promiscuous *trans*-acting transcription factors. Enhancers can increase transcriptional activity (after initiation by a promoter) independent of their genomic orientation and location. The enhancers for the different TCRs contain similar binding sites for transcription factors such as GATA-3, TCF-1, CREB proteins, core-binding factors (CBFs), and ets.[87] Ets expression is detected late in murine thymic ontogeny coinciding with TCRα gene expression and represents a candidate trigger factor for TCRα gene expression.[88, 89] GATA-3, a zinc finger protein, is expressed very early in T-cell development and may be one factor that determines T-lineage commitment in lymphoid precursor cells.[87] Promoters located in the 5′ flanking region of the Vβ gene segments (Vβ promoters) interact with a potent transcriptional enhancer located 3′ of the Cβ2 gene segment.[90, 91] The 3′ enhancer is therefore not deleted during the recombination events. Significant transcriptional activity of the promoters requires activation of the 3′ enhancers.[86] TCRβ gene expression might be limited to αβ T cells because it is only in that lineage that rearrangement brings Vβ promoters into proximity with the enhancer.[87] A set of *cis*-acting elements, termed "locus control region" (LCR), has been identified that regulates chromatin accessibility of the TCRαδ locus. Competitive expression of different LCRs may be involved in the differential regulation of TCRα versus TCRδ genes during development.[92] The presence of silencers has been postulated as limiting the enhancer activity. In mice, a *cis*-regulatory element localized between Cα and the TCRα enhancer silences the TCRα enhancer in a distance- and orientation-independent fashion in TCRγδ cells.[93] Downregulation of this silencer activates the TCRα enhancer and may initiate deletion of the TCRδ genes as circular DNA excision products during TCRα rearrangement. This could be another mechanism responsible for lineage determination in TCRαβ lymphocytes.

The human TCRα enhancer maps 4.5 kb downstream of the Cα gene and consists of two minimal transcription factor sequences (Tα1 and Tα2). Tα2 functions as a potent transcriptional activator in context with the TCRα enhancer but, depending on the localization to other regulatory elements, it can also function as an effective transcriptional repressor when positioned upstream or downstream of several promoter and enhancer elements.[94] In addition, a regulatory sequence designated "TEA" (T early α) is located between Vδ2 and the Jα gene cluster.[95] In cells of αβ lineage, TEA is deleted with the complete DJCδ locus on both chromosomes. TEA is also present in TCRγδ cells and may regulate lineage determination in this T-cell subset as well. A similar structure of the promoter/enhancer regions is also present in TCRα and γ genes.

T-CELL ONTOGENY AND THYMIC SELECTION

Growth of lymphocytes in the thymus depends on the interaction of various interleukins and other unknown growth signals. These events precede TCR expression and function independently of antigen-driven proliferation of mature peripheral T cells. Committed stem cells that enter the thymus have not initiated the process of gene rearrangement required for the production of functional TCRs for antigens. These early thymocytes may develop further along the γδ or αβ T-cell lineage. As discussed earlier, TCR genes undergo recombination events that generate a large repertoire of individual TCR V gene combinations. These join to their respective C region genes by RNA splicing.[58]

T-Cell Ontogeny

From gestational week 7 onward, putative prothymocytes have been identified with cytoplasmic CD3 positivity (cCD3+) in the fetal liver. They are TdT− but express CD7 and CD45 and no class II molecules.[96] Immature cCD3+ thymocytes are large blasts or intermediate-sized cells showing high TdT expression levels and very strong proliferative activity. They are CD4- and CD8-double negative (DN), CD2+, CD1−, and TCRβ− as the rearrangement of β genes likely takes place at this stage. More than 90% of CD3+ cells also express IL-2 receptor (IL-2R) at 8.5 weeks.[97] In the next stage of differentiation, common thymocytes also are cCD3+ and TdT+, have medium proliferative activity, and begin to show cytoplasmic TCRβ expression. Since these cortical thymocytes are in the process of rearranging α genes, TCRαβ is not yet expressed. Typically, these cells are CD4 and CD8 double positive (DP), CD1+ and CD2+. The last stage is characterized by mature thymocytes. They are either CD4 or CD8 single positive (SP), TdT−, CD1−, membrane CD3+, CD2+, and TCRαβ+.

The exact order in which the different TCR chain genes rearrange is unknown. Data mainly are derived from studies in the murine system and molecular analyses of thymic T-cell leukemias that supposedly have been arrested at different developmental stages. In mice, rearrangements in the TCRδ locus appear to precede recombination of the other TCR genes.[77, 98, 99] The TCRγ genes rearrange before the TCRβ genes. Productive TCRβ rearrangement on one allele leads to receptor protein translation. This blocks recombination of the TCRβ locus on the other chromosome, a phenomenon termed "allelic exclusion."[100] Rearrangement at the TCRβ locus occurs at the DN stage and precedes rearrangement at the TCRα locus.[38, 96, 101] Unlike the TCRβ protein, the TCRα protein does not feed back and prevent further TCRα rearrangement. Thus, mature human T cells can have two productive TCRα genes.[102] After expression of a functional TCR and during positive and negative selection a few thymocytes differentiate into mature SP cells.[103] From 9.5 weeks of gestation to birth TCRβ+ cells expand to include more than 90% of all CD7+ cells. Over the same time, TCRδ+ cell numbers fall from a peak of 11% of CD7+ cells to 1% of CD7+ cells at birth. These data suggest that human CD7+, CD2+, cCD3+ T-cell precursors produce both TCRδ T cells and T cells expressing αβ. Furthermore, DN and mCD3– thymocytes differentiate in culture into mature γδ T cells.[104] The separation between αβ and γδ lineages probably can occur during or after TCRβ rearrangement since the TCRβ gene is frequently rearranged in γδ T cells.[105]

Much has been learned about the importance of molecules involved in rearrangement events, accessory TCRs, and signal transduction elements from investigations of mice carrying germline mutations in the respective genes.[106] New findings include the following:

1. Inactivation of the *RAG1* or the *RAG2* gene leads to an absence of any V(D)J rearrangements. Thymocyte maturation is arrested at a very early DN stage, and mature T and B cells are missing.[55, 56]
2. Mice with a genomic deletion in the TCRβ locus spanning from Dβ1 to downstream Cβ2 have thymocytes arrested at an early stage before massive cell expansion.[107] This shows the importance of TCRβ rearrangement for the transition of DN to DP thymocytes and for the expansion of the DP cell pool. TCRβ–/– thymocytes lack any detectable TCR expression. However, substantial recombination of the TCRα was detected, suggesting that TCRβ rearrangement is not a prerequisite for TCRα rearrangement. Maturation of γδ cells did not depend on a functional TCRβ locus either. Expression of TCRβ chain thus may be necessary to drive DN IL-2R+ thymocytes to the DP stage and for expansion of this cell population.
3. A targeted disruption of the TCRδ gene causes the complete absence of γδ T cells but does not affect the development of thymocytes expressing TCRαβ receptors.[108] The thymocyte populations from TCRβ/TCRδ double knockout mice contain only DN thymocytes, and the number of thymocytes is lower than in TCR-deficient mice.[107] This suggests that DP cells in TCRβ–/– mice are committed to the γδ lineage.
4. The arrest in TCRα–/– mice occurs later in thymocyte ontogeny than in TCRβ-deficient mice.[107, 109] TCRα chain–mutated mice maturation ceases at the DP stage, and SP thymocytes are not detectable. The numbers of DN and DP thymocytes are normal, but

CD4 and CD8 SP cells are virtually absent. Expression of TCRα chain therefore does not limit the progression of thymocytes from the DN to the DP stage and the proper expansion of DP cells. TCRα is, however, required for the transition from the DP to the SP stage. Rearrangement of TCRα is observed in TCR Cα-disrupted thymocytes at reduced levels, but rearrangement of TCRβ in these mice occurs as extensively as in normal mice. The TCRα locus apparently does not need to be functional for TCRα or TCRβ rearrangement. Maturation of γδ T cells appears to proceed normally in these mice.

5. Mice lacking CD3ζ chains are almost devoid of DP thymocytes and have greatly reduced numbers of peripheral T cells.[110, 111] The few αβ T cells express only low levels of TCR and show impairment of their proliferation. This germline deletion does not obviously affect TCRγδ IELs. These results support the importance of the ζ chain for thymocyte differentiation; however, they also show that this molecule is not absolutely required for the generation of SP T cells and might be dispensable for γδ T-cell development.
6. CD4–/– mutant mice have markedly decreased helper cell activity but CD8+ T cells develop and function normally. This suggests that expression of CD4 on progenitor cells and CD4/8 DP thymocytes is not obligatory for development.[13] Normal mice have an extremely small proportion of DN T cells in the periphery, but in CD4-deficient mice up to 15% of peripheral T cells have this phenomenon. Cytotoxic T-cell activity against virus-infected cells is undetectable in CD8 knockout mice. Clearance of the virus from the host organism is strongly impaired and virus titers stay high after infection. Development and function of the CD4+ T lymphocytes is not affected.[112] Introduction of specific TCR transgenes in the CD8–/– mice made clear that CD8 expression is necessary for positive selection of thymocytes carrying the transgenes.[113]
7. CD45 is expressed in multiple isoforms that correlate with thymic selection events. The protein tyrosine phosphatase (PTPase) domain is believed to interact with the tyrosine kinases p56lck and p59fyn leading to dephosphorylation of negative regulatory sites of these src family members. This would assign CD45 a major role in thymic development and T-cell activation. Disruption of exon 6 of the CD45 gene in germline-mutated mice resulted in an impairment of thymocyte differentiation at the transition from DP to SP cells.[114] Expression of all CD45 isoforms was almost undetectable. These findings confirm the pivotal role of the CD45 PTPase activity at the transition from the DP to the SP stage in thymocyte development. This may at least be partially due to a lack of dephosphorylation of the tyrosine kinase p56lck. In CD45 exon 6–/– mice DP thymocytes have upregulated levels of CD4 and CD8. The maturational block of CD45 exon 6–/– thymocytes appears to be at a later stage as the block in p56lck–/– thymocytes. This suggests that different, until now unidentified PTPases mediate activation of p56lck in early thymic differentiation. Comparable with p56lck–/– mice, only a few T cells were present in

the periphery of CD45 exon 6–/– animals and CD8+ cytotoxic T cells were undetectable after infection with lymphocytic choriomeningitis virus. In contrast with p56lck–/–, T cells, mitogen activation and TCR cross-linking did not induce a proliferative response in T cells derived from CD45 exon 6–/– mice.

8. Targeted mutation of the p56lck gene[115] results in a dramatic reduction of thymocytes in p56lck-deficient mice (8×10^6). The number of DN cells is drastically reduced, thymocyte maturation is blocked at the early DP stage, and mature SP lymphocytes are almost undetectable. The amount of CD4 and CD8 expression on DP thymocytes is comparable with wild-type levels. Development of CD4–8– T cells bearing a transgenic γδ TCR is also severely impaired in p56lck-deficient mice.[116] Taken together this suggests a p56lck function in early thymocyte development that is independent from its association with CD4 and CD8.

9. Thymocytes upregulate their IL-2R during ontogeny, suggesting a role for IL-2 in thymic maturation.[117] In humans, the congenital defect of the IL-2Rγ chain leads to a severe combined immunodeficiency syndrome characterized by an absence or markedly reduced numbers of T cells with thymic hypoplasia, suggesting an essential role of IL-2Rγ in thymocyte maturation.[118] Mice deficient for IL-2 have apparently normal thymocyte development and peripheral T-cell populations. In vitro, proliferative responses after polyclonal T-cell stimulation are impaired. The addition of exogenous IL-2 restores this defect.[119] At a younger age, the in vivo immunoresponsiveness of IL-2–/– mice was surprisingly normal. Ig production of B cells was reduced but still efficient, and NK cell activity was detectable.[120] Other mediators seem to functionally substitute at least in part for IL-2. IL-2 binds to a cell surface receptor complex comprising at least three components (α, β, and γ).[117] IL-2R thus may have additional ligands, or individual components of the IL-2R can be used in different receptor complexes. The development of intestinal γδ TCR-bearing IELs seems not to be affected by the absence of p56lck, suggesting a differential dependency of p56lck for the thymus-derived and thymus-independent T cells.[116]

Thymic Selection

Thymocytes of the TCR αβ lineage are subject to thymic selection that shapes the TCR repertoire of the peripheral T-lymphocyte population for self-MHC restriction, self-tolerance, and immunocompetence. Selection ensures that only the most useful lymphocytes enter the peripheral pool. On their way to mature T cells, thymocytes go through a CD4 and CD8 DP stage (80% of thymocytes) and then finally become SP cells (about 10% of thymocytes).[103]

Thymic selection comprises two events. The intrathymic process that generates differentiated functional T cells competent to interact with antigen bound to MHC molecules is termed "positive selection." Negative selection eliminates thymocytes with high affinity to self-antigens, leaving behind those T cells with lower reactivity to self-MHC and the capability to recognize associated antigen.[121] T cells with no affinity to self-MHC and associated antigen (nonselection) usually undergo apoptosis. Positive selection occurs when the αβ TCR binds to a certain MHC molecule lacking the specific peptide that would be recognized by the TCR of mature T cells. Developing populations of CD4+8+ thymocytes continue to express new αβ TCRs until the individual cells are positively selected and the receptor is fixed or until the cell dies.

Two obvious candidates for cells that actually present TCR-reactive peptides or epitopes to the developing T cells are known: Epithelial cells that form the nonlymphoid framework of the thymus and specialized APCs known as dendritic cells, which invade the thymic rudiment from the bone marrow about halfway through intrauterine life. Bone marrow–derived accessory cells, mainly dendritic cells, can deliver the lethal signal in many instances.[122] Thymic epithelial cells are largely responsible for positive selection. Studies from thymic epithelial cell lines suggest, however, that the epithelial cells could also participate in negative selection of thymocytes.[123] A single thymocyte clone may be either negatively or positively selected by the same peptide-MHC complexes depending on the avidity of the interaction between the TCRs and the peptide-MHC complexes.[124] Underlying this so-called differential avidity model is the assumption that positive selection occurs when the avidity is relatively low. When the avidity exceeds this low range, the thymocytes undergo negative selection.

Different concepts exist to explain CD4 and CD8 lineage commitment. In a stochastic-selective model SP T cells are generated, irrespective of TCR specificity, and rescue from cell death requires coengagement of TCR and the matched coreceptor. Subsequent completion of positive selection is possible only for cells expressing the coreceptor that can bind to the MHC molecule recognized by the TCR. The instruction model postulates that coengagement of TCR, CD8, and MHC I on DP thymocytes leads to generation of a signal distinct from that generated by coengagement of TCR, CD4, and MHC II, resulting in a downregulation of the nonengaged coreceptor and selection.[40] The instruction model predicts that CD4 SP and CD8 SP thymocytes always have TCRs and coreceptors that recognize the same MHC molecule. The stochastic-selection model, on the other hand, predicts that some SP cells have mismatched TCRs and coreceptors and therefore fail to mature.

Analysis of thymocyte commitment of Iaβ–/– and β_2-microglobulin–/– mice provided evidence for the stochastic-selective model.[125, 126] An important MHC II–associated molecule is the invariant chain (Ii) that is believed to play a role in assembly, folding, and transport of MHC II heterodimers.[117] Cells from mutant animals lacking the Ii chain show aberrant transport of MHC II molecules that results in a moderately reduced level of MHC II heterodimer expression at the cell surface.[127] This suggests that without the Ii chain, MHC II molecules are not delivered to compartments that generate the appropriate antigenic peptides, which affects the CD4+ T-cell compartment in these mutant mice. Thymocyte development of SP CD4+ cells is disturbed and negative selection appears to be impaired. On the other hand, β_2-microglobulin–deficient mice express little if any functional MHC I antigen on the cell surface. Strikingly, CD8+ T cells are absent, showing that MHC I molecules are critical in a positive selection of

CD8+ T lymphocytes.[128] These MHC I knockout mice display similar functional losses in cytotoxicity as the CD8–/– mutant mice. CD8 is therefore necessary for the maturation and positive selection of MHC I–restricted cytotoxic T lymphocytes but not required for the MHC II–restricted T-helper cells.[14]

Positively selected cells eventually leave the thymus and patrol the body as long-lived resting lymphocytes that can generally be reactivated only by foreign peptides presented by self-MHC. Immune activation usually involves T cells leaving the G_0 state, entering the cell cycle, and creating a clone of progressively more differentiated immunologic effector cells, for example, cytokine-secreting T cells. This is called "clonal selection." By analogy, deletion of a self-reactive lymphocyte is termed "clonal deletion." However, lymphocytes can be functionally silenced by antigen without being killed, a phenomenon termed "clonal anergy."[129]

The selective processes acting on TCRγδ cells probably differ from those known for TCRαβ cells. They apparently belong to separate intrathymic lineages.[107] There is evidence for intrathymic selection of γδ cells in mice,[130, 131] but extrathymic expression of MHC or MHC-like molecules can also influence the repertoire of this T-cell population.[132, 133] The nonrandom pairing of protein products of the γδ chains thus could result from thymic or peripheral selection.[43]

SIGNAL TRANSDUCTION

Specific TCR-mediated interactions have to trigger a signal into the lymphocyte to induce proliferation and nonproliferative effector functions such as the production of cytokines or cytotoxic substances. Surface receptor stimulation has to be transduced to the cytoplasm and nucleus where it induces gene transcription. Signaling is organized in cascades and ultimately results in activation or inactivation of other regulatory molecules and transcription factors. TCR molecules are physically associated with a variety of coreceptor molecules. All these cooperate in their receptor and signal transducer function and determine the total response of a T cell on antigen recognition. Activation of T lymphocytes through the TCR results in progression of cells into the cell cycle (G_0/G_1) and the production of the growth factor IL-2 and its receptor.[134] The interaction of IL-2 with its receptor is essential for cell cycle progression from G_1 to S phase, and its commitment event in triggering T-cell proliferation. Induction of a proliferative T-cell response is therefore linked to the expression of the IL-2 and the IL-2R genes. Cytokines made by APCs or bystander T cells also influence signaling cascades. Antigen-capturing cells such as dendritic cells or macrophages ("professional APCs") have stimulatory capabilities not shared by other tissue cells. Recent work has suggested that one important molecular mechanism of costimulation results from B7 activation molecules expressed on APCs that bind CD28 or its homologue CTLA/4 on the T-cell surface. Without costimulatory signals, linking of TCR to an MHC epitope may deliver a downregulatory signal to the T cell.[135]

At least two signal transduction pathways are activated by TCR stimulation (Fig. 2–4). These are the inositol-phospholipid second-messenger pathway and a tyrosine-kinase pathway. Stimulation of T cells by antigen activates the intracellular enzyme PLC-γ1). Activation of PLC-γ1 by tyrosine phosphorylation and/or through guanosine triphosphate (GTP)-binding proteins results in the activation of protein kinase C (PKC).[136] This serine-threonine kinase, when activated, results in enhanced cell growth rates and can lead to tumor formation, suggesting that it functions upstream of growth effector molecules.[137, 138] PLC-γ1 hydrolyzes phosphatidylinositol-4,5-biphosphate (PIP_2) into inositol-1,4,5-trisphosphate (IP_3) and a minor membrane phospholipid termed "diacylglycerol" (DAG). These two second messengers are responsible for the rapid mobilization of intracellular calcium ions followed by further calcium ion accumulation due to an altered calcium influx across the plasma membrane and the activation of a serine-threonine kinase, PKC, respectively.[139] DAG in turn translocates a cytosolic protein kinase PKC to the plasma membrane where it acquires its calcium-dependent active form. Both the activation of PKC (the PKC signal) and the elevation of the intracellular calcium ion concentration (calcium signal) are believed to play central roles in the signal transduction of cytokine gene induction.[140] The balance between the activities of the two signaling pathways could contribute to cytokine expression. Active PKC was shown in vitro to phosphorylate the inhibitory subunit IκB of the pleiotropic transcription factor NK-κB, which then translocates to the nucleus to act as a transactivation factor for many genes, including the IL-2 gene.[141] Involvement of PKC as an upstream activator of p21ras appears to be unique to T cells[142] and occurs commonly after TCR/CD3, CD2, or IL-2 stimulation.[143]

P21ras, a GTP-binding protein, exists either as the activated GTP-bound form or the inactive guanosine diphosphate (GDP)-bound form after GTP hydrolysis. In nonactivated lymphocytes almost all p21ras is complexed to GDP. Molecules regulating the turnover of ras-GTP to ras-GDP control the activation state. One candidate for guanosine triphosphatase (GTPase)-activating enzyme is p21ras-GTPase-activating protein (GAP).[144] In fibroblasts p21ras was shown to control transcription factors such as c-*jun* and c-*fos*, together forming the activator protein-1 (AP-1) complex, which is involved in transcription of the IL-2 gene.[134, 145, 146] Mice lacking c-*fos* after homologous recombination have reduced numbers of peripheral T and B lymphocytes but increased numbers of macrophages.[147] Immature CD4/8 DP T cells are virtually absent from the thymus of adult c-*fos*–/– mice and the thymus size is vastly reduced.

Ras alone cannot activate IL-2 expression but must synergize with at least a calcium signal to stimulate IL-2 expression.[142] NF-AT is one, but probably not the only, target for the ras-dependent pathway. In T cells, PKC phosphorylates on serine the serine-threonine protein kinase p74raf.[148] Cytoplasmic p74raf may also translocate to the nucleus presumably to phosphorylate nuclear transcription factors and link cell membrane activation events with transcriptional activity.[145, 149] Presumably, p74raf functions downstream of protein tyrosine–activated PKC and p21ras.[143, 149] Raf binding to activated ras may serve as a mechanism to translocate to the membrane where it can act as a substrate for an upstream kinase and/or phosphorylate downstream targets. These complexes may then activate extracellular signal-regulated kinase (mitogen-activated erk

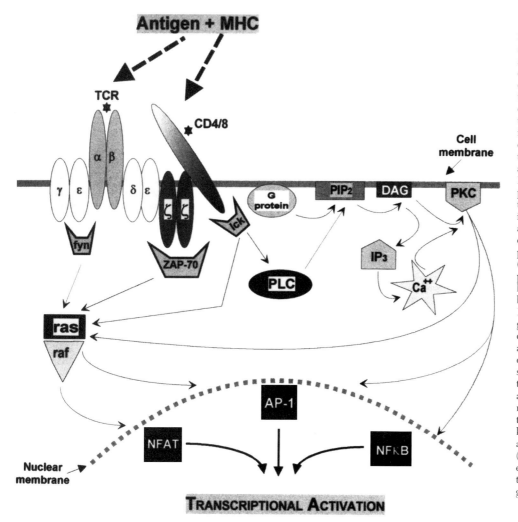

Figure 2–4. Signaling pathways on antigenic T-cell receptor (TCR) stimulation. The earliest response elicited by the TCR is the activation of protein tyrosine kinases (PTKs) that associate with the TCR/CD3 complex: the hematopoietic form of the PTK p59^{fyn} and ZAP-70, which interacts with the ζ chain homodimer. The cytoplasmic domains of the TCR coreceptors CD8 and CD4 are associated with the PTK p56^{lck}. Following ligation of the TCR complex, signaling can occur either through a protein kinase C (PKC)-independent PTK-induced p21^{ras} activation or through a PKC-dependent pathway. Tyrosine phosphorylation and/or GTP-binding (G) proteins induce phospholipase Cγ1 (PLCγ) activity. PLCγ hydrolizes phosphatidylinositol-4,5-biphosphate (PIP2) into inositol-1,4,5-triphosphate (IP3) and diacylglycerol (DAG). *IP3* mobilizes calcium ions that together with DAG activate PKC. This recruits among other transcription factors (TFs) such as NFκB or c-*jun*/c-*fos*, which together form the AP-1 complex, and activate p21^{ras}. Direct PTK-mediated *ras* activation leads to interaction with the serine/threonine kinase p74^{raf} and controls TFs such as nuclear factor of activated T cells (NFAT) and AP-1. These signal events are known to modulate the transcriptional activation of cytokine genes.

kinase [MEK]), which activates mitogen-activated protein (MAP) kinase.[150]

A second signal transduction group consists of tyrosine kinase pathways. PTKs are not intrinsic to the TCR but are recruited to the intracytoplasmic portion of the CD3, 4, and 8 receptors (see Fig. 2–1). Stimulation of the TCR with antigen results in the phosphorylation of tyrosine residues in several proteins, including the CD3ζ chain. PTKs not only activate or inactivate other kinases and phosphatases. An activation signal from TCR to PLCγ is believed to be mediated mainly through interactions between the TCRζ chain and members of the src family of PTKs such as p59fyn and/or p56lck.[151] Furthermore, PTKs induce PKC-independent p21ras activation mediated by tyrosine kinases. This alternative pathway is probably used by IL-2Rβ and TCR/CD3- or CD2-triggered activation.[143, 152] Two tyrosine kinases of the src family have been well characterized: p56lck and p59fyn. Src family genes encode proteins about 500 amino acids in length with similar design. They contain two noncatalytic, regulatory regions, known as src homology 2 and 3 (SH2, SH3) and the kinase domain with an autophosphorylation site. This site is next to a short carboxy-terminal region that negatively affects the kinase domain when tyrosine phosphorylates. Thus, src proteins are themselves regulated by tyrosine kinases and phosphatases.[153] Dephosphorylation at their regulatory residues during mitosis

activates both kinases. Their kinase activity increases during M phase and presumably promotes proliferation.[145] Membrane phosphotyrosine phosphatase CD45 activity represents 90% of the PTPase activity in lymphocyte membranes, which suggests that CD45 is probably responsible for p56lck and p59fyn activation. Cross-linking of TCR/CD3 or CD2 with different CD45 isoforms, however, may result in different signaling events, including inhibition of signaling.

P56lck is recruited via the CD4 or CD8 molecules. As much as 90% of membrane-associated p56lck interacts with CD4.[154] T lymphocytes containing mutant CD4 molecules, which either lack the carboxy tail or contain mutations at the intracellular cysteine residues mediating CD4-p56lck interaction, cannot be activated by specific antigen bound to MHC II molecules.[155, 156] Some substrates of p56lck specifically associate after TCR stimulation, including PLC-γ1 and ras-GAP.[157, 158] MAP-2 kinases in T cells also can be directly phosphorylated by p56lck.[159] Functional synergy of the TCR with CD4 in the activation of PLC-γ1 requires expression of the ζ chain, which probably reflects an interaction between p56lck and ζ-associated kinase ZAP-70. ZAP-70 is a 70-kD PTK exclusively expressed in T lymphocytes and NK cells.[160] It is not associated with the TCR in the basal state but is rapidly recruited to the ζ and CD3 chains following TCR stimulation. ZAP-70 associates only with tyrosine-phosphorylated antigen recognition activation motifs (ARAMs) of ζ that are found within the stimulated fraction of receptors. Patients with a selective T-cell defect due to a ZAP-70 gene mutation have no peripheral CD8+ T cells, and their peripheral T cells have an impaired signal transduction and function.[161] P56lck can also act independently from CD4 and CD8 molecules, and its association with CD4/8 might be relevant only in MHC I- or II-restricted TCR cells. In other cell types such as DN TCRγδ cells, NK cells, and possibly B cells, p56lck may act independently, or it could be associated with yet undefined surface molecules.[162]

The T-cell-specific isoform of p59fyn is required for TCR signaling, but less than 1% of the membrane-bound p59fynT may bind to TCR/CD3 complexes.[154] Fyn kinase associates with CD3ε and the ζ chain in T cells.[163] Based on experimental data the ζ protein appears to represent a novel guanosine nucleotide–binding structure. Since the GTP binding of ζ was found in functionally active TCR/CD3 complexes and also in intracellular ζ-ζ homodimers, an energetically driven conformational change of ζ is known to play a role in cell signal transduction.

TISSUE DISTRIBUTION AND FUNCTION OF PERIPHERAL T LYMPHOCYTES

T cells, which have a longer life span than B cells, are the major lymphocyte population in peripheral blood and in the lymphatic circulation. They recirculate and migrate to the secondary lymphoid organs such as spleen, lymph nodes, and the gut- and lung-associated lymphoid tissue. Lymphocyte recirculation through the spleen is predominantly from blood to blood. CD4+ T cells predominate over CD8+ cells in the white pulp, whereas an inverse relationship of the two lymphocyte subsets is found in the red pulp. Many T cells reach the lymph node in the afferent lymphatics that drain into the subcapsular sinus. Most lymphocytes enter the nodes from the blood across a specialized vascular endothelium in postcapillary venules, termed "high endothelial venules" (HEVs). These are located mainly at the junction of the cortical and paracortical regions.

T cells home to the paracortical regions of the lymph node and are also found in the medulla mixed with B lymphocytes and plasma cells. CD4+ T cells predominate over CD8+ lymphocytes and tend to cluster around interdigitating reticulum cells (IDCs). Scattered T cells with a helper phenotype also occur within germinal centers. All cells that have entered the node from either blood or lymph, and those produced because of clonal expansion within the node, leave the node in the efferent lymph via the medullary sinuses. Efferent lymphocytes are responsible for the establishment of immunologic memory and dissemination of the immune response to other lymphoid organs. Efferent lymph T cells are predominantly enriched for CD4 rather than CD8, implying that there is a preferential recirculation of the CD4+ cells into lymph node tissue.[164] Peripheral lymph nodes have a lower afferent input of T cells than do central nodes that receive all the efferent lymphocytes from the previous node in the chain.

Both T- and B-cell areas are readily identified within the Peyer's patch, with the T-cell area underlying the epithelial cells. HEVs are present in these areas. Nearly all T cells in tissues such as skin, in gut lamina propria, and on bronchial surfaces are of the memory phenotype (CD45RO^high). Memory cells prefer to migrate into both normal and inflamed nonlymphoid tissue, and they are biased to return to the tissue in which they were originally stimulated.[165] Conversely, naive T cells account for most of the cells entering the lymph node. T cells within the gut epithelium are predominantly CD8+, CD3+, αβ+, and CD45RO−.

In humans, TCRγδ cells are distributed as approximately 5% of the CD3+ cells in all organized lymphoid organs as well as in the skin- and gut-associated lymphoid tissues.[166] Lymphocytes expressing the γδ TCR represent a small subpopulation of the CD3+ T cells in the human gut, where they are randomly distributed within both the epithelium and the lamina propria.[167] TCRγδ T cells are preferentially located in the splenic sinusoids, whereas TCRαβ-bearing lymphocytes mostly occupy the periarteriolar sheaths of penicilliary arteries.[168] The preferential homing of γδ T cells to the epidermis seen in the mouse is undetectable in humans. However, the percentage of γδ T cells in epidermis is, on average, higher than in papillary dermis, suggesting a difference in migration of γδ versus αβ T cells.[169]

T-cell activation results in cell-mediated immunity dependent on effector cell clones that exert their influence, such as lymphokine secretion and cytotoxic killing, over a short range. The classic effector functions include delayed hypersensitivity, allograft rejections, graft-versus-host reactions, and cytotoxic reactions against virus-infected target cells. T cells also regulate the clonal expansion of both T and B cells. This regulatory lymphocyte subset consists mainly of TCRαβ+, CD3+, and CD4+ T helper cells. MHC-restricted cytotoxic activity is mainly exerted by peripheral CD8+ T cells. Antigenic peptides encountered by CD4 T cells on MHC II molecules are predominantly from extracellular sources. MHC I molecules, which present antigens to CD8 T cells and are expressed on essentially all nucleated cells, obtain their peptides primarily from the intracellular protein pool. It is advantageous to eliminate virally infected cells with their endogenously produced foreign proteins by CD8 cytotoxic T lymphocytes. It would not be appropriate, however, to generate cytotoxic T lymphocytes against cells that have endocytosed nonreplicating foreign proteins. Thus far, a T-helper response mainly mediated by CD4 T cells that leads to the production of antibodies against the extracellular antigen is more suited.

For the T-helper subset of T lymphocytes the relevant activities are carried out mostly by an array of secreted cytokines. They amplify specific immune responses by supporting the proliferation of small numbers of lymphocytes specific for any one antigen and by recruiting the multiple effector mechanisms required to eliminate foreign antigens.[140] Naive CD4+ T cells represent a set of relatively recent thymic emigrants that have not yet encountered or not yet responded to antigen. These cells express relatively large amounts of CD45RB. When stimulated by receptor engagement in the context of a costimulatory signal, naive CD4 cells produce IL-2 but little or no IL-4 or IFN-γ. They have been called precursors of T helper cells.[170] Compared with CD45RA+ naive T cells, CD45RO+ memory cells are functionally much more potent and can be stimulated by much lower amounts of antigen or anti-CD3 monoclonal antibodies. In the mouse, CD4, CD45, and the TCR complex are physically associated on memory T cells, whereas on naive T cells they are separate.[171] This physical association allows for a much greater efficiency in T-cell triggering and may form the molecular basis for T-cell memory. Memory T cells have many similarities to activated T cells or T-cell clones: both are CD45RO+ and express increased levels of adhesion molecules, MHC II molecules, and IL-2R. CD45RO+ T cells, although not as large as activated T cells, are larger than CD45RA+ T cells.[172]

Activated helper cells can differentiate into T-helper-1 cells that make predominantly tumor necrosis factor (TNF) and IFN-γ, or T-helper-2 cells that make predominantly IL-4, IL-5, IL-6, and IL-10. The T-helper-1 clones through their production of IFN-γ and TNF-β are well suited to induce enhanced microbicidal activity in macrophages (enhanced cellular immunity), whereas the T-helper-2 clones make products that are well adapted to act in helping B cells. They express CD40 ligand that binds to CD40 on the B-cell surface. Binding of CD40, together with the effect of cytokines, leads to B-cell proliferation, class switching, and the development of memory B cells.[173] T-helper-2-like response could control self-inflicted injury by opposing the effects of IFN-γ on macrophages through the actions of IL-10 and IL-4 and possibly by suppressing production of IFN-γ and other cytokines by T-helper-1 cells.

Cytotoxic T cells contain lytic granules that can destroy the integrity of most cell membranes. A principal component of these granules is the enzyme perforin, which produces pores in the membrane of target cells. In addition, it appears that serine proteases in the granules may initiate apoptosis when they gain access into target cells possibly via a perforin pore. Cytotoxicity may also involve contact-dependent signals from the killer to the target cells. One mechanism a T cell uses to kill, which is not dependent on extracellular calcium, requires the expression of fas on the target cell surface.[173] CD8+ T cells can also be subdivided into CD45RA+ and CD45RO+ subsets, which may reflect a functional dichotomy similar to the CD4+ T-lymphocyte subsets. The recognition process in the cytotoxic reaction against nonself-MHC antigens differs from the corecognition of self-MHC I molecules and endogenous antigen in virus-infected T cells. T cells bearing TCRαβ show a high frequency of reactivity to allelic variants of MHC I and II molecules, a phenomenon called "alloreactivity." CD4+ T cells are necessary and sufficient to initiate allograft rejection even in the absence of CD8+ lymphocytes. The host T cells probably recognize the differently shaped and charged grooves of the MHC complexes and the different peptide composition of the minor histocompatibility antigens on the allograft as numerous novel antigens.

About 0.5% of peripheral T cells are CD4–8– TCRαβ+. They may use APCs, restriction molecules, and selection routes different from those used by antigen-specific CD4+ T cells. These DN cells can recognize bacterial antigens, they are often oligoclonal, and the expanded clones may persist for several years.[174, 175]

Nearly all γδ T cells lack expression of CD4, and most lack CD8 or express it at relatively low levels. In contrast with the αβ T cells, no common restriction element such as MHC is presently known for γδ T cells. TCRγδ can potentially interact with MHC molecules, but this may be the exception rather than the rule. Candidates for other antigen-

presenting molecules are the products of so-called nonclassic MHC I genes. Human CD1 molecules represent perhaps the best characterized candidates for non-MHC-encoded antigen-presenting molecules for γδ T cells. Genes for CD1 molecules show a domain organization similar to that of MHC I genes. Another notable similarity between CD1 and MHC I molecules is the association of the heavy chain with β2-microglobulin, which is in both cases required for cell surface expression.

TCRγδ lymphocytes, which accumulate in reactive granulomatous lesions of leprosy and cutaneous leishmaniasis, appear to be genetically restricted and require self-antigen presentation.[176] On stimulation with antigen, they secrete lymphokines that cause macrophage adhesion, aggregation, and proliferation.[177] Comparison of cytokine secretion profiles for a series of γδ T cell clones with a series of αβ T cell clones reveals evidence of quantitative rather than qualitative differences. Many γδ T cell clones secrete lower or undetectable amounts of IL-2 and IL-4. This suggests that these cells may have a stronger requirement for exogenous growth factors than their αβ-bearing counterparts or that they produce and respond to different autocrine growth factors. No secreted factors have been identified thus far that are uniquely produced by γδ T cells.

B LYMPHOCYTES

B lymphocytes are the principal cell type involved in humoral immunity. B-effector cells, especially plasma cells, produce Igs. Igs are antibodies that bind antigen specifically with the N-terminal V domains of their heavy and light chains. The C-terminal region of the secreted Ig molecules binds to complement components and a multiplicity of Fc receptors. Resting naive or memory B cells carry membrane-bound Ig (mIg) receptors on their cell surface that are necessary for cellular activation and selection processes during B-cell maturation. Besides recognizing cell surface–bound antigen, mIgs also bind soluble antigens efficiently. B cells can internalize these antigens and process them for subsequent presentation to T cells.

Ig is associated with the CD79 molecules that have signal-transducing functions reminiscent of the CD3 molecules in T cells. The B-cell receptor (BCR) complex associates physically with coreceptor molecules such as the CD19/CD21 complex and CD22 that modify the B-cell response to antigen. This response leads to cellular activation and proliferation and to the induction of changes in the receptor specificity, depending on differences in the structural context of antigen recognition.

THE B-CELL RECEPTOR AND ITS CORECEPTORS

The B-Cell Receptor

The BCR complex consists of an mIg molecule noncovalently associated with heterodimers of Ig-α (CD79a; mb-1) and Ig-β (CD79b; B29).[178] Most B cells express IgM and IgD, and, rarely, other Ig isotypes as surface receptors. The coexpression of IgM and IgD on the same B cell seems to occur via alternative RNA splicing of either a Cμ or a Cδ segment to the same heavy chain variable (V_H) gene.

Membrane-associated Igs have extensive structural homology to secreted Igs. They differ in that mIgs possess a C-terminal spacer with an attached acidic transmembrane region of 12 to 14 residues and a short cytoplasmic domain of up to 28 amino acids (in γ and ε).[179] Regulation of the production of mIg versus secretory Ig likely occurs at the mRNA level by alternative splicing.[180]

Every Ig molecule is made of two heavy chains with a molecular weight ranging from 50 to 70 kD (depending on the IgH isoform) and two associated identical (κ or λ) light chains of approximately 23 kD. The chains are held together by noncovalent forces and by interchain disulfide bridges, giving the molecule ensemble its bilaterally symmetric structure. The heavy and light chains each form several 100 to 110 amino acid–long folded globular domains with single intrachain disulfide bonds. Light chains always contain two of these domains: an N-terminal V and one C domain. Heavy chains contain the V domain and three C domains with a hinge region between the heavy-chain constant region (C_H1) and the C_H2 domains. The hinge region is replaced by a fourth C_H domain in the μ and ε chains. The V domain consists of four relatively invariable framework regions of 15 to 30 amino acids separated by three 9 to 12 amino acid–long hypervariable or CDRs. The CDR3 region, furthest away from the N-terminus, is encoded by the D gene and the flanking J sequences. It is therefore more variable and usually longer than the CDR1 and CDR2 stretches.

Clonotypic surface Ig molecules are noncovalently associated with disulfide-linked heterodimers of a 41- to 47-kD Ig-α (CD79a; mb-1) and approximately 37-kD Ig-β (CD79b; B29) chain.[178] Both molecules are required for a complete signal transduction on antigen receptor engagement (Fig. 2–5). B29 mRNA is found throughout the B-cell lineage from pre-B to plasma cells, but mb-1 transcripts are undetectable in plasma cell stages. The CD79 heterodimer binds to the transmembrane spanning region and C_H3 and/or C_H4 domains of membrane-bound μ heavy (mμ) chains. Both CD79 molecules are structurally similar to CD3γ, δ, and ε. They have a single extracellular Ig-like domain and contain a single transmembrane region with an amino acid sequence motif called "ARAM." Like growth factor receptors, CD79 molecules show increased phosphorylation of their cytoplasmic domains after cross-linking. Ligation of mIg results in activation of the CD79-associated src-family PTKs, among others, p72syk. *Syc* also associates with the cytoplasmic tail of mμ, which has been implicated in receptor-mediated signal transduction.[181] In vitro studies suggest differences in the signaling capabilities of the two CD79 components. Ig-α, but not Ig-β, may directly associate with the PTK p53/p56lyn.

Coreceptors

Key accessory molecules known to modulate antigen receptor signaling in B cells are the CD19/CD21 complex, CD22, CD20, CD40, and CD45.

CD19 and CD21 noncovalently associate to form a multimolecular signal transduction complex on the B-cell surface. CD19 is a 95-kD Ig superfamily glycoprotein expressed from early stages of B-cell development until plasma cell differentiation. It first appears at the pro-B-cell stage before IgH gene rearrangements. CD21 is a 145-kD

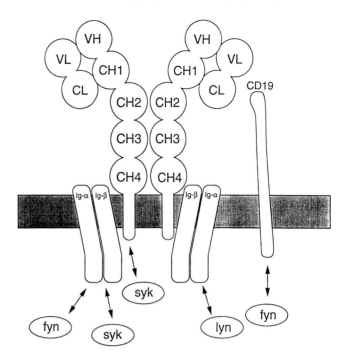

Figure 2–5. Structure of the B-cell receptor signaling complex. The membrane-bound immunoglobulin (Ig) molecule is assembled from a pair of identical light (L) and heavy (H) chains. H and L chains have a V domain (VH, VL) and in L chains one, in H chains four globular, folded C domains. Associated with the Ig molecule are heterodimers of Ig-α (CD79a) and Ig-β (CD79b). The cytoplasmic domains of the CD79 molecules, CD19, and also the cytoplasmic domains of at least some IgH isotypes are associated with src-like kinases fyn, lyn, and the tyrosine kinase syk.

glycoprotein member of the complement receptor family also known as "complement receptor type 2" (CR2). CD21 is expressed on mature B cells and is rapidly lost following cellular activation.[182] Engagement of CD19 in vitro is followed by increased tyrosine phosphorylation and activation of PLC; inositol phospholipid turnover; calcium ion mobilization; stimulation of serine-specific protein kinases, including PKC; and activation of NF-κB. Immunoprecipitation studies indicate an association of CD19 with PTKs such as p59fyn. Costimulatory signals can be delivered by activation of CD21. The short cytoplasmic domain of CD21, however, is unlikely to transduce signals and may require association to other receptor molecules such as CD19 for this purpose. CD21 interacts with several ligands, including C3 fragments of complement. Since complement associates with antigen-antibody complexes, this may provide a convenient mechanism of cocross-linking the CD19/CD21 complex with the antigen receptor for subsequent signal amplification. It may therefore be important for B-cell activation at low antigen concentrations.[183]

CD22 is a 135-kD glycoprotein and a member of the Ig superfamily that is first detected in the cytoplasm of pro-B cells shortly after CD19 expression. As the B cells differentiate, CD22 levels decline first, followed by CD19 and CD20, and are absent in plasma cells. CD22 surface expression tightly correlates with that of mIg, particularly of mIgD. Accordingly, CD22 expression is restricted mainly to mantle zone B cells and downregulated in germinal center B cells. Signaling through CD22 may function in lowering the threshold of BCR-mediated signals required for B-cell stimulation, but its in vivo functions are largely unknown. As discussed earlier, one of several possible CD22 ligands is CD45RO expressed on activated T lymphocytes and memory T cells. In vitro, CD22 might be an essential molecule for transducing mIgM-dependent signals arguing for a functional interaction between CD22 and the mIgM/BCR complex. The cytoplasmic domain of CD22 contains an ARAM sequence with tyrosine residues that becomes phosphorylated subsequently to BCR cross-linking and may enable p72syk to bind to this region, facilitating signal transduction.[184]

CD20 is a membrane-embedded protein of 33 to 37 KD, depending on its phosphorylation status. Its expression begins at the pre-B-cell stage and is downregulated on differentiation into plasma cells. The CD20 structure suggests a function as membrane transporter or ion channel. CD20 probably exists as a homooligomeric complex on the cell surface that associates with other surface or cytoplasmic molecules to form a multimeric cell surface receptor complex.[185] Binding of antibodies to CD20 generates transmembrane signals that result in enhanced phosphorylation of the molecule. CD20 may regulate cell cycle progression, playing a role in progression from the G_1 phase into the S/G_2 and M stages following stimulation. This could explain its relatively stronger expression on follicular center B cells than on mantle B cells.

CD40 is a 50-kD type I membrane protein belonging to the nerve growth factor receptor/TNF family. Signaling through CD40 in the presence of IL-10 induces isotype switching. The CD40 ligand (CD40L) gp39 is a type II membrane protein belonging to the TNF family. It is present on CD4+ T cells in the follicular mantle, the light zone of lymphoid follicles, and periarteriolar lymphatic sheaths (PALS) close to CD40+ B cells.[186] The binding of CD40L to CD40 on the B cells induces the B cell to move into the cell cycle and causes upregulation of other costimulatory molecules such as B7-1 (CD80) and B7-2 (CD86).[187] In contrast with naive B cells, memory B lymphocytes constitutively express B7 and therefore have the capacity to present antigen directly to T cells.[188] The role of the CD28-B7 interaction for Ig production and class switching is further elucidated in mice deficient for CD28 expression. Basal IgG1 and IgG2b antibody concentrations are drastically reduced, and Ig switching to IgG after infection is diminished.[189]

CD45 is most likely not physically associated with the BCR complex. The essential role of CD45 for normal BCR signaling function is implicated by studies of CD45-exon 6 knockout mice where B lymphocytes lack CD45 expression.[114] These B cells are unresponsive to BCR ligation and do not proliferate in response to mitogenic anti-Ig antibodies. Cocross-linking of mIg and CD45 enhances Ig-α and Ig-β dephosphorylation. This suggests that changes in CD45 or specific CD45 isoforms as a function of B-cell activation or differentiation may affect BCR-mediated signaling and its biologic effects.[178]

V REGION DIVERSITY OF IMMUNOGLOBULIN MOLECULES

The Ig V region assembly takes place during B lymphopoiesis and leads to an estimated primary Ig repertoire of more than 10^{10}. Mechanisms involved are recognition of conserved heptamer-spacer-nonamer sequence elements flanking the germline V, D, and J segments; the potential loss or addition of nucleotides at the coding junctions; introduction of double-strand breaks between the elements to be joined and the flanking recognition sequences; and ligation activities to complete the joining process. It is still unclear how transcription or transcriptional control elements act to promote recombination of V(D)J elements. Active transcription has been correlated with the degree of cytosine methylation at CpG residues within a given locus, and methylation status seems to have a significant effect on the VDJ recombination potential of substrate gene segments. Expressed loci generally are hypomethylated when compared with silent loci.

Genomic Organization of the Immunoglobulin Genes

Three separate Ig loci exist for Ig molecules: the heavy chain (IgH) locus and two light chain (IgL) loci, κ and λ. Each of the three loci is encoded by a separate autosomal chromosome (14q32.3, 2p12, and 22q11, respectively).

The IgH locus consists of a set of V, D, and J region segments that somatically rearrange and join to create the active IgH chain V domain. All V region genes have a similar organization containing a single large exon and an intron of about 100 to 150 bp near the end of the leader sequence. This sequence encodes a hydrophobic peptide that plays a role in directing synthesized Ig peptides to the outside of the cell. The 3′ end of the V segment is flanked by recombinase signals. It is estimated that about 50 functional and 50 nonfunctional V_H genes (grouped into seven families based on sequence homology) span a region of about 1100 kb upstream of the J_H segments on the telomeric region of chromosome 14.[190] The first functional V_H occurs 96 kb upstream of the Cμ, and the major cluster of D_H segments lies between this V_H and the six functional J_H segments. The D_H gene cluster consists of at least 10 segments and is only 35 kb 3′ to Cμ.[191] the IgH C region gene locus is rather complex (Fig. 2–6). Within about 200 kb, 11 C region segments are found. The Cμ region is closely followed by Cδ. Then come two clusters of C_H elements containing Cγ3, Cγ1, pseudogene ψε1, Cα1, and Cγ2, Cγ4, Cε, Cα2.[192] The precise position of the ψγ gene is not known. All but one C_H gene (Cδ) has immediately upstream a switch sequence responsible for the IgH chain class switch. The C_H gene segments contain several exons separated by intron sequences. Apart from their transmembrane domain, the Cμ and Cε genes have four domains, the Cδ gene has three, the Cγ genes have four (one of these being a hinge region that is quadruplicated in Cγ3), and the Cα genes have three, with the hinge as part of the second domain.

The two IgL loci lack D segments. V-J joining occurs to form functional V segments. A single Cκ gene resides about 3 kb downstream from the set of Jκ segments.[193] The Cκ element exists as a single exon with a splice acceptor site on its upstream side to which the rearranged Jκ segment joins by RNA splicing. The five Jκ segments follow about 3 kb upstream of the single Cκ gene on a 23-kb fragment (see Fig. 2–6). The first and second Vκ segment, located about 25 and 38 kb upstream of Jκ, have a reverse orientation. Rearrange-

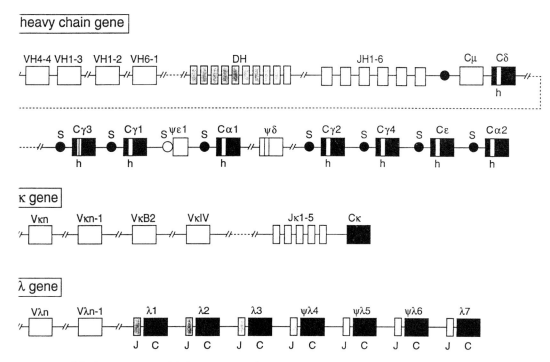

Figure 2–6. Organization of the human immunoglobulin (Ig) genes. The assembly of the Ig loci resembles the T-cell receptor (TCR) loci. The IgH and Igλ loci contain multiple C region segments with pseudogenes (ψ) among them. D segments are present only in the IgH locus. The CH genes contain hinge (h) regions and are preceded by a switch region (S), except Cδ. Some Vκ genes, such as VκB2 and VκIV, are in a reverse orientation to the only C gene.

ment of these inverted V region genes takes place via inversion rather than deletional joining. There is a total of about 80 Vκ genes, including a large duplicated region encompassing 28 Vκ genes, which belong to four distinct families.[194] No more than 50 of the Vκ genes are functional.

The λ L chain locus has a more complex C region cluster than the κ locus (see Fig. 2–6). The region of λ L chains are the products of at least four nonallelic (isotypic) genes and differ by small amino acid substitutions.[195] Three additional Cλ genes are pseudogenes.[196] In about 25% of people, even more than seven Cλ genes are present on one or both alleles. One Jλ segment lies approximately 1 kb upstream of each Cλ gene. The most 5' Vλ segment and the Cλ genes are separated by only 14 kb in germline configuration. Approximately 40 different Vλ gene segments are known that belong to at least seven families. The Vλ genes generally seem to have the same transcriptional orientation as the Jλ-Cλ gene segments.[197]

Regulatory Genes for Immunoglobulin Gene Rearrangements

Although a common recombinase system, including RAG products, mediates assembly of both Ig and TCR V regions, V(D)J recombination is differentially regulated in the two cell lineages. Complete Ig region gene rearrangements occur in B cells but not in T lymphocytes. The transcription of Ig genes is controlled by and is dependent on B-lymphocyte-specific V region gene promoters and enhancers. Intronic enhancer elements of the IgH and IgL genes target associated V region gene segments for V(D)J recombination.[198] Mice with homozygous deletion of the intronic Igκ enhancer exclusively contain λ light chain–positive B

cells. Rearrangement of the κ chain gene is completely abrogated.[199] Enhancers also have a critical role for somatic hypermutation in Ig V region genes.[200] Multiple B-cell-specific *cis*-acting regulatory elements, including the 3' and the intronic Ig enhancer and promoter elements, contain octamer-binding sites recognized by Oct-1 and Oct-2 proteins. Oct-2 comprises several isoforms, and their expression is largely B-cell restricted.[201] Studies in Oct-2–deficient mice have shown, however, that Oct-2 may not be necessary in the first, antigen-independent phase of B-cell differentiation.[202]

The Igμ enhancer is a *cis*-acting element functional from early B-cell stages on and contains both early and late regulatory components. These include multiple sites recognized by the ets transcription factor and basic helix-loop-helix (bHLH) transcription factor families.[203] The bHLH transcription factors, similar to ets proteins, recognize sequences in the regulatory elements of virtually all lymphoid-specific genes. Differentially spliced bHLH gene products may be important for stage-specific gene expression in differentiating B cells. The stage specificity of transcription factors involved in Ig rearrangement processes can also be determined at the levels of synthesis or association with other factors. One such molecule, Oct-binding factor-1 (OBF-1), has the properties of a B-cell-specific transcriptional coactivator protein.[204] It is possible that this type of factor without independent transcriptional activity influences cell lineage specificity of otherwise rather promiscuous DNA-binding transcription factors.

B-LYMPHOCYTE DEVELOPMENT

Commitment to the B-cell or T-cell lineage of lymphocytes occurs before or as progenitors enter the primary organs of lymphocyte differentiation. B-cell production starts in the fetal liver and continues in the bone marrow. B-lymphocyte development can be divided into two major stages: antigen-independent B lymphopoiesis, which takes place in fetal liver and adult bone marrow, and antigen-dependent B-cell maturation. B lymphopoiesis leads to naive B cells coexpressing IgM and IgD in a largely T-cell-independent and antigen-independent manner.

B-Cell Lymphopoiesis

The first descendant of the pluripotent stem cell committed to B lineage is termed a "pro-B cell." This pro-B cell does not express B-lineage-specific markers and has not yet begun to rearrange the Ig genes.[205] After colonizing the primary lymphoid organs, progenitors committed to B lineage probably first expand there. In bone marrow they fill the extravascular spaces between large sinus in the shaft of long bones. Proliferation of the most immature B lineage progenitors is highest near the inner surface of the bone in the subendosteal reticulum of the bone marrow.[206] As B lineage progenitors become more differentiated, they move toward the center of the marrow either to die in situ or to exit into the peripheral circulation via the sinus.[207] Bone marrow stromal cell–mediated cell contact and soluble mediators are mandatory for early murine B-cell development. In humans, bone marrow stromal cells and cytokines such as IL-7 or stem cell factor may not be absolutely required.[208]

In the earliest B-committed cell, the pro-B cell, the Ig genes are in germline configuration. From analyses of normal precursor B cells and precursor B-cell acute lymphoblastic leukemias, a model has arisen in which B cells develop from an HLA-DR+ precursor cell that acquires cell surface expression of the CD19 and subsequently the CD20 and CD10 molecule before cytoplasmic μ expression.[209, 210] Rearranging of the Ig heavy chain genes then leads to expression of cytoplasmic μ heavy chain that defines pre-B cells. Large pre-B cells are first seen in fetal liver at around 9 weeks of gestation, and small pre-B cells accumulate at 11 weeks. The pre-B cell pool expands, and some pre-B cells rearrange and express light chains. After surface Ig expression, CD10 is downregulated in immature B cells that now express surface IgM. They can recognize self-antigens, which leads to either deletion or a state of anergy. Non–self-reactive B cells are further induced to express IgD, defining them as naive B cells. In analogy to CD3 molecules in T cells, Ig-α (mb-1) and Ig-β (B29) molecules start to be expressed early during B-cell differentiation prior to cIgμ expression.[105]

In pro-B cells the Igμ gene starts to rearrange, with the D-to-J joining most likely preceding V-to-DJ joining.[211] Productive rearrangement on one allele arrests rearrangement on the second allele (allelic exclusion). This inhibition is dependent on the expression of mμ heavy chains in pre-B cells. Mice with deleted J_H gene loci (J_HEμT) lack transition from large to small pre-B cell stage, and IgH gene rearrangement does not occur.[212]

B cells with mμ chain express the products of two nonrearranging genes, one of which resembles an IgL V domain (termed "VpreB"), the other an IgL C domain (λ5 or 14.1).[213] These proteins assemble noncovalently to form a surrogate L chain, of which the λ5 protein can form a disulfide bond with the mμ chain. This assembly is likely to be anchored in the pre-B-cell membrane by the Ig-α/Ig-β protein complex, together forming the pre-BCR. The regulatory functions and ligands of the pre-B-cell mIg are still uncertain. Cross-linking of mIg in pre-B cells induces calcium ion mobilization and may have the potential for further signal transduction events.[214] Proteins from $D_H J_H C\mu$ recombinations in reading frame II may also bind to the surrogate light chain when joined by V_H germline transcription products such as the $V_H 5$ protein.[215] The importance of surrogate L chain expression for B-cell development becomes clear from mice with germline deletion of the λ5 gene. The pro-B-cell and early pre-B-cell development is not affected in these mice, but a drastic reduction in cell numbers is observed in late pre-B cells and immature B lymphocytes in the bone marrow. As development of B cells goes on, the λ5 and VpreB transcription ceases and the pre-BCR are replaced by the Ig receptor.

Nonproductive rearrangements (such as out-of-frame rearrangements, rearranged genes bearing stop codons or involving V_H pseudogenes) may be capable of secondary rearrangements on the other allele or, in cases of inversions, on the same allele. In most developing B cells $D_H J_H$ rearrangements are found on both chromosomes. Even when both alleles have rearranged nonproductively, a productive rearrangement can be generated by V_H gene replacement.[216] On the other hand, V_H replacement can also render a previously productive IgH rearrangement unproductive.[217] V_H replacement is mediated by heptamer joining sequences seven nucleotides upstream of the 3′ end of most V_H gene segments. The heptamer in the $V_H D_H J_H$-rearranged site aligns with the heptamer sequence in the unrearranged V_H.

Ig L chain rearrangement follows the IgH gene rearrangements accompanying the transition from small pre-B to immature B cells. The transmembrane expression of mμ chains may ease initiation of IgL rearrangements but is not absolutely required. Mice carrying germline-mutated forms of the Igμ gene in the transmembrane domain or of the λ5 gene are capable of IgL rearrangements.[218, 219] It is possible that two routes lead to the surface expression of an Ig receptor in B cells. If a productive rearrangement first occurs in an IgL locus, the cell will directly develop into a B cell following an in-frame IgH rearrangement. In most cells, the IgH locus is productively rearranged before an IgL locus, and such cells express a pre-BCR. Expression of the pre-BCR may then lead to an upregulation of L chain gene rearrangements.[212] Probably, light chain rearrangement preferably involves the κ locus first and subsequently the λ chain genes; in mice κ rearrangements are initially strongly preferred to λ rearrangements in immature B cells.[220] The κ genes are usually deleted in λ chain–producing cells, which is regulated by a sequence downstream of the Cκ gene, called the κ-deleting element (which replaces the Cκ gene or the whole Jκ-Cκ gene segment).[221] Simultaneous rearrangements at both L chain loci may, however, occur infrequently, which results in the production of κ+λ+ B cells and the formation of hybrid antibodies in some cases.[222] Nonproductive rearrangements of the Ig chain genes lead to surface Ig– B cells that die in situ by apoptosis. Functional IgL and IgH gene rearrangements result in B cells expressing either IgMκ or IgMλ on the surface. At this point, L chain gene rearrangements no longer occur and *RAG1* and *RAG2* gene expression is downregulated.[223]

B-Cell Maturation

Naive B cells enter the secondary lymphoid organs with a functional Igμ and Igδ receptor molecules on the surface. Antigen-induced B-cell activation and differentiation lead either to antibody formation or to production of a phenotypically and functionally separate population of memory B cells. Most induced B lymphocytes undergo an Ig class switch and express Ig receptor isotypes other than IgM and IgD. In this process, antigen-specific V_H region genes join to different downstream C_H regions. It involves recombination between repetitive switch (S) region sequences present 5′ of each germline C_H gene except for Cδ. Switch recombination likely occurs by looping-out and deletion.[224] Treatment of splenic B cells with different mitogens and cytokines generates different specific class switch events in mice.[225] Similar mechanisms play a role in human B cells and probably require interaction of the B cells with T cells and their products. Isotype switching is preceded by the expression of transcripts that initiate 5′ to every S region, proceeds through the S region, and end at the termination sites downstream of the involved C_H gene. It is possible that germline transcripts play a direct role in class switching by targeting the recombination event or serving as acceptor substrates in *trans*-splicing mechanisms that allow expression of downstream C_H genes without switch recombination.[226]

Another type of somatic variation can increase the affinity of Ig V region domains for specific antigens independent of receptor gene rearrangements. Point mutations are introduced throughout the IgH and IgL V region genes by a process called "somatic hypermutation." The density of base pair changes is about three times greater in CDRs, especially CDR3, than in FRs. As many as 90% of the peripheral B cells may express V_H genes that have undergone somatic mutation. Hypermutation is driven mainly by antigen selection processes but may also occur in pre-B cells without Ig surface expression.[227]

SELECTION

Immature B cells may undergo negative selection. Cell membrane–anchored self-antigens on adjacent bone marrow cells are suitable sources of such negative signals. B cells with the best-fitting receptors become eliminated or anergized.[228, 229] The others may be positively selected for exit from the primary lymphoid organ, which confers a longer life in the periphery, where they coexpress IgM and IgD. Anergy or a functionally silent stage may be acquired when binding occurs to self-antigen in soluble form and leads to downregulation of IgM in these B cells.[230] In a transgenic mouse model, however, immature B cells in the bone marrow can be rescued after an encounter with their autoantigen: They exchange the transgenic L chain in the Ig molecule with an endogenously encoded L chain.[231] This process, termed "receptor editing," could either silence unwanted specificity or salvage B cells with new, desirable specificity.

The B-cell repertoire that emerges from the bone marrow is shaped through positive selection by foreign antigens and negative selection by self-antigens. This is reminiscent of the thymic education of T lymphocytes. Limited-affinity maturation occurs in T-cell reactivity mainly by the selective amplification of best-fitting TCR clonotypes on repeated antigenic encounters. In B cells, however, affinity maturation generates an Ig V region diversity, which differs drastically from the original bone marrow–derived repertoire. Central to this amplification of receptor diversity is the somatic hypermutation in B-cell maturation involving specialized compartments of the secondary lymphoid tissues, the germinal centers (GCs).

Although a high frequency of B cells proliferating in GCs exhibits somatic mutations that confer high-affinity binding, the onset of the somatic hypermutation mechanism may not necessarily correlate with memory precursor cell proliferation within this site. It is possible that GC precursors are activated and start to undergo somatic mutation in the T-dependent areas of lymphoid tissues and PALS of the spleen. Further expansion and selection of high-affinity somatic mutants would then occur in the GC during further proliferation of these cells.[232] It is unknown what signals cause the cells to initiate or terminate somatic mutation in GC. A strong signal via surface Ig, indicating high-affinity interaction with antigen bound to FDCs, may cause the cells to stop hypermutation. The presence of unmutated and identically mutated sister cells in GCs suggests that proliferation may both precede and follow somatic mutation within the GCs. The GC B lymphocytes become extremely short-lived and are destined to die unless positively selected by antigen and other ligands.[233] Only those lymphocytes are rescued from apoptosis that have mutated Ig V genes coding for a receptor that binds most efficiently to antigen. The CD40 protein on the B cell (and FDC) surface appears to deliver a second signal required for the generation of long-lived memory B cells in GCs. Another set of signals (such as soluble CD23 and IL-1α) may alternatively drive the cells to plasmablast differentiation.[234]

SIGNAL TRANSDUCTION

In the BCR complex, the ligand-binding component is the membrane-bound Ig, whereas the Ig-α and Ig-β transmembrane proteins are the main signaling subunits (see Fig. 2–5). These molecules show sequence homology with the CD3 components and ζ chain of the TCR, which may explain why signal transduction is similar in each of these receptors. Desensitized Ig receptors may be reset by Ig-α and Ig-β dephosphorylation mediated by the predominant lymphocyte membrane tyrosine phosphatase CD45.

Signaling via the BCR involves as its most proximal step the activation of PTKs that propagate signals by phosphorylation of a variety of effector molecules. Immediately after receptor ligation, association to the BCR occurs with PTKs such as the src family members fyn, blk, and lyn. Lyn is expressed preferentially in B cells and physically associates with membrane-bound IgM and IgD.[235] Lyn and fyn bind to Ig-α via their SH3 domains. Lyn also binds to PLC-γ, GAP, and MAP kinase through a site within the first 27 residues of its N-terminal unique region.[178] Another kinase, syk, is also preferentially expressed in B cells. Like ZAP-70, it bears tandem SH2 domains that may mediate interaction with ARAMs, for example within the Ig-α or Ig-β molecules. It is possible that syk associates with the cytoplasmic domain of the mμ chain and that src family kinases operate upstream of syk activation analogous to the ZAP-70 activation pathway following TCR ligation.[178] After these initial events, the BCR signaling pathway appears to diverge into at least three biochemical cascades.

As in T cells, antigen receptor ligation in B cells leads to activation of the inositol-phospholipid second-messenger pathway that involves phosphorylation of PLC-γ2 as the predominant PLC-γ isoform in B cells.[236] The downstream events of the PKC signal and the calcium signal are not well characterized in B cells. Studies in other systems suggest that PKC modifies the transcriptional activity of the AP-1 complex and that the calcium signal is involved in the phosphorylation of the ets-1 DNA-binding protein.[237]

A second cytoplasmic signaling pathway involves the G-protein p21ras, which is primarily regulated by the GTP exchange protein p95vav, but may also be regulated by GAP. P21 regulation of c-*raf* initiates the MAP kinase pathway and may lead to phosphorylation of c-*jun*. Among the first substrates phosphorylated are the ARAM tyrosines of Ig-α and Ig-β. Their phosphorylation may lead to reorientation of associated src family kinases. Their SH2 domains would bind to the tyrosine-phosphorylated ARAMs by which they become activated.

A third cascade activated following BCR cross-linking involves the activation of phosphatidylinositol-3-kinase (PI3-k). This enzyme phosphorylates the position 3 in the inositol phospholipids. PI3-k can bind to the SH3 domains of lyn and fyn.[238] The precise effect and function of PI-3k products are unclear. It may play a role in the PKCζ-dependent pathway acting on downstream effectors such as NF-κB.[239, 240]

TISSUE DISTRIBUTION AND FUNCTION

In addition to the predominant conventional B-cell population in the spleen and lymph nodes, the CD5– or so-called B-2 cells, another largely CD5+ B lineage exists that arises early in ontogeny and gives rise to B-1 cells.[241] Murine B-1 lymphocytes do not seem to participate in conventional immune responses and appear to have the capacity for self-renewal. Human and murine B-1 cells frequently express V_H and V_L germline genes without somatic mutations, but they acquire some N-region diversity later in fetal development and may exhibit somatic mutations, arguing for an antigen-driven selection process. Human CD5+ B lymphocytes form a large population of the B cells in fetal lymphoid tissues but only a minor population of the B cells in adult lymphoid tissues. In lymph node and tonsil they are mainly localized in the inner mantle zone but not the follicle center of secondary follicles.[242] It is possible that the fetal-derived CD5+ B cells are selected based on germline-encoded self-reactivity into a long-lived pool.[243] It was proposed that a memory in form of an anti-idiotypic Ig V region becomes imprinted in adult-derived B-1 cells by somatic mutation in the V region CDRs and that this Ig expressed in a self-renewing CD5+ B-cell population acts as

a surrogate antigen keeping the repertoire of B-2 memory B cells alive even in the absence of specific antigen.[244]

The predominant, stable B-cell pool consists of recirculating follicular B cells constantly remigrating through T-dependent zones into follicles of secondary lymphoid organs and of nonrecirculating B cells, especially in the marginal zone.[245] Marginal zone and recirculating B cells contain both naive and memory B cells. The T zones and red pulp of the spleen are the sites for arrival of newly produced, short-lived naive B cells. In the murine spleen, first contact between antigen and specific T and B cells following immunization occurs in the outer PALS region of the white pulp, which is rich in T cells. If successful T-B collaboration occurs in the PALS, oligoclonal proliferative foci form that reach a maximum size within 3 to 4 days and then dissipate. Most B cells activated in T zones migrate to local sites of antibody production where they differentiate into short-lived plasma cells (spleen red pulp and lymph node medullary cords). Others migrate to the primary follicles and initiate GC formation.[246]

Under normal conditions, GCs develop oligoclonally from only a few antigen-activated IgD+ cells, which become IgD– within GC, as well as from IgM+ cells that have not yet expressed IgD. In the rat, first production of GC on immunization correlates with the appearance of FDCs. It is possible that antigen localized on the FDC surface in conjunction with adhesion molecules could serve to stimulate the antigen-specific B-cell proliferation directly. Alternatively, antigen could be taken up by GC B cells from FDCs via mIg receptors. It becomes endocytosed, processed, and presented with class II molecules to helper T cells in their vicinity, resulting in T-B cell interaction that leads to B-cell proliferation.

T dependence of GC formation is not only at the level of initial activation of B cells during primary antibody response. This is suggested by presence of CD4+ T cells within the GC, in particular in the apical light zone near the mantle zone area. Human CD40L (gp39) is expressed on CD4+ T cells in the mantle zone, the light zone of lymphoid follicles and PALS of the spleen, close to CD40+ B cells [186] and has an important role in GC formation. Germline mutated CD40–/– mice lack secondary immune responses and GC formation.[247] Defective CD40 expression may lead to apoptotic death or failure of further selection of centrocytes. In vitro exposure of GC B lymphocytes to anti-CD40, instead, increases *BCL2* expression along with survival of the cells. Antigenic T-cell activation leads to secretion of cytokines and induction of novel surface receptors, such as CD40L (gp39).[248] The binding of gp39 to CD40 on the B cells induces the B cell to move into cell cycle. This crucial receptor ligand interaction is nonfunctional in patients with congenital deficiency of CD40L expression, which results in the lack of GC formation.[249] CD40-CD40L association also causes upregulation of costimulatory molecules such as B7-1 and B7-2. B7 on the antigen-presenting B cell engages with CD28 on the T cell. Interaction between these cell surface ligands results in escalation of the response to antigen by increasing the expression of other receptors such as MHC II and CD54 (ICAM-1).[230] The absence of this second signal after the Ig receptor engagement may be one mechanism leading to B-cell death without T-cell help.

In an established GC, FDC networks become filled with B blasts, then transform into centroblasts forming the dark zone next to T zones. It is in this GC compartment where rapid division and presumably hypermutation occur. Between the tightly packed centroblasts a sparse network of CD23^{low} FDC processes is present. B cells within the dark zone have much downmodulated their Ig receptors, but when moving to the light zone they re-express them. Positive selection is believed to occur in the less populated light zone at the apex of the GC, which is rich in CD23^{high} FDCs, has high numbers of tingible body macrophages, and contains mainly centrocytes. Between the apical light zone and the mantle, an outer zone exists that is populated by T cells, centrocytes, B blasts, and plasmacytes.[246] Apoptosis provides a mechanism for positive recruitment of centrocytes into the memory cell pool. Presumably, this is based on the ability of the mIg to interact with antigen on FDC, and of antigen-specific T cells in the apical light zone to recognize processed Ag on B cells. The dying centrocytes are taken up by the tingible body macrophages. BCL2 protein expression in GC is consequently present on only a few B cells in the light zone. Susceptibility of GC cells to apoptosis could also contribute to negative selection processes at the centroblast stage in the dark zone, where the cells are not close to Ag-bearing FDCs or T cells.

B cells rescued from apoptosis may return to the dark zone and continue with hypermutation of their Ig V genes. Some may differentiate into plasma cells, and others become memory B cells. After stimulation in the follicles of the spleen, murine memory B cells usually colonize the splenic marginal zones after a period in the circulation. They then migrate from the marginal zone into the PALS, where they can be reactivated by subsequent antigenic challenge and the appropriate T-cell help.

CONCLUSION

Lymphocyte ontogeny and maturation are designed to keep the immune system alert for the presence of foreign peptides and neoantigens. This task requires the formation of a fully operational immune receptor for antigen, modulating coreceptors and ligands, and surface molecules for the interaction between immune accessory cells, B cells, and T lymphocytes. Quantitative and qualitative changes in the interaction of these receptors and ligands activate different intracellular signaling pathways, keeping the immune response focused and self-limited. Disturbance of this delicate system may result in autoimmune disease or malignant lymphoproliferations. B cells especially are at risk of chromosome instability in secondary lymphoid organs. Chromosome recombination is prominent in their postantigenic maturation, and their selection occurs continuously in GCs. Deregulated lymphocytes may become clonally expanded if they fail to enter apoptosis and escape immune surveillance. A more profound knowledge of B- and T-lymphocyte development, immune receptor interactions, and intracellular as well as intercellular signaling pathways is desirable. This will help to better understand the pathobiology in atypical or malignant immune disorders and to design novel therapeutic approaches.

REFERENCES

1. Georgopoulos K, Bigby M, Wang JH, et al: The Ikaros gene is required for the development of all lymphoid lineages. Cell 1994; 79:143–156.
2. Zinkernagel RM, Doherty PC: MHC-restricted cytotoxic T cells: Studies on the biological role of a polymorphic major transplantation antigen determining T-cell restriction-specificity, function, and responsiveness. Adv Immunol 1979; 27:52–142.
3. Brenner MB, Strominger JL, Krangel MS: The γδ T cell receptor. Adv Immunol 1988; 43:133–192.
4. Meuer SC, Fitzgerald KA, Hussey RE, et al: Clonotypic structures involved in antigen-specific human T-cell function: Relationship to the T3 molecular complex. J Exp Med 1983; 157:705–719.
5. Davis MM, Bjorkman PJ: T-cell antigen receptor genes and T-cell recognition. Nature 1988; 334:395–402.
6. Lefranc M-P, Rabbitts TH: The human T-cell receptor γ (TRG) genes. TIBS 1989; 14:214–218.
7. Klausner RD, Samelson LE: T-cell antigen receptor activation pathways: The tyrosine kinase connection. Cell 1991; 64:875–878.
8. Wegener A-MK, Letourneur F, Hoeveler A, et al: The T-cell receptor/CD3 complex is composed of at least two autonomous transduction modules. Cell 1992; 68:83–95.
9. Frank SJ, Niklinska BB, Orloff DG, et al: Structural mutations of the T-cell receptor zeta chain and its role in T-cell activation. Science 1990; 249:174–177.
10. Jin Y-J, Clayton LK, Howard FD, et al: Molecular cloning of the CD3η subunit identifies a CD3ε-related product in thymus-derived cells. Proc Natl Acad Sci U S A 1990; 87:3319–3323.
11. Norment AM, Salter RD, Parham P, et al: Cell-cell adhesion mediated by CD8 and MHC class I molecules. Nature 1988; 336:79–81.
12. Doyle C, Strominger JL: Interaction between CD4 and class II MHC molecules mediates cell adhesion. Nature 1988; 330:256–258.
13. Rahemtulla A, Fung-Leung WP, Schilham MW, et al: Normal development and function of CD8+ cells but markedly decreased helper cell activity in mice lacking CD4. Nature 1991; 353:180–184.
14. Fung-Leung WP, Schilham M, Rahemtulla A, et al: CD8 is needed for development of cytotoxic T cells but not helper T cells. Cell 1991; 65:443–449.
15. Parnes JR: Molecular biology and function of CD4 and CD8. Adv Immunol 1988; 44:265–311.
16. Janeway CA: The role of CD4 in T-cell activation: Accessory molecule or co-receptor. Immunol Today 1989; 10:234–238.
17. Robey E, Axel R: CD4: Collaborateur in immune recognition and HIV infection. Cell 1990; 60:697–700.
18. Fleury S, Lamarre D, Meloche S, et al: Mutational analysis of the interaction between CD4 and class II MHC: Class II antigens contact CD4 on a surface opposite the gp120 binding site. Cell 1991; 66:1037–1049.
19. Van Kerckhove C, Russell GJ, Deusch K, et al: Oligoclonality of human intestinal intraepithelial T cells. J Exp Med 1992; 175:57–63.
20. Salter RD, Benjamin RJ, Wesley PK, et al: A binding site for the T-cell co-receptor CD8 on the α3 domain of HLA-2. Nature 1990; 345:41–46.
21. Pingel JT, Thomas ML: Evidence that the leukocyte-common antigen is required for antigen-induced T-lymphocyte proliferation. Cell 1989; 58:1055–1065.
22. Klausner RD, Lippincott-Schwartz J, Bonifacino JS: The T-cell antigen receptor: Insights into organelle biology. Annu Rev Cell Biol 1990; 6:403–431.
23. Springer TA: Adhesion receptors and the immune system. Nature 1990; 346:425–434.
24. Meuer S, Resch K: Cellular signaling in T lymphocytes. Immunol Today 1989; 10:22–25.
25. Kanner SB, Damle NK, Blake J, et al: CD2/LFA-3 ligation induces phospholipase Cγ1 tyrosine phosphorylation and regulates CD3 signalling. J Immunol 1992; 148:2023–2029.
26. Thomas ML: The leukocyte common antigen family. Annu Rev Immunol 1989; 7:339–369.
27. Hathcock KS, Lazlo G, Dickler HB, et al: Expression of variable exon A-, B-, and C-specific CD45 determinants on peripheral and thymic T-cell populations. J Immunol 1992; 148:19–28.
28. Wallace VA, Fung-Leung WP, Gray D, et al: CD45RA and CD45RB high expression induced by thymic selection events. J Exp Med 1992; 176:1657–1663.

29. Stamenkovic I, Sgroi D, Aruffo A, et al: The B lymphocyte adhesion molecule CD22 interacts with leukocyte common antigen CD45RO on T cells and a 2-6 sialyltransferase, CD75, on B cells. Cell 1991; 66:1133–1144.

30. Dianziani U, Redoglia V, Malavasi F, et al: Isoform-specific association of CD45 with accessory molecules in human T lymphocytes. Eur J Immunol 1992; 22:365–371.

31. Townsend A, Bodmer H: Antigen recognition by class I–restricted T lymphocytes. Annu Rev Immunol 1989; 7:601–624.

32. Rothbard JB, Gefter ML: Interactions between immunogenic peptides and MHC proteins. Annu Rev Immunol 1991; 9:527–565.

33. Falk K, Rotzschke O, Rammensee HG: Cellular peptide composition governed by major histocompatibility complex class I molecules. Nature 1990; 348:248–251.

34. Hood L, Kronenberg M, Hunkapiller T: T-cell antigen receptors and the immunoglobulin supergene family. Cell 1985; 40:225–229.

35. Behlke MA, Chou HS, Huppi K, Loh DY: Murine T-cell receptor mutants with deletions of β-chain variable region genes. Proc Natl Acad Sci U S A 1986; 83:767–771.

36. Kotzin BL, Barr VL, Palmer E: A large deletion within the T-cell receptor beta-chain gene complex in New Zealand white mice. Science 1985; 229:167–171.

37. Noonan DJJ, Kofler R, Singer PA, et al: Delineation of a defect in T-cell receptor β genes of NZW mice predisposed to autoimmunity. J Exp Med 1986; 163:644–653.

38. Ferrick DA, Ohashi PS, Wallace V, et al: Thymic ontogeny and selection of αβ and γδ T cells. Immunol Today 1989; 10:403–407.

39. Kappler JW, Roehm N, Marrack P: T-cell tolerance by clonal elimination in the thymus. Cell 1987; 49:273–280.

40. von Boehmer H, Teh HS, Kisielow P: The thymus selects the useful, neglects the useless, and destroys the harmful. Immunol Today 1989; 10:57–61.

41. Kappler JW, Staerz U, White J, Marrack PC: Self-tolerance eliminates T cells specific for mls-modified products of the major histocompatibility complex. Nature 1988; 332:35–40.

42. Schwartz RH: Acquisition of immunological self-tolerance. Cell 1989; 57:1073–1081.

43. Raulet DH: The structure, function, and molecular genetics of the gamma/delta T cell receptor. Annu Rev Immunol 1989; 7:175–208.

44. Bjorkman PJ, Saper MA, Samraoui B, et al: The foreign antigen binding site and T-cell recognition regions of class I histocompatibility antigens. Nature 1987; 329:512–518.

45. Katayama CD, Eidelman FJ, Duncan A, et al: Predicted complementarity-determining regions of the T-cell antigen receptor determine antigen specificity. EMBO J 1995; 14:927–938.

46. Yancopoulos GD, Blackwell TK, Suh H, et al: Introduced T-cell receptor variable region gene segments recombine in pre-B cells: Evidence that B and T cells use a common recombinase. Cell 1986; 44:251–259.

47. Boehm T, Rabbitts TH: A chromosomal basis of lymphoid malignancy in man. Eur J Biochem 1989; 185:1–17.

48. Lafaille JJ, DeCloux A, Bonneville M, et al: Junctional sequences of T-cell receptor γδ genes: Implications for γδ T-cell lineages and for a novel intermediate of V-(D)-J joining. Cell 1989; 59:859–870.

49. Landau NR, Schatz PG, Rosa M, Baltimore D: Increased frequency of N-region insertion in a murine pre-B cell line infected with a terminal deoxynucleotidyl transferase retroviral expression vector. Mol Cell Biol 1987; 7:3237–3243.

50. Alt FW, Oltz EM, Young F, et al: VDJ recombination. Immunol Today 1992; 13:306–314.

51. Roth D, Zhu C, Gellert M: Characterization of broken DNA molecules associated with V(D)J recombination. Proc Natl Acad Sci U S A 1993; 90:10788–10792.

52. Lin W-C, Desiderio S: Regulation of V(D)J recombination activator protein RAG-2 by phosphorylation. Science 1993; 260:953–959.

53. Schatz DG, Oettinger MA, Schlissel MS: V(D)J recombination: Molecular biology and regulation. Annu Rev Immunol 1992; 10:359–383.

54. Yoneda N, Tatsumi E, Kawano S, et al: Human recombination activating gene-1 in leukemia/lymphoma cells: Expression depends on stage of lymphoid differentiation defined by phenotype and genotype. Blood 1993; 82:207–216.

55. Mombaerts P, Iacomini J, Johnson RS, et al: RAG-1 deficient mice have no mature B and T lymphocytes. Cell 1992; 68:869–877.

56. Shinkai Y, Rathbun G, Lam K-P, et al: *RAG-2*–deficient mice lack mature lymphocytes owing to inability to V(D)J rearrangement. Cell 1992; 68:855–867.

57. Hochstenbach F, Brenner MB: T-cell receptor δ-chain can substitute for α to form a βδ heterodimer. Nature 1989; 340:562–565.

58. Kronenberg M, Siu G, Hood L, Shastri N: The molecular genetics of the T-cell antigen receptor and T-cell antigen recognition. Annu Rev Immunol 1986; 4:529–591.

59. Caccia N, Bruns GAP, Kirsch IR, et al: T-cell receptor α chain genes are located on chromosome 14 at 14q11-14q12 in humans. J Exp Med 1985; 161:1255–1260.

60. Yoshikai Y, Kimura N, Toyonaga B, Mak TW: Sequences and repertoire of human T-cell receptor alpha chain variable region genes in mature lymphocytes. J Exp Med 1986; 164:90–103.

61. Griesser H, Champagne E, Tkachuk D, et al: Mapping of the human α–δ region: A locus with a new constant region gene and prone to multiple chromosomal translocations. Eur J Immunol 1988; 18:641–644.

62. Hayday AC, Diamond DJ, Tanigawa G, et al: Unusual organization and diversity of T-cell receptor α-chain genes. Nature 1985; 316:828–832.

63. Toyonaga B, Mak TW: Genes of the T-cell antigen receptor in normal and malignant T cells. Annu Rev Immunol 1987; 5:585–620.

64. Baer R, Boehm T, Yssel H, et al: Complex rearrangements within the human Jδ-Cδ/Jα-Cα locus and aberrant recombination between Jα segments. EMBO J 1988; 7:1661–1668.

65. Champagne E, Sagman U, Biondi A, et al: Structure and rearrangement of the T-cell receptor J α locus in T cells and leukemia T-cell lines. Eur J Immunol 1988; 18:1033–1036.

66. Takihara Y, Tkachuk D, Michalopoulos E, et al: Sequence and organization of the diversity, joining, and constant region genes of the human T-cell δ-chain locus. Proc Natl Acad Sci U S A 1988; 85:6097–6101.

67. Takihara Y, Champagne E, Ciccone E, et al: Organization and orientation of a human T-cell receptor δ chain V gene segment that suggests an inversion mechanism is utilized in its rearrangement. Eur J Immunol 1989; 19:571–574.

68. Krangel MS, Yssel H, Brocklehurst C, Spits H: A distinct wave of human T-cell receptor γδ lymphocytes in the early fetal thymus: Evidence for controlled gene rearrangements and cytokine production. J Exp Med 1990; 172:847–859.

69. Guglielmi P, Davi F, D'Auriol L, et al: Use of a variable α region to create a functional T-cell receptor δ chain. Proc Natl Acad Sci U S A 1988; 85:5634–5638.

70. Loh EY, Cwirla S, Serafini AT, et al: Human T-cell receptor δ chain: Genomic organization, diversity, and expression in populations of cells. Proc Natl Acad Sci U S A 1988; 85:9714–9718.

71. Davodeau F, Peyrat M-A, Hallet M-M, et al: Characterization of a new functional TCR Jδ segment in humans. J Immunol 1994; 153:137–142.

72. Caccia N, Kronenberg M, Saxe D, et al: The T-cell receptor β chain genes are located on chromosome 6 in mice and chromosome 7 in humans. Cell 1984; 37:1091–1099.

73. Kimura N, Toyonaga B, Yoshikai Y, et al: Sequences and diversity of human T-cell receptor β chain variable region genes. J Exp Med 1986; 164:739–750.

74. Lai E, Concannon P, Hood L: Conserved organization of the human and murine T-cell receptor β-gene families. Nature 1988; 331:543–546.

75. Yuuki H, Yoshikai Y, Kishihara K, et al: The expression and sequences of the T-cell antigen receptor β-chain genes in the thymus at an early stage after sublethal irradiation. J Immunol 1989; 142:3683–3691.

76. Toyonaga B, Yoshikai Y, Vadasz V, et al: Organization and sequences of the diversity, joining, constant region genes of the human T-cell receptor β chain. Proc Natl Acad Sci U S A 1985; 82:8624–8628.

77. Leiden JM, Strominger JL: Generation of diversity of the β chain of the human T-lymphocyte receptor for antigen. Proc Natl Acad Sci U S A 1986; 83:4456–4460.

78. Strauss WM, Quertermous T, Seidman JG: Measuring the human T cell receptor γ-chain locus. Science 1987; 237:1217–1219.

79. Forster A, Huck S, Ghanem N, et al: New subgroups in the human T cell rearranging Vγ gene locus. EMBO J 1987; 6:1945–1950.

80. Chen Z, Font MP, Loiseau P, et al: The human T-cell Vγ gene locus: Cloning of new segments and study of Vτ rearrangements in neoplastic T and B cells. Blood 1988; 72:776–783.

81. Quertermous T, Murre C, Dialynas D, et al: Human T-cell γ chain

genes: Organization, diversity, and rearrangement. Science 1986; 231:252–255.

82. LeFranc M-P, Forster A, Baer R, et al: Diversity and rearrangement of the human T-cell rearranging γ genes: Nine germline variable genes belonging to two subgroups. Cell 1986; 45:237–246.

83. Krangel MS, Band H, Hata S, et al: Structurally divergent human T-cell receptor τ proteins encoded by distinct Cγ genes. Science 1987; 237:64–67.

84. Hochstenbach F, Parker C, McLean J, et al: Characterization of a third form of the human T-cell receptor γ/δ. J Exp Med 1988; 168:761–776.

85. Clevers HC, Owen MJ: Towards a molecular understanding of T-cell differentiation. Immunol Today 1991; 12:167–173.

86. Gottschalk LR, Leiden JM: Identification and functional characterization of the human T-cell receptor β gene transcriptional enhancer: Common nuclear proteins interact with the transcriptional regulatory elements of the T-cell receptor α and β genes. Mol Cell Biol 1990; 10:5486–5495.

87. Leiden JM: Transcriptional regulation of T-cell receptor genes. Annu Rev Immunol 1993; 11:539–570.

88. Bhat NK, Komschlies KL, Fisher RJ, et al: Expression of *ets* genes in mouse thymocyte subsets and T cells. J Immunol 1989; 142:672–678.

89. Ho I-C, Bhat NK, Gottschalk LR, et al: Sequence-specific binding of human *ets-1* to the T-cell receptor α gene enhancer. Science 1990; 250:814–818.

90. McDougall S, Peterson CL, Calame K: A transcriptional enhancer 3′ of Cβ2 in the T-cell receptor β locus. Science 1988; 241:205–208.

91. Anderson SJ, Miyake S, Loh DY: Transcription from a murine T-cell receptor Vβ promoter depends on a conserved decamer motif similar to the cyclic AMP response element. Mol Cell Biol 1989; 9:4835–4845.

92. Diaz P, Cado D, Winoto A: A locus control region in the T-cell receptor α/δ locus. Immunity 1994; 1:207–217.

93. Winoto A, Baltimore D: αβ lineage-specific expression of the T-cell receptor gene by nearby silencers. Cell 1989; 59:649–655.

94. Ho IC, Leiden ML: The Tα2 nuclear protein binding site from the human T-cell receptor α enhancer functions as both a T-cell specific transcriptional activator and repressor. J Exp Med 1990; 172:1443–1449.

95. de Villartay JP, Hockett RD, Coran D, et al: Deletion of the human T-cell receptor δ-gene by a site-specific recombination. Nature 1988; 335:170–174.

96. Campana D, Janossy G, Coustan-Smith E, et al: The expression of T-cell receptor–associated proteins during T-cell ontogeny in man. J Immunol 1989; 142:57–66.

97. Haynes BF, Singer KH, Denning SM, Martin ME: Analysis of expression of CD2, CD3, and T-cell antigen receptor molecules during early human fetal thymic development. J Immunol 1988; 141:3776–3784.

98. Bories JC, Loiseau P, d'Auriol L, et al: Regulation of the transcription of the human T-cell antigen receptor δ chain gene: A T-lineage–specific enhancer element is located in the Jδ3-Cδ intron. J Exp Med 1990; 171:75–83.

99. De Villartay JP, Pullmann AB, Anrade R, et al: γ/δ lineage relationship within a consecutive series of human precursor T-cell neoplasms. Blood 1989; 74:2508–2518.

100. Uematsu Y, Ryser S, Dembic Z, et al: In transgenic mice the introduced functional T-cell receptor β gene prevents expression of endogenous β genes. Cell 1988; 52:831–841.

101. Chien Y, Iwashima M, Kaplan KB, et al: A new T-cell receptor gene located within the alpha locus and expressed early in T-cell differentiation. Nature 1987; 327:677–682.

102. Padovan E, Casorati G, Dellabona P, et al: Frequent expression of two TCRα chains in human αβ lymphocytes creates dual receptor cells. Science 1993; 262:422–424.

103. Shortman K: Cellular aspects of early T-cell development. Curr Opinion Immunol 1992; 4:140–146.

104. Haas W, Kaufman S, Martinez AC: The development and function of γδ T cells. Immunol Today 1990; 11:340–343.

105. Borst J, Brouns GS, de Vries E, et al: Antigen receptors on T and B lymphocytes: Parallels in organization and function. Immunol Rev 1993; 132:49–84.

106. Pfeffer K, Mak TW: Knockout mice: Insights into the ontogeny and activation of T cells. Immunologist 1993; 1:191–197.

107. Mombaerts P, Clarke AR, Rudnicki MA, et al: Mutations in T-cell antigen receptor genes α and β block thymocyte development at different stages. Nature 1992; 360:225–231.

108. Itohara S, Mombaerts P, Lafaille J, et al: T-cell receptor delta gene mutant mice: Independent generation of alpha beta T cells and programmed rearrangements of gamma delta TCR genes. Cell 1993; 72:337–348.

109. Philcott KL, Viney JL, Kay G, et al: Lymphoid development in mice congenitally lacking T cell receptor alpha-beta-expressing cells. Science 1992; 256:1448–1452.

110. Love PE, Shores EW, Johnson MD, et al: T-cell development in mice that lack the zeta chain of the T cell antigen receptor complex. Science 1993; 261:918–921.

111. Ohno H, Aoe T, Taki S, et al: Development and functional impairment of T cells in mice lacking CD3 zeta chains. EMBO J 1993; 12:4357–4366.

112. Fung-Leung WP, Kündig TM, Zinkernagel RM, Mak TW: Immune response against lymphocytic choriomeningitis virus infection in mice without CD8 expression. J Exp Med 1991; 174:1425–1429.

113. Fung-Leung WP, Wallace VA, Gray D, et al: CD8 is needed for positive selection but differentially required for negative selection of T cells during thymic ontogeny. Eur J Immunol 1993; 23:212–216.

114. Kishihara K, Penninger J, Wallace VA, et al: Normal B lymphocyte development but impaired T cell maturation in CD45-Exon 6 protein tyrosine phosphatase–deficient mice. Cell 1993; 74:143–156.

115. Molina TJ, Kishihara K, Siderovski DP, et al: Profound block in thymocyte development in mice lacking p56lck. Nature 1992; 357:161–164.

116. Penninger J, Kishihara K, Molina T, et al: Requirement for tyrosine kinase p56lck for thymic development of transgenic γδ T cells. Science 1993; 260:358–361.

117. Taniguchi T, Minami Y: The IL-2/IL-2 receptor system: A current overview. Cell 1993; 73:5–8.

118. Griscelli C, Lisowska-Grospierre B: Combined immunodeficiency with defective expression in MHC class II genes. Immunodeficiency Rev 1989; 1:135–153.

119. Schorle H, Holtschke T, Hünig T, et al: Development and function of T cells in mice rendered interleukin-2 deficient by gene targeting. Nature 1991; 352:621–624.

120. Kündig TM, Schorle H, Bachmann MF, et al: Immune responses in interleukin-2–deficient mice. Science 1993; 262:1059–1061.

121. Kappler J, Wade T, White J, et al: A T-cell receptor Vβ segment that imparts rectivity to a class II major histocompatibility complex product. Cell 1987; 49:263–271.

122. Miller JFAP, Heath WR: Self-ignorance in the peripheral T cell pool. Immunol Rev 1993; 133:131.

123. Hugo P, Kappler JW, Godfrey DI, Marrack PC: Thymic epithelial cell lines that mediate positive selection can also induce thymocyte clonal deletion. J Immunol 1994; 152:1022.

124. Ashton-Rickardt PG, Bandeira A, Delaney JR, et al: Evidence for a differential avidity model of T cell selection in the thymus. Cell 1994; 76:651.

125. Chan SH, Cosgrove D, Waltzinger C, et al: Another view of the selective model of thymocyte selection. Cell 1993; 73:225.

126. Davis CB, Killeen N, Crooks MEC, et al: Evidence for a stochastic mechanism in the differentiation of mature subsets of T lymphocytes. Cell 1993; 73:237.

127. Viville S, Neefjes J, Lotteau V, et al: Mice lacking the MHC class II–associated invariant chain. Cell 1993; 72:635.

128. Zijlstra M, Li E, Sajjadi F, et al: Germline transmission of a disrupted beta₂-microglobulin gene produced by homologous recombination in embryonic stem cells. Nature 1989; 342:435–438.

129. Nossal GJV, Pike BL: Claonal anergy: Persistence in tolerant mice of antigen-binding B lymphocytes incapable of responding to antigen or mitogen. Proc Natl Acad Sci U S A 1980; 77:1602–1606.

130. Dent AL, Matis LA, Hooshmand F, et al: Self-reactive τδ T cells are eliminated in the thymus. Nature 1990; 343:714–719.

131. Bonneville M, Ishida I, Itohara S, et al: Self-tolerance to transgenic γδ T cells by intrathymic inactivation. Nature 1990; 344:163–165.

132. Sim GK, Augustin A: Extrathymic-positive selection of γδ T cells. J Immunol 1991; 146:2439–2445.

133. Lefrancois L, LeCorre R, Mayo J, et al: Extrathymic selection of TCRγδ+ T cells by class II major histocompatibility complex molecules. Cell 1990; 63:333–340.

134. Crabtree G: Contingent genetic regulatory events in T lymphocyte activation. Science 1989; 243:355–361.

135. Linsley PS, Brady W, Grosmaire L, et al: Binding of the B-cell activation antigen B7 to CD28 costimulates T-cell proliferation and interleukin-2 mRNA accumulation. J Exp Med 1991; 173:721–730.

136. Weiss A, Koretzky G, Schatzman RC, Kadlecek T: Functional activation of the T-cell antigen receptor induces tyrosine phosphorylation of PLCγ-1. Proc Natl Acad Sci U S A 1991; 88:5484–5488.

137. Cantley LC, Auger KR, Carpenter C, et al: Oncogenes and signal transduction. Cell 1991; 64:281–302.

138. Gschwendt M, Kittstein W, Marks F: Protein kinase C activation by phorbol esters: Do cystein-rich regions and pseudosubstrate motifs play a role? TIBS 1991; 16:167–169.

139. Weiss A, Imboden J, Hardy K, et al: The role of the T3/antigen receptor complex in T-cell activation. Annu Rev Immunol 1986; 4:593–679.

140. Arai KI, Lee F, Miyajima A, et al: Cytokines: Coordinators of immune and inflammatory responses. Annu Rev Biochem 1990; 59:783–836.

141. Ghosh S, Baltimore D: Activation in vitro of NF-κB by phosphorylation of the inhibitor IκB. Nature 1990; 344:678–682.

142. Rayter SI, Woodrow M, Lucas SC, et al: P21ras mediates control of IL-2 gene promoter function in T-cell activation. EMBO J 1992; 11:4549–4556.

143. Downward J, Graves JD, Cantrell DA: The regulation and function of p21ras in T cells. Immunol Today 1992; 13:89–92.

144. Hanley MR, Jackson TJ: The *ras* gene: Transformer and transducer. Nature 1987; 328:668–669.

145. Hunter T: Cooperation between oncogenes. Cell 1991; 64:249–270.

146. Jamal S, Ziff E: Transactivation of c-*fos* and β-actin genes by raf as a step in early response transmembrane signals. Nature 1990; 344:463–466.

147. Wang Z-Q, Ovitt C, Grigoriadis AE, et al: Bone and hematopoietic defects in mice lacking c-*fos*. Nature 1992; 360:741–745.

148. Siegel JN, Klausner RD, Rapp UR, Samelson LE: T-cell antigen receptor engagement stimulates c-*raf* phosphorylation and induces c-*raf*-associated kinase activity via a protein kinase–dependent pathway. J Biol Chem 1990; 265:18472–18480.

149. Bruder JT, Heidecker G, Rapp UR: Serum TPA- and ras-induced expression from AP1/ets-driven promoters requires raf-1 kinase. Genes Develop 1992; 6:545–556.

150. Crews CM, Erikson RL: Extracellular signals and reversible protein phosphorylation: What to make of it all. Cell 1993; 74:215–217.

151. Perlmutter RM, Levin SD, Appleby MW, et al: Regulation of lymphocyte function by protein phosphorylation. Annu Rev Immunol 1993; 11:451–499.

152. Izquierdo M, Downward J, Otani H, et al: Interleukin activation of p21ras in murine myeloid cells transfected with the human IL-2 receptor β-chain. Eur J Immunol 1992; 22:817–821.

153. Varmus HE, Lowell CA: Cancer genes and hematopoiesis. Blood 1994; 83:5–9.

154. Rudd CE: CD4, CD8, and the TCR-CD3 complex: A novel class of protein-tyrosine kinase receptor. Immunol Today 1990; 11:400–410.

155. Glaichenhaus N, Shastri N, Littman DR, Turner JM: Requirement for association of p56lck with CD4 in antigen-specific signal transduction in T cells. Cell 1991; 64:511–520.

156. Collins TL, Uniyal S, Shin J, et al: P56lck association with CD4 is required for the interaction between and the TCR/CD3 complex and for optimal antigen stimulation. J Immunol 1992; 148:2159–2162.

157. Weber JR, Bell GM, Han MY, et al: Association of the tyrosine kinase lck with phospholipase C-γ1 after stimulation of the T-cell antigen receptor. J Exp Med 1992; 176:373–379.

158. Amrein KE, Flint N, Panholzer B, Burn P: Ras GTPase-activating protein: A substrate and a potential binding protein of the protein tyrosine kinase p56lck. Proc Natl Acad Sci U S A 1992; 89:3343–3346.

159. Ettehadieh E, Sanghera JS, Pelech SL, et al: Tyrosyl phosphorylation and activation of MAP kinases by p56lck. Science 1992; 255:853–856.

160. Chan AC, Iwashima M, Turck CW, Weiss A: ZAP-70 kd protein tyrosine kinase that associates with the TCRζ chain. Cell 1992; 71:649–662.

161. Arpaia E, Shahar M, Dadi H, et al: Defective T-cell receptor signaling and CD8+ thymic selection in humans lacking Zap-70 kinase. Cell 1994; 76:947–958.

162. Veillette A, Davidson D: Src-related protein tyrosine kinases and T-cell receptor signalling. TIBS 1992; 8:61–66.

163. Sancho J, Choi MS, Dasgupta JD, et al: Stimulation of T cells through the TCR/CD3 complex induces tyrosine phosphorylation of a 70-kDa polypeptide chain associated with the CD3-zeta chain. J Biol Chem 1992; 267:7871–7879.

164. Mackay CR, Kimpton WG, Brandom MR, Cahill RNP: Lymphocyte subsets show marked differences in their distribution between blood and the afferent and efferent lymph of peripheral lymph nodes. J Exp Med 1988; 167:1755–1756.

165. Shimizu Y, Newman W, Tanaka Y, Shaw S: Lymphocyte interactions with endothelial cells. Immunol Today 1992; 13:106–112.

166. Groh V, Porcelli S, Fabbi M, et al: Human lymphocytes bearing T-cell receptor γ/δ are phenotypically diverse and evenly distributed throughout the lymphoid system. J Exp Med 1989; 169:1277–1294.

167. Inghirami G, Zhu BY, Chess L, Knowles DM: Flow cytometric and immunohistochemical characterization of the γ/δ T-lymphocyte population in normal human lymphoid tissue and peripheral blood. Am J Pathol 1990; 136:357–367.

168. Falini B, Flenghi L, Pileri S, et al: Distribution of T cells bearing different forms of the T-cell receptor γ/δ in normal and pathological human tissues. J Immunol 1989; 143:2480–2488.

169. Bos JD, Kapsenberg ML: The skin immune system: Progress in cutaneous biology. Immunol Today 1993; 14:75–78.

170. Paul WE, Seder RA: Lymphocyte responses and cytokines. Cell 1994; 76:241–251.

171. Dianzani U, Luqman M, Rojo J, et al: Molecular associations on the T-cell surface correlate with immunological memory. Eur J Immunol 1990; 20:2249–2257.

172. Beverley PCL: Human T-cell memory. Curr Topics Microbiol Immunol 1990; 159:111–122.

173. Janeway CA, Golstein P: Lymphocyte activation and effector functions. Curr Opinion Immunol 1993; 5:313–323.

174. Dellabona P, Casorati G, Friedli B, et al: In vivo persistence of expanded clones specific for bacterial antigens within the human T-cell receptor α/β CD4–8– subset. J Exp Med 1993; 177:1763–1771.

175. Porcelli S, Yockey CE, Brenner MB, Balk SP: Analysis of T-cell antigen receptor (TCR) expression by human peripheral blood CD4–8– α/β+ T cells demonstrates a preferential use of several Vβ genes and an invariant TCRα chain. J Exp Med 1993; 178:1–16.

176. Uyemura K, Deans RJ, Band H, et al: Evidence for clonal selection of γ/δ T cells in response to a human pathogen. J Exp Med 1991; 174:683–692.

177. Modlin RL, Pirmez C, Hofman FM, et al: Lymphocytes bearing antigen-specific γ/δ T-cell receptors accumulate in human infectious disease lesions. Nature 1989; 339:544–548.

178. Cambier JC, Pleiman CM, Clark MR: Signal transduction by the B-cell antigen receptor and its coreceptors. Annu Rev Immunol 1994; 12:457–486.

179. Reth M: Antigen receptors on B lymphocytes. Annu Rev Immunol 1992; 10:98–121.

180. Early P, Rogers J, Davis M, et al: Two mRNAs can be produced from a single immunoglobulin μ gene by alternative RNA processing pathways. Cell 1980; 20:313–319.

181. Taniguchi T, Kobayashi T, Kondo J, et al: Molecular cloning of porcine gene *syk* that encodes a 72-kDa protein tyrosine kinase showing high susceptibility to proteolysis. J Biol Chem 1991; 266:15790–15796.

182. Tedder TF, Zhou L-J, Engel P: The CD19/CD21 signal transduction complex of B lymphocytes. Immunol Today 1994; 15:437–442.

183. Carter RH, Fearon DT: Lowering the threshhold for antigen receptor stimulation of B lymphocytes. Science 1992; 256:105–107.

184. Law C-L, Sidorenko SP, Clark EA: Regulation of lymphocyte activation by the cell surface molecule CD22. Immunol Today 1994; 15:442–449.

185. Tedder TF, Engel P: CD20: A regulator of cell cycle progression of B lymphocytes. Immunol Today 1994; 15:450–454.

186. Lederman S, Yellin MJ, Inghirami G, et al: Molecular interactions mediating T-B lymphocyte collaboration in human lymphoid follicles: Roles of T cell–B cell activating molecule (5c8 antigen) and CD40 in contact-dependent help. J Immunol 1992; 149:3817–3826.

187. Laman JD, Claassen E, Noelle RJ: Immunodeficiency due to faulty interaction between T cells and B cells. Curr Opinion Immunol 1994; 6:636–641.

188. Liu Y-J, Barthélémy C, de Bouteiller O, et al: Memory B cells from human tonsils colonize mucosal epithelium and directly present antigen to T cells by rapid up-regulation of B7-1 and B7-2. Immunity 1995; 2:239–248.

189. Shahinian A, Pfeffer K, Lee KP, et al: Differential T-cell costimulatory requirements in CD28-deficient mice. Science 1993; 261:609–612.

190. Cook GP, Tomlinson IM, Walter G, et al: A map of the human immunoglobulin V_H locus completed by analysis of the telomeric region of chromosome 14q. Nature Genet 1994; 7:162–168.

191. Buluwela L, Albertson DG, Sherrington P, et al: The use of chromosomal translocations to study human immunoglobulin gene organization: Mapping D_H segments within 35 kb of the $C\mu$ gene and identification of a new D_H locus. EMBO J 1988; 7:2003–2010.

192. Flanagan JG, Rabbitts TH: The sequence of a human immunoglobulin epsilon heavy chain constant region gene, and evidence for three non-allelic genes. EMBO J 1982; 1:655–660.

193. Hieter PA, Max EE, Seidman JG, et al: Cloned human and mouse kappa immunoglobulin constant and J region genes conserve homology in functional segments. Cell 1980; 22:197–207.

194. Meindl A, Klobeck H-G, Ohnheiser R, Zachau HG: The Vκ gene repertoire in human germline. Eur J Immunol 1990; 20:1855–1863.

195. Dariavach P, Lefranc G, Lefranc M-P: Human immunoglobulin Cλ6 gene encodes the Kern+Oz+1 chain and Cλ4 and Cλ5 are pseudogenes. Proc Natl Acad Sci U S A 1987; 84:9074–9078.

196. Vasicek TJ, Leder P: Structure and expression of the human immunoglobulin λ genes. J Exp Med 1990; 172:609–620.

197. Combriato G, Klobeck H-G: Vλ and Jλ-Cλ gene segments of the human immunoglobulin λ light chain locus are separated by 14 kb and rearrange by a deletion mechanism. Eur J Immunol 1991; 21:1513–1522.

198. Staudt LM, Lenardo MJ: Immunoglobulin gene transcription. Annu Rev Immunol 1991; 9:373–398.

199. Takeda S, Zou Y, Bluethmann H, et al: Deletion of the immunoglobulin κ chain intron enhancer abolishes κ chain gene rearrangement in *trans*. EMBO J 1993; 12:2329–2336.

200. Betz AG, Milstein C, González-Fernández A, et al: Elements regulating somatic hypermutation of an immunoglobulin κ gene: Critical role for the intron enhancer/matrix attachment region. Cell 1994; 77:239–248.

201. Wirth T, Priess A, Annweiler A, et al: Multiple *oct-2* isoforms are generated by alternative splicing. Nucleic Acid Res 1991; 19:43–51.

202. Corcoran L, Karvelas M, Nossal GJ, et al: *Oct-2*, although not required for early B-cell development, is critical for later B-cell maturation and for postnatal survival. Genes Develop 1993; 7:570–582.

203. Hagman J, Grosschedl R: Regulation of gene expression at early stages of B-cell differentiation. Curr Opinion Immunol 1994; 6:222–230.

204. Strubin M, Newell JW, Matthias P: OBF-1, a novel B-cell-specific coactivator that stimulates immunoglobulin promoter activity through association with octamer-binding proteins. Cell 1995; 80:497–506.

205. Rolink A, Melchers F: Molecular and cellular origins of B lymphocyte diversity. Cell 1991; 66:1081–1094.

206. Jacobson K, Tepper J, Osmond DG: Early B-lymphocyte precursor cells in mouse bone marrow: Substeal localization of B220+ cells during post-irradiation regeneration. Exp Hematol 1990; 18:304–310.

207. Banchereau J, Rousset F: Human B lymphocytes: Phenotype, proliferation, and differentiation. Adv Immunol 1992; 52:125–262.

208. Punnonen J, Aversa G, de Vries J: Human pre-B cells differentiate into Ig-secreting plasma cells in the presence of interleukin-4 and activated CD4+ T cells or their membranes. Blood 1993; 82:2781–2789.

209. Hokland P, Ritz J, Schlossman SF, Nadler LM: Orderly expression of B-cell antigens during the in vitro differentiation of nonmalignant human pre-B cells. J Immunol 1985; 135:1746–1751.

210. Nadler LM, Korsmeyer SJ, Anderson KC, et al: B-cell origin of non-T-cell acute lymphoblastic leukemia. J Clin Invest 1984; 74:332–340.

211. Alt FW, Yancopoulos GD, Blackwell TK, et al: Ordered rearrangement of immunoglobulin heavy chain variable region segments. EMBO J 1984; 3:1209–1219.

212. Ehlich A, Schaal S, Gu H, et al: Immunoglobulin heavy and light chain genes rearrange independently at early stages of B-cell development. Cell 1993; 72:695–704.

213. Nishimoto N, Kubagawa H, Ohno T, et al: Normal pre-B cells express a receptor complex of μ heavy chains and surrogate light chain proteins. Proc Natl Acad Sci U S A 1991; 88:6284–6288.

214. Takemori T, Mizuguchi J, Miyazoe I, et al: Two types of μ chain complexes are expressed during differentiation from pre-B to mature B cells. EMBO J 1990; 9:2493–2500.

215. Melchers F, Karasuyama H, Haasner D, et al: The surrogate light chain in B-cell development. Immunol Today 1993; 14:60–68.

216. Reth M, Alt FW: Novel immunoglobulin heavy chains are produced from DJ$_H$ gene segment rearrangements in lymphoid cells. Nature 1984; 312:418–423.

217. Maeda T, Sugiyama H, Tani Y, Kishimoto S: The DJ$_H$ complex remains active in recombination to V$_H$ segments after the loss of μ chain expression in μ-positive pre-B cells. J Immunol 1989; 142:3652–3656.

218. Kitamura D, Kudo A, Schaal S, et al: A critical role of λ5 protein in B-cell development. Cell 1992; 69:823–831.

219. Kitamura D, Roes J, Kühn R, Rajewsky K: A B-cell-deficient mouse by targeted disruption of the membrane exon of the immunoglobulin μ chain gene. Nature 1991; 350:423–426.

220. Melchers F, Haasner D, Grawunder U, et al: Roles of IgH and L chains and of surrogate H and L chains in the development of cells of the B-lymphocyte lineage. Annu Rev Immunol 1994; 12:209–225.

221. Graninger WB, Goldman PL, Morton CC, et al: The κ-deleting element: Germline and rearranged, duplicated, and dispersed forms. J Exp Med 1988; 167:488–501.

222. Giachino C, Padovan E, Lanzavecchia A: $\kappa+\lambda+$ dual receptor B cells are present in the human peripheral repertoire. J Exp Med 1995; 181:1245–1250.

223. Storb U: Transgenic mice with immunoglobulin genes. Annu Rev Immunol 1987; 5:151–174.

224. Von Schwedler U, Jäck H-M, Wabl M: Circular DNA is a product of immunoglobulin class switch rearrangement. Nature 1990; 345:452–455.

225. Purkerson JM, Isakson PC: Independent regulation of DNA recombination and immunoglobulin (Ig) secretion during isotype switching in IgG1 and IgE. J Exp Med 1994; 179:1877–1883.

226. Chen J, Alt FW: Gene rearrangement and B-cell development. Curr Opinion Immunol 1993; 5:194–200.

227. Wabl M, Burrows PD, von Gabain A, Steinberg C: Hypermutation at the immunoglobulin heavy chain locus in pre-B-cell lines. Proc Natl Acad Sci U S A 1985; 82:479–482.

228. Goodnow CC, Crosbie J, Jorgensen H, et al: Induction of self-tolerance in mature peripheral B lymphocytes. Nature 1989; 342:385–391.

229. Nemazee DA, Bürki K: Clonal deletion of B lymphocytes in transgenic mice bearing anti-MHC class I antibody genes. Nature 1989; 337:562–566.

230. Hodgkin PD, Basten A: B-cell activation, tolerance, and antigen-presenting function. Curr Opinion Immunol 1995; 7:121–129.

231. Gay D, Saunders T, Camper S, Weigert M: Receptor editing: An approach by autoreactive B cells to escape self-tolerance. J Exp Med 1993; 177:999–1008.

232. Thorbecke GJ, Amin AR, Tsiagbe VK: Biology of germinal centers in lymphoid tissue. FASEB J 1994; 8:832–840.

233. Liu YJ, Joshua DE, Williams GT, et al: Mechanism of antigen-driven selection in germinal centers. Nature 1989; 342:929–931.

234. Liu YJ, Cairns JA, Holder MJ, et al: Recombinant 25-kDa CD34 and interleukin-1 alpha promote the survival of germinal center B cells: Evidence for bifurcation in the development of centrocytes rescued from apoptosis. Eur J Immunol 1991; 21:1107–1114.

235. Yamamoto T, Yamanashi Y, Toyoshima K: Association of src-family kinase lyn with B-cell antigen receptor. Immunol Rev 1993; 132:187–206.

236. Coggeshall KM, McGugh JC, Altman A: Predominant expression and activation-induced tyrosine phosphorylation of phospholipase C-γ2 in B lymphocytes. Proc Natl Acad Sci U S A 1992; 89:5660–5664.

237. Boyle WM, Smeal T, Defize LHK, et al: Activation of protein kinase C decreases phosphorylation of c-*jun* sites that negatively regulate its DNA binding activity. Cell 1991; 64:573–584.

238. Pleiman CM, Clark MR, Winitz S, et al: Mapping of sites on src-family protein tyrosine kinases p55blk, p59fyn, and p56lyn which interact with effector molecules PLC-γ2, MAP kinase, GAP, PI 3-kinase. Mol Cell Biol 1993; 13:5877–5887.

239. Nakanishi H, Brewer KA, Exton JH: Activation of the ζ isozyme of protein kinase C by phosphatidylinositol 3,4,5-triphosphate. J Biol Chem 1993; 268:13–16.

240. Diaz-Meco MT, Berra E, Municio MM, et al: A dominant negative protein kinase C ζ subspecies blocks NF-kB activation. Mol Cell Biol 1993; 13:4770–4775.

241. Kantor A: A new nomenclature for B cells. Immunol Today 1991; 12:388.

242. Abe M, Tominaga K, Wakasa H: Phenotypic characterization of human B-lymphocyte subpopulations, particularly human CD5+ B-lymphocyte subpopulations within the mantle zones of secondary follicles. Leukemia 1994; 8:1039–1044.

243. Haughton G, Arnold LW, Whitmore AC, Clarke SH: B-1 cells are made, not born. Immunol Today 1993; 14:84–87.

244. UytdeHaag F, van der Heijden R, Osterhaus A: Maintenance of immunological memory: A role for CD5+ B cells. Immunol Today 1991; 12:439–442.

245. MacLennan I, Chan E: The dynamic relationship between B-cell populations in adults. Immunol Today 1993; 14:29–34.

246. MacLennan IC: Germinal centers. Annu Rev Immunol 1994; 12:117–139.

247. Kawabe T, Naka T, Yoshida K, et al: The immune responses in CD40-deficient mice: Impaired immunoglobulin class switching and germinal center formation. Immunity 1994; 1:167–178.

248. Castle BE, Kishimoto K, Stearns C, et al: Regulation of expression of the ligand for CD40 on T-helper lymphocytes. J Immunol 1993; 151:1777–1788.

249. Korthauer U, Graf D, Mages HW, et al: Defective expression of T-cell CD40 ligand causes X-linked immunodeficiency with hyper-IgM. Nature 1993; 361:539–543.

Three

——— Epidemiology of Hodgkin's ——— Disease and Non-Hodgkin's Lymphoma

Albert Y. Lin
Margaret A. Tucker

The term "malignant lymphoma" was originally introduced by Billroth[1] to describe neoplasms of lymphoid tissue. It has been traditional to divide lymphomas into Hodgkin's disease (HD) and non-Hodgkin's lymphoma (NHL) because of their difference in histology and patterns of behavior. However, HD and NHL may occur as synchronous or metachronous double primaries.[2–5] In this chapter, we discuss recent findings in the epidemiology of HD and NHL, and related issues.

HODGKIN'S DISEASE

HD, first described by Dr. Thomas Hodgkin in 1832, is a relatively uncommon malignancy. It is characterized by the presence of Reed-Sternberg cells, which are multinucleated giant cells described by Drs. Sternberg, in 1898, and Reed, in 1902. As late as the 1940s, HD was classified as an infectious disease by the *Manual of the International List of Causes of Death, Fourth Edition.*[6, 7]

INCIDENCE, MORTALITY RATES, AND TRENDS

International Data

Age-Adjusted Rates by Gender. Around the world, from 1968 to 1972, the age-adjusted rates in men varied widely from 0.8 per 100,000 person-years in Asia to 4 per 100,000 person-years in North America (Fig. 3–1A), with intermediate rates in Europe. However, these rates dropped to 0.4 and 3.7 per 100,000 person-years during the 1983 to 1987 period.[8] In every geographic area, the incidence rates are lower in women than in men (Fig. 3–1B), and they range from 0.2 per 100,000 person-years in Asia to 3 per 100,000 person-years in North America from 1968 to 1972. Similar to the rates in men, the rates in women have decreased slightly over time in most areas.[8]

Age-Adjusted Rates by Race and Geographic Areas. Although the largest variation in international rates is between different racial groups, the racial differences do not explain all the variance. Rates in white men range from 2.1 per 100,000 person-years (in Warsaw) to 3.7 per 100,000 person-years (in the United States), and the rates in black men range from 0.2 (in Gambia) to 2.0 (in the United States). The rates appear to vary less among Asian men, with the same age-adjusted rate of 0.6 in Chinese men in Singapore and Los Angeles.[9]

U.S. Data

Age-Adjusted Rates by Gender. The current U.S. age-adjusted incidence rate for HD is 2.9 per 100,000 person-years in both sexes combined (Table 3–1). Over the past 18 years, the age-adjusted incidence rates for HD range from 2.6 to 3.0 per 100,000 person-years (Fig. 3–2).[10] Incidence is higher in men than in women. An overall decrease of 12% was observed from 1973 to 1991 (Fig. 3–3), but an increase of 2% in the same period was noted in women younger than 65 years of age, especially among black women, for which there is no clear explanation. Overall decline may be partially explained by changing diagnostic criteria (see the section on trends by subtype).[11] Owing to the development of effective treatment, the mortality rates have declined in both men and women at a rate of 4.5% per year in the same period (see Figs. 3–2 and 3–3).

Age-Adjusted Rates by Race and Geographic Areas. In the data gathered by the Surveillance, Epidemiology, and End Results (SEER) program of the National Cancer Institute (NCI), the incidence is highest in whites (men, 3.5 per 100,000 person-years; women, 2.6), lower in blacks (men; 3.0 per 100,000 person-years; women 2.5), and lowest in Asians (Chinese in Los Angeles: men, 0.6 per 100,000 person-years; women, 0.4) (Fig. 3–4). Within SEER areas, there is some variance, but it is not as great as the international variation (Table 3–2). The rates in Connecticut are the highest (3.6 per 100,000 person-years in 1990), whereas those in Hawaii are the lowest (1.7 per 100,000 person-years). These differences imply that both racial and geographic factors are important in the incidence rates.

Age-Specific Incidence Rates. MacMahon was the first to describe the bimodal distribution of HD, with one peak being at adolescence to young adulthood (15 to 34 years) and the other peak at older age (>50 years).[12] This observation stimulated a series of investigations that have greatly increased our understanding of HD. Over the past 3 decades, the pattern of age-specific incidence has changed with a flattening of the bimodal age distribution (Fig. 3–5). Since the late 1940s, the incidence rates at ages 15 to 24 have been increasing. In the 25- to 34-year-old group, the incidence rate started to plateau from 1960 to the 1970s. In the group older than 55 years of age, the incidence rates have decreased since the early 1970s. The bimodal distribution appears more distinct among women (Fig. 3–6). In addition, among young adults, the recent rates in women have been at least as high as those in men, whereas among older people the rates are lower in women than in men. This finding may imply a hormonal effect (see the section on gender).[13]

In the developing countries, such as India, the age-specific incidence rates of HD present a different pattern. In these areas incidence starts to rise in childhood, and the rates are slightly higher than those in developed countries. In contrast with westernized countries, there is no clear peak in young adulthood. The incidence rate continues to rise with age, and in late adult life approaches the age-specific rates of westernized countries (Fig. 3–7). This difference in age-specific patterns has led to investigators exploring the environmental risk factors for HD (see the section on infectious agents).[14]

Age-Specific Incidence Rates by Gender. Regardless of geographic region, men generally have a higher incidence rate of HD than women.[15] This excess is more pronounced during childhood and in people older than 35

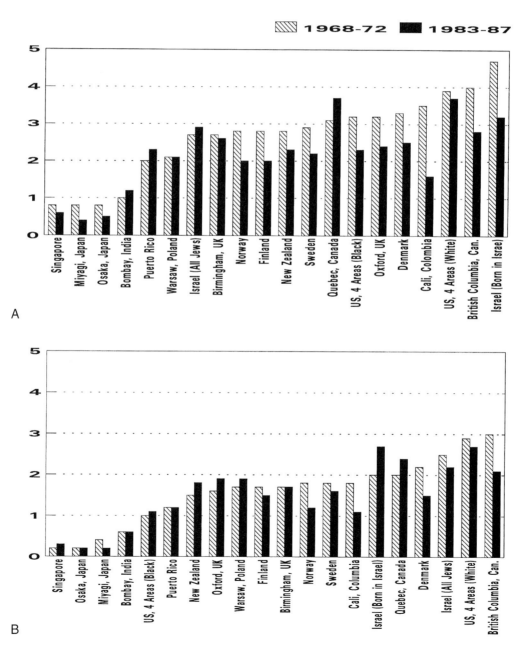

Figure 3–1. Age-adjusted incidence rates (per 100,000 person-years, age-adjusted to world standard population) for Hodgkin's disease in selected populations, from 1968–1972 and 1983–1987: men (A) and women (B). (Data from reference 9.)

Table 3–1. Comparison of Some Epidemiologic Features Between Hodgkin's Disease and Non-Hodgkin's Lymphoma According to Data from the SEER Program, 1987 to 1991

	Hodgkin's Disease	Non-Hodgkin's Lymphoma
Frequency (number of cases)	3540	17,568
Age-adjusted incidence rate (per 100,000 person-years) in 1991	2.9	15.1
Median age at diagnosis	33	65
Age (yr) distribution (%)		
<20	12.7	1.8
20–34	40.3	7.1
35–44	16.1	10.4
45–54	8.2	11.7
55–64	7.4	17.9
65–74	8.3	25.7
75–84	5.4	19.4
>84	1.5	6.0
5-year relative survival rates (%) by year of diagnosis		
1974–1976	71.1	47.1
1977–1979	73.0	48.1
1980–1982	74.3	51.1
1983–1990	78.9°	52.0°

°The difference in rates between 1974–1976 and 1983–1990 is statistically significant.

Data from Ries LAG, Miller BA, Hankey BF, et al (eds): SEER Cancer Statistics Review, 1973–1991: Tables and Graphs, National Cancer Institute. NIH Publication No. 94-2789. Bethesda, MD, US Department of Health and Human Services, 1994.

years of age (see Fig. 3–6), but in late adolescence and the 20- to 30-year-old group there is a female excess. In a case-control study, Abramson and coworkers[13] observed that women with HD had a lower parity than did their control group. The relative risk associated with parity of less than three was 1.9 ($P < 0.05$). The data were substantiated by a recent Norwegian study.[16] This registry-based study examined 695 men and 441 women patients with HD born between 1935 and 1974. The data suggested that the incidence of HD in women was inversely related to parity. Among 215 women patients with HD of the nodular sclerosis subtype, the relative incidence decreased as parity increased ($P < 0.03$). This relationship was not observed in other histologic subtypes. Over time, as the age at first birth has increased, the female excess has persisted to a later age. Prior to 1970 in the Connecticut tumor registry, the excess was seen only in the 15- to 19-year-old group. In the 1986 to 1990 SEER data, the female excess begins in the 15- to 19-year-old group and persists until the 25- to 29-year-old group.[10]

Trends by Subtype. Reviewing data from SEER program, Medeiros and Greiner[17] noted an increase from 1.1 to 1.6 per 100,000 in age-adjusted incidence in the nodular sclerosis subtype of HD from the period of 1973 to 1977 to the period of 1983 to 1987. This increase in incidence over time was most dramatic in young adult women. During the same interval, the incidence of the lymphocyte depletion subtype decreased from 0.2 to 0.1 per 100,000. The decrease has been attributed to changes in diagnostic criteria, with the lymphocyte depletion currently being classified as NHL.[18] It

White

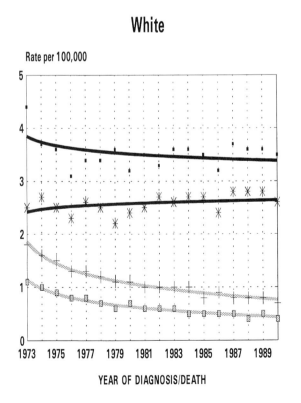

Black

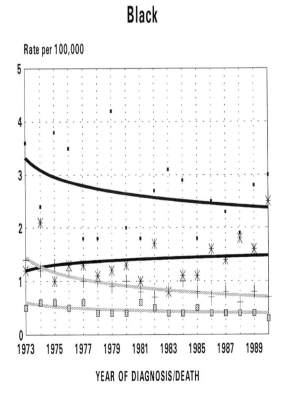

✱ MALE, INCIDENCE   ✝ MALE, MORTALITY   ✻ FEMALE, INCIDENCE   ▨ FEMALE, MORTALITY

Figure 3–2. Age-adjusted incidence and mortality rates for Hodgkin's disease, by race. (Data from reference 10.)

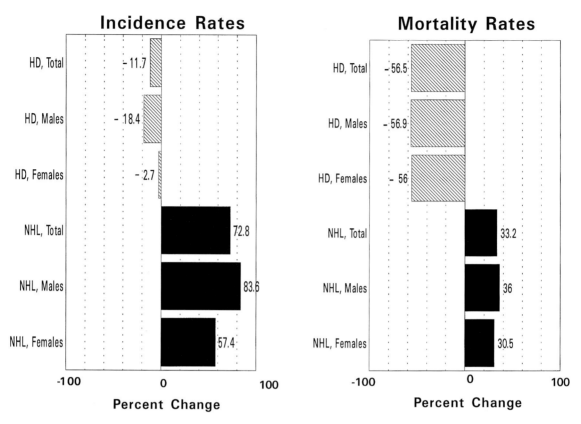

Figure 3–3. Trends in U.S. age-adjusted incidence and mortality rates for Hodgkin's disease (HD) and non-Hodgkin's lymphoma (NHL) by sex, 1973–1991. (Data from SEER Program, reference 188.)

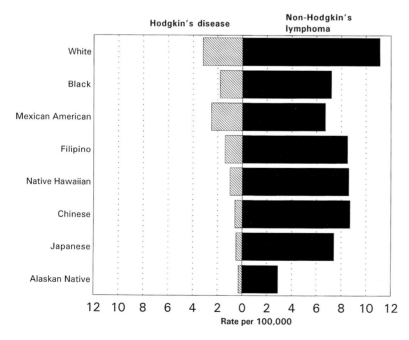

Figure 3–4. Age-adjusted (1970 U.S. Standard) U.S. cancer incidence rates, by race, both sexes, 1977–1983. (Data from reference 10.)

Table 3–2. Age-Adjusted Incidence of Hodgkin's Disease (HD) and Non-Hodgkin's Lymphoma (NHL) in Nine U.S. Areas, 1987–1991

Geographic Area	HD Incidence per 100,000	HD Percentage of All Cancers	NHL Incidence per 100,000	NHL Percentage of All Cancers
San Francisco	3.1	0.74	17.2	4.37
Connecticut	3.6	0.83	14.9	3.72
Detroit	3.1	0.70	14.4	3.37
Hawaii	1.7	0.57	10.5	3.19
Iowa	2.9	0.63	14.5	3.82
New Mexico	2.0	0.64	10.0	3.11
Seattle	2.9	0.69	14.9	3.57
Utah	2.4	0.88	13.1	4.10
Atlanta	2.4	0.84	12.8	3.55
TOTAL	2.9	0.73	14.4	3.71

Data from Ries LAG, Miller BA, Hankey BF, et al (eds): SEER Cancer Statistics Review, 1973–1991: Tables and Graphs, National Cancer Institute. NIH Publication No. 94-2789. Bethesda, MD, US Department of Health and Human Services, 1994.

is estimated that the accuracy of original histologic classification, which was confirmed subsequently by experts in the field, was 83.2% for nodular sclerosis subtype, 51.7% for mixed cellularity, 22.1% for lymphocyte depletion, and 17.1% for lymphocyte predominance.[11] Although the incidence of mixed cellularity subtype was noted to be increased in areas associated with prevalent human immunodeficiency virus (HIV) infections such as San Francisco County, the overall incidence rates of mixed cellularity and lymphocyte predominance subtypes have been stable over time.

Pediatric Hodgkin's Disease

The age-adjusted incidence rates for HD in children younger than 15 years of age over the past 17 years (1973 to 1990) were relatively stable, ranging from 0.5 to 0.9 per 100,000 person-years.[10] Since pediatric HD in the United States comprises only 5% of the total cases, the rates are less stable than adult rates because of the small numbers on which the rates are based. In contrast, childhood HD mortality rates have declined substantially between 1973 and 1990. Mortality rates for those younger than 15 years of age were reduced by more than one half, from 0.1 per 100,000

person-years to 0.0, but this change is based on relatively small numbers. Decline in mortality occurred in both whites and blacks, though it was statistically significant only for whites.

RISK FACTORS ASSOCIATED WITH HODGKIN'S DISEASE

Infectious Agents

Epstein-Barr Virus. Certain parallels between HD and paralytic poliomyelitis have been noted.[19] This observation led to the suggestion that late onset of exposure to a common infectious agent could result in adolescent and young-adult HD. The epidemiologic evidence suggesting that HD may have an infectious etiology is strongest for the young-adult age group. Since the first study to suggest an association between infectious mononucleosis and HD was reported in 1973,[20] Epstein-Barr virus (EBV) has become a major focus of epidemiologic studies in HD. EBV was originally discovered in a cell line derived from an African Burkitt's lymphoma. An initial seroepidemiologic study[21] suggested an association between mixed cellularity and lymphocyte depletion subtypes of HD and EBV infection. Numerous

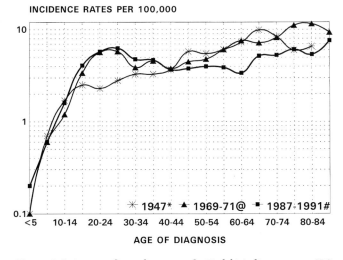

Figure 3–5. Age-specific incidence rates for Hodgkin's disease among U.S. white males over time. °Morbidity from cancer in the United States. (Data from references 15 [@] and 10 [#].)

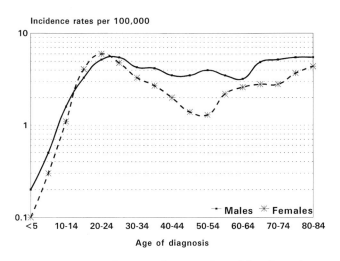

Figure 3–6. Age-specific U.S. incidence rates for Hodgkin's disease by sex, 1986–1991. (Data from reference 10.)

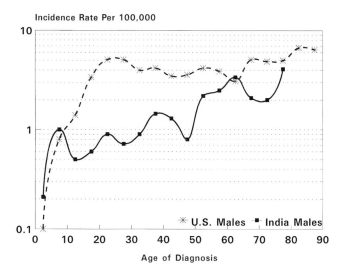

Figure 3–7. Comparison of age-specific incidence rates between U.S. and India males. (Data from references 8 and 10.)

case-control studies suggested that a prior diagnosis of infectious mononucleosis carries a two-fold to 13-fold risk of HD (Table 3–3). Subsequent investigations[22, 23] demonstrated a significant elevation of antibody titers against EBV preceding the diagnosis of HD.

Recent advances in molecular biology have allowed investigators to examine the EBV genome and gene products by Southern blot, in situ hybridization, and polymerase chain reaction in Reed-Sternberg cells. Evidence of EBV can be identified in the Reed-Sternberg cells of approximately 20% to 50% of cases, depending on the population and method of study.[24] It is generally believed that the prevalence of EBV in Reed-Sternberg cells varies by age,[25] histologic subtype, and geographic distribution of the cases.[26] The cases most likely to have EBV present in the Reed-Sternberg cells are those at younger age of onset, in less developed countries, with mixed cellularity histologic subtype. These factors may reflect the underlying socioeconomic status of the affected patients.[27] The results of the in situ hybridization studies suggest that young-adult HD (ages 15 to 34) is less likely to

be EBV associated.[25] It is still unclear whether EBV is a pathogen or a passenger in Reed-Sternberg cells.[28]

There is thus an apparent dichotomy in results. EBV was initially investigated because of the hypothesized viral etiology of young-adult HD. EBV, however, appears to be more related to either childhood or late-onset HD but not young-adult HD. It seems plausible that EBV is an important cofactor or possibly etiologic agent in a subset of HD, such as mixed cellularity and lymphocyte predominant subtypes, in some areas. The putative virus suggested by epidemiologic studies responsible for young-adult nodular sclerosis has yet to be identified.

A recent study, designed to examine the role of EBV among HD kindreds with several affected members as a possible factor from "shared environment,"[29] showed no association between EBV and familial aggregation of HD.[30] As in many other studies, this finding may indicate that an interaction of genetic and environmental factors is required in a disease with multifactorial etiology.

Human Herpesvirus-6. Human herpesvirus-6 (HHV-6) was first isolated from the peripheral blood cells of six patients with immunosuppressive disorders and/or lymphoproliferative disorders.[31] HHV-6 is generally accepted as the primary cause of exanthem subitum.[32] Shortly after HHV-6 was isolated, it was evaluated as a possible cause of early-adult–onset HD. An initial seroepidemiologic study[33] suggested a link between HHV-6 and HD on the basis of elevated IgG antibody titers to the viral capsid antigen. Subsequent studies[34, 35] identified 8% to 10% of HD tumor tissue carrying HHV-6 by polymerase chain reaction, which, unfortunately, did not allow localization of virus in the Reed-Sternberg cells. A longitudinal study[36] indicated that elevation of antibody titers was most likely associated with therapy, since untreated patients had titers similar to those of their age- and sex-matched control subjects. The role of HHV-6 in the etiology of HD remains elusive and speculative. It is plausible that it simply reflects reactivation of latent viruses.

Human Immunodeficiency Virus. The first report of HD associated with HIV infection was published in 1984.[37–39] The occurrence of HIV-associated HD has been overshadowed by the highly prevalent HIV-associated NHL. There is a growing body of evidence to suggest that HIV

Table 3–3. Case-Control Studies on Infectious Mononucleosis (IM) as a Risk Factor for Hodgkin's Disease

Study, Year	Location, Time Period	Study Size	Findings: RR (95% CI)
Connelly, 1974[177]	Connecticut, 1948–1964	Case°: 4529 Control: 0.9-population rates	4 (N/A)
Carter, 1977[178]	United States, 1949–1969	Case†: 2282 Control: 2455	2 (N/A)
Munoz, 1978[179]	Scotland and Sweden, 1957–1971	Case: 9454 Control: 1.8-population rates	4 (1.6–8.0)
Kvale, 1979[180]	Norway, 1961–1972	Case: 5840 Control: 1.2-population rates	4 (N/A)
Serraino, 1991[49]	Italy, 1985–1990	Case: 152 Control: 613	8.2 (0.8–81.4) 13.1‡ (1.0–176.7)

°Cases with a medical history of IM.
†Students from five universities.
‡Nodular sclerosis.
N/A, not available; RR, relative risk; CI, confidence interval.

Table 3–4. Epidemiologic Studies on HIV Exposure as a Risk Factor for Lymphomas

Study, Year	Diagnosis	Observed Number of Lymphoma Cases	Expected Number of Lymphoma Cases	Ratio of Observed/Expected Cases (95% CI)
Hessol, 1992[44]	HD	7	1.4	5.0 (2.0–10.3)
Tirelli, 1993[181]	HD	167	125	4.0° (2.9–5.1); 12.0† (7.0–18.0)
Hessol, 1992[44]	NHL	87	2.3	37.7 (30.3–46.7)
Biggar, 1994[182]	NHL	168	0.8	198‡ (169–232)

°Mixed cellularity subtype.
†Lymphocyte depletion subtype.
‡Risk of developing NHL among 4946 patients with AIDS-related Kaposi's sarcoma.
HD, Hodgkin's disease; NHL, non-Hodgkin's lymphoma; CI, confidence interval.

carriers have a fivefold to eightfold greater risk of HD[40–45] (Table 3–4). Mixed cellularity and lymphocyte depletion subtypes are more prevalent among these cases, compared with HD patients without HIV infection. The virus has not been localized to Reed-Sternberg cells and does not appear to be directly causal, but rather a significant risk factor. Clinicians should be aware that HD, not only NHL, is a risk in HIV-infected patients. The case definition for acquired immunodeficiency syndrome (AIDS) may have to be changed to include HD.[44]

Occupation

Several investigations have evaluated the role of occupational exposures in HD. However, no conclusive evidence has emerged from these studies.

A moderate association between HD and exposure to a woodworking environment has been demonstrated in a number of studies conducted using a variety of methods.[46, 47] Chronic antigen stimulation, by particles or other heterogeneous contact with unknown agents through woodworking processes, has been suggested as a mechanism.[48]

The relationship between HD and potential occupational exposures as teachers or physicians has been examined as part of the viral etiology of HD, but no convincing evidence of an increased risk for HD has been found.[47] Occupational risk factors among HD cases were assessed in a case-control study that found that people who were farmers for more than 10 years had a twofold (95% confidence interval [CI]:1.1–3.7) risk.[49] The risk increased to 3.2-fold or 3.4-fold in farmers with pesticide or livestock and meat processing exposures, respectively.[49] Because of the small number of cases in this study, however, the data require further confirmation.

Genetic Predisposition

There have been numerous case reports of familial aggregations of HD. Most epidemiologic studies indicate that about 1% of patients with HD have a family history of HD. In an attempt to measure the relative risk for HD among first-degree relatives of HD patients, Razis and associates estimated a three-fold increase.[50] A population-based study also suggested a seven-fold increased risk among siblings.[29] An interesting finding from that study was an excess of sex-concordant pairs. In contrast with earlier reports, a recent prospective followup study showed no predilection for the same gender among sibling pairs.[51] This prospective followup study, with 48 families and 10-year median followup, demonstrated a six-fold increase, though not statistically significant, of HD and four-fold increase (95% CI:1.2–11.0) of NHL among their first-degree or second-degree relatives.

HD was the first disease in which susceptibility was reported to be associated with the human leukocyte antigen (HLA) region.[52] Several investigations have suggested weak and inconsistent associations between HD and HLA class I antigens.[53] Genes encoded for HLA are located on chromosome 6, in a region designated the major histocompatibility complex. The primary function of HLA molecules is to bind and present antigen fragments to T cells. The most convincing evidence of HLA involvement in the etiology of HD was generated in studies on affected sibling pairs.[54, 55] Using a restriction fragment length polymorphism analysis, Bodmer and colleagues showed an association of HD with the DPB1 locus.[56] A recent study examining HLA class II loci among 196 cases with HD suggested that a genetic propensity to develop nodular sclerosis HD is associated with the HLA DR-DQ subregion, with an odds ratio of 4.5 for the DRB1 locus.[57]

Among 41 multiplex families, Chakravarti and colleagues found that, under a recessive model of inheritance, the proportion of cases due to HLA linkage is 0.6 ± 0.08 (95% CI: 0.44–0.76), with maximum lod score of 3.67. On the other hand, under a dominant model, the proportion of HLA-linked cases is 0.68 ± 0.11 (95% CI: 0.45–0.90) with a maximum lod score of 2.59.[58] The study demonstrates not only that both models reject no linkage but also that etiologic heterogeneity exists, irrespective of genetic model. In this study, the recessive model appears much more likely than the dominant. Using a sib-pair analysis of 33 multiple-case families, Hors and Dausset found a highly significant distortion of segregation of HLA haplotypes in pairs of affected siblings ($P < 0.00025$).[54] The lod score analysis suggested maximum lod scores of 2.12 (at 8% recombination) and 2.18 (at 14% recombination) with a 60% and 10% penetrance, respectively, in dominant and recessive models.[54] In a study of 16 families, Berberich and colleagues demonstrated that there was a significant increase in the concordance rate of HLA haplotype among patients, as compared with what would be expected by chance alone ($P < 0.0015$).[59] Overall, it appears that a subset of families is genetically linked. However, the exact location of this susceptibility or association locus within the HLA region is not yet known.

The notion of genetic susceptibility of HD was further supported by a recent twin study. Mack and associates[60] followed 172 sets of monozygotic and 181 dizygotic twins, in whom one of them was diagnosed with HD, between 1980 and 1990. Prospectively, among monozygotic twins five incident cases developed in their twin siblings, but none occurred among dizygotic twins. This rendered a relative risk of 128 (95% CI:42–299). The phenomenon was not found in other cancers. If confirmed, the data strongly suggest a genetic basis of HD. However, the fact that only 5 (3%) of 172 siblings developed concordant HD also indicates a low penetrance rate of such a susceptibility gene.

Clusters

For years, cancer clustering has intrigued epidemiologists and clinicians because of the hope that causal explanations may be derived from such investigations. As classified by Alexander,[61] many different methods have been applied to examine clusters, including spatial-temporal cluster,[62–67] social linkage studies,[68–72] and spatial clustering.[65, 73–75] Together, "shared social experience in school" in some of the social linkage studies and residence at diagnosis in some of the spatial clustering studies have been suggested as weak exposures. No definitive links, however, between potential causes and HD were established among these clusters.

Other Factors

Tonsillectomy. Studies on the association between HD and tonsillectomy have produced inconsistent results. Recent studies have suggested that tonsillectomy does not increase the risk for HD.[47, 48, 76] The conflicting data may well be confounded by socioeconomic status.

Hormonal Effect. Because of the difference in age-specific incidence by gender, as mentioned earlier (see Fig. 3–6), it is intriguing to hypothesize that there is an element of reproductive and hormonal factors in the pathogenesis of HD in women.[77] However, opposing data exist.[77] Further study is needed to elucidate this issue.

NON-HODGKIN'S LYMPHOMA

NHLs are a heterogeneous group of lymphoproliferative malignancies that are much less predictable than HD and have a far greater predilection to disseminate to extranodal tissues.

INCIDENCE, MORTALITY RATES, AND TRENDS

International Data

In general, age-adjusted incidence rates of NHL are higher in the more developed countries. The geographic patterns for NHL are thus somewhat similar to those for HD, although the incidence rates are higher (Fig. 3–8). For example, the age-adjusted incidence rates for men varied from 3.7 to 14.0 per 100,000 person-years from 1983 to 1987 for NHL. In the same period, the rates for HD among men were from 0.4 to 3.7 per 100,000 person-years. In contrast

with HD, the age-adjusted incidence rates in 20 countries increased by about 50% or more within 2 decades.[8] This phenomenon was observed in both men and women. The rates by subtype also vary widely in differing geographic areas; for example, Burkitt's lymphoma, human T-cell lymphotropic virus, type I (HTLV-I)-related lymphoma/leukemia, and HIV-related lymphomas are much more frequent in endemic areas.

U.S. Data

The current U.S. age-adjusted rate for NHL is 15.1 per 100,000 person-years for both sexes combined (see Table 3–1). The incidence of NHL has been increasing much more rapidly than that of most other cancers.[10] The increase in incidence has been noted since the 1940s, but since the 1970s, the annual age-adjusted incidence rates have been increasing at 3% per year among women and 4% per year among men. Among the SEER areas, the incidence rates vary from 10.0 per 100,000 in New Mexico to 17.2 in San Francisco (see Table 3–2). Overall, the incidence of NHL has increased more than 73% between 1973 and 1991 (Fig. 3–9; see also Fig. 3–3). The increases in all age groups were significant, except among black men 65 years of age and older.[10] Changes in the rates of diagnosis, the percentage of tumors discovered at autopsy, or diagnostic criteria do not account for the large increase over time. Mortality rates for NHL have also increased significantly in each race/sex group (see Figs. 3–3 and 3–9). Recent data suggest that 5-year survival rates are higher among whites than blacks. Women have a better survival outcome than men as do patients younger than 65 years of age, compared with those aged 65 and older.[10] The rates of change in mortality are highest in areas where HIV is epidemic and in farming areas.

Trends by Site

Extranodal disease increased more rapidly than nodal disease over the past 2 decades. Brain and eye involvement increased 10% and 6% per year, respectively.[78] This is most likely due to AIDS, although central nervous system (CNS) lymphomas are also increasing in the non-AIDS population.[79] Better imaging techniques and improved surgical techniques that have allowed biopsies of lesions that previously were not possible to perform may have contributed to these increases.

Trends by Subtype

The increase in incidence of NHL has been partially attributed to a change in classification of lymphomas, which account for 10% to 15% of the shift of HD to NHL.[80] However, absolute increases have been noted in most of the subtypes of NHL (Fig. 3–10). Between 1978 and 1990, the incidence of high-grade lymphomas increased much more than that of low-grade lymphoma. The most dramatic increase was reported in diffuse large cell lymphoma by the Working Formulation (see Fig. 3–10).[81] Diffuse small cleaved was the only subtype that clearly decreased over time, which may be the result of changes in diagnostic criteria. Other entities, including T-cell lymphomas, such as angiocentric T-cell lymphoma, subcutaneous T-cell lymphoma, γδ T-cell lymphoma, angioimmunoblastic lymphadenopathy, and Ki-1 lymphoma; and B-cell lymphomas, such as mucosal-associated lymphoid tissue–derived lymphoma, monocytoid B-cell lymphoma, T-cell-rich B-cell lymphoma, and mantle zone lymphoma, represent less than 10% of all NHLs. There is no appreciable impact on the NHL trends by reclassification of these rare tumors due to newly developed techniques, because they comprise such a small percentage of NHL.[82, 83]

Age

Age greatly affects the risk of developing NHL. The incidence rate increases exponentially with age between 20 and 79 years (Fig. 3–11).[10] Incidence rates for NHL in men aged 20 to 54, especially unmarried men, are particularly high in recent years among HIV epidemic areas, such as in the San Francisco/Oakland area. At least part of the increase in NHL can be explained by the influence of HIV infection.

Race

The incidence of NHL varies by race, as noted in Figures 3–4 and 3–8. Whites have higher rates than do blacks or Asians. Data from the SEER registry demonstrated that rates in white men are 49% greater than in blacks, 54% greater than in Japanese Americans, and 27% greater than in Chinese Americans. The differences also apply to women, with a magnitude of 43%, 54%, and 39%, respectively.[82]

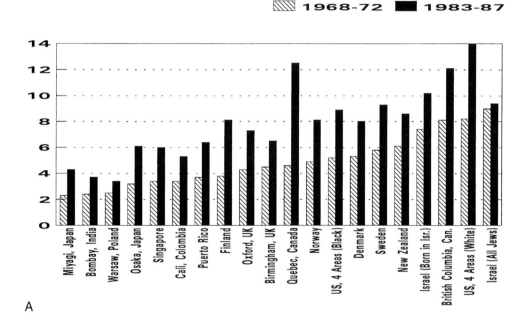

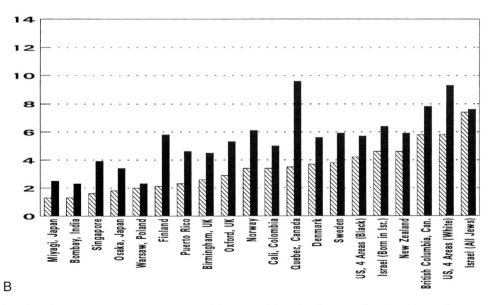

Figure 3–8. Age-adjusted incidence rates (per 100,000 person-years) for non-Hodgkin's lymphoma in selected populations from 1968–1972 (hatched bar) and 1983–1987 (solid bar): male *(A)* and female *(B)*. (Data from reference 8.)

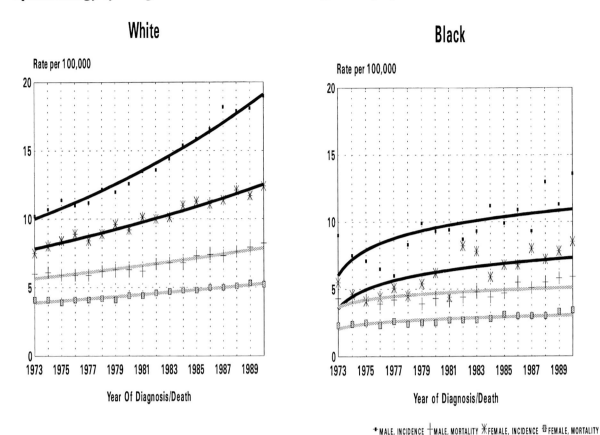

Figure 3–9. Age-adjusted U.S. incidence and mortality rates for non-Hodgkin's lymphoma by race. (Data from reference 10.)

Pediatric Non-Hodgkin's Lymphoma

The age-adjusted incidence rates for childhood NHL (age younger than 15 years), over the past 17 years (1973 to 1990) ranged from 0.6 to 1.1 per 100,000 person-years with a significant increase over time.[10] Incidence rates were slightly higher when age range was expanded to include those younger than 20 years of age. As with pediatric HD, childhood NHL mortality rates have declined substantially between 1973 and 1990, among both whites and blacks. Mortality rates for those younger than age 15 were reduced by one half, from 0.4 per 100,000 person-years to 0.2 with 4.8% estimated annual percentage change. The decrease in mortality is also likely the result of improved treatment.

RISK FACTORS ASSOCIATED WITH NON-HODGKIN'S LYMPHOMA

Infectious Agents

Epstein-Barr Virus. It is well recognized that EBV is associated with so-called classic or endemic Burkitt's lymphoma in the malaria-endemic areas, particularly those in Africa. It is essentially a pediatric disease, with a median age of diagnosis about 8 years. Most patients are in the 6- to 9-year-old range, with a predilection in boys (boy-to-girl ratio is 2:1 to 3:1). In endemic areas, the average annual incidence for children younger than 15 years of age is 4 per 100,000 per year. EBV genome has been identified in 100% of cases with chromosome 8 breakpoints generally within the

c-*myc* oncogene. In contrast, so-called sporadic Burkitt's lymphoma, constituting a high proportion of Burkitt's lymphoma in the United States, occurs less frequently, with 0.2 per 100,000 per year; is less likely to be involved with EBV (< 15%); and has different genomic alterations.[84] The age distribution is older than endemic Burkitt's lymphoma, with a median age at diagnosis of 10 years. Burkitt's lymphoma is also seen in patients in their sixth or seventh decade in nonendemic areas.

Overall, EBV DNA has been shown in 10% to 30% of NHL tumors.[85] Seroepidemiologic studies show that elevated titers against viral capsid antigen preceding the diagnosis of NHL were associated with a twofold or threefold increased risk of developing NHL. This suggested the hypothesis that endogenous immunosuppression, prior to the development of NHL, leads to EBV reactivation. EBV may have a direct role in the development of a subset of NHL, or it may be a surrogate marker for immune dysfunction.

Human Immunodeficiency Virus. Although AIDS was first reported in 1981, the significant increase in frequency of AIDS NHL was not recognized until 1985.[86] The definition of AIDS was changed to include the high-grade, B-cell lymphomas at the same time.[87] Several epidemiologic studies have tried to estimate the risk of AIDS NHL among HIV carriers. A study examining "unmarried males" in San Francisco as a risk group demonstrated a 412-fold increase in NHL.[88] Reviewing the

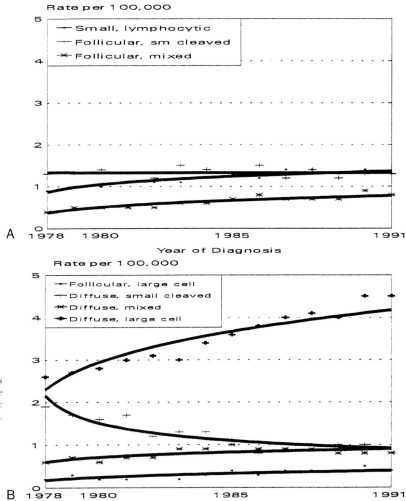

Figure 3–10. Trends of age-adjusted U.S. incidence rates by non-Hodgkin's lymphoma subtype (according to the Working Formulation) and year of diagnosis, 1978–1991: low grade (*A*); intermediate grade (*B*); and high grade (*C*). (Data from reference 10.)

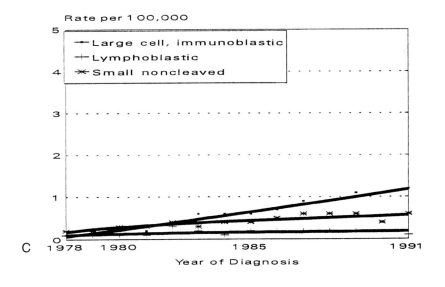

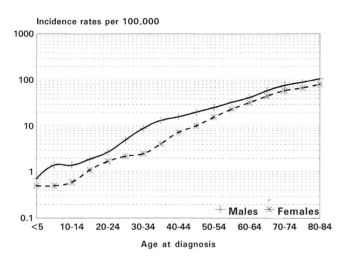

Figure 3–11. Age-specific U.S. incidence rates for non-Hodgkin's lymphoma by sex, 1986–1991. (Data from reference 10.)

incidence of NHL among prisoners in New York State facilities, Ahmed and associates showed an 18-fold increase in NHL in this population and a 40-fold increase in the prisoners with a drug abuse history.[89] A study by Beral and colleagues among almost 100,000 unselected AIDS patients during 1981 to 1989 found that 3% of them had NHL and that there was a 60-fold greater risk compared with the general population.[90] The role of EBV in the pathogenesis of HIV-associated lymphomas continues to be debated. In a case-control study, Levine and coworkers demonstrated by in situ hybridization that EBV genome was present in 68% of HIV-positive lymphoma patients, compared with 15% of HIV-negative patients.[84] EBV early-region RNA has been shown in 100% of primary CNS lymphoma tumors from patients with AIDS.[91] Again, it is not clear whether the EBV is a reactivated carrier virus or important in the etiology.

In 1985, the NCI began to follow a cohort of patients with AIDS or symptomatic HIV infection.[92] One hundred sixteen patients were treated with either zidovudine or dideoxyinosine and followed through 1991. Twelve patients developed NHL. Overall, patients in this cohort had an 8% risk of NHL 2 years after initiation of antiviral therapy and 19% risk at 3 years. The incidence rate of developing an NHL was 5.6% per patient-year, which is substantially higher than 0.015% (15 per 100,000 person-years) in the general population. The risk was not constant but rather increased over time. As indicated earlier, data from the San Francisco/Oakland area suggest that incidence rates in this area account for only a small impact of the overall recent rise in reported cases of NHL. However, as HIV infection increases, the incidence of lymphoma will continue to rise further throughout the world.[43, 45, 93, 94] It is estimated that more than one fourth of NHL cases occurring in the next decade may be secondary to HIV infection.[95] Although HIV does not appear to be causal in NHL, the immunosuppression related to HIV infection appears to be a major risk factor for NHL.

Human T-Cell Lymphotropic Virus Type I. HTLV-I was first isolated by Gallo and associates.[96] The virus was subsequently linked to adult T-cell leukemia/lymphoma

(ATL), which was described by Dr. Uchiyama and colleagues in the early 1970s.[97] HTLV-I is an RNA-containing C-type virus with low infectivity that now accounts for a small fraction of lymphomas in the United States but is a major fraction of lymphomas in endemic areas. Unlike HIV, HTLV-I, as indicated by epidemiologic studies, has a unique, restricted geographic distribution. The endemic area with highest prevalence of HTLV-I infection, suggested by seroepidemiologic studies, is in Japan. The endemic area is located in the southern islands of Kyushu, Shikoku, and Okinawa, with seroprevalence rates ranging from 10% to 20%. The rates of ATL are also increased in these islands. Other endemic areas include the Caribbean basin, Trinidad, Africa, and the southeastern region of United States. These reported "hot spots" are shown in Figure 3–12. In the southeastern United States, ATL cases have also been reported among blacks. Seroepidemiologic studies reveal that the age-specific infection rate increases in men and women, starting in adolescence. The rate, however, levels off in men about age 40 while it continues to rise in women.[98, 99] Studies from Japan suggest that infection with HTLV-I clusters in families. Vertical transmission through infected lymphocytes in breast milk and horizontal transmission through frequent sexual exposure over several years have been hypothesized. Transmission through blood donors has also been documented.[100] Cross-sectional[101, 102] and prospective[103] studies have suggested that the infectivity of HTLV-I has two periods: one is in the initial viremic stage and the other requires an extended latency.[104] Overall, HTLV-I carriers have a 2% to 5% lifetime risk of developing characteristic ATL in the endemic areas.[105] The epidemiology and clinical features of ATL have been extensively described.[106–109] Monoclonal integration of viral genome into tumor cells and the concordance of seroprevalence of HTLV and distribution of ATL strongly support the link between HTLV-I and ATL. Interruption of breastfeeding in endemic areas is being studied and suggested as a measure of prevention.[110]

Human Herpesvirus-6. Detection of HHV-6 in NHL tissues has been infrequent.[111, 112] Up to 18% of NHL tissues have been observed in a series from China[113] to harbor HHV-6 genome by in situ hybridization, but some of them were found in nontumor tissue. Taken together, the role of HHV-6 in NHL remains speculative.

Environmental Factors

Occupational Factors. A number of different occupations have been linked to NHL risk, including anesthesiology, carpentry, chemistry, construction, engineering, farming, fishing, forestry, leather work, mechanics, metal working, road transport working, rubber working, sales and clerical work, vinyl chloride working, and working in the food industry.[114–120] However, most of these associations are weak or inconsistent. A recent case-control study, examining 622 NHL cases from Iowa or Minnesota, concluded that no significant excesses were found among occupational groups, except "special industrial machinery (odds ratio [OR] = 9.6; 95% CI: 1.1–80.6), real estate (OR = 3.9; 95% CI: 1.01–14.8), and personal service (OR = 1.9; 95% CI: 1.1–3.2)."[121, 122] Exposure is a complicated issue, in that it is difficult to pinpoint the effects of particles or solvents in a given occupational exposure. Specific chemical exposures (discussed in the following section) are becoming the focus of interest. Other studies have suggested residential proximity to certain industries,[117] or paternal occupational exposures as risk factors for the cases' or their children's cancer, respectively. However, further studies are needed to confirm these data.

Pesticides. The increase in mortality in the United States for NHL and other hematologic cancers from 1950 to 1980 has been reported mainly in farming states.[123] Agricultural workers, who are in contact with a host of exposures, including pesticides, animal viruses, dusts, fuels, and oils, have been consistently noted to have increased risks for NHL and other hematologic malignancies.[124] Pesticides include herbicides (weed killers), insecticides, fungicides, and other agents.[125] The first epidemiologic study suggesting an association between cancer and herbicides was reported by Hardell.[126] In this hospital-based case-control study, the investigators found 105 cases who were exposed to phenoxy acids or chlorophenols. An OR of 6.0 (95% CI: 3.7–9.7) was observed. These results were confirmed in a subsequent study,[127] which analyzed 106 cases exposed to phenoxy acids. An OR of 4.9 (95% CI: 1.0–27.0) was reported. Most studies of farmers, agricultural workers, and other exposed populations showed an association between NHL and pesticide exposure; however, only some were significant. For example, 2,4-dichlorophenoxyacetic acid (2,4-D) has been associated with twofold to eightfold risks of NHL in several studies.[125, 128–131] Canine NHL has also been linked to dog owner use of 2,4-D and commercial lawn care pesticide treatments.[132] The National Academy of Science, in response to the U.S. Congress's request concerning potential

health effects of herbicides and the contaminant dioxin, conducted a comprehensive review and evaluation in period of 1992 to 1993. A report, which summarized all the studies, was issued in 1993 from the Institute of Medicine and concluded that "evidence is sufficient that there is a positive association between exposure to herbicides (2,4-D; 2,4,5-T and its contaminant TCDD; cacodylic acid; picloram) and NHL."[133] It is generally believed that veterans exposed to herbicides in Vietnam do not have a higher risk of NHL.[134] Pesticide exposures are not limited to farmers. In the United States, the use of lawn care pesticides is increasing 5% to 8% each year.[125] Thus, pesticide exposure may be important in identifying a subset of the population at risk of NHL.

In an attempt to identify populations at risk, Kirsch and others designed a novel polymerase chain reaction-based assay.[135, 136] Among patients with ataxia-telangiectasia, who have higher risk of lymphoid malignancy, their V(D)J (variable-[diversity]-joining) recombination between different antigen receptor genes is 100-fold higher than baseline. Among 12 agriculture workers, the group with the higher pesticide exposures had a 10-fold to 20-fold increase over baseline in interlocus V(D)J recombination. This phenomenon can be reversed when pesticide exposures are avoided among these workers. If confirmed, this assay could be used as a marker to detect genomic instability among high-risk populations.[135, 136]

Hair Dyes. After Ames and colleagues reported in 1975[137] that hair dyes and some of their constituents were mutagenic in the in vitro assay, the issue of hair dyes as carcinogens has been the subject of many occupational and epidemiologic studies, since hair dyes are used by an estimated 20% to 60% of the U.S. population. Most of the occupational studies linking hair dyes and NHL have

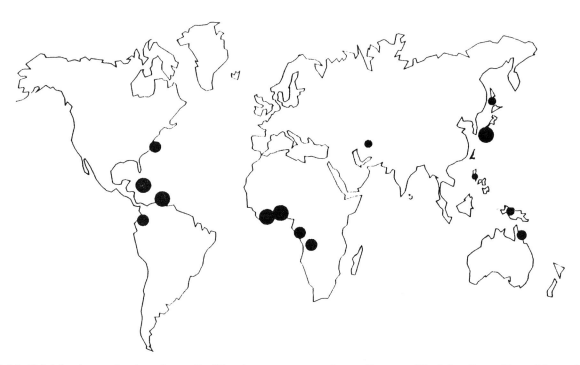

Figure 3–12. Global distribution of endemic human T-cell lymphotropic virus, type I areas. (Courtesy of Dr. Robert Bigger, National Cancer Institute.)

reported negative results (Table 3–5). Cantor and coworkers, in a population-based, case-control study, found that hair dye users had a two-fold (95% CI: 1.3–3.0) increased risk of NHL.[138] This study, however, only involved adult men. Women hair dye users in another case-control study were estimated to have a relative risk of 1.5 (95% CI: 1.1–2.2).[139] In addition, women who used permanent dyes or darker-colored products appeared to have a greater risk. Among men, the risk was not significantly increased. Two other recent cohort studies[140, 141] (see Table 3–5) showed no increased risk among permanent hair dye users. A subset analysis in one study[140] found that women black hair dye users had a significantly increased risk of fatal NHL, although the number of cases was small. Taken together, it is plausible that a subset of hair dye users, particularly those who use permanent dark-colored dyes over a prolonged period (such as >20 years), might have an increased risk for NHL. This association, however, needs to be confirmed. Nevertheless, this variable does not explain the recent rising incidence of NHL.

Radiation. Ionizing radiation appears to have little or no role in the risk of NHL.[142] The association between electromagnetic-fields exposure and NHL in children is weak and inconsistent.[124, 142, 143] The role of ultraviolet exposure in the causation of NHL is highly speculative but interesting. A number of studies are underway to investigate this hypothesis.

Primary and Secondary/Iatrogenic Immunodeficiency

Primary Immunodeficiency. Studies of genetic immunodeficiency syndromes, such as ataxia-telangiectasia, common variable immunodeficiency, Wiskott-Aldrich syndrome, and X-linked lymphoproliferative syndrome, have documented a clear association between immune dysfunction and NHL. It is estimated that as many as 25% of patients with certain genetically determined immunodeficiencies will develop cancers, and NHL accounts for more than 50% of such malignancies.[144] Among survivors of HD the risk of NHL is approximately 20-fold increased,[145] and the cumulative risk continues to increase until at least 20 years after the treatment of HD.[146] The risk of NHL does not appear

Table 3–5. Epidemiologic Studies of Hair Dyes as Occupational Exposure or Personal Use and Non-Hodgkin's Lymphoma

Author, Year	Study Design	Relative Risk (95% CI or *P*)
Occupational Exposure		
Teta, 1984[183]	Cohort; 11,845 female cosmetologists; Connecticut, 1925–1974	1.29 (*P* > 0.05)
Lynge, 1988[184]	Cohort; 9497 female and 4874 male hairdressers and barbers; Denmark, 1970–1980	Male: 1.30 (*P* > 0.05) Female: 2.01 (*P* > 0.05)
Persson, 1989[127]	Case-control; 106 NHL cases; Sweden, 1964–1986	2.2 (*P* > 0.05)
Shibata, 1989[185]	Cohort; 3701 female and 4615 male barbers; Aichi Prefecture, Japan, 1976–1987	Male: 0.44 (*P* > 0.05); Female: 1.37 (*P* > 0.05)
Blair, 1993[122]	Case-control; 622 male NHL cases; Iowa and Minnesota, 1980–1983	2.1°–2.7† (*P* > 0.05)
Boffetta, 1994[186]	Case-control; cancer registry, Denmark, Sweden, Norway, Finland, 1970–1987	1.2 (0.8–1.7); Denmark: 1.92; Sweden: 0.63
Personal Use		
Hennekens, 1979[187]	Cohort; 120,557 female nurses, 11 U.S. states, 1972–1976	0.59 (*P* > 0.05)
Cantor, 1988[138]	Population-based, case-control; 633 male NHL cases; Iowa and Minnesota, 1980–1983	2.0 (1.3–3.0)
Zahm, 1992[139]	Population-based, case-control; 201 male and 184 female NHL cases; 725 male and 707 female population controls; Nebraska, 1983–1986	Females: 1.5 (1.1–2.2), 1.7 (1.1–2.8)‡; Male: 0.8 (0.4–1.6)
Thun, 1994[140]	Cohort; 573,369 females; American Cancer Society study, 1982–1989	0.93§ (0.89–0.98), 4.37¶ (1.3–15.2)
Grodstein, 1994[141]	Cohort; 99,067 females; Nurses' Health Study; 1976–1990	1.1 (0.8–1.6)

°Barbers.
†Barbers/cosmetologists.
‡Use of permanent hair coloring products.
§Ever used.
¶Use of black hair dye >20 years.
CI, confidence interval; N/A, not available; NHL, non-Hodgkin's lymphoma.

Table 3–6. Selected Epidemiologic Studies on Medical Conditions as Risk Factors for NHL

Study, Year	Medical Condition	Observed Number of Lymphoma Cases	Expected Number of Lymphoma Cases	Ratio of Observed/ Expected Cases	95% CI	Comments
Kassan, 1978[167]	Sjögren's disease					Pooled data
	Without IST	5	0.14	36.0	11.5–83.3	
	With IST	2	0.02	100.0	12.0–361.2	
Kinlen, 1992[151]	Rheumatoid arthritis					Pooled data
	Without IST	56	22.67	2.5	1.9–3.2	
	With IST	21	2.1	10	6.2–15.3	
Gridley, 1994[153]	Felty's syndrome	19	1.5	12.8	7.7–20.0	

IST, immunosuppression therapy, such as azathioprine or cyclophosphamide; CI, confidence interval.

to be associated with a specific type of treatment but may be related to the underlying immune defects of HD.

Secondary/Iatrogenic Immunodeficiency. Similar to genetic immunodeficiency, immunosuppressive therapy in organ transplant recipients has also been reported to substantially increase the risk for NHL.[147–150] This risk can be as high as 46-fold, as compared with the general population.[151] It appears that the risk was higher among early transplant patients who received a transplant with poorer matches and more immunosuppressive medications. The rates among recent recipients seem to be decreasing with better tissue matching and use of less immunosuppressive drugs.[152] One hypothesis is that the development of lymphoma may be related to the chronic antigen stimulation of the graft combined with immunosuppression.[153] This conclusion is based on the observation that even among patients who received immunosuppressive agents without grafts, there was an 11-fold increase for NHL. Immunodeficiency-related lymphomas are usually large cell lymphomas with an aggressive nature and a relative overrepresentation of distribution in the CNS.

Familial Aggregation

Familial lymphoma is relatively rare. In an extensive literature review, Greene identified 38 multiple-case families with NHL.[114] Among the family members, there was a total of 111 cases of NHL, with an average of 3 cases per family. Almost 80% were sib pairs with either sibs alone (63%), including one pair of monozygotic twins, or sibs plus other relatives (13%). Among the familial cases, the male/female ratio was 1.8 versus 1.4 in the general population. The average age at diagnosis was 23.5 years versus 42.3 in the general population. Of interest, two subtypes of high-risk families were noted. One group consisted of primarily male preadolescent sibships with extranodal NHL, with gastrointestinal tract predominance. Another group of families consisted of primarily nodal NHL predominantly in adult women. These data are not free of selection bias, since the cases were collected from case reports, not from population-based surveys.

Socioeconomic Status

Between the 1950s and 1970s, data on mortality rates from NHL suggested a gradual decline of differences by urbanization, education, and income.[66, 154] Other population-based data have not consistently illustrated this association. Recent data suggest that socioeconomic status does not play a major role in the development of NHL.[78]

Other Factors

Medication. Medication-induced lymphadenopathy was noted in the 1960s. Phenytoin (Dilantin) was reported to be associated with "pseudolymphoma," which histologically resembles, but fails to be diagnostic of, lymphoma. Subsequent reports[155, 156] suggested a small increased risk of NHL associated with phenytoin usage. This finding, however, was not confirmed in a population-based study.[157] Since then, many studies have linked medication usage, such as commonly taken steroidal drugs,[158, 159] and some more common conditions, such as asthma, allergies, arthritis, rheumatic fever, tuberculosis, and infectious mononucleosis,[159, 160] with NHL, although only weak associations was reported in most of the studies. Some cancer chemotherapeutic agents moderately increase the risk of NHL.[114]

Autoimmune Disorders. A host of autoimmune disorders has been linked to NHL, with variable significance (Table 3–6). Patients with rheumatoid arthritis have a twofold or threefold increase in risk.[150, 151, 161–166] However, in the subset of patients with Felty's syndrome, the risk increased from twofold or threefold to 13-fold.[153] One caveat is that it is difficult to separate the effects of immunosuppressive drugs and chronic immune system stimulation associated with the underlying autoimmune disease. A synergistic effect between these two factors was demonstrated by Kinlen.[151] It is generally accepted that among patients with rheumatoid arthritis, the risk of developing NHL is 2.5-fold, compared with the control group. This risk increases to 10-fold among patients with rheumatoid arthritis and immunosuppressive therapy. A similar observation was also made among patients with Sjögren's disease[167]; that is, immunosuppressive therapy is associated with a 100-fold increase of NHL risk as compared with a 35-fold increase among patients with the same diagnosis but no immunosuppressive therapy (see Table 3–6). Eczema and other skin conditions have been recent topics of interest as risk factors for NHL in several reports.[159, 166, 168, 169] However, no consistent results have been found among these studies. Chronic fatigue syndrome does not increase NHL risk, based on relatively limited data.[170]

Dietary Factors. There is little epidemiologic evidence to support an etiologic link between dietary factors and NHL. Although dairy product, coffee, cola, and liver consumption have been reported as risk factors,[171–173] the evidence is only suggestive. It is generally accepted that smoking and alcohol do not have a major role in NHL.[124, 174, 175]

CONCLUSIONS

HODGKIN'S DISEASE

The incidence rates of HD, depending on geographic area, vary from 0.5 to 3.4 per 100,000 person-years. Recently, the incidence rates have been stable or have slightly declined in most cancer registries worldwide. Clearly, improvement in the treatment of HD has prolonged survival and decreased mortality. Despite years of effort, the etiology of HD remains an enigma. EBV may have a role in the pathogenesis of a subset of HD and is the subject of intense research. Future efforts will be directed to studies of other possible causal agents, such as new viruses, or genes, such as susceptibility genes.

NON-HODGKIN'S LYMPHOMA

The incidence and mortality rates of NHL have been increasing steadily during the past few decades in several countries. In the United States, the incidence rate has increased more than 50% in the last 16 years with a 3%-to 4%-per-year increment.[10] Despite improvements in treatment, NHL mortality rates in the United States are increasing at 2% per year.[10] Epidemiologic studies have provided several clues regarding etiologic factors. Pesticides and hair dyes may explain part of the observed increase in NHL, but more research is required to confirm their contributions. Clearly, HIV infection increases the risk of NHL. However, HIV-related lymphoma has been responsible for only a small portion of the recent increase. Diagnostic improvements and changes in HD and NHL classification[176] have been noted to have some impact on changing trends. Little of the increase in NHL over the last 40 years can be explained by known risk factors. Multidisciplinary approaches should be used to identify new viruses, genetic-environmental interactions, and exposures that alter susceptibility. In particular, studies on molecular epidemiology, such as genomic instability,[136] may shed some light in identifying new molecular markers leading to cancer prevention.

REFERENCES

1. Billroth T: Multiple lymphoma: Erfogreiche Behandlung mit Arsenik. Wien Med Wochenschr 1871; 21:1066.
2. Travis LB, Curtis RE, Hankey BF, Fraumeni JJ: Second cancers in patients with chronic lymphocytic leukemia. J Natl Cancer Inst 1992; 84:1422.
3. Travis LB, Gonzalez CL, Hankey BF, Jaffe ES: Hodgkin's disease following non-Hodgkin's lymphoma. Cancer 1992;69:2337.
4. Strom HH, Prener A: Second cancer following lymphatic and hematopoietic cancers in Denmark, 1943–80. Natl Cancer Inst Monogr 1985; 68:389.
5. Greene MH, Wilson J: Second cancer following lymphatic and hematopoietic cancers in Connecticut, 1935–82. Natl Cancer Inst Monogr 1985; 68:191.
6. Bureau of Census: Manual of the International List of Causes of Death, Fourth Edition, 1939. Washington, DC, US Government Printing Office, 1940.
7. Grufferman G: Hodgkin's disease. In Schottenfeld D, Fraumeni JJ (eds): Cancer Epidemiology and Prevention. Philadelphia, WB Saunders, 1982, pp 739–753.
8. Hartge P, Devesa SS, Fraumeni JFJ: Hodgkin's and non-Hodgkin's lymphomas. In Doll R, Fraumeni J, Muir C (eds): Trends in Cancer Incidence and Mortality Cancer Surveys. Cold Spring, Cold Spring Harbor Laboratory Press, 1994, pp 423–453.
9. Parkin DM, Muir CS, Whelan SL, et al (eds): Cancer Incidence in Five Continents, vol 6. IARC Scientific Publication No. 120. Lyon, IARC, 1992.
10. Ries LAG, Miller BA, Hankey BF, et al (eds): SEER Cancer Statistics Review, 1973–1991: Tables and Graphs, National Cancer Institute. NIH Publication No. 94-2789. Bethesda, MD, US Department of Health and Human Services, 1994.
11. Glaser SL, Swartz WG: Time trends in Hodgkin's disease incidence: The role of diagnostic accuracy. Cancer 1990; 66:2196.
12. MacMahon B: Epidemiological evidence on the nature of Hodgkin's disease. Cancer 1957;10:1045.
13. Abramson JH, Pridan H, Sacks MI, et al: A case-control study of Hodgkin's disease in Israel. J Natl Cancer Inst 1978; 61:307.
14. Correa P, O'Conor GT: Epidemiologic patterns of Hodgkin's disease. Int J Cancer 1971; 8:192.
15. Cutler SJ, Young JL: Third National Cancer Survey: Incidence data. National Cancer Institute. NIH Publication No. 75-787. Bethesda, MD, US Department of Health and Human Services, 1975.
16. Kravdal O, Hansen S: Hodgkin's disease: The protective effect of childbearing. Int J Cancer 1993; 55:909.
17. Medeiros LJ, Greiner TC: Hodgkin's disease. Cancer 1995; 75:357.
18. Levine PH, Pallesen G, Ebbesen P, et al: Evaluation of Epstein-Barr virus antibody patterns and detection of viral markers in the biopsies of patients with Hodgkin's disease. Int J Cancer 1994; 59:48.
19. Gutensohn N, Cole P: Childhood social environment and Hodgkin's disease. N Engl J Med 1981; 304:135.
20. Miller RB, Beebe GW: Infectious mononucleosis and the empirical risk of cancer. J Natl Cancer Inst 1973; 50:315.
21. Levine PH, Ablashi DV, Berard CW, et al: Elevated antibody titers to Epstein-Barr virus in Hodgkin's disease. Cancer 1971; 27:416.
22. Evans AS, Comstock GW: Presence of elevated antibody titers to Epstein-Barr virus. Lancet 1981; 1:1183.
23. Mueller N, Evans A, Harris NL, et al: Hodgkin's disease and Epstein-Barr virus: Altered antibody pattern before diagnosis. N Engl J Med 1989; 320:689.
24. Weiss LM, Chang KL: Molecular biologic studies of Hodgkin's disease. Semin Diagn Pathol 1992; 9:272.
25. Jarrett RF, Gallagher A, Jones DB, et al: Detection of Epstein-Barr virus genomes in Hodgkin's disease: Relation to age. J Clin Pathol 1991; 44:844.
26. Ambinder RF, Browning PJ, Lorenzana I, et al: Epstein-Barr virus and childhood Hodgkin's disease in Honduras and the United States. Blood 1993; 81:462.
27. Jarrett RF: Viruses and Hodgkin's disease. Leukemia 1993; 7:S78.
28. O'Grady J, Stewart S, Elton RA, Krajewski AS: Epstein-Barr virus in Hodgkin's disease and site of origin tumour. Lancet 1994; 343:265.
29. Grufferman S, Cole P, Smith PG, Lukes R: Hodgkin's disease in siblings. N Engl J Med 1977; 296:248.
30. Lin A, Kingma D, Lennette E, et al: Epstein-Barr virus is not associated with familial Hodgkin's disease. Proc Annu Meet Am Soc Clin Oncol 1994; 13:5.
31. Salahuddin SZ, Ablashi DV, Markham PD, et al: Isolation of a new virus, HBLV, in patients with lymphoproliferative disorders. Science 1986; 234:596.
32. Yamanishi K, Okuno T, Shiraki K, et al: Identification of human herpesvirus-6 as a causal agent for exanthem subitum. Lancet 1988; 1:1065.
33. Clark DA, Alexander FE, McKinney PA, et al: The seroepidemiology of human herpesvirus-6 (HHV-6) from a case-control study of leukemia and lymphoma. Int J Cancer 1990; 45:829.
34. Torelli G, Marasca R, Luppi M, et al: Human herpesvirus-6 in human lymphomas: Identification of specific sequences in Hodgkin's lymphomas by polymerase chain reaction. Blood 1991; 77:2251.

35. Gompels UA, Carrigan DR, Carss AL, et al: Two groups of human herpesvirus 6 identified by sequence analyses of laboratory strains and variants from Hodgkin's lymphoma and bone marrow transplant patients. J Gen Virol 1993; 74:613.

36. Levine PH, Ebbesen P, Ablashi DV, et al: Antibodies to human herpesvirus type 6 and clinical course. Int J Cancer 1992; 51:53.

37. Ioachim HL, Cooper MC, Hellman GC: Hodgkin's disease and the acquired immunodeficiency syndrome. Ann Intern Med 1984; 101:876.

38. Robert NJ, Schneiderman H: Hodgkin's disease and the acquired immunodeficiency syndrome. Ann Intern Med 1984; 101:142.

39. Andrieu JM, Roithmann S, Tourani JM, et al: Hodgkin's disease during HIV1 infection: The French registry experience—French Registry of HIV-associated Tumors. Ann Oncol 1993; 4:635.

40. Tirelli U, Vacher E, Rezza G, et al: Hodgkin's disease and infection with the human immunodeficiency virus in Italy. Ann Intern Med 1988; 108:309.

41. Roithmann S, Tourani JM, Andrieu JM: Hodgkin's disease in HIV-infected intravenous drug abusers. N Engl J Med 1990; 323:275.

42. Garnier G, Michiels JF: HIV-associated Hodgkin's disease. Ann Intern Med 1991; 115:233.

43. Rabkin CS, Biggar RJ, Horm JW: Increasing incidence of cancers associated with human immunodeficiency virus epidemic. Int J Cancer 1991; 47:692.

44. Hessol NA, Katz MH, Liu JY, et al: Increased incidence of Hodgkin's disease in homosexual men with HIV infection. Ann Intern Med 1992; 117:309.

45. Rabkin CS, Hilgartner MW, Hedberg KW, et al: Incidence of lymphomas and other cancer in HIV-infected and HIV-uninfected patients with hemophilia. JAMA 1992; 267:1090.

46. Greene MH, Brinton LA, Fraumeni JJ, D'Amico R: Familial and sporadic Hodgkin's disease associated with occupational wood exposure. Lancet 1978; 2:626.

47. Grufferman S, Delzell E: Epidemiology of Hodgkin's disease. Epidemiol Rev 1984; 6:76.

48. Gutensohn N, Cole P: Epidemiology of Hodgkin's disease. Semin Oncol 1980; 7:92.

49. Serraino D, Franceschi S, Talamini R, et al: Socio-economic indicators, infectious diseases, and Hodgkin's disease. Int J Cancer 1991; 47:352.

50. Razis DV, Diamond HD, Carver LF: Familial Hodgkin's disease: Its significance and implications. Ann Intern Med 1959; 51:933.

51. Lin A, Whitehouse J, Shaw G, Tucker M: Familial aggregation of Hodgkin's disease in a cohort of 48 families [Meeting abstract]. Proc Annu Meet Am Soc Clin Oncol 1993; 12:184.

52. Amiel JL: Study of the leukocyte phenotype in Hodgkin's disease. *In* Curtoni ES, Matting PL, Tosi MR (eds): Histocompatibility Testing. Copenhagen, Denmark, Ejnar Munksgaard, 1967, pp 79–81.

53. Greene MH, McKeen EA, Li FP, et al: HLA antigens in familial Hodgkin's disease. Int J Cancer 1979; 23:777.

54. Hors J, Dausset J: HLA and susceptibility to Hodgkin's disease. Immunol Rev 1983; 70:167.

55. Kalidi I, Masset M, Gony J, et al: MHC-related genetic susceptibility to Hodgkin's disease. Nouv Rev Fr Hematol 1989; 31:149.

56. Bodmer JG, Tonks S, Oza AM, et al: HLA-DP–based resistance to Hodgkin's disease [Letter]. Lancet 1989; 1:1455.

57. Klitz W, Aldrich CL, Fildes N, et al: Localization of predisposition to Hodgkin's disease in the HLA class II region. Am J Hum Genet 1994; 54:497.

58. Chakravarti A, Halloran S, Bale SJ, Tucker MA: Etiological heterogeneity in Hodgkin's disease: HLA linked and unlinked determinants of susceptibility independent of histological concordance. Genet Epidemiol 1986; 3:407.

59. Berberich FR, Berberich MS, King MC, et al: Hodgkin's disease susceptibility: Linkage to the HLA locus demonstrated by a new concordance method. Hum Immunol 1983; 6:207.

60. Mack T, Cozen W, Shibata DK, et al: Concordance for Hodgkin's disease in identical twins suggesting genetic susceptibility to the young-adult form of the disease. N Engl J Med 1995; 332:413.

61. Alexander FE: Clustering and Hodgkin's disease [Editorial]. Br J Cancer 1990; 62:708.

62. Fraumeni JF, Li FP: Hodgkin's disease in childhood: An epidemiologic study. J Natl Cancer Inst 1969; 42:681.

63. Alderson MR, Mayak R: A study of space-time clustering of Hodgkin's disease in the Manchester region. Br J Prev Soc Med 1971; 25:253.

64. Kryscio RJ, Myers MH, Prusiner ST, et al: The space-time distribution of Hodgkin's disease in Connecticut. J Natl Cancer Inst 1973; 50:1107.

65. Abramson JH, Goldblum N, Avitzur M, et al: Clustering of Hodgkin's disease in Israel: A case-control study. Int J Epidemiol 1980; 9:137.

66. Greenberg MR: Urbanization and Cancer Mortality—The United States experience, 1950–1975. New York, Oxford University Press, 1983.

67. Mangoud A, Hillier VF, Leck I, Thomas RW: Space-time interaction in Hodgkin's disease in greater Manchester. J Epidemiol Community Health 1985; 39:58.

68. Vianna NJ, Polan AK: Epidemiologic evidence for transmission of Hodgkin's disease. N Engl J Med 1973;289:499.

69. Pike MC, Smith PG: Clustering of cases of Hodgkin's disease and leukemia. Cancer 1974; 34:1390.

70. Paffenberger RS, Wing AL, Hyde RT: Characteristics in youth indicative of adult-onset Hodgkin's disease. J Natl Cancer Inst 1977; 58:1489.

71. Zack MM Jr, Heath CW Jr, Andrews MD, et al: High school contact among persons with leukemia and lymphoma. J Natl Cancer Inst 1977; 59:1343.

72. Grufferman S, Cole P, Levitan T: Evidence against transmission of Hodgkin's disease in high schools. N Engl J Med 1979; 300:1006.

73. Alexander FE, Williams J, McKinney PA, et al: A specialist leukaemia/lymphoma registry in the UK: II. Clustering of Hodgkin's disease. Br J Cancer 1989; 60:948.

74. McKinney PA, Alexander FE, Ricketts TJ, et al: A specialist leukaemia/lymphoma registry in the UK: I. Incidence and geographical distribution of Hodgkin's disease: Leukaemia Research Fund Data Collection Study Group. Br J Cancer 1989; 60:942.

75. Glaser SL: Spatial clustering of Hodgkin's disease in the San Francisco Bay area. Am J Epidemiol 1990; 132:S167.

76. Gledovic Z, Radovanovic Z: History of tonsillectomy and appendectomy in Hodgkin's disease. Eur J Epidemiol 1991; 7:612.

77. Glaser SL: Reproductive factors in Hodgkin's disease in women: A review. Am J Epidemiol 1994; 139:237.

78. Devesa SS, Fears T: Non-Hodgkin's lymphoma time trends: United States and international data. Cancer Res 1992; 52:5432s.

79. Eby NL, Grufferman S, Flannelly CM, et al: Increasing incidence of primary brain lymphoma in the U.S. Cancer 1988; 62:2461.

80. Banks PM: Changes in diagnosis of non-Hodgkin's lymphomas over time. Cancer Res 1992; 52:5453s.

81. Non-Hodgkin's Lymphoma Pathology Classification Project: National Cancer Institute sponsored study of classification of non-Hodgkin's lymphomas. Cancer 1982; 49:2112.

82. Rabkin CS, Devesa SS, Zahm SH, Gail MH: Increasing incidence of non-Hodgkin's lymphoma. Semin Hematol 1993; 30:286.

83. Greiner TC, Medeiros LJ, Jaffe ES: Non-Hodgkin's lymphoma. Cancer 1995; 75:370.

84. Levine AM, Shibata D, Sullivan HJ, et al: Epidemiological and biological study of acquired immunodeficiency syndrome–related lymphoma in the County of Los Angeles: Preliminary results. Cancer Res 1992; 52:5482s.

85. Ott G, Ott MM, Feller AC, Seidl S, Muller-Hermelink HK: Prevalence of Epstein-Barr virus DNA in different T-cell entities in a European population. Int J Cancer 1992; 51:562.

86. Ross RK, Dworsky RL, Paganini HA, et al: Non-Hodgkin's lymphomas in never married men in Los Angeles. Br J Cancer 1985; 52:785.

87. CDC: Revision of the case definition of acquired immunodeficiency. MMWR Morb Mortal Wkly Rep 1985; 34:373.

88. Biggar RJ, Horm J, Goedert JJ, Melbye M: Cancer in a group at risk of acquired immunodeficiency syndrome (AIDS) through 1984. Am J Epidemiol 1987; 126:578.

89. Ahmed T, Wormser GP, Stahl RE, et al: Malignant lymphomas in a population at risk for acquired immune deficiency syndrome. Cancer 1987; 60:719.

90. Beral V, Peterman T, Berkelman R, Jaffe H: AIDS-associated non-Hodgkin's lymphoma. Lancet 1991; 337:805.

91. MacMahon EMF, Glass JD, Hayward SD, et al: Epstein-Barr virus in AIDS-related primary central nervous system lymphoma. Lancet 1991; 338:969.

92. Pluda JM, Venzon DJ, Tosato G, et al: Parameters affecting the development of non-Hodgkin's lymphoma in patients with severe human immunodeficiency virus infection receiving antiretroviral therapy. J Clin Oncol 1993; 11:1099.

93. Obrams GI, Grufferman S: Epidemiology of HIV-associated non-Hodgkin lymphoma. Cancer Surv 1991; 10:91.

94. Serraino D, Salamina G, Franceschi S, et al: The epidemiology of AIDS-associated non-Hodgkin's lymphoma in the World Health Organization European Region. Br J Cancer 1992; 66:912.

95. Gail MH, Pluda JM, Rabkin CS, et al: Projections of the incidence of non-Hodgkin's lymphoma related to acquired immunodeficiency syndrome. J Natl Cancer Inst 1991; 83:695.

96. Poiesz BJ, Ruscetti FW, Gazdar AF, et al: Detection and isolation of type-C retrovirus particles from fresh and cultured lymphocytes of a patient with cutaneous T-cell lymphoma. Proc Natl Acad Sci USA 1980; 77:7415.

97. Uchiyama T, Sagawa K, Takatsuki K, et al: Adult T-cell leukemia: Clinical and hematologic features of 16 cases. Blood 1977; 50:481.

98. Kajiyama W, Kashiwagi S, Nomura H, et al: Seroepidemiologic study of antibody to adult T-cell leukemia virus in Okinawa, Japan. Am J Epidemiol 1986; 123:41.

99. Murphy EL, Figueroa JP, Gibbs WN, et al: Human T-lymphotropic virus type I (HTLV-I) seroprevalence in Jamaica: I. Demographic determinants. Am J Epidemiol 1991; 133:1114.

100. Okochi K, Sato H, Hinuma Y: A retrospective study on transmission of adult T cell leukemia virus by blood transfusion: Seroconversion in recipients. Vox Sang 1984; 46:245.

101. Tajima K, Kamura S, Ito S, et al: Epidemiological features of HTLV-I carriers and incidence of ATL in an ATL-endemic island: A report of the community-based co-operative study in Tsushima, Japan. Int J Cancer 1987; 40:741.

102. Kajiyama W, Kashiwaga S, Ikematsu H, et al: Intrafamilial transmission of adult T-cell leukemia virus. J Infect Dis 1986; 154:851.

103. Mueller N, Tachibana N, Stuver SO, et al: Epidemiologic perspectives of HTVL-1. *In* Blattner, WA (ed): Human Retrovirology: HTLV. New York, Raven, 1990, pp 281–293.

104. Okayama A, Ishizaki J, Tachibana N, et al: The particle agglutination (PA) assay and its use in detection of lower-titer HTLV-1 antibodies. *In* Blattner WA (ed): Human Retrovirology: HTLV-1. New York: Raven, 1990, pp 401–407.

105. Murphy EL, Hanchard B, Figueroa JP, et al: Modelling the risk of adult T-cell leukemia/lymphoma type I. Int J Cancer 1989; 43:250.

106. The T- and B-cell Malignancy Study Group: Statistical analysis of immunologic, clinical, and histopathologic data on lymphoid malignancies in Japan. Jpn J Clin Oncol 1981; 11:15.

107. The T- and B-cell Malignancy Study Group: Statistical analyses of clinico-pathological, virological, and epidemiological data on lymphoid malignancies with special reference to adult T-cell leukemia/lymphoma: A report of the second nationwide study of Japan. Jpn J Clin Oncol 1985; 15:517.

108. The T- and B-cell Malignancy Study Group: The third nationwide study on adult T-cell leukemia/lymphoma (ATL) in Japan: Characteristic patterns of HLA antigen and HTLV-I infection in ATL patients and their relatives. Int J Cancer 1988; 41:505.

109. Tajima K, The T- and B-cell Malignancy Study Group, et al: The Fourth Nation-wide Study of Adult T-cell Leukemia/Lymphoma (ATL) in Japan: Estimates of risk of ATL and its geographical and clinical features. Int J Cancer 1990; 45:237.

110. Mueller N: The epidemiology of HTLV-1 infection. Cancer Causes Controls 1991; 2:37.

111. Jarrett RF, Gledhill S, Qureshi F, et al: Identification of human herpesvirus 6-specific sequences in two patients with non-Hodgkin's lymphoma. Leukemia 1988; 2:496.

112. Josephs SF, Buchbinder A, Streicher HZ, et al: Detection of human B-lymphotropic virus (human herpesvirus 6) sequences in B-cell lymphoma tissues of three patients. Leukemia 1988; 2:132.

113. Yin SY, Ming HA, Jahan N, et al: In situ hybridization detection of human herpesvirus 6 in biopsy specimens from Chinese patients with non-Hodgkin's lymphoma. Arch Pathol Lab Med 1993; 117:502.

114. Greene MH: Non-Hodgkin's lymphoma and mycosis fungoides. *In* Schottenfeld D, Fraumeni JF Jr (eds): Cancer Epidemiology and Prevention. Philadelphia, WB Saunders, 1982, pp 754–778.

115. Cantor KP: Farming and mortality from non-Hodgkin's lymphoma: A case-control study. Int J Cancer 1982; 29:239.

116. Armenian HK, Hamadeh RR: Epidemiology of non-Hodgkin's lymphomas. *In* Lilienfeld AM (ed): Reviews in Cancer Epidemiology. New York, Elsevier/North-Holland Biomedical, 1983, pp 141–169.

117. Linos A, Blair A, Gibson RW, et al: Leukemia and non-Hodgkin's lymphoma and residential proximity to industrial plants [published erratum appears in Arch Environ Health 1991 Sep-Oct; 46(5):305]. Arch Environ Health 1991; 46:70.

118. Pasqualetti P, Casale R, Colantonio D, Collacciani A: Occupational risk for hematological malignancies. Am J Hematol 1991; 38:147.

119. Cantor KP, Blair A, Everett G, et al: Pesticides and other agricultural risk factors for non-Hodgkin's lymphoma among men in Iowa and Minnesota. Cancer Res 1992; 52:2447.

120. Scherr PA, Hutchison GB, Neiman RS: Non-Hodgkin's lymphoma and occupational exposure. Cancer Res 1992; 52:5503S.

121. Blair A, Linos A, Stewart PA, et al: Comments on occupational and environmental factors in the origin of non-Hodgkin's lymphoma. Cancer Res 1992; 52:5501S.

122. Blair A, Linos A, Stewart PA, et al: Evaluation of risks for non-Hodgkin's lymphoma by occupation and industry exposures from a case-control study. Am J Ind Med 1993; 23:301.

123. Pickle LW, Mason TJ, Howard N, et al: Atlas of US Cancer Mortality Among Whites: 1950–1980, DHHS (NIH) Publication No. 87-2900. Bethesda, MD, National Cancer Institute, 1987.

124. Pearce N, Bethwaite P: Increasing incidence of non-Hodgkin's lymphoma: Occupational and environmental factors. Cancer Res 1992; 52:5496s.

125. Zahm SH, Blair A: Pesticides and non-Hodgkin's lymphoma. Cancer Res 1992; 52:5485s.

126. Hardell L: Malignant lymphoma of histiocytic type and exposure to phenoxyacetic acids or chlorophenols. Lancet 1979; 1:55.

127. Persson B, Dahlander AM, Fredriksson M, et al: Malignant lymphomas and occupational exposures. Br J Ind Med 1989; 46:516.

128. Hardell L, Eriksson M, Lenner P, Lundgren E: Malignant lymphoma and exposure to chemicals, especially organic solvents, chlorophenols, and phenoxy acids: A case-control study. Br J Cancer 1981; 43:169.

129. Hoar SK, Blair A, Holmes FF, et al: Agricultural herbicide use and risk of lymphoma and soft-tissue sarcoma. JAMA 1986; 256:1141.

130. Zahm SH, Weisenburger DD, Babbitt PA, et al: A case-control study of non-Hodgkin's lymphoma and the herbicide 2,4-dichloro-phenoxyacetic acid (2,4-D) in eastern Nebraska. Epidemiology 1990; 1:349.

131. Wigle DT, Semenciw RM, Wilkins K, et al: Mortality study of Canadian male farm operators. J Natl Cancer Inst 1990; 82:575.

132. Hayes HM, Tarone RE, Cantor KP, et al: Case-control study of canine malignant lymphoma: Positive association with dog owner's use of 2,4-dichlorophenoxyacetic acid herbicides. J Natl Cancer Inst 1991; 83:1226.

133. Veterans and Agent Orange: Health effects of herbicides used in Vietnam. Washington, DC, National Academy of Science, 1994.

134. Dalager NA, Kang HK, Burt WL: Non-Hodgkin's lymphoma among Vietnam veterans. J Occupat Med 1991; 33:774.

135. Lipkowitz S, Garry VF, Kirsch IR: Interlocus V-J recombination measures genomic instability in agriculture workers at risk for lymphoid malignancies. Proc Natl Acad Sci USA 1992; 89:5301.

136. Kirsch IR, Lipkowitz S: A measure of genomic instability and its relevance to lymphomagenesis. Cancer Res 1992; 52:5545s.

137. Ames BN, Kammen HO, Yamasaki E: Hair dyes are mutagenic: Identification of a variety of mutagenic ingredients. Proc Natl Acad Sci USA 1975; 72:2423.

138. Cantor KP, Blair A, Everett G, et al: Hair dye use and risk of leukemia and lymphoma. Am J Public Health 1988; 78:570.

139. Zahm SH, Weisenburger DD, Babbitt PA, et al: Use of hair coloring products and the risk of lymphoma, multiple myeloma, and chronic lymphocytic lymphoma. Am J Public Health 1992; 82:990.

140. Thun MJ, Altekruse SF, Namboodiri MM, et al: Hair dye use and risk of fatal cancers in U.S. women. J Natl Cancer Inst 1994; 86:210.

141. Grodstein F, Hennekens CH, Colditz GA, et al: A prospective study of permanent hair dye use and hematopoietic cancer. J Natl Cancer Inst 1994; 86:1466.

142. Boice JJ: Radiation and non-Hodgkin's lymphoma. Cancer Res 1992; 52:5489s.

143. Milham SJ: Increased mortality in amateur radio operators due to lymphatic and hematopoietic malignancies. Am J Epidemiol 1988; 127:50.

144. Filipovich AH, Mathur A, Kamat D, et al: Primary immunodeficiencies: Genetic risk factors for lymphoma. Cancer Res 1992; 52:5465s.

145. Tucker M, Coleman C, Cox R, et al: Risk of second cancers after treatment for Hodgkin's disease. N Engl J Med 1988; 318:76.

146. van Leeuwen FE, Klokman WJ, Hagenbeek A, et al: Second cancer risk following Hodgkin's disease: A 20-year follow-up study. J Clin Oncol 1994; 12:312.

147. Penn I, Starzl J: Malignant tumors arising *de novo* in immunosuppressed organ transplant recipients. Transplantation 1972; 11:407.

148. Hoover R, Fraumeni JF: Risk of cancer in renal transplant recipients. Lancet 1973; 2:55.

149. Anderson JL, Bieber CP, Fowles RE, et al: Idiopathic cardiomyopathy, age, and suppressor-cell dysfunction as risk determinants of lymphoma after cardiac transplantation. Lancet 1978; 2:1174.

150. Kinlen LJ, Shiel AG, Peto J, et al: A collaborative study of cancer in patients who have received immunosuppressive therapy. Br Med J 1979; 2:1461.

151. Kinlen L: Immunosuppressive therapy and acquired immunological disorders. Cancer Res 1992; 52:5474S.

152. Penn I: Malignancy. Surg Clin North Am 1994; 75:1247.

153. Gridley G, Klippel JH, Hoover RN, Fraumeni JJ: Incidence of cancer among men with the Felty syndrome. Ann Intern Med 1994; 120:35.

154. Hoover R, Mason TJ, McKay FW, et al: Geographic patterns of cancer mortality in the US. *In* Jr FJ (ed): Persons at High Risk of Cancer. New York, Academic Press, 1975, pp 343–360.

155. Hyman GA, Sommers SC: The development of Hodgkin's disease and lymphoma during anticonvulsant therapy. Blood 1966; 28:416.

156. Li FP, Willard DR, Goodman R, et al: Malignant lymphoma after diphenylhydantoin (Dilantin). Cancer 1975; 36:1359.

157. Clemmesen J: Are anticonvulsants oncogenic? Lancet 1974; 1:705.

158. Bernard SM, Cartwright RA, Bird CC, et al: Aetiologic factors in lymphoid malignancies: A case-control epidemiologic study. Leuk Res 1984; 8:681.

159. Cartwright RA, McKinney PA, O'Brien C, et al: Non-Hodgkin's lymphoma: Case-control epidemiologic study in Yorkshire. Leuk Res 1988; 12:81.

160. Tielsch JM, Linet MS, Szklo M: Acquired disorders affecting the immune system and non-Hodgkin's lymphoma. Prev Med 1987; 16:96.

161. Hakulinen T, Isamaki H, Knekt P: Rheumatoid arthritis and cancer studies based on linking nationwide registries in Finland. Am J Med 1985; 7:2.

162. Gridley G, McLaughlin JK, Ekbom A, et al: Incidence of cancer among patients with rheumatoid arthritis. J Natl Cancer Inst 1993; 85:307.

163. Kinlen LJ: Incidence of cancer in rheumatoid arthritis and other disorders after immunosuppressive treatment. Am J Med 1985; 78:44.

164. Symmons DPM: Second cancer following lymphatic and hematopoietic cancer. Nat Cancer Inst Monogr 1985; 68:389.

165. Symmons D: Neoplasia in rheumatoid arthritis [Editorial]. J Rheumatol 1988; 15:1319.

166. Doody MM, Linet MS, Glass AG, et al: Leukemia, lymphoma, and multiple myeloma following selected medical conditions. Cancer Causes Control 1992; 3:449.

167. Kassan SS, Thomas TL, Moutsopolos HM, et al: Increased risk of lymphoma in sicca syndrome. Ann Intern Med 1978; 89:888.

168. McWhorter W: Allergy and risk of cancer: A prospective study using NHANESI followup data. Cancer 1988; 62:451.

169. Bernstein L, Ross RK: Prior medication use and health history as risk factors for non-Hodgkin's lymphoma: Preliminary results from a case-control study in Los Angeles County. Cancer Res 1992; 52:5510S.

170. Levine PH, Peterson D, McNamee FL, et al: Does chronic fatigue syndrome predispose to non-Hodgkin's lymphoma? Cancer Res 1992; 52:5516S.

171. Franceschi S, Serraino D, Carbone A, et al: Dietary factors and non-Hodgkin's lymphoma: A case-control study in the northeastern part of Italy. Nutr Cancer 1989; 12:333.

172. Ursin G, Bjelke E, Heuch L, Vollset SE: Milk consumption and cancer incidence: A Norwegian prospective study. Br J Cancer 1990; 61:456.

173. Davis S: Nutritional factors and the development of non-Hodgkin's lymphoma: A review of the evidence. Cancer Res 1992; 52:5492s.

174. Brown LM, Gibson R, Burmeister LF, et al: Alcohol consumption and risk of leukemia, non-Hodgkin's lymphoma, and multiple myeloma. Leuk Res 1992; 16:979.

175. Brown LM, Everett GD, Gibson R, et al: Smoking and risk of non-Hodgkin's lymphoma and multiple myeloma. Cancer Causes Control 1992; 3:49.

176. Hartge P, Devesa SS: Quantification of the impact of known risk factors on time trends in non-Hodgkin's lymphoma incidence. Cancer Res 1992; 52:5566s.

177. Connelly RR, Christine BW: A cohort study of cancer following infectious mononucleosis. Cancer Res 1974; 34:1172.

178. Carter CD, Brown TMJ, Herbert J, et al: Cancer incidence following infectious mononucleosis. Am J Epidemiol 1977; 105:30.

179. Munoz N, Davidson RJL, Wirthoff B, et al: Infectious mononucleosis and Hodgkin's disease. Int J Cancer 1978; 22:10.

180. Kvale G, Hiby EA, Pedersen F: Hodgkin's disease in patients with previous infectious mononucleosis. Int J Cancer 1979; 23:593.

181. Tirelli U, Seraino D, Carbone A: Hodgkin's disease and HIV. Ann Intern Med 1993; 118:313.

182. Biggar BJ, Curtis RE, Cote TR, et al: Risk of other cancers following Kaposi's sarcoma: Relation to acquired immunodeficiency syndrome. Am J Epidemiol 1994; 139:362.

183. Teta MJ, Walrath J, Meigs JW, et al: Cancer incidence among cosmetologists. J Natl Cancer Inst 1984; 72:1051.

184. Lynge E, Thygesen L: Use of surveillance systems for occupational cancer: Data from the Danish national system. Int J Epidemiol 1988; 17:493.

185. Shibata A, Sasaki R, Hamajima N, Aoki K: Mortality of hematopoietic disorders and hair dye use among barbers. Acta Haematol 1989; 52:116.

186. Boffetta P, Andersen A, Lynge E, et al: Employment as hairdresser and risk of ovarian cancer and non-Hodgkin's lymphomas among women. J Occup Med 1994; 36:61.

187. Hennekens CH, Speizer FE, Rosner B, et al: Use of permanent hair dyes and cancer among registered nurses. Lancet 1979; 1:1390.

188. National Cancer Institute Initiatives for Special Populations 1993–1994. Bethesda, MD, US Department of Health and Human Services, 1994.

Chapter Four

Epstein-Barr Virus and Human Lymphomas

George Klein
Eva Klein

The renaissance of viral oncology in the 1950s and 1960s was due to the discovery that a large number of retroviruses can cause a variety of malignancies in birds, mice, cats, and other vertebrates. Many of the retroviruses caused leukemias or lymphomas under experimental conditions, and a few of them could be proven to do so under natural conditions as well. In contrast, DNA tumor viruses do not cause lymphomas or leukemias in experimental animals, as a rule. Marek's disease virus, a member of the herpesvirus family that can cause epizootic lymphomas in chickens, is the most notable exception.

The subsequent extensive search for leukemogenic human retroviruses has been disappointing. Only one such virus, human T-cell lymphotropic virus type I (HTLV-I), was found.[1] A member of the lentivirus group like human immunodeficiency virus (HIV), HTLV-I can cause adult T-cell leukemia/lymphoma (ATL) and can immortalize normal T cells in vitro. Such lines are not immediately tumorigenic, however. Frank malignant transformation requires additional changes that have not been defined. HTLV-I is believed to create a preleukemic condition, probably by inducing the potential target cells to divide and thereby expanding the target cell population at risk. The likelihood of the ultimate cytogenetic change increases with the number of cell divisions. Chromosomal aberrations in ATL often involve chromosome 7, but no single, consistent cytogenetic aberration has been identified.

Epstein-Barr virus (EBV), a human lymphotropic herpesvirus, is presently the best known viral contributor to the development of human lymphomas. It is a highly powerful transforming agent for B lymphocytes, which it can convert into immortalized cell lines in vitro.[2] Morphologically, the transformed cells correspond to activated immunoblasts. They secrete immunoglobulins and a variety of cytokines, similarly to mitogen-activated or antigen-activated immunoblasts.

The virus transforms normal resting B cells into immunoblasts in vivo, just as it does in vitro. This transformation can be most readily observed in infectious mononucleosis (IM), a self-limiting lymphoproliferative disease that can be regarded as a pathologic form of primary EBV infection. In most young children and in about half of the adolescents and adults with the primary infection, there are no disease symptoms at all. The other half of the older group comes down with mononucleosis, in which dividing virus-carrying B blasts can be detected in the blood and the lymphoid organs.[3] This proliferation and the reactions it provokes are responsible for the disease symptoms. The reasons for the age-related difference between silent and pathogenic infection are not known.

Only a few of the atypical cells that appear in the blood during IM are EBV-carrying B cells. Most are T cells and other immune effectors that kill the virally infected B blasts with a high degree of efficiency. During the convalescent phase of mononucleosis, the EBV-positive immunoblasts disappear but the virus persists, probably largely if not exclusively in the small resting B-cell fraction.[4] The reasons for the rejection of the virus-carrying immunoblasts and the persistence of the resting cells may be sought in the cell phenotype–dependent differences in viral expression. Infected immunoblasts express nine virally encoded proteins. Six of them are nuclear antigens, designated as EBNA1 to 6, and three are membrane antigens (latent membrane protein 1 [LMP1], 2A, and 2B). Resting B cells express EBV-determined nuclear antigen 1 (EBNA1) only and do not seem to generate cytotoxic T cells (CTLs) (for review, see references 6 to 8). The difference is due to the differential usage of promoters and splicing programs. Owing to its exclusive expression of EBNA1, the virus-harboring, resting B cell apparently remains unrecognizable to the immune system. The virus persists throughout life (without causing any disease in most instances) in all infected people.

These and other features of EBV biology make the virus and its normal and neoplastic host cells highly interesting for molecular and biologic studies. The interaction of EBV with one of its main host cells, the B lymphocyte, is best known. The virus has adapted to the B cell at several levels. It uses a B-cell–specific surface moiety, CD21, also known as CR2, a complement (C3d) receptor, as its receptor. Normally, CD21 is involved in the activation of B cells by antigen–antibody complement complexes. The virus is a polyclonal B-cell activator in itself, and its attachment to CD21 may provide it with a particularly favorable point of entry that can facilitate the activation of the host cell.

The virally encoded growth transformation–associated EBNAs and LMPs participate in this activation in a cascadelike fashion that has not been clarified in detail. It is clear, however, that the expression of EBNA2 is an essential prerequisite for activation. LMP1, the main membrane antigen, is known to prevent apoptotic death, a frequent fate of B lymphocytes, probably through its ability to activate the apoptosis-antagonizing *bcl*-2 gene.[8, 9] The virally activated immunoblasts produce a variety of cytokines, including B-cell growth factors, and express corresponding receptors, such as CD23. An autocrine loop is generated that may stimulate the proliferation of the virally infected B cells in vivo, as it certainly does in vitro. In consequence, the number of virally infected cells may reach a sufficiently high level, prior to the onset of the rejection response, to secure the persistence of the virus and its spreading to new hosts.

Eight of the nine virally encoded proteins expressed in the transformed immunoblasts are competent to induce a rejection response. The predominant rejection target is determined by the human leukocyte antigen (HLA) constitution of the host.[10] In immunocompetent persons, the response is powerful: It clears away the virally infected blasts within a few days. Persons with congenital or acquired immunodeficiencies may succumb to progressive lymphoproliferative disease, however.

In spite of the efficient immune response, the virus persists in resting B cells. It probably does so by switching to the "EBNA1 only" program. EBV-carrying resting B cells show no tendency to expand and are probably long lived. It may be surmised that their activation and subsequent immunoblastic proliferation are prevented by the switch-on of the highly immunogenic EBNAs. It is not known how the latently infected cells that express only EBNA1 manage to maintain themselves at an apparently constant level throughout life.

How did the virtually watertight surveillance that prevents the proliferation of the virally transformed blasts evolve? This question must be seen in relation to the fact that closely related viruses are present in all Old World, but not in New World, primates. In the immunologically naive New World monkeys, the virus can cause fatal lymphoproliferative disease, quite like in immunodefective humans.[2] It may be surmised that humans and other Old World primates have reached the present state of an essentially nonpathogenic coexistence with this potentially dangerous virus family only after having been selected for the efficient recognition of the virus-carrying immunoblasts. The HLA class I allotype spectrum is obviously highly competent to deal with the problem. Analyses performed at various laboratories have shown that different responders target their CTLs against peptides derived from eight of the nine virally encoded, transformation-associated proteins, with the notable exception of EBNA1 (for review, see reference 7). The precise choice of the target depends on the immunodominant HLA class I restriction element. The total major histocompatibility complex (MHC) equipment of the human species, in combination with the eight virally encoded target proteins, apparently provides full protection against the unlimited proliferation of the virally transformed immunoblasts in virtually all normal immunocompetent people.

EBV AND HUMAN MALIGNANCY

It follows from what has been stated earlier about the stable, nonpathogenic equilibrium between EBV and the human host that EBV-induced or EBV-associated disease arises only as a biologic accident. The nature of this accident is fairly well known for some but not all EBV-associated neoplastic diseases.

IM is caused by a primary viral infection after the age of approximately 10 years, as already mentioned. The reasons for the age-related difference in viral pathogenicity are not known. However, symptom-free early childhood infection is the rule in all developing countries and in low socioeconomic groups throughout the world.[11] The virus is believed to spread largely, if not exclusively, through the saliva. Postponement of the regular early childhood infection by good hygienic conditions is thus one "accident" that may disrupt the normal "rejection-geared" immune response that prevents proliferative disease in young children and in half of the adolescents and adults as well. The IM syndrome may be viewed as a delayed and, initially at least, quite disorganized rejection reaction that permits a considerable degree of immunoblast proliferation, perhaps because of the remarkably strong T-cell suppression that precedes it.[12] Nevertheless, the rejection reaction is unerringly efficient, unless the host is immunocompromised. The following is the next accident.

Lymphoproliferative Disease in Immunodefective Hosts. Congenital, iatrogenic (posttransplant), and infectious (acquired immunodeficiency syndrome [AIDS]) immunodeficiencies may be accompanied by the fatal proliferation of EBV-transformed immunoblasts.[13, 14] It starts as polyclonal growth, as in mononucleosis, but it fails to regress. It may turn into oligoclonal and later monoclonal growth in the course of time.[15, 16] The cells maintain their immunoblastic phenotype in the course of this progression. They resemble the lymphoblastoid cell lines in vitro and express the full set of EBNAs and LMPs accordingly.[17, 18] Apparently, the cells proliferate because the host response has broken down. Initially at least, no cellular change is required over and above the EBV-induced transformation.

At least 90% of the posttransplant lymphoproliferative diseases (PT-LPDs) were found to carry EBV.[19, 20] On the basis of their immunoglobulin rearrangement patterns, the lesions can be subdivided into polymorphic (oligoclonal or polyclonal) and monomorphic (monoclonal) types. The polymorphic group is often associated with polyclonal EBV infection. As discussed in a subsequent section, part of the HIV-infected group, but not other groups, consists of monoclonal lymphomas that have a rearranged c-*myc* gene, due to an Ig/*myc* translocation, that corresponds to sporadic Burkitt's lymphoma (BL) in its details. About 70% of this group are EBV negative. It is important, for conceptual and clinical reasons, to distinguish between lymphomas with and without *myc* rearrangement in the HIV-infected group.

The occurrence and clinical features of PT-LPD have been summarized by Nalesnik and associates,[21] and its EBV aspects have been reviewed by Ho and colleagues.[22] In the Pittsburgh-Denver organ transplant series, the total detection rate was 1.7%. Kidney recipients had the lowest (1.0%) and heart/lung recipients had the highest (4.6%) frequency of PT-LPD. Bone marrow transplant cases were not included. The main clinical categories included a mononucleosis-like syndrome, gastrointestinal/abdominal disease, and solid organ disease. In cyclosporin A (CSA)-treated patients, the median time of onset was 4.4 months after transplantation, regardless of tumor clonality. The histologic spectrum ranged from polymorphic to monomorphic. Polymorphic lesions could be either clonal or nonclonal, whereas monomorphic lesions were clonal. Clonal and nonclonal lesions were about equally frequent. All nonclonal and about half of the clonal lesions responded to reduced immunosuppression and supportive surgery. Patients who received other forms of immunosuppression developed lymphoproliferative disease after significantly longer intervals.[23]

Patients with a preferentially localized symptomatology show head and neck, gastrointestinal, and other organ involvement. The allografted organ is also frequently affected. The most famous case of multiple PT-LPD presentation is the "bubble boy," who had concurrent clonal and nonclonal tumors, including more than 20 lesions, with polymorphic lymphoid tumor histology.[24] Some of the phenotypically polymorphic proliferations were genotypically oligoclonal, and one had a monoclonal component. This case is consistent with a progression series in which monoclonal tumors evolve from a polyclonal background. Clonal B-cell infiltrates can also be observed in fatal mononucleosis,[21] although the proliferation associated with mononucleosis is generally polyclonal. As Nalesnik pointed out, it is often difficult to clearly separate malignant from nonmalignant PT-LPD. Many lesions that would be self-limiting in immunocompetent hosts may act in a malignant fashion in immunosuppressed hosts. Monoclonal tumors capable of invasion and distant metastasis are considered malignant, regardless of whether they regress. The concepts of malignancy and progressive disease must be obviously dissociated in this system. This is not surprising, in view of the highly immunogenic nature of EBV-transformed cells, the potentiality of tumor progression by genetic changes in the EBV-generated polyclonal lymphoproliferative lesion, and the counteracting influence of the host response that may, depending on the EBV expression phenotype of the tumor cell, act more or less efficiently. The three independent variables—progression of the tumor by genetic changes, EBV expression phenotype that strongly influences the potential immunogenicity of the cells, and pharmacologically modulated host response—can obviously produce a large variety of clinical phenotypes.

The precarious balance between progression and regression and the potential strength of the immune response, unparalleled in other tumor systems, is well brought out by the early experience that kidney transplant recipients who developed PT-LPD may reject their immunoblastomas, even of recipient origin, if immunosuppression is lifted. Following the rejection of the kidney and return to dialysis, a second kidney may be grafted. Renewed immunosuppression does not lead to recurrence of the immunoblastoma.

Hickey and colleagues have studied a large material that is relevant in this context.[25] Renal transplant patients who lost their allografts during the management of a previous PT-LPD were drawn from a total of 1226 transplant patients

managed at the University of Pittsburgh. They had all been treated with CSA. Fourteen patients (1.1%) developed PT-LPD during a 7-year period. Following the reduction of immunosuppression, the immunoblastomas regressed. Six of the 14 patients retained their allografts, 3 were retransplanted, and 2 died. All retransplanted patients were treated with CSA with no adverse effects. Two of the 3 second transplants were still functioning 18 to 26 months after retransplantation.

In this study, the simple expedient of stopping or reducing immunosuppression in CSA- and prednisone-treated patients led to prompt and apparently permanent resolution of the lymphoproliferative disease, provided that infection and other complications could be controlled. Monoclonal and polyclonal immunoblastomas regressed equally easily.

Special risk factors that promote the development of PT-LPD in bone marrow transplant recipients include T-cell depletion of the graft, HLA mismatching between donor and recipient, and treatment of acute graft-versus-host disease (GVHD) with T-cell antibodies.[26, 27]

Recently, Papadopoulos and coworkers[28] infused donor leukocytes in five bone marrow transplant recipients who had developed EBV-carrying lymphoproliferative disease after allogeneic bone marrow transplant. Unirradiated donor leukocytes were infused in doses calculated to provide approximately 10^6 CD3+ T cells per kilogram of body weight. Each of the four immunoblastoma specimens that could be evaluated were of donor cell origin. EBV DNA was detected by polymerase chain reaction (PCR) in all five samples. In all five patients, complete clinically and histologically documented regression occurred within 8 to 21 days after infusion. Clinical remissions were achieved 14 to 30 days after the infusions and were sustained without further therapy in the three surviving patients for 10, 16, and 16 months.

BURKITT'S LYMPHOMA

In contrast with the immunoblastomas that arise in immunodefective hosts, both high endemic and sporadic BL develops in immunocompetent persons. Its progressive growth is not due to the breakdown of immune surveillance but to the escape of the BL cell from immune rejection. It is not driven by the growth transformation–associated, EBV-encoded proteins as the immunoblast but by the juxtaposition of c-*myc* to immunoglobulin sequences. The chromosomal translocation accident generates a permanent stimulus for cell proliferation, owing to the constitutive activation of c-*myc*. Moreover, it positions the BL cell in a phenotypic window where it is prone to escape rejection, owing to the downregulation of the potentially immunogenic EBNA2 to 6 and LMP proteins, the low expression of cellular adhesion molecules, and a relative deficiency of MHC class I antigen expression.

Only 97% of the high endemic BLs, prevalent in the rain forest areas of Africa and New Guinea, and not more than 20% of the sporadic BLs that occur at a lower frequency all over the world, carry EBV (for reviews, see references 6 and 10). One of the three alternative forms of the

Ig/*myc* translocation—8;14 (*myc*/IgH), 2;8 (κ/*myc*),and 8;22 (*myc*/λ)—are regularly present in all BLs, whether EBV positive or negative (for review, see reference 29). The subordination of c-*myc* to one of the continuously active immunoglobulin regions interferes with the normal regulability of the gene. As a result, the cells are prevented from leaving the cycling compartment.

Thus, the translocation, rather than EBV, must be considered as the main rate-limiting event in the development of BL. EBV may increase the probability of this event by expanding the target cell population at risk, prolonging the life span of the target cells, and increasing the number of their divisions. The risk of genetic accidents is proportional to the number of consecutive mitoses.

The BL Cell Phenotype. Nilsson and Pontén found in 1975 that BL-derived cell lines differ from EBV-transformed lymphoblastoid cell lines (LCLs) of nonneoplastic origin in several respects.[30] The ultrastructure and surface glycoprotein pattern of the LCLs resembled mitogen-transformed immunoblasts, whereas BL cells were more like resting B cells. Later, surface marker analysis confirmed and further emphasized these differences (for review, see reference 31). BL cells express CD10 (CALLA) and CD77 (BLA), but they do not express the numerous "activation markers" and adhesion molecules associated with mitogen-induced blast transformation. LCLs showed the opposite pattern. The difference in the expression of the adhesion molecules explains why LCLs grow as large clusters, whereas BL cell lines proliferate as single cell suspensions.

The phenotype of the BL tumor cells in vivo is faithfully reproduced within the freshly established cell lines, as a rule. They are designated as type I or group I BL lines. In the course of serial propagation in vitro, most EBV-carrying but not EBV-negative BL lines tend to "drift" phenotypically, that is, to convert spontaneously into more "LCL-like" (type III) cultures.[32] Their drift is reflected by the appearance of activation markers and adhesion molecules and the gradual disappearance of the BL type I–associated CD10 and CD77 markers. Concurrently, the EBV expression of the cells changes dramatically. Type I BL cells express EBNA1 only, alone among the EBV-encoded, growth transformation–associated proteins. Type II/III BL cells express all six EBNAs and the LMP1 and 2 membrane antigens.

The differential EBNA expression of the BL cells can be related to the alternative use of promoters and splicing programs. In EBV-transformed normal B cells, and in type II/III BL cells, one of two alternative promoters (designated as Wp and Cp, respectively), is used to generate a giant, approximately 85-kilobase-long message, out of which all six EBNAs are spliced.[33] In type I BL cells, and in all other EBV-carrying cells that do not have an immunoblastic phenotype, the W/C promoter system is inactive. An alternative promoter is used, located in the F-Q region. It generates a short message that encodes EBNA1 only.[34] Promoter usage and the corresponding antigen expression can be shifted experimentally in both directions.[35] Type I BL cells that express EBNA1 only can switch on the W/C program either in connection with the phenotypic drift mentioned earlier or on exposure to 5-azacytidine. The latter finding indicates that DNA methylation is involved in the downregulation of the missing proteins, as also shown by more direct experimental evidence.[36, 37]

W/C usage can be switched to the F-Q program by hybridizing LCLs with non-B cells, whereupon the expression of EBNA2 to 6 is eclipsed, and the exclusive EBNA1 program is switched on.[38]

We and others have suggested that the differential usage of alternative viral programs in immunoblasts and in type I BL cells reflects the viral life cycle in corresponding normal cells. Although the lymphoproliferative diseases of the immunodefective hosts are due to the progressive growth of the virally transformed immunoblasts, the type I BL cell appears to represent the neoplastic counterpart of latently infected resting B cells. The latter provides one, if not the only, reservoir of the persisting virus in normal seropositive persons, as already discussed. We have recently obtained evidence that such cells express EBNA1 only.[5] This is probably one reason for the nonrejectability of the BL cell in immunocompetent hosts. There are two other reasons as well: the allele-specific HLA class I antigen suppression, characteristic for type I BL cells,[39] and the deficient expression of adhesion molecules.[31] Together with the downregulation of the immunogenic EBV proteins, these phenotypic traits all may stem from the fact that the Ig/*myc* translocation "fixes" the cellular phenotype in a state in which it resembles resting, rather than dividing, cells. It is a peculiar coincidence that the two most important features of the EBV-carrying BL cell—the presence of the latent virus in a regulated state where it expresses only EBNA1 and the proliferation driving force of the illegitimate Ig/*myc* translocation—have the resting B cell as their common target. The former is due to the fact that the resting B cell serves as the main, if not the only, reservoir of latently persisting virus, whereas the Ig/*myc* translocation generates monoclonal neoplastic growth by preventing the resting (virgin or memory) B cell from leaving the cycling compartment.

Etiologic Considerations. Among the two potentially important etiologic factors considered so far—EBV and the Ig/*myc* translocation—the former is obviously a contributory step, particularly in the high endemic forms of the lymphoma, whereas the latter is an essential, rate-limiting factor, as indicated by its virtually 100% association with the tumor.

Among the environmental factors that can be related to the high endemic form, chronic hyperendemic or holoendemic malaria occupies a dominating position, for geographic and climate-related reasons.[40] It may act by stimulating chronic cell proliferation within the target cell population at risk. Prolonged stimulation of cell division is also involved in the development of the rodent Ig/*myc* translocation–carrying tumors.[29] Chronic local granuloma formation and high genetic susceptibility are the two most prominent requirements for the induction of mouse plasmacytoma. Hypersensitization to helminths in the ileocecal region may play a similar role in the induction of the Louvain rat immunocytoma. Chronic proliferation involves a long series of cell divisions in the tumor precursor cells. The probability of genetic accidents increases with the number of divisions. The development of autonomously growing tumors is promoted when the translocation accident happens to juxtapose the coding exons of c-*myc* and immunoglobulin sequences, as already discussed. Additional genetic changes are probably required before the tumor clone reaches full autonomy.

The "molecular anatomy" of the Ig/*myc* translocation shows certain differences between endemic and sporadic BL (for review, see reference 10). In the high endemic, largely EBV-associated form, the break of chromosome 8 hits usually upstreams of the intact c-*myc* gene. In the largely EBV-negative sporadic tumors, the break occurs usually within the first intron or the first exon, or immediately upstreams of the gene. There are also certain differences in the immunoglobulin sequences involved. In the sporadic form, a switch region within the IgH locus, usually Smu, is the most common recipient site. The breaks are more variable in the high endemic form. They are higher upstreams, as a rule, in a J or a V region. This finding implies that the distance between the *myc* and the Ig sequences is often greater in the EBV-carrying than in the EBV-negative form. Conceivably, activating and activated sequences may have to be closer to each other in the absence of EBV. This would be understandable if EBV contributed to the constitutive activation of *myc* in a positive way.

The *myc* breakpoint difference between endemic and sporadic tumors implies, furthermore, that the gene is transcribed from its own promoters in the high endemic tumors, whereas in the sporadic tumors transcription starts at a cryptic promoter within the first intron. These differences between the high endemic and the sporadic tumors with regard to breakpoint location, together with several differences in primary localization, bone marrow involvement, and other clinical features, suggest that the precursor cells of the two tumor forms may represent different stages of maturity, perhaps because of the involvement of different etiologic factors reviewed by Magrath.[10]

The accidental nature of the translocation is confirmed by the fact that the c-*myc*–carrying chromosome can break at many different points, upstreams or within the c-*myc* gene in the typical (IgH/*myc*) translocation, or downstreams of the gene, in the variant translocations that involve the light chain genes. No breakpoint clusters, fragile sites, or hot spots are involved. This indicates that the break occurs at random. The immunoglobulin locus–carrying chromosomes break at more specific points, corresponding to sites that serve as targets for the recombinases involved in physiologic Ig rearrangement.

Although the Ig/*myc* juxtaposition is thus a common molecular feature of all BLs, irrespective of geographic origin or EBV-carrying status, it is probably not the only change. Evidence on immunoglobulin enhancer/c-*myc* construct–carrying transgenic mice[41] and examination of preneoplastic tissues during the development of mouse plasmacytoma[52a] concur in suggesting that constitutive activation of c-*myc* by its juxtaposition to immunoglobulin sequences is not sufficient to cause a lymphoma by itself. Secondary changes may include point mutations in the c-*myc* locus itself, affecting some probably critical phosphorylation sites.[43, 44] Additional oncogene activation events and suppressor gene losses may be involved as well. Mutation of p53 may be one such event.[45–47] Further changes, including a deletion of 6q and mutation of K-*ras*, have been found in HIV-infected patients with non-Hodgkin's lymphoma (NHL), as described in the next section.

High endemic BLs present usually as well-circumscribed, solid tumors, whereas sporadic BLs may be more generalized, with lymph node and bone marrow involvement.

African BLs appear often as jaw tumors around the age of dental development, as gonadal tumors in prepubertal children, and as long bone tumors in adolescents. Bilateral breast tumors were found in a lactating woman.[48] These characteristics indicate that local growth factors may play a promoting role.

Immunologic Features. BL cells are relatively or completely resistant to CTL-mediated killing, in comparison with LCLs, derived from the same patient.[49, 50] The phenotypic features responsible for this finding have already been discussed. BL cells are also less able to process antigen[51] and less effective in stimulating allogeneic T cells.[52] The reduced expression of adhesion molecules[53] is consistent with the resemblance between BL cells and resting B cells. This may also contribute to CTL resistance, together with the downregulation of certain class I HLAs.[54]

These features of the EBV-carrying BL cell provide an adequate explanation for its ability to grow in immunocompetent persons, in contrast with the EBV-carrying immunoblast. The observations that EBV-carrying BLs are more localized than their EBV-negative counterparts and are more curable by chemotherapy nevertheless indicate that the specific immune response of the patient can affect the former more than the latter.

NON-HODGKIN'S LYMPHOMA IN HIV-INFECTED PATIENTS

AIDS-related NHL is 60 times more prevalent than NHL in the general population.[55] Seventy percent of the tumors are high-grade NHL. They are almost exclusively B cell derived. They belong to a variety of types, such as small noncleaved cell lymphoma (SNCCL), large cell immunoblastic plasmacytoid lymphoma (LC-IBPL), and large noncleaved cell lymphoma (LNCCL), reviewed by Ballerini and associates.[56] In the reviewed material, 42% carried EBV, 29% had c-*myc* rearrangement, 15% had a *ras* mutation, and 37% had lost or carried mutated p53. The frequency of each of these changes varies with the type of AIDS NHL. All LC-IBPLs carried EBV and were similar to, if not identical with, the immunoblastic lymphomas seen in congenital and iatrogenic (posttransplant) T-cell deficiencies. It may be surmised that the immunoblasts proliferate as a result of immune breakdown in all these cases. Only about 30% to 40% of the SNCCLs carry EBV, however. Virtually all of them carry an Ig/*myc* translocation. Unlike the sharp association of the Ig/*myc* translocation with both high endemic and sporadic BL, the translocations carried by the HIV-associated lymphomas are present in a variety of histologic types. Many of them would not be normally classified as BL by the pathologist, but the presence of the Ig/*myc* translocation may be taken to indicate that they all originate from a similar oncogene activation event. Conceivably, they may diversify phenotypically as a result of the T-cell immunodeficiency.

According to the review of Gaidano and Dalla-Favera,[19] EBV is present in 30% to 40% of HIV-associated SNCCL and LNCCL and in 100% of systemic LC-IBPL and central nervous system (CNS)NHL.[20]

EBV-carrying and c-*myc*–rearranged B cells can thus undergo oligoclonal expansion that may give rise to monoclonal neoplasia in the context of AIDS.[57] A positive correlation has been found between the appearance of detectable EBV-carrying B-cell clones in patients with HIV-associated, persistent generalized lymphadenopathy (PGL) and the later development of EBV-carrying NHL.[58] The clonal expansion was preceded by EBV infection, as shown by EBV termini analysis.[56, 59]

EBV infection is a universal feature of systemic AIDS LC-IBPL, as already mentioned. A subgroup in this category originates in the CNS and was found to carry EBV in 100%.[60, 61] This is reminiscent of our early finding, showing that EBV-transformed LCLs of normal origin do not grow subcutaneously in nude mice, in contrast with BL cells, but can grow progressively in the nude mouse brain.[62, 63]

The EBV-carrying status of 128 AIDS-related lymphomas (ARLs) has been also surveyed by Hamilton-Dutoit and colleagues.[64] The presence of EBV in the tumor cells was detected by in situ hybridization for the virally encoded small RNA, EBER1. EBV was present in 85 (66%) of the 128 lymphomas, but the frequency of virus-carrying tumors differed according to the histologic type. EBER1 expression was detected in all 11 HIV-positive Hodgkin's disease (HD) cases (100%), 15 (94%) of 16 NHLs originating in the CNS, and 46 (77%) of 60 immunoblastomas, but only 12 (34%) of 35 of the Burkitt-type (SNCCL) lymphomas. One of 6 diffuse LNCCLs carried the virus as well. Patients with EBV-carrying immunoblastoma showed more severe immunosuppression, as indicated by the level of CD4+ cells, than patients with BLs.[42]

The authors concluded that all AIDS-related HD, virtually all primary CNS-derived ARLs, and most immunoblastomas carry EBV, but only a few BLs and monomorphic centroblastic lymphomas are EBV positive. Similar conclusions were reached by other authors.[64, 65] It is noteworthy that primary CNS lymphomas that arise in immunocompetent HIV-negative persons only infrequently carry EBV.[66] The presence of EBV in virtually all tumor cells in the EBV-positive ARLs was taken to indicate that EBV infection preceded clonal expansion. This suggests that it plays a pathogenic role in the EBV-positive tumors.

Hamilton-Dutoit and coworkers have studied the expression of EBV genes in relation to the tumor cell phenotype in AIDS-associated NHLs.[67] Forty-nine cases were examined by Southern blotting, in situ hybridization, and immunophenotyping. The choice of the viral program by the EBV-carrying cells was assessed by measuring the expression of EBNA2 and LMP1. As already discussed in the section on EBV biology, immunoblastic cells express both proteins within their "latency III" program. BLs express neither (latency I), whereas cells with a non-B phenotype express LMP1 but not EBNA2 (latency II). All three patterns were found in the 22 EBV-positive immunoblast-rich, large cell lymphomas. EBNA2 and LMP1 were expressed in 9 lymphomas, corresponding to the type III latency of the in vitro LCLs. They carried activation markers, as expected. Extranodal lymphomas belonged to this category. A BL-like, EBER-positive, EBNA2-negative, LMP1-negative type I latency was found in 6 lymphomas. The 7 remaining lymphomas were EBER1 positive, EBNA2 negative, but LMP1 positive, as in latency II. The latter category is particularly interesting, because latency II was previously seen only in EBV-carrying tumors of non-B-cell origin, such as HD, T-cell lymphomas, and nasopharyngeal carcinoma.

It thus appears that the ARLs belong to at least three major, pathogenetically distinct groups. The EBV-carrying immunoblastomas are phenotypically similar to the proliferative lesions that arise in organ transplant recipients. They arise owing to the deficiency of the immune surveillance mechanisms that keeps EBV-infected B cells under control in normal EBV-carrying persons but can evolve toward oligoclonality and monoclonality by further cellular changes. The BLs and other Ig/*myc* translocation–carrying lymphomas correspond phenotypically to the sporadic, largely EBV-negative BLs. Only one third of them carry EBV. The latter express EBNA1 only, according to the type I latency model, characteristic for the high endemic BLs. This is in contrast to their *myc* rearrangement pattern that resembles the sporadic BLs (for review, see reference 10). There is also a group of Hodgkin's lymphomas (HLs). They carry EBV in 100%, unlike their non-AIDS–associated counterparts, which are only 50% EBV positive (see following section).

The LCL-like type III latency is a general characteristic of all immunoblastomas, also observed in transplant recipients, as already mentioned. It is also found in the EBV-induced lymphoproliferative lesions in tamarins[68] and in LCLs or EBV-carrying normal B cells that grow progressively in SCID mice.[69]

In contrast with the immunoblastomas that are believed to arise due to immunosuppression and deficient surveillance, the Ig/*myc* translocation–carrying Burkitt's or Burkitt-like tumors in HIV-infected patients have a more complex pathogenesis. It is basically comparable to what has been discussed earlier for high endemic BLs, with only some differences. BL and other Ig/*myc* translocation–carrying lymphomas are not observed in transplant recipients or in patients with congenital T-cell deficiencies. Chronic stimulation of cell division in the B-cell population at risk must be an essential requirement for facilitating the translocation. This stimulation may be provided by the HIV itself or by the many AIDS-associated opportunistic infections, or both. HIV-associated lymphadenopathy is known to involve chronic stimulation of the B-cell population, leading to high proliferative activity and hypergammaglobulinemia. This may predispose the cell to translocations and other genetic accidents. Activated cells may also act by increased cytokine production, providing autocrine and paracrine stimulation for the target cells at risk. T cells, monocytes, bone marrow, and stromal cells are known to respond to HIV infection by increased cytokine production. The B cells of HIV-infected persons secrete tumor necrosis factor-α and interleukin-6 without in vitro stimulation. They may promote the expansion of oligoclonal B-cell populations.

HODGKIN'S DISEASE

The idea that EBV may play an important role in the genesis of BL and also nasopharyngeal carcinoma (NPC) came originally from serologic studies. The interpretation of the frequently elevated EBV antibody titers in HD patients remained ambiguous, in contrast with the association of the virus with African BL and with NPC of any geographic origin occurred exclusively in EBV-seropositive persons. The small EBV-seronegative subpopulation was uniquely absent in BL and NPC, in contrast with all other groups, and most patients had high EBV titers. Detection of viral genomes in the tumor cells of BL and NPC has confirmed the postulated association (for review, see reference 70).

EBV seropositivity in HD was not equally regular. HD patients were more frequently seropositive than matched control subjects, and their mean antibody titers were higher, but a substantial minority of the HD patients was seronegative. The titer elevations were therefore written off as probable secondary consequences of the HD-associated immune defects. In particular, the antiviral (EA and VCA) antibody titers were known to increase in T-cell deficiencies.

The detection of EBV at the cellular level by immunohistologic techniques has brought the possible role of EBV in HD again to the forefront of interest after a dormancy of 2 decades (for review, see reference 71). Improved techniques of in situ hybridization and the use of probes for the highly transcribed EBV-encoded small RNA (EBER) cells opened the field for the detection and identification of virally infected cells in complex tissues. Mixed cellularity (MC) and nodular sclerosis (NS) were found to be the most frequent EBV-positive forms of HD, in that order.[72] Lymphocyte predominance is largely EBV negative. This is in line with earlier serologic findings.[73]

The detection of EBV DNA in HD tissues has provoked much discussion. Are the viral genomes harbored by the neoplastic cells? If so, are all of them positive in a given tumor, or only some? Are the viral genomes also present in reactive normal cells?

Localization of EBV DNA to Reed-Sternberg cells is shown by many authors.[74–83] The episomal EBV in HD is clonal, as indicated by the terminal repeat hybridization method. This supports the idea that the virus may play an etiologic role in the EBV-positive HLs.[74, 82–87]

The variable appearance and the complexity of HD, its approximately 50% overall association with the virus, and the differences in the positivity of the morphologic subtypes create problems. The immunohistochemical distinction made between EBV-carrying HD cells and normal lymphocytes, using a highly sensitive single-stranded EBER antisense probe, was an important improvement.[72] In contrast with the uniform EBER expression of all neoplastic cells in the EBV-harboring HD cases, only a small number of normal B cells were positive. They were also present in EBV-negative HD lesions. These distinctions have brought the possible role of the virus in the EBV-positive HD lesions into much sharper focus, but that does not mean that the relationship has been explained.

Mutatis mutandis, the partial EBV positivity of the HLs is not entirely unlike the much better known relationship between EBV and BL. The regular association of EBV with high endemic BL has been taken to indicate that the virus must play some role in the etiology of the tumor, perhaps by expanding or immortalizing a subset of Ig/*myc* translocation–prone B cells, as already discussed. In the absence of any information on the steps involved in generating HD, many questions remain enigmatic. If the neoplastic HL cells belong to the B-cell series, why does their viral antigen expression (EBNA2 negative, LMP positive)[88] resemble the epithelial cells of NPC rather than BL cells (EBNA1 only) or the EBV-carrying immunoblastomas that arise in immunodefective hosts (EBNA1 to 6 and LMP)?

Critical studies excluded the possible presence of EBNA2 in HL cells.[79, 88–92]

The overall prevalence of EBV-positive HD, as well as the subtype distribution (more MC than NS) of Chinese EBV-positive HD, was similar to what was found in the developing countries.[93] Immunodeficiency-associated HD cases are rare.[76, 78, 84, 86, 94–96]

Is there any relationship between IM and HL? Such a relationship has been postulated on the basis of certain epidemiologic similarities, the preferential appearance of both diseases in high socioeconomic groups, and the documented appearance of HD in the wake of IM. Cohort studies have shown two to four times increased risk for HD after IM, with the greatest risk within 3 years after IM.[97, 98]

Does the delayed EBV infection of hygienically protected subpopulations increase the risk of HD in a similar way as it increases the likelihood of clinically manifest mononucleosis, or is this relatively slight epidemiologic similarity of the two diseases mainly coincidental, perhaps related to the EBV-like socioepidemiology of some unknown infectious agent in HD? Comparative epidemiologic studies on EBV-carrying and EBV-negative cases of HD would be of great interest in this context.

Since the EBV-encoded LMP1 protein is potentially immunogenic and is regularly expressed by EBV-carrying cases of HD, the question arises as to how such cells escape immune surveillance. The findings of Knecht and associates[99] may provide a clue. In five cases of EBV-carrying HD, deletions were found near the 3′ end of the LMP1 gene. Similar deletions were seen in nasopharyngeal carcinoma. Conceivably, these deletions may impair the immunogenicity of the LMP1 protein.

EBV AND T-CELL LYMPHOMAS

The unexpected association of EBV with some T-cell lymphomas was initially found by Jones and colleagues,[100] who found EBV DNA by Southern blotting and in situ hybridization in three cases. Subsequently, EBV genomes were detected in a certain proportion of human postthymic T-cell malignancies and related lymphoproliferative disorders.[67, 93, 101–107] Surprisingly, the virus was more frequently associated with T-cell than with B-cell lymphomas in immunocompetent patients with NHL. The EBV-carrying neoplastic T cells belonged to a range of immunophenotypically different cell types, indicating that functionally distinct subpopulations of neoplastic T cells are involved. T-cell lymphomas arising in the upper aerodigestive tract are particularly frequent carriers of EBV. They include sinonasal peripheral T-cell lymphoma, lethal midline granuloma, lymphomatoid granulomatosis, and angiocentric lymphoproliferative lesions. According to Pallesen and coworkers,[108] EBV is particularly often associated with angioimmunoblastic lymphadenopathy, pleomorphic medium and large cell type, and Lennert's lymphoma.

De Bruin and colleagues[109] showed that the association of EBV with T-cell lymphomas differs, depending on the site of presentation. Nasal T-cell tumors are invariably EBV positive; those of the skin are predominantly negative. Tokunaga and associates[110] found that ATL carried EBV DNA in 21 cases according to PCR. EBER hybridization confirmed this in 16 cases. De Bruin and colleagues[111] studied 46 nodal T-cell lymphomas for EBV DNA by PCR and EBER1 and 2, and LMP1 by in situ hybridization and immunohistochemistry. Twenty-one of 45 cases had EBV DNA by PCR. Eight of 15 cases showed clusters of EBER-positive cells. These lymphomas were therefore considered to be strongly EBV associated.

Kumar and coworkers[112] reported an EBV-associated T-cell immunoblastic lymphoma that occurred in a renal transplant recipient after 7 years. Tien and associates[113] found chromosomal anomalies in EBV-carrying T-cell lymphomas, affecting particularly chromosome 7, as in other T-cell lymphomas.

Su and associates[114] found that 10 of 35 subcutaneous T-cell lymphomas were EBV associated. Three distinct clinical pathologic subgroups could be recognized. The most consistent EBV association was seen with angiocentric T-cell lymphoma or lymphomatoid granulomatosis. EBV-associated T-cell lymphomas were quite resistant to therapy and had a poor prognosis.

Monoclonal proliferation of cytotoxic T cells containing the EBV genome was also seen in a young child with sporadic fatal IM.[115]

The pattern of latent gene expression in EBV-carrying T-cell lymphomas corresponded to latency II, with EBNA1 and LMP1 but without EBNA2 to 6. However, two cases have been reported with latency III.[116]

Most of the EBV-positive T lymphomas contained monoclonal EBV episomes, indicating that EBV infection had occurred prior to the clonal expansion of the lymphoma. This finding is consistent with the possibility that EBV plays a direct or indirect pathogenetic role.

T-cell lymphomas are rare in AIDS patients and in organ transplant recipients. There is thus no strong evidence to suggest that defects of EBV immunity are involved in their genesis.

CONCLUSIONS

EBV is a highly transforming virus. For human B cells, its transforming (immortalizing) ability is superior to any other known transforming virus. In spite of this, it lives in a virtually nonpathogenic equilibrium with the normal human host.

Following primary infection, the virus transforms a fraction of the B-cell population into proliferating immunoblasts. Similar to their in vitro transformed counterparts, they express nine viral proteins. Several of them are required for the stimulation of B-cell proliferation. Eight of the nine proteins are potentially immunogenic and can generate powerful CTLs. They are targeted against peptides derived from one or several of these proteins. The choice of the target in the newly infected young child depends on the HLA class I constitution of the host. This process usually goes unnoticed. If primary infection is delayed until adolescence or to adulthood by modern hygienic conditions, it leads to mononucleosis in about half of the cases. Rejection may fail in immunodeficient hosts, whereupon the proliferation of B blasts may take a lethal course. EBV-carrying blasts may also grow progressively. Immunodeficiency states of congenital (e.g., X-linked lymphoproliferative syndrome), iatrogenic (e.g., organ transplant recipients), and infectious (HIV) origin all are at risk. Immunoblastic disease usually starts as a polyclonal proliferation, but it may progress to

oligoclonal and then to monoclonal disease by as yet undefined events.

The origin of EBV-carrying BL is fundamentally different. It occurs in immunocompetent persons and is monoclonal from its inception. BL cells do not resemble immunoblasts but are more like resting B cells with regard to ultrastructure and marker equipment. They invariably carry a chromosomal translocation that has juxtaposed the c-*myc* protooncogene to one of the three immunoglobulin loci. Although the precise relationship and the relative timing of EBV infection and chromosomal translocation have not been defined in association with the developmental history of the BL precursor cells, both the biology of translocation and the EBV latency can be seen in a scenario where the CTL-mediated rejection of the virally transformed immunoblasts is followed by the silent persistence of the virus in the resting B-cell fraction. There, it expresses EBNA1 only, required for viral episome maintenance, but no potentially immunogenic proteins.[5] EBNA1 is apparently unable to induce a CTL response. As long as the cell maintains a resting phenotype, akin to a virgin or memory B cell, it is not recognized by the host rejection response. Following blast transformation, it expresses the highly immunogenic EBNA2 to 6 and LMPs and is promptly rejected. Such periodic activation may explain the maintenance of a sensitized state to the growth transformation–associated proteins in healthy seropositive persons.

It appears likely that most of the high endemic BLs originate in EBV-carrying resting cells where a chromosomal translocation has occurred during the immunoglobulin rearrangement process, accidentally juxtaposing c-*myc* to one of the three Ig loci. This leads to the deregulated, constitutive expression of c-*myc* that prevents the cell from leaving the cycling compartment. A phenotypically resting B cell that is not resting has a number of properties that prevent immune elimination. In addition to the previously mentioned eclipse of EBNA2 to 6 and LMP, adhesion molecules and certain MHC class I antigens are downregulated as well. In addition, BL cells process antigen much less effectively than do immunoblasts. All this contributes to the "cellular escape" of BL.

This scenario, and the added fact that some of the high endemic and most of the sporadic BLs are EBV negative, raises questions about the way in which EBV may contribute to the etiology of the lymphoma. The fact that EBV-carrying B cells represent only a small minority of the total B-cell population even in persons with high EBV antibody titers who live in the endemic region, the 97% EBV positivity of the African BLs must mean, ipso facto, that the probability of the lymphomatous transformation is greater in the EBV-carrying than in the EBV-negative B cell. This implies that the virus contributes to the etiology of the high endemic African form. The same argument does not apply equally to the HIV-associated BLs that carry EBV in about 30% and exhibit the molecular geometry of the sporadic rather than the high endemic BL-associated Ig/*myc* translocations (for review, see reference 10). This suggests that different cofactors act on different B-cell subcompartments. Chronic holoendemic or hyperendemic malaria is the most likely cofactor in the high endemic African form, whereas HIV itself or the opportunistic infections associated with it may act in the ARLs.

By what mechanism could the EBV carrier status increase the probability of BL development? It could act directly or indirectly. In an indirect scenario, it would expand the target cell population at risk by extending the life span of the infected lymphocyte and increasing the number of cell divisions prior to its elimination from the B-cell pool. Alternatively, it could contribute to the oncogenic process directly. This effect would have to be mediated by EBNA1, the only virally encoded protein expressed in the BL cell. This possibility is supported by two findings: EBNA1 transgenic mice were found to develop B-cell lymphomas with a high frequency.[117] Preliminary experiments by Magrath have suggested, moreover, that EBNA1 may exert a transactivating effect on compounded Ig/*myc* sequences (Magrath, I, personal communication, 1995).

Little can be said about the involvement of EBV in HD and T-cell lymphomas. The fact that the neoplastic cell clones carry EBV that has infected the cells on a single occasion, as indicated by the terminal repeat hybridization test, is in line with the assumption that the viral infection preceded the appearance of the neoplastic clone and that the virus is, therefore, somehow involved in the causation of the tumor. Since the interaction of the virus with the normal precursor cells of these tumors has not been defined, it is premature to speculate about the nature of this involvement.

REFERENCES

1. Hunsmann G, Hinuma Y: Human adult T-cell leukemia virus and its association with disease. Adv Viral Oncology 1985; 5:147.
2. Miller G: Biology of Epstein-Barr virus. *In* Klein G (ed): Viral Oncology. New York, Raven Press, 1980, pp 713–738.
3. Klein G, Svedmyr E, Jondal M, et al: EBV-determined nuclear antigen (EBNA)-positive cells in the peripheral blood of infectious mononucleosis patients. Int J Cancer 1976; 17:26.
4. Lewin N, Aman P, Masucci MG, et al: Characterization of EBV-carrying B-cell populations in healthy seropositive individuals with regard to density, release of transforming virus, and spontaneous outgrowth. Int J Cancer 1987; 39:472.
5. Chen F, Zou J-Z, Di Renzo L, et al: A subpopulation of latently EBV-infected normal B cells resembles Burkitt lymphoma (BL) cells in expressing EBNA1 but not EBNA2 or LMP1. Submitted for publication.
6. Klein G: Epstein-Barr virus (EBV) strategy in normal and neoplastic B cells [Minireview]. Cell 1994; 77:791.
7. Masucci MG, Ernberg I: Epstein-Barr virus: Adaptation to a life within the immune system. Trends Microbiol 1994; 2:125.
8. Gordon J, Cairns JA: Autocrine regulation of normal and malignant B lymphocytes. Adv Ca Res 1991; 56:313.
9. Henderson S, Rowe M, Gregory C, et al: Induction of *bcl*-2 expression by Epstein-Barr virus latent membrane protein 1 protects infected B cells from programmed cell death. Cell 1991; 65:1107.
10. Magrath I: The pathogenesis of Burkitt's lymphoma. Adv Cancer Res 1990; 55:133.
11. Henle G, Henle W: The virus as the etiologic agent of infectious mononucleosis. *In* Epstein MA, Achong BG (eds): The Epstein-Barr Virus. Berlin, Springer-Verlag, 1979, pp 297–320.
12. Svedmyr E, Ernberg I, Seeley J, et al: Virologic, immunologic, and clinical observations on a patient during the incubation, acute, and convalescent phases of infectious mononucleosis. Clin Immunol Immunopathol 1984; 30:437.
13. Purtilo DT, Sakamoto K, Barnabei V, et al: Epstein-Barr virus–induced diseases in boys with the X-linked lymphoproliferative syndrome (XLP). Am J Med 1982; 73:49.
14. Rickinson AB, Murray RJ, Brooks J, et al: T-cell recognition of Epstein-Barr virus–associated lymphomas. Cancer Surv 1992; 13:53.
15. Cleary ML, Sklar J: Lymphoproliferative disorders in cardiac transplant recipients are multiclonal lymphoma. Lancet 1993; 2:489.
16. Kaplan MA, Ferry JA, Harris NL, et al: Clonal analysis of posttransplant lymphoproliferative disorders, using both episomal Epstein-Barr virus and immunoglobulin genes as markers. Am J Clin Pathol 1994; 101:590.
17. Gratama JW, Zutter MM, Minarovits J, et al: Expression of Epstein-Barr virus–encoded growth transformation–associated proteins in lymphoproliferations of bone marrow transplant recipients. Int J Cancer 1991; 47:188.
18. Young LC, Alfieri C, Hennesey K, et al: Expression of Epstein-Barr virus transformation-associated genes in tissues of patients with EBV lymphoid proliferative diseases. N Engl J Med 1989; 321:1080.
19. Gaidano G, Dalla-Favera R: Molecular biology of lymphoid neoplasms. *In* Mendelsohn J, Howley PM, Israel MA, Liotta LA (eds): The Molecular Basis of Cancer. Philadelphia, WB Saunders, 1995, pp 251–279.
20. Gaidano G, Parsa NZ, Tassi V, et al: In vitro establishment of AIDS-related lymphoma cell lines: Phenotypic characterization, oncogene and tumor suppressor gene lesions, and heterogeneity in Epstein-Barr virus infection. Leukemia 1993; 7:1621.
21. Nalesnik MA, Jaffe R, Starzl TE, et al: The pathology of host transplant lymphoproliferative disorders occurring in the setting of cyclosporin A–prednisone immunosuppression. Am J Pathol 1988; 133:173.
22. Ho M, Jaffe R, Miller G, et al: The frequency of Epstein-Barr virus infection and associated lymphoproliferative syndrome after transplantation and its manifestation in children. Transplantation 1988; 45:719.
23. Penn I: Cancers following cyclosporine therapy. Transplantation 1987; 43:32.
24. Shearer WT, Ritz J, Finegold MJ, et al: Epstein-Barr virus–associated B-cell proliferations of diverse clonal origins after bone marrow transplantation in a 12-year-old patient with severe combined immunodeficiency. N Engl J Med 1985; 312:1151.
25. Hickey DP, Nalesnik MA, Vivas CA, et al: Renal retransplantation in patients who lost their allografts during management of previous post-transplant lymphoproliferative disease. Clin Transplant 1990; 4:187.
26. Shapiro RS, McClain K, Frizzera G, et al: Epstein-Barr virus–associated B-cell lymphoproliferative disorders following bone marrow transplantation. Blood 1988; 71:1234.
27. Leblond V, Sutton L, Dorent R, et al: Lymphoproliferative disorders after organ transplantation. J Clin Oncol 1995; 13:961.
28. Papadopoulos EB, Ladanyi M, Emanuel D, et al: Infusions of donor leukocytes to treat Epstein-Barr virus–associated lymphoproliferative disorders after allogeneic bone marrow transplantation. N Engl J Med 1994; 330:1185.
29. Klein G: Multiple phenotypic consequences of the Ig/*myc* translocation in B-cell–derived tumors. Genes Chromosom Cancer 1989; 1:3.
30. Nilsson K, Pontén J: Classification and biological nature of established human hematopoietic cell lines. Int J Cancer 1975; 15:321.
31. Gregory CD: Epstein-Barr virus and B-cell survival. Med Virol 1992; 2:205.
32. Rowe M, Rowe DT, Gregory CD, et al: Differences in B-cell growth phenotype reflect novel patterns of Epstein-Barr virus latent gene expression in Burkitt's lymphoma cells. EMBO J 1987; 6:2743.
33. Woisetschlaeger M, Strominger JL, Speck SH: Mutually exclusive use of viral promoters in Epstein-Barr virus latently infected lymphocytes. Proc Natl Acad Sci U S A 1989; 86:6489.
34. Sample J, Henson EBD, Sample C: The Epstein-Barr virus nuclear protein 1 promoter active in type I latency is autoregulated. J Virol 1992; 66:4654.
35. Hu LF, Chen F, Altiok E, et al: Cell phenotype–dependent alternative splicing of EBNA mRNAs in EBV-carrying cells. J Gen Virol, in press.
36. Hu LF, Minarovits J, Cao SL, et al: Variable expression of latent membrane protein in nasopharyngeal carcinoma can be related to methylation status of the Epstein-Barr virus BNLF-1 5′-flanking region. J Virol 1991; 65:1558.
37. Minarovits J, Minarovits-Kormuta S, Ehlin-Henriksson B, et al: Host cell phenotype–dependent methylation patterns of Epstein-Barr virus DNA. J Gen Virol 1991; 72:1591.
38. Contreras-Brodin B, Anvret M, Imreh S, et al: B cell phenotype–dependent expression of the Epstein-Barr virus nuclear antigens EBNA-2 to EBNA-6: Studies with somatic cell hybrids. J Gen Virol 1991; 72:3025.
39. Andersson ML, Stam NJ, Klein G, et al: Aberrant expression HLA class I antigens in Burkitt lymphoma cells. Int J Cancer 1991; 47:544.

40. Burkitt D: Etiology of Burkitt's lymphoma—an alternative hypothesis to a vectored virus. J Natl Ca Inst 1969; 42:19.

41. Adams JM, Harris AW, Pinker CA, et al: The c-*myc* oncogene driven by immunoglobulin enhancers induces lymphoid malignancy in transgenic mice. Nature 1985; 318:533.

42. Pedersen C, Gerstoft J, Lundgren JD, et al: HIV-associated lymphoma: Histopathology and association with Epstein-Barr virus genome related to clinical, immunological, and prognostic features. Eur J Cancer 1991; 27:1416.

43. Axelson H, Henriksson M, Wang Y, et al: The amino-terminal phosphorylation sites of c-*myc* are frequently mutated in lymphomas but not in mouse plasmacytomas. Submitted for publication.

44. Henriksson M, Bakardjiev A, Klein G, et al: Phosphorylation site mutants in the transactivating domain of c-*myc* modulate its function. Oncogene 1993; 8:3199.

45. Farrel P, Allan GJ, Shanahan F, et al: p53 is frequently mutated in Burkitt's lymphoma cell lines. EMBO J 1991; 10:2879.

46. Gaidano G, Ballerini P, Gong JZ, et al: p53 mutations in human lymphoid malignancies: Association with Burkitt lymphoma and chronic lymphocytic leukemia. Proc Natl Acad Sci U S A 1991; 88:5413.

47. Wiman KG, Magnusson KP, Ramqvist T, et al: Mutant p53 detected in a majority of Burkitt lymphoma cell lines by monoclonal antibody PAb240. Oncogene 1991; 6:1633.

48. Burkitt DP, Kyalwazi SK: Spontaneous remission of African lymphoma. Br J Cancer 1967; 21:14.

49. Rooney CM, Edwards CF, Lenoir GM, et al: Differential activation of cytotoxic responses by Burkitt's lymphoma (BL) cell lines: Relationship to the BL-cell surface phenotype. Cell Immunol 1986; 102:99.

50. Rooney CM, Rickinson AB, Moss DJ, et al: Paired Epstein-Barr virus–carrying lymphoma and lymphoblastoid cell lines from Burkitt's lymphoma patients: Comparative sensitivity to non-specific and to allo-specific cytotoxic responses in vitro. Int J Cancer 1984; 34:339.

51. de Campos-Lima PO, Torsteinsdottir S, Cuomo L, et al: Antigen processing and presentation by EBV-carrying cell lines: Cell-phenotype dependence and influence of the EBV-encoded LMP1. Int J Cancer 1993; 53:856.

52. Avila-Carino J, Torsteinsdottir S, Ehlin-Henriksson B, et al: Paired Epstein-Barr virus (EBV)-negative and EBV-converted Burkitt lymphoma lines: Stimulatory capacity in allogeneic mixed lymphocyte cultures. Int J Cancer 1987; 40:691.

52a. Janz S, Müller J, Shaughnessy J, et al: Detection of recombinations between c-*myc* and immunoglobulin switch alpha in murine plasma cell tumors and preneoplastic lesions by polymerase chain reaction. Proc Natl Acad Sci U S A 1993; 90:7361.

53. Gregory CD, Murray RJ, Edwards CF, et al: Down regulation of cell adhesion molecules LFA-3 and ICAM-1 in Epstein-Barr virus–positive Burkitt's lymphoma underlies tumour cell escape from virus-specific T-cell surveillance. J Exp Med 1988; 167:1811.

54. Masucci MG, Torsteinsdottir S, Colombani J, et al: Down-regulation of class I HLA antigens and of the Epstein-Barr virus-encoded latent membrane protein in Burkitt lymphoma lines. Proc Nat Acad Sci U S A 1987; 84:4567.

55. Beral V, Peterman T, Berkelman R, et al: AIDS-associated non-Hodgkin lymphoma. Lancet 1991; 337:805.

56. Ballerini P, Gaidano G, Gong JZ, et al: Multiple genetic lesions in acquired immunodeficiency syndrome–related non-Hodgkin's lymphoma. Blood 1993; 81:166.

57. Pelicci P-G, Knowles DM II, Arlin ZA, et al: Multiple monoclonal B cell expansions and c-*myc* oncogene rearrangements in acquired immunodeficiency syndrome–related lymphoproliferative disorders: Implications for lymphomagenesis. J Exp Med 1986; 164:2049.

58. Shibata D, Weiss LM, Nathwani BN, et al: Epstein-Barr virus in benign lymph node biopsies from individuals infected with the human immunodeficiency virus is associated with concurrent or subsequent development of non-Hodgkin's lymphoma. Blood 1991; 77:1527.

59. Neri A, Barriga F, Inghirami G, et al: Epstein-Barr virus infection precedes clonal expansion in Burkitt's and acquired immunodeficiency syndrome–associated lymphoma. Blood 1991; 77:1092.

60. Karp JE, Broder S: Acquired immunodeficiency syndrome and non-Hodgkin's lymphomas. Cancer Res 1991; 51:4743.

61. MacMahon EME, Glass JD, Hayward SD, et al: Epstein-Barr virus in AIDS-related primary central nervous system lymphoma. Lancet 1991; 338:969.

62. Giovanella BC, Nilsson K, Zech L, et al: Growth of diploid, Epstein-Barr virus–carrying human lymphoblastoid cell lines heterotransplanted into nude mice under immunologically privileged conditions. Int J Cancer 1979; 24:103.

63. Nilsson K, Giovanella BC, Stehlin JS, et al: Tumorgenicity of human hematopoietic cell lines in athymic nude mice. Int J Cancer 1977; 19:337.

64. Hamilton-Dutoit SJ, Raphael M, Audouin J, et al: In situ demonstration of Epstein-Barr virus small RNAs (EBER 1) in acquired immunodeficiency syndrome–related lymphomas: Correlation with tumor morphology and primary site. Blood 1993; 82:619.

65. Hamilton-Dutoit SJ, Rea D, Raphael M, et al: Epstein-Barr virus latent gene expression and tumor cell phenotype in AIDS-related non-Hodgkin's lymphoma: Correlation of lymphoma phenotype with three distinct patterns of viral latency. Am J Pathol 1993; 143:1072.

66. Geddes JF, Bhattacharjee MB, Savage K, et al: Primary cerebral lymphomas: A study of 47 cases probed for Epstein-Barr virus genome. J Clin Pathol 1992; 45:587.

67. Hamilton-Dutoit SJ, Pallesen G: A survey of Epstein-Barr virus (EBV) gene expression in sporadic non-Hodgkin's lymphomas: Detection of EBV in a subset of peripheral T-cell lymphomas. Am J Pathol 1992; 140:1315.

68. Young LS, Finerty S, Brooks L, et al: Epstein-Barr virus gene expression in malignant lymphomas induced by experimental virus infection of cottontop tamarins. J Virol 1989; 63:1967.

69. Rowe M, Young LS, Crocker J, et al: Epstein-Barr virus (EBV)-associated lymphoproliferative disease in the SCID mouse model: Implications for the pathogenesis of EBV-positive lymphomas in man. J Exp Med 1991; 173:147.

70. Klein G: The Epstein-Barr virus. *In* Kaplan AS (ed): The Herpesviruses. New York, Academic Press, 1973, pp 521–555.

71. Klein G: Epstein-Barr virus–carrying cells in Hodgkin's disease. Blood 1992; 80:299.

72. Herbst H, Steinbrecher E, Niedobitek G, et al: Distribution and phenotype of Epstein-Barr virus–harboring cells in Hodgkin's disease. Blood 1992; 80:484.

73. Johansson B, Klein G, Henle W, et al: Epstein-Barr virus (EBV)-associated antibody patterns in malignant lymphoma and leukemia. I: Hodgkin's disease. Int J Cancer 1970; 6:450.

74. Anagnostopoulos I, Herbst H, Niedobitek G, et al: Demonstration of monoclonal EBV genomes in Hodgkin's disease and Ki-1-positive anaplastic large cell lymphoma by combined Southern blot and in situ hybridization. Blood 1989; 74:810.

75. Brousset P: Detection of Epstein-Barr virus messenger RNA in Reed-Sternberg cells of Hodgkin's disease by in situ hybridization with biotinylated probes on sections. Blood 1991; 77:1781.

76. Coates PJ, Slavin G, D'Ardenne AJ: Persistence of Epstein-Barr virus in Reed-Sternberg cells throughout the course of Hodgkin's disease. J Pathol 1991; 164:291.

77. Guarner J, del Rio C, Hendrix L, et al: Composite Hodgkin's and non-Hodgkin's lymphoma in a patient with acquired immune deficiency syndrome: In-situ demonstration of Epstein-Barr virus. Cancer 1990; 66:796.

78. Herbst H, Niedobitek G, Kneba M, et al: High incidence of Epstein-Barr virus genomes in Hodgkin's disease. Am J Pathol 1990; 137:13.

79. Niedobitek G, Deacon EM, Young LS, et al: Epstein-Barr virus gene expression in Hodgkin's disease. Blood 1991; 78:1628.

80. Uccini S, Monardo F, Stoppacciaro A, et al: High frequency of Epstein-Barr virus genome detection in Hodgkin's disease in HIV-positive patients. Int J Cancer 1990; 46:581.

81. Uhara H, Sato Y, Mukai K, et al: Detection of Epstein-Barr virus DNA in Reed-Sternberg cells of Hodgkin's disease using the polymerase chain reaction and in situ hybridization. Jpn J Cancer Res 1990; 81:272.

82. Weiss LM, Strickler JG, Warnke RA, et al: Epstein-Barr viral DNA in tissues of Hodgkin's disease. Am J Pathol 1987; 129:86.

83. Weiss LM, Movahed LA, Warnke RA, et al: Detection of Epstein-Barr viral genomes in Reed-Sternberg cells of Hodgkin's disease. N Engl J Med 1989; 320:502.

84. Boiocchi M, Carbone A, De Re V, et al: Is the Epstein-Barr virus involved in Hodgkin's disease? Tumori 1989; 75:345.

85. Gledhill S, Gallagher A, Jones DB, et al: Viral involvement in Hodgkin's disease: Detection of clonal type A Epstein-Barr virus genomes in tumour samples. Br J Cancer 1991; 64:227.

86. Jarrett RF, Gallagher A, Jones DB, et al: Detection of Epstein-Barr virus genomes in Hodgkin's disease: Relation to age. J Clin Pathol 1991; 44:844.

87. Staal SP, Ambinder R, Beschorner WE, et al: A survey of Epstein-Barr virus DNA in lymphoid tissue: Frequent deletion in Hodgkin's disease. Am J Clin Pathol 1989; 91:1.

88. Pallesen G, Hamilton-Dutoit SJ, Rowe M, et al: Expression of Epstein-Barr virus (EBV) latent gene products in tumour cells of Hodgkin's disease. Lancet 1991; 337:320.

89. Deacon EM, Pallesen G, Niedobitek G, et al: Epstein-Barr virus and Hodgkin's disease: Transcriptional analysis of virus latency in the malignant cells. J Exp Med 1993; 177:339.

90. Delsol G, Brousset P, Chittal S, et al: Correlation of the expression of Epstein-Barr virus latent membrane protein and in situ hybridization with biotinylated BamHI-W probes in Hodgkin's disease. Am J Pathol 1992; 140:247.

91. Herbst H, Dallenbach F, Hummel M, et al: Epstein-Barr virus latent membrane protein expression in Hodgkin and Reed-Sternberg cells. Proc Natl Acad Sci U S A 1991; 88:4766.

92. Poppema S, van Imhoff G, Torensma M, et al: Lymphadenopathy morphologically consistent with Hodgkin's disease associated with Epstein-Barr virus infection. Am J Clin Pathol 1985; 84:385.

93. Zhou X, Hamilton-Dutoit SJ, Yan Q-H, et al: The association between Epstein-Barr virus and Chinese Hodgkin's disease. Int J Cancer 1993; 55:359.

94. Libetta CM, Pringle JH, Angel CA, et al: Demonstration of Epstein-Barr viral DNA in formalin-fixed, paraffin-embedded samples of Hodgkin's disease. J Pathol 1990; 161:255.

95. Vestlev PM, Pallesen G, Sandvej K, et al: Prognosis of Hodgkin's disease is not influenced by Epstein-Barr virus latent membrane protein. Int J Cancer 1992; 50:670.

96. Weinreb M, Day PJ, Murray PG, et al: Epstein-Barr virus (EBV) and Hodgkin's disease in children: Incidence of EBV latent membrane protein in malignant cells. J Pathol 1992; 168:365.

97. Munoz N, Davidson RJ, Witthoff B, et al: Infectious mononucleosis and Hodgkin's disease. Int J Cancer 1978; 22:10.

98. Rosdahl N, Larsen SO, Clemmesen J: Hodgkin's disease in patients with previous infectious mononucleosis: 30 years' experience. Br Med J 1974; 2:253.

99. Knecht H, Bachmann E, Brousset P, et al: Deletions within the LMP1 oncogene of Epstein-Barr virus are clustered in Hodgkin's disease and identical to those observed in nasopharyngeal carcinoma. Blood 1993; 82:2937.

100. Jones CH, Shurin S, Aabramowsky C, et al: T-cell lymphomas containing Epstein-Barr viral DNA in patients with chronic Epstein-Barr virus infections. N Engl J Med 1988; 318:733.

101. Anagnostopoulos I, Hummel M, Finn T, et al: Heterogeneous Epstein-Barr virus infection patterns in peripheral T-cell lymphoma of angioimmunoblastic lymphadenopathy type. Blood 1992; 80:1804.

102. Chan JKC, Ng CS, Lau WH, et al: Most nasal/nasopharyngeal lymphomas are peripheral T-cell neoplasms. Am J Surg Pathol 1987; 11:418.

103. Chott A, Rappersberger K, Schlossarek W, et al: Peripheral T-cell lymphoma presenting primarily as lethal midline granuloma. Hum Pathol 1988; 19:1093.

104. Hastrup N, Hamilton-Dutoit S, Ralfkiaer E, et al: Peripheral T-cell lymphomas: An evaluation of reproducibility of the updated Kiel classification. Histopathology 1991; 18:99.

105. Ohshima K, Kikkuchi M, Eguchi F, et al: Analysis of Epstein-Barr viral genomes in lymphoid malignancy using Southern blotting, polymerase chain reaction, and in situ hybridization. Virchows Arch B Cell Pathol Incl Mol Pathol 1990; 59:383.

106. Ott G, Ott MM, Feller AC, et al: Prevalence of Epstein-Barr virus DNA in different T-cell lymphoma entities in a European population. Int J Cancer 1992; 51:562.

107. Su IJ, Tsai TF, Cheng AL, Chen CC: Cutaneous manifestations of Epstein-Barr virus–associated T-cell lymphoma. J Am Acad Dermatol 1993; 29:685.

108. Pallesen G, Hamilton-Dutoit SJ, Zhou X: The association of Epstein-Barr virus (EBV) with T-cell lymphoproliferations and Hodgkin's disease: Two new developments in the EBV field. Adv Cancer Res 1993; 62:179.

109. De Bruin PC, Jiwa M, Oudejans JJ, et al: Presence of Epstein-Barr virus in extranodal T-cell lymphomas: Differences in relation to site. Blood 1994; 83:1612.

110. Tokunaga M, Land CE, Uemura Y, et al: Epstein-Barr virus in gastric carcinoma. Am J Pathol 1993; 143:1250.

111. De Bruin PC, Jiwa NM, Van der Valk P, et al: Detection of Epstein-Barr virus nucleic acid sequences and protein in nodal T-cell lymphomas: Relation between latent membrane protein-1 positivity and clinical course. Histopathology 1993; 23:509.

112. Kumar S, Kumar D, Kingma DW, et al: Epstein-Barr virus–associated T-cell lymphoma in a renal transplant patient. Am J Surg Pathol 1993; 17:1046.

113. Tien H-F, Su I-J, Chuang S-M, et al: Cytogenetic characterization of Epstein-Barr virus–associated T-cell malignancies. Cancer Genet Cytogenet 1993; 69:25.

114. Su I-J, Hsiech H-C, Lin K-H, et al: Aggressive peripheral T-cell lymphomas containing Epstein-Barr viral DNA: A clinicopathologic and molecular analysis. Blood 1991; 77:799.

115. Mori M, Kurozumi H, Akagi K, et al: Monoclonal proliferation of T cells containing Epstein-Barr virus in fatal mononucleosis. N Engl J Med 1992; 327:58.

116. Minarovits J, Hu L-F, Imai S, et al: Clonality, expression, and methylation patterns of the Epstein-Barr virus genomes in lethal midline granulomas classified as peripheral angiocentric T cell lymphomas. J Gen Virol 1994; 75:77.

117. Wilson JB, Levine AJ: The oncogenic potential of Epstein-Barr virus nuclear antigen 1 in transgenic mice. Curr Top Microbiol Immunol 1992; 182:375.

PATHOLOGY

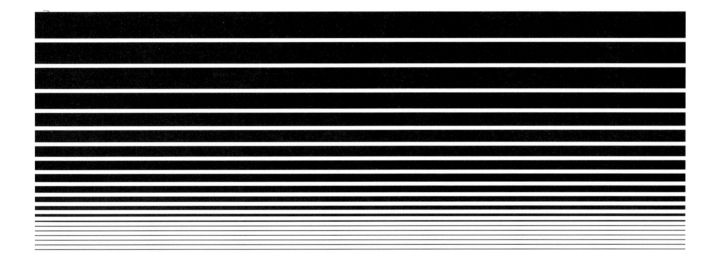

Histopathology of the Non-Hodgkin's Lymphomas and Hodgkin's Disease

Elaine S. Jaffe

The classification of the malignant lymphomas has undergone significant reappraisal over the past 40 years. These changes have resulted from insights gained through the application of immunologic and molecular techniques, as well as a better understanding of the clinical aspects of lymphoma through advances in diagnosis, staging, and treatment. At one point lymphomas were seen as no more than four generic types: lymphosarcoma, reticulum cell sarcoma, giant follicle lymphoma, and Hodgkin's disease (HD); however, many additional distinct entities are now recognized. Each variant can be distinguished by a combination of morphologic, immunophenotypic, and genotypic analyses, and each is associated with a characteristic clinical behavior, pattern of spread, and response to therapy.

NON-HODGKIN'S LYMPHOMAS[1]

Historically, the Rappaport classification, first introduced in 1956, divided lymphomas according to pattern, either nodular or diffuse, and then according to cell type, based on the degree to which the lymphoid cells morphologically resembled either normal lymphocytes or histiocytes.[1] The advances in immunology that occurred in the 1970s made it apparent that this approach was flawed and that the cells termed "histiocytic" were mostly transformed lymphocytes. In addition, the recognition of T cells, B cells, and various other subsets made it reasonable to see lymphomas in functional terms, each deriving from a unique cell type. Both the Kiel classification, proposed by Karl Lennert and colleagues,[2, 3] and the Lukes-Collins scheme[4] were immunologically based, although at the time immunologic techniques were still in their infancy, and monoclonal antibodies as a diagnostic tool were not yet available.

By the 1970s, six different classifications had been proposed, and at least four were in general use: the Rappaport (Table 5–1) and Lukes-Collins schemes in the United States; the Kiel classification (Table 5–2) in Europe;

and the classification of the British National Lymphoma Investigation (BNLI) in Great Britain.[5] Although several meetings attended by pathologists and clinicians were held in an attempt to reach consensus (in London, England; Florence, Italy; and Airlie, Virginia), no agreement could be reached. The National Cancer Institute (NCI) responded by sponsoring a study to test each of the classification schemes, using a data base containing clinical data from approximately 1200 cases of lymphoma treated on prospective clinical trials from four different institutions.[6]

This NCI study indicated that each of the schemes could segregate the tumors into broad groups of low, intermediate, and high clinical grade, as determined by survival in the test group of cases.[6] No one scheme appeared superior to any other. Moreover, the study demonstrated both a relatively high lack of reproducibility by individual pathologists (0.53 to 0.93), when confronted by the same slides on a second review, as well as a low rate of concordance among the various pathologists (0.21 to 0.65) in trying to reproduce diagnoses within a given scheme. The pathologists were restricted to only routine hematoxylin and eosin–stained sections and limited clinical information (age, sex, and anatomic site). Nevertheless, the clinicians involved in this study reached the conclusion that "clinical outcome" was a reasonable basis for a lymphoma classification scheme, since agreement could not be achieved regarding the individual pathologic entities.

The participants proposed the Working Formulation (WF) for the non-Hodgkin's lymphomas (NHLs) based on the clinical and pathologic findings (Table 5–3). The original intent was to have the WF serve as a common language to translate among classifications and not to serve a free-standing classification scheme. However, because it was a convenient guide to therapy, it quickly became popular among clinicians and was adopted for use in many centers in the United States for clinical trials. In reality the WF was in essence the Rappaport scheme. It substituted the term "large cell" for "histiocytic" and divided the histiocytic lymphomas of the Rappaport scheme into two subgroups:

Table 5–1. Modified Rappaport Classification

Nodular

Lymphocytic, poorly differentiated
Mixed lymphocytic-histiocytic
Histiocytic

Diffuse

Lymphocytic, well-differentiated
Lymphocytic, intermediate differentiation
Lymphocytic, poorly differentiated
Mixed lymphocytic-histiocytic
Undifferentiated, Burkitt's type
Undifferentiated, non-Burkitt's type
Histiocytic
Lymphoblastic

large cell and large cell immunoblastic. This separation split the histiocytic lymphomas among the intermediate- and high-grade categories, a division that has been controversial and not supported as justified by subsequent analyses.

Another more basic flaw in the WF is that it is a classification based on treatment outcome, not the recognition of individual disease entities or cell of origin for a malignant neoplasm. This conceptual approach is a significant deviation from the way in which classification systems have been developed for other organ systems. It lumps diseases that share a similar cell size and survival into single categories and splits diseases with variations in cytologic composition and clinical grade into separate categories.

It is apparent that major differences exist in the incidence of lymphoma subtypes, as well as other cancers, in different geographic regions and among different racial and ethnic populations. To pursue these epidemiologic differences, standardized classifications of disease should be employed on a worldwide basis. More important, precise identification of disease entities is required to gain insight into pathogenesis. Although the WF is a useful scheme for the oncologist in providing clinical groupings as a guide to therapy, it does not for the most part delineate disease entities. In recent years there have been many advances in lymphoma patho-

Table 5–2. Kiel Classification, 1974

Low-Grade Malignancy

Lymphocytic
Lymphoplasmacytoid
Centrocytic
Centroblastic-centrocytic
    Follicular
    Follicular and diffuse
    Diffuse

High-Grade Malignancy

Centroblastic
Lymphoblastic
    Burkitt's type
    Convoluted cell type
Immunoblastic

Table 5–3. Working Formulation for Clinical Usage

Low Grade

A. Malignant lymphoma, small lymphocytic
        Consistent with CLL
        Plasmacytoid
B. Malignant lymphoma, follicular, predominantly small cleaved cell
        Diffuse areas
        Sclerosis
C. Malignant lymphoma, follicular, mixed, small cleaved and large cell
        Diffuse areas
        Sclerosis

Intermediate Grade

D. Malignant lymphoma, follicular, predominantly large cell
        Diffuse areas
        Sclerosis
E. Malignant lymphoma, diffuse, small cleaved cell
        Sclerosis
F. Malignant lymphoma, diffuse, mixed, small and large cell
        Sclerosis
        Epithelioid cell component
G. Malignant lymphoma, diffuse, large cell
        Cleaved cell
        Noncleaved cell
        Sclerosis

High Grade

H. Malignant lymphoma, large cell, immunoblastic
        Plasmacytoid
        Clear cell
        Polymorphous
        Epithelioid cell component
I. Malignant lymphoma, lymphoblastic
        Convoluted cell
        Nonconvoluted cell
J. Malignant lymphoma, small noncleaved cell
        Burkitt's
        Follicular areas

Miscellaneous

Composite
Mycosis fungoides
Histiocytic
Extramedullary plasmacytoma
Unclassifiable
Other

CLL, chronic lymphocytic leukemia.

genesis (Table 5–4). Most of these diseases, other than follicular lymphoma and Burkitt's lymphoma, are not identified in the WF. Therefore, clinical and epidemiologic studies employing the WF are limited in their ability to identify differences in the clinical behavior and incidence of individual lymphoma subtypes and hamper further studies of lymphoma biology.

Of the classifications originally tested in the NCI study,[6] only the Kiel classification has remained in widespread use, mainly in Europe and Asia. It is a functionally based classification, which divides tumors mainly according to their cell of origin, as well as other cytologic features. Several revisions have been published in recent years, with the addition of some of the more newly described entities, such as anaplastic large cell lymphoma (ALCL) (Table 5–5).

Table 5–4. Pathogenic Insights Based on a Disease-Oriented Approach to Lymphoma Classification

Disease	Pathogenesis/Cofactor	Epidemiology
Burkitt's	EBV, malaria, immunodeficiency, *cMYC* aberrations	Endemic vs. sporadic in North America
Adult T-cell leukemia/lymphoma	HTLV-I	SW Japan, Caribbean
MALT lymphomas	*Helicobacter*, genetic predisposition	Feltre, Italy
Nasal T/NK lymphoma	Genetics, EBV	Asia, Central and South America
Follicular lymphoma	*BCL2* overexpression, ? genetic predisposition	United States and Western Europe
Mantle cell lymphoma	*PRAD1* overexpression	Southern Europe
Anaplastic large cell lymphoma	*NPM/ALK* fusion	Unknown

NK, natural killer; EBV, Epstein-Barr virus; MALT, mucosal-associated lymphoid tissue.

However, several aspects of the Kiel scheme have not been universally accepted. For one, it is intended for nodal lymphomas only. It has become apparent that lymphomas arising in extranodal sites, whether they be of T-cell or B-cell origin, are often distinct and do not represent simply secondary spread of nodal disease. Moreover, its adherence to a relatively pure cytologic approach limits its usefulness in the delineation of certain diseases, such as nasal T/natural killer (NK) cell lymphoma, and adult T-cell leukemia/lymphoma, both of which are distinguished in part by their modes of presentation, epidemiology, and respective etiologic agents, Epstein-Barr virus (EBV) and the human T-cell lymphotropic virus type I (HTLV-I).[7, 8] Moreover, its failure to subclassify or grade follicular lymphomas has made it unpopular in the United States, where follicular lymphoma is the most common single disease, accounting for at least 40% of all NHLs. By contrast, it attempts to delineate several different subtypes of large B-cell lymphoma and several morphologic variants of node-based peripheral T-cell lymphoma. It remains to be shown that these distinctions are reproducible by others and whether they are biologically or clinically relevant.

This chapter uses the classification scheme proposed by the International Lymphoma Study Group (ILSG), which is a revision of former European and American schemes (Table 5–6). This scheme recognizes that the cell of origin, principally T cell or B cell, must be the starting point of any modern classification scheme. Stage of differentiation is also important, although in many instances the precise stage of differentiation is unknown. The classification delineates individual disease entities, based on morphologic features, immunophenotype and/or stage of differentiation, genotype, etiology, epidemiology, and clinical behavior. In many instances several different entities are contained within a single WF category and share some clinical characteristics, such as an indolent (low-grade) or aggressive (intermediate- or high-grade) natural history. Many of the entities are also recognized in the Kiel classification. Therefore, both the designation adopted by the ILSG as well as the most equivalent terms in the WF and Kiel classification are provided.

The ILSG classification recognizes that many distinct lymphoma entities have a range in histologic grade and clinical aggressiveness. This point is exemplified by the follicle center lymphomas (FCLs) (follicular lymphoma in the WF). FCL is recognized as a single disease entity, with a common molecular pathogenesis, in most instances. However, variations in cytologic grade are a valid basis for stratifying patients for therapy. A similar point can be made for many of the entities in the ILSG scheme. As a guide to therapy, the predominant clinical behavior for each of the subtypes is provided (Table 5–7). Patients could be stratified according to these clinical groupings for clinical trials, as is commonly done for the low-, intermediate-, and high-grade

Table 5–5. Updated Kiel Classification of Non-Hodgkin's Lymphomas, 1992

B-Cell	T-Cell
Low-Grade Malignant Lymphomas	
Lymphocytic	Lymphocytic
Chronic lymphocytic leukemia	Chronic lymphocytic leukemia
Prolymphocytic leukemia	Prolymphocytic leukemia
Hairy cell leukemia	Small cell, cerebriform
Lymphoplasmacytic/cytoid (immunocytoma)	Mycosis fungoides/Sézary syndrome
Plasmacytic	Lymphoepithelioid (Lennert's lymphoma)
Centroblastic-centrocytic (follicular ± diffuse; diffuse)	Angioimmunoblastic
Centrocytic (mantle cell)	T-zone lymphoma
Monocytoid, including marginal zone cell	Pleomorphic, small cell (HTLV-I±)
High-Grade Malignant Lymphomas	
Centroblastic	Pleomorphic, medium-sized and large cell (HTLV-I±)
Immunoblastic	Immunoblastic (HTLV-I±)
Burkitt's lymphoma	Large cell anaplastic (Ki1+)
Large cell anaplastic (Ki1+)	
Lymphoblastic	Lymphoblastic

Other rare types of lymphoma may be separately identified for T-cell and B-cell lymphomas, respectively.

Table 5–6. Revised European-American Lymphoma Classification from the International Lymphoma Study Group

B-Cell Neoplasms

Precursor B-Cell Neoplasm
Precursor B-lymphoblastic leukemia/lymphoma

Peripheral B-Cell Neoplasms
1. B-cell CLL/PLL/SLL
2. Lymphoplasmacytoid lymphoma/immunocytoma
3. Mantle cell lymphoma
4. Follicle center lymphoma, follicular
   Provisional cytologic grades: I (small), II (mixed), III (large)
   Provisional subtype: diffuse, predominantly small cell
5. Marginal zone B-cell lymphoma
   Extranodal (MALT ± monocytoid B cells)
   Provisional category: Nodal (± monocytoid B cells)
6. Provisional entity: Splenic marginal zone lymphoma
7. Hairy cell leukemia
8. Plasmacytoma/myeloma
9. Diffuse large B-cell lymphoma
10. Burkitt's lymphoma
11. Provisional entity: High-grade B-cell lymphoma, Burkitt's-like

T-Cell and Putative NK-Cell Neoplasms

Precursor T-Cell Neoplasm
Precursor T-lymphoblastic leukemia/lymphoma

Peripheral T-Cell and NK-Cell Neoplasms
1. T-cell CLL/PLL
2. Large granular lymphocyte leukemia
3. Mycosis fungoides/Sézary syndrome
4. Peripheral T-cell lymphomas, unspecified
   Provisional categories: medium, mixed, large, lymphoepithelioid
   Provisional subtypes:
      Hepatosplenic γδT-cell lymphoma
      Subcutaneous panniculitic T-cell lymphoma
5. Adult T-cell lymphoma/leukemia
6. Angioimmunoblastic T-cell lymphoma
7. Angiocentric lymphoma/nasal T/NK-cell lymphoma
8. Intestinal T-cell lymphoma (± enteropathy)
9. Anaplastic large cell lymphoma (T/Null)
10. Provisional: ALCL Hodgkin's-like

Hodgkin's Disease

1. Lymphocyte predominance (nodular ± diffuse)
2. Nodular sclerosis
3. Mixed cellularity
4. Lymphocyte depletion
5. Lymphocyte-rich classic HD (provisional subtype)

See text for abbreviations.

categories of the WF, and yet analyzed separately to observe differences in response to therapy, patterns of relapse, or biologic parameters.

The ILSG classification also includes HD. Although the classification of HD has undergone relatively few revisions since the institution of the Rye modification of the Lukes-Butler scheme, it has become apparent that the cell of origin of HD is almost certainly a lymphoid cell. Moreover, identifying a sharp distinction between HD and NHL is often not possible. Instances of composite HD/NHL and sequential HD/NHL further indicate a close relationship.[9] Therefore, although for clinical purposes we segregate HD and NHL, conceptually it is appropriate for them to be included in any classification scheme of lymphomas. The

ILSG classification includes all lymphoid neoplasms. However, for the purposes of this chapter those entities other than the malignant lymphomas are touched on only briefly or are not discussed.

The ILSG classification is a significant achievement in that it represents a consensus achieved by 19 hematopathologists from diverse schools of thought. Many prior attempts at consensus over the past 25 years have been unsuccessful. We now have the objective immunophenotypic, molecular, and clinical data to resolve many former areas of controversy. However, even the ILSG classification must be regarded as provisional. Over the next few years, more than 50 hematopathologists will work together to arrive at a new classification to be sponsored by the World Health Organization. It is hoped that that document will produce a classification that not only will be widely accepted but will be capable of withstanding the test of time.

Table 5–7. Suggested Clinical Groupings of Entities Recognized by the International Lymphoma Study Group Classification

I. Indolent Lymphomas and Lymphoid Leukemias

B cell
   B-CLL/SLL
   Lymphoplasmacytoid lymphoma
   Follicle center lymphoma, follicular (small and mixed)
   Marginal zone B-cell lymphoma
   Hairy cell leukemia
   Plasmacytoma/myeloma
T cell
   Large granular lymphocyte leukemia
   ATL/L (smoldering)
   Mycosis fungoides/Sézary syndrome

II. Moderately Aggressive Lymphomas and Lymphoid Leukemias

B cell
   B-PLL
   Mantle cell lymphoma
   Follicle center lymphoma (follicular large cell)
T cell
   T-CLL/PLL
   ATL/L (chronic)
   Angiocentric lymphoma
   Angioimmunoblastic lymphoma

III. Aggressive Lymphomas

B cell
   Large B-cell lymphoma
T cell
   Peripheral T-cell lymphomas
   Intestinal T-cell lymphoma
   Anaplastic large cell lymphoma

IV. Highly Aggressive Lymphomas and Lymphoid Leukemias

B cell
   Precursor B-LBL/L
   Burkitt's lymphoma
   High-grade B-cell lymphoma, Burkitt's-like
T cell
   Precursor T-LBL/L
   ATLL (acute and lymphomatous)

See text for abbreviations.

B-CELL NEOPLASMS

Precursor B-Lymphoblastic Leukemia/Lymphoma (PB-LBL/L)

WF: malignant lymphoma, lymphoblastic
Kiel: lymphoblastic, B-cell type

Although most PB-LBL/Ls present as leukemia, lymphomatous presentations occur in approximately 5% to 10% of patients.[10–12] Frequent sites of involvement include lymph nodes, skin, and bone. Skin lesions in children frequently present in the head and neck region, including the scalp (Fig. 5–1).[10] Progression to leukemia occurs in most patients if a complete remission is not obtained. The disease is most common in children and young adults. This disease is considered the solid tumor equivalent of common acute lymphoblastic leukemia and pre-B-cell acute lymphoblastic leukemia.

Cytologically, it is composed of lymphoblasts that are usually somewhat larger than a small lymphocyte but smaller than the cells of large B-cell lymphoma.[13] The cells have

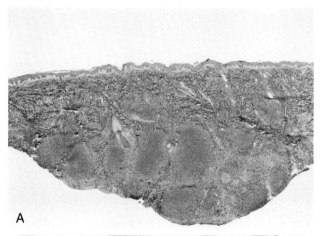

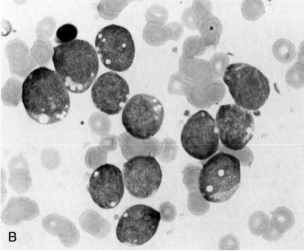

Figure 5–1. Precursor B-lymphoblastic leukemia/lymphoma. *A,* This scalp lesion was the initial presenting site of disease in this 10-year-old boy. The tumor infiltrates the reticular dermis but leaves a Grenz zone beneath the epidermis (hematoxylin-eosin, ×11.5). *B,* Peripheral blood involvement developed in this patient who presented with cutaneous disease (Giemsa-Wright, ×1000).

finely stippled chromatin with very sparse cytoplasm and inconspicuous nucleoli. The nuclei may be round or convoluted, and the presence or absence of nuclear convolutions is not useful in predicting immunophenotype in lymphoblastic malignancies. Mitotic figures are frequent, in keeping with the high-grade nature of this neoplasm.

The differential diagnosis of PB-LBL/L includes the blastic variant of a mantle cell lymphoma (MCL).[14] The cells of MCL usually have more abundant cytoplasm and some evidence of chromatin clumping. The clinical presentation is useful in that MCL is much more common in adults. In some patients immunophenotypic studies are required for the differential diagnosis. The blastic variant of MCL is negative for terminal deoxynucleotidyl transferase and has a mature B-cell phenotype, in contrast with PB-LBL/L.

B-Cell Chronic Lymphocytic Leukemia (B-CLL)
Prolymphocytic Leukemia (B-PLL)
Small Lymphocytic Lymphoma (B-SLL)

WF: small lymphocytic, consistent with CLL
Kiel: B-CLL, B-PLL, immunocytoma, lymphoplasmacytoid type

B-CLL usually presents in adults with generalized lymphadenopathy, frequent bone marrow and peripheral blood involvement, and often hepatosplenomegaly. Presentation as leukemia, that is, B-CLL, is more common than as lymphoma, that is, B-SLL. Even in patients with a lymphomatous presentation, careful examination of the peripheral blood may disclose a circulating monoclonal B-cell component. Nevertheless, there are some patients who present with generalized lymphadenopathy, and although progression to leukemia is frequent, it does not necessarily occur in all instances.[15]

Histologically, the lymph nodes involved by B-CLL show diffuse architectural effacement, although occasional residual naked germinal centers may be present (Fig. 5–2). In this regard, the process may simulate MCL but usually can be readily distinguished from MCL on cytologic grounds. Although the predominant cell is a small lymphocyte with clumped nuclear chromatin, usually a spectrum of nuclear morphology may be seen. Pseudofollicular growth centers or proliferation centers are present in most cases.[16] These proliferation centers contain a spectrum of cells ranging from small lymphocytes to larger prolymphocytes and paraimmunoblasts. The prolymphocytes and paraimmunoblasts have somewhat more dispersed chromatin and usually centrally placed prominent nucleoli. There is a moderate amount of amphophilic cytoplasm. Paraimmunoblasts are larger than prolymphocytes but in other respects are similar.

In some instances, the small lymphoid cells may show nuclear irregularity. This feature has caused confusion with MCL. However, the presence of pseudofollicles and paraimmunoblasts argues strongly in favor of a diagnosis of B-CLL over MCL. It has been shown that cases with cleaved nuclear morphology and pseudofollicles retain the indolent clinical behavior of B-CLL and not the more aggressive clinical course of MCL.[17, 18] If needed, immunophenotypic studies can be helpful in this differential diagnosis, since the cells of B-CLL are usually CD23+, whereas the cells of MCL are usually CD23−.

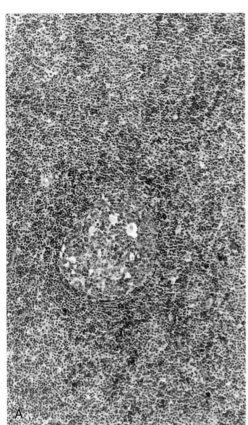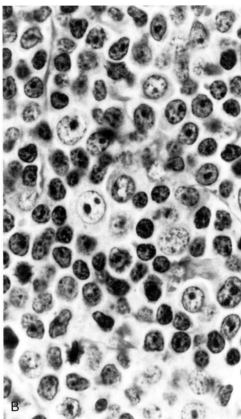

Figure 5–2. B-cell chronic lympho-cytic leukemia, lymph node. *A,* A residual naked germinal center is seen surrounded by a diffuse infil-trate (hematoxylin-eosin, ×200). *B,* Small lymphocytes are admixed with larger cells (prolymphocytes and paraimmunoblasts). Occasional cells show plasmacytoid differentia-tion (hematoxylin-eosin, ×1000).

Mitotic rate has been shown to be prognostically impor-tant in B-CLL/SLL. Although the presence of pseudofol-licles does not necessarily indicate a more aggressive clinical course, a high mitotic rate (>30 mitoses per 20 high-powered fields) is associated with more aggressive disease and shortened survival.[19] As with B-CLL, prolymphocytic trans-formation may occur in lymph nodes, and the endpoint in this process is an aggressive large B-cell lymphoma, so-called Richter's syndrome.[20] However, some of the large B-cell malignancies occurring in B-CLL/SLL appear to be second-ary, derived from a separate B-cell clone.

A Hodgkin's-like transformation has also been described in B-CLL/SLL. This transformation can take one of two forms. In some instances Reed-Sternberg cells and mono-nuclear variants are seen in a background of small, round B lymphocytes, consistent with B-CLL.[21] The process lacks the rich inflammatory background characteristic of HD, such as eosinophils, plasma cells, and histiocytes. However, patients with this type of Hodgkin's transformation appear to progress to a process that is more typical of HD, with loss of the B-cell small lymphocytic component. In other instances classic HD of the mixed cellularity or nodular sclerosis subtype may be seen in patients with a history of B-CLL.[22] Studies have implicated EBV in the HD type of Richter's transformation.[23] The Reed-Sternberg cells and variants are positive for EBV, and the implication is that they are derived from the underlying B-cell clone.

In some cases of B-CLL/SLL, limited plasmacytoid differentiation may occur.[24] The overall cytology may resemble that of B-CLL/SLL, but the cells contain moderate amounts of cytoplasmic immunoglobulin. In such cases a small monoclonal immunoglobulin spike may be detected in the serum. These cases conform to the lymphoplasmacytoid subtype of immunocytoma in the Kiel classification.[25] However, because such cases retain the immunophenotype of classic B-CLL, they are regarded in the ILSG classifica-tion as a variant of B-CLL.[26]

Lymphoplasmacytoid Lymphoma/Immunocytoma (LPL)

WF: small lymphocytic, plasmacytoid
Kiel: immunocytoma, lymphoplasmacytic type

LPL conforms in most patients to the clinical picture of Waldenström's macroglobulinemia. This is a disease of adult life that usually presents with generalized lymphadenopathy, vague constitutional symptoms, anemia, and splenomegaly. Autoimmune hemolytic anemia is a common complication. Immunoglobulin M (IgM) monoclonal gammopathy may be associated with increased serum viscosity leading to neuro-logic and vascular complications. Peripheral blood involve-ment with an absolute lymphocytosis is less common in LPL than in B-cell CLL/SLL.

The neoplastic cells in LPL show evidence of plasmacytic differentiation.[27, 28] They have been referred to as "lympho-plasmacytoid" because, while the cytoplasm assumes a distinctly plasmacytic appearance with amphophilic cyto-plasm and a perinuclear *HOF,* the nucleus retains the condensed nuclear chromatin characteristic of a lymphocyte (Fig. 5–3). Usually, a spectrum of plasmacytoid differentia-tion is seen, with the most plasmacytoid-appearing cells found in a perivascular and perisinusoidal location. Dutcher bodies are another characteristic cytologic feature of LPL. An interesting architectural feature of LPL is the tendency for lymphoid sinuses to be preserved and even congested and distended. This apparent preservation of nodal architecture may cause problems in diagnosis. However, careful examination usually reveals an absence of follicles and paracortical regions, indicating architectural effacement by the lymphoid neoplasm.

Those cells showing plasmacytoid differentiation can usually be demonstrated to contain cytoplasmic immunoglobulin, even in paraffin section immunohistochemistry. Immunophenotypically, this tumor lacks CD5 and by analogy can be related to a late stage in B-cell differentiation, just prior to the plasma cell stage.[29, 30] Conceptually, it can be related to a postfollicular medullary cord B cell, in contrast with B-CLL/SLL, which appears to be prefollicular in its stage of differentiation.[27]

Mantle Cell Lymphoma (MCL)

WF: diffuse or follicular, small cleaved cell (rarely diffuse large cleaved cell)
Kiel: centrocytic lymphoma

MCL is a distinct clinical pathologic entity that has been more precisely defined in recent years through the integration of immunophenotypic, molecular genetic, and clinicopathologic studies.[31, 32] This tumor had been recognized in the Kiel classification as centrocytic lymphoma and in the modified Rappaport scheme as lymphocytic lymphoma of

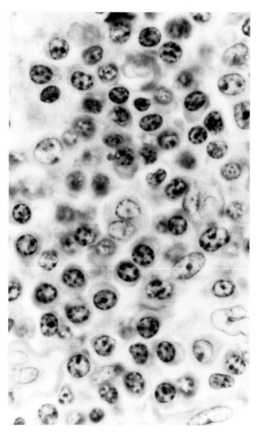

Figure 5–3. Lymphoplasmacytoid lymphoma. Cells have a marked plasmacytoid appearance, with eccentric nuclei and amphophilic cytoplasm (hematoxylin-eosin, ×1000).

intermediate differentiation. Early on it was noted that this tumor tended to surround residual naked germinal centers, and a derivation from the follicular lymphoid cuff was postulated.[33] Tumors with a conspicuous mantle zone pattern of growth were also termed "mantle zone lymphoma."[34] This tumor is not recognized in the WF, but most cases would fall within the category of diffuse small cleaved cell. However, a vaguely follicular pattern may lead to a diagnosis of follicular, small cleaved cell. The blastic variant, described later, would be considered large cleaved cell in the WF in some cases.

MCL occurs in adults, with a high male-to-female ratio. Most patients present with stage III or IV disease at diagnosis.[35, 36] Common sites of involvement include the lymph nodes, spleen, bone marrow, and lymphoid tissue of Waldeyer's ring. Gastrointestinal tract involvement is frequent and is associated with the picture of lymphomatous polyposis.[37] As in the low-grade lymphomas in the WF, this tumor appears to be incurable with available treatment. Although initial complete remissions may be obtained, the relapse rate is high. However, the median survival is shorter than for most other low-grade lymphomas in the WF and is in the range of 3 to 5 years. The relatively short median survival places this tumor in the intermediate-grade category in the WF.

The hallmark of MCL is a monotonous cytologic composition. Within a given case the cells are usually of comparable size and share similar cytologic features. In the typical case, the cells are slightly larger than a normal lymphocyte with finely clumped chromatin, scant cytoplasm, and inconspicuous nucleoli (Fig. 5–4). The nuclear contour is usually irregular or cleaved. However, in some instances nuclear irregularities may be minimal, leading to a diagnosis of SLL in the WF. Transformed cells resembling centroblasts or immunoblasts are essentially absent, providing an important distinction from FCLs. In addition, transformation to a large cell lymphoma, a common event in many other low-grade lymphomas, is not seen.

Approximately 25% of cases of MCL have cells with large nuclei, more dispersed chromatin, and a higher proliferation fraction. This cytologic variant has been termed the "blastic" variant, because of the resemblance of the cells to lymphoblasts.[14] Indeed, immunophenotypic studies may be required to differentiate this process from lymphoblastic lymphoma. Cases with similar cytologic features had been termed "anaplastic centrocytic" or "centrocytoid centroblastic" in the Kiel classification.[38] Epithelioid histiocytes with pale pink cytoplasm are frequent in MCL and usually more numerous in the blastic variant.[27] These cells differ from the typical so-called starry sky histiocytes of Burkitt's lymphoma, in that they usually do not contain nuclear debris. Nevertheless, their presence appears to correspond to a higher mitotic rate. As noted earlier, the blastic variant is associated with a more aggressive clinical course and a median survival of 2 years.

The presence or absence of a mantle zone pattern of growth also appears to have prognostic implications. Cases with a pure mantle zone growth pattern have a longer median survival, perhaps an indication that the process was diagnosed at an earlier stage.[14, 39] Cases with a vaguely nodular growth pattern may represent the next level of architectural effacement. As noted earlier, such cases may be

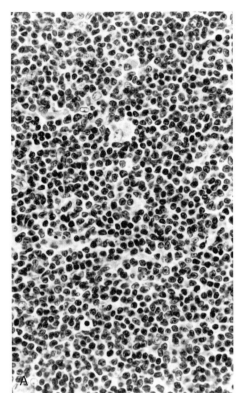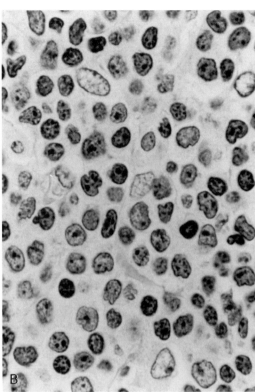

Figure 5–4. Mantle cell lymphoma. *A*, The infiltrate is exceedingly monotonous, without pseudofollicular growth centers. Scattered single epithelioid histiocytes are admixed (hematoxylin-eosin, ×400). *B*, The lymphoid cells are slightly angulated and cleaved (hematoxylin-eosin, ×1000).

distinguished from FCLs by the absence of large cells or centroblasts.

A controversy in the past has been the categorization of cases containing cleaved lymphocytes but also showing pseudofollicular growth centers. Some authors have considered such cases as part of the spectrum of CLL,[17, 33] whereas others have classified such cases as intermediate lymphocytic lymphoma,[39] the category in the modified Rappaport classification closest to MCL. Further analysis has indicated that cases with pseudofollicular growth centers have the clinical course of CLL, and inclusion of such cases alters the clinical profile of true MCL, which is an aggressive disease.[18]

Immunophenotypic and genotypic studies have been helpful in precisely defining MCL. For example, cases of B-CLL with or without cleaved cells usually express CD23, in contrast with true MCL.[40] In addition, the chromosomal translocation t(11;14) causing rearrangement of the *BCLl/PRAD1* locus on chromosome 11 is highly associated with MCL but is absent in most other low-grade and high-grade B-cell malignancies.[41, 42] *PRAD1* encodes cyclin D1. By Northern analysis, virtually 100% of cases of MCL have shown overexpression of *PRAD1*, but overexpression has not been identified to the same degree in other B-cell malignancies.[43, 44] Very low levels of overexpression have been identified in hairy cell leukemia.[44]

Follicle Center Lymphoma (FCL)

WF: follicular, small cleaved, mixed small cleaved and large cell, large cell
Kiel: centroblastic/centrocytic follicular, follicular centroblastic

FCL is the most common subtype of NHL within the United States and accounts for approximately 45% of all

newly diagnosed patients. It has a peak incidence in the fifth and sixth decades and is rare in patients younger than 20 years of age. Men and women are equally affected. FCL is less common in black and Asian populations. Most patients have stage III or IV disease at diagnosis, with generalized lymphadenopathy.[6] Staging evaluation usually detects bone marrow involvement. Approximately 10% of patients have circulating malignant cells.[45] However, careful immunophenotypic or molecular analyses may disclose peripheral blood involvement in a higher proportion of patients.[46]

FCL is indolent but currently incurable with available therapeutic modalities. The natural history of the disease is associated with histologic progression in both pattern and cell type. A heterogeneous cytologic composition is one of the hallmarks of FCL. Usually, all types of follicle center cells are represented, but in varying proportions, accounting for the classification of this tumor as centroblastic/centrocytic in the Kiel scheme.[3] This variation in cytologic composition has been the basis for the subclassification of follicular lymphoma in the WF. The ILSG classification has provisionally adopted cytologic grades equivalent to the three major subtypes of the WF: grade 1 (predominantly small cleaved cell), grade 2 (mixed small cleaved and large cell), and grade 3 (predominantly large cell). However, the variation in cytologic grade is a continuum, and precise morphologic criteria for subclassification are difficult to establish (Fig. 5–5). Most studies have shown that subclassification of follicular lymphoma is difficult to reproduce among groups of pathologists. However, methods that rely on the enumeration of large transformed cells or mitotic figures appear more reproducible than those using techniques based on estimating the proportion of various cell types present.[47]

Follicular small cleaved and follicular mixed lymphomas are considered low grade in the WF. Although many studies have shown subtle differences in the complete remission rate and median survival between these two subtypes, they share a generally indolent clinical course and an absence of long-term complete remissions. By contrast, the subset of FCL classified as predominantly large cell type has a more aggressive natural history. These tumors account for only 10% of all FCLs.[6] They more commonly present with stage I disease, and it is in this subtype that some long-term complete remissions have been seen.

Most FCLs (approximately 85%) are associated with a t(14;18) involving rearrangement of the *BCL2* gene.[48] This translocation appears to result in constitutive expression of *BCL2* protein, which is capable of inhibiting apoptosis in lymphoid cells.[49] The cells of FCL accumulate and are at risk to undergo secondary mutations that may be associated with histologic progression. It is interesting that the small subset of follicular large cell lymphomas are less commonly associated with the *BCL2* translocation.[50] Thus, this subset may have a different pathogenesis. It is believed that the *BCL2* translocation occurs at a very early stage of B-cell development, during immunoglobulin gene rearrangement. This fact may contribute to the difficulty in eradicating the neoplastic clone with chemotherapy. If follicular large cell lymphoma lacks the *BCL2* translocation, this observation might explain its more frequent curability with aggressive therapy.

Nearly all FCLs have a follicular growth pattern that may predominate or be seen only focally within the lymph node.

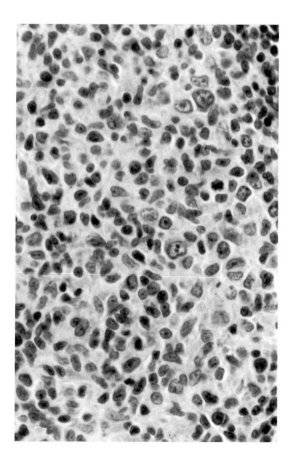

Figure 5–5. Follicle center lymphoma. These tumors usually have an admixture of cell types, including centrocytes (small cleaved cells) and centroblasts (large cells) (hematoxylin-eosin, ×400).

Rare FCLs may have an entirely diffuse growth pattern and be composed predominantly of small cleaved cells. Such cases should be considered low grade, along with their more diffuse counterparts.[51] Diffuse lymphomas composed of small cleaved and large follicle center cells are rare but should be considered clinically aggressive. They comprise some of the cases included in the WF category of diffuse mixed small and large cell type.[52]

Most FCLs present in lymph nodes. A subset of cases with the morphologic features of FCL may present in skin.[53] Clinically, these tumors are usually localized and infrequently associated with lymph node involvement. They have an excellent prognosis, and complete remissions may be obtained with either surgical excision or local radiation therapy.[54] These cutaneous FCLs frequently lack the *BCL2* translocation associated with nodal FCLs. Biologically, the cutaneous FCL may be part of the mucosal-associated lymphoid tissue (MALT) lymphoma spectrum (see below).[27]

Marginal Zone B-Cell Lymphoma

Extranodal low-grade B-cell lymphoma of MALT
Nodal marginal zone B-cell lymphoma with monocytoid B cells (provisional)

WF: small lymphocytic, small lymphocytic plasmacytoid, small cleaved or mixed small and large cell, follicular and/or diffuse
Kiel: monocytoid B-cell lymphoma (MALT lymphomas discussed but not included in classification scheme)

Most lymphomas of marginal zone derivation present in extranodal sites and have the histopathologic and clinical features identified by Isaacson and colleagues as part of the spectrum of MALT lymphomas.[55, 56] MALT lymphomas are characterized by a heterogeneous cellular composition that includes marginal zone or centrocyte-like cells, monocytoid B cells, small lymphocytes, and plasma cells. In most cases, large transformed cells are infrequent. Reactive germinal centers are nearly always present (Fig. 5–6). Therefore, it is not surprising that based on the heterogeneous cellular composition and presence of reactive follicles, most MALT lymphomas were diagnosed in the past as pseudolymphomas or atypical hyperplasias. However, recent studies have shown most to be composed of monoclonal B cells. The follicles usually contain reactive germinal centers, but the germinal centers may become colonized by neoplastic cells. When follicular colonization occurs, the process may simulate follicular lymphoma.[57] The plasma cells are usually found in the subepithelial zones and are monoclonal in up to 50% of cases.

MALT lymphomas have been described in nearly every anatomic site but are most frequent in the stomach, lung, thyroid, salivary gland, and lacrimal gland.[30, 58] Other less common sites of involvement include the orbit, breast, conjunctiva, bladder and kidney, and thymus gland.[59] Most patients present with localized disease, although regional lymph node involvement is common in gastric and salivary gland MALT lymphoma. The involved lymph nodes in those cases resemble monocytoid B-cell lymphoma, and it is believed that monocytoid B-cell lymphoma is the nodal equivalent of a MALT lymphoma.[60–63] Widespread nodal involvement is infrequent, as is bone marrow involvement.

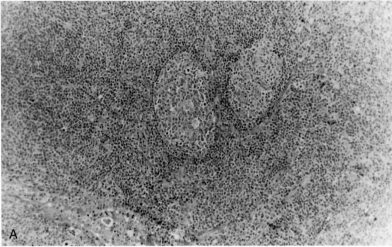

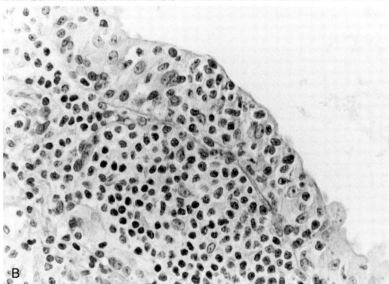

Figure 5–6. Mucosal-associated lymphoid tissue lymphoma, lung. *A,* Residual germinal centers with an attenuated cuff are surrounded by a polymorphous infiltrate. The cells have a moderate amount of indistinct cytoplasm (hematoxylin-eosin, ×200). *B,* Centrocyte-like cells infiltrate the bronchial epithelium (hematoxylin-eosin, ×400).

The clinical course is usually quite indolent, and many patients are asymptomatic. MALT lymphomas tend to relapse in other MALT-associated sites. For example, a patient with a salivary gland lymphoma may relapse with lacrimal gland involvement or conjunctival disease.[30]

MALT lymphomas of the salivary gland are usually associated with Sjögren's syndrome and a history of autoimmune disease. Similarly, MALT lymphomas of the thyroid are associated with Hashimoto's thyroiditis. *Helicobacter pylori* gastritis is frequent in most patients with gastric MALT lymphomas, and it has been suggested that antigen stimulation is critical to both the development of MALT lymphoma and the maintenance of the neoplastic state.[64] Indeed, antibiotic therapy for the eradication of *H. pylori* has led to the spontaneous remission of gastric MALT lymphoma in some patients.

The therapy of MALT lymphomas is still controversial. Isolated lesions readily amenable to surgical excision should be removed. Systemic chemotherapy may be warranted for more widespread disease, and local radiation therapy may play a role in the control of localized tumor masses, especially for gastric and orbital MALT lymphomas.

As noted earlier, most MALT lymphomas are clinically low grade and contain a paucity of large transformed cells.

However, histologic progression may occur, and the endpoint in this progression is a diffuse large B-cell lymphoma.

Monocytoid B-cell lymphoma is seen most often in association with an extranodal MALT lymphoma.[65] However, the existence of the primary extranodal disease may not be immediately apparent. Relapses in nodal sites may occur many years after primary diagnosis. A morphologically similar but different phenomenon is monocytoid B-cell differentiation in a primary nodal lymphoma. Cells resembling monocytoid B lymphocytes have been described in many low-grade lymphomas, most commonly FCL.[66] The monocytoid B-cell component appears to occupy the marginal zone. Nevertheless, the immunophenotype and genotype of the neoplastic cells is that of FCL. The monocytoid differentiation is an interesting morphologic variant but does not appear to have independent clinical or biologic significance.

Splenic Marginal Zone Lymphoma (provisional category)

WF: small lymphocytic, small lymphocytic plasmacytoid
Kiel: not listed

Recent studies have shown that small lymphocytic lymphomas presenting with predominant splenomegaly and minimal lymphadenopathy differ in their immunophenotype from those presenting primarily with lymph node and bone marrow involvement. Whereas typical B-CLL/SLLs are CD5+, splenic small lymphocytic lymphomas are usually CD5–.[67] Careful attention to the cytologic features in these cases indicates that the cells have somewhat more abundant cytoplasm than those of typical B-CLL/SLL and resemble the lymphocytes of the normal splenic marginal zone. The nuclei are usually predominantly round but may be slightly irregular. They have a moderate amount of pale cytoplasm (Fig. 5–7). Histologically, the spleen shows expansion of the white pulp, but usually some infiltration of the red pulp is present as well.[68] In early cases, preferential involvement of the marginal zone may be seen.[69]

Splenic marginal zone lymphomas present in adults and are slightly more frequent in women than men. The clinical presentation is splenomegaly, usually without peripheral lymphadenopathy. Most patients have bone marrow involvement, but there is usually only a modest lymphocytosis, with elevations in the lymphocyte count usually less than seen in B-CLL. Some evidence of plasmacytoid differentiation may be seen, and patients may have a small M component. The abundant pale cytoplasm evident in tissue sections may also be seen in peripheral blood smears. The cytologic features may be mistaken for hairy cell leukemia. The disorder described as splenic lymphoma with villous lymphocytes appears equivalent to splenic marginal zone lymphoma.[70] The course is reported to be indolent, and splenectomy may be followed by a prolonged remission.

Plasmacytoma/Plasma Cell Myeloma

WF: extramedullary plasmacytoma
Kiel: plasmacytic lymphoma

Plasmacytomas are rare in lymph nodes but occur with some frequency in extranodal sites. Patients with localized plasmacytomas involving lymph nodes or other organs are at risk to develop systemic disease, that is, plasma cell myeloma. Most localized plasmacytomas are well-differentiated, clinically low grade, and morphologically composed of normal-appearing plasma cells.[71]

Some plasma cell malignancies are composed of immature cells with prominent central nucleoli and abundant deeply amphophilic cytoplasm.[72] Marked nuclear irregularity may be seen in rare cases.[73] This morphologic appearance has been termed "anaplastic myeloma." Patients with this high-grade histology are at greater risk to develop disease outside the bone marrow, such as in the lymph nodes, spleen, and liver. In addition, anaplastic myeloma may be difficult to distinguish from large cell immunoblastic lymphoma exhibiting plasmacytoid differentiation. The cells contain abundant monoclonal cytoplasmic immunoglobulin and may lack B-cell–associated antigens. The clinical behavior of these high-grade malignancies is more similar to aggressive lymphoma than to typical multiple myeloma.

Diffuse Large B-Cell Lymphoma

WF: diffuse mixed small and large cell, diffuse large cell, large cell immunoblastic

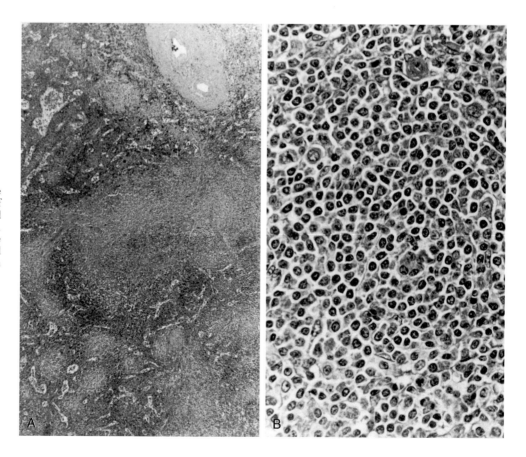

Figure 5–7. Splenic marginal zone lymphoma. *A,* There is expansion of white pulp and infiltration of red pulp (hematoxylin-eosin, ×25). *B,* The cells resemble the cells of the normal splenic marginal zone and have a pale rim of cytoplasm (hematoxylin-eosin, ×400).

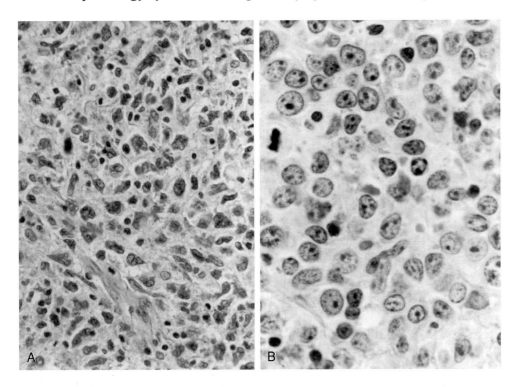

Figure 5–8. Large B-cell lymphoma. *A,* In this primary tumor of bone, the cells are irregular and associated with marked sclerosis (hematoxylin-eosin, ×400). *B,* In this example the cells resemble centroblasts or large noncleaved cells and have membrane-bound nucleoli (hematoxylin-eosin, ×1000).

Kiel: centroblastic, immunoblastic, large cell anaplastic (B cell)

Diffuse large B-cell lymphomas are composed of large, transformed lymphoid cells with nuclei at least twice the size of a small lymphocyte. The nuclei generally have vesicular chromatin, prominent nucleoli, basophilic cytoplasm, and a moderate to high proliferation fraction (Fig. 5–8). The cells have been likened by Lukes and Collins to either large cleaved or large noncleaved follicular center cells.[4] Marked variation in the nuclear contour may be seen. In most instances, the cells are round to oval. However, in some instances the cells may be polylobated or cleaved.[74]

Diffuse large B-cell lymphomas may be associated with sclerosis, particularly in extranodal sites.[6, 75] Sclerosis is more common in those tumors with a large cleaved cell morphology and is also seen in mediastinal or thymic large B-cell lymphoma (see later).[76]

Some large B-cell lymphomas are rich in either small T lymphocytes or histiocytes or both. Histologically, they may resemble peripheral T-cell lymphomas or HD (Fig. 5–9).[77–79] In the WF most such cases would be classified as diffuse mixed small and large cell lymphoma.[52] They are clinically aggressive with a prognosis comparable to that of diffuse large B-cell lymphoma.[80] The admixture of small lymphocytes and histiocytes is a variable phenomenon, and the inflammatory background may be absent on second biopsies. These tumors have been referred to in the literature as "pseudoperipheral T-cell lymphomas,"[77] or T-cell–rich B-cell lymphoma.[81] T-cell–rich B-cell lymphoma, as currently defined, does not appear to be a distinct clinical pathologic entity but a variant that can be seen in association with several different subtypes of diffuse large B-cell lymphoma.[82]

The WF subdivided the histiocytic lymphomas of Rappaport into two major subgroups: large cell and large cell immunoblastic.[6] Based on minor differences in median survival, the large cell group was placed in the intermediate-grade category and the large cell immunoblastic group placed in the high-grade category. Subsequent studies have not been able to justify the validity of this subclassification.[83]

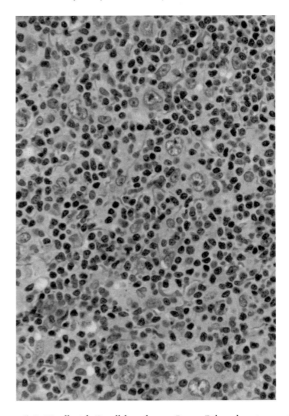

Figure 5–9. T-cell–rich B-cell lymphoma. Large B lymphocytes are in a background of small normal T cells. In this example the large cells resemble L & H cells (hematoxylin-eosin, ×400).

Moreover, it is exceedingly difficult for pathologists to make this distinction reliably and reproducibly.[84, 85] Most aggressive lymphomas show a spectrum in cytologic appearance, and in any given field the predominant cell could be large cell or large cell immunoblastic. Similarly, the Kiel classification describes four different variants of centroblastic lymphoma: monomorphic, polymorphic, multilobated, and centrocytoid.[86] The designation of immunoblastic lymphoma of B-cell type is reserved for cases in which more than 90% of the cells have an immunoblastic appearance. If only 10% of the cells resemble centroblasts, the case is classified as a centroblastic lymphoma. Using these criteria, only 4% of all NHLs are classified as B immunoblastic.[86]

Diffuse large B-cell lymphoma is one of the more common subtypes of NHL, representing up to 40% of cases. It has an aggressive natural history but responds well to chemotherapy. The complete remission rate with modern regimens is 75% to 80%, with long-term disease-free survival approaching 50% or more in most series.[87] This lymphoma may present in lymph nodes or in extranodal sites. Frequent extranodal sites of involvement include bone, skin, thyroid, gastrointestinal tract, and lung. Some of these extranodal diffuse large cell B-cell lymphomas may be MALT lymphomas with histologic progression, in which the low-grade component is not recognized. Nevertheless, once progression has occurred to a diffuse large B-cell lymphoma, the clinical approach is equivalent to that of node-based large B-cell lymphoma.

Because there is variation in the responsiveness to chemotherapy, and because large B-cell lymphoma is one of the more common subtypes, there has been great interest over the years in identifying morphologic or immunophenotypic features that might be prognostically important. In most studies there is some suggestion that tumors composed of large cleaved or large noncleaved follicular center cells have a slightly better prognosis than those composed predominantly of immunoblasts.[6, 84] However, the differences have been neither statistically significant nor consistently reproducible. Most data suggest that growth fraction is an important prognostic marker.[88] It is likely that in the future the use of immunophenotypic and genotypic markers may yield useful information in the subclassification of large B-cell lymphoma.[88–91] Although morphologic features are useful in identifying the spectrum of appearances that one may encounter diagnostically, morphologic features do not appear to be important prognostically.

Primary Mediastinal (Thymic) Large B-Cell Lymphoma

WF: large cell, large cell immunoblastic
Kiel: discussed as "rare and ambiguous subtype"

Primary mediastinal large B-cell lymphoma has emerged in recent years as a distinct clinicopathologic entity.[76, 92, 93] Cytologically, it resembles many other large B-cell lymphomas and is composed of large transformed cells that can resemble large noncleaved cells, large cleaved cells, multilobated cells, and even immunoblasts. A constant feature is relatively abundant pale cytoplasm, often with distinct cytoplasmic membranes (Fig. 5–10).[93] Many patients have fine compartmentalizing sclerosis, which may even lead to misdiagnosis as an epithelial tumor, such as thymoma. The

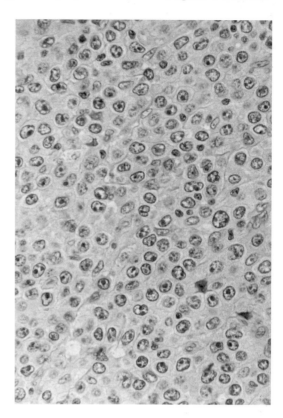

Figure 5–10. Thymic B-cell lymphoma. The cells have abundant clear cytoplasm, and there is a fine compartmentalizing fibrosis (hematoxylin-eosin, ×400).

tumor appears to be derived from medullary B cells within the thymus gland.[92, 94, 95]

Clinically, mediastinal large B-cell lymphoma is much more common in women than men.[96] It is common in adolescents and young adults, with a median age at presentation in the fourth decade. The clinical presentation is that of a rapidly growing anterior mediastinal mass with frequent superior venacaval syndrome and/or airway obstruction. Nodal involvement is uncommon at presentation and also at relapse. Frequent extranodal sites of involvement, particularly at relapse, include the liver, kidneys, adrenal glands, ovaries, gastrointestinal tract, and central nervous system (CNS). Some studies suggested that the tumor was associated with an unusually aggressive clinical course with poor responses to conventional chemotherapy. More recent studies have reported cure rates similar to those seen for other large B-cell lymphomas.

Burkitt's Lymphoma

WF: small noncleaved cell, Burkitt's type
Kiel: Burkitt's lymphoma

Burkitt's lymphoma is most common in children and accounts for up to one third of all pediatric lymphomas in the United States.[97] It is the most rapidly growing of all lymphomas, with 100% of the cells in cell cycle at any time. It usually presents in extranodal sites. In nonendemic regions, such as the United States, frequent sites of presentation are the ileocecal region, ovaries, kidneys, or breasts. Jaw presentations, as well as involvement of other facial bones, are common in African or endemic cases and are seen occasionally in nonendemic regions. Rare cases present as acute leukemia with diffuse bone marrow infiltration and circulating Burkitt's tumor cells (acute lymphoblastic leukemia). Even in patients with typical extranodal disease, bone marrow involvement is a poor prognostic sign.

Burkitt's lymphoma is one of the more common tumors associated with the human immunodeficiency virus (HIV).[98] It can present at any time during the clinical course. In some patients with HIV infection, Burkitt's lymphoma may be the initial acquired immunodeficiency syndrome (AIDS)-defining illness.

The pathogenesis of Burkitt's lymphoma is undoubtedly related to the translocations involving the *cMYC* oncogene, which are seen in virtually 100% of cases.[99, 100] Most cases involve the immunoglobulin heavy-chain gene on chromosome 14. Less commonly, the light-chain genes on chromosomes 2 and 22 are involved in the translocation. African Burkitt's lymphoma occurs in regions endemic for malaria, and it has been postulated that immunosuppression associated with malaria infection places patients at increased risk for Burkitt's lymphoma.[48] In this regard, the pathogenesis appears similar to that seen with HIV infection.

EBV is closely linked to Burkitt's lymphoma in endemic regions but is less frequently seen (15% to 20%) in European and North American patients.[97] In other regions characterized by low socioeconomic status and EBV infection at an early age, Burkitt's lymphoma is often EBV positive, in the range of 50% to 70%.[101] These data support the concept that

EBV is a cofactor for the development of Burkitt's lymphoma. Differences in EBV strain type have also been shown in sporadic and endemic EBV-positive Burkitt's lymphomas.[102]

Cytologically, Burkitt's lymphoma is exceedingly monomorphic. The cells are medium in size with round nuclei, moderately clumped chromatin, and multiple two to five basophilic nucleoli (Fig. 5–11). The cytoplasm is deeply basophilic and moderately abundant. These cells contain cytoplasmic lipid vacuoles, which are probably a manifestation of the high rates of proliferation and spontaneous cell death. Lipid vacuoles are usually evident on imprints or smears but not in tissue sections. The starry sky pattern characteristic of Burkitt's lymphoma is a manifestation of the numerous benign macrophages that have ingested karyorrhectic or apoptotic tumor cells.

Some cases of Burkitt's lymphoma are associated with a marked granulomatous reaction, which may even obscure the lymphoma in some instances. This reaction is often seen in patients with early stage, but, despite the stage at presentation, these patients usually have an excellent prognosis.[103] Thus, this granulomatous reaction may be a manifestation of host immune response to the disease. The reaction has also been described in Burkitt's-like lymphomas.[103]

High-Grade B-Cell Lymphoma, Burkitt's-Like (provisional)

WF: small noncleaved cell, non-Burkitt's
Kiel: not listed (centroblastic)

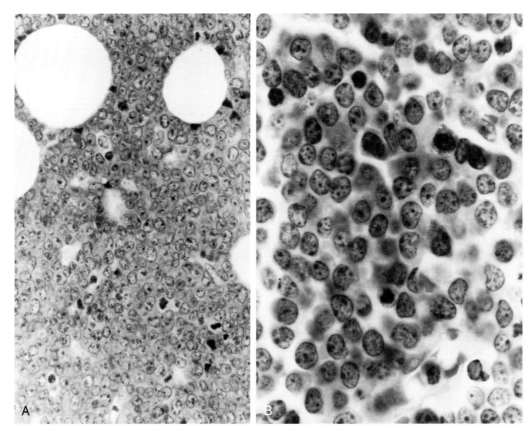

Figure 5–11. Burkitt's lymphoma. *A,* The cells diffusely infiltrate omental fat (hematoxylin-eosin, ×400). *B,* The cells are uniform, round to oval, with multiple small basophilic nucleoli (hematoxylin-eosin, ×1000).

The WF includes in the small noncleaved cell category tumors with cells similar in size and appearance to Burkitt's lymphoma, but with greater pleomorphism.[6] These lymphomas lack the monotonous cytology of Burkitt's lymphoma but are composed of cells that have nuclei roughly equivalent to the size of the nuclei of the starry sky macrophages. However, there is usually some variation in cell size and shape. There may be multiple nucleoli or a single distinct, prominent nucleolus.

In the WF, small noncleaved cell, non-Burkitt's is a heterogeneous category and includes both B-cell and T-cell lymphomas. For example, some cases of adult T-cell leukemia/lymphoma are composed of cells conforming to this description. However, in the ILSG classification high-grade B-cell lymphoma, Burkitt's-like, is reserved for tumors with a B-cell phenotype. However, even in the ILSG scheme, this category is probably heterogeneous. A number of clinical studies have suggested that small noncleaved cell lymphomas, whether or not they conform to classic Burkitt's lymphoma, have a high growth fraction and an aggressive clinical course.[88, 104] It was believed that the separation of such tumors from diffuse large B-cell lymphoma may be warranted on clinical grounds. When immunocytochemistry is used to detect the Ki67 or MIB1 antigen, such tumors usually are found to have a growth fraction in excess of 80%, which places them in a highly aggressive category.

On clinical grounds Burkitt's-like lymphomas share more similarities with large B-cell lymphomas than with true Burkitt's lymphomas. They usually present in adults, often with nodal as well as extranodal disease.[105] Review of data from the original WF project data base indicated a median survival of 1.5 years for large cell lymphoma, 1.3 years for small noncleaved, non-Burkitt's lymphoma, but only 0.5 year for Burkitt's lymphomas (Berard, CW, personal communication, 1982). Similarly the 5-year survival rates for large cell lymphoma and small noncleaved, non-Burkitt's lymphoma were 35% and 41%, respectively, in contrast with 20% for Burkitt's lymphoma, with complete remission rates of 59%, 57%, and 42%, respectively. Therefore, based on these data, categorization of the Burkitt's-like lymphomas with other large B-cell lymphomas would seem appropriate.

Biologically, these tumors appear to be more closely related to large noncleaved or centroblastic lymphomas than true Burkitt's lymphoma. A recent study showed that cases classified as small noncleaved non-Burkitt's lacked *CMYC* rearrangement but contained *BCL2* rearrangement with a frequency equivalent to that of large B-cell lymphoma.[100] Given the improvement in prognosis with third-generation regimens, a distinction from large B-cell lymphoma may not be warranted in the future.[104]

Burkitt's-like lymphomas occurring in the setting of HIV infection, by contrast, are biologically comparable to true Burkitt's lymphoma. They frequently contain *CMYC* rearrangements, despite their greater nuclear pleomorphism.[98]

T-CELL AND PUTATIVE NK CELL NEOPLASMS

Although the definition of precursor T-cell or lymphoblastic neoplasms is straightforward, the classification of peripheral T-cell lymphomas has been controversial. Most classification schemes for the malignant lymphomas published in the United States or Europe have been based on B-cell malignancies, because these are far more common than their T-cell counterparts. The Rappaport classification and the original Kiel and Lukes-Collins classifications focus primarily on B-cell lymphomas. The WF, being based on the Rappaport scheme, also focuses almost exclusively on B-cell malignancies. Only mycosis fungoides is delineated as a specific entity, and it is included in the miscellaneous category. Most peripheral T-cell lymphomas in the WF are classified as either diffuse, mixed, small, and large cell or large cell immunoblastic. T-cell lymphomas composed predominantly of small atypical cells would be included in the diffuse small cleaved cell category or remain unclassified.

The revised Kiel classification does include T-cell lymphomas.[86, 106] However, the ILSG classification differs from the approach used in the Kiel scheme in several respects. For one, the ILSG classification recognizes adult T-cell leukemia/lymphoma as a distinct clinicopathologic entity.[8] The Kiel classification describes T-cell lymphomas in morphologic terms and notes independently the status as HTLV-I positive or negative.

The ILSG classification also recognizes the distinctive nature of many extranodal T-cell lymphomas. These include the nasal and nasal-type angiocentric lymphomas, enteropathy-associated T-cell lymphoma, and subcutaneous panniculitic T-cell lymphoma. Clinical features play an important role in the definition of many T-cell lymphoma entities, as it is believed that cytologic features alone are not sufficient to delineate many of these diseases.

Additionally, the Kiel classification divides T-cell lymphomas into low-grade and high-grade forms based on the cytologic features of the neoplastic cells. Low-grade lymphomas are composed of small- to medium-sized atypical cells, whereas large transformed cells predominate in the high-grade lymphomas. Although these distinctions are valid cytologically, they do not necessarily relate to a more aggressive clinical course for the tumors composed of large cells.[107] For this reason, the ILSG classification does not divide T-cell lymphomas into low-grade and high-grade variants.

Finally, T-zone lymphoma and lymphoepithelioid cell lymphoma were not believed to be distinct clinicopathologic entities, although they do represent morphologic variations that can be seen in peripheral T-cell lymphoma. In addition, previous studies have suggested that they are difficult to reliably distinguish from other nodal T-cell lymphomas.[108] Cytogenetic studies also have suggested overlap among these categories of low-grade T-cell lymphoma in the Kiel classification.[109] Therefore, they were left within the category of peripheral T-cell lymphomas, unspecified.

Precursor T-Lymphoblastic Leukemia/Lymphoma (PT-LBL/ALL)

WF: lymphoblastic
Kiel: T lymphoblastic

Most PT-LBLs are cytologically indistinguishable from their B-cell counterparts. The cells usually are convoluted, but nonconvoluted forms also exist.[13, 110] The cells have finely distributed chromatin, inconspicuous nucleoli, and sparse, pale cytoplasm (Fig. 5–12). Eighty-five percent of

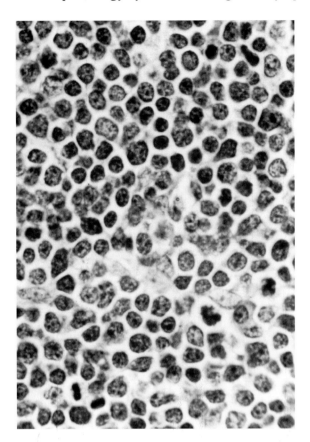

Figure 5–12. Precursor-T lymphoblastic leukemia/lymphoma. In this case the cells are not convoluted. The chromatin is finely distributed with inconspicuous nucleoli and sparse cytoplasm (hematoxylin-eosin, ×650).

patients with lymphoblastic lymphoma have a tumor of precursor T-cell phenotype. This is a disease of adolescents and young adults, with an increased male-to-female ratio. Fifty to 80% of patients present with an anterior mediastinal mass, usually with involvement of the thymus gland. This tumor is a high-grade lymphoma; the rapidly growing mass may be associated with airway obstruction. Bone marrow involvement is common, and progression to a leukemic picture occurs in the absence of effective therapy. The tumor also has a high frequency of involvement of the CNS, which is a poor prognostic sign. PT-LBL is closely related to T-cell acute lymphoblastic leukemia although the lymphomatous forms usually exhibit a more mature T-cell phenotype.[111]

In lymph nodes PT-LBL has a diffuse leukemic pattern of infiltration. There is little stromal reaction, and the cells diffusely infiltrate the lymph node parenchyma. Streaming of cells in the medullary cords may be prominent, especially around vascular structures. Some residual follicles may be present, but ultimately architectural effacement is the rule. A starry sky pattern is seen in approximately one third of cases. Mitotic figures are readily observed.

Histologically, it is not possible to differentiate PT-LBL from PB-LBL. Immunophenotypic studies performed in paraffin or frozen sections can usually identify the cell of origin. PT-LBL may also simulate the blastic variant of MCL. The cells of MCL usually show more chromatin clumping and have more abundant cytoplasm than either PT-LBL or PB-LBL.

T-Cell Chronic Lymphocytic Leukemia/Prolymphocytic Leukemia (T-CLL/PLL)

WF: small lymphocytic, consistent with CLL, diffuse small cleaved cell, unclassified
Kiel: T-cell CLL/PLL

T-CLL/PLL presents with leukemia, with or without lymphadenopathy, usually with markedly elevated white blood cell counts.[112, 113] Instances of primary lymph node involvement are exceedingly rare. The lymph node involvement is diffuse, primarily paracortical, with sparing of the follicles. The cellular infiltrate is usually more monotonous than that of B-CLL and lacks pseudofollicular proliferation centers. Involvement of the spleen is associated with diffuse red pulp infiltration. Hepatomegaly is frequently present. Clinically, T-CLL/PLL is much more aggressive than B-CLL. In most cases, some cytologic atypia is present, so that the cells do not resemble small, round, normal-appearing lymphocytes. On this basis, they are more accurately classified as T-PLL.

Large Granular Lymphocyte (LGL) Leukemia, T-Cell and NK Cell Types

WF: small lymphocytic, consistent with CLL
Kiel: T-CLL

These disorders are not generally considered with the malignant lymphomas and are discussed only briefly. The cells have more abundant pale cytoplasm than those of T-CLL. In smear preparations azurophil granules are readily identified. Most cases of T-LGL have been shown to be clonal, based on analysis of T-cell receptor gene rearrangement.[114] Clonality has not been convincingly shown in most cases of low-grade NK-LGL leukemia. In some cases, this may represent an atypical reactive, nonneoplastic lymphoproliferative disorder. Clonal disorders of T-LGL are more common. In addition to peripheral blood involvement, the cells infiltrate the marrow, splenic red pulp, and liver. Lymphadenopathy is uncommon, and the clinical course is indolent.

Two high-grade variants of NK cell leukemia have been described. One resembles acute myeloid leukemia.[115] The cells have a blastic or monomorphic appearance and are usually negative for EBV. The second variant is EBV positive and may represent a leukemic form of angiocentric nasal T/NK-cell lymphoma (see later).[116] It is much more common in Asian than in Western countries and pursues an aggressive clinical course. The cells are medium to large in size, contain hyperchromatic nuclei, and demonstrate nuclear pleomorphism. Azurophil granules can be seen on smears, but the marked cytologic atypia readily permits distinction from the more indolent forms of T-LGL and NK-LGL.

Mycosis Fungoides/Sézary Syndrome (MF/SS)

WF: mycosis fungoides
Kiel: small cell, cerebriform

MF/SS, by definition, presents with cutaneous disease. Skin involvement may be manifested as multiple cutaneous plaques or nodules, or with generalized erythroderma.

Lymphadenopathy is usually not found at presentation and, when identified, is associated with a poor prognosis.[117] In early stages enlarged lymph nodes may show only dermatopathic changes (LN1 or LN2 according to the NCI-Navy grading scheme).[118, 118a] If malignant cells are present in significant numbers and are associated with architectural effacement (LN3 and LN4), the prognosis is significantly worse.

Cytologically, the small cells of MF/SS demonstrate cerebriform nuclei with clumped chromatin, inconspicuous nucleoli, and sparse cytoplasm. The larger cells may be hyperchromatic or have more vesicular nuclei with prominent nucleoli. Nuclear pleomorphism is usually evident in the large cells. Epidermotropism is usually a prominent feature of the cutaneous infiltrates (Fig. 5–13).

Peripheral T-Cell Lymphomas (PTLs), Unspecified

Provisional Cytologic Grades: Medium-sized Cell, Mixed Medium and Large Cell, Large Cell

WF: diffuse small cleaved, diffuse mixed small and large cell, large cell immunoblastic
Kiel: T-zone lymphoma; lymphoepithelioid cell lymphoma; pleomorphic small, medium, and large cell (HTLV-I negative); immunoblastic (HTLV-I negative)

PTLs account for only 10% to 15% of all NHLs. Angioimmunoblastic T-cell lymphoma is the most common specific form. Most other PTLs arising in lymph nodes would fall in the unspecified category. PTLs are characterized by a heterogeneous cellular composition. There is usually a mixture of small and large atypical lymphoid cells. An inflammatory background is common, consisting of eosinophils, plasma cells, and histiocytes. If the epithelioid histiocytes are numerous and clustered, it fulfills criteria for lymphoepithelioid cell lymphoma or Lennert's lymphoma.[119, 120] In the ILSG classification lymphoepithelioid cell lymphoma was considered a morphologic variant of PTL and not a distinctive clinicopathologic entity. It has not been associated with

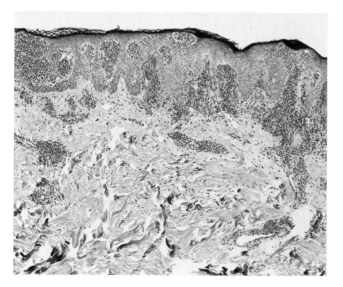

Figure 5–13. Mycosis fungoides/Sézary syndrome. The infiltrate shows prominent epidermotropism (hematoxylin-eosin, ×25).

any immunophenotypic, cytogenetic, or molecular features permitting distinction from other PTLs.[109]

PTLs may show preferential involvement of the paracortical region of lymph nodes. In some instances this architectural pattern is striking, with sparing of follicles. Such cases have been referred to as "T-zone lymphoma."[106] However, on cytologic grounds they resemble other peripheral T-cell lymphomas of medium or mixed cytologic types. The neoplastic cells usually have a moderate amount of pale cytoplasm. A conspicuous clear cell component is more characteristic of angioimmunoblastic T-cell lymphoma than PTL, unspecified.

Clinically, PTLs present in adults. Most patients exhibit generalized lymphadenopathy, hepatosplenomegaly, and frequent bone marrow involvement. Constitutional symptoms, including fever and night sweats, are common, as is pruritus. The clinical course is aggressive, although complete remissions may be obtained with combination chemotherapy.[121–123] However, the relapse rate is higher in PTLs than in B-cell lymphomas of comparable histologic grade.[123]

PTL, as defined in the ILSG classification, is heterogeneous. It is likely that individual clinicopathologic entities will be delineated in the future from this broad group of malignancies.

Subcutaneous Panniculitic T-Cell Lymphoma

WF: diffuse mixed small and large cell, large cell immunoblastic, small cleaved cell
Kiel: pleomorphic medium mixed and large cell (HTLV-I negative)

Subcutaneous panniculitic T-cell lymphoma is sufficiently distinct to warrant separation from other forms of peripheral T-cell lymphoma.[124] The disease usually presents with subcutaneous nodules, primarily affecting the extremities (Fig. 5–14). The nodules range from 0.5 cm to several centimeters in diameter. Larger nodules may become necrotic. In its early stages the infiltrate may appear deceptively benign, and lesions are often misdiagnosed as panniculitis.[124, 125] However, histologic progression usually occurs, and subsequent biopsies show more pronounced cytologic atypia, permitting the diagnosis of malignant lymphoma.

As noted earlier, the cytologic composition of subcutaneous panniculitic T-cell lymphoma is extremely variable. The lesions may contain a predominance of small atypical lymphoid cells, large transformed cells with hyperchromatic nuclei, or an admixture of several different cell types. Admixed reactive histiocytes are frequently present, particularly in areas of fat infiltration and destruction. The histiocytes are frequently vacuolated owing to ingested lipid material. Vascular invasion may be seen in some cases, and necrosis and karyorrhexis are common.

A hemophagocytic syndrome is a frequent complication of subcutaneous panniculitic T-cell lymphoma.[124] Patients present with fever, pancytopenia, and hepatosplenomegaly. It is most readily diagnosed in bone marrow aspirate smears where histiocytes containing phagocytozed erythrocytes and occasionally platelets may be observed. The hemophagocytic syndrome usually precipitates a fulminant downhill clinical

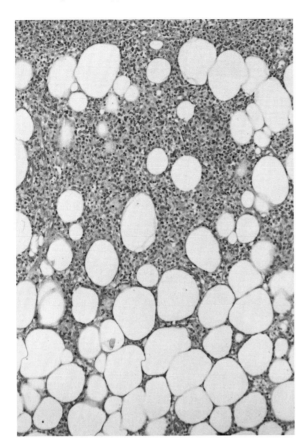

Figure 5–14. Subcutaneous panniculitic T-cell lymphoma. A lacelike infiltrate extensively infiltrates subcutaneous tissue (hematoxylin-eosin, ×60).

course. However, if therapy for the underlying lymphoma is instituted and is successful, the hemophagocytic syndrome may remit. A hemophagocytic syndrome is the cause of death in most patients with subcutaneous panniculitic T-cell lymphoma. Dissemination to lymph nodes and other organs is uncommon and usually occurs late in the clinical course. The cause of hemophagocytic syndrome appears related to cytokine production by the malignant cells. Both interferon-γ as well as granulocyte-monocyte colony-stimulating factor have been identified.[125]

It is likely that subcutaneous panniculitic T-cell lymphoma is the process previously described as histiocytic cytophagic panniculitis. It had been believed that histiocytic cytophagic panniculitis was a malignant histiocytic proliferation.

γδ T-Cell Lymphoma

WF: diffuse small cleaved cell, unclassified
Kiel: pleomorphic small cell, medium size cell (HTLV-I negative)

Most peripheral T lymphocytes belong to the αβ subset, whereas only a few are γδ T cells. Similarly, most peripheral T-cell lymphomas are of αβ T-cell derivation. However, there is a unique subtype of peripheral T-cell lymphoma that is derived from γδ T cells.

γδ T-cell lymphoma presents with marked hepatosplenomegaly.[126] This tumor has also been referred to in the literature as "hepatosplenic T-cell lymphoma." The homing pattern manifested by the malignant cells is similar to that of normal γδ T cells, which preferentially involve the sinusoidal areas of the spleen and also the intestinal mucosa.

γδ T-cell lymphomas show a marked male predominance. Most patients are young adults. The clinical presentation is that of marked hepatosplenomegaly in the absence of lymphadenopathy. Abnormal cells are usually present in the bone marrow but may be difficult to identify. They selectively infiltrate the bone marrow sinusoids and can be most easily recognized with immunohistochemical stains of bone marrow biopsy sections. A variant of γδ T-cell lymphoma with cutaneous disease has also been reported.[125]

The cells of γδ T-cell lymphoma are usually moderate in size, with a rim of pale cytoplasm (Fig. 5–15). The nuclear chromatin is loosely condensed with small, inconspicuous nucleoli. Usually some irregularity of the nuclear contour can be seen. The liver and spleen show marked sinusoidal infiltration, with sparing of both portal triads and white pulp, respectively.

Clinically, γδ T-cell lymphoma is aggressive.[127, 128] Although patients may respond initially to chemotherapy, relapse has been seen in most cases, and the median survival is less than 3 years.

Angioimmunoblastic T-Cell Lymphoma (AILD)

WF: diffuse mixed small and large cell, large cell immunoblastic, AILD
Kiel: angioimmunoblastic

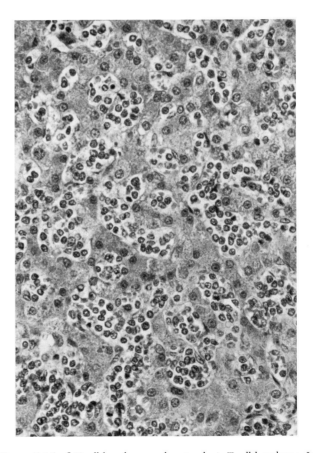

Figure 5–15. γδ T-cell lymphoma or hepatosplenic T-cell lymphoma. In this liver biopsy the cells extensively infiltrate the sinusoids. They are of moderate size, round, with a rim of pale cytoplasm. The infiltrate is uniform, without admixed inflammatory cells (hematoxylin-eosin, ×400).

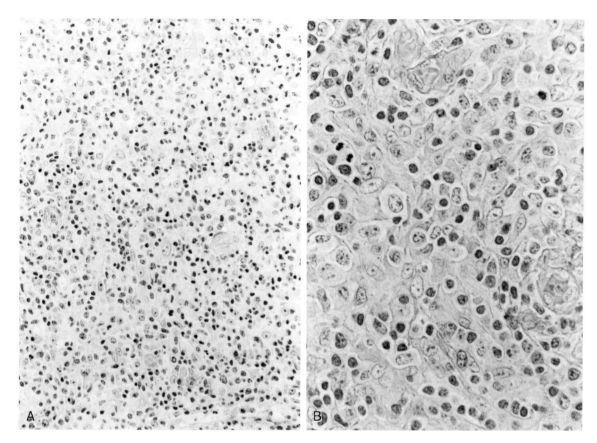

Figure 5–16. Angioimmunoblastic T-cell lymphoma. *A,* A diffuse polymorphous infiltrate effaces the architecture (hematoxylin-eosin, ×200). *B,* The atypical cells have abundant pale cytoplasm. A postcapillary venule with plump endothelial cells is in the lower portion of the field (hematoxylin-eosin, ×400).

AILD was initially proposed as an abnormal immune reaction or a form of atypical lymphoid hyperplasia with a high risk of progression to malignant lymphoma.[128] Because most cases show clonal rearrangements of T-cell receptor genes, it is now regarded as a variant of T-cell lymphoma.[129] The median survival is generally less than 5 years, so that the designation as lymphoma is warranted on clinical grounds as well.[130]

The nodal architecture is generally effaced, but peripheral sinuses are often open and even dilated. The abnormal infiltrate usually extends beyond the capsule into the surrounding adipose tissue. Hyperplastic germinal centers are absent. However, there may be regressed follicles containing a proliferation of dendritic cells and blood vessels. These regressed follicles are referred to as "burned out."

At low power there is usually a striking proliferation of postcapillary venules with prominent arborization (Fig. 5–16). The cellularity of the lymph node usually appears reduced or depleted at low power. Clusters of lymphoid cells with clear cytoplasm may be seen. Their nuclei exhibit moderately condensed chromatin and a slightly irregular nuclear contour. These are admixed with a polymorphous cellular background containing small normal-appearing lymphocytes, basophilic immunoblasts, plasma cells, and histiocytes, with or without eosinophils.

AILD presents in adults. Most patients have generalized lymphadenopathy and prominent systemic symptoms with fever, weight loss, and skin rash. There is usually a polyclonal hypergammaglobulinemia. Patients may respond initially to steroids or mild cytotoxic chemotherapy, but progression usually occurs. More aggressive combination chemotherapeutic regimens have led to a higher remission rate, but patients are prone to secondary infectious complications. Progression to a more high-grade T-cell immunoblastic lymphoma occurs in some patients. Rarely, B-cell immunoblastic lymphomas positive for EBV are seen.[131] These latter malignancies appear secondary to the underlying immunodeficiency.

Adult T-Cell Leukemia/Lymphoma (ATLL)

WF: diffuse small cleaved, diffuse mixed small and large cell, large cell, large cell immunoblastic, small noncleaved non-burkitt

Kiel: pleomorphic small cell, medium sized and large cell, immunoblastic (HTLV-I positive)

ATLL is a distinct clinicopathologic entity, originally described in southwestern Japan, that is associated with the retrovirus HTLV-I.[132, 133] HTLV-I is found clonally integrated in the T cells of this lymphoma. HTLV-I is also endemic in the Caribbean, where clusters of ATLL have been described, predominantly among blacks.[134, 135] It is seen with lesser frequency in blacks in the southeastern United States.[136] The median age of affected people is 45 years. Patients in the Caribbean tend to be slightly younger than those in Japan.[137] Patients may present with leukemia or with generalized lymphadenopathy. The leukemic form predominates in Japan, whereas lymphomatous presentations are more common in the Western hemisphere. Other clinical findings include lymphadenopathy, hepatospleno-megaly, lytic bone lesions, and hypercalcemia.[5] The acute form of the disease is associated with a poor prognosis and a median survival of less than 2 years.[136] Complete remissions may be obtained, but the relapse rate is nearly 100%.

Chronic and smoldering forms of the disease are seen less commonly.[138] These types are associated with a much more indolent clinical course. There is usually minimal lymphad-enopathy. The predominant clinical manifestation is skin rash, with only small numbers of atypical cells in the peripheral blood. In the chronic and smoldering forms, HTLV-I virus is also found integrated within the atypical lymphoid cells.

The cytologic spectrum of ATLL is extremely diverse. The cells may be small with condensed nuclear chromatin and markedly polylobated nuclear appearance.[136, 139] Larger cells with dispersed chromatin and small nucleoli may be admixed and predominate in some cases. Reed-Sternberg–like cells can be seen, simulating HD.[140] In the smoldering form of ATLL, the cells may show minimal cytologic atypia and may even be diagnosed as small lymphocytic lymphoma in the WF. The larger cells usually show abundant cytoplas-mic basophilia. Skin involvement is seen in approximately two thirds of patients, and the cutaneous infiltrates often show prominent epidermotropism, simulating mycosis fun-goides (Fig. 5–17).

Angiocentric T/NK-Cell Lymphoma

> WF: *diffuse small cleaved, mixed small and large cell, large cell immunoblastic*
> Kiel: *pleomorphic small cell, medium and large cell (HTLV-I negative)*

Angiocentric T/NK-cell lymphoma is a distinct clinico-pathologic entity highly associated with EBV.[141, 142] The most common clinical presentation is with a destructive nasal or midline facial tumor. Palatal destruction, orbital swelling, and edema may be prominent.[143] Angiocentric lymphomas have been reported in other extranodal sites, including skin,

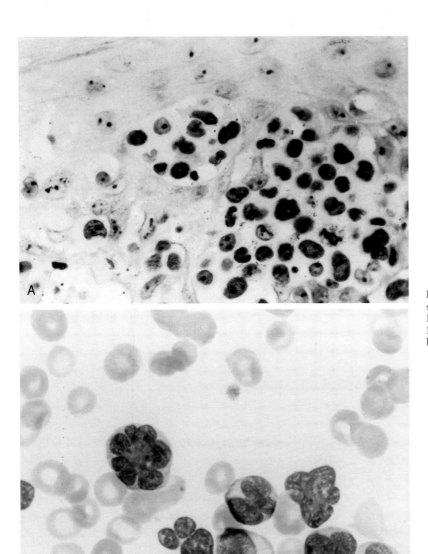

Figure 5–17. Adult T-cell leukemia/lymphoma. *A,* In the skin the cells frequently infiltrate the epidermis, producing Pautrier microabscesses (hematoxylin-eosin, ×650). *B,* Markedly polylobated cells circulate in the peripheral blood (Giemsa-Wright, ×1000).

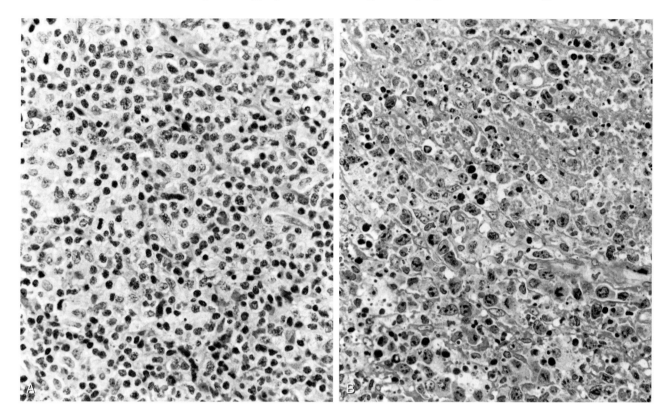

Figure 5–18. Angiocentric nasal T/natural killer cell lymphoma. *A,* In this example the cells are small to medium in size, without pronounced atypia. Mitotic figures provide a clue to the neoplastic nature of the infiltrate. Nearly all of the lymphoid cells are positive for EBV sequences (hematoxylin-eosin, ×400). *B,* In this case the cells are large and pleomorphic. There is extensive necrosis (hematoxylin-eosin, ×400).

soft tissue, testis, upper respiratory tract, and gastrointestinal tract. A leukemic form of the disease also has been reported with similar morphologic, immunophenotypic, and genotypic features.[116]

Angiocentric T/NK-cell lymphoma is characterized by a broad cytologic spectrum (Fig. 5–18). The atypical cells may be small or medium in size. Large atypical and hyperchromatic cells may be admixed, or they may predominate. If the small cells are in the majority, the disease may be difficult to distinguish from an inflammatory or infectious process. In early stages there may also be a prominent admixture of inflammatory cells, further causing difficulty in diagnosis.[144]

Because virtually all cases of nasal T/NK-cell lymphoma are positive for EBV, in situ hybridization studies with probes to EBV-encoded small nuclear RNA (EBER 1/2) may be helpful in diagnosis and can detect even small numbers of neoplastic cells.[145, 146]

Angiocentric T/NK-cell lymphoma is much more common in Asians than in people of European background. Clusters of the disease have also been reported in Central and South America in people of Native American heritage.[147] Thus, a racial predisposition appears to play a role in the pathogenesis of angiocentric T/NK-cell lymphoma.

Nasal disease may be controlled with radiation therapy, but the relapse rate is high. Chemotherapy is generally used in conjunction with radiation therapy. The most common site of relapse is skin and subcutaneous tissue.

A hemophagocytic syndrome is a common clinical complication, which adversely affects survival in angiocentric T/NK-cell lymphoma.[148] It is likely that EBV plays a role in the pathogenesis of the hemophagocytic syndrome.

Lymphomatoid granulomatosis (LYG) exhibits many similarities clinically and pathologically to angiocentric T/NK-cell lymphoma.[144] Only recently it was considered to be part of the same disease spectrum, angiocentric immunoproliferative lesions. However, recent data indicate that LYG is an EBV-positive B-cell proliferation associated with an exuberant T-cell reaction.[149] LYG also presents in extranodal sites, but the most common site of involvement is the lung.[150] The kidney and CNS are also frequently involved, as are skin and subcutaneous tissue. The pattern in necrosis in both LYG and T/NK-cell lymphoma is similar, emphasizing the likely importance of EBV in mediating the vascular damage.

Intestinal T-Cell Lymphoma (+/− enteropathy) (EATL)

WF: diffuse small cleaved, diffuse mixed small and large cell, diffuse large cell immunoblastic
Kiel: pleomorphic small, medium, and large

EATL was originally termed "malignant histiocytosis of the intestine."[151] However, the demonstration of clonal T-cell gene rearrangement indicated that it was a T-cell lymphoma. The small bowel usually shows ulceration, frequently with perforation. A mass may or may not be present. The infiltrate shows a varying cytologic composition with an admixture of small, medium, and larger atypical lymphoid cells. The adjacent small bowel may show villous atrophy associated with celiac disease.[152]

This disease occurs in adults, most of whom have a history of gluten-sensitive enteropathy. Patients usually present with abdominal symptoms such as pain, small bowel perforation, and associated peritonitis. The clinical course is aggressive.

Anaplastic Large Cell Lymphoma (ALCL)

WF: large cell, large cell immunoblastic
Kiel: ALCL (Ki1 + T cell)

ALCL is characterized by pleomorphic cells that have a propensity to invade lymphoid sinuses.[153] Because of the sinusoidal location of the tumor cells and their lobulated nuclear appearance, this disease was previously interpreted as a variant of malignant histiocytosis (Fig. 5–19). Misdiagnosis as metastatic carcinoma or melanoma is also common.

A consistent feature is the expression of the CD30 antigen, which is a hallmark of this disease. It has been referred to as "Ki-1+ lymphoma."[154] However, antigen expression is not specific for ALCL and is also seen in other forms of malignant lymphoma, including HD.[155]

ALCL can present in all age groups but is relatively more common in children and young adults. A high incidence of cutaneous disease has been reported.[156] A primary cutaneous form of ALCL is associated with lymphomatoid papulosis, and differs clinically, immunophenotypically, and at the molecular level.[157–159] Classic ALCL is associated with a characteristic chromosomal translocation, t(2;5)(p23;q35).[160, 161] Recently, the genes involved in this translocation have been identified, and a polymerase chain reaction method has been developed to detect cells containing the fused genes.[162]

The cells of classic ALCL have large, often lobated nuclei. Nucleoli are present but are usually not prominent and frequently basophilic. In some cases the nuclei may be round. The cytoplasm is usually abundant, amphophilic, with distinct cytoplasmic borders. A prominent Golgi region is usually apparent. Immunohistochemistry is valuable in the correct diagnosis of ALCL. The prominent Golgi region usually shows intense staining for CD30 and epithelial membrane antigen.[163]

Recently, histologic variants of classic ALCL have been described. These may contain a prominent admixture of histiocytes, which may lead to misdiagnosis as an inflammatory condition.[164] In some cases the cells are small to medium in size with abundant cytoplasm.[165] Again, staining with antibodies to CD30 can serve to highlight the malignant cells.

Primary cutaneous ALCL is a different disease that is closely related to lymphomatoid papulosis.[166] Indeed, lymphomatoid papulosis and cutaneous ALCL appear to represent a histologic and clinical continuum.[158, 167] Small lesions are likely to regress. Patients with large tumor masses may develop disseminated disease with lymph node involvement (Fig. 5–20). Patients with disseminated ALCL may relapse following therapy with skin lesions characteristic of lymphomatoid papulosis; these recurrent lesions may undergo spontaneous resolution.[166] Most patients with primary cutaneous ALCL have multiple skin lesions. Because the skin nodules may show spontaneous regression, usually a period of observation is warranted before the institution of any chemotherapy. Cutaneous ALCL is CD30+ but usually epithelial membrane antigen negative. It also appears to lack the t(2;5) translocation.[159]

ALCL Hodgkin's-Like (provisional)

WF: Hodgkin's disease, large cell immunoblastic
Kiel: ALCL, Hodgkin's disease

Hodgkin-related ALCL has been described as a provisional form of lymphoma that is difficult to distinguish from HD.[168] In many cases this process appears to be part of the spectrum of nodular-sclerosing Hodgkin's disease (NSHD).[169] It usually presents in young adults, often with a mediastinal mass. Skin lesions are not described. At low power, involved lymph nodes may show fibrous bands or capsular fibrosis resembling NSHD. An inflammatory background may be present focally, but elsewhere there is sheeting out of the malignant cells in a monomorphic fashion. In these monomorphic areas, the cells may lack the prominent eosinophilic nucleoli of Reed-Sternberg cells. Intrasinusoidal growth of the malignant cells may also be present.

It is still uncertain whether Hodgkin-like ALCL is part of the spectrum of HD or a variant of NHL.[170] It has been suggested that these patients respond poorly to conventional therapy for HD but do respond to third-generation chemotherapy regimens used in the treatment of aggressive NHL.[168]

HODGKIN'S DISEASE

SUBTYPES

The classification of HD has changed little since the introduction of the Lukes-Butler classification.[171] The original Lukes-Butler scheme contained six histologic subtypes (Table 5–8), which were reduced to four at the Rye Conference.[172] The elimination of the nodular lymphocyte predominant category is regrettable in that the lymphocyte-predominant category of HD as defined by the Rye scheme is heterogeneous.[173]

HD is somewhat unique among the malignant lymphomas in that the Reed-Sternberg cells and variants, the malignant cells, constitute the minority of cells present in the tumor mass (Fig. 5–21). These are associated with a rich inflammatory background containing lymphocytes, eosinophils, neutrophils, histiocytes, and plasma cells in varying proportions.

Nodular Sclerosis

NSHD is the most common subtype of HD, accounting for approximately 75% of cases in the United States.[171] This subtype is the only one that is more common in females than males. It tends to occur in young adults, usually younger than 50 years of age. Anterior mediastinal involvement is exceedingly common, with subsequent involvement of cervical and supraclavicular lymph nodes, upper abdominal lymph nodes, and spleen. Most patients present with stage 2 disease. Bulky mediastinal masses occur and are a poor prognostic sign. The disease may also directly extend into the adjacent lung.

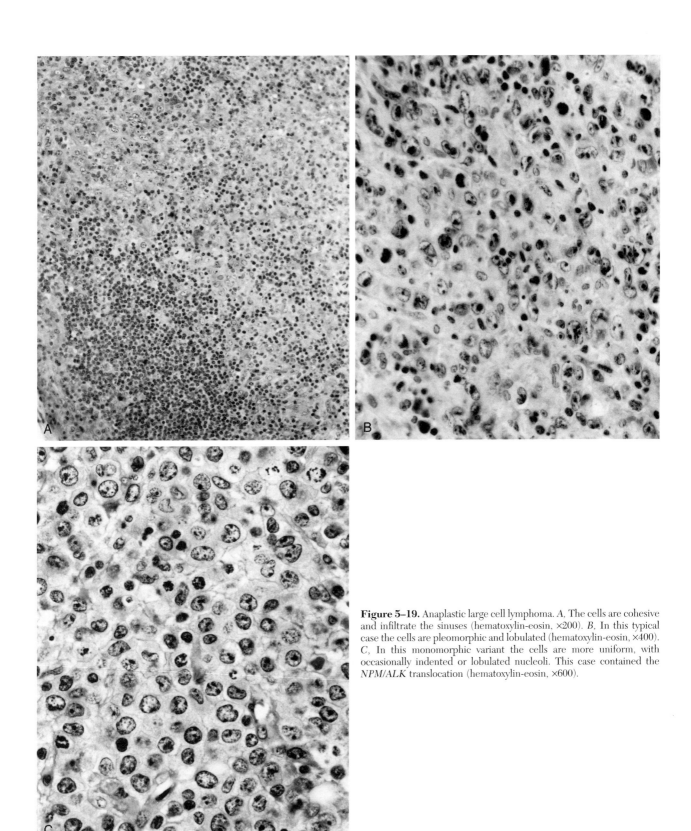

Figure 5–19. Anaplastic large cell lymphoma. *A*, The cells are cohesive and infiltrate the sinuses (hematoxylin-eosin, ×200). *B*, In this typical case the cells are pleomorphic and lobulated (hematoxylin-eosin, ×400). *C*, In this monomorphic variant the cells are more uniform, with occasionally indented or lobulated nucleoli. This case contained the *NPM/ALK* translocation (hematoxylin-eosin, ×600).

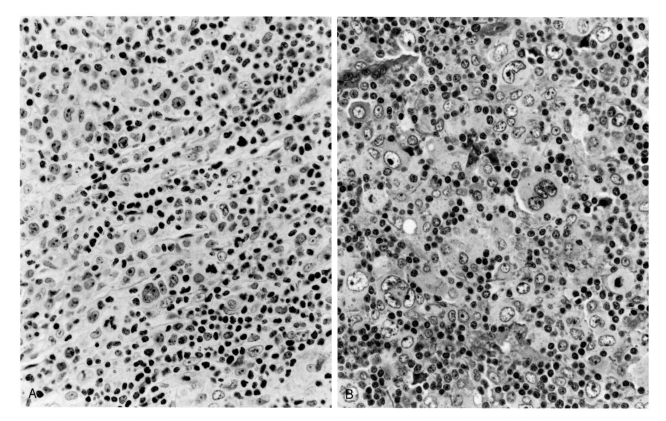

Figure 5–20. Lymphomatoid papulosis *(A)* and cutaneous anaplastic large cell lymphoma (ALCL) *(B)* are closely related. In this case both lesions were diagnosed in the same patient 5 years apart. The ALCL spread to lymph nodes (hematoxylin-eosin, ×400).

The diagnosis of NSHD requires the presence of (1) a nodular growth pattern, (2) broad bands of fibrosis, and (3) a characteristic variant of the Reed-Sternberg cell known as a "lacunar cell." The lacunar cell has abundant, clear cytoplasm with a sharply demarcated cell membrane. In formalin-fixed tissue a characteristic artifact often occurs; the cytoplasm of the cell retracts, leaving a clear space, or lacunus. The lacunar cell may be mononuclear, hyperlobated, or multinucleated. The nucleoli of the lacunar cell are generally smaller than those seen in classic Reed-Sternberg cells. The cellular phase of NSHD is defined as containing a nodular growth pattern with lacunar cells but with absent or minimal fibrous bands. The cellular phase of NSHD is not associated with unique clinical features and is a phase in the development of NSHD.

NSHD may be subclassified based on the frequency of the malignant cells and the presence of other histologic features such as necrosis and fibroblastic proliferation. The lymphocyte-depleted variant of NSHD contains numerous malignant cells that sheet out, often surrounding areas of necrosis.[174] This variant of NSHD is comparable to type 2 NSHD as defined in the classification of the BNLI.[170] The lymphocyte-depleted variant of NS and type 2 NSHD are associated with more aggressive clinical course. Type 2 NSHD also includes a fibrohistiocytic variant, rich in fibroblasts and histiocytes. The syncytial variant of NSHD, which lacks necrosis, is not generally associated with a poor prognosis.[175]

Mixed Cellularity Hodgkin's Disease

Mixed cellularity Hodgkin's disease (MCHD) as originally defined in the Lukes-Butler scheme is a category of exclusion that does not fulfill criteria for any of the other five histologic subtypes. It is usually associated with diffuse architectural effacement, but many cases of MCHD show an interfollicular pattern of involvement, with residual hyperplastic follicles. MCHD contains a rich inflammatory background with numerous eosinophils, plasma cells, and histiocytes. The Reed-Sternberg cells are of the classic type with prominent inclusion-like nucleoli. Lacunar cells are inconspicuous.

MCHD is more common in men than women.[172] It is frequently associated with disseminated disease at presentation.[176] B symptoms are also common.[177] It is one of the variants of HD, along with lymphocyte depletion, that is seen

Table 5–8. Classifications of Hodgkin's Disease

Lukes and Butler	Rye Modification	ILSG Scheme
Lymphocytic and/or histiocytic	Lymphocytic predominance	Lymphocyte predominance, nodular +/- diffuse
Nodular		Lymphocyte rich, classical HD
Diffuse		
Nodular sclerosis	Nodular sclerosis	Nodular sclerosis
Mixed cellularity	Mixed cellularity	Mixed cellularity
Diffuse fibrosis	Lymphocytic depletion	Lymphocytic depletion
Reticular		

ILSG, International Lymphoma Study Group.

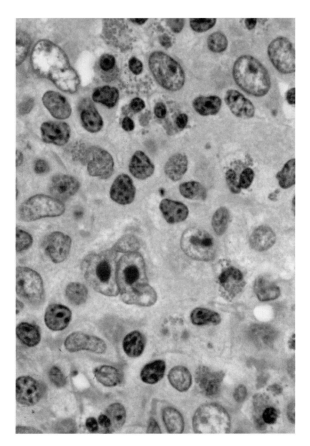

Figure 5–21. Hodgkin's disease, mixed cellularity. Classic Reed-Sternberg cells are admixed with lymphocytes, plasma cells, and eosinophils (hematoxylin-eosin, ×1000).

in association with HIV infection. MCHD is the subtype most often positive for EBV sequences.[178, 179]

Lymphocyte Depletion Hodgkin's Disease

Lymphocyte depletion Hodgkin's disease (LDHD) is the most uncommon subtype of HD, accounting for fewer than 5% of cases.[174] It is more common in men than women. Most patients with LDHD present with advanced-stage disease and B symptoms. Historically, many cases of high-grade NHL were misdiagnosed as LDHD. With improvements in diagnostic criteria, including immunohistochemical techniques, LDHD is diagnosed with much less frequency. Although it is still considered an aggressive form of HD, complete remissions can be obtained. The exceedingly poor prognosis of LDHD was most likely the result of the misdiagnosis of aggressive NHL as HD.

In the original Lukes-Butler scheme, LDHD consisted of two subtypes: diffuse fibrosis and reticular. Most cases of reticular LDHD were probably high-grade NHLs, although some cases can be seen in association with HIV infection or histologic progression. Most cases of LDHD diagnosed now would conform to the diffuse fibrosis subtype. In this form of HD there is a diffuse fibroblastic proliferation, abundant collagen deposition, and a paucity of inflammatory cells. Reed-Sternberg cells and variants are seen interspersed among the fibrous and inflammatory reaction.

Lymphocyte Predominance Hodgkin's Disease, Nodular and/or Diffuse

Lymphocyte predominance Hodgkin's disease (LPHD), a subtype of HD, has undergone significant reappraisal in recent years. Most cases have a nodular growth pattern, conforming to nodular paragranuloma in the Kiel scheme. However, mostly diffuse forms with identical cytologic features do exist, but are rare.

LPHD differs from classic HD in its immunophenotypic profile, histologic characteristics, and clinical behavior. Classic Reed-Sternberg cells are not seen or are exceedingly rare. The neoplastic cells are referred to as "L & H cells" or "popcorn cells." They have a lobulated nuclear contour, dispersed chromatin, and inconspicuous nucleoli (Fig. 5–22). They generally cluster within nodules associated with lymphocytes and histiocytes. Early on, the background lymphocytes are predominantly of B-cell phenotype, but T cells may predominate in later stages. The neoplastic cells, the popcorn cells, stain for CD20 and are generally negative for CD15 and negative or weakly positive for CD30.

LPHD is more common in men than women. It presents in young adults with a median peak incidence in the fourth and fifth decades. Most patients present with stage I disease. There is a high frequency of involvement of axillary, cervical, periparotid, and inguinal lymph nodes. Mediastinal lymphadenopathy is rare, in contrast with other forms of HD.

LPHD has an indolent clinical course but, paradoxically, a high relapse rate. However, relapses are not necessarily associated with clinical progression, and survival remains excellent, even in patients with recurrent disease. Progression to a large cell lymphoma of B-cell phenotype occurs in a small proportion of cases. The large cell lymphomas occasionally disseminate and pursue an aggressive clinical course.

Lymphocyte-Rich Classic Hodgkin's Disease (provisional)

Lymphocyte-rich classic HD is a provisional subtype defined in the ILSG classification. It is included in the lymphocyte predominant category of the Rye classification. It may be diffuse or nodular.[179a]

This tumor contains infrequent Reed-Sternberg cells, but the Reed-Sternberg cells have the classic morphology and immunophenotype. Popcorn cells are not seen; however, lacunar cells may be present. The background contains a predominance of small lymphocytes. However, there are usually small numbers of eosinophils and/or plasma cells. Eosinophils and plasma cells are rare in typical LPHD. This subtype of HD includes "lymphocyte predominant mixed cellularity" of Lennert and Mohri.[180] Recognition of this variant of LPHD is important because it carries the clinical behavior of classic HD rather than LPHD. If a complete remission is obtained, late relapses are exceedingly rare, in contrast with LPHD. Because it has not been widely diagnosed, however, data concerning its clinical behavior and prognosis are not widely available.

STAGING

The pathologist plays an important role in the staging of patients with HD. Although staging laparotomies are less

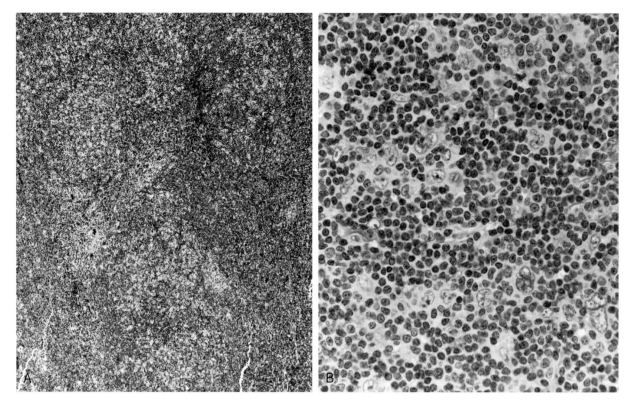

Figure 5–22. Nodular lymphocyte predominance Hodgkin's disease. *A*, Large, vague nodules replace the lymph node (hematoxylin-eosin, ×60). *B*, L & H cells have lobulated nuclei and inconspicuous nucleoli. Classic Reed-Sternberg cells are not seen (hematoxylin-eosin, ×500).

frequently performed now, needle-core biopsies of bone marrow are nearly always obtained.[181] Involved bone marrows usually have a fibrotic background with interspersed inflammatory cells, including plasma cells, eosinophils, and neutrophils. Reed-Sternberg cells and mononuclear variants may be difficult to observe. One does not require diagnostic Reed-Sternberg cells to interpret such a specimen as positive, although atypical mononuclear cells should be seen. Even in the absence of atypical mononuclear cells, a diffusely fibrotic bone marrow in a patient with HD should be regarded as highly suspicious for involvement. Serial sections may be needed to detect atypical mononuclear cells.

Similar criteria are used for the diagnosis of HD in needle-core biopsies of other sites, such as the liver. Fine-needle aspirates are also being performed for the diagnosis of HD and are particularly valuable in the diagnosis of relapse following therapy.[182] Immunocytochemistry may improve diagnostic accuracy when dealing with limited material, such as that obtained through needle biopsy.

Patients with a mediastinal mass often may present with a pleural effusion. However, it is extremely uncommon to observe malignant cells in such a specimen. The fluid usually accumulates secondary to obstruction and not secondary to pleural seeding by HD.

If a staging laparotomy is performed, careful examination of the spleen is required. The spleen should be sectioned at intervals of 3 to 4 mm to detect small foci of disease. Multiple splenic nodules are associated with an increased risk of hepatic involvement. Liver involvement virtually never occurs in the absence of splenic disease. HD involves the splenic white pulp. The involved malpighian corpuscles may be widely separated. If foci are not identified grossly, it is unlikely that occult microscopic disease will be found.

The criteria for involvement by lymphocyte predominance differ from those of classic HD. In LPHD popcorn cells or L & H cells will be identified in a background of normal lymphocytes with admixed histiocytes. Although bone marrow involvement is uncommon in LPHD, it does occur, especially in patients with progressive disease following multiple relapses. However, if bone marrow involvement is detected, the diagnosis of a T-cell–rich B-cell lymphoma should be suspected. In some instances this distinction is extremely difficult, and indeed, the neoplastic cells in some cases of T-cell–rich B-cell lymphoma are morphologically and phenotypically identical to those of LPHD.[78, 79]

SECOND HEMATOLOGIC MALIGNANCIES FOLLOWING HODGKIN'S DISEASE

Among the second malignancies following treatment for HD, acute nonlymphocytic leukemias and NHLs are the most common.[183] Acute leukemias occur usually 2 to 5 years after initial therapy but can be seen as late as 12 years. Patients receiving both radiation therapy and chemotherapy are at increased risk. The NHLs occur later in the course of disease, most often 10 or more years after diagnosis. The risk is relatively small (< 2% of cases of classic HD).[184] Most such NHLs are large cell lymphomas of B-cell type and Burkitt's-like lymphomas, often presenting as abdominal mass with involvement of the gastrointestinal tract. Rare cases of T-cell lymphoma have been described.[184] It had been postulated that these tumors might be secondary to the immunodeficiency of HD, possibly aggravated by additional immunosuppressive therapy.[185] Therefore, a role for EBV seemed likely. However, fewer than 20% of these tumors are EBV positive.[186]

Large B-cell lymphomas also occur in patients with LPHD. In large series this phenomenon occurs in fewer than 5% of cases.[187] It is postulated that these tumors most likely represent clonal progression of the original malignancy, since composite LCL and LPHD are observed with some frequency.[188] In both tumors the cells express a B-cell phenotype, but clonal identity by immunoglobulin gene rearrangement has not yet been shown. LCL in patients with LPHD often does not pursue an aggressive clinical course, especially if detected simultaneously with LPHD.[188]

REFERENCES

1. Rappaport H: Tumors of the hematopoietic system. *In* Atlas of Tumor Pathology. Washington, DC, Armed Forces Institute of Pathology, 1966.
2. Gerard-Marchant R, Hamlin I, Lennert K, et al: Classification of non-Hodgkin's lymphomas. Lancet 1974; 2:406.
3. Lennert K, Mohri N, Stein H, et al: The histopathology of malignant lymphoma. Br J Haematol 1975; 31 [suppl]:193.
4. Lukes R, Collins R: Immunologic characterization of human malignant lymphomas. Cancer 1974; 34:1488.
5. Bennett MH, Farrer-Brown, G, Henry K, et al: Classification of non-Hodgkin's lymphomas. Lancet 1974; 2:405.
6. Non-Hodgkin's Lymphoma Pathologic Classification Project: National Cancer Institute–sponsored study of classifications of non-Hodgkin's lymphomas: Summary and description of a Working Formulation for clinical usage. Cancer 1982; 49:2112.
7. Chan JK, Yip TT, Tsang WY, et al: Detection of Epstein-Barr viral RNA in malignant lymphomas of the upper aerodigestive tract. Am J Surg Pathol 1994; 18(9):938.
8. Levine PH, Cleghorn F, Manns A, et al: Adult T-cell leukemia/lymphoma: A working point-score classification for epidemiological studies. Int J Cancer 1994; 59(4):491.
9. Jaffe ES, Zarate OA, Medeiros LJ: The interrelationship of Hodgkin's disease and non-Hodgkin's lymphomas—lessons learned from composite and sequential malignancies. Semin Diagn Pathol 1992; 9(4):297.
10. Sander C, Medeiros L, Abruzzo L, et al: Lymphoblastic lymphoma presenting in cutaneous sites: A clinicopathologic analysis of six cases. J Am Acad Dermatol 1991; 25:1023.
11. Haddy TB, Kennan AM, Jaffe ES, et al: Bone involvement in young patients with non-Hodgkin's lymphoma: Efficacy of chemotherapy without local radiotherapy. Blood 1988; 72:1141.
12. Borowitz M, Croker B, Metzgar R: Lymphoblastic lymphoma with the phenotype of common acute lymphoblastic leukemia. Am J Clin Pathol 1983; 79:387.
13. Nathwani B, Diamond L, Winberg C, et al: Lymphoblastic lymphoma: A clinicopathologic study of 95 patients. Cancer 1981; 48:2347.
14. Lardelli P, Bookman M, Sundeen J, et al: Lymphocytic lymphoma of intermediate differentiation: Morphologic and immunophenotypic spectrum and clinical correlations. Am J Surg Pathol 1990; 14:752.
15. Pangalis G, Nathwani B, Rappaport H: Malignant lymphoma, well-differentiated lymphocytic: Its relationship with chronic lymphocytic leukemia and macroglobulinemia of Waldenström. Cancer 1977; 39:999.
16. Dick F, Maca R: The lymph node in chronic lymphocytic leukemia. Cancer 1978; 41:283.
17. Pombo de Oliveira MS, Jaffe ES, Catovsky D: Leukemic phase of mantle zone (intermediate) lymphoma: Its characterization in 11 cases. J Clin Pathol 1989; 42:962.
18. Perry D, Bast M, Armitage J, et al: Diffuse intermediate lymphocytic lymphoma: A clinicopathologic study and comparison with small lymphocytic lymphoma and diffuse small cleaved cell lymphoma. Cancer 1990; 66:1995.
19. Evans H, Butler J, Youness E: Malignant lymphoma, small lymphocytic type: A clinicopathologic study of 84 cases with suggested criteria for intermediate lymphocytic lymphoma. Cancer 1978; 41:1440.
20. Richter M: Generalized reticular cell sarcoma of lymph nodes associated with lymphocytic leukemia. Am J Pathol 1982; 4:285.
21. Williams J, Schned A, Cotelingam JD, et al: Chronic lymphocytic leukemia with coexistent Hodgkin's disease: Implications for the origin of the Reed-Sternberg cell. Am J Surg Pathol 1991; 15:33.
22. Brecher M, Banks P: Hodgkin's disease variant of Richter's syndrome: Report of eight cases. Am J Clin Pathol 1990; 93:333.
23. Momose H, Jaffe ES, Shin SS, et al: Chronic lymphocytic leukemia/small lymphocytic lymphoma with Reed-Sternberg–like cells and possible transformation to Hodgkin's disease: Mediation by Epstein-Barr virus. Am J Surg Pathol 1992; 16(9):859.
24. Ben-Ezra J, Burke J, Swartz W, et al: Small lymphocytic lymphoma: A clinicopathologic analysis of 268 cases. Blood 1989; 73:579.
25. Lennert K, Tamm I, Wacker HH: Histopathology and immunocytochemistry of lymph node biopsies in chronic lymphocytic leukemia and immunocytoma. Leuk Lymphoma 1991; 7(Suppl):157.
26. Hall PA, D'Ardenne AJ, Richards MA, et al: Lymphoplasmacytoid lymphoma: An immunohistological study. J Pathol 1987; 153(3):213.
27. Jaffe ES, Raffeld M, Medeiros LJ: Histopathologic subtypes of indolent lymphomas: Caricatures of the mature B-cell system. Semin Oncol 1993; 20:3.
28. Harris N, Bhan A: B-cell neoplasms of the lymphocytic, lymphoplasmacytoid, and plasma cell types: Immunohistologic analysis and clinical correlation. Hum Pathol 1985; 16:829.
29. Zukerberg L, Medeiros L, Ferry J, et al: Diffuse low-grade B-cell lymphomas: Four clinically distinct subtypes defined by a combination of morphologic and immunophenotypic features. Am J Clin Pathol 1993; 100:373.
30. Sundeen J, Longo D, Jaffe E: CD5 expression in B-cell small lymphocytic malignancies: Correlations with clinical presentation and sites of disease. Am J Surg Pathol 1992; 16:130.
31. Raffeld M, Jaffe ES: *bcl-1*, t(11;14), and mantle cell–derived neoplasms. Blood 1991; 78:259.
32. Banks P, Chan J, Cleary M, et al: Mantle cell lymphoma: A proposal for unification of morphologic, immunologic, and molecular data. Am J Surg Pathol 1992; 16:637.
33. Jaffe E, Bookman M, Longo D: Lymphocytic lymphoma of intermediate differentiation: Mantle zone lymphoma. Hum Pathol 1987; 18:877.
34. Weisenburger DD, Kim H, Rappaport H: Mantle zone lymphoma: A follicular variant of intermediate lymphocytic lymphoma. Cancer 1982; 49:1429.
35. Bookman MA, Lardelli P, Jaffe ES, et al: Lymphocytic lymphoma of intermediate differentiation: Morphologic, immunophenotypic, and prognostic factors. J Natl Cancer Inst 1990; 82:742.
36. Meusers P, Engelhard M, Bartels H, et al: Multicentre randomized therapeutic trial for advanced centrocytic lymphoma: Anthracycline does not improve the prognosis. Hematol Oncol 1989; 7:365.
37. O'Brian D, Kennedy M, Daly P, et al: Multiple lymphomatous polyposis of the gastrointestinal tract: A clinicopathologically distinctive form of non-Hodgkin's lymphoma of centrocytic type. Am J Surg Pathol 1989; 13:691.
38. Lennert K: Histopathology of non-Hodgkin's lymphomas: Based on the Kiel classification. New York, Springer-Verlag, 1981.
39. Weisenburger DD, Nathwani BN, Diamond LW, et al: Malignant lymphoma, intermediate lymphocytic type: A clinicopathologic study of 42 cases. Cancer 1981; 48:1415.
40. Zukerberg L, Medeiros L, Ferry J, et al: Diffuse low-grade B-cell lymphomas: Identification of four major immunophenotypic subtypes [Abstract]. Lab Invest 1991; 62:87A.
41. Medeiros L, van Krieken J, Jaffe E, et al: Association of *bcl-1* rearrangements with lymphocytic lymphoma of intermediate differentiation. Blood 1990; 76:2086.
42. Raffeld M, Sander CA, Yano T, et al: Mantle cell lymphoma: An update. Leuk Lymphoma 1992; 8(3):161.
43. Rosenberg C, Wong E, Petty E, et al: Overexpression of *PRAD1*, a candidate *BCL1* breakpoint region oncogene, in centrocytic lymphomas. Proc Natl Acad Sci U S A 1991; 88:9638.
44. Bosch F, Jares P, Campo E, et al: *PRAD-1* cyclin D1 gene overexpression in chronic lymphoproliferative disorders: A highly specific marker of mantle cell lymphoma. Blood 1994; 84(8):2726.
45. Come FS, Jaffe ES, Andersen JC, et al: Non-Hodgkin's lymphomas

in leukemic phase: Clinicopathologic correlations. Am J Med 1980; 69:667.

46. Hu E, Trela M, Thompson J, et al: Detection of B-cell lymphoma in peripheral blood by DNA hybridisation. Lancet 1985; 2:1092.

47. Mann R, Berard C: Criteria for the cytologic subclassification of follicular lymphomas: A proposed alternative method. Hematol Oncol 1982; 1:187.

48. Croce C, Nowell P: Molecular basis of human B-cell neoplasia. Blood 1985; 65:1.

49. Hockenbery D, Zutter M, Hickey W, et al: BCL2 protein is topographically restricted in tissues characterized by apoptotic cell death. Proc Natl Acad Sci U S A 1991; 88:6961.

50. Gaulard P, d'Agay M, Peuchmaur M, et al: Expression of the *bcl-2* gene product in follicular lymphoma. Am J Pathol 1992; 140:1089.

51. Garvin AJ, Simon R, Young RC, et al: The Rappaport classification of non-Hodgkin's lymphomas: A closer look using other proposed classifications. Semin Oncol 1980; 7:234.

52. Medeiros L, Lardelli P, Stetler-Stevenson M, et al: Genotypic analysis of diffuse, mixed cell lymphomas: Comparison with morphologic and immunophenotypic findings. Am J Clin Pathol 1991; 95:547.

53. Garcia CF, Weiss LM, Warnke RA, et al: Cutaneous follicular lymphoma. Am J Surg Pathol 1986; 10:454.

54. Santucci M, Pimpinelli N, Arganini L: Primary cutaneous B-cell lymphoma—a unique type of low-grade lymphoma: Clinicopathologic and immunologic study of 83 cases. Cancer 1991; 67:2311.

55. Isaacson P, Wright D: Malignant lymphoma of mucosa associated lymphoid tissue: A distinctive B-cell lymphoma. Cancer 1983; 52:1410.

56. Isaacson P, Spencer J: Malignant lymphoma of mucosa-associated lymphoid tissue. Histopathology 1987; 11:445.

57. Isaacson P, Wotherspoon A, Diss T, et al: Follicular colonization in B-cell lymphoma of mucosa-associated lymphoid tissue. Am J Surg Pathol 1991; 15:819.

58. Pelstring R, Essell J, Kurtin P, et al: Diversity of organ site involvement among malignant lymphomas of mucosa-associated tissues. Am J Clin Pathol 1991; 96:738.

59. Parveen T, Navarro-Roman L, Medeiros L, et al: Low-grade B-cell lymphoma of mucosa-associated lymphoid tissue arising in the kidney. Arch Pathol Lab Med 1993; 117:780.

60. Shin S, Sheibani K, Fishleder A, et al: Monocytoid B-cell lymphoma in patients with Sjögren's syndrome: A clinicopathologic study of 13 patients. Hum Pathol 1991; 22:422.

61. Cogliatti S, Lennert K, Hansmann M, et al: Monocytoid B-cell lymphoma: Clinical and prognostic features of 21 patients. J Clin Pathol 1990; 43:619.

62. Ortiz-Hidalgo C, Wright DH: The morphological spectrum of monocytoid B-cell lymphoma and its relationship to lymphomas of mucosa-associated lymphoid tissue. Histopathology 1992; 21:555.

63. Nizze H, Cogliatti S, von Schilling C, et al: Monocytoid B-cell lymphoma: Morphological variants and relationship to low-grade B-cell lymphoma of the mucosa-associated lymphoid tissue. Histopathology 1991; 18:403.

64. Hussell T, Isaacson P, Crabtree J, et al: The response of cells from low-grade B-cell gastric lymphomas of mucosa-associated lymphoid tissue to *Helicobacter pylori.* Lancet 1993; 342:571.

65. Sheibani K, Burke J, Swartz W, et al: Monocytoid B-cell lymphoma: Clinicopathologic study of 21 cases of a unique type of low-grade lymphoma. Cancer 1988; 62:1531.

66. Ngan BY, Warnke R, Wilson M, et al: Monocytoid B-cell lymphoma: A study of 36 cases. Hum Pathol 1991; 22:409.

67. Hollema H, Visser L, Poppema S: Small lymphocytic lymphomas with predominant splenomegaly: A comparison of immunophenotypes with cases of predominant lymphadenopathy. Mod Pathol 1991; 4:712.

68. Neiman R, Sullivan A, Jaffe R: Malignant lymphoma simulating leukaemic reticuloendotheliosis: A clinicopathologic study of ten cases. Cancer 1979; 43:329.

69. Schmid C, Kirkham N, Diss T, et al: Splenic marginal zone cell lymphoma. Am J Surg Pathol 1992; 16:455.

70. Melo J, Hegde U, Parreira A, et al: Splenic B-cell lymphoma with circulating villous lymphocytes: Differential diagnosis of B-cell leukaemias with large spleens. J Clin Pathol 1987; 40:642.

71. Callihan TT, Holbert JM, Berard CW: Neoplasms of terminal B-cell differentiation: The morphological basis of functional diversity. *In* Sommers SC, Rosen PP (eds): Malignant Lymphomas, Pathology Annual. Norwalk, CT, Appleton-Century-Crofts, 1983, p. 169.

72. Falini B, De Solas I, Levine A, et al: Emergence of B-immunoblastic sarcoma in patients with multiple myeloma: A clinicopathologic study of 10 cases. Blood 1982; 59:923.

73. Zukerberg L, Ferry J, Conlon M, et al: Plasma cell myeloma with cleaved, multilobated, and monocytoid nuclei. Am J Clin Pathol 1990; 93:657.

74. O'Hara C, Said J, Pinkus G: Non-Hodgkin's lymphoma, multilobated B cell type. Hum Pathol 1986; 17:593.

75. Pettit C, Zukerberg L, Gray M, et al: Primary lymphoma of bone: A B-cell tumor with a high frequency of multilobated cells. Am J Surg Pathol 1990; 14:329.

76. Lamarre L, Jacobson J, Aisenberg A, et al: Primary large cell lymphoma of the mediastinum. Am J Surg Pathol 1989; 13:730.

77. Jaffe E: Post-thymic lymphoid neoplasia. *In* Jaffe E (ed): Surgical Pathology of the Lymph Nodes and Related Organs. Philadelphia, WB Saunders, 1985, p 218.

78. Chittal S, Brousset P, Voigt J, et al: Large B-cell lymphoma rich in T cells and simulating Hodgkin's disease. Histopathology 1991; 19:211.

79. Delabie J, Vandenberghe E, Kennes C, et al: Histiocyte-rich B-cell lymphoma: A distinct clinicopathologic entity possibly related to lymphocyte predominant Hodgkin's disease, paragranuloma subtype. Am J Surg Pathol 1992; 16:37.

80. Macon W, Williams M, Greer J, et al: T-cell-rich B-cell lymphomas: A clinicopathologic study of 19 cases. Am J Surg Pathol 1992; 16(4):351.

81. Ramsay A, Smith W, Isaacson P: T-cell-rich B-cell lymphoma. Am J Surg Pathol 1988; 12:433.

82. Krishnan J, Wallberg K, Frizzera G: T-cell-rich large B-cell lymphoma: A study of 30 cases supporting its histologic heterogeneity and lack of clinical distinctiveness. Am J Surg Pathol 1994; 18:455.

83. Nathwani B, Dixon D, Jones S, et al: The clinical significance of the morphological subdivision of diffuse "histiocytic" lymphoma: A study of 162 patients treated by the Southwest Oncology Group. Blood 1982; 60:1068.

84. Warnke RA, Strauchern JA, Burke JS, et al: Morphologic types of diffuse large cell lymphoma. Cancer 1982; 50:690.

85. Harris NL, Jaffe ES, Stein H, et al: A revised European-American classification of lymphoid neoplasms: A proposal from the International Lymphoma Study Group [see comments]. Blood 1994; 84(5):1361.

86. Lennert K, Feller A: Histopathology of Non-Hodgkin's Lymphomas, 2nd ed. New York, Springer-Verlag, 1992.

87. Longo DL, Duffey PL, DeVita VJ, et al: Treatment of advanced-stage Hodgkin's disease: Alternating noncross-resistant MOPP/CABS is not superior to MOPP. J Clin Oncol 1991; 9(8):1409.

88. Miller TP, Grogan TM, Dahlberg S, et al: Prognostic significance of the Ki-67–associated proliferative antigen in aggressive non-Hodgkin's lymphomas: A prospective Southwest Oncology Group trial. Blood 1994; 83:1460.

89. Hall PA, Richards MA, Gregory WM, et al: The prognostic value of Ki-67 immunostaining in non-Hodgkin's lymphoma. J Pathol 1988; 154(3):223.

90. Gerdes J, Stein H, Pileri S, et al: Prognostic relevance of tumour cell growth fraction in malignant non-Hodgkin's lymphomas [letter] [published erratum appears in Lancet 1987 Sep 26;2(8561):756]. Lancet 1987; 2(8556):448.

91. Piris MA, Pezzella F, Martinez MJ, et al: p53 and *bcl-2* expression in high-grade B-cell lymphomas: Correlation with survival time [published erratum appears in Br J Cancer 1994 May;69(5):978]. Br J Cancer 1994; 69(2):337.

92. Addis B, Isaacson P: Large cell lymphoma of the mediastinum: A B-cell tumor of probable thymic origin. Histopathology 1986; 10:379.

93. Moller P, Moldenhauer G, Momburg F, et al: Mediastinal lymphoma of clear cell type is a tumor corresponding to terminal steps of B-cell differentiation. Blood 1987; 69:1087.

94. Hofmann WJ, Momburg F, Moller P: Thymic medullary cells expressing B-lymphocyte antigens. Hum Pathol 1988; 19:1280.

95. Kanavaros P, Gaulard P, Charlotte F, et al: Discordant expression of immunoglobulin and its associated molecule mb-1/CD79a is frequently found in mediastinal large B-cell lymphomas. Am J Pathol 1995; 146(3):735.

96. Jacobson J, Aisenberg A, Lamarre L, et al: Mediastinal large cell lymphoma: An uncommon subset of adult lymphoma curable with combined modality therapy. Cancer 1988; 62:1893.

97. Magrath I, Shiramizu B: Biology and treatment of small noncleaved cell lymphoma. Oncology 1989; 3:41.

98. Ballerini P, Gaidano G, Gong J, et al: Multiple genetic lesions in AIDS-related non-Hodgkin's lymphoma. Blood 1993; 81:166.

99. Pelicci P, Knowles D, Magrath I, et al: Chromosomal breakpoints and structural alterations of the c-*myc* locus differ in endemic and sporadic forms of Burkitt's lymphoma. Proc Natl Acad Sci U S A, 1986; 83: 2984.

100. Yano T, van Krieken J, Magrath IT, et al: Histogenetic correlations between subcategories of small noncleaved cell lymphomas. Blood 1992; 79(5):1282.

101. Cavdar AO, Gozdasoglu S, Yavuz G, et al: Burkitt's lymphoma between African and American types in Turkish children: Clinical, viral (EBV), and molecular studies. Med Pediatr Oncol 1993; 21(1):36.

102. Goldschmidts WL, Bhatia K, Johnson JF, et al: Epstein-Barr virus genotypes in AIDS-associated lymphomas are similar to those in endemic Burkitt's lymphomas. Leukemia 1992; 6(9):875.

103. Hollingsworth HC, Longo DL, Jaffe ES: Small noncleaved cell lymphoma associated with florid epithelioid granulomatous response: A clinicopathologic study of seven patients. Am J Surg Pathol 1993; 17(1):51.

104. Longo DL, Duffey PL, Jaffe ES, et al: Diffuse small noncleaved cell, non-Burkitt's lymphoma in adults: A high-grade lymphoma responsive to ProMACE-based combination chemotherapy. J Clin Oncol 1994; 12(10):2153.

105. Miliauskas JR, Berard CW, Young RC, et al: Undifferentiated non-Burkitt's lymphomas (Burkitt's and non-Burkitt's types): The relevance of making this histologic distinction. Cancer 1982; 50:2115.

106. Suchi T, Lennert K, Tu LY: Histopathology and immunohistochemistry of peripheral T-cell lymphomas: A proposal for their classification. J Clin Pathol 1987; 40:995.

107. Noorduyn LA, Van der Valk P, Van Heerde P, et al: Stage is a better prognostic indicator than morphologic subtype in primary noncutaneous T-cell lymphoma. Am J Clin Pathol 1990; 93:49.

108. Hastrup N, Hamilton-Dutoit S, Ralfkiaer E, et al: Peripheral T-cell lymphomas: An evaluation of reproducibility of the updated Kiel classification. Histopathology 1991; 18:99.

109. Schlegelberger B, Himmler A, Godde E, et al: Cytogenetic findings in peripheral T-cell lymphomas as a basis for distinguishing low-grade and high-grade lymphomas. Blood 1994; 83:505.

110. Nathwani B, Kim H, Rappaport H: Malignant lymphoma, lymphoblastic. Cancer 1976; 38:964.

111. Gouttefangeas C, Bensussan A, Boumsell L: Study of the CD3-associated T-cell receptors reveals further differences between T-cell acute lymphoblastic lymphoma and leukemia. Blood 1990; 74:931.

112. Matutes E, Brito-Babapulle V, Swansbury J, et al: Clinical and laboratory features of 78 cases of T-prolymphocytic leukemia. Blood 1991; 78:3269.

113. Brouet J, Sasportes M, Flandrin G, et al: Chronic lymphocytic leukemia of T-cell origin. Lancet 1975; 2:890.

114. Loughran T: Clonal diseases of large granular lymphocytes. Blood 1993; 82:1.

115. Scott AA, Head DR, Kopecky KJ, et al: HLA-DR–, CD33+, CD56+, CD16– myeloid/natural killer cell acute leukemia: A previously unrecognized form of acute leukemia potentially misdiagnosed as French-American-British acute myeloid leukemia-M3 [see comments]. Blood 1994; 84(1):244.

116. Imamura N, Kusunoki Y, Kawa-Ha K, et al: Aggressive natural killer cell leukaemia/lymphoma—report of four cases and review of the literature: Possible existence of a new clinical entity originating from the third lineage of lymphoid cells [see comments]. Br J Haematol 1990; 75(1):49.

117. Colby T, Burke J, Hoppe R: Lymph node biopsy in mycosis fungoides. Cancer 1981; 47:351.

118. Burke J, Khalil S, Rappaport H: Dermatopathic lymphadenopathy: An immunophenotypic comparison of cases associated and unassociated with mycosis fungoides. Am J Pathol 1986; 123:256.

118a. Sausville EA, Eddy JL, Makuch RW, et al: Histopathologic staging at initial diagnosis of mycosis fungoides and the Sézary syndrome: Definition of three distinctive prognostic groups. Ann Intern Med 1988; 109(5):372.

119. Patsouris E, Noel H, Lennert K: Histological and immunohistological findings in lymphoepithelioid cell lymphoma (Lennert's lymphoma). Am J Surg Pathol 1988; 12(5):341.

120. Kim H, Jacobs C, Warnke R, et al: Malignant lymphoma with a high content of epithelioid histiocytes: A distinct clinicopathologic entity and a form of so-called "Lennert's lymphoma." Cancer 1978; 41:620.

121. Armitage J, Greer J, Levine A, et al: Peripheral T-cell lymphoma. Cancer 1989; 63:158.

122. Lippman S, Miller T, Spier C, et al: The prognostic significance of the immunotype in diffuse large cell lymphoma: A comparative study of the T-cell and B-cell phenotype. Blood 1988; 72:436.

123. Coiffier B, Brousse N, Peuchmaur M, et al: Peripheral T-cell lymphomas have a worse prognosis than B-cell lymphomas: A prospective study of 361 immunophenotyped patients treated with the LNH-84 regimen. Ann Oncol 1990; 1:45.

124. Gonzalez C, Medeiros L, Braziel R, et al: T-cell lymphoma involving subcutaneous tissue: A clinicopathologic entity commonly associated with hemophagocytic syndrome. Am J Surg Pathol 1991; 15:17.

125. Burg G, Dummer R, Wilhelm M, et al: A subcutaneous delta-positive T-cell lymphoma that produces interferon gamma [see comments]. N Engl J Med 1991; 325(15):1078.

126. Farcet J, Gaulard P, Marolleau J, et al: Hepatosplenic T-cell lymphoma: Sinusal/sinusoidal localization of malignant cells expressing the T-cell receptor γδ. Blood 1990; 75:2213.

127. Cooke CB, Greiner T, Raffeld M, et al: Gamma/delta T-cell lymphoma: A distinct clinico-pathological entity. Mod Pathol 1994; 7:106A.

128. Cooke CB, Krenacs L, Stetler-Stevenson M, et al. Hepatosplenic T cell lymphoma: a distinct clinicopathologic entity of cytotoxic γδ T-cell origin, Blood 1996; 88:4265.

129. Frizzera G, Moran E, Rappaport H: Angio-immunoblastic lymphadenopathy with dysproteinemia. Lancet 1974; 1:1070.

130. Weiss L, Strickler J, Dorfman R, et al: Clonal T-cell populations in angioimmunoblastic lymphadenopathy and angioimmunoblastic lymphadenopathy-like lymphoma. Am J Pathol 1986; 122:392.

131. Feller A, Griesser H, Schilling C, et al: Clonal gene rearrangement patterns correlate with immunophenotype and clinical parameters in patients with angioimmunoblastic lymphadenopathy. Am J Pathol 1988; 133:549.

132. Abruzzo LV, Schmidt K, Weiss LM, et al: B-cell lymphoma after angioimmunoblastic lymphadenopathy: A case with oligoclonal gene rearrangements associated with Epstein-Barr virus. Blood 1993; 82(1):241.

133. Uchiyama T, Yodoi J, Sagawa K, et al: Adult T-cell leukemia: Clinical and hematologic features of 16 cases. Blood 1977; 50:481.

134. Poiesz B, Ruscetti F, Gazdar A: Detection and isolation of type C retrovirus particles from fresh and cultured lymphocytes of a patient with cutaneous T-cell lymphoma. Proc Natl Acad Sci U S A 1980; 77:7415.

135. Swerdlow S, Habeshaw J, Rohatiner A, et al: Caribbean T-cell lymphoma/leukemia. Cancer 1984; 54:687.

136. Manns A, Cleghorn FR, Falk RT, et al: Role of HTLV-I in the development of non-Hodgkin's lymphoma in Jamaica and Trinidad and Tobago: The HTLV Lymphoma Study Group. Lancet 1993; 342(8885):1447.

137. Jaffe E, Blattner W, Blayney D, et al: The pathologic spectrum of adult T-cell leukemia/lymphoma in the United States. Am J Surg Pathol 1984; 8:263.

138. Levine PH, Manns A, Jaffe ES, et al: The effect of ethnic differences on the pattern of HTLV-I–associated T-cell leukemia/lymphoma (HATL) in the United States. Int J Cancer 1994; 56(2):177.

139. Abrams M, Sidawy M, Novich M: Smoldering HTLV-associated T-cell leukemia. Arch Intern Med 1985; 145:2257.

140. Kikuchi M, Mitsui T, Takeshita M, et al: Virus-associated adult T-cell leukemia (ATL) in Japan: Clinical, histological, and immunological studies. Hematol Oncol 1987; 4:67.

141. Duggan D, Ehrlich G, Davey F, et al: HTLV-I–induced lymphoma mimicking Hodgkin's disease: Diagnosis by polymerase chain reaction amplification of specific HTLV-I sequences in tumor DNA. Blood 1988; 71:1027.

142. Chan J, Ng C, Lau W, et al: Most nasal/nasopharyngeal lymphomas are peripheral T-cell neoplasms. Am J Surg Pathol 1987; 11:418.

143. Ho F, Choy D, Loke S, et al: Polymorphic reticulosis and conventional lymphomas of the nose and upper aerodigestive tract: A clinicopathologic study of 70 cases, and immunophenotypic studies of 16 cases. Hum Pathol 1990; 21:1041.

144. Ferry J, Sklar J, Zukerberg L, et al: Nasal lymphoma: A clinicopathologic study with immunophenotypic and genotypic analysis. Am J Surg Pathol 1991; 15:268.

145. Lipford E, Margolich J, Longo D, et al: Angiocentric immunoproliferative lesions: A clinicopathologic spectrum of post-thymic T-cell proliferations. Blood 1988; 5:1674.

146. Jaffe E, Chan J, Su I, et al: Report of the workshop on nasal and related extranodal angiocentric T/NK cell lymphomas: Definitions, differential diagnosis, and epidemiology. Am J Surg Pathol 1996; 20:103.

147. Tsang WY, Chan JK, Yip TT, et al: In situ localization of Epstein-Barr virus–encoded RNA in non-nasal/nasopharyngeal CD56-positive and CD56-negative T-cell lymphomas. Hum Pathol 1994; 25(8):758.

148. Arber DA, Weiss LM, Albujar PF, et al: Nasal lymphomas in Peru: High incidence of T-cell immunophenotype and Epstein-Barr virus infection. Am J Surg Pathol 1993; 17(4):392.

149. Jaffe ES, Costa J, Fauci AS, et al: Malignant lymphoma and erythrophagocytosis-simulating malignant histiocytosis. Am J Med 1983; 75(5):741.

150. Guinee DJ, Jaffee E, Kingma D, et al: Pulmonary lymphomatoid granulomatosis: Evidence for a proliferation of Epstein-Barr virus–infected B lymphocytes with a prominent T-cell component and vasculitis. Am J Surg Pathol 1994; 18(8):753.

151. Katzenstein AL, Peiper S: Detection of Epstein-Barr genomes in lymphomatoid granulomatosis: Analysis of 29 cases by the polymerase chain reaction. Mod Pathol 1990; 3:435.

152. Isaacson P, Spencer J, Connolly C, et al: Malignant histiocytosis of the intestine: A T-cell lymphoma. Lancet 1985; 2:688.

153. Chott A, Dragosics B, Radaszkiewicz T: Peripheral T-cell lymphomas of the intestine. Am J Pathol 1992; 141:1361.

154. Stein H, Mason D, Gerdes J, et al: The expression of the Hodgkin's disease–associated antigen Ki-1 in reactive and neoplastic lymphoid tissue: Evidence that Reed-Sternberg cells and histiocytic malignancies are derived from activated lymphoid cells. Blood 1985; 66:848.

155. Agnarsson B, Kadin M: Ki-1–positive large cell lymphoma: A morphologic and immunologic study of 19 cases. Am J Surg Pathol 1988; 12:264.

156. Piris M, Brown D, Gatter K, et al: CD30 expression in non-Hodgkin's lymphoma. Histopathology 1990; 17:211.

157. Kaudewitz P, Stein H, Dallenbach F, et al: Primary and secondary cutaneous Ki-1+ (CD30+) anaplastic large cell lymphomas: Morphologic, immunohistologic, and clinical characteristics. Am J Pathol 1989; 135(2):359.

158. de Bruin P, Beljaards R, van Heerde P, et al: Differences in clinical behaviour and immunophenotype between primary cutaneous and primary nodal anaplastic large cell lymphoma of T-cell or null cell phenotype. Histopathology 1993;23:127.

159. Willemze R, Beljaards RC: Spectrum of primary cutaneous CD30 (Ki-1)-positive lymphoproliferative disorders: A proposal for classification and guidelines for management and treatment. J Am Acad Dermatol 1993;28(6):973.

160. Wellman A, Otsuki T, Vogelbruch M, et al: Analysis of the t(2;5) (p23;q35) by RT-PCR in CD30-positive anaplastic large cell lymphomas, in other non-Hodgkin's lymphomas of T-cell phenotype, and in Hodgkin's disease. Blood 1995; 86:2321.

161. Mason D, Bastard C, Rimokh R, et al: CD30-positive large cell lymphomas ("Ki-1 lymphoma") are associated with a chromosomal translocation involving 5q35. Br J Haematol 1990; 74:161.

162. Bitter MA, Franklin WA, Larson RA, et al: Morphology in Ki-1(CD30)-positive non-Hodgkin's lymphoma is correlated with clinical features and the presence of a unique chromosomal abnormality, t(2;5)(p23;q35). Am J Surg Pathol 1990; 14(4):305.

163. Morris SW, Kirstein MN, Valentine MB, et al: Fusion of a kinase gene, ALK, to a nucleolar protein gene, NPM, in non-Hodgkin's lymphoma [published erratum appears in Science 1995 Jan 20;267(5196):316]. Science 1994; 263(5151):1281.

164. Delsol G, Al Saati T, Gatter K, et al: Coexpression of epithelial membrane antigen (EMA), Ki-1, and interleukin-2 receptor by anaplastic large cell lymphomas: Diagnostic value in so-called malignant histiocytosis. Am J Pathol 1988; 130:59.

165. Pileri S, Falini B, Delsol G, et al: Lymphohistiocytic T-cell lymphoma (anaplastic large cell lymphoma CD30+/Ki1+) with a high content of reactive histiocytes. Histopathology 1990; 16:383.

166. Kinney M, Collins R, Greer J, et al: A small cell–predominant variant of primary Ki-1 (CD30)+ T-cell lymphoma. Am J Surg Pathol 1993; 17:859.

167. McCarty MJ, Vukelja SJ, Sausville EA, et al: Lymphomatoid papulosis associated with Ki-1–positive anaplastic large cell lymphoma: A report of two cases and a review of the literature. Cancer 1994; 74 (11):3051.

168. Kaudewitz P, Burg G, Stein H: Ki-1 (CD30)-positive cutaneous anaplastic large cell lymphomas. Curr Probl Dermatol 1990; 19(150): 150.

169. Pileri S, Bocchia M, Baroni C, et al: Anaplastic large cell lymphoma (CD30+/Ki-1+): Results of a prospective clinicopathologic study of 69 cases. Br J Haematol 1994; 86:513.

170. Leoncini L, Del Vecchio M, Kraft R, et al: Hodgkin's disease and CD30-positive anaplastic large cell lymphomas—a continuous spectrum of malignant disorders. Am J Pathol 1990; 137:1047.

171. MacLennan K, Bennett M, Tu A, et al: Relationship of histopathologic features to survival and relapse in nodular sclerosing Hodgkin's disease. Cancer 1989;64:1686.

172. Lukes R, Butler J, Hicks E: Natural history of Hodgkin's disease as related to its pathological picture. Cancer 1966; 19:317.

173. Kaplan HS: Hodgkin's Disease, 2nd ed. Cambridge, MA, Harvard Press, 1980.

174. Mason DY, Banks PM, Chan J, et al: Nodular lymphocyte predominance Hodgkin's disease: A distinct clinicopathological entity [Editorial]. Am J Surg Pathol 1994; 18(5):526.

175. Kant J, Hubbard S, Longo D, et al: The pathologic and clinical heterogeneity of lymphocyte-depleted Hodgkin's disease. J Clin Oncol 1986; 4:284.

176. Ferry JA, Linggood RM, Convery KM, et al: Hodgkin's disease, nodular sclerosis type: Implications of histologic subclassification. Cancer 1993; 71(2):457.

177. Axtell L, Myers M, Thomas L, et al: Prognostic indicators in Hodgkin's disease. Cancer 1972; 29:1481.

178. Colby T, Hoppe R, Warnke R: Hodgkin's disease: A clinicopathologic study of 659 cases. Cancer 1981; 49:1848.

179. Brousset P, Chittal S, Schlaifer D, et al: Detection of Epstein-Barr virus messenger RNA in Reed-Sternberg cells of Hodgkin's disease by in situ hybridization with biotinylated probes on specially processed modified acetone methyl benzoate xylene (ModAMeX) sections. Blood 1991; 77:1781.

180. Weiss L, Chen Y, Liu X, et al: Epstein-Barr virus and Hodgkin's disease: A correlative in situ hybridization and polymerase chain reaction study. Am J Pathol 1991; 139:1259.

179a. Ashton-Key M, Thorpe PA, Allen JP, Isaacson PG: Follicular Hodgkin's disease. Am J Surg Pathol 1995; 19:1294.

181. Lennert K, Mohri N: Histologische Klassifizierung und Vorkommen des M. Hodgkin. Internist 1974; 15:57.

182. Lister TA, Crowther D, Sutcliffe SB, et al: Report of a committee convened to discuss the evaluation and staging of patients with Hodgkin's disease: Cotswolds meeting [published erratum appears in J Clin Oncol 1990 Sep; 8(9):1602] [see comments]. J Clin Oncol 1989; 7(11):1630.

183. Dmitrovsky E, Martin S, Krudy A, et al: Lymph node aspiration in the management of Hodgkin's disease. J Clin Oncol 1986; 4:306.

184. Kaufman D, Longo D: Hodgkin's disease. Crit Rev Oncol Hematol 1992; 13:135.

185. Bennett M, MacLennan K, Hudson G, et al: Non-Hodgkin's lymphoma arising in patients treated for Hodgkin's disease in the BNLI: A 20-year experience. Ann Oncol 1991; 2 (Suppl 2):83.

186. Zarate OA, Medeiros LJ, Longo DL, et al: Non-Hodgkin's lymphomas arising in patients successfully treated for Hodgkin's disease: A clinical, histologic, and immunophenotypic study of 14 cases. Am J Surg Pathol 1992; 16(9):885.

187. Kingma DW, Medeiros LJ, Barletta J, et al: Epstein-Barr virus is infrequently identified in non-Hodgkin's lymphomas associated with Hodgkin's disease. Am J Surg Pathol 1994; 18(1):48.

188. Hansmann M, Stein H, Fellbaum C, et al: Nodular paragranuloma can transform into high-grade malignant lymphoma of B type. Hum Pathol 1989; 20:1169.

189. Sundeen J, Cossman J, Jaffee E: Lymphocyte predominant Hodgkin's disease, nodular subtype with coexistent "large cell lymphoma": Histological progression or composite malignancy? Am J Surg Pathol 1988; 12:599.

Chapter Six

Major Cytogenetic Findings in Non-Hodgkin's Lymphoma

Krzysztof Mrózek
Clara D. Bloomfield

Methodologic advances in cytogenetic and molecular genetic studies of human leukemia, lymphoma, and solid tumors during the last 25 years have led to an accumulation of experimental data supporting the view that cancer is a genetic disease. Both the initiation and progression of a neoplasm can be directly related to mutations, that is, acquired alterations of the genetic material in somatic cells. Many of these mutations are detectable microscopically as changes of either the structure or the number of the chromosomes (structural and numerical chromosome aberrations). Extensive cytogenetic analyses of human tumors have revealed the nonrandom nature of most chromosome aberrations and their remarkable specificity in certain types of malignant and benign lesions.[1–3] However, for technical reasons, most karyotypic data have been obtained from the study of leukemias and myelodysplastic and myeloproliferative syndromes. These disorders account for approximately two thirds of more than 17,000 human tumors with abnormal karyotypes published.[3]

The first aberrant karyotypes in malignant lymphomas were reported only a few years after the discovery of the first consistent chromosome abnormality in cancer, the Philadelphia chromosome of chronic myelocytic leukemia (CML) in 1960,[4, 5] and the first structural abnormality specific for a particular histology, that is, Burkitt's lymphoma (BL), a 14q+ marker, was identified soon after the introduction of chromosome banding methods.[6] Even so, the accrual of cytogenetic data on non-Hodgkin's lymphoma (NHL) has been substantially slower than for other hematologic disorders. To date, clonal chromosome aberrations (an identical structural rearrangement or the same extra chromosome present in at least two cells and monosomy detected in three or more cells[7]) have been reported in approximately 1700 NHLs studied with chromosome banding techniques.[3] However, because the NHLs represent disparate groups of diseases that, despite their common origin from lymphoid cells, possess distinct morphologic, immunologic, and genetic features, few categories of NHL have been well defined cytogenetically. Moreover, the concurrent use of various morphologic classification systems of NHL has made

comparison between results obtained by researchers from different institutions difficult. For example, among 1456 NHLs with clonal aberrations listed in the fourth edition of the *Catalog of Chromosome Aberrations in Cancer,*[8] 908 tumors have been classified by the Working Formulation for Clinical Usage[9] and 266 tumors by the Kiel classification[10]; the remaining tumors have been histologically subdivided according to other morphologic classifications.

Another factor limiting our knowledge of cytogenetics in lymphoma is the high degree of complexity of karyotypes, which sometimes contain marker chromosomes of unknown origin. In addition, cytogenetic results are presented in various ways: in some reports full descriptions of the karyotypes are provided, whereas in others only selected data are available, and they are often displayed differently. Furthermore, most reports correlating cytogenetic and clinical features include patients studied at diagnosis and relapse, and those studies that deal with newly diagnosed patients alone differ in the ways of grouping karyotypic, histologic, and treatment data.

The aforementioned limitations notwithstanding, specific aberrations and chromosome bands or regions rearranged in nonrandom fashion have been identified, and important correlations between karyotype and histology, immunology, and clinical outcome of NHL have been made. This chapter presents what has been learned over the past 2 decades about nonrandom chromosome aberrations characteristic of lymphomas and their significance in the diagnosis and management of patients with NHL.

SUCCESS RATES, NORMAL KARYOTYPES, AND MODAL CHROMOSOME NUMBER

Successful cytogenetic analysis can be performed in most NHLs. In large series of NHLs that include all histologic subtypes, sufficient numbers of good quality metaphase cells have been obtained in 56% to 96% of cases analyzed, with the average success rate slightly higher than 80%.[11–18] Some researchers have reported that rates of cytogenetic failure decreased in the later years of investigation.[10, 17] There seem

This work was supported by the Coleman Leukemia Research Fund.

to be differences in the success rates between low-grade and high-grade lymphomas. In a study of 60 patients with indolent (low-grade) NHL, Speaks and associates[19] obtained analyzable karyotypes in 65% of samples. This success rate is lower than the average rate for studies comprising intermediate- and high-grade tumors as well. Likewise, researchers from Sloan-Kettering Cancer Center,[17] who cytogenetically studied 434 patients with NHL, observed a trend toward an increased proportion of failures in low-grade lymphomas as compared with high-grade tumors (21.5% versus 13.2% failures, $P = .09$).

It has been shown that almost all successfully karyotyped lymphomas display clonal chromosome aberrations. Sometimes abnormal karyotypes have been reported in all patients studied.[11, 13] However, in most large series, tumors with exclusively normal karyotypes have constituted from 4% to 20% of cytogenetically characterized cases.[12, 14–17, 20] A normal chromosome complement can be found in lymphomas of all histologies, but the frequencies with which solely normal karyotypes occur in particular histologies seem to vary. Table 6–1 presents the distribution of tumors without clonal chromosome aberrations among histologic subgroups in nearly 500 patients who have been studied cytogenetically before any antineoplastic therapy. In both studies included in this table,[17, 21] the finding of a normal karyotype was most frequent in diffuse, small cleaved cell (DSC) lymphoma (on average 32%); lymphoblastic lymphoma (LBL) (31%); follicular, predominantly small cleaved cell (FSC) lymphoma (25%); and diffuse, mixed small and large cell (DM) lymphoma (25%). In contrast, the very high incidence of small lymphocytic lymphomas (SLLs) with a normal karyotype (41%) in the study of Offit and colleagues[17] was not observed at the Fifth International Workshop on Chromosomes in Leukemia/Lymphoma.[21] Only 5% to 9% of small noncleaved cell (SNC), diffuse, large cell (DLC), and follicular, predominantly large cell (FL) tumors had solely normal metaphases.

The finding of a normal karyotype in preparations from lymphoma specimens may be attributed in some instances to the presence of nonneoplastic, reactive cells that may preferentially divide in vitro. Normal results also may be obtained when only bone marrow aspirates instead of lymph nodes or other tumor masses are cytogenetically studied, especially in cases in which the degree of marrow infiltration by neoplastic cells is low.[22] However, it has been demonstrated that apparently normal karyotypes may be detected in tumor cells that have been identified as neoplastic by their morphology and reaction with a specific antiidiotype antibody.[23] Findings of this kind suggest that sometimes the degree of resolution of standard cytogenetic analysis, even when the quality of preparations is excellent, may be too low to visualize subtle rearrangements, such as small interstitial deletions, paracentric inversions, or reciprocal translocations of tiny fragments between similarly banded regions. Indeed, in a BL cell line, a subtle deletion of the long arm of chromosome 6 could be discovered exclusively by the loss of heterozygosity analysis.[24] In other tumors with a normal karyotype, genomic alterations occur at the gene level and cannot be demonstrated by cytogenetic techniques. For example, rearrangements of the *ALL1 (MLL)* gene, which is located in band 11q23 and frequently disrupted by structural chromosome abnormalities in acute leukemias and, with lower frequency, in NHL,[25, 26] have been detected also in patients with normal karyotypes.[27, 28] In one of these cases, *ALL1* rearrangement has been shown to result from a direct tandem duplication of a portion of the gene.[29]

Early studies, performed in the prebanding era, demonstrated that, in contrast with Hodgkin's disease, most NHLs had near-diploid modal chromosome numbers (see reference 30 for review). These observations have been confirmed by later analyses. Approximately one third of lymphomas with chromosome abnormalities exhibit the pseudodiploid modal chromosome number of 46. Notably, pseudodiploid tumors have been significantly more often found in patients studied at diagnosis than at relapse.[31] Hypodiploidy (a modal chromosome number of 45 or less) is seen rarely, in no more than 8% of tumors. In several large studies, most cases (54% to 65%) had karyotypes containing

Table 6–1. Incidence of Tumors with Normal Karyotypes in Histologic Subgroups in the Two Largest Published Series of NHL°

Histologic Subgroup	5th IWCLL[21]		Offit et al[17]		Total	
	No./All†	*Percentage*	*No./All†*	*Percentage*	*No./All†*	*Percentage*
SLL	3/21	14	11/27	41	14/48	29
FSC	7/25	28	6/28	21	13/53	25
FM	3/33	9	5/20	25	8/53	15
FL	0/6	0	1/5	20	1/11	9
DSC	3/10	30	4/12	33	7/22	32
DM	9/36	25	6/23	26	15/59	25
DLC	1/36	3	8/76	11	9/112	8
IBL	5/42	12	6/25	24	11/67	16
LBL	6/16	38	2/10	20	8/26	31
SNC	1/32	3	1/11	9	2/43	5
MISC	0/3	0	—	—	0/3	0
Total	**38/260**	15	**50/237**	21	**88/497**	18

°Only patients studied at diagnosis, before any treatment was administered, are included.
†Number of cytogenetically normal cases among the total number of successfully karyotyped cases.
NHL, non-Hodgkin's lymphoma; IWCLL, International Workshop on Chromosomes in Leukemia-Lymphoma; SLL, small lymphocytic lymphoma; FSC, follicular, predominantly small cleaved cell; FM, follicular, mixed small cleaved and large cell; FL, follicular, predominantly large cell; DSC, diffuse, small cleaved cell; DM, diffuse, mixed small and large cell; DLC, diffuse, large cell; IBL, diffuse, large cell, immunoblastic lymphoma; LBL, lymphoblastic lymphoma; SNC, small noncleaved cell; MISC, miscellaneous.

47 or more chromosomes. Among hyperdiploid tumors the most frequent chromosome number has been 47, followed by 48 and 49.[11–15, 21] Levine and coworkers[20] correlated ploidy with histologic subtypes and found that SLL, LBL, and SNC lymphoma tended to be pseudodiploid; FSC, DM, and immunoblastic (IBL) lymphomas were associated with modal chromosome numbers of 47 to 48, and most FL, and DLC lymphomas had a modal chromosome number of 49 or more.

RECURRENT CHROMOSOME ABNORMALITIES IN NHL

Compared with leukemia, the karyotypic picture of cytogenetically abnormal NHLs is generally much more complex. Tumors with a single clonal aberration are detected infrequently; more often than not, numerous chromosome aberrations are found concurrently. For instance, in the two large series from Minnesota[11–13, 20] and in the multinational collaborative study,[21] karyotypes with only one chromosome aberration were found in 24 (29%) of 83 cases,[11, 13] in 22 (18%) of 120 cases,[12, 20] and in 27 (10%) of 260 patients,[21] respectively. On the whole, structural abnormalities such as reciprocal and unbalanced translocations, duplications, interstitial and terminal deletions, ring chromosomes, and isochromosomes are more common than gains or losses of entire chromosomes.

Many, but not all, of the aberrations detected as a part of complex karyotypes represent unique changes that are probably of little significance for either pathogenesis or progression of the neoplastic process. Most important are abnormalities observed repeatedly. They have been divided with regard to their specificity and assumed significance into two main classes: primary and secondary changes. Those chromosome aberrations that are strongly associated with a given tumor type, and are occasionally detected as the only karyotypic change, have been postulated to play a key role in initiating the neoplasm. They have been classified as primary aberrations. The secondary abnormalities are less specific; they are believed to be later events that reflect clonal karyotypic evolution during tumor progression.[1–3]

Abnormalities that have been recurrently found as solitary changes in NHL, and consequently appear most likely to be primary aberrations, are listed in Table 6–2. Most of the aberrations recorded in Table 6–2 have been seen more frequently than is indicated by their status, since cases with complex karyotypes have not been included in this listing. Indeed, the molecular dissection of several of these abnormalities, predominantly reciprocal translocations, has confirmed their important role in lymphomagenesis.

The molecular investigation of t(8;14)(q24;q32), the translocation typical for most BLs, and of its less frequent variants t(8;22)(q24;q11) and t(2;8)(p12;q24), resulted in elucidation of mechanisms of oncogene activation by chromosome translocation. A protooncogene *MYC*, residing at 8q24, is juxtaposed to the immunoglobulin heavy chain (*IGH*) locus at 14q32 or, as a result of variant translocations, one of the immunoglobulin light chain genes, assigned to bands 22q11 (λ) and 2p12 (κ), is translocated to a telomeric region of the *MYC* oncogene. Likewise, in T-cell leukemias and lymphomas carrying the t(8;14)(q24;q11), *MYC* is

Table 6–2. Chromosome Aberrations Recurrently Detected as the Solitary Change in NHL[a]

Aberration	Status[b]	Aberration	Status[b]
del(1)(q32)	III	del(11)(q14-23)[e]	III
t(2;5)(p23;q35)	II	t(11;18)(q21;q21)[g]	II
t(2;8)(p12;q24)[c]	II	+12	I
+3	I	−14	III
del(3)(p21-25)	III	inv(14)(q11q32)	I
del(6)(q13-24-q21-27)[d]	I	del(14)(q11-24-q22-32)	II
+7	III	t(14;18)(q32;q21)	I
i(7)(q10)	III	t(14;19)(q32;q13)	III
t(8;14)(q24;q32)[c]	I	del(16)(q22)	III
t(8;14)(q24;q32)	II	−17	III
t(8;22)(q24;q11)[c]	II	+20	III
t(9;17)(q34;q23)[f]	III	+22	III
t(9;22)(q34;q11)	III	−X	II
t(11;14)(q13;q32)	I	+X	I
dup(11)(q13q23-25)	III	−Y	I

[a]Reported in Chromosome Coordinating Meeting, 1992 (CCM92).[3]
[b]Status categories depend on the number of tumors with individual abnormality seen as a sole change at the time of CCM92[3]: I, >10 cases; II, 5–10 cases; III, <5 cases.
[c]Burkitt's lymphoma.
[d]del (6)(q21) most common.
[e]del (11)(q23) most common.
[f,g]Translocations published recently (f = refs 166, 171; g = refs 82–85) not included in CCM92.[3]
NHL, non-Hodgkin's lymphoma.
Modified from Mrózek K, Bloomfield CD: Cytogenetics of indolent lymphoma. Semin Oncol 1993; 20(5, Suppl 5):47.

juxtaposed to the α or δ locus of the T-cell receptor (*TCR*), mapped to 14q11. In all of the aforementioned conditions, *MYC* is "activated" and expressed at high levels. The product of the *MYC* gene, a nuclear DNA binding protein, is implicated in the regulation of a number of other critical genes. Hence, its constitutive production may result in uncontrolled proliferation of B or T cells containing one of the translocations.[25, 32]

Molecular studies of other translocations, such as t(11; 14)(q13;q32), t(14;18)(q32;q21), and t(14;19)(q32;q13), have led to the identification of the putative oncogenes *BCL1* on chromosome 11, *BCL2* on chromosome 18, and *BCL3* on chromosome 19, which are also deregulated when translocated into the vicinity of the *IGH* gene at 14q32.[3, 32] Interestingly, in most instances, the protein products of genes activated by juxtaposition to the loci for immunoglobulin or *TCR* genes remain unchanged and are identical to their nontranslocated counterparts. In contrast, the molecular consequences of less frequent translocations in NHL that do not involve the immunoglobulin or *TCR* genes are different. Translocations (9;22)(q34;q11) and (2;5)(p23;q35) result in gene fusion leading to the production of hybrid proteins with excessive tyrosine kinase activity. Specifically, the oncogene *ABL* on chromosome 9 at q34 is fused to the *BCR* locus mapped to 22q11,[3, 25] and the nuclear phosphoprotein gene (*NPM*) located at 5q35 is fused to a protein tyrosine kinase gene *ALK* on chromosome 2 at p23.[33] The t(9;22) found in NHL is at the molecular level similar to that in Philadelphia chromosome–positive acute lymphoblastic leukemia (ALL). This differs from the t(9;22) in CML by the more proximal breakpoint in *BCR* and a smaller-sized bcr-abl protein.[34]

A different mechanism of tumorigenesis is involved in tumors in which loss of genetic sequences due to chromosome deletion takes place. Consistently lost chromosome bands or regions may harbor tumor suppressor genes (TSGs), the inactivation of which promotes the neoplastic process by causing disturbances in the cell's growth control. To date, nine TSGs have been cloned, and another six putative TSGs have been mapped but not cloned. These TSGs have been shown to be lost or mutated in a wide spectrum of human neoplasms.[35, 36] Perhaps the most frequently affected gene in human oncogenesis is *p53*, a TSG that is located at 17p13.[37] Recently, studies of the *p53* gene in NHL have been reported. Gaidano and associates[38] described loss and inactivation of *p53* in more than 30% of BL; these alterations were not found in other B-cell lymphomas. In contrast, *p53* mutations were detected in 9 of 48 clinically advanced Japanese patients with diffuse and follicular lymphomas.[39] Gaidano and Dalla-Favera[40] have suggested that the discrepancy between their results and the findings of Ichikawa and colleagues[39] may reflect ethnic or geographic differences such as have already been proposed to influence the distribution of the t(14;18). However, several recent studies[41–45] have revealed mutations of the *p53* gene and/or abnormal expression of the p53 protein in a substantial number of American and European patients with diffuse and follicular lymphomas, thus challenging the existence of geographic and racial factors affecting the distribution of *p53* lesions.

Abnormalities of the retinoblastoma gene and/or its aberrant expression have been demonstrated in a small percentage of low-grade B-cell lymphoid malignancies[46] and in as many as 58% of high-grade lymphomas.[47] Whether alterations of other TSGs play a role in lymphomagenesis is unknown. The nonrandom occurrence of deletions of 1q, 3p, 6q, 11q, 14q, and 16q as the only changes (see Table 6–2), or in conjunction with other aberrations in NHL,[8] suggests that these chromosome arms contain loci of TSGs. To date, however, no such genes have been characterized. In their molecular and cytogenetic analysis of B-cell NHL, Gaidano and coworkers[24] have identified two distinct regions of minimal deletion at 6q25-27 and at 6q21-23, and concluded that they most likely contain TSGs. In a subsequent report, Offit and associates[48] postulated the existence of a third TSG at 6q23. They also correlated sites of commonly deleted bands or regions with clinicopathologic subsets of NHL. They suggested that deletions including band 6q23 are frequent in low-grade lymphomas without t(14;18), that deletions encompassing 6q25-27 occur preferentially in intermediate-grade NHL, and that a missing band 6q21 is associated with high-grade lymphomas. However, further analysis is necessary to determine the specificity of associations reported by Offit and associates,[48] since the cytogenetic literature contains examples of NHL with deletions of 6q in which bands postulated to be lost in a given histologic subtype were retained.[8] Such studies will be facilitated once the involved genes are identified.

Table 6–3 contains a list of recurring structural abnormalities that have been observed in two or more NHL cases, usually with coexisting chromosome changes. Most of these aberrations probably represent secondary abnormalities. However, some of them have already proved to be of primary significance pathogenetically. The best example of the latter

Table 6–3. Recurrent Structural Chromosome Aberrations in NHL that Have Predominantly Occurred as Additional Abnormalities[a,b]

Aberration	Aberration
del(1)(p32-36)	i(6)(p10)
t(1;1)(p36;p11-12)	t(7;14)(p15;q32)[g]
der(1)t(1;2)(p36;q31)[c]	del(7)(p13-14)
del(1)(p13)	del(7)(q32)
i(1)(q10)	t(8;14)(q22;q32)
t(1;17)(p11orq11;q11orp11)	t(8;9)(q24;p13)[h]
dup(1)(q12q31)	del(9)(p13)
del(1)(q21)	t(9;14)(p13;q32)[j]
t(1;6)(q21;q25)[d]	del(10)(q23-24)
t(1;14)(q21-25;q32)	t(11;14)(p13;q11)[g]
del(1)(q42)	t(11;14)(q21;q32)
t(1;14)(q42;q32)	t(11;14)(q23;q32)
del(2)(p21)	del(12)(p11-12)
t(2;18)(p12;q21)	dup(12)(q13q21-22)
t(2;3)(p12;q27)[e]	del(12)(q22)
t(2;3)(q21-23;q27)	del(13)(q22)
del(2)(q32)	t(14;15)(q32;q15)[h]
t(3;14)(p21;q32)	i(17)(q10)
t(3;14)(q27;q32)[f]	der(22)t(17;22)(q11;p11)[h]
t(3;22)(q27-28;q11)	i(18)(q10)
del(4)(p13-14)	t(18;22)(q21;q11)[k]
del(5)(p13)	del(22)(q11-12)
del(6)(p21-23)	

[a]Reported in Human Gene Mapping 10.5 (HGM10.5).[209]
[b]Abnormalities included in Table 6–2 are not repeated here.
[c–h; j,k]Recurrent abnormalities not included in HGM10.5[209]: c = refs 109; d = ref 17; e = refs 18,211; f = refs 18,50; g = ref 166; h = ref 82; j = refs 94,95; k = refs 54,55. NHL, non-Hodgkin's lymphoma.
Modified from Mrózek K, Bloomfield CD: Cytogenetics of indolent lymphomas. Semin Oncol 1993; 20(5, Suppl 5):47.

category are the following translocations involving 3q27: t(3;14)(q27;q32), t(3;22)(q27;q11), and t(2;3)(p12;q27). Recently, a novel zinc finger–encoding oncogene, *BCL6/LAZ3*, sharing homology with several transcription factors has been isolated from the 3q27 breakpoint region of t(3;14) and other translocations involving 3q27 (see later).[49–51] Another translocation of primary importance appears to be the t(2;18)(p12;q21),[19, 52, 53] because in all three cases with this rearrangement studied by Hillion and colleagues,[53] the *BCL2* gene was juxtaposed to J segments of the immunoglobulin κ gene, indicating that the t(2;18) is a variant form of the well-known t(14;18)(q32;q21). Likewise, a second variant translocation, the t(18;22)(q21;q11), has been recently reported in two cases of B-cell lymphoma.[54, 55] Molecular genetic studies of other recurrent, albeit not very frequent, translocations involving loci of immunoglobulin genes, such as t(11;14)(q23;q32),[3, 56] may eventually result in identification of new cellular oncogenes implicated in lymphomagenesis.

CORRELATIONS BETWEEN HISTOLOGY AND KARYOTYPES

Although initial attempts to correlate chromosome aberrations with histologic subtypes of NHL were made in the late 1970s,[57] it was not until 1982 that systematic cytogenetic analyses of large numbers of lymphomas classified morphologically according to the Working Formulation for Clinical Usage began to be published. Since then, many associations

Table 6–4. Associations Between Nonrandom Chromosome Aberrations and Histologic Subgroups of NHL°

Histologic Group	Chromosome Abnormality†
SLL	+3, *del(6q)*, del(11)(q14-23),‡ **+12,**‡ **del(14)(q22-24)**
SLL, extranodal	*t(11;18)(q21;q21)*
SLL, plasmacytoid	*t(9;14)(p13;q32)*
FSC	del(6q), t(6p) or i(6)(p10), **t(14;18)(q32;q21)**
FM	del(2q), +3/3q§, +8, **t(14;18)(q32;q21)**
FL	+7, **t(14;18)(q32;q21)**
DSC	del(8p), t(11;14)(q13;q32), del(20q)
ILL/MCL	*t(11;14)(q13;q32)*
DM	+3, +5, +14
DLC	**+X,** *t(3;14)(q27;q32)*, *t(3;22)(q27;q11)*, **+4,** del(6q), +7, +9, **+12, +21**
Ki1 + ALCL	*t(2;5)(p23;q35)*
IBL	**+X,** +3, del(3p), +5, del(5q), **del(6q),** +7, +18
LBL	*t(9;17)(q34;q23)*
SNC	**t(8;14)(q24;q32), t(2;8)(p12;q24), t(8;22)(q24;q11)**

°From references 3, 8, 15–17, 19–21, 72, 73, 78, 82–85, 89, 94, 106, 161, 166, and 171.

†Abnormalities in **bold** type represent correlations confirmed by statistical methods in at least two independent studies; *italics* denote aberrations that have been more frequently observed in a given histologic subtype but no statistical analysis was conducted; ***italic bold*** type is used when a nonstatistical correlation has been observed in at least two independent studies.

‡As a sole abnormality.

§Trisomy 3 or structural changes of 3q.[19]

ILL/MCL, intermediate lymphocytic/mantle cell lymphoma; Ki1 + ALCL, Ki1-positive anaplastic large cell lymphoma; see Table 6–1 for other abbreviations.

have been reported, some of which have been well substantiated, whereas others, reported in only single studies, await confirmation. Chromosome changes that have been significantly associated with histologic subtypes of NHL are presented in Table 6–4. However, essentially none of these correlations is absolute, that is, specific abnormalities are almost never exclusively seen in a given histologic subtype. This may be explained in part by the fact that most of the Working Formulation categories do not represent individual diseases[58]; some types of lymphoma may be classified within two or even more different Working Formulation groups. At the same time, one Working Formulation category may contain several entities that have distinct etiology, karyotypic and phenotypic features, and clinical behavior.

SMALL LYMPHOCYTIC LYMPHOMA

SLL is the best example of a Working Formulation category that comprises several different entities. These include nodal B-cell SLL, extranodal SLL, SLL with plasmacytoid differentiation, low-grade B-cell lymphoma of mucosa-associated lymphoid tissue (MALT), a subset of mantle cell lymphoma, small cell T-cell neoplasms, monocytoid B-cell lymphoma, and primary splenic SLL.[59] Al-

though the number of cytogenetically characterized cases classified as SLL is still limited, several cytogenetic subgroups of SLL have been delineated. Moreover, in a few instances, specific cytogenetic changes seem to be closely associated with some of the earlier mentioned diseases included in the SLL category.

Because morphologic and immunophenotypic features of nodal SLL and B-cell CLL are identical, it has been suggested that these diseases represent different clinical presentations of the same neoplastic process.[59] This notion is supported by the results of cytogenetic analyses in SLL and CLL, since all major types of chromosome abnormalities representative for SLL have been repeatedly found in its leukemic counterpart. However, deletions and translocations involving band q14 of chromosome 13, frequently seen in CLL (in as many as 16% of cytogenetically abnormal cases),[60] which is known to contain both a retinoblastoma gene and another newly discovered TSG called *DBM* (disrupted in B-cell malignancy),[61] have rarely been detected in SLL.[13, 62]

The most common chromosome change in nodal SLL is trisomy of chromosome 12, detected in approximately 20% of cases.[8] In one half of these tumors, trisomy 12 occurs as a sole abnormality. This phenomenon seems to be limited to SLL histology, because, with the exception of two cases of IBL and one case of intermediate lymphocytic lymphoma,[8, 13, 63] trisomy 12 alone does not appear to have been reported in any other histologic subtype of NHL.[8] The significance of trisomy 12 as a primary abnormality in neoplastic processes is further substantiated by its consistent occurrence as a sole abnormality not only in SLL and CLL but also in benign nonhematologic disorders, such as uterine leiomyoma,[64] and ovarian sex cord/stromal tumors.[65–67] It is thus possible that the gain of an additional copy of chromosome 12 may represent a general mechanism through which uncontrolled, chronic proliferation of cells from different tissues may be achieved.

The exact manner whereby trisomy 12 contributes to the pathogenesis of SLL, B-cell CLL, and benign solid tumors is unknown. Studies of restriction fragment length polymorphisms of genes localized on the 12q arm performed on several B-cell CLL cases with trisomy 12 have revealed that this trisomy is a result of simple nondysjunction and duplication of one of the homologues and that the second copy of chromosome 12 is always retained in leukemic cells.[68, 69] No further evolution of trisomic cells, analogous to that observed in the murine lymphoma cell line TIKAUT with trisomy 15 and submicroscopic rearrangements of *MYC*, where initial duplication of one chromosome 15 with molecular alteration was followed by a triplication of this chromosome and loss of a normal chromosome 15,[70] has been observed in any of the CLL cases studied to date.[68, 69] The discovery of structural aberrations leading to partial trisomies of chromosome 12 in rare CLL cases suggests that the gene or genes that might be rearranged at the submicroscopical level and subsequently duplicated by trisomy are localized in the long arm of chromosome 12 between bands q13 and q24.[71] It is hoped that future molecular genetic studies will identify such genes and elucidate whether the same genes are involved in the pathogenesis of SLL, CLL, and benign solid tumors with trisomy 12.

A second cytogenetic group of SLL displays interstitial or terminal deletions of the long arm of chromosome 11. These deletions have been detected in approximately 13% of SLL,[8] and when not accompanied by additional changes, seem to be highly specific for SLL.[72] The breakpoints vary, but in all cases, a band 11q22 or its part has been lost, making this the most likely location of a potential TSG. However, no such gene has yet been identified. In no case of SLL with a complex karyotype have deletion 11q and trisomy 12 been seen together, suggesting that these abnormalities represent independent pathways of SLL tumorigenesis.

Another group of SLLs that might be associated with the loss of a second unidentified TSG is characterized by deletions of the long arm of chromosome 14. Initial observations of Levine and coworkers[20] linking breaks in 14q22-24 due to deletions or translocations with SLL histology have been corroborated by subsequent studies.[62, 73, 74] Kristoffersson and associates[73] described four new cases and reviewed an additional 43 published cases of NHL and other lymphoproliferative disorders with del(14)(q22-24). They confirmed that these deletions occurred significantly more frequently in SLL as compared with tumors of other histologies (*P* < .001). Moreover, since SLL may undergo transformation to high-grade DLC or IBL lymphoma (Richter's syndrome), and all high-grade tumors with del(14)(q22-24) had either of these histologies, the authors suggested that at least some of the high-grade lymphomas with del(14q) might have originated from previous SLL. If true, this would make the association between del(14)(q22-24) and SLL even stronger. Analysis of chromosome 14 breakpoints has indicated that the commonly deleted region contains part of band q24.[73] Of interest, the *MAX* gene encoding a protein that cooperates with the myc protein in regulating gene transcription is located at 14q23.[40, 75] However, whether the function of the *MAX* gene is changed as a result of del(14)(q22-24) in SLL, other NHL subtypes or CLL has not yet been determined. As in the case of trisomy 12 and del(11q), 14q deletions as a sole anomaly appear to be restricted to SLL histology.[8] In a few SLL cases, del(14q) has been seen together with trisomy 12.[62, 73, 74]

In most large series of NHL, deletions of 6q have either not been observed or only sporadically in SLL patients.[11-13, 76, 77] Recently, Offit and colleagues[78] reported an unusually high frequency (25%) of 6q abnormalities among 55 SLL cases, three of which had del(6q) as the only change. Since two other patients with a solitary del(6q) have been previously reported,[21, 76] the investigators suggested that del(6q) plays an important pathogenetic role in a subset of SLL. Moreover, they associated del(6q) with the presence of larger prolymphocytoid cells in the blood. The clinical course of their SLL patients with del(6q) did not differ from that in patients with other low-grade diffuse NHL.[78]

Other cytogenetic subgroups of SLL are defined by the presence of reciprocal translocations that involve chromosomes 9, 11, 14, and 18. The t(11;14)(q13;q32) has been described in 10% of SLL cases.[8] Additionally, this translocation, or its molecular equivalent—the *BCL1* rearrangement—has been described sporadically in a wide variety of lymphoproliferative disorders including B-cell CLL, follicular lymphomas, lymphomas of DSC, DM, DLC, and SNC type, and prolymphocytic leukemia.[79]

The strongest correlation, however, has been observed between t(11;14) or *BCL1* rearrangements and intermediate lymphocytic/mantle cell lymphomas (ILL/MCLs), 50% of which display the t(11;14) or *BCL1* changes (see later). In the Working Formulation, cases of ILL/MCL are predominantly placed within the DSC category, but occasionally ILL/MCL cases may be classified as SLL.[59] It is thus possible that some cases with the t(11;14) reported to be SLL were in fact mantle cell lymphomas. On the other hand, the t(11;14) has been repeatedly demonstrated in a subset of low-grade splenic lymphoma with villous lymphocytes,[80] a disease that might be misdiagnosed as CLL or hairy cell leukemia but does not resemble ILL/MCL, and also in one fifth of B-cell prolymphocytic leukemia, a well-recognized pathologic entity that is separate from ILL/MCL.[79] Consequently, it has been suggested that the presence of t(11;14) in morphologically and immunophenotypically distinct lymphomas and leukemias[81] of mature B cells indicates that these entities may be more closely related pathogenetically than hitherto anticipated.[79]

A second translocation involving chromosome 11, t(11;18)(q21;q21), seems to be nonrandomly associated with a subset of extranodal B-cell SLL. All patients with this translocation have had remarkably similar immunopathologic and clinical features, including a mature B-cell immunophenotype with the absence of CD5 expression which occurs in most SLLs, λ light chain expression, indolent clinical course, and extranodal involvement, particularly of the stomach (three of six cases had gastric involvement).[82–85] In all six cases thus far reported, the t(11;18) was the only cytogenetic change seen in the abnormal clone, emphasizing its pathogenetic importance. The molecular consequences of the t(11;18) are at present unknown. Even though the breakpoint in chromosome 18 is identical cytogenetically to that in the t(14;18)(q32;q21) typical for follicular lymphomas, no evidence of rearrangements of the *BCL2* gene at either the major breakpoint region or the minor cluster region has been shown in any of the four tumors studied at the molecular level.[83–85] Additionally, the involvement of the *FVT1* (follicular variant translocation) gene that is located 10 kilobases (kb) upstream of the *BCL2* locus, and appears to be implicated in the variant translocation t(2;18)(p12;q21),[86] has been excluded in one case of SLL with the t(11;18).[85] In spite of the consistent involvement of extranodal sites in patients with the t(11;18), only one of the six cases with this translocation has been classified as a lymphoma of MALT.[84] Because careful pathologic examination of the case studied by Leroux and coworkers[85] ruled out MALT lymphoma as a diagnostic possibility, and none of 24 successfully karyotyped lymphomas of MALT had the t(11;18),[23, 78, 87, 88] it is likely that tumors with solitary t(11;18) represent a disease that is different from both MALT lymphoma and other forms of SLL.

Cytogenetic studies of MALT lymphoma have failed to identify a specific chromosome change. The only recurring abnormality has been trisomy of chromosome 3 or its short arm, which has been seen in 6 (40%) of 15 karyotypically abnormal tumors, always accompanied by other aberrations.[23, 78, 87, 88] In this context, findings of Offit and associates[17] are interesting. They observed a significantly higher frequency of trisomy 3 in SLL. Seven (30%) of 23 patients with SLL in their series had an additional copy of chromosome 3, whereas this trisomy was present in 7.5% of lymphomas of other histologic types (*P* < .05). However, the increased frequency of trisomy 3 in SLL has not been observed in other large published series of NHL.[11–13, 15, 16] Instead, trisomy 3 has been nonrandomly related to DM NHL,[21, 89] to high-grade NHL,[16] and to adult T-cell leukemia/lymphoma in Japanese patients.[90] As the sole abnormality, trisomy 3 has been found predominantly in T-cell lymphomas.[1, 21, 91, 92]

Although rearrangements of band q32 of chromosome 14 are the most frequently encountered structural changes in B-cell NHLs regardless of their histology, abnormalities involving 14q32 have been detected in SLL less than half as often as in tumors of other histologic types[20]; they account for approximately 30% of SLL cases.[8] The t(14;18)(q32; q21)[15, 17, 21, 93] and t(14;19)(q32;q13)[12, 19] and the presence of extra material of unknown origin at 14q32 have each been reported in a few SLL cases, and chromosomes 1, 2, 6, 8, 14, and 15 have been found to be the translocation partners of 14q32 in single patients.[8]

Recently, t(9;14)(p13;q32) has been associated with SLL with plasmacytoid differentiation.[94] In a series of nine lymphomas with t(9;14)(p13;q32), five cases were diagnosed as SLL of the plasmacytoid subtype at the time of cytogenetic analysis. Furthermore, the same diagnosis was also documented on retrospective review of histologic slides from prior lymph node biopsies in an additional two DLC lymphomas that demonstrated the t(9;14). The clinical course of patients with the t(9;14) did not differ significantly from that typical of patients with low-grade

lymphoma and other chromosome aberrations. The gene on chromosome 9 involved in the t(9;14) is presently unknown. It is also unknown whether the same DNA sequences of chromosome 9 are rearranged in plasmacytoid SLL and cases of follicular, mixed small cleaved and large cell (FM) and Ki1-positive large-cell lymphomas with the same translocation.[94, 95]

A recent study provided cytogenetic characterization of another disease that is classified within the SLL category. Oscier and colleagues[80] karyotyped 31 cases of low-grade splenic lymphoma with villous lymphocytes and identified clonal abnormalities in 87% of cases, 15 of which had complex cytogenetic changes. Although no unique aberration could be found, certain abnormalities were observed recurrently: t(11;14)(q13;q32) in five patients; i(17)(q10) in four, mostly as a sole aberration; translocations involving band 2p11 in another four; and deletions and translocations involving the long arm of chromosome 7 at q22 or q35 in five patients. Notably, trisomy 12 and del(13)(q14q22) were seen in only one patient each.

FOLLICULAR LYMPHOMAS

The B-cell follicular lymphomas are the most common type of lymphoma in the United States and Europe, accounting for nearly half of all NHL cases.[59] They are strongly associated with the reciprocal translocation t(14; 18)(q32;q21) (Fig. 6–1). It is thus not surprising that the t(14;18) is the single most frequently observed chromosome aberration in NHL. In most large published series comprising NHLs of all histologic types, the t(14;18) has been

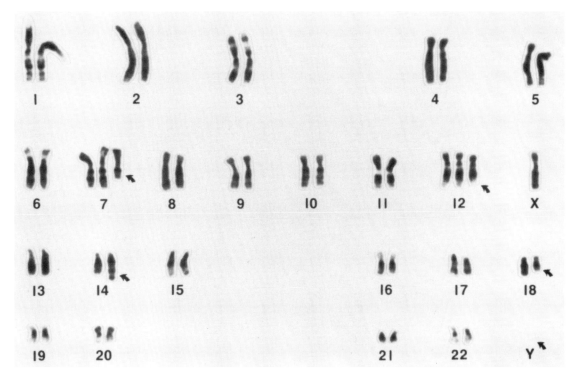

Figure 6–1. G-banded karyotype of a patient with FL lymphoma (case S15 in the report of Levine and associates[20]). In this karyotype, a primary abnormality typical for follicular histology, t(14;18)(q32;q21), is accompanied by secondary numerical and structural changes such as −Y, +12, and an extra copy of del(7)(q22q32). *Arrows* indicate chromosome abnormalities.

Table 6–5. Incidence of Translocations t(14;18) and t(8;14) in Histologic Subgroups Based on Cytogenetic Findings in Large Published Series of NHL from the United States,[11–13, 16, 17, 20] Australia,[15] and Japan[52, 106]

Histologic Subgroup	t(14;18)(q32;q21)				t(8;14)(q24;q32)			
	US and Australia		Japan		US and Australia		Japan	
	No./All	Percentage	No./All	Percentage	No./All	Percentage	No./All	Percentage
SLL	2/100	2	0/2	0	2/100	2	0/2	0
FSC	102/135	76	2/3	67	3/135	2	0/3	0
FM	36/60	60	2/7	29	5/60	8	0/7	0
FL	20/38	53	0/8	0	1/38	3	0/8	0
DSC	9/57	16	1/10	10	0/57	0	0/10	0
DM	6/68	9	0/28	0	3/68	4	0/28	0
DLC	52/199	26	0/43	0	20/199	10	1/43	2
IBL	11/74	15	0/21	0	7/74	9	1/21	5
LBL	0/24	0	0/8	0	1/24	4	0/8	0
SNC	2/29	7	0/7	0	22/29	76	5/7	71
MISC	2/11	18	1/6	17	0/11	0	0/6	0
Total	**242/795**	**30**	**6/143**	**4**	**64/795**	**8**	**7/143**	**5**

See Table 6–1 for abbreviations.

observed in 22%[21] to 47%[15] of all cases, with an average of about 30% in Western series (Table 6–5). Recognized for the first time in 1978 by Fukuhara and Rowley,[96] this translocation was significantly correlated with lymphomas of a follicular growth pattern 1 year later,[57] and this correlation has been confirmed by numerous studies.[11–17, 19–21] By applying a cell synchronization technique, Yunis and co-workers[11] achieved a high-resolution banding pattern of chromosomes and were able to sublocalize the translocation breakpoints to bands 14q32.3 and 18q21.3. Subsequently, a candidate oncogene named *BCL2* was cloned from the region 18q21.3, and was shown to be activated through juxtaposition with the *IGH* locus.[25, 32] Recent studies have indicated that BCL2 is a novel type of oncogene whose product may be an inner mitochondrial membrane protein and plays a role in blocking programmed cell death (apoptosis) of B lymphocytes within lymph node follicular centers, as well as of progenitor and long-lived cells in other hematopoietic lineages and epithelium.[97] Therefore, the elevated levels of BCL2 proteins would result in extended survival of cells bearing the t(14;18).[97] The primary importance of the t(14;18) is further underlined by its occurrence as the sole cytogenetic abnormality in some patients and by cytogenetic investigations of sequential lymph node biopsies, indicating that in patients who had this translocation at diagnosis, it was always retained during the course of their disease.[98, 99]

Although the t(14;18) has been detected in lymphomas of all histologic types,[8] the frequency with which it is found in different morphologic subgroups varies greatly (see Table 6–5). In large Western series, t(14;18) is seen in 45%[16] to 89%[15] of follicular lymphomas, with the highest incidence (on average, 76%) among FSC, and the lowest (on average 53%) among FL lymphomas (see Table 6–5). In addition, about 20% of diffuse lymphomas demonstrate this translocation; at least half of these cases have had evidence of histologic transformation from previous follicular histologies.[20, 100] The distribution of cases with the t(14;18) appearing as a sole karyotypic change among histologic subtypes is also nonrandom. Approximately 15% of cytoge-

netically aberrant FSC cases have had a solitary t(14;18), compared with only 7% of FM, 4% of FL, and 0.5% of diffuse lymphomas.[8]

Several numerical and structural changes have been recurrently found in association with t(14;18). These changes include trisomy of chromosomes X, 3, 5, 7, 8, 9, 12, 17, 18, 20, and 21; missing sex chromosomes; partial deletion of the long arm of chromosome 6; isochromosome for the long arm of chromosomes 17 and 18; an extra copy of der(18)t(14;18); duplication of the long arm of chromosome 1; and abnormalities of regions Xp22, 1p21-22, 1p36, 3q21-27, 7q32, and 10q23-25.[12, 13, 17, 19, 100–105] Of these, trisomies of chromosomes 7, 12, and 17 or i(17)(q10) were found to be significantly more common in intermediate- and high-grade tumors than in low-grade lymphomas.[17, 100–102] With regard to deletions of the long arm of chromosome 6, Offit and coworkers[48] have suggested that in low-grade NHL with t(14;18), commonly deleted segments usually encompass 6q23 and 6q25-27, but not 6q21, deletion of which has been proposed to be specific for high-grade NHL, particularly of the IBL type. On the other hand, structural changes of chromosome 1 seem to be randomly distributed among histologic subsets.[17, 102]

Possible geographic and racial differences in the frequency of t(14;18)-carrying lymphomas in the United States, Australia, and Western Europe compared with Japan have been suggested.[21, 52, 106] The overall lower frequency of lymphomas displaying t(14;18) in Japan can be explained partly by the fact that low-grade follicular lymphomas are uncommon in this region of the world.[21, 106] Since the numbers of patients studied in the Japanese series have been relatively small, large-scale prospective studies will be necessary to confirm the existence of geographical and racial differences in the distribution of the t(14;18). Likewise, whether the absence of this translocation in a Russian series[76] reflects a genuine geographic diversity, or is related to the small number of cases analyzed, remains to be determined.

Despite the fact that t(14;18) is the most common chromosome abnormality in follicular lymphoma, many tumors do not demonstrate this translocation (see Table 6–5). Ladanyi and associates[107] recently described a subset of follicular lymphomas (one FSC, four FM, and one FL) showing t(8;14)(q24;q32) in the absence of t(14;18). The breakpoints in the t(8;14), studied both molecularly and cytogenetically, were located outside the commonly affected sites in the t(8;14) of BL. Based on this observation and the indolent clinical course of all of their cases, the authors proposed that the t(8;14) in follicular lymphoma, if not accompanied by t(14;18), is distinct from that encountered in high-grade NHL. Other examples of recurrent abnormalities in follicular lymphoma that are not accompanied by t(14;18) or rearrangements of *BCL2* gene have been provided by Wlodarska and colleagues[108] and Bajalica and coworkers.[109] In the former study, two cases of FSC lymphoma with duplication of the region 12q13-qter were reported.[108] In the latter, two FM lymphomas had an apparently identical der(1)t(1;2)(p36;q31), which in one case was the only abnormality in a stemline.[109]

In other follicular lymphomas, the extra material at 14q32 has been translocated from chromosomes different than 18 or 8. Translocations (3;14)(q27;q32), (11;14)(q13;q32), (1;14)(q42;q32), and (1;14)(q21-25;q32) have been detected in a few cases, and chromosomes 2, 3, 5, 10, 12, 16, and 17 have been found sporadically to be chromosome 14 translocation partners.[8] In about 4% of follicular tumors, the origin of extra chromatin in 14q+ markers could not be established by conventional cytogenetic techniques.[8] This failure may be the result of the loss of the other partner in the reciprocal translocation or further structural rearrangements of the marker chromosomes precluding their proper identification. Alternatively, some of these cases may represent variant translocations with possible involvement of more than two chromosomes and transposition of submicroscopic segments of chromatin in a manner similar to that detected in variant translocations of t(9;22) in CML.[1, 110] Indeed, rearrangements of the *BCL2* gene have been demonstrated in three of seven follicular lymphomas with an unidentified 14q+ marker chromosome using molecular genetic techniques.[111, 112] However, since molecular studies indicate that rearrangements and activation of the *BCL2* gene cannot be detected in all follicular lymphomas,[113] other chromosome translocations without involvement of chromosome 18 probably represent alternative, as yet not fully characterized, mechanisms of lymphomagenesis.

DIFFUSE SMALL CLEAVED CELL LYMPHOMA AND INTERMEDIATE LYMPHOCYTIC/MANTLE CELL LYMPHOMA

The intermediate-grade lymphomas with a diffuse growth pattern have not been associated with a characteristic chromosome aberration typical for most tumors. However, recent discoveries shed light on the cytogenetic constitution and the molecular genetic events in the pathogenesis of some lymphomas belonging to this heterogeneous subset. The first cytogenetic abnormality that appears to identify a subgroup of DSC lymphomas designated as ILL/MCL is t(11;14)(q13;q32). The t(11;14) was originally reported more than 15 years ago.[114, 115] It was subsequently described in a broad range of B-cell lymphoid malignancies, including CLL; SLL; follicular lymphomas; DSC, DM, and SNC lymphomas; and acute prolymphocytic leukemia, in most instances with rather low frequency. The findings of Weisenburger and associates,[116] who described the presence of t(11;14)(q13;q32) in 3 of their 12 cases of intermediate lymphocytic lymphoma in 1987, prompted several groups of investigators to examine the distribution of the t(11;14) among histologic subtypes in large series of lymphomas. In a series of 163 karyotypically abnormal NHLs of various histologies, Leroux and colleagues[117] identified 13 lymphomas with this rearrangement, 12 of which, after reexamination of histologic slides, met the diagnostic criteria for ILL/MCL. The same diagnosis was reached in 3 of 4 tumors with the t(11;14) found in a large Japanese study,[52] and the t(11;14) was present in 8 of 12 leukemic intermediate lymphocytic lymphomas[22] as well as in all 9 ILL/MCLs described by Vandenberghe and coworkers.[118] All tumors reported in the latter study and one half of the ILL/MCL cases analyzed by Leroux and associates[117] had been initially diagnosed as DSC lymphoma. ILL/MCL frequently imitates other lymphoma subtypes, and most such tumors have been originally classified as DSC lymphoma.[119] It is thus possible that the nonrandom association between t(11;14) and DSC histology, described by Juneja and colleagues,[15] may be attributed to the presence of unrecognized ILL/MCL cases in their material. Likewise, some of the additional DSC lymphomas carrying the t(11;14) reported by other researchers,[8] mostly before recognition of ILL/MCL as a separate entity, may have been cases of ILL/MCL. Notably, the t(11;14) has never been observed together with the t(14;18), nor has the latter translocation been found in any ILL/MCL case. Therefore, the finding of one of these translocations, or their molecular counterparts, may be useful in differential diagnosis, especially between ILL/MCL cases with a vaguely nodular growth pattern and FSC lymphomas.

The availability of genomic probes permitting detection of *BCL1* rearrangements at the DNA level has made possible studies of large numbers of patients with ILL/MCL that were not analyzed cytogenetically. *BCL1* rearrangements have been found in 41 of 81 cases (51%) studied by five groups.[120–124] Because only one group[124] used probes capable of detecting both major and minor breakpoint cluster regions, it is likely that the real overall incidence of *BCL1* rearrangements is higher and close to the 73% shown by Williams and coworkers.[124]

Recent studies have provided evidence that the oncogene which is deregulated and overexpressed as a result of the t(11;14) is identical to *PRAD1* or the cyclin D1 gene. This gene is closely linked to the *BCL1* breakpoint locus, and its protein product is involved in controlling the cell cycle.[125–127] Rosenberg and associates[125] found increased expression of *PRAD1* mRNA in all seven ILL/MCLs studied even though only three of them had detectable rearrangements of *BCL1* DNA. Overexpression of *PRAD1* also has been demonstrated in a case of ILL/MCL with a variant translocation t(11;22)(q13;q11).[128]

No chromosome abnormality has been shown as specific for DSC lymphoma. As many as 16% of DSC cases demonstrate the presence of t(14;18)(q32;q21) (see Table 6–5). In the study of Koduru and colleagues,[89] del(8p) and del(20q) were found to be more frequent in DSC histology than expected; however, they were seen in only two cases each, and with the exception of an additional case with 8p–[96] have not been observed by other investigators. Recently, Vandenberghe and coworkers[129] reported six DSC cases with complex karyotypes that included various deletions, inversions, and a translocation involving region p34-36 of chromosome 1. They suggested that genes located in this region may be important in tumor initiation or progression of a subgroup of DSC lymphomas.[129] However, the repetitive occurrence of 1p34-36 abnormalities in all histologic types of both B-cell and T-cell lymphoma[8, 21] as well as in many types of solid tumors with complex karyotypes[8] suggests that these changes play an evolutionary rather than a causative role in a wide spectrum of human neoplasms.

DIFFUSE LYMPHOMAS WITH LARGE CELL COMPONENTS

The most spectacular recent breakthrough in the genetics of NHL has been the characterization of a novel oncogene, *BCL6* or *LAZ3*, that is located at band q27 of chromosome 3 and implicated in the genesis of DLC lymphoma.[49–51, 128–133] As in the case of other oncogenes involved in lymphomagenesis, the discovery of *BCL6/LAZ3* stems from preceding cytogenetic studies. Structural aberrations of the distal part of the long arm of chromosome 3 had been observed in sporadic cases of NHL during the 1970s, but these anomalies did not attract much attention until 1983, when Kaneko and associates[134] noted an association between 3q abnormalities and DLC histology. In their series of 30 karyotypically abnormal tumors,

seven displayed 3q27-29 rearrangements, including a t(3;6)(q29;q15) and six translocations of an unidentified segment onto the terminal region of 3q. Six of these patients had DLC lymphoma, and the remaining one had a composite lymphoma with follicular and diffuse small cleaved cell components. Thereafter, several other cases of structural aberrations affecting 3q27-29 were reported, including two DLC lymphomas with the t(3;14)(q27;q32)[13] and one case with t(3;22)(q29;q11).[135]

Despite reports of structural abnormalities of chromosome 3 in as many as approximately 25% of all cytogenetically aberrant NHLs,[1] the observations of rearrangements of this chromosome at several different bands throughout its length, together with the lack of statistically significant correlations with histology,[20, 21, 89] suggested that structural changes of chromosome 3 represented secondary events in lymphomagenesis.[136] In 1989, however, Offit and colleagues[137] and in 1990 Leroux and coworkers[138] described the presence of t(3;22)(q27-28;q11) in a total of 11 NHLs, mostly of DLC type. The authors of the former study estimated that in their series the t(3;22) was the third most common nonrandom translocation in diffuse lymphomas. Subsequently, Bastard and associates[18] reported 3 further cases of t(3;22)(q27;q11), as well as 15 cases of t(3;14)(q27; q32), and 2 cases of t(2;3)(p12;q27); a t(3;14) and a t(2;3) were seen as sole anomalies. This suggested that 3q27 abnormalities might be of primary significance in lymphomagenesis. As in the previous studies, the histologic distribution of lymphomas with 3q27 changes was nonrandom. Table 6–6 collates results from 103 cases pub-

Table 6–6. Distribution of 103 Tumors with Rearrangements Involving Region 3q27-29 Among Histologic Subtypes of NHL°

Histologic Subgroup	t(3;14)(q27;q32)	t(3;22)(q27;q11)	t(2;3)(p12;q27)	add(3)(q27-29)	t(3;A)†	[Breakpoints in Translocation Partners of Chromsome 3 in Column to Left]	Total
SLL	—	—	—	1			1
FSC	—	1	—	2	4	[2q11, 2q14, 2q21, 5q14]	7
FM	3	1	1	1	6	[3p21, 3q29, 6p21, 6q15, 9p13, 9q21]	12
FL	2	—	—	3	1	[10q24]	6
DSC	1	1	—	3	—		5
DM	2	2	—	3	—		7
DLC	14	8	2	13	16	[1q11, 1q21, 1q25, 1q25, 1q32, 2q21, 2q23, 5q31, 6q15, 6q21, 9q13, 11p13, 11q13, 12q11, 12q24, 19q13]	53
IBL	—	2	—	3	1	[2q23]	6
LBL	—	—	—	—	—		—
SNC	—	2	—	—	—		2
MISC	1	2	—	—	1	[2q11]	4
Total	**23**	**19**	**3**	**29**	**29**		**103**

°From references 8, 12, 13, 18, 20, 50, 51, 76, 77, 80, 92, 98, 106, 109, 134, 137, 138, 144, and 210–212.
†Translocations with chromosomes other than 14, 22 or 2 at p12.
See Table 6–1 for abbreviations.

lished with microscopically detectable rearrangements of the region 3q27-29 that have been morphologically classified according to the Working Formulation. More than 70% of these lymphomas had a diffuse growth pattern, and more than half of all cases were diagnosed as DLC lymphoma. Among follicular lymphomas, 3q27 changes were found mainly in tumors with a large cell component (FM and FL).

Although several different chromosomes were found to be 3q27 translocation partners, the consistent involvement of bands 14q32, 22q11, and 2p12 in translocations with chromosome 3 implied that band 3q27 is a site of a novel oncogene that might be involved in the pathogenesis of B-cell NHL. It appeared that it might be activated by juxtaposition with the one of the three immunoglobulin genes in a mode parallel to the molecular consequences of well-characterized translocations such as t(8;14), t(11;14), t(14;18), and their variants. Indeed, molecular probes encompassing a major translocation cluster region at band 3q27 have been independently cloned by several groups,[128–133] and a novel zinc-finger encoding gene called *BCL6/LAZ3*, which shares amino-terminal homology with several transcription factors, has been isolated.[49–51] By using cDNA and genomic probes, Ye and colleagues[50] screened a panel of 17 DLC cases with translocations between band 3q27 and various chromosomes. Rearrangements of *BCL6/LAZ3* were found in 12 tumors, including all 4 carrying t(3;14), 2 of 3 with t(3;22), and single cases with translocations not involving an immunoglobulin gene, specifically t(1;3)(q21;q27), t(2;3)(q23;q27), der(3)t(3;5)(q27;q31), t(3;11)(q27;q13), t(3;12)(q27;q11), and add(3)(q27). Almost identical results were obtained by another group,[132] who showed that *BCL6/LAZ3* was rearranged in 13 of 17 NHLs with 3q27 translocations, including a t(3;4)(q27;p11) and a t(3;7)(q27;p12). Whether the absence of *BCL6/LAZ3* rearrangements in one fourth of tumors with cytogenetic changes of 3q27 indicates the presence of another, as yet uncharacterized, oncogene near *BCL6/LAZ3* or is the result of the existence of additional breakpoint cluster regions that are not detectable by the probes used remains to be elucidated.

The true incidence of aberrations involving *BCL6/LAZ3* in NHL, and particularly among DLC tumors, is at present uncertain. On the basis of karyotype analysis alone, the overall frequency of 3q27 alterations has been estimated to be between 8% and 13% of all NHL cases.[49, 50] However, the t(3;14)(q27;q32) is quite subtle and can be difficult to recognize, especially if cytogenetic preparations are of suboptimal quality. It has already been reported that in some cases the t(3;14) was initially misinterpreted as a del(3)(q27) and a translocation of unknown material onto 14q32.[18, 131] Therefore, the earlier mentioned incidences may be underestimates. This conclusion appears to be supported by molecular analyses of the *BCL6/LAZ3* rearrangements in large series of NHL. Alterations of the gene were found in 27 of 151 tumors (18%)[139] and in 18 of 125 NHL (14%)[140]; if additional breakpoint cluster regions exist, the actual frequencies may be even higher. In the study of Ye and colleagues,[50] *BCL6/LAZ3* changes were found in 33% of DLC lymphomas and no rearrangement was detected in any SLL, follicular, or BLs. In contrast, Otsuki and coworkers[139] reported *BCL6/LAZ3*

changes in 20% of both de novo and transformed (from follicular histology) diffuse lymphomas but also in 13% of indolent follicular tumors. The latter finding is compatible with the cytogenetic demonstration of 3q27 translocations in a proportion of low-grade NHL (see Table 6–6) and with the results of a second molecular study from New York.[140] The frequency of *BCL6/LAZ3* rearrangements in DLC lymphomas in this report[140] was 45%, the highest thus far reported. Further studies are required to determine the specificity and histologic distribution of 3q27/*BCL6/LAZ3* alterations, as well as whether they have prognostic significance.

Approximately one fourth of DLC lymphomas in large Western series, and 9% and 15% of DM and IBL lymphomas, respectively, have had the t(14;18) in their karyotype (see Table 6–5). Although a proportion of these tumors have evolved from a preceding follicular histology, the t(14;18) or its molecular equivalent, the *BCL2* rearrangement, was also demonstrated in de novo diffuse lymphomas with a large-cell component.[141] Additionally, the t(8;14)(q24;q32) (Fig. 6–2) has been recurrently observed in diffuse histologies other than BL, albeit with significantly lower frequency (see Table 6–5).

Two new cytogenetic subgroups of diffuse lymphomas with a large-cell component, both involving the long arm of chromosome 9, have been recently identified.[142] The presence of mainly interstitial 9q deletions with the commonly lost region being 9q31-32 was ascertained in seven cases. These findings, together with 10 previously reported DM and DLC lymphomas with deletions of 9q,[12, 76, 77, 96, 106, 134, 143, 144] indicate that a TSG may be involved in such tumors. Interestingly, a TSG *BCNS*, thus far implicated in medulloblastoma and basal cell carcinoma of the skin, has been mapped to 9q31.[35] A second subset of diffuse lymphomas with large-cell components comprised 12 tumors with different translocations involving bands 9q11 and 9q13.[142] The significance of these aberrations in lymphomagenesis is presently obscure.

T-cell lymphomas are heterogeneous and consist of several clinicopathologic entities, including lymphomas of low- and high-grade types. Morphologically, most postthymic or peripheral T-cell lymphomas are classified within two Working Formulation categories: DM and IBL.[58] Apart from a t(2;5) (see later), no abnormality has been found to be specific to T-cell NHL. A relatively common cytogenetic feature in T-cell NHL is the presence of cells with nonclonal aberrations, which are particularly common in angioimmunoblastic lymphadenopathy with dysproteinemia.[145, 146] Some tumors display translocations disrupting *TCR* genes (Table 6–7), but in general such rearrangements are observed more frequently in T-cell ALL than in T-cell NHL.[31] Other aberrations frequently occurring in T-cell lymphomas include trisomy of chromosomes X, 3, 5, 19, and 7 or 7q and structural rearrangements of the following chromosome arms or regions: 1p, 1q, 1q21, 2p11-14, 2p23-25, 2q21, 3q27, 4q21, 6p21-23, 6q, 9p21-23, 10p13-15, 13q, 14q32, 17q10, and 17q21.[52, 91, 106, 145–148] Among T-cell diffuse NHL, Ki1-positive anaplastic large cell lymphoma represents a morphologically, immunologically, and clinically distinct subset. Characteristic features of these cases include bimodal age distribution with the

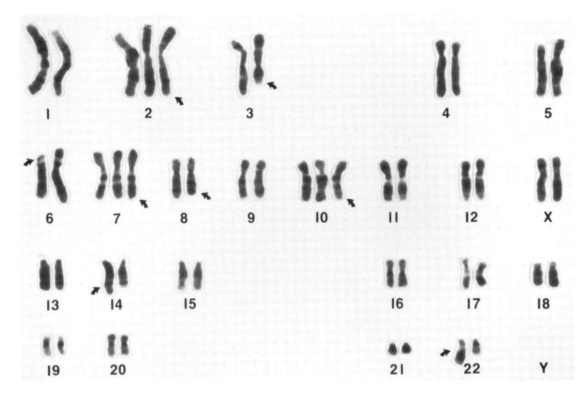

Figure 6–2. G-banded complex karyotype of a patient with diffuse large cell lymphoma (case 69 in the report of Bloomfield and associates[12]). This case demonstrates that the t(8;14)(q24;q32), a primary abnormality characteristic of Burkitt's lymphoma, also can be seen in lymphomas of other histologic types. Additional aberrations include trisomies of chromosomes 2, 7, and 10; an interstitial deletion of the chromosome 6 short arm [del(6)(p22p24)]; and a reciprocal translocation t(3;22)(q23;q13). *Arrows* indicate chromosome aberrations.

predominance of young age at presentation, frequent skin infiltration by large pleomorphic lymphoma cells, which in lymph nodes preferentially involve sinuses and paracortical areas, infrequent marrow involvement, and better survival than other non–B-cell lymphomas.[149, 150] Within the Working Formulation, cases of Ki1-positive anaplastic large cell lymphoma are usually classified as IBL, DLC, or DM lymphomas. Recent cytogenetic studies indicate that Ki1-positive lymphomas are strongly associated with a particular chromosome anomaly, namely t(2;5)(p23;q35). Initially, this translocation, or its variant t(5;6)(q35;p12), were reported in 10 cases diagnosed as malignant histiocytosis.[151–156] However, following the publications linking t(2;5)(p23;q35) to Ki1-positive lymphoma,[157–160] Mason and associates[161] reexamined the morphologic appearance of eight of these

cases and performed immunophenotypic studies of Ki1, CD3, and CD68 antigens. The results unequivocally indicated that all reexamined neoplasms with the t(2;5), originally diagnosed as malignant histiocytosis, were of lymphoid origin and showed typical features of Ki1-positive lymphoma. To date, more than 30 cases with the t(2;5) have been reported,[33, 149–161] and most of them have had similar immunologic, histologic, and clinical features. Hence, the specificity of the t(2;5) appears to be the highest among NHL, and it is comparable to that of t(12;16)(q13;p11) and t(X;18)(p11;q11), which are pathognomonic for myxoid liposarcoma[162] and synovial sarcoma,[163] respectively. Thus, the results of cytogenetic analyses were crucial in delineating a small-cell variant of Ki1-positive lymphoma. All 4 predominantly small cell Ki1-positive lymphomas that were karyotyped in a study of nine such cases displayed the t(2;5)(p23;q35).[164]

The molecular consequences of the t(2;5) have been recently elucidated. By using chromosome walking techniques, Morris and colleagues[33] cloned genes involved in this translocation: a previously unidentified protein tyrosine kinase gene, designated *ALK* (anaplastic lymphoma kinase), residing at 2p23, and the nuclear phosphoprotein gene *(NPM)* located at 5q35. They showed the expression of *NPM-ALK* fusion gene mRNA in all seven specimens studied, that is, three cell lines and four tumor samples of anaplastic large cell lymphoma with the t(2;5). Such expression was absent in several cell lines without the translocation. Since the *ALK* gene is not expressed in human normal lymphoid cells, its deregulation and overexpression

Table 6–7. Structural Aberrations Involving TCR Genes That Have Been Reported in at Least One Case of T-Cell NHL[3, 8, 167]

Aberration	Gene	Gene
t(1;14)(p32;q11)	*TAL1*	*TCRD*
inv(7)(p15q35)	*TCRG*	*TCRB*
t(7;11)(q35;p13)	*TCRB*	*RBTNL1*
t(8;14)(q24;q11)	*MYC*	*TCRA*
t(10;14)(q24;q11)	*HOX11*	*TCRD*
t(11;14)(p13;q11)	*RBTNL1*	*TCRD*
t(14;14)(q11;q32)	*TCRA*	
inv(14)(q11q32.3)	*TCRA*	IGH

NHL, non-Hodgkin's lymphoma.

owing to fusion with *NPM* may lead to malignant transformation.[33]

Despite a strong correlation between the t(2;5) and Ki1-positive anaplastic lymphoma, not all lymphomas that are Ki1-positive display this translocation.[146, 149, 150, 165] Bitter and coworkers[165] suggested that those Ki1-positive NHLs that do not possess t(2;5) are morphologically and clinically different from anaplastic large cell lymphoma with the translocation. Future studies should verify this hypothesis and determine whether the presence of t(2;5) has prognostic utility.

LYMPHOBLASTIC LYMPHOMA

LBL is a morphologic entity distinct from other NHL subtypes. Most tumors have an immature T-cell phenotype, although precursor B-cell phenotypes have been described.[58] Cytogenetically, T-cell LBL is similar to T-cell ALL. A substantial proportion of tumors have had a normal karyotype (see Table 6–1), a phenomenon also noted in ALL. The largest subgroup of cytogenetically aberrant lymphomas comprises tumors with inv(14)(q11q32) and various translocations involving bands 14q11, 7p15, and 7q35 known to harbor α and δ, γ, and β loci of *TCR*, respectively. Two of these translocations, t(11;14)(p13;q11) and t(7;14)(p15;q32), have been observed recurrently in LBL,[166] and identical rearrangements have also been detected in several cases of T-cell ALL.[8, 166] Similarly, the recurrent ALL translocations t(1;14)(p32-34;q11), t(7;11)(q35;p13), and t(10;14)(q24;q11)[167] have been reported in single cases of LBL.[8, 166, 168, 169] A few LBLs have had deletions of 9p[170] that encompass the locus (9p21) of a newly cloned TSG called *MTS1* (multiple tumor suppressor 1).[36] Deletions of 6q, commonly seen in ALL of both B and T lineage, as well as in other types of NHL, were also noted in LBL.[8] There are, however, LBLs that do not share common karyotypic features with ALL. Among such cases are six Japanese children with a rapidly progressive disease and fatal outcome who exhibited t(9;17)(q34;q23) in their karyotype.[166, 171] Additionally, a subset of T-cell LBL with other rearrangements of band 9q34 may exist.[142] However, the involvement of band 9q34 has been repeatedly noted in NHL of other histologic types.[8]

SMALL NONCLEAVED CELL LYMPHOMA

SNC lymphoma comprises two main groups: SNC of the Burkitt's and non-Burkitt's types. BL occurs mainly in young children and presents in extranodal sites.[58] Two forms of this disease, endemic and nonendemic, have been distinguished. The former occurs in equatorial Africa and is almost invariably associated with Epstein-Barr virus (EBV) infections. In the latter, the presence of EBV has been detected in the minority of cases—20% to 30% in the United States.[172] Both forms, however, display high incidences of *MYC* gene rearrangements owing to the presence of the t(8;14)(q24;q32) or its variants, which are regarded as primary genetic abnormalities in the generation of BL. It has been demonstrated that the breakpoints in the t(8;14) and variant translocations are different in endemic and nonendemic BLs at the molecular level,[172] but these translocations are indistinguishable cytogenetically.

The exact nature of the 14q+ marker seen consistently for the first time in both cell lines and BL biopsies by Manolov and Manolova[6] was elucidated by Zech[173] in 1976. They determined that additional material on 14q originated from the long arm of chromosome 8. These investigators also described one case with a t(8;22); 3 years later this was shown to be one of the variant translocations in BL.[174] A second variant translocation, the t(2;8), was concurrently described by Van Den Berghe and associates[175] and Miyoshi and colleagues.[176] Subsequent high-resolution cytogenetic studies allowed assigning the breakpoints in the t(8;14) to 8q24.1 and 14q32.3.[11] Despite their relative infrequency, BL and its leukemic counterpart, ALL L3, are among those human malignancies that have been most extensively characterized cytogenetically. Karyotypes of more than 200 cases of BL have been reported, and the largest series include those investigated by Douglass and coworkers,[177] Knuutila and associates,[178] and Kornblau and colleagues.[179] The last authors presented 22 of their own cases and reviewed 148 adult and pediatric patients with nonendemic BL or ALL L3. In this patient population, only 4% (6) patients had a normal karyotype, 62% displayed the t(8;14)(q24;q32), 12% and 9% of cases had the t(8;22)(q24;q11) and t(2;8)(p12;q24), respectively, and 14% had aberrant karyotypes without any of the classic translocations. A few patients in this last group had 14q+ markers, which may have involved rearrangements of *MYC*, as shown by Nakamine and colleagues.[112] Patients with acquired immunodeficiency syndrome (AIDS) who develop BL (which may occur in as many as 4% of all AIDS patients) had one of the classic translocations in their tumors more frequently than other patients (91% versus 81% of cases), although this difference was not statistically significant. Furthermore, the incidence of t(8;22) was significantly higher in patients with AIDS.[179] In approximately 30% of BL cases, one of the classic translocations has been the only chromosome abnormality.[8] Among secondary aberrations, the most frequent have been duplications of the long arm of chromosome 1, followed by trisomies of chromosomes 7, 12, 8, and 18, i(17)(q10) and structural aberrations affecting chromosome 17, with breakpoints predominantly localized in 17p.[8, 179]

In contrast with BL, the number of cytogenetically investigated cases with the non-Burkitt's type of SNC lymphoma is much smaller. In a subset of these tumors the t(14;18) or *BCL2* rearrangements were found.[21, 111, 141, 144] Although the t(8;14) or 8q24 abnormalities were also detected in some cases,[11, 21] most non-Burkitt's SNC lymphomas, unlike BLs, have not demonstrated 8q24 changes.[21, 144] These observations have been confirmed by a molecular genetic study performed on carefully selected BL and non-Burkitt's SNC lymphomas.[180] Whereas 17 (94%) of 18 BLs contained *MYC* rearrangements, none of 11 non-Burkitt's SNC tumors had *MYC* rearrangements in Southern blot analysis. *BCL2* changes were found in 3 of 10 evaluable non-Burkitt's SNC lymphomas and in none of the BLs studied. These results support the notion that BL and non-Burkitt's SNC lymphoma represent entities that are distinct not only morphologically, and to some extent clinically, but also with regard to pathogenetic mechanisms.[180]

GENETIC CHANGES IN TUMOR PROGRESSION OF NHL

Tumor progression, defined as a stepwise acquisition of new phenotypic properties by cancer cells leading to more aggressive biologic and clinical behavior of a tumor over time, has been observed in many different types of neoplasia. There is growing evidence that accumulation of nonrandom, secondary chromosome aberrations may contribute to this process.[181, 182]

Analyses of the natural history of NHL have indicated that indolent lymphomas eventually undergo histologic transformation to an intermediate- or high-grade tumor in 40% to 70% of patients at 8 to 10 years after initial diagnosis.[183] In other patients clinical progression may occur without a change in tumor morphology. Therefore, several groups have attempted to identify the chromosome aberrations that could be responsible for the accelerated course of the disease. Yunis and coworkers[101] on the basis of cytogenetic analysis of 71 patients with follicular lymphoma, proposed a model for the evolution of t(14;18)-bearing tumors. They suggested that progression from FSC to higher-grade NHL was associated with the appearance of additional chromosome aberrations, in particular del(6q), +7 or dup(7p), or +12 or dup(12q). Moreover, a gain of extra copies of chromosomes 3, 18, or 21 was correlated with FL and DLC lymphomas in their model. Subsequent studies have confirmed that intermediate- and high-grade tumors with t(14;18) have significantly higher frequencies of trisomy 7,[17, 100, 102] trisomy 12,[17] and del(6q) or monosomy 6[100] as compared with low-grade lymphomas.

Conclusive evidence that histologic transformation can in fact be brought about by the aforementioned abnormalities could be provided only by sequential cytogenetic studies in patients who have had two or more biopsies over the course of their disease. Such sequential analyses have been performed in only about 50 patients with various types of NHL, and change in morphologic features of lymphoma has been observed in one half of them.[14, 17, 98, 99, 101, 102, 134, 144] Indeed, in four cases with t(14;18), an additional copy or two copies of chromosome 7, not present in the initial biopsy, have been found in the karyotype of the transformed lymphoma.[98, 99, 102, 144] Furthermore, a minor clone with +7 present at diagnosis in another patient with FSC became predominant after 25 months associated with a transformation to FM histology.[101] However, because most transformed tumors do not display trisomy 7, the acquisition of this chromosome, albeit important in a subset of t(14;18)-positive tumors, does not seem to represent the major cytogenetic route of tumor progression.

Another mechanism of tumor progression of follicular lymphomas has been demonstrated in rare tumors in which the t(8;14) is superimposed on a t(14;18).[54, 184–187] A secondary dysregulation of *MYC* in such lymphomas has led to histologic transformation and rapid advance to high-grade disease. This scenario, however, is also not a frequent one, as shown by Yano and associates,[187] who detected *MYC* rearrangements in only 3 (8%) of 38 histologically transformed NHLs. In one case of SNC lymphoma, the sequence of events was apparently reversed, that is, the t(18;22) occurred in a clone already bearing the t(8;14).[54] This case lends support to the view that in some instances it is not the sequential order of genetic events but their cumulative effect that is critical in tumor evolution.[182]

Recent studies indicate that transformation of a significant proportion of follicular lymphomas to higher grade NHL is associated with mutations of the *p53* gene. That loss and rearrangements of this gene may be implicated in clonal evolution of some lymphomas has been suggested by previous cytogenetic findings in large cell lymphoma[11, 12, 20, 92] and in serial biopsies of transformed lymphomas.[99] Monosomy 17 or structural aberrations of 17p have been consistently observed in 30% to 45% of large cell NHL,[11, 12, 20, 92] and similar aberrations were acquired in three of seven sequentially studied follicular lymphomas that underwent histologic transformation.[99] Moreover, Rodriguez and colleagues[188] detected allelic losses of the *p53* gene by the Southern blot technique in three of eight cell lines and large cell lymphoma samples with cytogenetic abnormalities of 17p. Further molecular genetic studies have revealed mutations of the *p53* gene or overexpression of p53 protein in 5 of 6,[42] and in 10 of 34[41] aggressive NHLs that transformed from preceding follicular histologies. Sander and coworkers[41] estimate that mutations of *p53* are associated with histologic transformation in approximately 25% to 30% of follicular lymphomas. They observed *p53* mutations in 3 of 25 patients with low-grade follicular lymphomas. Two of these patients subsequently developed transformed NHL; the third achieved a long-lasting remission after treatment on an intensive chemotherapy regimen (ProMACE/MOPP°).[41] These data and those obtained by others[42] suggest that the finding of *p53* mutations in indolent lymphoma indicates an increased risk for progression and may justify more aggressive therapy.

It has been recently shown that mutations in the *p53* gene disturb cell cycle control and increase the rate at which genetic alterations accumulate within cells.[189] Therefore, Sander and coworkers[41] have proposed a model for a *p53*-dependent progression pathway in follicular lymphoma, in which histologic transformation is not caused directly by *p53* mutations, but changes in the tumor phenotype are associated with other genetic rearrangements that accumulate in cells defective in *p53*. The nature of such transforming mutations is unknown. The absence of *MYC* gene rearrangements in *p53*-positive transformed lymphomas[41, 42] indicates that these mutations may be independent events in lymphoma progression. However, given the high complexity of karyotypes and the heterogeneity of chromosome changes encountered in advanced lymphomas, it is quite likely that there will be no single genetic rearrangement that is responsible for progression in *p53*-positive or the twice as frequent *p53*-negative lymphomas.

The number of patients with non-follicular NHL that have been analyzed serially is smaller than that of patients with FSC, FM, and FL. Of eight SLL cases, four did not exhibit

---

°ProMACE/MOPP = prednisone, methotrexate (with leucovorin rescue), Adriamycin, cyclophosphamide, etoposide/mechlorethamine, Oncovin, procarbazine, prednisone.

any change in the tumor karyotype over time, even though in one of these patients transformation to DLC lymphoma had occurred.[98, 99] In the remaining four patients, followup analyses showed signs of the karyotypic evolution, but acquired aberrations were different in each case.[99] So few NHL of other histologies have been studied sequentially that no conclusions can be drawn.

CLINICAL RELEVANCE OF CHROMOSOME ABERRATIONS IN NHL

The prognostic utility of chromosome aberrations in the acute leukemias and myelodysplastic syndromes (MDSs) is well-established.[2, 167, 190–192] In NHL, however, only limited data are available. Although in recent years several groups have reported correlations between particular cytogenetic features of NHL and clinical outcome (Table 6–8), many of these relationships have been detected in relatively small groups of patients, and frequently associations significant in one series have not been significant in others. Furthermore, to obtain enough cases for statistical analysis, many studies have included lymphomas of various histologic subtypes, as well as patients studied at diagnosis and at relapse.

Studies that provide information on the prognostic importance of karyotypes detected exclusively in untreated NHL patients include reports by Levine and associates[193] and Offit and colleagues.[194] In the former study, comprising 68 patients, the presence of normal metaphases in tumor material was predictive for an increased rate of complete remission (CR) and longer survival. Among 30 patients with follicular lymphoma, the CR rate was higher and the survival was significantly longer in the group with more than 20% cytogenetically normal cells in tumor material.[193] Correspondingly, prolonged survival of patients without any cytogenetically abnormal clone, but not of those with normal metaphase cells present in addition to abnormal ones, was demonstrated in a Swedish series of NHL containing lymphomas of both low- and high-grade malignancy,[195] as well as in a smaller Polish series.[196] However, others[16, 194] have not found any difference in survival duration between patients with NHL who had entirely normal karyotypes, abnormal karyotypes alone, or a combination of both. Thus, it is uncertain whether the finding of normal metaphases in a lymphoma specimen confers a favorable prognosis.

Hyperdiploidy, with the number of chromosomes exceeding 50, has been found to constitute a favorable prognostic factor in childhood ALL, especially in cases with only numerical chromosome changes.[167, 191] Initial study of a relatively small number of patients suggested that a similar phenomenon may also exist in NHL[134]; six patients with a near-tetraploid modal chromosome number had the longest median survival among 30 karyotypically abnormal patients. However, larger cytogenetic[195] and flow cytometric[197] analyses did not find correlations between increased ploidy of lymphoma and overall survival.

Although Levine and associates[193] did not demonstrate the influence of more complex karyotypes on survival of patients with NHL, two studies found a negative impact of multiple chromosome changes on clinical outcome.[194, 195] Kristoffersson and coworkers[195] in 106 NHLs of various histologies, found that survival was significantly shorter for patients with 10 or more aberrations compared with patients with normal karyotypes or only one to four aberrations. Similarly, among 104 patients with DM and DLC lymphomas and IBL who had abnormal karyotypes at diagnosis, the presence of more than four marker chromosomes was associated with a shortened median survival.[194] These preliminary results indicate that the complexity of the patient's karyotype may become an important prognostic indicator in NHL as it already has in acute myeloid leukemia[190] and MDS.[192]

The observation, made in a small group of 20 cases with FM or FL lymphoma, that the presence of the t(14;18) or BCL2 rearrangement was correlated with a poor response to therapy and shortened survival,[198] has not been substantiated in several larger studies.[16, 193–195, 199] Instead, an adverse prognosis seems to be associated with the addition of other chromosome changes in a follicular lymphoma karyotype. Yunis and colleagues[101] observed that while patients with FSC lymphoma and a solitary t(14;18) had an indolent course, all four patients with an additional del(13)(q32) had an acceleration of the disease with a poor response to chemotherapy. Furthermore, trisomy of chromosomes 7 and 12, as well as deletions of 6q, were found more often in clinically more aggressive mixed and large cell subtypes of follicular lymphoma, and trisomy 3, 18, and 21 correlated almost exclusively with FL lymphoma. In addition, trisomy of chromosome 2 or its short arm and homogeneously staining regions or double minutes were found to correlate with a poor prognosis in patients with follicular lymphoma.[101]

Not all these observations have been confirmed by subsequent studies. In a group of 53 karyotypically abnormal patients with low-grade lymphomas, Offit and associates[194] did not find any correlation between clinical outcome and the presence of trisomy 2 or deletions of 2p; aberrations involving band 13q32 were detected too infrequently in this study to be analyzed. On the other hand, the survival of patients with trisomy 7 or trisomy 12 or structural abnormalities involving region 1p32-36 was shorter than that of patients without these aberrations.[194]

The t(14;18) or BCL2 gene rearrangements can be found in 18% to 40% of DLC lymphomas (see Table 6–5).[111, 141, 200–202] Several groups have demonstrated that the overall survival of patients with DLC lymphoma does not correlate with the presence or absence of the t(14;18) or BCL2 gene rearrangements or bcl-2 protein expression.[193, 194, 200–203] However, in three independent studies,[198, 201, 204] the disease-free survival of t(14;18)/BCL2-positive DLC patients was significantly shorter than that of DLC patients without 18q21 rearrangements. Although in one study there was no such difference,[200] in another, comprising 83 cases of DLC lymphoma or IBL, BCL2 rearrangements were significantly associated with shorter disease-free duration among patients with extranodal presentation.[202] Thus, the presence of t(14;18)/BCL2 changes seems to delineate a subgroup of DLC lymphoma patients who demonstrate a decreased remission duration but respond well to therapy; therefore, their overall survival is not significantly diminished.

Table 6–8. Cytogenetic Features Reported to Have Prognostic Significance in NHL

Cytogenetic Feature*	Prognostic Relevance
Exclusively normal karyotype	Longer survival[195, 196]; no correlation[16, 194]
Normal metaphase cells in NHL specimen	Increased CR rate and longer survival[193]; no correlation[16, 194]
More than 20% of normal metaphases in follicular NHL	Increased CR rate and longer survival[193]; no correlation[16, 194]
Near-tetraploidy	Longer survival[134]; no correlation[195, 197]
Hypodiploidy	Shorter survival[195]
>Four aberrations in DM, DLC, and IBL	Shorter survival[194]; no correlation[193]
>10 aberrations	Shorter survival[195]; no correlation[193]
1p+	Shorter survival[195]
Break at 1p32	Shorter disease-free interval[193]
Break at 1p32-36 in low-grade NHL†	Shorter survival[194]
Break at 1p32-36 in DM, DLC, and IBL	Shorter duration of CR[194]
Break at 1q21-23 in DM, DLC, and IBL	Shorter duration of CR and shorter survival[194]
+2 or dup(2p) in FM, FL, DM and DLC	Poor response to treatment and shorter survival[101, 198]; no correlation[16, 194]
Break in 2p in DLC and IBL	Longer survival[193]; no correlation[194]
+3 or dup(3p) in FM, FL, DM, and DLC	Longer survival[198]; no correlation[16]; no correlation in DM, DLC, and IBL[194]
+5	Shorter survival[16]; no correlation in DM, DLC, and IBL[194]
Any abnormality of 5	Shorter survival[16]
+6	Shorter survival[16]; no correlation in DM, DLC, and IBL[194]
Break at 6q21-25 in DM, DLC, and IBL	Shorter survival and diminished probability of achieving CR[194]; no correlation between del(6q) and survival in DLC and IBL[200]
−7 or structural abnormality of 7p	Poor response to chemotherapy, shorter disease-free and overall survival[205]; no correlation between −7 and survival in DM, DLC, and IBL[194]
+7	Shorter survival[195]
+7 in low-grade NHL†	Shorter survival[194]
t(8;14) in low-grade NHL and in DM, DLC, and IBL	No significant difference in survival as compared with patients without the translocation in a given subset[194]
+12 in low-grade NHL†	Shorter survival[194]
del(13)(q32) in FSC with t(14;18)	Poor response to treatment and shorter survival[101]
Break at 14q11-12	Shorter survival[16]
t(14;18)/*BCL2* rearrangement in FM and FL	Poor response to treatment and shorter survival[198]; no correlation with survival in FSC, FM, and FL,[16, 193–195, 199]
t(14;18)/*BCL2* rearrangement in DM and DLC	Shorter disease-free survival[198]
t(14;18)/*BCL2* rearrangement in DLC	Shorter disease-free survival[204]; no correlation with overall survival[204]
BCL2 rearrangement in de novo DLC	Shorter disease-free period[201]; no correlation with overall survival[201]
t(14;18)/*BCL2* rearrangement in DLC and IBL	Shorter disease-free period in extranodal NHL[201]; no correlation with overall[200, 202] and disease-free survival[200]
−17 or del(17q) in DLC and IBL	Poor response to treatment and shorter survival[198]
−17 or structural abnormality of 17p	Poor response to chemotherapy, shorter disease-free and overall survival[205]
Structural abnormality of 17	Shorter survival[16]
Structural abnormality of 17 in follicular NHL	Shorter survival[193]
+18	Shorter survival[16]; no correlation in DM, DLC, and IBL[194]

*The molecular equivalent of the t(14;18), *BCL2* rearrangement, is also included.
†Statistically significant when breaks at 1p32–36, +7, and +12 combined.
NHL, non-Hodgkin's lymphoma; CR, complete remission.

Several other specific chromosome abnormalities have been reported to be markers whose presence in the tumor karyotype may affect clinical outcome. Among them, structural changes of chromosome 17 have been repeatedly shown to correlate with an adverse prognosis. In a study of Levine and colleagues,[193] 8 patients with follicular lymphoma and various structural changes of either the short or long arm of chromosome 17 had significantly shorter survival than 22 patients without breaks in this chromosome. Poor clinical outcome of patients with structural changes of chromosome 17 or monosomy 17 has also been demonstrated in series that included all histologic subtypes of NHL[16, 205] and in subsets of patients with diffuse lymphomas with large cell components,[194, 198] as well as in patients with BL.[179] In some of these studies,[16, 205] multivariate analyses were conducted, and abnormalities of chromosome 17 were shown to be a risk factor independent from other unfavorable prognostic features such as tumor grade, increased lactic dehydrogenase (LDH) level or tumor burden. These findings are in good agreement with the recently demonstrated role of *p53* mutations in tumor progression of NHL.[41, 42, 45] Additionally, in a recent analysis of 119 patients with high-grade B-cell NHL, increased *p53* expression in tumor cells correlated significantly with a decreased life expectancy during the first months after diagnosis.[203] Therefore, detection of chromosome 17 abnormalities or *p53* changes may identify patients who require more intensive treatment.

Additional chromosome abnormalities have been reported to influence clinical outcome in single studies. Poor prognosis has been associated with the presence of trisomies of chromosomes 5, 6, and 18[16]; any abnormality of chromosome 5[16]; monosomy 7 and structural changes of 7p[205]; breaks at 14q11-12[16]; and, only in DM, DL, and IBL patients, breaks at 1q21-23 or 6q21-25.[194] Among patients with DLC lymphomas, those with breaks in 2p[193] or trisomy 3 or duplication of 3p[198] had prolonged survival. All these correlations still require corroboration.

Likewise, associations of karyotypic features with clinical sites of disease and other characteristics require confirmation. Levine and coworkers[193] demonstrated, in a small number of patients, significant correlations between structural changes of 11q13 and tumorous involvement of the gastrointestinal tract, and between trisomy 11 and del(6)(q23) and meningeal involvement. Deletions of chromosome 6 at q21-25 or translocations involving this region correlated with bone marrow involvement in another study.[206] In addition, bone marrow involvement was associated with breaks at 1p32-36, and this correlation remained significant when patients with follicular and diffuse histologies were grouped separately.[206] On the other hand, Schouten and colleagues[16] associated structural changes of chromosome 1 with the absence of bone marrow involvement, but in their analysis the breakpoints clustered between bands q21-q25 in the long arm of chromosome 1. Moreover, splenic involvement has been associated with monosomy 14 or del(14)(q22-24), pulmonary involvement with trisomy or structural changes of chromosome 9, and bone involvement with monosomy 11.[206]

Other clinical correlations with karyotype have been published. Schouten and colleagues[16] have associated structural changes involving regions 3q21-25 or 13q21-24 with bulky disease, abnormalities of 6q11-16 with the presence of B symptoms, and the t(11;14)(q13;q32) with increased levels of LDH.

CONCLUSIONS

Cytogenetic analyses of NHL have revealed several specific chromosome abnormalities associated with the initiation and progression of the malignant process. Mapping of breakpoints in recurring translocations have led to the cloning and characterization of genes involved in lymphomagenesis and to identification of the mechanisms whereby their expression has been altered. Recent studies, pursuing cytogenetic reports on repeatedly lost chromosome bands or regions, have demonstrated that TSGs may also take part in the multistage evolution of lymphoma cells. Moreover, correlations between karyotypic changes and histology, disease characteristics, and clinical outcome have been made. Chromosome aberrations have proved to be important biologic markers that together with immunophenotypic, morphologic, and molecular genetic data have helped to delineate individual diseases within particular Working Formulation categories. Conversely, the presence of the same nonrandom karyotypic abnormality in entities thus far regarded as not closely related, have indicated their closer than anticipated pathogenetic associations. However, many of the reported correlations between karyotype and other features of lymphoma are still preliminary and require corroboration by large prospective studies.

The recent development of fluorescence in situ hybridization (FISH) techniques that use chromosome-specific DNA probes has provided valuable supplementation to classic cytogenetics. Chromosome painting can increase the accuracy of cytogenetic investigation of metaphase cells. This method is particularly advantageous in determining the origin of unidentified material adjoined to chromosome arms, a phenomenon that is often encountered in NHL.[109] Additionally, FISH studies of selected chromosome abnormalities can be performed on a large number of nondividing individual tumor cells (interphase cytogenetics).[207] Since it has been shown that such investigations can be performed successfully on archival tumor tissues as old as 25 years,[208] not only prospective but also large retrospective studies have become feasible. Although increasingly important, FISH techniques have only limited applications and in the foreseeable future will probably not substitute for conventional cytogenetic analyses. It is hoped that continuing cytogenetic studies will not only lead to a better understanding of lymphomagenesis but also result in delineation of both karyotypic and molecular genetic markers that are helpful in clinical management of patients with NHL.

Acknowledgments

We are indebted to Dr. Kenneth Offit for making available a preprint of his article.[78]

REFERENCES

1. Heim S, Mitelman F: Cancer Cytogenetics. New York, Alan R Liss, 1987.

2. Sandberg AA: The Chromosomes in Human Cancer and Leukemia, 2nd ed. New York, Elsevier, 1990.

3. Mitelman F, Kaneko Y, Berger R: Report of the Committee on Chromosome Changes in Neoplasia, Chromosome Coordinating Meeting (1992). *In* Cuticchia AJ, Pearson PL, Klinger HP (eds): Genome Priority Reports, vol 1. Basel, Karger, 1993, p 700.

4. Nowell PC, Hungerford DA: A minute chromosome in human chronic granulocytic leukemia. Science 1960; 132(3438):1497.

5. Rowley JD, Fukuhara S: Chromosome studies in non-Hodgkin's lymphomas. Semin Oncol 1980; 7(3):255.

6. Manolov G, Manolova Y: Marker band in one chromosome 14 from Burkitt lymphomas. Nature 1972: 237(5349):33.

7. Mitelman F (ed): ISCN (1991): Guidelines for Cancer Cytogenetics, Supplement to An International System for Human Cytogenetic Nomenclature. Basel, Karger, 1991.

8. Mitelman F: Catalog of Chromosome Aberrations in Cancer, 4th ed. New York, Wiley-Liss, 1991.

9. The Non-Hodgkin's Lymphoma Pathologic Classification Project: National Cancer Institute sponsored study of classifications of non-Hodgkin's lymphomas: Summary and description of a working formulation for clinical usage. Cancer 1982; 49(10):2112.

10. Gerard-Marchant R, Hamlin I, Lennert K, et al: Classification of non-Hodgkin's lymphomas. Lancet 1974; 2(7877):406.

11. Yunis JJ, Oken MM, Kaplan ME, et al: Distinctive chromosomal abnormalities in histologic subtypes of non-Hodgkin's lymphoma. N Engl J Med 1982; 307(20):1231.

12. Bloomfield CD, Arthur DC, Frizzera G, et al: Nonrandom chromosome abnormalities in lymphoma. Cancer Res 1983; 43(6):2975.

13. Yunis JJ, Oken MM, Theologides A, et al: Recurrent chromosomal defects are found in most patients with non-Hodgkin's lymphoma. Cancer Genet Cytogenet 1984; 13(1):17.

14. Kristoffersson U, Heim S, Olsson H, et al: Cytogenetic studies in non-Hodgkin lymphomas—Results from surgical biopsies. Hereditas 1986; 104(1):1.

15. Juneja S, Lukeis R, Tan L, et al: Cytogenetic analysis of 147 cases of non-Hodgkin's lymphoma: Non-random chromosomal abnormalities and histological correlations. Br J Haematol 1990; 76(2):231.

16. Schouten HC, Sanger WG, Weisenburger DD, et al: Chromosomal abnormalities in untreated patients with non-Hodgkin's lymphoma: Associations with histology, clinical characteristics, and treatment outcome. Blood 1990; 75(9):1841.

17. Offit K, Jhanwar SC, Ladanyi M, et al: Cytogenetic analysis of 434 consecutively ascertained specimens of non-Hodgkin's lymphoma: Correlations between recurrent aberrations, histology, and exposure to cytotoxic treatment. Genes Chromosom Cancer 1991; 3(3):189.

18. Bastard C, Tilly H, Lenormand B, et al: Translocations involving band 3q27 and Ig gene regions in non-Hodgkin's lymphoma. Blood 1992; 79(10):2527.

19. Speaks SL, Sanger WG, Linder J, et al: Chromosomal abnormalities in indolent lymphoma. Cancer Genet Cytogenet 1987; 27(2):335.

20. Levine EG, Arthur DC, Frizzera G, et al: There are differences in cytogenetic abnormalities among histologic subtypes of the non-Hodgkin's lymphomas. Blood 1985; 66(6):1414.

21. Fifth International Workshop on Chromosomes in Leukemia-Lymphoma: Correlation of chromosome abnormalities with histologic and immunologic characteristics in non-Hodgkin's lymphoma and adult T-cell leukemia-lymphoma. Blood 1987; 70(5):1554.

22. Criel A, Billiet J, Vandenberghe E, et al: Leukaemic intermediate lymphocytic lymphomas: Analysis of twelve cases diagnosed by morphology. Leuk Lymphoma 1992; 8(4-5):381.

23. Wotherspoon AC, Pan L, Diss TC, et al: Cytogenetic study of B-cell lymphoma of mucosa-associated lymphoid tissue. Cancer Genet Cytogenet 1992; 58(1):35.

24. Gaidano G, Hauptschein RS, Parsa NZ, et al: Deletions involving two distinct regions of 6q in B-cell non-Hodgkin lymphoma. Blood 1992; 80(7):1781.

25. Croce CM: Molecular biology of lymphomas. Semin Oncol 1993; 20(5, Suppl 5):31.

26. Thirman MJ, Gill HJ, Burnett RC, et al: Rearrangement of the *MLL* gene in acute lymphoblastic and acute myeloid leukemias with 11q23 chromosomal translocations. N Engl J Med 1993; 329(13):909.

27. Cimino G, Lo Coco F, Biondi A, et al: *ALL-1* gene at chromosome 11q23 is consistently altered in acute leukemia of early infancy. Blood 1993; 82(2):544.

28. Caligiuri MA, Schichman SA, Strout MP, et al: Molecular rearrangement of the *ALL-1* gene in acute myeloid leukemia without evidence of 11q23 chromosomal translocations. Cancer Res 1994; 54(2):370.

29. Schichman SA, Caligiuri MA, Strout MP, et al: *ALL-1* tandem duplication in acute myeloid leukemia with a normal karyotype involves homologous recombination between *Alu* elements. Cancer Res 1994; 54(16):4277.

30. Mark J: Chromosomal abnormalities and their specificity in human neoplasms: An assessment of recent observations by banding techniques. Adv Cancer Res 1977; 24:165.

31. Mrózek, Bloomfield CD: Cytogenetics of non-Hodgkin's lymphoma and Hodgkin's disease. *In* Wiernik PH, Canellos GP, Dutcher JP, Kyle RA (eds): Neoplastic Diseases of the Blood, 3rd ed. New York, Churchill Livingstone, 1996, p 835.

32. Nowell PC, Croce CM: Chromosome translocations and oncogenes in human lymphoid tumors. Am J Clin Pathol 1990; 94(2):229.

33. Morris SW, Kirstein MN, Valentine MB, et al: Fusion of a kinase gene, *ALK*, to a nucleolar protein gene, *NPM*, in non-Hodgkin's lymphoma. Science 1994; 263(5151):1281.

34. Mitani K, Sato Y, Tojo A, et al: Philadelphia chromosome positive B-cell–type malignant lymphoma expressing an aberrant 190 kDa *bcr-abl* protein. Br J Haematol 1990; 76(2):221.

35. Knudson AG: Antioncogenes and human cancer. Proc Natl Acad Sci U S A 1993; 90(23):10914.

36. Kamb A, Gruis NA, Weaver-Feldhaus J, et al: A cell cycle regulator potentially involved in genesis of many tumor types. Science 1994; 264(5157):436.

37. Marshall CJ: Tumor suppressor genes. Cell 1991; 64(2):313.

38. Gaidano G, Ballerini P, Gong JZ, et al: p53 mutations in human lymphoid malignancies: Association with Burkitt lymphoma and chronic lymphocytic leukemia. Proc Natl Acad Sci U S A 1991; 88(12):5413.

39. Ichikawa A, Hotta T, Takagi N, et al: Mutations of p53 gene and their relation to disease progression in B-cell lymphoma. Blood 1992; 79(10):2701.

40. Gaidano G, Dalla-Favera R: Biologic and molecular characterization of non-Hodgkin's lymphoma. Curr Opin Oncol 1993; 5(5):776.

41. Sander CA, Yano T, Clark HM, et al: p53 mutation is associated with progression in follicular lymphomas. Blood 1993; 82(7):1994.

42. Lo Coco F, Gaidano G, Louie DC, et al: p53 mutations are associated with histologic transformation of follicular lymphoma. Blood 1993; 82(8):2289.

43. Pezzella F, Morrison H, Jones M, et al: Immunohistochemical detection of p53 and *bcl-2* proteins in non-Hodgkin's lymphoma. Histopathology 1993; 22(1):39.

44. Farrugia MM, Duan L-J, Reis MD, et al: Alterations of the p53 tumor suppressor gene in diffuse large cell lymphomas with translocations of the c-*MYC* and *BCL-2* proto-oncogenes. Blood 1994; 83(1):191.

45. Chang H, Benchimol S, Minden MD, et al: Alterations of p53 and c-*myc* in the clonal evolution of malignant lymphoma. Blood 1994; 83(2):452.

46. Ginsberg AM, Raffeld M, Cossman J: Inactivation of the retinoblastoma gene in human lymphoid neoplasms. Blood 1991; 77(4):833.

47. Weide R, Tiemann M, Pflüger K-H, et al: Altered expression of the retinoblastoma gene product in human high-grade non-Hodgkin's lymphomas. Leukemia 1994; 8(1):97.

48. Offit K, Parsa NZ, Gaidano G, et al: 6q deletions define distinct clinico-pathologic subsets of non-Hodgkin's lymphoma. Blood 1993; 82(7):2157.

49. Kerckaert J-P, Deweindt C, Tilly H, et al: *LAZ3*, a novel zinc-finger encoding gene, is disrupted by recurring chromosome 3q27 translocations in human lymphomas. Nature Genet 1993; 5(1):66.

50. Ye BH, Lista F, Lo Coco F, et al: Alterations of a zinc finger–encoding gene, *BCL-6*, in diffuse large-cell lymphoma. Science 1993; 262(5134):747.

51. Miki T, Kawamata N, Hirosawa S, et al: Gene involved in the 3q27 translocation associated with B-cell lymphoma, *BCL5*, encodes a Krüppel-like zinc-finger protein. Blood 1994; 83(1):26.

52. Konishi H, Sakurai M, Nakao H, et al: Chromosome abnormalities in malignant lymphoma in patients from Kurashiki: Histological and immunophenotypic correlations. Cancer Res 1990; 50(9):2698.

53. Hillion J, Mecucci C, Aventin A, et al: A variant translocation t(2;18) in follicular lymphoma involves the 5′ end of *bcl*-2 and Igκ light chain gene. Oncogene 1991; 6(1):169.

54. Koduru PRK, Offit K: Molecular structure of double reciprocal translocations: Significance in B-cell lymphomagenesis. Oncogene 1991; 6(1):145.

55. Leroux D, Hillion J, Monteil M, et al: t(18;22)(q21;q11) with rearrangement of *BCL2* as a possible secondary change in a lymphocytic lymphoma. Genes Chromosom Cancer 1991; 3(3):205.

56. Meerabux JM, Cotter FE, Kearney L, et al: Molecular cloning of a novel 11q23 breakpoint associated with non-Hodgkin's lymphoma. Oncogene 1994; 9(3):893.

57. Fukuhara S, Rowley JD, Variakojis D, et al: Chromosome abnormalities in poorly differentiated lymphocytic lymphoma. Cancer Res 1979; 39(8):3119.

58. Jaffe ES, Raffeld M, Medeiros LJ, et al: An overview of the classification of non-Hodgkin's lymphomas: An integration of morphological and phenotypical concepts. Cancer Res 1992; 52(19, Suppl):5447s.

59. Jaffe ES, Raffeld M, Medeiros LJ: Histopathologic subtypes of indolent lymphomas: Caricatures of the mature B-cell system. Semin Oncol 1993; 20(5, Suppl 5):3.

60. Juliusson G, Oscier DG, Fitchett M, et al: Prognostic subgroups in B-cell chronic lymphocytic leukemia defined by specific chromosomal abnormalities. N Engl J Med 1990; 323(11):720.

61. Brown AG, Ross FM, Dunne EM, et al: Evidence for a new tumour suppressor locus *(DBM)* in human B-cell neoplasia telomeric to the retinoblastoma gene. Nature Genet 1993; 3(1):67.

62. Tilly H, Bastard C, Halkin E, et al: Del(14)(q22) in diffuse B-cell lymphocytic lymphoma. Am J Clin Pathol 1988; 89(1):109.

63. Brusamolino E, Bernasconi P, Pasquali F, et al: Trisomy 12 in a case of large cell, immunoblastic, polymorphous non-Hodgkin's lymphoma with IgGκ monoclonal paraprotein. Cancer Genet Cytogenet 1984; 13(3):279.

64. Nilbert M, Heim S: Uterine leiomyoma cytogenetics. Genes Chromosom Cancer 1990; 2(1):3.

65. Mrózek K, Nedoszytko B, Babinska M, et al: Trisomy of chromosome 12 in a case of thecoma of the ovary. Gynecol Oncol 1990; 36(3):413.

66. Pejovic T, Heim S, Mandahl N, et al: Trisomy 12 is a consistent chromosomal aberration in benign ovarian tumors. Genes Chromosom Cancer 1990; 2(1):48.

67. Fletcher JA, Gibas Z, Donovan K, et al: Ovarian granulosa-stromal cell tumors are characterized by trisomy 12. Am J Pathol 1991; 138(3):515.

68. Crossen PE, Horn HL: Origin of trisomy 12 in B-cell chronic lymphocytic leukemia. Cancer Genet Cytogenet 1987; 28(1):185.

69. Einhorn S, Burvall K, Juliusson G, et al: Molecular analyses of chromosome 12 in chronic lymphocytic leukemia. Leukemia 1989; 3(12):871.

70. Wirshubsky Z, Wiener F, Spira J, et al: Triplication of one chromosome no. 15 with an altered *c-myc* containing EcoRI fragment and elimination of the normal homologue in a T-cell lymphoma line of AKR origin (TIKAUT). Int J Cancer 1984; 33(4):477.

71. Juliusson G, Gahrton G: Chromosome aberrations in B-cell chronic lymphocytic leukemia: Pathogenetic and clinical implications. Cancer Genet Cytogenet 1990; 45(2):143.

72. Mrózek K, Bloomfield CD: Cytogenetics of indolent lymphomas. Semin Oncol 1993; 20(5, Suppl 5):47.

73. Kristoffersson U, Heim S, Johnsson A, et al: Deletion of 14q in non-Hodgkin's lymphoma. Eur J Haematol 1990; 44(4):261.

74. Hammond DW, Goepel JR, Aitken M, et al: Cytogenetic analysis of a United Kingdom series of non-Hodgkin's lymphomas. Cancer Genet Cytogenet 1992; 61(1):31.

75. Wagner AJ, Le Beau MM, Diaz MO, et al: Expression, regulation, and chromosomal localization of the *Max* gene. Proc Natl Acad Sci U S A 1992; 89(7):3111.

76. Fleischman EW, Prigogina EL, Ilynskaya GW, et al: Chromosomal characteristics of malignant lymphoma. Hum Genet 1989; 82(4):343.

77. Schouten HC, Sanger WG, Weisenburger DD, et al: Abnormalities involving chromosome 6 in newly diagnosed patients with non-Hodgkin's lymphoma. Cancer Genet Cytogenet 1990; 47(1):73.

78. Offit K, Louie DC, Parsa NZ, et al: Clinical and morphologic features of B-cell small lymphocytic lymphoma with del(6)(q21q23). Blood 1994; 83(9):2611.

79. Brito-Babapulle V, Ellis J, Matutes E, et al: Translocation t(11;14)(q13;q32) in chronic lymphoid disorders. Genes Chromosom Cancer 1992; 5(2):158.

80. Oscier DG, Matutes E, Gardiner A, et al: Cytogenetic studies in splenic lymphoma with villous lymphocytes. Br J Haematol 1993; 85(3):487.

81. Newman RA, Peterson B, Davey FR, et al: Phenotypic markers and BCL-1 gene rearrangements in B-cell chronic lymphocytic leukemia: A Cancer and Leukemia Group B Study. Blood 1993; 82(4):1239.

82. Levine EG, Arthur DC, Machnicki J, et al: Four new recurring translocations in non-Hodgkin lymphoma. Blood 1989; 74(5):1796.

83. Griffin CA, Zehnbauer BA, Beschorner WE, et al: t(11;18)(q21;q21) is a recurrent chromosome abnormality in small lymphocytic lymphoma. Genes Chromosom Cancer 1992; 4(2):153.

84. Horsman D, Gascoyne R, Klasa R, et al: t(11;18)(q21;q21.1): A recurring translocation in lymphomas of mucosa-associated lymphoid tissue (MALT)? Genes Chromosom Cancer 1992; 4(2):183.

85. Leroux D, Seité P, Hillion J, et al: t(11;18)(q21;q21) may delineate a spectrum of diffuse small B-cell lymphoma with extranodal involvement. Genes Chromosom Cancer 1993; 7(1):54.

86. Rimokh R, Gadoux M, Bertheas M-F, et al: FVT-1, a novel human transcription unit affected by variant translocation t(2;18)(p11;q21) of follicular lymphoma. Blood 1993; 81(1):136.

87. Robledo M, Benitez J, Rivas C, et al: Cytogenetic study of B-cell lymphoma of mucosa-associated lymphoid tissue. Cancer Genet Cytogenet 1992; 62(2):208.

88. Wlodarska I, De Wolf-Peeters C, Dierick H, et al: Detection of amplified sequences at 5q11-q13 in a homogenously staining region found by fluorescent in situ hybridization in a case of B-cell non-Hodgkin's lymphoma. Cytogenet Cell Genet 1994; 65(3):179.

89. Koduru PRK, Filippa DA, Richardson ME, et al: Cytogenetic and histologic correlations in malignant lymphoma. Blood 1987; 69(1):97.

90. Kamada N, Sakurai M, Miyamoto K, et al: Chromosome abnormalities in adult T-cell leukemia/lymphoma: A Karyotype Review Committee report. Cancer Res 1992; 52(6):1481.

91. Lakkala-Paranko T, Franssila K, Lappalainen K, et al: Chromosome abnormalities in peripheral T-cell lymphoma. Br J Haematol 1987; 66(4):451.

92. Cabanillas F, Pathak S, Trujillo J, et al: Frequent nonrandom chromosome abnormalities in 27 patients with untreated large cell lymphoma and immunoblastic lymphoma. Cancer Res 1988; 48(19):5557.

93. Franssila KO, Lindholm C, Teerenhovi L, et al: A method combining morphological, immunocytochemical, and chromosomal examinations of the same cell in the study of lymphoproliferative diseases. Eur J Haematol 1988; 40(4):332.

94. Offit K, Parsa NZ, Filippa D, et al: t(9;14)(p13;q32) denotes a subset of low-grade non-Hodgkin's lymphoma with plasmacytoid differentiation. Blood 1992; 80(10):2594.

95. Ohno H, Furukawa T, Fukuhara S, et al: Molecular analysis of a chromosomal translocation, t(9;14)(p13;q32), in a diffuse large cell lymphoma cell line expressing the Ki-1 antigen. Proc Natl Acad Sci U S A 1990; 87(2):628.

96. Fukuhara S, Rowley JD: Chromosome 14 translocations in non-Burkitt lymphomas. Int J Cancer 1978; 22(1):14.

97. Korsmeyer SJ: Bcl-2 initiates a new category of oncogenes: Regulators of cell death. Blood 1992; 80(4):879.

98. Sanger WG, Armitage JO, Bridge J, et al: Initial and subsequent cytogenetic studies in malignant lymphoma. Cancer 1987; 60(12):3014.

99. Levine EG, Juneja S, Arthur D, et al: Sequential karyotypes in non-Hodgkin lymphoma: Their nature and significance. Genes Chromosom Cancer 1990; 1(4):270.

100. Richardson ME, Chen Q, Filippa DA, et al: Intermediate- to high-grade histology of lymphomas carrying t(14;18) is associated with additional nonrandom chromosome changes. Blood 1987; 70(2):444.

101. Yunis JJ, Frizzera G, Oken MM, et al: Multiple recurrent genomic defects in follicular lymphoma: A possible model for cancer. N Engl J Med 1987; 316(2):79.

102. Armitage JO, Sanger WG, Weisenburger DD, et al: Correlation of secondary cytogenetic abnormalities with histologic appearance in non-Hodgkin's lymphomas bearing t(14;18)(q32;q21). J Natl Cancer Inst 1988; 80(8):576.

103. Fukuhara S, Ohno H, Amakawa R, et al: Significance of extra 18q− chromosome in Japanese t(14;18)-positive lymphoma. Blood 1988; 71(6):1748.

104. Speaks SL, Sanger WG, Masih AS, et al: Recurrent abnormalities of chromosome bands 10q23-25 in non-Hodgkin's lymphoma. Genes Chromosom Cancer 1992; 5(3):239.

105. Goyns MH, Hammond DW, Harrison CJ, et al: Structural abnormalities of the X chromosome in non-Hodgkin's lymphoma. Leukemia 1993; 7(6):848.

106. Maseki N, Kaneko Y, Sakurai M, et al: Chromosome abnormalities in malignant lymphoma in patients from Saitama. Cancer Res 1987; 47(24 Pt1):6767.

107. Ladanyi M, Offit K, Parsa NZ, et al: Follicular lymphoma with t(8;14)(q24;q32): A distinct clinical and molecular subset of t(8;14)-bearing lymphomas. Blood 1992; 79(8):2124.

108. Wlodarska I, Mecucci C, Vandenberghe E, et al: dup(12)(q13→qter) in two t(14;18)-negative follicular B–non-Hodgkin's lymphomas. Genes Chromosom Cancer 1992; 4(4):302.

109. Bajalica S, Sørensen A-G, Tinggaard Pedersen N, et al: Chromosome painting as a supplement to cytogenetic banding analysis in non-Hodgkin's lymphoma. Genes Chromosom Cancer 1993; 7(4):231.

110. Dubé I, Dixon J, Beckett T, et al: Location of breakpoints within the major breakpoint cluster region *(bcr)* in 33 patients with *bcr* rearrangement-positive chronic myeloid leukemia (CML) with complex or absent Philadelphia chromosomes. Genes Chromosom Cancer 1989; 1(1):106.

111. Lee M-S, Blick MB, Pathak S, et al: The gene located at chromosome 18 band q21 is rearranged in uncultured diffuse lymphomas as well as follicular lymphomas. Blood 1987; 70(1):90.

112. Nakamine H, Masih AS, Chan WC, et al: Oncogene rearrangement in non-Hodgkin's lymphoma with a 14q+ chromosome of unknown origin. Leuk Lymphoma 1993; 10(1-2):79.

113. Pezzella F, Ralfkiaer E, Gatter KC, et al: The 14;18 translocation in European cases of follicular lymphoma: Comparison of Southern blotting and the polymerase chain reaction. Br J Haematol 1990; 76(1):58.

114. Fleischman EW, Prigogina EL: Karyotype peculiarities of malignant lymphomas. Hum Genet 1977; 35(3):269.

115. Van Den Berghe H, Parloir C, David G, et al: A new characteristic karyotypic anomaly in lymphoproliferative disorders. Cancer 1979; 44(1):188.

116. Weisenburger DD, Sanger WG, Armitage JO, et al: Intermediate lymphocytic lymphoma: Immunophenotypic and cytogenetic findings. Blood 1987; 69(6):1617.

117. Leroux D, Le Marc'Hadour F, Gressin R, et al: Non-Hodgkin's lymphomas with t(11;14)(q13;q32): A subset of mantle zone/intermediate lymphocytic lymphoma? Br J Haematol 1991; 77(3):346.

118. Vandenberghe E, De Wolf-Peeters C, Van Den Oord J, et al: Translocation (11;14): A cytogenetic anomaly associated with B-cell lymphomas of non-follicle centre cell lineage. J Pathol 1991; 163(1):13.

119. Raffeld M, Jaffe ES: bcl-1, t(11;14), and mantle cell–derived lymphomas. Blood 1991; 78(2):259.

120. Medeiros LJ, Van Krieken JH, Jaffe ES, et al: Association of bcl-1 rearrangements with lymphocytic lymphoma of intermediate differentiation. Blood 1990; 76(10):2086.

121. Rimokh R, Berger F, Cornillet P, et al: Break in the BCL1 locus is closely associated with intermediate lymphocytic lymphoma subtype. Genes Chromosom Cancer 1990; 2(3):223.

122. Wotherspoon AC, Pan L, Diss TC, et al: A genotypic study of low grade B-cell lymphomas, including lymphomas of mucosa-associated lymphoid tissue (MALT). J Pathol 1990; 162(2):135.

123. Athan E, Foitl DR, Knowles DM: BCL-1 rearrangement: Frequency and clinical significance among B-cell chronic lymphocytic leukemias and non-Hodgkin's lymphomas. Am J Pathol 1991; 138(3):591.

124. Williams ME, Swierdlow SH, Rosenberg CL, et al: Characterization of chromosome 11 translocation breakpoints at the bcl-1 and PRAD1 loci in centrocytic lymphoma. Cancer Res 1992; 52(19, Suppl):5541s.

125. Rosenberg CL, Wong E, Petty EM, et al: PRAD1, a candidate BCL1 oncogene: Mapping and expression in centrocytic lymphoma. Proc Natl Acad Sci U S A 1991; 88(21):9638.

126. Seto M, Yamamoto K, Iida S, et al: Gene rearrangement and overexpression of PRAD1 in lymphoid malignancy with t(11;14)(q13;q32) translocation. Oncogene 1992; 7(7):1401.

127. Akiyama N, Tsuruta H, Sasaki H, et al: Messenger RNA levels of five genes located at chromosome 11q13 in B-cell tumors with chromosome translocation t(11;14)(q13;q32). Cancer Res 1994; 54(2):377.

128. Komatsu H, Yoshida K, Seto M, et al: Overexpression of PRAD1 in a mantle zone lymphoma patient with a t(11;22)(q13;q11) translocation. Br J Haematol 1993; 85(2):427.

129. Vandenberghe E, De Wolf-Peeters C, Louwagie A, et al: Chromosome 1p abnormalities in B non-Hodgkin's lymphoma. Leuk Lymphoma 1991; 5(2-3):193.

130. Ye BH, Rao PH, Chaganti RSK, et al: Cloning of *bcl-6*, the locus involved in chromosome translocations affecting band 3q27 in B-cell lymphoma. Cancer Res 1993; 53(12):2732.

131. Baron BW, Nucifora G, McCabe N, et al: Identification of the gene associated with the recurring chromosomal translocations t(3;14)(q27; q32) and t(3;22)(q27;q11) in B-cell lymphomas. Proc Natl Acad Sci U S A 1993; 90(11):5262.

132. Deweindt C, Kerckaert J-P, Tilly H, et al: Cloning of a breakpoint cluster region at band 3q27 involved in human non-Hodgkin's lymphoma. Genes Chromosom Cancer 1993; 8(3):149.

133. Miki T, Kawamata N, Arai A, et al: Molecular cloning of the breakpoint for 3q27 translocation in B-cell lymphomas and leukemias. Blood 1994; 83(1):217.

134. Kaneko Y, Rowley JD, Variakojis D, et al: Prognostic implications of karyotype and morphology in patients with non-Hodgkin's lymphoma. Int J Cancer 1983; 32(6):683.

135. Berger R, Bernheim A, Valensi F, et al: 22q- and 8q- in a non-Burkitt lymphoma. Cancer Genet Cytogenet 1983; 8(1):91.

136. Heim S: Cytogenetics in the investigation of haematological disorders. Bailliere's Clin Haematol 1990; 3(4):921.

137. Offit K, Jhanwar S, Ebrahim SAD, et al: t(3;22)(q27;q11): A novel translocation associated with diffuse non-Hodgkin's lymphoma. Blood 1989; 74(6):1876.

138. Leroux D, Stul M, Sotto JJ, et al: Translocation t(3;22)(q28;q11) in three patients with diffuse large B cell lymphoma. Leukemia 1990; 4(5):373.

139. Otsuki T, Yano T, Clark H, et al: Rearrangement of the LAZ3 gene locus in human B-cell lymphomas [abstract]. Proc Am Assoc Cancer Res 1994; 35:238.

140. Lo Coco F, Ye BH, Lista F, et al: Rearrangements of the BCL6 gene in diffuse large cell non-Hodgkin's lymphoma. Blood 1994; 83(7): 1757.

141. Weiss LM, Warnke RA, Sklar J, et al: Molecular analysis of the t(14;18) chromosomal translocation in malignant lymphomas. N Engl J Med 1987; 317(19):1185.

142. Offit K, Parsa NZ, Jhanwar SC, et al: Clusters of chromosome 9 aberrations are associated with clinico-pathologic subsets of non-Hodgkin's lymphoma. Genes Chromosom Cancer 1993; 7(1):1.

143. Mark J, Dahlenfors R, Ekedahl C: Recurrent chromosomal aberrations in non-Hodgkin and non-Burkitt lymphomas. Cancer Genet Cytogenet 1979; 1(1):39.

144. Chenevix-Trench G, Brown JA, Tyler GB, et al: Chromosome analysis of 30 cases of non-Hodgkin's lymphoma. Med Oncol Tumor Pharmacother 1988; 5(1):17.

145. Kaneko Y, Maseki N, Sakurai M, et al: Characteristic karyotypic pattern in T-cell lymphoproliferative disorders with reactive "angio-immunoblastic lymphadenopathy with dysproteinemia-type" features. Blood 1988; 72(2):413.

146. Schlegelberger B, Himmler A, Gödde E, et al: Cytogenetic findings in peripheral T-cell lymphomas as a basis for distinguishing low-grade and high-grade lymphomas. Blood 1994; 83(2):505.

147. Levine EG, Arthur DC, Gajl-Peczalska KJ, et al: Correlations between immunological phenotype and karyotype in malignant lymphoma. Cancer Res 1986; 46(12 Pt1):6481.

148. Berger R, Baranger L, Bernheim A, et al: Cytogenetics of T-cell malignant lymphoma: Report of 17 cases and review of the chromosomal breakpoints. Cancer Genet Cytogenet 1988; 36(1):123.

149. Greer JP, Kinney MC, Collins RD, et al: Clinical features of 31 patients with Ki-1 anaplastic large-cell lymphoma. J Clin Oncol 1991; 9(4):539.

150. Offit K, Ladanyi M, Gangi MD, et al: Ki-1 antigen expression defines a favorable clinical subset of non-B cell non-Hodgkin's lymphoma. Leukemia 1990; 4(9):625.

151. Kristoffersson U, Heim S, Heldrup J, et al: Cytogenetic studies of childhood non-Hodgkin lymphomas. Hereditas 1985; 103(1):77.

152. Morgan R, Hecht BK, Sandberg AA, et al: Chromosome 5q35 breakpoint in malignant histiocytosis. N Engl J Med 1986; 314(20): 1322.

153. Soulie J, Rousseau-Merck M-F, Mouly H, et al: Cytogenetic study of malignant histiocytosis transplanted into nude mice: Presence of translocation between chromosomes 5 and 6 and a unique marker (13q+). Virchows Arch B Cell Pathol 1986; 50(4):339.

154. Vannier JP, Bastard C, Rossi A, et al: Chromosomal t(2;5) and hematologic malignancies. Pediatr Hematol Oncol 1987; 4(2):177.

155. Bloomfield CD, Levine EG, Machnicki J, et al: Recurring chromosome translocations in B-cell malignant lymphoma [Abstract]. Cytogenet Cell Genet 1987; 46(1-4):583.

156. Benz-Lemoine E, Brizard A, Huret J-L, et al: Malignant histiocytosis: A specific t(2;5)(p23;q35) translocation? Review of the literature. Blood 1988; 72(3):1045.

157. Fisher P, Nacheva E, Mason DY, et al: A Ki-1 (CD30)-positive human cell line (Karpas 299) established from a high-grade non-Hodgkin's lymphoma, showing a 2;5 translocation and rearrangement of the T-cell receptor β-chain gene. Blood 1988; 72(1):234.

158. Kaneko Y, Frizzera G, Edamura S, et al: A novel translocation, t(2;5)(p23;q35), in childhood phagocytic large T-cell lymphoma mimicking malignant histiocytosis. Blood 1989; 73(3):806.

159. Rimokh R, Magaud J-P, Berger F, et al: A translocation involving a specific breakpoint (q35) on chromosome 5 is characteristic of anaplastic large cell lymphoma ("Ki-1 lymphoma"). Br J Haematol 1989; 71(1):31.

160. Le Beau MM, Bitter MA, Larson RA, et al: The t(2;5)(p23;q35): A recurring chromosomal abnormality in Ki-1–positive anaplastic large cell lymphoma. Leukemia 1989; 3(12):866.

161. Mason DY, Bastard C, Rimokh R, et al: CD30-positive large cell lymphomas ("Ki-1 lymphoma") are associated with a chromosomal translocation involving 5q35. Br J Haematol 1990; 74(2):161.

162. Sreekantaiah C, Karakousis CP, Leong SPL, et al: Cytogenetic findings in liposarcoma correlate with histopathologic subtypes. Cancer 1992; 69(10):2484.

163. Limon J, Mrózek K, Mandahl N, et al: Cytogenetics of synovial sarcoma: Presentation of ten new cases and review of the literature. Genes Chromosom Cancer 1991; 3(5):338.

164. Kinney MC, Collins RD, Greer JP, et al: A small-cell–predominant variant of primary Ki-1 (CD30) + T-cell lymphoma. Am J Surg Pathol 1993; 17(9):859.

165. Bitter MA, Franklin WA, Larson RA, et al: Morphology in Ki-1 (CD30)-positive non-Hodgkin's lymphoma is correlated with clinical features and the presence of a unique chromosomal abnormality, t(2;5)(p23;q35). Am J Surg Pathol 1990; 14(4):305.

166. Kaneko Y, Frizzera G, Shikano T, et al: Chromosomal and immunophenotypic patterns in T-cell acute lymphoblastic leukemia (T-ALL) and lymphoblastic lymphoma (LBL). Leukemia 1989; 3(12):886.

167. Raimondi SC: Current status of cytogenetic research in childhood acute lymphoblastic leukemia. Blood 1993; 81(9):2237.

168. Dubé ID, Raimondi SC, Pi D, et al: A new translocation, t(10;14)(q24;q11), in T-cell neoplasia. Blood 1986; 67(4):1181.

169. Kagan J, Finger LR, Letofsky J, et al: Clustering of breakpoints on chromosome 10 in acute T-cell leukemias with the t(10;14) chromosome translocation. Proc Natl Acad Sci U S A 1989; 86(11):4161.

170. Pollak C, Hagemeijer A: Abnormalities of the short arm of chromosome 9 with partial loss of material in hematological disorders. Leukemia 1987; 1(7):541.

171. Shikano T, Ishikawa Y, Naito H, et al: Cytogenetic characteristics of childhood non-Hodgkin lymphoma. Cancer 1992; 70(3):714.

172. Magrath I: Molecular basis of lymphomagenesis. Cancer Res 1992; 52(19, Suppl):5529s.

173. Zech L, Haglund U, Nilsson K, et al: Characteristic chromosomal abnormalities in biopsies and lymphoid-cell lines from patients with Burkitt and non-Burkitt lymphomas. Int J Cancer 1976; 17(1):47.

174. Berger R, Bernheim A, Weh H-J, et al: A new translocation in Burkitt's tumor cells. Hum Genet 1979; 53(1):111.

175. Van Den Berghe H, Parloir C, Gosseye S, et al: Variant translocation in Burkitt lymphoma. Cancer Genet Cytogenet 1979; 1(1):9.

176. Miyoshi I, Hiraki S, Kimura I, et al: 2/8 translocation in a Japanese Burkitt's lymphoma. Experientia 1979; 35(6):742.

177. Douglass EC, Magrath IT, Lee EC, et al: Cytogenetic studies in non-African Burkitt lymphoma. Blood 1980; 55(1):148.

178. Knuutila S, Elonen E, Heinonen K, et al: Chromosome abnormalities in 16 Finnish patients with Burkitt's lymphoma or L3 acute lymphocytic leukemia. Cancer Genet Cytogenet 1984; 13(2):139.

179. Kornblau SM, Goodacre A, Cabanillas F: Chromosomal abnormalities in adult non-endemic Burkitt's lymphoma and leukemia: 22 new reports and a review of 148 cases from the literature. Hematol Oncol 1991; 9(2):63.

180. Yano T, van Krieken JHJM, Magrath IT, et al: Histogenetic correlations between subcategories of small noncleaved cell lymphomas. Blood 1992; 79(5):1282.

181. Nowell PC: Cytogenetics of tumor progression. Cancer 1990; 65(10):2172.

182. Heim S: Tumor progression: Karyotypic keys to multistage pathogenesis. *In* Iversen OH (ed): Cancer Causation: Exploring New Frontiers. Washington, Hemisphere Scientific Productions, 1993, p 247.

183. Horning SJ: Natural history of and therapy for the indolent non-Hodgkin's lymphomas. Semin Oncol 1993; 20(5, Suppl 5):75.

184. De Jong D, Voetdijk BMH, Beverstock GC, et al: Activation of the c-*myc* oncogene in a precursor-B-cell blast crisis of follicular lymphoma, presenting as composite lymphoma. N Engl J Med 1988; 318(21):1373.

185. Gauwerky CE, Hoxie J, Nowell PC, et al: Pre–B-cell leukemia with a t(8;14) and a t(14;18) translocation is preceded by follicular lymphoma. Oncogene 1988; 2(5):431.

186. Lee JT, Innes DJ Jr, Williams ME: Sequential *bcl*-2 and c-*myc* oncogene rearrangements associated with the clinical transformation of non-Hodgkin's lymphoma. J Clin Invest 1989; 84(5):1454.

187. Yano T, Jaffe ES, Longo DL, et al: *MYC* rearrangements in histologically progressed follicular lymphomas. Blood 1992; 80(3):758.

188. Rodriguez MA, Ford RJ, Goodacre A, et al: Chromosome 17p and p53 changes in lymphoma. Br J Haematol 1991; 79(4):575.

189. Hartwell L: Defects in a cell cycle checkpoint may be responsible for the genomic instability of cancer cells. Cell 1992; 71(4):543.

190. Arthur DC, Berger R, Golomb HM, et al: The clinical significance of karyotype in acute myelogenous leukemia. Cancer Genet Cytogenet 1989; 40(2):203.

191. Bloomfield CD, Secker-Walker LM, Goldman AI, et al: Six-year follow-up of the clinical significance of karyotype in acute lymphoblastic leukemia. Cancer Genet Cytogenet 1989; 40(2):171.

192. Pierre RV, Catovsky D, Mufti GJ, et al: Clinical-cytogenetic correlations in myelodysplasia (preleukemia). Cancer Genet Cytogenet 1989; 40(2):149.

193. Levine EG, Arthur DC, Frizzera G, et al: Cytogenetic abnormalities predict clinical outcome in non-Hodgkin lymphoma. Ann Intern Med 1988; 108(1):14.

194. Offit K, Wong G, Filippa DA, et al: Cytogenetic analysis of 434 consecutively ascertained specimens of non-Hodgkin's lymphoma: Clinical correlations. Blood 1991; 77(7):1508.

195. Kristoffersson U, Heim S, Mandahl N, et al: Prognostic implication of cytogenetic findings in 106 patients with non-Hodgkin lymphoma. Cancer Genet Cytogenet 1987; 25(1):55.

196. Haus O, Kozlowska J, Zubkiewicz L, et al: Cytogenetic studies in patients with non-Hodgkin's lymphoma (NHL) [in Polish]. Pol Arch Med Wewn 1991; 86(3):132.

197. Cowan RA, Harris M, Jones M, et al: DNA content in high and intermediate grade non-Hodgkin's lymphoma: Prognostic significance and clinicopathological correlations. Br J Cancer 1989; 60(6):904.

198. Yunis JJ, Mayer MG, Arnesen MA, et al: *bcl*-2 and other genomic alterations in the prognosis of large-cell lymphoma. N Engl J Med 1989; 320(16):1047.

199. Pezzella F, Jones M, Ralfkiaer E, et al: Evaluation of bcl-2 protein expression and 14;18 translocation as prognostic markers in follicular lymphoma. Br J Cancer 1992; 65(1):87.

200. Romaguera JE, Pugh W, Luthra R, et al: The clinical relevance of t(14;18)/BCL-2 rearrangement and DEL 6q in diffuse large cell lymphoma and immunoblastic lymphoma. Ann Oncol 1993; 4(1):51.

201. Jacobson JO, Wilkes BM, Kwiatkowski DJ, et al: *bcl*-2 rearrangements in de novo diffuse large cell lymphoma: Association with distinctive clinical features. Cancer 1993; 72(1):231.

202. Tang SC, Visser L, Hepperle B, et al: Clinical significance of *bcl*-2-MBR gene rearrangement and protein expression in diffuse large-cell non-Hodgkin's lymphoma: An analysis of 83 cases. J Clin Oncol 1994; 12(1):149.

203. Piris MA, Pezzella F, Martinez-Montero JC, et al: p53 and *bcl*-2 expression in high-grade B-cell lymphomas: Correlation with survival time. Br J Cancer 1994; 69(2):337.

204. Offit K, Koduru PRK, Hollis R, et al: 18q21 rearrangement in diffuse large cell lymphoma: Incidence and clinical significance. Br J Haematol 1989; 72(2):178.

205. Cabanillas F, Pathak S, Grant G, et al: Refractoriness to chemotherapy and poor survival related to abnormalities of chromosomes 17 and 7 in lymphoma. Am J Med 1989; 87(2):167.

206. Offit K, Richardson ME, Chen Q, et al: Nonrandom chromosomal aberrations are associated with sites of tissue involvement in non-Hodgkin's lymphoma. Cancer Genet Cytogenet 1989; 37(1):85.

207. Younes A, Pugh W, Goodacre A, et al: Polysomy of chromosome 12 in 60 patients with non-Hodgkin's lymphoma assessed by fluorescence in situ hybridization: Differences between follicular and diffuse large cell lymphoma. Genes Chromosom Cancer 1994; 9(3):161.

208. Schofield DE, Fletcher JA: Trisomy 12 in pediatric granulosa-stromal cell tumors. Am J Pathol 1992; 141(6):1265.

209. Mitelman F, Kaneko Y, Trent JM: Report of the Committee on Chromosome Changes in Neoplasia. Human Gene Mapping 10.5 (1990): Update to the 10th International Workshop on Human Gene Mapping. Cytogenet Cell Genet 1990; 55(1-4):358.

210. Hebert J, Romana SP, Hillion J, et al: Translocation t(3;22)(q27;q11) in non-Hodgkin's malignant lymphoma: Chromosome painting and molecular studies. Leukemia 1993; 7(12):1971.

211. Yoshizawa K, Kiyosawa K, Yamada S, et al: Establishment of Epstein-Barr virus–associated lymphoma cell line SUBL with t(2;3)(p11;q27) from a liver transplant patient. Cancer Genet Cytogenet 1993; 71(2):155.

212. Ohno H, Akasaka T, Ohmura K, et al: Non-Hodgkin's lymphomas with chromosomal translocations involving 3q27 band and immunoglobulin gene loci: Report of two cases. Cancer Genet Cytogenet 1994; 72(1):33.

Chapter Seven

Molecular Diagnosis of Lymphoma and Related Disorders

Jeffrey L. Sklar

Among all forms of cancer, lymphomas stand out for the special problems and opportunities they present with regard to diagnosis and detection. Much of the difficulty stems from the fact that cytologically malignant lymphocytes may resemble normal lymphocytes at various stages of differentiation and activation. Furthermore, the histologic features that distinguish the many different subtypes of lymphomas can be subtle and rather subjective, even to the experienced pathologist. Over the past 25 years, these difficulties have motivated intensive efforts to develop and refine additional diagnostic modalities that might assist the morphologic evaluation of lymphoid tissue specimens for the presence and classification of lymphoma. Immunohistochemistry was the first of these ancillary modalities applied to the diagnosis of lymphoma, and over the years it has gained an important role in the diagnostic evaluation of lymphoid biopsy specimens. Classic cytogenetics has also sometimes provided valuable diagnostic information about lymphoma, although its application has been relatively limited in most centers. More recently, molecular genetic methods of diagnosis have begun to contribute significantly to improved accuracy in the diagnostic evaluation of lymphoid tissue specimens. This chapter reviews the principles, techniques, and major findings of molecular genetic diagnosis applied to lymphomas and related disorders. (For background in general molecular genetics and the essentials of molecular genetic techniques, see Chapter 1, "Introduction to Molecular Biology.")

The application of molecular genetics to the diagnosis of lymphoma and other cancers has often been referred to as "molecular diagnosis," a term that has had varying meanings in different contexts. For the purposes of the present discussion, molecular diagnosis is defined as diagnostic testing directed at markers consisting of nucleotide sequences within DNA and RNA. Such tests have been applied in lymphoma for the full range of diagnostic purposes for which other forms of tests have been employed, including the primary distinction of malignant from benign processes, the staging of tumors, the determination of prognosis, and the monitoring of residual disease following therapy. Additionally, subtyping of lymphoma into the various classifications of lymphoma, an activity closely related to the determination of prognosis, has been an important objective of molecular diagnosis.

In addition to offering another diagnostic dimension to be added to that of histology and immunohistochemistry, molecular diagnosis has at least three general advantages that account at least in part for the growing interest in and use of this approach to diagnosis.[1] First, the results of molecular tests tend to be more objective than histology or even immunohistochemistry. Second, molecular tests have the potential of being considerably more sensitive than histology or immunohistochemistry to detect small numbers of malignant cells. A third, but less consistent, advantage with molecular diagnosis is that the DNA (much more so than RNA) is relatively stable in devitalized tissues, and often interpretable results can be obtained when inadequate or suboptimal handling of specimens has compromised histologic or immunohistochemical evaluation. On the other hand, like all forms of diagnostic testing, molecular diagnosis has its own disadvantages and is subject to certain artifacts, as is pointed out later.

The remainder of this chapter reviews molecular diagnosis of lymphoma from the perspective of the markers analyzed. These fall into three groups: antigen receptor gene rearrangements, chromosome translocations, and viral genomes. As is evident in the following discussion, these markers pertain almost exclusively to non-Hodgkin's lymphomas and related lymphocytic cancers. No reliable nucleic acid marker of molecular method for Hodgkin's disease has been yet demonstrated for the diagnosis of Hodgkin's disease.

ANTIGEN RECEPTOR GENE REARRANGEMENTS

Rearrangements of antigen receptor genes comprise the most general molecular diagnostic marker in lymphoma, being relevant to all lymphocytic cancers (including lymphocytic leukemias).[2, 3] Antigen receptor genes encode the amino acid sequences of the polypeptide subunits that make up immunoglobulins and T-cell receptors (Fig. 7–1).[4] These are the structurally and functionally homologous glycopro-

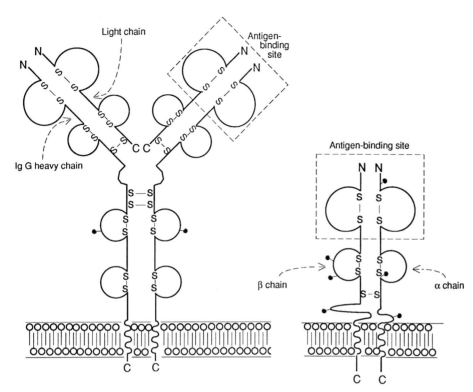

Figure 7–1. Structure of the immunoglobulin (Ig) and T-cell receptor (TCR) proteins. On the left is shown a prototypic membrane-bound IgG molecule; on the right a TCR molecule. The plasma membrane is illustrated near the bottom of the figure. The area above the membrane represents extracellular space, and the area below represents the cytoplasm. The variable regions of the polypeptide subunits are contained within the portions of the molecules making up the antigen binding sites. N and C indicate the amino and carboxy ends of the subunits. S-S indicates a disulfide bond. The lollipop-like structures indicate carbohydrate groups.

teins that mediate the recognition of antigens and account for the specificity of the normal immune responses.[5, 6] Immunoglobulins, the products of B-lineage lymphocytes, consist of a core tetramer containing two identical heavy-chain subunits, each about 440 amino acids long, linked by disulfide bonds and noncovalent forces to two identical light chains of about 215 amino acids. The light chains occur as two isotypes, κ and λ, with about two thirds of immunoglobulins containing κ light chains and the rest λ. Immunoglobulins may be expressed by B lymphocytes as cell surface proteins anchored in the plasma membrane by a short hydrophobic transmembrane domain located near the carboxy terminus of the two heavy chains. Changes in the alternative splicing of the heavy-chain mRNA as B lymphocytes differentiate into plasma cells shift expression exclusively to a secreted form lacking the transmembrane domain.[7, 8] Other changes in the carboxy terminal portion of the heavy chains that distinguish five separate classes of immunoglobulin—α, γ, δ, ε, and μ—together with two subclasses of α and four of γ, occur during differentiation of B lymphocytes over time and at certain anatomic sites or in response to various kinds of antigens.[9] However, the antigenic specificity of the immunoglobulin produced by a B lymphocyte and its clonal descendants remains the same as long as that line of cells persists.

T-cell receptors, on the other hand, are expressed by T lymphocytes only as membrane-bound heterodimers consisting of one α and one β chain, or on a small percentage of T lymphocytes, dimers of a γ and δ chain.[10] Each of these chains is about 300 amino acids long. Like immunoglobulins, the antigenic specificities of the T-cell receptors produced by a T lymphocyte are fixed throughout the life of that cell and any clonal descendants it may generate.

A portion of each antigen receptor subunit chains, termed the "variable region," differs widely among antigen receptors produced by different lymphocytes. This region extends about one fifth of the distance along the chain from the amino terminus of the immunoglobulin heavy chain and for slightly less than one half of the length of the other chains. In all antigen receptor proteins, the variable regions of two chains collaborate to form the antigen binding site (hence, a typical immunoglobulin molecule contains two identical antigen binding sites, and a T-cell receptor contains one). The portions of the antigen receptor subunits that do not show the high degree of variability found in the variable region are termed "constant regions."

The seven different subunits that make antigen receptors are encoded in separate genes scattered throughout the genome but having the same overall structure (Fig. 7–2).[4] In the germline and all nonhematopoietic cells, coding sequences for the genes are divided among at least three sets of nonidentical but related segments termed "V" (for variable), "J" (for joining), and "C" (for constant). The immunoglobulin heavy-chain gene and β and δ T-cell receptor genes also include a fourth set of segments termed "D" (for diversity). Collectively, V, D, and J segments contain the repertoire of sequence information for the synthesis of all possible variable regions within expressed antigen receptor subunits. The number and distribution of segments within each set of segments differ among the genes, but generally there are numerous V segments and a smaller number of J segments clustered near one or several C segments. Several families of V segments sharing more closely related sequences can be discerned among some genes, especially that of the immunoglobulin heavy-chain locus. If D segments are present, their number is usually intermediate between that of V and J segments, and they lie within the DNA between these two groups of segments. V segments contain about 300 to 400 base pairs (as do C segments, except for those in immunoglobulin heavy-chain genes, which are roughly three times as long), and both D and J segments contain about 10 to 50 base pairs. With the rare exception of a few individual V segments, all segments within a gene are oriented in the same 5'-to-3' direction.

Early in lymphocyte development, segments of antigen receptor genes are joined together by DNA recombination in attempts to assemble intact functional coding sequences for these genes (Fig. 7–3).[11–18] In B-lineage cells, rearrangements of the immunoglobulin genes take place within prelymphocytes of the bone marrow. In T-lineage cells, rearrangement of T-cell receptor genes is delayed until prelymphocytes of this lineage migrate from the bone marrow to the cortex of the thymus. Either in the bone marrow or in the thymus, the result of

rearrangement is that a particular V segment becomes joined to one J segment, or if D segments are included in the gene, a D segment becomes joined to a J segment, followed by joining of a V segment to the DJ sequences. DNA originally lying between the rearranged segments is excised and eventually lost from the cell.[19, 20] Concurrently with the rearrangement of the V segment, a promoter upstream of this segment is significantly up-regulated, leading to transcription of the continuous V(D)J sequences, together with a downstream C segment, into a single transcript. DNA sequences transcribed between the end of the rearranged J segment and the beginning of the C segment are spliced out of the initial transcription product to yield a mature V(D)JC mRNA, which can then be transported to the cytoplasm of the cell for translation into protein.

Immunoglobulin heavy chain gene (chromosome 14q32)

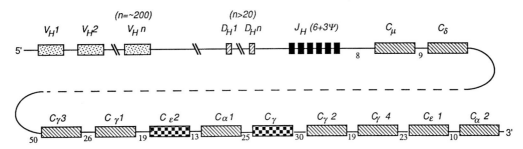

Immunoglobulin kappa light chain gene (chromosome 2p12)

Immunoglobulin lambda light chain gene (chromosome 22q11)

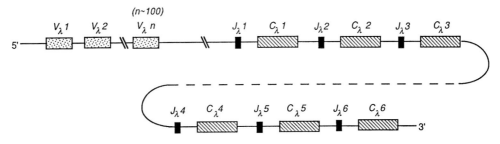

Figure 7–2. Schematic representation of the seven germline antigen receptor genes. The chromosome sites of these genes are indicated. ψ stands for pseudogene segments; illustrated pseudogene segments are checkered. The distances between the constant region gene segments in the immunoglobulin heavy-chain gene are shown in kilobases. Introns within constant region segments have been omitted. The δ T-cell-receptor gene is embedded within the α gene and contains one inverted V segment (V$_δ$4).

Illustration continued on following page

Beta T cell receptor gene (chromosome 7q34)

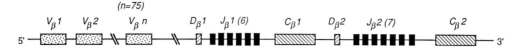

Alpha T cell receptor gene (chromosome 14q11)

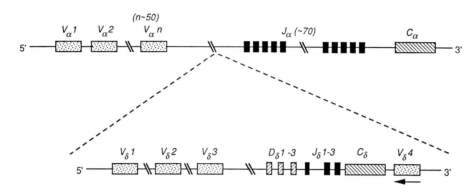

Delta T cell receptor gene (chromosome 14q11)

Gamma T cell receptor gene (chromosome 7p15)

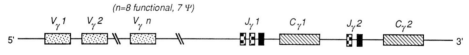

Figure 7–2 *Continued*

The almost random inclusion of different V, D, and J segments in rearrangements of antigen receptor genes accounts for much of the variability among immunoglobulins and T-cell receptors for the binding of antigens. This combinatorial diversity is augmented by a high degree of sequence heterogeneity at the junctions of rearranged segments caused by frequent deletion of short stretches of base pairs from the ends of the segments and the addition of up to about 30 base pairs (so-called N region nucleotides) of largely arbitrary sequence (with a bias toward G and C) between the segments prior to joining.[21, 22] Not infrequently, major errors occur in the rearrangement process, and more often, sequences of DNA created at the junction of rearranged segments put the coding sequence downstream of the rearranged V segment out of frame, so that a full-length antigen receptor polypeptide cannot be synthesized. If a defective rearrangement occurs in one allele, the second allele undergoes rearrangement; however, only one allele for an antigen receptor gene is rearranged when that rearrangement produces a functional gene. Among immunoglobulin genes, there is a hierarchy of rearrangement such that a functional heavy-chain gene rearrangement seems to be necessary in most instances before κ light-chain alleles rearrange, and λ light-chain alleles rearrange only if both κ alleles fail to assemble a functional product (thus explaining expression of either κ or λ light chains by the cell).[23–27] Whether there is a similar order to rearrangement among T-cell receptor genes (or whether normal α-β T cells have γ or δ rearrangements) is less clear, although lymphocytes containing γ and δ gene rearrangements appear earlier during thymic development than do lymphocytes with rearranged α and β genes.[25–34]

After rearrangement is completed, a final process of diversification, termed "affinity maturation," fine-tunes the sequences of the variable regions within the subunits of expressed immunoglobulins to maximize the strength of antigen binding (this process is restricted to immunoglobulins and does appear to take place among T-cell-receptor genes). As B lymphocytes encounter antigen within the germinal centers of activated lymph nodes, the nucleotide sequences in and around the rearranged V segment are subjected to intensive mutation owing to base substitutions.[35, 36] The mutated immunoglobulins are displayed on the surface of the cells, such that lymphocytes bearing immunoglobulin with the increased affinity for antigen undergo more efficient mitogenic stimulation by antigen and preferential expansion. As expected from this mechanism of selective proliferation, most mutations found in the immunoglobulins of postgerminal center B lymphocytes accumulate predominantly in three complement-determining regions (CDRs) of the V segment, which correspond to those regions of the immunoglobulin proteins that contact the antigen within the binding site.

The primary step in affinity maturation, usually referred to as "somatic hypermutation," probably produces changes that reduce affinity as often as changes that improve it. Other mutations may disrupt essential features of immunoglobulin structure or even produce nonsense codons. Recently, evidence has been reported to suggest a way that B lymphocytes may rescue genes having deleterious mutations and possibly certain faulty rearrangements as well. It was found that the two principal enzymes RAG1 and RAG2 that mediate breakage of the DNA at sites of gene rearrangement are reexpressed within the germinal center of lymph nodes and spleen.[37–40] On the basis of this finding, it is suggested

that B lymphocytes with bad rearrangements of κ genes can rearrange λ genes within the lymph nodes. Furthermore, some disadvantageous V segments may be replaced by recombination of an unrearranged, upstream V segment into the VDJ sequence. Such replacement rearrangements would be dependent on the presence of the characteristic nonamer sequence of base pairs recognized by RAG1 and RAG2 at the sites of cleavage in all antigen receptor gene rearrangements.[16, 18, 40, 41] In fact, certain V segments have such nonamer sequences near their 3' ends, and replacement rearrangements of these V segments have been observed in cultured cell lines over time.[42, 43]

From the standpoint of diagnosis, the most important feature of antigen receptor gene rearrangement is that, with some qualifications to be discussed later, the sequences of DNA in a rearranged gene marks the lymphocyte in which that rearrangement occurs and any clonal progeny of that cell. Consequently, since all neoplasms are clonal, lymphocytes making up a neoplasm generally carry uniform rearrangements. In contrast, most lymphocytes in benign, reactive processes are not clonal and carry diverse rearrange-

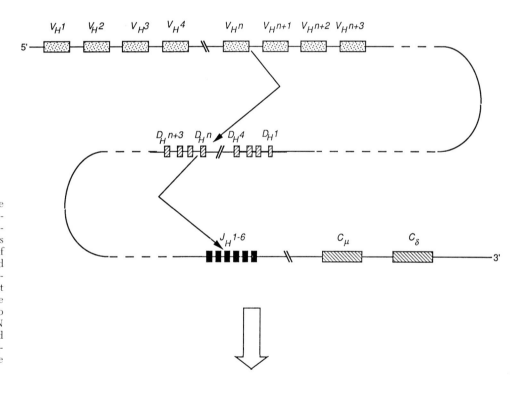

Figure 7–3. Antigen receptor gene rearrangement. A schematic representation of VDJ joining in the immunoglobulin heavy-chain gene is shown. The germline configuration of the gene is illustrated at the top and the resulting rearranged configuration below it. At the bottom, the part of the rearranged gene containing the VDJ junction has been expanded to illustrate the position of the two N regions usually found in expressed copies of this gene. The gene segments shown to undergo joining are arbitrary.

ments. Given the fact that the distinction of neoplastic from reactive processes within biopsy tissues is a primary goal of diagnosis, detection of uniform rearrangements in a significant fraction of cells in a tissue specimen provides a useful indication of malignancy.

ANALYSIS OF ANTIGEN RECEPTOR GENE REARRANGEMENTS BY SOUTHERN BLOT HYBRIDIZATION

The uniformity of rearrangements in antigen receptor genes can be analyzed in several ways. The original method used for this purpose, and still the most reliable, is Southern blot hybridization.[3, 44–52] The precise marker in this test is the configuration of rearranged V and J segments; that is, which V and J segments were brought together during rearrangement of the gene under analysis (for Southern blot analysis, the rearrangement of a D segment is irrelevant unless VD joining has not taken place, as may occur in some nonproductive alleles or in lymphoblastic neoplasms derived from immature lymphocytic precursors). In Southern blot procedure, total cellular DNA extracted from a biopsy specimen is digested with one or two bacterial restriction enzymes that produce fragments spanning the J segments, and the membrane is hybridized with a probe containing sequences complementary to DNA lying between the 3' of the last J segment and the restriction site flanking that side of the J segments (Fig. 7–4). The autoradiogram generated after hybridization shows one or two rearranged, nongermline bands, depending on whether one or both alleles for that gene have rearranged, but only if more than about 1% to 5% of the cells in the biopsy specimen represent clonal lymphocytes that happen to have rearrangements of that gene. Additionally, bands corresponding to unrearranged, germline genes almost always are found at characteristic and predictable positions within the autoradiogram because one of the alleles in the lymphocytes of the tissues may be unrearranged and/or the specimen contains nonlymphocytic cells, such as stromal cells, macrophages, and granulocytes, which lack the capacity for rearrangement of antigen receptor genes. Most important, although polyclonal lymphocytes in a biopsy possess many different rearrangements of antigen receptor DNA, these cells do not contribute a visible band to the autoradiogram because non-neoplastic clones rarely constitute more than a small percentage of the total cells in the tissue sample.

A single Southern blot analysis with one enzyme-probe combination requires about 5 million cells or 0.5 mm^3 of wet tissue (the equivalent of 5 μg of total cellular DNA). Disaggregated cells, such as those obtained from aspiration of solid tissues or in body fluids, also produce good results as long as enough can be collected. DNA used in the analysis must be fairly intact to yield the 5- to 25-kilobase (kb) fragments usually detected in the procedure, but DNA in most tissues and cells is sufficiently stable to produce satisfactory results even when specimens are left at room temperature for several hours after removal from the body. Specimens can routinely be stored indefinitely prior to extraction in freezers at −20°C without using any sort of storage medium. Alternatively, high-quality DNA has been extracted from tissue that has been fixed in ethanol and retained for long periods at room temperature. On the other hand, formalin fixation crosslinks protein to DNA and

prevents extraction of large enough pieces of DNA free of protein to give reliable results.[53, 54]

Although, theoretically, all antigen receptor genes are potential markers for analysis by Southern blot hybridization, only the three immunoglobulin genes and the β gene are generally tested. The α T-cell receptor gene contains too many widely distributed J segments (about 70) to be analyzed feasibly with a reasonable number of probes. The γ and δ genes are rearranged in a few lymphomas, and because they have a small number of V segments, frequent rearrangement of the same segments within reactive tissues can produce nongermline bands. Nevertheless, when the lymphocytes in a specimen are rather homogeneously clonal, detection of a predominant rearrangement can be helpful.

Even among the immunoglobulin genes, it is common to test only the heavy-chain gene and the κ gene, since the λ gene rearranges only after κ. (Rearrangement of λ genes is often accompanied by deletion of the C κ segment by recombination between a specific site between the J segment and another site far downstream of C^{55}; however, this deletion leaves intact the VJ join, and detection of abortive κ rearrangements can still be detected with probes complementary to sequence just 3' of J.) In most instances, when adequate amounts of DNA are available, each gene is independently analyzed with different enzymes, since not infrequently rearrangements are detected with one enzyme and not with another (probably owing to superimposition of rearranged and germline bands or to fragments too small or too large to be analyzed by Southern blot hybridization). Similarly, rearrangement in one gene may not be detected in a second gene. Therefore, when little DNA is obtained from a sample and a single enzyme can be used for two genes, a Southern blot may be stripped of probe by boiling and rehybridized with a probe for the second gene.

Using the principles discussed earlier, Southern blot hybridization analysis of antigen receptor genes is now regularly applied for the detection of clonality among lymphocytes in specimens that are equivocal by histologic and immunohistochemical criteria. Additionally, this test has been historically useful in establishing the neoplastic nature of certain types of lesions that were formally regarded as reactive. Examples of such lesions include angioimmunoblastic lymphadenopathy and lethal midline granuloma, both now considered most often to be T-cell lymphomas[56]; pseudolymphomas of lung and gut, now considered to be low-grade B-cell lymphomas[57–59]; and non-Hodgkin's lymphomas arising in immunosuppressed patients, once believed to be reactive, virally induced hyperplasias but now understood to autonomous B-cell neoplasms, at least late in the course of the disease.[60]

Besides detecting clonality of lymphocytes for the purpose of distinguishing neoplastic from reactive processes, another, less frequent application of Southern blot analysis of antigen receptor gene rearrangements is the determination of cell lineage when the basic neoplastic nature of the lesion is not in question (e.g., B versus T differentiation based on rearrangement of immunoglobulin or T-cell receptor genes, or in certain situations, lymphocytic derivation as opposed to origin from nonlymphocytic cells). Disorders for which lineage has been redefined in large part as a result of Southern blot analysis of antigen receptor gene rearrangements include hairy cell leukemia (reclassified as a B-cell neoplasm)

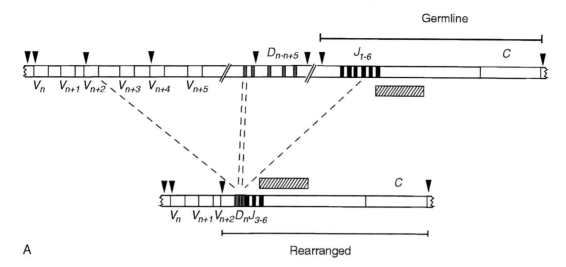

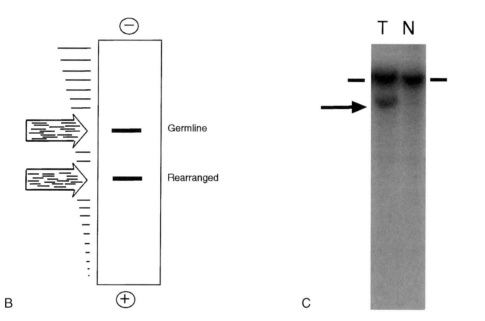

Figure 7–4. Southern blot hybridization analysis of antigen receptor gene rearrangement. *A,* Schematic representation of a possible rearrangement in the immunoglobulin heavy-chain gene. The germline positions of the V, D, J, and C gene segments are shown on the top line of the figure; the configuration of segments after rearrangement is shown below. *Downward arrowheads* indicate the positions within the DNA of potential sites of cleavage by a particular restriction enzyme. The bracketed lines above and below the DNA indicate the size of the germline and rearranged fragments that span the J-segment region (or what remains of it) and are released as a consequence of cleavage by the restriction enzyme. A probe represented by a cross-hatched rectangle has been placed adjacent to complementary sequence within the DNA of the heavy-chain gene. *B,* Schematic representation of an autoradiogram produced by analysis of a biopsy specimen in which at least 5000 lymphocytes contain the rearrangement illustrated in *A.* The distribution of polyclonal rearranged fragments, clonal rearranged fragments (contained within the *lower arrow*), and germline fragments (within the *upper arrow*) are shown to the left of the autoradiogram. After hybridization with the probe, only the germline and clonal rearranged fragments are sufficiently abundant to be detected as discrete bands in the autoradiogram. *C,* Autoradiogram resulting from analysis of the immunoglobulin heavy-chain gene in a B-cell non-Hodgkin's lymphoma. T indicates the lane containing tumor DNA; N is the lane containing normal lymph node DNA. Dashes have been placed beside the germline band; an *arrow* has been placed beside the clonal rearranged band.

and many so-called true histiocytic lymphomas (most of which are now recognized to be T-cell lymphomas).[61, 62]

Although Southern blot hybridization analysis of antigen receptor gene rearrangements has improved the diagnosis and characterization of lymphoid neoplasms, application of this test is not without complications and interpretive challenges, some of which have changed our understanding

of the biology of certain types of lymphoma and related disorders. For instance, some rare lymphoproliferative disorders regarded as clinically benign may contain clonal lymphocytes. Among these disorders are lymphomatoid papulosis,[63, 64] T-γ lymphocytosis,[65] lymphoepithelial lesions of the salivary gland in Sjögren's disease,[66] and systemic Castleman's disease[67] (the first two disorders contain clonal

T lymphocytes; the latter two clonal B lymphocytes). The simplest interpretation is that these entities represent benign tumors of the lymphocytes, a category of disease not generally recognized to exist before Southern blot analyses of antigen receptor genes were performed. However, it is also possible that these disorders are in reality very-low-grade malignancies, since patients with these conditions seem generally to be at increased risk for the development of lymphoid cancers. Perhaps the most accurate view is that the clonal populations in these disorders, although not fully malignant, contain one or more genetic alterations that render them neoplastic and more readily susceptible to malignant transformation through the acquisition of additional mutations. This interpretation is consistent with the current prevailing notions about the multistep mutational pathogenesis of cancer. In any event, the clonality of lymphocytes in some clinically benign diseases indicates that clonality does not necessarily imply malignancy. Furthermore, clonality in benign disorders underscores the message that diagnosis should not rely solely on analysis of antigen receptor gene rearrangements but should take into consideration all relevant information, including any histologic, immunohistochemical, and clinical data available. At the same time, it seems reasonable to suggest that the detection of clonal populations within a biopsy specimen should always alert the pathologist and the oncologist to the chance of progression to lymphoma.

Another source of diagnostic ambiguity in the application of Southern blot analysis of antigen receptor gene rearrangements is that occasionally, bona fide lymphomas lack detectable gene rearrangements.[68, 69] These tumors constitute a small fraction of all lymphomas, but their malignant nature is clear from the fact that many metastasize and have pursued a fatal course. Based on immunohistochemistry, most seem to be T-lineage tumors, and histologically, many show angiocentric features. The midline and upper respiratory passages seem to be preferential sites of involvement. Some of these cases have been shown to bear antigenic markers of natural killer cells, a lineage that normally does not rearrange antigen receptor genes.[70, 71] In other cases, technical reasons may account for failure to detect rearrangements in some tumors having lymphocytic markers, although the search for rearrangements in many of these cases has been thorough, including analysis of most antigen receptor genes using numerous restriction enzyme digests. Taken together, these findings indicate that the apparent absence of clonal antigen receptor gene rearrangements does not preclude the diagnosis of lymphoma.

The diagnosis of lymphoma by Southern blot analysis of antigen receptor gene rearrangements can be also be complicated by the appearance in autoradiograms of more than two clonal bands, the maximum expected from a monoclonal lymphocytic population. A related finding is the change in the positions of bands within the autoradiogram when analyses are performed on multiple specimens from individual patients undergoing biopsy at several sites or at different times. These kinds of results have a number of possible explanations. In some cases of B-lineage lymphomas, somatic hypermutations may occur in or around rearranged immunoglobulin genes, destroying or creating restriction sites in a portion of the lymphocytes. The resulting changes in the sizes of restriction fragments shift the position of

bands in Southern blot autoradiograms, thereby simulating the presence of additional clones in the biopsy tissues.[72–74] This mechanism probably occurs predominantly among follicular lymphomas, in which ongoing somatic hypermutation of rearranged immunoglobulin genes is common.[75] Other cases that yield more than two rearranged bands probably represent tumors that arise from lymphocytes or their precursors containing incomplete DJ joins or genes in the unrearranged, germline configuration. As these tumor progenitors proliferate, rearrangement may occur in daughter cells, generating subclones with additional rearrangements not present in the progenitor. This probably occurs in some lymphomas but is most often seen in lymphoblastic leukemias, from which 10 or more detectable nongermline heavy-chain bands are often obtained in Southern blot autoradiograms.[76–78] Rare examples of lymphomas with both B- and T-lineage clones have been reported, and it may be that such tumors develop from the elusive prelymphocytic stem cell or, alternatively, from independent transformation events in separate tumor progenitors.[79] Another phenomenon that takes place in lymphoblastic leukemia, and probably in occasional B-lineage lymphomas as well, is V-segment replacement, as discussed earlier. Again, this process produces subclones with altered bands in Southern blot analyses of immunoglobulin genes.[78, 80]

True multiclonality of tumors seems to form the basis for finding more than two rearranged bands in immunosuppressed patients, such as organ transplant recipients and patients with acquired immunodeficiency syndrome (AIDS).[81, 82] Non-Hodgkin's lymphomas arising in these patients often harbor genomes of the Epstein-Barr virus (EBV), which presumably provides the primary mitogenic stimulus in the cells of these tumors. EBV genomes in these cells appear to be indistinguishable from those of latently infected lymphoblastoid cells present in low numbers within the peripheral blood of most normal adults. Presumably, in the absence of cytolytic immunity, lymphoblastoid cells proliferate unchecked and, over time, cells with faster rates of growth come to dominate at particular sites, so that different clones may be detected in separate biopsy specimens or in specimens acquired at various times.[83, 84] Southern blot analysis of tissue specimens has provided evidence consistent with the progression from polyclonality to oligoclonality to monoclonality in lymphomas of immunosuppressed patients.

Oligoclonality documented by Southern blot analyses also occurs in some patients with no obvious underlying immunodeficiency or likely instability in antigen receptor gene sequences (e.g., oligoclonality of T lymphocytes, in which neither somatic hypermutation or V-segment replacement is a plausible explanation for the extra bands in Southern blot autoradiograms). These results frequently cause consternation with regard to diagnosis since no long-term followup studies have been reported to determine the outcome in such cases. The author has personally followed a patient with an unchanging oligoclonal pattern of T-cell-receptor gene rearrangements in the peripheral blood and bone marrow for more than 5 years without evidence for progression to monoclonality or overt malignancy. However, in view of the information available on lymphoproliferative disorders in immunosuppressed patients and from those clonal, clinically benign conditions that predispose to malignancy, it seems prudent to assume that patients with oligoclonal processes may be at risk for evolution to clear-cut monoclonal cancer and should be followed carefully.

The determination of lineage by Southern blot analysis of antigen receptor genes can also be less than straightforward. Some leukemias and lymphomas contain both immunoglobulin and T-cell-receptor gene rearrangements, and as many as 20% of acute myeloid leukemias may have such rearrangements.[85–89] Whether or not normal lymphocytes ever have rearrangements of both immunoglobulin and T-cell receptor genes is an unresolved question. In light of these data, a consistent pattern of rearrangements (i.e., only immunoglobulin-gene rearrangements and no T-cell-receptor gene rearrangements, or vice versa) may constitute evidence strongly supporting differentiation along one or the other lymphocytic line, but lineage should be assigned only in conjunction with immunohistochemical and histologic findings.

ANALYSIS OF ANTIGEN RECEPTOR GENE REARRANGEMENTS BY POLYMERASE CHAIN REACTION AMPLIFICATION

Southern blot hybridization analysis of antigen receptor gene rearrangements has become a valuable technique in the diagnosis of lymphocytic cancers, yet three major disadvantages still limit its use: (1) the length of time necessary to obtain the analysis (about 5 days or longer); (2) the requirement for radioactivity; and (3) the sensitivity restricted to detecting no less than 1% of clonal lymphocytes within a tissue specimen. Since the introduction of the polymerase chain reaction (PCR), attempts have been made to adapt this technique for the analysis of antigen receptor gene rearrangements to overcome the inconveniences of the Southern blot approach. A fourth limitation of Southern blot hybridization for which PCR offers a potential solution is the lack of direct correlation with histology.

The application of PCR to the detection of clonal antigen receptor gene rearrangements is based on the same general biologic principles as the the application of Southern blot hybridization; however, the specific marker analyzed by PCR is actually different. In Southern blot analysis, the marker is the configuration of rearranged gene segments in an antigen receptor gene (i.e., which V and J segments have been joined), whereas in PCR the marker is the sequence at the junction of rearranged segments (Fig. 7–5). As discussed earlier, unique nucleotide sequences are created at these sites by the combined effects of the joining of different gene segments, small deletions of base pairs from the ends of the segments, and the insertion of N region sequence between the ends prior to joining. The net result is a clonotypic marker even more specific than the configuration of rearranged gene segments.[90]

Application of PCR for the primary detection of clonality involves amplifying DNA across the V(D)J junction within a rearranged antigen receptor gene and then assaying the uniformity of the products by some form of gel electrophoresis. Oligonucleotide primers used in these amplifications are constructed to complement sequences in V and J segments common to as many rearrangements as possible. The need to find such conserved sequences among V

segments and, to a lesser extent, among J segments is the principal handicap of PCR for clonal antigen receptor gene rearrangements. In practice, this restricts the technique to immunoglobulin heavy-chain[91–95] and γ and δ T-cell-receptor genes.[96] Even then, only about 50% to 70% of immunoglobulin heavy-chain gene rearrangements in lymphocytic tumors can be amplified by PCR, although this number varies among types of tumors owing to preferential rearrangement of certain V-segment families within these cases.[97, 98] The likelihood of amplification may be somewhat improved by performing multiple reactions with primers for each of the six V-segment families[78] but is still very low in certain types of lymphomas (such as follicular lymphomas; in contrast, clonal immunoglobulin heavy-chain gene rearrangements can be amplified from about 50% of acute lymphoblastic leukemias using a V-segment primer complementary to sequence near the conserved nonamer recombinase recognition site near the 3′ end of many V segments). Detection of clonality by analysis of γ and δ genes is less problematic because of the smaller number of V segments in the gene and the ability of a small set of V-segment primers to cover amplification of all or most of the rearrangements in these genes.

The electrophoretic system generally used to analyze the PCR products depends on the size of the junctional region sequence amplified. Most immunoglobulin heavy-chain gene rearrangements have relatively large junctional regions that usually include one D segment with N region nucleotides on either side. As a result, PCR across the VDJ junction of immunoglobulin heavy-chain genes generates a broad range of differently sized products that are well separated by electrophoresis in a standard agarose or polyacrylamide gel. PCR of DNA from a tissue specimen containing clonal population of lymphocytes having a uniform heavy-chain gene rearrangement generates a predominant product of a single size. This product is manifest by a discrete band in the gel viewed under ultraviolet light after staining with ethidium bromide. PCR products derived from polyclonal cells are diverse in size and form a diffuse smear within the gel. No products are generated from unrearranged genes because of the distances lying between the segments in the germline configuration. The threshold for detecting a clonal population by gel electrophoresis of PCR products is about 1%.

The junctional regions of rearranged δ T-cell-receptor gene are even more complex and variable than those of immunoglobulin heavy-chain genes (many have two D segments and three N regions, and some only one or even no D segments). Consequently, clonality of lymphocytes containing rearrangements of these genes should by analyzable in the same way as immunoglobulin heavy-chain genes, although far less work using these genes has been reported.

In comparison with immunoglobulin heavy-chain and δ T-cell-receptor genes, the junctional regions of γ T-cell-receptor genes are short, containing no D segments and a single N region. Polyacrylamide gels of polyclonal tissues show a relatively simple ladder of bands, sometimes with one or more bands having increased intensity, the significance of which is unclear. If blood from normal control subjects is assessed in this manner, the dominant bands often change over time. Based on these observations, size alone is an inadequate criterion with which to evaluate the PCR prod-

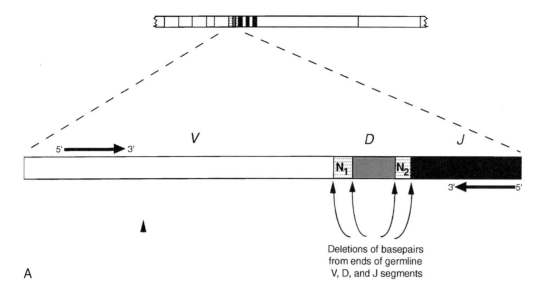

Figure 7–5. Analysis of rearranged antigen receptor genes by PCR. *A*, Schematic diagram of sequence encompassing the VDJ junction within a rearranged immunoglobulin heavy chain. The rearrangement illustrated contains one D segment and two N regions. The positions in the DNA to which V- and J-segment primers anneal are shown. *B*, Photograph of an ethidium bromide–stained agarose gel in which PCR products amplified from the immunoglobulin heavy-chain genes of two tissue specimens have been separated by agarose gel electrophoresis. T indicates the lane containing products amplified from the DNA of a B-cell non-Hodgkin's lymphoma; N is the lane containing products amplified from the DNA of a hyperplastic lymph node.

ucts amplified from γ T-cell-receptor genes. Therefore, gradient denaturing gel electrophoresis has been adapted to detect clonal rearrangements among these genes, since this technique discriminates differences in DNA fragments by both size and nucleotide sequence.[96] Following electrophoresis of the PCR products amplified from the γ T-cell genes, staining of the gradient gel with ethidium bromide reveals a discrete band under ultraviolet light, provided that 1% or more of the fragments in the PCR products contain uniform sequence and therefore stopped at the same position within the gel. In contrast, PCR products amplified from polyclonal gene rearrangements form a diffuse smear along the length of the gel.

The virtues of PCR combined with gel electrophoresis to assess clonality of lymphocytes include the fact that the whole procedure can be completed in 1 or 2 days and does not employ radioactivity. Additionally, since the product of PCR is frequently less than several hundred kilobases in length, amplifications can be performed on DNA extracted from formalin-fixed, paraffin-embedded tissues.[95, 99] Furthermore, it is applicable in certain situations in which Southern blot hybridization is not; namely, when the numbers of lymphocytes in a specimen are very low, such as in early phases of cutaneous T-cell lymphoma[100] or lymphocytosis within cerebrospinal fluid.

The capability of PCR to amplify clonal antigen receptor gene rearrangements from isolated single cells also has potential diagnostic applications in lymphoma. Unlike disorders such as early cutaneous T-cell lymphoma in which the absolute number of lymphocytes within a specimen is small, there are conditions in which lymphoid cells suspicious for malignancy constitute a fraction of the total lymphocytes, below the 1% threshold for detection by Southern blot analysis or simple PCR. A frequently encountered example is the diagnosis of T-cell-rich B-cell lymphoma. Unfortunately, the dilemma in this situation is the distinction between non-Hodgkin's lymphoma and Hodgkin's disease, and numerous reports in recent years have documented the finding of clonal immunoglobulin-gene rearrangements in Reed-Sternberg cells and their variants of some (but not all) cases of Hodgkin's disease, including by PCR of DNA isolated from single cells microdissected from paraffin sections.[101–103] At the same time, the proportion of Hodgkin's cases lacking rearrangements that are clonal and amplifiable is sufficiently high to discourage routine-application, single-cell PCR for the diagnosis of Hodgkin's disease. Nevertheless, PCR for analysis of gene rearrangements in single cells may have diagnostic usefulness under certain circumstances when direct correlation of clonality and histology is desired, particularly if convenient methods for microdissection of individual cells are available.[104]

MONITORING OF RESIDUAL DISEASE BY POLYMERASE CHAIN REACTION OF ANTIGEN RECEPTOR GENES

Like all gel-based detection systems, PCR of junctional sequence combined with gel electrophoresis is limited to detecting clonal lymphocytes in excess of 1%—a level too high to provide meaningful information about residual disease after therapy or possibly for identifying small numbers of disseminated tumor cells in sensitive staging procedures. In response to this deficiency, several strategies have been devised for monitoring of residual lymphocytic cancer by detecting clonotypic junctional sequences among the rearranged antigen receptor genes of tissue specimens. These strategies invariably involve a two-step format: in the first step, junctional sequence is amplified by PCR from the antigen receptor genes of diagnostic reference specimens, and then in a second step, other specimens from the same patient are screened for the junctional region found in the reference specimen (Fig. 7–6). Usually, the nucleotide sequence is determined for the PCR product of the clonal gene rearrangement, and a tumor-specific oligonucleotide complementary to the junctional sequence is synthesized. In one strategy, the oligonucleotide is used as a primer with a general V-segment primer to attempt amplification of DNA from test specimens.[90, 105] In the second method, the oligonucleotide is radiolabeled and used as a probe to detect the specific junctional sequence among the PCR products amplified from test specimens with general V- and J-segment primers for the gene under analysis.[106]

Oligonucleotide used as probes can be hybridized directly to the PCR products of the test specimen after immobilizing these products on nylon membranes (so-called dot-blot analysis). Rough quantitation of the clonotypic junctional sequence within the test specimen can be achieved by comparing the intensity in an autoradiogram of the hybridization signal from the PCR products of the test specimen to that of PCR products amplified from test-specimen DNA diluted with normal DNA from an unrelated source. Alternatively, the PCR products can be molecularly cloned in M13 viral vectors that are then used to produce plaques on lawns of *Escherichia coli* grown on the surface of agar plates. A nylon membrane is briefly laid on the surface of the plate to transfer DNA in the plaques to the membrane, and the oligonucleotides probes are hybridized to the mem-

brane. This maneuver, although tedious, probably permits more accurate quantitation than does dot-blot analysis and also allows for sequence analysis of DNA within positive plaques (which are not destroyed by the transfer procedure) to confirm the identity of the junctional sequences inserted into the viruses. Both the dot-blot and plaque hybridization methods are capable of detecting tumor cells at the level of 10^{-5} in a single assay. This figure represents detection of one gene in 1 μg of total cellular DNA—about the limit of total DNA that can be conveniently amplified in a single standard PCR reaction.

An obvious disadvantage of the strategies described earlier is that they require sequence analysis and construction of tumor-specific oligonucleotides. To circumvent these requirements, a method for analysis of δ T-cell-receptor gene rearrangements has been developed in which a probe is directly synthesized for the junctional region by PCR amplification of δ gene DNA from a diagnostic specimen, followed by restriction cleavage of the PCR product to yield a small subfragment containing the junctional sequence.[107] The fragment is then hybridized to dot-blots of PCR-amplified δ genes from test specimens. The method has comparable sensitivity to the earlier methods, but it is only applicable to the δ gene because of the crucial position of a conserved restriction site in the V segments of this gene.

A more general method that also avoids sequence analysis and synthesis of tumor-specific oligonucleotides relies on PCR using general V- and J-segment primers to which have been appended sequences for the RNA polymerase promoter from the bacteriophage T7.[108] Rearranged gene DNA is amplified from both diagnostic and test specimens using one such primer and a second standard V- or J-segment primer. Presence of the T7 promoter at one end of the PCR product from the diagnostic specimen and at the other end of the test PCR product permits rapid transcription of radiolabeled riboprobe from one strand of the diagnostic PCR product and nonradioactive target RNA from the opposite strand of the test PCR product. Probe and test RNAs are hybridized together, and the hybrids are subjected to digestion by ribonucleases (RNases) A and T1. RNases cleave any single-stranded sequence of the hybrid (especially that at the junction region) but do not affect double-stranded RNA. Tumor cells within the test specimen result in test RNA matching the probe RNA and protection of the probe from RNase digestion. Full-length, protected probe is revealed as a band in a polyacrylamide gel. This RNase protection method seems to be as sensitive as any other method and is applicable to any antigen receptor gene that can be reliably amplified from lymphoid neoplasms.

Highly sensitive monitoring of residual disease is most likely to be useful in potentially curable disorders, for which it may be important to adjust therapy to maximize the chance for cure while minimizing the likelihood of serious side effects. Acute lymphoblastic leukemias are the paradigm of such disorders and, in fact, are the diseases for which sensitive monitoring by PCR of antigen receptor genes was devised. Intermediate- and high-grade non-Hodgkin's lymphomas are possibly other diseases on which such strategies may be tried. The type of test specimens appropriate for such monitoring is not established, but preliminary studies indicate that a high percentage of patients with overt

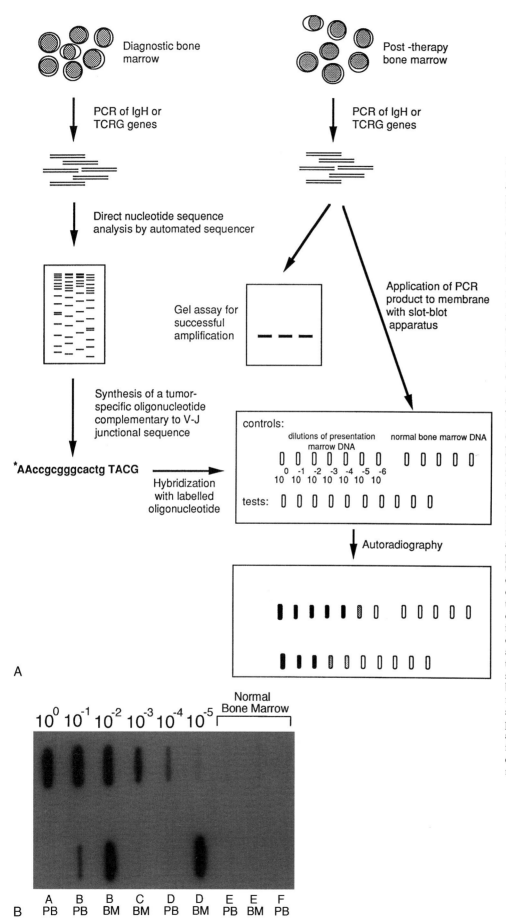

Figure 7–6. Test for minimal residual disease in lymphocytic leukemia. *A,* Schematic representation of the procedure. The left portion of the figure illustrates the steps performed to prepare a tumor-specific oligonucleotide probe containing an N region (arbitrarily indicated to be CCGCGGGCACTG) found within the DNA of a rearranged antigen receptor gene amplified from a diagnostic bone marrow specimen. The right portion of the figure illustrates the preparation of a membrane on which polymerase chain reaction (PCR) products amplified from post-therapy specimens have been spotted, along with negative controls and standards for quantitation of results. *B,* Autoradiogram demonstrating the results of the procedure in *A* for a patient with acute lymphoblastic leukemia. Normal bone marrow DNAs were derived from specimens of unrelated people. Rough quantitation of residual leukemia is possible by comparing the intensity of the signals obtained from test specimens *(bottom row)* with those obtained from dilutions of diagnostic DNA into normal bone marrow DNA *(top row).* Analyses were performed on both peripheral blood (PB) and bone marrow (BM) at various time points (**A,** 1 month after initiation of therapy; **B,** 2 months after initiation of therapy; **C,** 7 months after initiation of therapy; **D,** 1 year after initiation of therapy; **E,** 2 years after initiation of therapy; and **F,** 27 months after initiation of therapy). Fluctuating levels of residual disease, as found here, are not infrequently detected during the consolidation phases of therapy. As suggested by the results, peripheral blood is often negative when bone marrow is positive; the reverse is seldom true. The patient was in complete clinical remission from shortly after the start of therapy and remained free of disease by PCR and all other criteria 4 years later. TCRG, T-cell receptor γ.

intermediate-grade lymphomas, even in early-stage disease, have large numbers of circulating tumor cells in their peripheral blood.[109] Therefore, the effects of therapy may be investigated by monitoring peripheral blood in some forms of lymphoma.

Monitoring of residual disease by screening of clonotypic junctional sequences of antigen receptor gene rearrangements must contend with the possibility of changes that may occur in these sequences over time. The events that can lead to some of these changes (discussed earlier) include V-segment substitution, origin of the tumor from a lymphocyte precursor lacking rearrangements, and somatic mutation (the first and last applying only to immunoglobulin heavy-chain genes). Failure to detect residual disease because of the first two processes has been documented in acute lymphoblastic leukemia.[110–112] The problem of V-segment replacement within immunoglobulin heavy-chain genes can at least be partially overcome by using junctional sequence oligonucleotides complementary to the DNJ part of the region, since recombination of the upstream V segment occurs into the 3′ end of the previously rearranged V segment, often affecting the first N region but not the second.[113]

A central issue associated with sensitive monitoring of residual disease, aside from that of its technical feasibility, is its clinical value. In acute lymphoblastic leukemia, which has been studied in this regard for some years, the data are inconsistent. Some investigators have argued that the rate of elimination of detectable tumor cells during early therapy is an indicator of disease-free survival, whereas others have found that in prospective studies there is not a strong correlation between the detection of low levels of disease and clinical outcome. In fact, fluctuating levels of disease have been encountered in numerous patients who have not relapsed for several years after therapy has been discontinued.[114]

CHROMOSOME TRANSLOCATIONS

Rearrangements of antigen receptor genes found in lymphomas represent genetic alterations that probably occur before the malignant transformation of the progenitor that gives rise to these tumors. In any event, no outstanding features of these rearrangements distinguish them from those found in normal lymphocyte precursors, and they serve merely as markers of clonality rather than of malignancy. Lymphocytic tumors also contain numerous other genetic alterations with a more direct role in the malignant phenotype of the cells. Some of these alterations involve tumor suppressor genes and oncogenes, as well as probably other less well-defined types of genes with functions that affect properties such as the rate of cellular proliferation and the propensity to spread to nonlymphoid sites. For diagnostic purposes, the most important of these genetic alterations are chromosome translocations.

Interest in chromosome translocations as diagnostic markers is based on several considerations. Chromosome translocations are common in lymphoma.[115] The oncogenes that are modified in structure or expression as a result of the translocation have in most instances been directly implicated in some aspect of the malignant behavior of the cells

containing them. Therefore, chromosome translocations are good (but not absolute) markers of malignancy and tend to be stable genetic changes that remain constant throughout the course of the disease. Different types of translocations are associated with different subtypes of lymphoma, so that evidence for their presence within a tissue biopsy gives specific prognostic information about the likely clinical course and response to therapy, akin to and frequently coinciding with the information obtained from histologic classification of tumors. Finally, chromosome translocations are markers that are relatively easy to detect by sensitive molecular methods (as opposed to point mutations within tumor suppressor genes, which are generally far harder to identify). On the other hand, the principal limitation of chromosome translocations as diagnostic markers is that their specificity for tumor subtypes makes them a poor general marker with which to distinguish neoplastic from reactive processes, as can be done, for instance, using antigen receptor gene rearrangements, regardless of the subtype of the tumor.

Chromosome translocations exert their oncogenic effects by somehow affecting the function of a gene or genes located at or near the breakpoint on one or both of the chromosomes involved in the translocation.[116] This result may occur through the overexpression of the gene without any structural change in the gene product, through inappropriate expression of the gene relative to the various phases of the cell cycle, or through heterotopic expression of the gene in a tissue in which it is not normally active. Sometimes the mechanism for altered expression is straightforward, such as breakage in the nontranslated portion of the transcription template or substitution of one promoter for another. In other examples, the mechanism is more obscure and is presumably related to the proximity brought about between the translocated gene in one chromosome and regulatory elements in the second chromosome on the opposite side of the breakpoint. Structural changes in genes also result from certain translocations. For instance, the coding sequence of some genes is simply truncated by the translocation. More commonly, a chimeric protein product is created by breakage within the introns of a gene in each participating chromosome, transcription across the breakpoint, and joining of exons from different genes within the RNA. Whatever genetic change wrought by translocations and the functional consequence of these changes, it is generally true that the precise positions of the breakpoints within the DNA of either chromosome vary to one degree or another among tumors containing a specific type of translocation. This fundamental feature of chromosome translocations is the most important technical consideration that must be taken into account when these markers are used for molecular diagnosis.

Molecular detection of chromosome translocations can generally be achieved using three techniques. First, Southern blot hybridization can be performed using probes constructed from cloned DNA of one chromosome lying near the breakpoint.[117] A rearranged, nongermline band within the autoradiogram (in addition to the germline band derived from the untranslocated allele and any contaminated normal tissue), indicates the presence of a translocation. This method depends on the breakpoints in one of the chromosomes among different tumors being sufficiently closely clustered in the DNA that a breakpoint in any one tumor can predictably be contained in one or a few restriction fragments (each restriction fragment requiring a separate probe). The sensitivity of Southern blot hybridization for detecting cells with chromosome translocation is the same as that for cells with clonal antigen receptor gene rearrangements—one cell in a total of 20 to 100.

A second method of testing for chromosome translocations is PCR. Primers complementary to DNA of the two participating chromosomes are used to amplify a product from the translocation, whereas no product is obtained from the DNA of normal tissue in which the sequences complementary to the primers remain on separate chromosomes. PCR can be performed directly on DNA if the breakpoints in both chromosomes in different tumors are distributed over a cumulative distance of no more than 1 or 2 kb, the limit that can be amplified into a single PCR product by conventional PCR.[118] However, PCR is still possible in some translocations with widely scattered breakpoints by using reverse-transcription PCR (RT-PCR) of RNA.[119] RT-PCR depends on consistent breakage within the same introns of the two genes. Under these conditions, primers are selected to be complementary to exonic sequence near the breakpoints from each of the two genes. A PCR product is generated only if a translocation within the tissues places both exons within a single transcription unit. Standard and RT-PCR both are capable of detecting a single cell containing a translocation in 10^5 total cells, making this method of detection well suited for monitoring residual disease.

A last method for detecting chromosome translocations is fluorescence in situ hybridization (FISH).[120] FISH performed on metaphase chromosomes involves almost all of the procedural steps that are necessary for conventional cytogenetics (namely, the requirement for viable biopsy tissues, the successful growth of tumor cells in culture, and the preparation of high-quality spreads of metaphase chromosomes), which has mitigated against extensive use of metaphase FISH for routine cancer diagnosis. However, FISH performed on interphase nuclei avoids these steps and can truly be considered a molecular method of diagnosis. The basic concept in interphase FISH

is to hybridize the nuclei with two differentially labeled probes derived from DNA on either side of the breakpoint in one or the other chromosome (Fig. 7–7; see also color section). In normal nuclei, the hybridized probes produce coincident or overlapping signals, but in nuclei containing the translocation, the signals are split. Untranslocated chromosome homologues give separate signals, serving as internal controls. Alternatively, probes from the regions of recombination in the two participating chromosomes can be used, and the fusion of two signals can be monitored in cells containing the translocation. Since overlapping fluorescence from the two probes yields a color distinguishable from either probe alone (e.g., the red of rhodamine and the green of fluorescein combine to give a pale orange), the presence of a translocation is indicated by chromatic as well as numerical changes in the signal.

Although FISH has not yet been widely exploited for cancer diagnosis, its potential is great. Hybridization can be performed on nuclei extracted from paraffin blocks, and a large variety of probes consisting of yeast or bacterial artificial chromosomes (YACs and BACs, respectively) or cosmids containing chromosome DNA mapped to the appropriate regions are available for this purpose. FISH may reveal translocation equivalents not evident from conventional cytogenetics owing to complicated or microscopically occult rearrangements, and the method is relatively fast (<1 day). The scatter of breakpoints within the chromosomes among different tumors is not an issue in this technique since the probes can be directed against DNA sequences widely separated on a molecular scale. The major problem with interphase FISH is artifacts in the signal, either in the form of extra or deficient fluorescent spots, created presumably by the effects on the binding of probe owing to the large amount of protein content of the nuclei, even after treatment with trypsin prior to hybridization. To some degree, false-positive and negative signals can be reduced by digitalization and computer processing of the images. Direct labeling of probe DNA rather than indirect labeling by detection of chemically tagged probes with fluorescent antibodies, as is usually practiced, may also lower background. Nevertheless, an ample number of nuclei must be

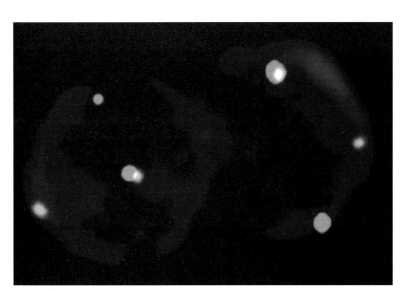

Figure 7–7. Detection of chromosome translocations by interphase fluorescence in situ hybridization (FISH). The figure shows a digitized image of two nuclei that were isolated from a paraffin section of a gastric lymphoma of mucosa-associated lymphoid tissue (MALT) and then analyzed for the presence of the t(11;18)(q21;q21), a translocation found in about 20% of MALT lymphomas. Two bacterial artificial chromosomes (BACs) that flank the chromosome 11 breakpoint on either side were used as hybridization probes and appear as red or green dots. The normal chromosome 11q21 region is identified by closely lying or superimposed red and green dots. The discrete green and red dots identify the two translocation derivatives and demonstrate that the translocation breakpoint in chromosome 11 occurred between the sequences contained within the two BACs. (See also color section.)

Table 7–1. Major, Molecularly Characterized and Diagnostically Useful Chromosome Translocations Associated with Lymphomas

Translocation	Subtype	Incidence (%)	Genes	Activation Mechanism	Methods of Detection
B-Cell					
t(14;18)(q32;q11)	Follicular	>90	*IgH;*<u>*BCL-2*</u>	Overexpression	SB, PCR, FISH
	Transformed DLCL	>90			
	De novo DLCL	20			
t(8;14)(q24;q32)	Burkitt's	80	<u>*MYC*</u>*;IgH*	Constitutive expression	FISH, SB
or t(2;8)(p11;q24)		20	*IgK;*<u>*MYC*</u>		
or t(8;22)(q24;q11)		5	<u>*MYC*</u>*;IgL*		
t(11;14)(q13;q32)	Mantle cell	70	*BCL-1;IgH*	Constitutive expression	SB, PCR, FISH
t(3;N)(q27;N)	De novo DLCL	40	<u>*BCL-6;*</u> *IgH or IgL* *or* ?	Overexpression; ? induced mutation	SB, FISH
T-Cell					
t(2;5)(p23;q35)	Anaplastic large cell	80	<u>*ALK*</u>*;NPM*	Chimeric gene (*NPM-ALK*)	RT-PCR, FISH, SB

The genes proximal to the breakpoints in the translocation are indicated to correspond to the order of the breakpoints designated by the nomenclature for translocation. The underlined gene is the presumed oncogene altered by the translocation in a way critical to the development of the tumor.

DLCL, diffuse large cell lymphoma; SB, Southern blot hybridization; PCR, polymerase chain reaction; FISH, fluorescence in situ hybridization; RT-PCR, reverse-transcriptase PCR; N, numerous cytogenetic sites.

examined to obtain convincing evidence for the presence or absence of the translocation. Consequently, the method is not likely to be useful for monitoring residual disease.

In addition to Southern blot hybridization, PCR, and FISH, immunohistochemistry offers another option for inferring the presence of chromosome translocations in biopsy samples. Since immunohistochemistry is not strictly a molecular method of diagnosis as defined earlier, it is not considered in detail here. However, in those chromosome translocations leading to overexpression of a gene or gene fragment within a chimeric protein, antibodies directed against epitopes within the translocation-associated protein can be valuable reagents for diagnosing and classifying tumors. This technique has the significant advantage of permitting direct correlation with histology but is probably not sufficiently sensitive to be as useful in monitoring of residual disease as are molecular techniques.

Table 7–1 lists the major molecularly characterized chromosome translocations found in lymphomas, along with the genes proximal to the breakpoints and the frequency of these translocations in the subtypes with which they are associated. Etiologic aspects of these translocations are discussed in other chapters, and the following review concentrates primarily on diagnostic matters.

As is evident from Table 7–1, among those translocations associated with B-lineage lymphomas, recombination in one of the two chromosomes commonly occurs within an immunoglobulin gene. Similar observations have been made with respect to chromosome translocations of T-lineage leukemias, in which recombination often occurs in T-cell-receptor genes. Usually recombination takes place adjacent to a J segment, leading to the hypothesis that the mechanism of chromosome translocation involves an aberrant attempt at immunoglobulin-gene rearrangement, with the oncogene replacing the D or V segment in the normal rearrangement process.[121–124] In support of this notion, intergenic rearrangements between various antigen receptor genes can be found relatively frequently in presumably normal lymphocytes.[125] The site of recombination in sporadic Burkitt's

lymphomas is different than in endemic cases, with joining of DNA in the *MYC* gene to DNA within the switch region of the immunoglobulin heavy-chain gene.[126–128] In any case, Southern blot analysis of immunoglobulin-gene rearrangements often detect a nongermline band owing to translocation besides the band arising from VDJ joining within the immunoglobulin gene.

The t(14;18)(q32;q11) of follicular B-cell lymphoma joins the 3′ untranslated region of the *BCL-2* gene on chromosome 18 to a J segment of the immunoglobulin heavy-chain gene on chromosome 14 (Fig. 7–8A).[129–132] The *BCL-2* product dimerizes with and thereby inhibits the action of a second protein, bax, and possibly other proteins, which regulate cell death, or apoptosis.[133] Apparently, expression of *BCL-2* in the normal germinal center of lymph nodes plays a part in the selection of long-lived memory B cells.[134, 135] Constitutive overexpression of *BCL-2* by the translocation antagonizes apoptosis and prolongs the survival of the follicular lymphoma cells. Breakpoints in the *BCL-2* gene occur in two discrete, relatively short cluster regions: MBR containing breakpoints in about 70% of tumors and MCR containing breakpoints in the remainder.[117, 136] No prognostic significance has been ascribed to differences in recombination among these two cluster regions. Separate probes for the two cluster regions are employed in Southern blot analyses for this translocation.[117] Both regions are sufficiently short that a product can be generated from most cases containing the translocation by PCR using one consensus primer to the J segments and a second primer complementary to DNA flanking one or the other cluster region on its 5′ side.[118, 137, 138]

The feasibility of detecting the t(14;18)(q32;q11) by PCR has led to many studies of residual disease in follicular lymphoma, despite the fact that there is no evidence that any current form of therapy affects the ultimate fatal outcome in this lymphoma. Failure to amplify product from the blood or bone marrow of patients in remission apparently indicates only the reduction in levels of disease below the threshold for detection by PCR. Absence of amplifiable product from

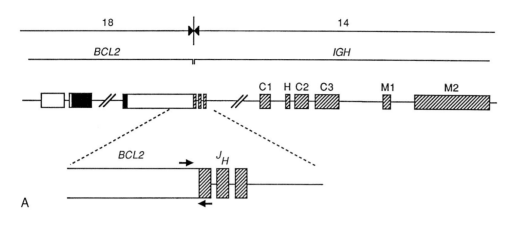

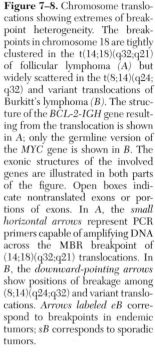

Figure 7–8. Chromosome translocations showing extremes of breakpoint heterogeneity. The breakpoints in chromosome 18 are tightly clustered in the t(14;18)(q32;q21) of follicular lymphoma (*A*) but widely scattered in the t(8;14)(q24;q32) and variant translocations of Burkitt's lymphoma (*B*). The structure of the *BCL-2-IGH* gene resulting from the translocation is shown in *A*; only the germline version of the *MYC* gene is shown in *B*. The exonic structures of the involved genes are illustrated in both parts of the figure. Open boxes indicate nontranslated exons or portions of exons. In *A*, the *small horizontal arrows* represent PCR primers capable of amplifying DNA across the MBR breakpoint of (14;18)(q32;q21) translocations. In *B*, the *downward-pointing arrows* show positions of breakage among (8;14)(q24;q32) and variant translocations. *Arrows labeled eB* correspond to breakpoints in endemic tumors; *sB* corresponds to sporadic tumors.

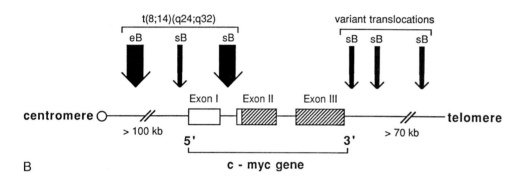

autografts used for autologous bone marrow transplantation correlates with prolonged disease-free survival but probably not with cure.[139]

Hyperplastic tonsils lacking any histologic features of lymphoma have been shown repeatedly to contain one or more (14;18)(q32;q11) translocations by PCR.[140, 141] These data are consistent with the interpretation that overexpression of *BCL-2* is not by itself sufficient for malignant transformation and that additional mutations or even epigenetic alterations are necessary for full oncogenesis. Similar interpretations have been made from the finding that transgenic mice containing B lymphocytes overexpressing *BCL-2* develop hyperplastic, polyclonal lymphoid tissues in which a dominant clone emerges later in life only in a fraction of animals.[142–144] The implication of these observations for diagnosis would seem to be that detection of a product by PCR for the t(14;18)(q32;q11) in a single analysis, particularly of DNA from hyperplastic lymph node, must not be taken to be indicative of lymphoma. Some assessment of the size of the population containing the translocation is advisable, either by Southern blot hybridization, by repetitive PCR on multiple aliquots of DNA, or by PCR on DNA of the lesion after dilution with normal control DNA.

The t(8;14)(q24;q32) and its variant forms join DNA in or near the *MYC* gene on chromosome 8 to the J region of an immunoglobulin gene (the exception among sporadic Burkitt's lymphoma is discussed earlier) (Fig. 7–8B).[145–147] The shared consequence of all these translocations is the altered expression of the *MYC* gene product, which participates in the regulation of genes controlling the cell cycle, differentiation, and apoptosis. Myc normally competes with two other proteins, mad and mxi1, for binding to a third protein, max.[148–151] Abundance of myc favors formation of myc-max dimers, which are transcriptional activators, over formation of mad-max and mad-mxi1, which sequester mad from myc and block the DNA binding sites recognized by myc-max.

Chromosome translocations involving *MYC* are highly heterogeneous with respect to the sites of recombination about this gene. Recombination in (8;14)(q24;q32) translocations occurs either far 5′ of the gene (endemic Burkitt's) or near the 5′ end and within the gene before the second of three exons (sporadic Burkitt's). Recombination in the variant translocations occurs far 3′ of the gene.[126] The breakpoints are clearly too widely distributed for detection of the translocation by PCR. Southern blot hybridization with a series of probes for the 5′ end may pick up most (8;14)(q24;q32) translocations in sporadic cases; however, overall, FISH would seem to be the best option for detection of these translocations.

The t(11;14)(q13;q32) leads to constitutive expression of *BCL-1* (also known as *CCND1* or *PRAD1*), which encodes cyclin D1, one of the D cyclins that promotes passage through the G_1 phase of the cell cycle.[152–154] It is the only oncogene of those in Table 7–1 implicated in other tumors (by translocation in parathyroid adenomas and by amplification in some breast carcinomas). The breakpoints are scattered relative to *BCL-1*, but most are confined to a small region that can be evaluated both by Southern blot hybridization and by PCR.[155, 156]

The molecular characterization of translocations involving *BCL-6* is still incomplete at this time. The product of this gene appears to be a transcriptional repressor normally expressed in B lymphocytes of lymph node germinal centers.[157–160] The gene partner to which *BCL-6* DNA becomes joined is variable, including at least 10 sites within the genome in addition to the three immunoglobulin genes. Recombination occurs primarily within the 5′ portion of the *BCL-6* gene, effectively removing the first exon (which is noncoding) and putting the remaining part of the gene under the control of the promoter from the partner gene. Additionally, there is evidence that in all translocations, *BCL-6* acquires point mutations similar to those associated with somatic hypermutation of rearranged immunoglobulin genes.[161] Cases containing translocations involving this gene may have a better prognosis than other diffuse large cell lymphomas.[162] The clustering of most breakpoints within a single intron suggests that Southern blot hybridization should detect many translocations involving *BCL-6*.[163] However, the promiscuity of the translocations with respect to partner genes probably precludes application of PCR. Cases of large cell lymphoma lacking translocations of this gene may still have point mutations, possibly expanding the relevance of *BCL-6* as a diagnostic marker, if good screening methods for base substitutions can be developed.

The only common and consistent translocation in T-lineage lymphomas, the t(2;5)(p23;q35), joins the 5′ portion of the *NPM* gene to the 3′ portion of the *ALK* gene.[164] The result is a chimeric protein with the amino terminus of a gene coding for a nucleolar phosphoprotein and a carboxy terminus of a gene coding for a previously unknown protein tyrosine kinase. Replacement of the 5′ part of the *ALK* gene

switches transcription regulation of the catalytic sequences of *ALK* to the *NPM* promoter, thereby apparently causing heterotopic expression of this kinase, which is not normally present in T lymphocytes. Furthermore, the structural alteration of *ALK* may redirect the phosphorylation to abnormal substrates.

Experience with the detection of t(2;5)(p23;q35) in anaplastic T-cell lymphoma has so far been that the breakpoints in *NPM* and *ALK* are tightly clustered and that the translocation can be identified in most cases containing a cytogenetic abnormality by both Southern blot hybridization and RT-PCR.[165–167] A matter of some controversy has been the amplification of products from the t(2;5)(p23;q35) by RT-PCR of RNA from tissues of Hodgkin's disease. More recent data suggest that the t(2;5)(p23;q35) is restricted to anaplastic T-cell lymphoma and that positive results reported in earlier studies of RT-PCR in Hodgkin's disease were due to artifact or errors in histologic diagnosis.

VIRAL GENOMES

Three viruses have potential diagnostic relevance to lymphoma: EBV; human T-cell leukemia/lymphoma virus, type I (HTLV-I); and human herpesvirus, type 8 (HHV-8).[168] The lymphomas associated with these viruses and the state of the genome in latently infected cells are described in Table 7–2.

The mechanisms by which these viruses contribute to the malignant transformation of cells in lymphoma are reviewed elsewhere in this volume. Briefly, EBV DNA is maintained in the nuclei of latently infected cells as extracellular DNA circles, or episomes, of about 150 kb. These episomes express five genes for nuclear antigens (EBNAs) and latent membrane protein (LMP1) that appear to promote cellular proliferation.[169] EBNAs are transcriptional activators, the function of which requires the DNA binding capacity of a coactivator, RBPJκ (also called CBP-1).[170] LMP1 is an integral plasma membrane protein that forms aggregates with itself and TRAF1 and TRAF2 cytoplasmic proteins.[171, 172] TRAF2 possesses a kinase activity that phosphorylates IκB

Table 7–2. Viruses Associated with Tumor Cells in Lymphomas

Virus	Lymphoma	Lineage	Incidence (%)	Status of Genome in Infected Cells
Epstein-Barr (EBV)	Burkitt's (endemic)	B	>95	Mostly episomal DNA; occasionally integrated into the host cell genome
	Burkitt's (sporadic)	B	30	
	Immunosuppressed transplant recipients (various histologies)	Mostly B	>80	
	AIDS-associated			
	Burkitt's-like	B	100	
	DLCL	B	70	
	Hodgkin's disease	?	20–50	Episomal DNA in Reed-Sternberg cell
Human T-cell leukemia/lymphoma, type I (HTLV-I)	Adult T-cell lymphoma	T	100	Integrated DNA provirus
Human herpesvirus, type 8 (HHV-8)	Body-cavity–based lymphoma (AIDS-associated)	B	100	Probably episomal DNA
	Multicentric Castleman's disease	B		
	AIDS-associated		100	
	Non-AIDS-associated		50	

AIDS, acquired immunodeficiency syndrome; DLCL, diffuse large cell lymphoma.

proteins, which then release active NFκB, a transcriptional activator that regulates a series of growth-related genes.

Despite the small size and simple structure of the HTLV-I genome (8.6 kb; five genes), the oncogenic mechanism of this virus in adult T-cell lymphoma (ATL) is still not well understood.[173] Several processes may be involved. After infection of the cell, the RNA genome is converted into a double-stranded DNA, or provirus, which inserts at random sites into the host genome, where it continues to express viral proteins for the life of the cell. One of these proteins, tax, appears to interact with numerous transcription factors to activate many cellular genes, including the gene for interleukin-2 (IL-2) and its receptor.[174–176] The latter proteins, in turn, may act in an autocrine fashion to stimulate the proliferation of infected cells. Autocrine-stimulated growth does not account completely for ATL, however, because only low levels of tax are expressed by T lymphocytes in the premalignant carrier stages of the disease. Presumably, in addition to HTLV-I infection, other mutations within infected cells are necessary for complete malignant transformation. Other tax-independent mechanisms have also been suggested for HTLV-I–mediated lymphomagenesis, including up-regulation of the Jak-STAT system of transcriptional activation by events not fully elucidated at this time[177] and mitogenic stimulation of T lymphocytes by virion envelope proteins.[178]

HHV-8 has only recently been discovered by the analysis of DNA in the tissues of Kaposi's sarcoma from patients with AIDS.[179] Subsequently, DNA sequences of this virus were found in two rare lymphoproliferative disorders, body-cavity–based lymphoma of the peritoneal and pleural spaces, a condition encountered so far only in AIDS patients,[180] and multicentric Castleman's disease.[181] Little is known of its biologic aspects, except that its DNA resembles that of EBV and herpesviruses and that it is lymphotropic, as evidenced by the identification of viral sequences within latently infected lymphocytes.[182]

From the technical point of view, viral genomes in general represent ideal markers for detection. Unlike the other diagnostic markers reviewed in this chapter, the viral genomes represent entirely foreign nucleotide sequences rather than rearrangements of sequences native to normal human cells. Therefore, all methods for detecting specific nucleic acids are potentially applicable to these markers, although to the extent that FISH may be ever be used for this purpose, HTLV-I genomes would be somewhat smaller targets than are ordinarily investigated by this technique. Additionally, immunologic detection of viral antigens offers an often simpler alternative to nucleic acid–based techniques to reveal the presence of infected cells, combining the advantages of direct histologic correlation.

The major qualification in using viral genomes as markers is that the presence of virus is not synonymous with lymphoma, since viral infection is apparently not sufficient for complete transformation of the cells. Viral infection precedes lymphomagenesis, and at least in the examples of EBV and HTLV-I, most carriers never develop those tumors with which the viruses are associated. Therefore, highly sensitive, nonquantitative detection methods, such as procedures using straightforward, nonquantitative PCR, run the risk of producing positive results that may mistakenly be interpreted as indicating malignancy. One solution to this problem is to rely on methods, such as

Southern blot hybridization, which only detect large numbers of infected cells within a lesion, consistent with the presence of a virus-associated tumor. A second solution is to use viral genomes as markers of clonality, which can be done with both EBV and HTLV-I, and possibly with HHV-8 as well.

Since HTLV-I proviruses integrate virtually randomly into the DNA of the host cell, a malignant clone of T lymphocytes carries one or a few copies of the proviral DNA at uniform sites unique to the transformed progenitor cell from which the tumor arose.[183] The uniformity of insertion sites in the cells of a biopsy sample can be assessed by Southern blot hybridization using probes for the HTLV-I sequence and restriction enzymes that create fragments including host DNA sequence and sequence complementary to the probe. In this situation, a specimen in which more than 1% to 5% of cells consist of malignant T lymphocytes containing ATL yields one or more discrete bands, depending on how many proviruses are present within each cell.

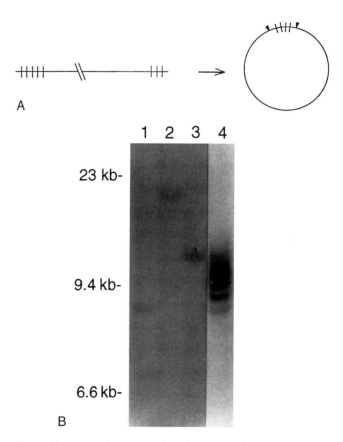

Figure 7–9. Detection of clonal proliferations of Epstein-Barr virus (EBV)-infected cells by analysis of the terminal repeat region of EBV DNA. *A,* Schematic representation of circularization of the linear EBV genome on entry into the cell, with inclusion of variable numbers of terminal repeat sequences in the resulting episome of latently infected cells. The *arrowheads* indicate positions of cleavage by a restriction enzyme such as Bam HI at sites flanking the region of terminal repeats within the episome. *B,* Southern blot autoradiogram of DNA from four tissue specimens. The DNA was digested with Bam HI and hybridized with a probe containing sequences of the terminal repeat. The positions to which marker fragments of defined size migrated within the gel are indicated. Cases 1 to 3 were from lymphomas containing EBV DNA; case 4 was from a case of fatal mononucleosis. The single band obtained in cases 1 to 3 reflects a monoclonal population of EBV-infected cells.

EBV genomes introduced from the infecting virions into the cell are originally linear but are quickly circularized by ligation of the two free ends (Fig. 7–9). These circles are maintained within the nuclei of infected cells as extrachromosome episomes that replicate along with the cell cycle of the host. The linear genomes of different virions are polymorphic with respect to the number of 500 base pair–long repeated sequences at both ends of the DNA.[184] Circularization of the genome is accomplished by homologous recombination at some point among the repeated sequences, leaving different numbers of repeated sequences in each episome. Since most cells are infected by a single virion, the number of repeated sequences within an infected cell marks that cell. Since the viral DNA within a clone of cells is relatively structurally stable throughout successive replicative cycles, the number of repeated sequences within the episome is characteristic of that clone, even though an episome may be represented by 30 or more copies per infected cell. Therefore, the clonality of the infected cells within a biopsy sample can be determined by Southern blot hybridization using a probe complementary to the terminal genomic repeats of EBV and restriction enzymes that cut within EBV DNA flanking the region of the fused repeats.[185, 186] A clone of infected lymphocytes is identified by a discrete band in the autoradiogram at a position reflecting the number of repeats within the episome DNA of that clone. Usually only one band is seen; however, occasionally several bands are found, presumably because of homologous recombinations between repeated sequences in some progeny cells within the clone. In contrast, normal tissues produce no bands, and polyclonal infected tissues, such as those in some cases of early posttransplant lymphoproliferative disorders or fatal infectious mononucleosis, produce a ladder of bands, with each band separated by a distance corresponding to the length of a single terminal repeat.

REFERENCES

1. Sklar JL, Costa JC: Principles of cancer management: Molecular pathology. *In* DeVita VTJ, Hellman S, Rosenberg SA (eds): Cancer: Principles and Practice of Oncology, 5th ed. Philadelpia, Lippincott-Raven, 1997, p 259.
2. Sklar J, Weiss L, Cleary ML: Diagnostic molecular biology of non-Hodgkin's lymphomas. *In* Berard CW, Dorfman RF (eds): Malignant Lymphoma. Baltimore, Williams & Wilkins, 1987, p 204.
3. Sklar J, Weiss LM: Applications of antigen receptor gene rearrangements to the diagnosis and characterization of lymphoid neoplasms. Ann Rev Med 1988; 39:315.
4. Sklar J: Antigen receptor genes: Structure, function, and techniques for analysis of their rearrangements. *In* Knowles DM (ed): Neoplastic Hematology. Baltimore, Williams & Wilkins, 1992, p 215.
5. Hasemann CA, Capra JD: Immunoglobulins: Structure and function. *In* Paul WE (ed): Fundamental Immunology. New York, Raven Press, 1989, p 209.
6. Abbas AK, Lichtman AH, Pober JS: Cellular and Molecular Immunology. Philadelphia, WB Saunders, 1991.
7. Alt F, Bothwell ALM, Knapp M, et al: Synthesis of secreted and membrane-bound immunoglobulin mu heavy chains is directed by mRNAs that differ at their 3' ends. Cell 1980; 20:293.
8. Rogers J, Earl P, Carter C, et al: Two mRNAs with different 3' ends encode membrane-bound and secreted forms of immunoglobulin mu chain. Cell 1980; 20:330.
9. Honjo T, Shimizu A, Yaoita Y: Constant-region genes of the immunoglobulin heavy chain and the molecular mechanism of class switching. *In* Honjo T, Alt FW, Rabbitts TH (eds): Immunoglobulin Genes. San Diego, Academic Press, 1989, p 123.
10. Hedrick SM: T-lymphocyte receptors. In Paul WE (ed): Fundamental Immunology. New York, Raven Press, 1989, p 291.
11. Hozumi N, Tonegawa S: Evidence for somatic rearrangement of immunoglobulin genes coding for variable and constant regions. Proc Natl Acad Sci U S A 1976; 73:3628.
12. Bernard O, Hozumi N, Tonegawa S: Sequences of mouse immunoglobulin light chain genes before and after somatic changes. Cell 1978; 15:1133.
13. Seidman J, Leder P: The arrangement and rearrangement of antibody genes. Nature 1978; 276:790.
14. Davis MM, Calame K, Early PW, et al: An immunoglobulin heavy-chain gene is formed by at least two recombinational events. Nature 1980; 283:733.
15. Alt F, Rosenberg N, Lewis S, et al: Organization and reorganization of immunoglobulin genes in A-MuLV-transformed cells: Rearrangement of heavy but not light chain genes. Cell 1981; 127:381.
16. Tonegawa S: Somatic generation of antibody diversity. Nature 1983; 302:575.
17. Alt FW, Blackwell TK, DePinko RA, et al: Regulation of genome rearrangement events during lymphocyte differentiation. Immunol Rev 1986; 89:5.
18. Early P, Huang H, Davis M, et al: An immunoglobulin heavy chain variable region gene is generated from three segments of DNA: V_H, D, and J_H. Cell 1980; 19:981.
19. Okazaki K, Davis MM, Sakano H: T-cell receptor β gene sequences in the circular DNA of thymocyte nuclei: Direct evidence for intramolecular DNA deletion in V-D-J joining. Cell 1987; 49:477.
20. Alt FW, Baltimore D: Joining of immunoglobulin heavy chain gene segments: Implications from a chromosome with evidence of three D-J_H fusions. Proc Natl Acad Sci U S A 1982; 167:4118.
21. Desiderio SV, Yancopoulos GD, Paskind M, et al: Insertion of N regions into heavy-chain genes is correlated with expression of terminal deoxytransferase in B cells. Nature 1984; 311:752.
22. Landau NR, Schatz DG, Rosa M, Baltimore D: Increased frequency of N-region insertion in a murine pre-B-cell line infected with a terminal deoxynucleotidyl transferase retroviral expression vector. Mol Cell Biol 1987; 7:3237.
23. Alt FW, Yancopoulos GD, Blackwell TK, et al: Ordered rearrangement of immunoglobulin heavy chain variable region segments. EMBO J 1984; 3:1209.
24. Korsmeyer SJ, Hieter PA, Ravetch JV, et al: Developmental hierarchy of immunoglobulin gene rearrangements in human leukemic pre-B-cells. Proc Natl Acad Sci U S A 1981; 78:7096.
25. Hieter PA, Korsmeyer SJ, Waldmann TA, Leder P: Human immunoglobulin κ light-chain genes are deleted or rearranged in λ-producing B cells. Nature 1981; 290:368.
26. Korsmeyer SJ, Hieter PA, Sharrow SO, et al: Normal human B cells display ordered light chain gene rearrangements and deletions. J Exp Med 1982; 156:975.
27. Coleclough C, Perry RP, Karjalainen K, Weigert M: Aberrant rearrangements contribute significantly to the allelic exclusion of immunoglobulin gene expression. Nature 1981; 290:372.
28. Chien Y, Iwashima M, Wettstein DA, et al: T-cell receptor δ gene rearrangements in early thymocytes. Nature 1987; 330:722.
29. Born W, Yage J, Palmer E, et al: Rearrangement of T-cell receptor β-chain genes during T-cell development. Proc Natl Acad Sci U S A 1985; 82:2925.
30. Born W, Rathbun G, Tucker P, et al: Synchronized rearrangement of T-cell γ and β chain genes in fetal thymocyte development. Science 1985; 234:479.
31. Raulet DH, Garman RD, Saito H, Tonegawa S: Developmental regulation of T-cell receptor gene expression. Nature 1985; 314:103.
32. Snodgrass HR, Dembic Z, Steinmetz M, Von Boehmer H: Expression of T-cell antigen receptor genes during fetal development in the thymus. Nature 1985; 315:232.
33. Pardoll DM, Fowlkes BJ, Bluestone JA, et al: Differential expression of two distinct T-cell receptors during thymocyte development. Nature 1987; 326:79.
34. Havran WL, Allison JP: Developmentally ordered appearance of thymocyte development. Nature 1987; 335:443.
35. Berek C, Milstein C: Mutation drift and repertoire shift in the maturation of the immune response. Immunol Rev 1987; 96:23.
36. French DL, Laskov R, Scharff MD: The role of somatic hypermutation in the generation of antibody diversity. Science 1989; 244:1152.
37. Oettinger MA, Schata DG, Gorka C, Baltimore D: RAG-1 and RAG-2, adjacent genes that synergistically activate V(D)J recombination. Science 1990; 248:1517.

38. van Gent D, McBlane J, Ramsden D, et al: Initiation of V(D)J recombination in a cell-free system. Cell 1995; 81:925.

39. Hikida M, Mori M, Takai T, et al: Reexpression of RAG-1 and RAG-2 genes in activated mature mouse B cells. Science 1997; 274:2092.

40. Han S, Zheng B, Schatz DG, et al: Neoteny in lymphocytes: *Rag1* and *Rag2* expression in germinal center B cells. Science 1997; 274:2094.

41. Akira S, Okazaki K, Sakano H: Two pairs of recombination signals are sufficient to cause immunoglobulin V-(D)-J joining. Science 1987; 238:1134.

42. Kleinfield R, Hardy RR, Tarlinton D, et al: Recombination between an expressed immunoglobulin heavy-chain gene and a germline variable gene segment in a Ly-1+ B-cell lymphoma. Nature 1986; 322:843.

43. Reth MG, Jackson S, Alt FW: $V_H DJ_H$ formation and DJ_H replacement during pre-B differentiation: Nonrandom usage of gene segments. EMBO J 1986; 5:2131.

44. Cleary ML, Chao J, Warnke R, Sklar J: Immunoglobulin gene rearrangement as a diagnostic criterion of B-cell lymphoma. Proc Natl Acad Sci U S A 1984; 81:593.

45. Arnold A, Cossman J, Bakhshi A, et al: Immunoglobulin-gene rearrangements as unique clonal markers in human lymphoid neoplasms. N Engl J Med 1983; 309:1593.

46. Bertness V, Kirsch I, Hollis G, et al: T-cell receptor gene rearrangements as clinical markers of human T-cell lymphomas. N Engl J Med 1985; 313:534.

47. Weiss LM, Hu E, Wood GS, et al: Clonal rearrangements of T-cell receptor genes in mycosis fungoides and dermatopathic lymphadenopathy. N Engl J Med 1985; 313:539.

48. Flug F, Pelicci PG, Bonetti R, et al: T-cell receptor gene rearrangements as markers of lineage and clonality in T-cell neoplasms. Proc Natl Acad Sci U S A 1985; 82:3460.

49. O'Connor NTJ, Wainscoat JS, Weatherall DJ, et al: Rearrangement of the T-cell-receptor β-chain gene in the diagnosis of lymphoproliferative disorders. Lancet 1985; 1:1295.

50. Waldmann TA, Davis MM, Bongiovanni KF, Korsmeyer SJ: Rearrangements of genes for the antigen receptor on T cells as markers of lineage and clonality in human lymphoid neoplasms. N Engl J Med 1985; 313:776.

51. Minden MD, Toyonaga B, Ha K, et al: Somatic rearrangement of the T-cell antigen receptor gene in human T-cell malignancies. Proc Natl Acad Sci U S A 1985; 82:1224.

52. Korsmeyer SJ: Antigen receptor genes as molecular markers of lymphoid neoplasms. J Clin Invest 1987; 79:1291.

53. Dubeau L, Weinberg K, Jones PA, Nichols PW: Studies on immunoglobulin gene rearrangement in formalin-fixed, paraffin-embedded pathology specimens. Am J Pathol 1988; 180:588.

54. Wu AM, Ben-Ezra J, Winberg C, et al: Analysis of antigen receptor gene rearrangements in ethanol and formaldehyde-fixed, paraffin-embedded specimens. Lab Invest 1990; 63:107.

55. Siminovitch KA, Bakhshi A, Goldman P, Korsmeyer SJ: A uniform deleting element mediates the loss of kappa genes in human B cells. Nature 1985; 316:260.

56. Weiss ML, Strickler J, Dorfman R, et al: Clonal T-cell populations in angioimmunoblastic lymphadenopathy and angioimmunoblastic lymphadenopathy-like lymphoma. Am J Pathol 1986; 122:392.

57. Sigal SH, Saul SH, Auerbach HE, et al: Gastric small lymphocytic proliferation with immunoglobulin gene rearrangement in pseudolymphoma versus lymphoma. Gastroenterology 1989; 97:195.

58. Knowles DM, Athan E, Ubriaco A, et al: Extranodal noncutaneous lymphoid hyperplasias represent a continuous spectrum of B-cell neoplasia: Demonstration by molecular genetic analysis. Blood 1989; 73:1635.

59. Wechsler J, Bagot M, Henni T, Gaulard P: Cutaneous pseudolymphomas: Immunophenotypical and immunogenotypical studies. Curr Probl Dermatol 1990; 19:183.

60. Cleary ML, Warnke R, Sklar J: Monoclonality of lymphoproliferative lesions in cardiac transplant recipients: Clonal analysis based on immunoglobulin gene rearrangements. N Engl J Med 1984; 310:477.

61. Cleary ML, Wood GS, Warnke R, et al: Immunoglobulin gene rearrangement in hairy cell leukemia. Blood 1984; 64:99.

62. Cleary ML, Trela M, Weiss LM, et al: Frequent immunoglobulin and T-cell receptor gene rearrangements in "histiocytic" neoplasms. Am J Pathol 1985; 121:369.

63. Weiss LM, Wood G, Treis M, et al: Clonal T-cell populations in lymphomatoid papulosis: Evidence for a lymphoproliferative origin for a clinically benign disease. N Engl J Med 1986; 315:475.

64. Kadin ME, Vonderheid EC, Sako D, et al: Clonal composition of T cells in lymphomatoid papulosis. Am J Pathol 1987; 126:13.

65. Foa R, Pelicci PG, Migone M, et al: Analysis of T-cell receptor beta chain (T-beta) gene rearrangements demonstrates the monoclonal nature of T-cell chronic lymphoproliferative disorders. Blood 1986; 67:247.

66. Fishleder A, Tubbs R, Hesse B, Levine H: Uniform detection of immunoglobulin gene rearrangements in benign lymphoepithelial lesions. N Engl J Med 1987; 316:1118.

67. Hanson CA, Frizzera G, Patton DF, et al: Clonal rearrangement for immunoglobulin and T-cell receptor genes in systemic Castleman's disease: Association with Epstein-Barr virus. Am J Pathol 1988; 131:84.

68. Weiss LM, Picker LJ, Grogan TM, et al: Absence of clonal beta and gamma T-cell receptor gene rearrangements in a subset of peripheral T-cell lymphomas. Am J Pathol 1988; 130:436.

69. Ferry JA, Sklar J, Zukerberg LR, Harris NL: Nasal lymphoma: A clinicopathologic study with immunophenotypic and genotypic analysis. Am J Pathol 1991; 15:268.

70. Emile J-F, Boulland M-L, Haioun C, et al: CD5− and CD56+ T-cell receptor silent peripheral T-cell lymphomas are natural killer cell lymphomas. Blood 1996; 87:1466.

71. Jaffe E: Classification of natural killer (NK) cell and NK-like T-cell malignancies. Blood 1996; 87:1207.

72. Sklar J, Cleary ML, Thielemanns K, et al: Biclonal B-cell lymphoma. N Engl J Med 1984; 311:20.

73. Siegelman M, Cleary R, Warnke R, Sklar J: Frequent biclonality and immunoglobulin gene alterations among B cell lymphomas that show multiple histologic forms. J Exp Med 1985; 161:850.

74. Cleary ML, Galili N, Trela M, et al: Single cell origin of bigenotypic and biphenotypic B-cell proliferations in human follicular lymphomas. Blood 1988; 72:349.

75. Cleary M, Meeker T, Levy S, et al: Clustering of extensive somatic mutations in the variable region of an immunoglobulin heavy chain gene from a human B-cell lymphoma. Cell 1986; 44:97.

76. Kitchingman GR, Mirro J, Stass S, et al: Biologic and prognostic significance of the presence of more than two mu heavy-chain genes in childhood acute lymphoblastic leukemia of B precursor cell origin. Blood 1986; 67:698.

77. Bird J, Galili N, Link M, et al: Continuing rearrangement but absence of somatic hypermutation in immunoglobulin genes in human B-cell precursor leukemias. J Exp Med 1988; 168:229.

78. Davi F, Gocke C, Smith S, Sklar J: Lymphoid stem cell origin of human precursor B-lineage acute leukemia. Blood 1996; 88:609.

79. Hu E, Weiss LM, Warnke R, Sklar J: Non-Hodgkin's lymphoma containing both B- and T-cell clones. Blood 1987; 70:287.

80. Wasserman R, Yamada M, Ito Y, et al: VH gene rearrangement events can modify the immunoglobulin heavy chain during progression of B-lineage acute lymphoblastic leukemia. Blood 1992; 79:223.

81. Cleary ML, Sklar J: Lymphoproliferative disorders in cardiac transplant recipients are multicellular lymphomas. Lancet 1984; 2:489.

82. Pelicci P-G, Knowles DMI, Arlin ZA, et al: Multiple monoclonal B-cell expansions and c-*myc* oncogene rearrangements in acquired immune deficiency syndrome–related lymphoproliferative disorders. J Exp Med 1986; 164:2049.

83. Shearer WT, Ritz J, Finegold MJ, et al: Epstein-Barr virus–associated B-cell proliferations of diverse clonal origins after bone marrow transplantation in a 12-year-old patient with severe combined immunodeficiency. N Engl J Med 1985; 312:1151.

84. Seiden MV, Sklar J: Virally induced B cell tumors. *In* Rich RR (ed): Clinical Immunology. St. Louis, CV Mosby, 1996, p 1768.

85. Ha K, Minden M, Hozumi N, Gelfand EW: Immunoglobulin gene rearrangement in acute myelogenous leukemia. Cancer Res 1984; 44:4658.

86. Kitchingman GR, Rovigatti U, Mauer AM, et al: Rearrangement of immunoglobulin heavy chain genes in T-cell acute lymphoblastic leukemia. Blood 1985; 654:725.

87. Greaves MF, Chan LC, Furley SM, et al: Lineage promiscuity in hemopoietic differentiation and leukemia. Blood 1986; 67:1.

88. Cheng G, Minden M, Toyonaga B, et al: T-cell receptor and immunoglobulin gene rearrangements in acute myeloblastic leukemia. J Exp Med 1986; 163:414.

89. Greaves MF, Furley AJW, Chain LC, et al: Inappropriate rearrangement of immunoglobulin and T-cell receptor genes. Immunol Today 1987; 8:115.

90. Tycko B, Palmer JD, Link MP, et al: Polymerase chain reaction amplification of rearranged antigen receptor genes using junction-

specific oligonucleotides: Possible application for detection of minimal residual disease in acute lymphoblastic leukemia. Cancer Cells 1989; 7:47.

91. McCarthy KP, Sloane JP, Wiedemann LM: Rapid method for distinguishing clonal from polyclonal B-cell populations in surgical biopsy specimens. J Clin Pathol 1990; 43:429.

92. Trainor KJ, Brisco MJ, Story CJ, Morley AA: Monoclonality in B-lymphoproliferative disorders detected at the DNA level. Blood 1990; 75:2220.

93. Wan JH, Sykes PJ, Orell SR, Morley AA: Rapid method for detecting monoclonality in B-cell lymphoma in lymph node aspirates using the polymerase chain reaction. J Clin Pathol 1992; 45:420.

94. Segal GH, Wittwer CT, Fishleder AJ, et al: Identification of monoclonal B-cell populations by rapid-cycle polymerase chain reaction: A practical screening method for the detection of immunoglobulin gene rearrangements. Am J Pathol 1992; 141:1291.

95. Inghirami G, Szabolcs MJ, Yee HT, et al: Detection of immunoglobulin gene rearrangement of B-cell non-Hodgkin's lymphomas and leukemias in fresh, unfixed and formalin-fixed, paraffin-embedded tissue by polymerase chain reaction. Lab Invest 1993; 68:746.

96. Bourguin A, Tung RM, Galili N, Sklar J: Rapid, nonradioactive detection of clonal T-cell—receptor gene rearrangements in lymphoid neoplasms. Proc Natl Acad Sci U S A 1990; 87:8536.

97. Humphries CG, Shen A, Kuziel WA, et al: A new human immunoglobulin VH family preferentially rearranged in immature B-cell tumors. Nature 1988; 331:446.

98. Pratt LF, Rassenti L, Larrick J, et al: Ig V region gene expression in small lymphocytic lymphoma with little or no somatic hypermutation. J Immunol 1989; 143:699.

99. Wan JH, Trainor KJ, Brisco MJ, Morley AA: Monoclonality in B-cell lymphoma detected in paraffin wax–embedded sections using the polymerase chain reaction. J Clin Pathol 1990; 43:888.

100. Wood GS, Tung RM, Crooks CF, et al: Cutaneous lymphoid infiltrates: Analysis of T-cell receptor γ gene rearrangements by polymerase chain reaction and denaturing gradient gel electrophoresis (PCR/DGGE). J Invest Dermatol 1994; 103:34.

101. Weiss LM, Warnke RA, Sklar J: Clonal antigen receptor gene rearrangements and Ebstein-Barr viral DNA in tissues of Hodgkin's disease. Hematol Oncol 1988; 6:233.

102. Kuppers R, Rajewsky K, Zhao M, et al: Hodgkin disease: Hodgkin and Reed-Sternberg cells picked from histological sections show clonal immunoglobulin gene rearrangements and appear to be derived from B cells at various stages of development. Proc Natl Acad Sci U S A 1994; 91:10962.

103. Kamel OW, Chang PP, Hsu FJ, et al: Clonal VDJ recombination of the immunoglobulin heavy chain gene by PCR in classical Hodgkin's disease. Am J Clin Pathol 1995; 104:419.

104. Emmert-Buck MR, Bonner RF, Smith PD, et al: Laser capture microdissection. Science 1996; 274:998.

105. D'Auriol L, Macintyre E, Galibert F, Sigaux F: In vitro amplification of T-cell gene rearrangements: A new tool for the assessment of minimal residual disease in acute lymphoblastic leukemias. Leukemia 1989; 3:155.

106. Yamada M, Hudson S, Tournay O, et al: Detection of minimal disease in hematopoietic malignancies of B-cell lineage by using third-complementary–determining region (CDR-III)-specific probes. Proc Natl Acad Sci U S A 1989; 86:5123.

107. Hansen-Hagge TE, Yokota S, Bartram CR: Detection of minimal residual disease in acute lymphoblastic leukemia by in vitro amplification of rearranged T-cell receptor delta sequences. Blood 1989; 74:1762.

108. Veelken H, Tycko B, Sklar J: Sensitive detection of clonal antigen receptor gene rearrangements for the diagnosis and monitoring of lymphoid neoplasia by a PCR-mediated ribonuclease protection assay. Blood 1991; 78:1318.

109. Herrera ML, Reynolds C, Mashal R, Sklar J: Unpublished results.

110. Tycko B, Ritz J, Sallan S, Sklar J: Changing antigen receptor gene rearrangements in a case of early pre-B cell leukemia: Evidence for a malignant lymphoid stem cell and its implications for monitoring residual disease. Blood 1992; 79:481.

111. Steward C, Goulden F, Katz F, et al: A polymerase chain reaction study of the stability of Ig heavy-chain and T-cell receptor delta gene rearrangements between presentation and relapse of childhood B-lineage acute lymphoblastic leukemia. Blood 1994; 83:1355.

112. Beishuizen A, Verhoeven M, van Wering E, et al: Analysis of Ig and T-cell receptor genes in 40 childhood acute lymphoblastic leukemias at diagnosis and subsequent relapse: Implications for the detection of minimal residual disease by polymerase chain reaction analysis. Blood 1994; 83:2238.

113. Yamada M, Wasserman R, Lange B, et al: Minimal residual disease in childhood B-lineage lymphoblastic leukemia: Persistence of leukemic cells during the first months of treatment. N Engl J Med 1990; 323:448.

114. Herrera ML, Reynolds C, Sklar J: Unpublished results.

115. Offit K, Jhanwar SC, Ladanyi M, et al: Cytogenetic analysis of 434 consecutively ascertained specimens of non-Hodgkin's lymphoma: Correlations between recurrent aberrations, histology, and exposure to cytotoxic treatment. Genes Chromosomes Cancer 1991; 3:189.

116. Rabbitts TH: Chromosomal translocations in human cancer. Nature 1994; 372:143.

117. Weiss LM, Warnke R, Sklar J, Cleary ML: Molecular analysis of the t(14;18) chromosomal translocation in malignant lymphoma. N Engl J Med 1987; 317:1185.

118. Lee M-S, Chang K-S, Cabanillas F, et al: Detection of minimal residual cell carrying the t(14;18) by DNA sequence amplification. Science 1987; 237:175.

119. Kawasaki ES, Clark SS, Coyne MY, et al: Diagnosis of chronic myelogenous leukemia and acute leukemia by detection of leukemia-specific mRNA sequences amplified in vitro. Proc Natl Acad Sci U S A 1988; 85:5689.

120. Tkachuk D, Westbrook C, Andreeff M, et al: Detection of *bcr-abl* fusion in chronic myelogenous leukemia by in situ hybridization. Science 1990; 250:559.

121. Tsujimoto Y, Gorham J, Cossman J, et al: The t(14;18) chromosome translocation involved in B-cell malignancies results from mistakes in V-D-J joining. Science 1985; 229:1390.

122. Haluska FG, Finger S, Tsijimoto Y, Croce CM: The t(8;14) chromosomal translocation occurring in B-cell malignancies results from mistakes in V-D-J joining. Nature 1986; 324:158.

123. Tycko B, Reynolds TC, Smith SD, Sklar J: Consistent breakage between consensus recombinase heptamers of chromosome 9 DNA in a recurrent chromosomal translocation of human T-cell leukemia. J Exp Med 1989; 169:369.

124. Tycko B, Sklar J: Chromosomal translocation in lymphoid neoplasia: A reappraisal of the recombinase model. Cancer Cells 1990; 2:1.

125. Tycko B, Palmer JD, Sklar J: T-cell receptor gene trans-rearrangements: Chimeric delta-gamma genes in normal lymphoid tissues. Science 1989; 245:1242.

126. Croce CM, Nowell PC: Molecular basis of B-cell neoplasia. Blood 1985; 65:1.

127. Pelicci P-G, Knowles DMI, McGrath I, et al: Chromosomal breakpoints and structural alterations of the c-*myc* locus differ in endemic and sporadic forms of Burkitt lymphoma. Proc Natl Acad Sci U S A 1986; 83:2984.

128. Showe LC, Croce CM: The role of chromosomal translocation in B- and T-cell neoplasia. Annu Rev Immunol 1987; 5:253.

129. Tsujimoto Y, Finger LR, Yunis J, et al: Cloning of the chromosome breakpoints of neoplastic B cells with the t(14;18) chromosomal translocation. Science 1984; 226:1097.

130. Cleary ML, Sklar J: Nucleotide sequence of a t(14;18) chromosomal bp in follicular lymphoma and demonstration of a breakpoint cluster region near a transcriptionally active locus on chromosome 18. Proc Natl Acad Sci U S A 1985; 82:7439.

131. Bakhshi A, Jensen JP, Goldman P, et al: Cloning the chromosome bp of t(14;18) in human lymphomas: Clustering around JH on chromosome 14 and near a transcriptional unit on chromosome 18. Cell 1985; 41:899.

132. Cleary ML, Smith SD, Sklar J: Cloning and structural analysis of cDNAs for the *bcl-2* and a hybrid *bcl-2*/immunoglobulin transcript resulting from t(14;18) chromosomal translocation. Cell 1986; 47:19.

133. Oltvai ZN, Milliman CL, Korsmeyer SJ: *Bcl-2* heterodimerizes in vivo with a conserved homolog, Bax, that accelerates programmed cell death. Cell 1993; 74:609.

134. Vaux DL, Cory S, Adams JM: *Bcl-2* gene promotes hematopoietic cell survival and cooperates with c-*MYC* to immortalize pre-B cells. Nature 1988; 335:440.

135. Nunez G, Hockenbery D, McDonnel TM, et al: *Bcl-2* maintains B-cell memory. Nature 1991; 353:71.

136. Cleary ML, Galili N, Sklar J: Detection of a second t(14;18) breakpoint cluster region in follicular lymphoma. J Exp Med 1986; 164:305.

137. Crescenzi M, Seto M, Herzig GP, et al: Thermostable DNA polymerase chain amplification of t(14;18) chromosome breakpoints and detection of minimal residual disease. Proc Natl Acad Sci U S A 1988; 85:4869.

138. Ngan BY, Nourse J, Cleary ML: Detection of chromosomal translocation t(14;18) within the minor cluster region of *bcl-2* by polymerase chain reaction and direct genomic sequencing of the enzymatically amplified DNA in follicular lymphomas. Blood 1989; 73:1759.

139. Gribben J, Freedman A, Neuberg D, et al: Immunologic purging of marrow assessed by PCR before autologous bone marrow transplantation for B-cell lymphoma. N Engl J Med 1991; 325:1525.

140. Limpens J, de Jong D, Voetdijk AMH, et al: Translocation t(14;18) in benign B lymphocytes. Blood 1990; 76:2379.

141. Aster JC, Kobayashi Y, Shiota M, et al: Detection of the t(14;18) at similar frequencies in follicular lymphoid hyperplasia from American and Japanese patients. Am J Pathol 1992; 141:291.

142. Vaux DL, Cory S, Adams JM: Bcl-2 gene promotes hemopoietic cell survival and cooperates with c-myc to immortalize pre-B cells. Nature 1988; 335:440.

143. McDonnell TJ, Deane N, Platt FM, et al: *bcl-2*-immunoglobulin transgenic mice demonstrate extended B-cell survival and follicular lymphoproliferation. Cell 1989; 57:79.

144. McDonnel TJ, Korsmeyer SL: Progression from lymphoid hyperplasia to high-grade lymphoma in mice transgenic for the t(14;18). Nature 1991; 349:254.

145. Dalla-Favera R, Bregni M, Erickson J, et al: Human c-*myc* oncogene is located on the region of chromosome 8 that is translocated in Burkitt lymphoma cells. Proc Natl Acad Sci U S A 1982; 79:7824.

146. Taub R, Kirsch I, Morton C, et al: Translocation of c-*myc* gene into the immunoglobulin heavy chain locus in human Burkitt lymphoma and murine plasmacytoma cells. Proc Natl Acad Sci U S A 1982; 79:7837.

147. Davis M, Malcom S, Rabbits TH: Chromosome translocations can occur on either side of the c-*myc* oncogene in Burkitt lymphoma cells. Nature 1984; 30:286.

148. Blackwood EM, Eisenman RN: Max: A helix-loop-helix zipper protein that forms a sequence-specific DNA binding complex with *myc*. Science 1991; 251:1211.

149. Amati B, Dalton S, Brooks MW, et al: Transcriptional activation by the human c-*myc* oncoprotein in yeast requires interaction with Max. Nature 1992; 359:423.

150. Ayer DE, Kretzner L, Eisenman RN: Mad: A heterodimeric partner for max that antagonizes *myc* transcriptional activity. Cell 1993; 72:211.

151. Zervos AS, Gyuris J, Brent R: Mxi1, a protein that specifically interacts with Max to bind Myc-Max recognition sites. Cell 1993; 72:223.

152. Tsujimoto Y, Yunis J, Onorato-Showe L, et al: Molecular cloning of the chromosomal breakpoint on chromosome 11 in human B-cell neoplasms with the t(11;14) chromosome translocation. Science 1984; 224:1403.

153. Motokura T, Bloom T, Goo KH, et al: A novel cyclin encoded by a *bcl-1*-linked candidate oncogene. Nature 1991; 350:512.

154. Rosenberg CL, Wong E, Petty EM, et al: PRAD1, a candidate *BCL1* oncogene: Mapping and expression in centrocytic lymphoma. Proc Natl Acad Sci U S A 1991; 88:9638.

155. Williams ME, Meeker TC, Swerdlow SH: Rearrangement of the chromosome 11 *bcl-1* locus in centrocytic lymphoma: Analysis with multiple breakpoint probes. Blood 1991; 78:493.

156. Rimokh R, Berger F, Delsol G, et al: Detection of the chromosomal translocation t(11;14) by polymerase chain reaction in mantle cell lymphomas. Blood 1994; 83:1871.

157. Ye BH, Rao PH, Chaganti RSK, Dalla-Favera R: Cloning of *BCL-6*, the locus involved in chromosome translocations affecting band 3q27 in B-cell lymphoma. Cancer Res 1993; 53:2732.

158. Ye BH, Lista F, Lo Coco F, et al: Alterations of *BCL-6*, a novel zinc-finger gene, in diffuse large cell lymphoma. Science 1993; 262:747.

159. Baron BW, Nucifora G, McNabe N, et al: Identification of the gene associated with the recurring chromosomal translocations t(3;14)(q27;q32) and t(3;22)(q27;q11) in B-cell lymphoma. Proc Natl Acad Sci U S A 1993; 90:5262.

160. Kerckaert J-P, Deweindt C, Tilly H, et al: *LAZ3*, a novel zinc-finger encoding gene, is disrupted by recurring chromosome 3q27 translocations in human lymphoma. Nat Genet 1993; 5:66.

161. Migliazza A, Martinotti S, Chen W, et al: Frequent somatic hypermutation of the 5′ noncoding region of the *BCL-6* gene in B-cell lymphoma. Proc Natl Acad Sci U S A 1995; 92:12520.

162. Offit K, Lo Coco F, Louie DC, et al: Rearrangements of the *bcl-6* gene as a prognostic marker in diffuse large cell lymphoma. N Engl J Med 1994; 331:74.

163. Lo Coco F, Ye BH, Lista F, et al: Rearrangements of the *BCL-6* gene in diffuse large cell non-Hodgkin's lymphoma. Blood 1994; 83:1757.

164. Morris SW, Kirstein MN, Valentine MB, et al: Fusion of a kinase gene, *ALK*, to a nucleolar protein gene, *NPM*, in non-Hodgkin's lymphoma. Science 1994; 263:1281.

165. Downing JR, Shurtleff SA, Zielenska M, et al: Molecular detection of the (2;5) translocation of non-Hodgkin's lymphoma by reverse transcriptase–polymerase chain reaction. Blood 1995; 85:3416.

166. Yee HT, Ponzoni M, Merson A: Molecular characterization of the t(2;5)(p23;q35) translocation in anaplastic large cell lymphoma (Ki-1) and Hodgkin's disease. Blood 1996; 87:1081.

167. Lamant L, Meggetto F, al Saati T, et al: High incidence of the t(2;5)(p23;q35) translocation in anaplastic large cell lymphoma and its lack of detection in Hodgkin's disease. Comparison of cytogenetic analysis, reverse transcriptase–polymerase chain reaction, and P-80 immunostaining. Blood 1996; 87:284.

168. Zur Hausen H: Viruses in human cancers. Science 1991; 254:1167.

169. Howley PM, Ganem D, Kieff E: Etiology of cancer: Viruses–DNA viruses. *In* DeVita VTJ, Hellman S, Rosenberg SA (eds): Principles and Practice of Oncology, 5th ed. Philadelphia, Lippincott-Raven, 1997, p 168.

170. Robertson E, Grossman S, Johannsen E, et al: Epstein-Barr virus nuclear protein 3C modulates transcription through interaction with the sequence-specific DNA-binding protein J kappa. J Virol 1995; 69:3108.

171. Kaye K, Izumi K, Mosialos G, Kieff E: The Epstein-Barr virus LMP1 cytoplasmic carboxy terminus is essential for B lymphocyte transformation: Fibroblast co-cultivation complements a critical function within the terminal 155 residues. J Virol 1995; 69:6.

172. Mosialos G, Birkenbach M, Yalamanchili R, et al: The Epstein-Barr virus–transforming protein LMP1 engages signaling proteins for the tumor necrosis factor receptor family. Cell 1995; 80:389.

173. Poeschla EM, Wong-Staal F: Etiology of cancer: Viruses–RNA viruses. *In* DeVita VTJ, Hellman S, Rosenberg SA (eds): Cancer: Principles and Practice of Oncology, 5th ed. Philadelphia, Lippincott-Raven, 1997, p 153.

174. Gallo RC: Human retroviruses: A decade of discovery and link with human disease. J Infect Dis 1991; 164:235.

175. Perini G, Wagner S, Green MR: Recognition of bZIP proteins by the GTLV transactivator Tax. Nature 1995; 376:602.

176. Baranger AM, Palmer CR, Hamm MK, et al: Mechanism of the DNA-binding enhancement by the HTLV transactivator Tax. Nature 1995; 376:606.

177. Migone T, Lin J, Cereseto A, et al: Constitutively activated Jak-STAT pathway in T cells transformed with HTLV-I. Science 1995; 269:79.

178. Gazzolo L, Duc Dodon M: Direct activation of resting T lymphocytes by HTLV-I. Nature 1987; 326:714.

179. Chang Y, Cesarman E, Pessin MS, et al: Identification of herpesvirus-like DNA sequences in AIDS-associated Kaposi's sarcoma. Science 1994; 266:1865.

180. Cesarman E, Chang Y, Moore PS, et al: Kaposi's sarcoma–associated herpesvirus-like DNA sequences in AIDS-related body-cavity–based lymphomas. N Engl J Med 1995; 332:1186.

181. Soulier J, Grollet L, Oksenhendler E, et al: Kaposi's sarcoma–associated herpesvirus-like DNA sequences in multicentric Castleman's disease. Blood 1995; 86:1276.

182. Whitby D: Detection of Kaposi's sarcoma–associated herpesvirus in peripheral blood of HIV-infected individuals and progression to Kaposi's sarcoma. Lancet 1995; 346:799.

183. Reitz MSJ, Kalyanarraman VS, Robert-Gurnoff M, et al: Human T-cell leukemia/lymphoma virus: The retrovirus of adult T-cell leukemia/lymphoma. J Infect Dis 1983; 147:399.

184. Raab-Traub N, Flynn K: The structure of the termini of the Epstein-Barr virus as a marker of clonal cellular proliferation. Cell 1986; 47:883.

185. Weiss LM, Movahed LA, Warnke RA, Sklar J: Detection of Epstein-Barr virus genomes in Reed-Sternberg cells of Hodgkin's disease. N Engl J Med 1989; 320:502.

186. Cleary ML, Nalesnik MA, Shearer WT, Sklar J: Clonal analysis of transplant-associated lymphoproliferations based on the structure of the genomic termini of the Epstein-Barr virus. Blood 1988; 72:349.

Chapter Eight

Immunohistochemistry of Lymphomas

Thomas M. Grogan

Much of the biology of the lymphomas has been elucidated by studying their antigenic features and immunologic properties. The understanding of lymphomas has been greatly enhanced by new reagents (such as monoclonal antibodies), new techniques (such as tissue section immunohistochemistry [IHC] and immunofluorescence), and new instruments (such as the cytocentrifuge, epifluorescence microscopes, flow cytometers, and automated immunostainers).[1, 2] With the use of cell suspensions or tissue section methods with a battery of monoclonal and polyclonal antibodies, virtually all lymphoid lesional tissue demonstrates diagnostically useful phenotypic data. Although a full immunophenotypic profile may be determined by using serial tissue sections, serial cytocentrifuge slides, or flow cytometry coplots, this chapter has as its focal point the use of serial tissue section IHC. The major advantages of tissue-section IHC are that the topography of the tissue is intact and that morphologic and immunologic features can be integrated to allow analysis of tissue immunoarchitecture.[1, 2] By this means, morphologically obvious neoplastic and reactive components can be analyzed for their separate chemistries. Delineation of the microanatomic context and immunologic topography are the strengths of tissue section IHC and the point of emphasis of this discussion. Indeed, the thesis is that distinctive, combined microanatomic and immunotopographic features specifically characterize many of the lymphomas as biologic entities. This integration of morphologic and immunologic findings is pivotal to the proper diagnosis of lymphomas, as emphasized in the 1994 Revised European-American Lymphoma (REAL) classification, which is used throughout.[3]

IMMUNOHISTOCHEMISTRY METHODS

TISSUE HANDLING AND PREPARATION

The quality of the histologic and immunophenotypic data is highly dependent on the manner in which the tissue is handled and prepared.[1] In histologic and tissue section IHC, it is the technically poor slide that defeats diagnosis. High-quality slides begin with timely, adept gross tissue examination, appropriate tissue preservation (snap freezing and fixation), followed by proper cutting and staining. Since absolutely fresh tissue is required for specialized procedures (such as IHC, genotyping, flow cytometry, and Southern blotting), we place a premium on the pathologist going to the operating room or clinic to receive the specimen within minutes of its removal. This act alone may represent the most difficult and important component of lymphoma diagnosis and IHC.[1]

After touch preparations are made, tissue preparation should include fixation for histology. We fix dime-thickness (2-mm) tissue slides in 10% neutral buffered formalin for 4 hours and snap freeze tissue for IHC phenotyping. Since many of the specialized procedures detailed earlier are needed for full lymphoma characterization, the practice of placing lymphoid biopsy specimens entirely into formalin is no longer acceptable.

Snap freezing entails placing a pea- to almond-sized portion of tissue in ornithine transcarbamoylase compound and freezing at −150°C for 10 seconds in either isopentane quenched in liquid nitrogen or liquid nitrogen alone.[1] The tissue is then stored at −80°C in airtight containers. Sectioning tissue as thin as possible entails the use of sharp knives (e.g., disposable blades) to give 3-μ sections. For serial frozen section IHC, the sections are fixed in ice cold (4°C) acetone for 10 minutes and then stained. For most lymphoma typing, snap frozen material is favored, because it ensures maximum antigen preservation without epitope masking due to cross-linking fixatives. Although snap freezing involves more time initially, it results in fewer antigen false-negative results compared with paraffin sections.[1] Full antigen preservation gives more reliable results.

In some instances paraffin-section IHC provides superior results. Certain antigens, such as cytoplasmic immunoglobulin (Ig) in plasma cells, benefit from the fixation process.[1] Paraffin IHC assays also benefit from superior morphologic detail, which may be critical in delineating single cells (e.g., CD15+ Reed-Sternberg cells). The major deficiency of paraffin IHC assays—the masking of epitopes by cross-linking fixatives—has been greatly obviated by the recent addition of new antibodies to fixative-resistant epitopes (e.g., L26 and CD20) and new methods of antigen unmasking.[4]

Recently, tissue enzyme digests (such as trypsin and protease digestions) and tissue acid hydrolysis via microwaving have greatly enhanced detection of many antigens in paraffin sections, as illustrated later. Reviews suggest that specific combinations of enzyme and microwaving are relevant to specific epitopes and specific antibodies.[4] This arcane bit of immunoarchaeology affords the prospect of returning to stored banks of archival lymphomas and performing retrospective IHC analysis or allowing phenotyping of tissue fixed without additional frozen tissue.

IMMUNOHISTOCHEMISTRY DETECTION METHODS

A variety of detection reagents and methodologies are available for IHC analyses. As illustrated in Figure 8–1, we use a four-step multichromogen detection method in kinetic mode (Ventana Medical Systems, Tucson, AZ) that allows, as previously described, rapid and sensitive immunoassay in multiple colors (brown, red, and blue).[5] The multichromogen capability facilitates antigen colocalizations, as demonstrated throughout this chapter.

The first IHC detection step entails applying the primary antibody that is either a monoclonal mouse antihuman hybridoma antibody or a polyclonal heteroserum from rabbit or goat. Table 8–1 lists according to cluster designation (CD) the primary antibodies used in lymphoma IHC studies. If the primary antibody is directly linked to a chromogen or fluorochrome, specific detection is the result. Sensitivity, however, is limited. If, as in Figure 8–1, a secondary antibody and linked-enzyme complex are added, in the indirect method, then sensitivity is greatly increased. The specific signal is multiplied by the added secondary antibody and the large size of the streptavidin-linked enzyme complex, which serves as a platform for chromogen dye precipitation and amplification.[5]

Table 8–1. Key Human Leukocyte Antigens

CD	Additional Names	Cell Type	Function
CD1	T6, Leu-6	Thy, LC	Unknown
CD2	T11, Leu-2	T, NK	$CD58_R$, sheep RBC_R
CD3	T3, Leu-4	T	TC_R-associated
CD4	T4, Leu-3	T subset	Class II MHC; HIV_R
CD5	T1, Leu-1	T, B subset	Ligand to CD72
CD7	Leu-9	T, NK	Unknown
CD8	T8, Leu-2	T subset, NK subset	Class I MHC_R
CD10	CALLA	Pre-B, G	Neutral endopeptidase
CD11a	LFA-1 α chain	Leukocytes	Ligand for ICAM; β chain CD18
CD11b	Mo1, Mac1, OKM1	NK, M, G	$C3bi_R$, β chain, CD18
CD11c	Leu-M5	NK, B subset, M, G	Unknown; β chain, CD18
CD15	Leu-M1, X-hapten	G, Reed-Sternberg	Unknown
CD16	Leu-11	NK, G	$Fc\alpha_RIII$
CD18	LFA-1 β-chain	Leukocytes	β chain to CD11a, 11b, 11c; $ICAM_R$
CD19	B4, Leu-12	B	Unknown
CD20	B1, Leu-16, Leu-26	B	? Ion channel
CD21	B2, CR2	B subset, DRC	C3d and EBV_R
CD22	Bgp 135, Leu-14	B	Ligand for CD45RO
CD23	Blast-2	B subset, M subset, Eo	Fc_R II
CD25	Tac	ACT T, B, M	β chain of IL-2_R
CD28	Tp44	T subset, ACT B	B7 ligand
CD30	Ki1	ACT T, B; Reed-Sternberg	Unknown
CD34	My10	Progenitors, endothelial	Unknown
CD38	T10	Plasma, T	Unknown
CD43	Leukosialin	WBC except B	Ligand for CD54
CD44	Pgp-1, Hermes-1	WBC, RBC	Homing receptors
CD45	T200, LCA	WBC	Tyrosine phosphatase
CD45RO	UCHL-1	T, B, M, M	Ligand for CD22
CD45RA	ALB11	B, T, M	Unknown
CDw49a	VLAα1	Thy, PL	Laminin
CDw49b	VLAα2	Thy, PL	Collagen
CDw49c	VLAα3	B, T	Collagen laminin, fibronectin R
CDw49d	VLAα4	M, B, T	Unknown
CDw49e	VLAα5	PL	Fibronectin R
CDw49f	VLAα6	PL, Meg	Laminin R
CD54	ICAM	Broad activation	Ligand for LFA-1
CD56	NKH1, Leu-19	NK, ACT lymphs	Isoform of NCAM
CD57	Leu-7, HNK1	NK, T subset, B subset	Unknown
CD58	LFA3	Leukocytes, epithel	Ligand for CD2
CD72	10B72	Pan B	Ligand for CD5
CD77	CB3	Burkitt's ML	Unknown

Thy, thymocyte; LC, Langerhans' cell; NK, natural killer; R subscript, receptor; G, granulocytes; mo, monocytes/macrophages; PL, platelets; ACT, activated; epithel, epithelial cells; ML, malignant lymphoma; Eo, eosinophil; Meg, megakaryocyte; WBC, white blood cell; RBC, red blood cell; TC_R, T-cell receptor; HIV, human immunodeficiency virus; EBV, Epstein-Barr virus; IL, interleukin; DRC, dendritic reticulum cell; MHC, major histocompatibility complex.

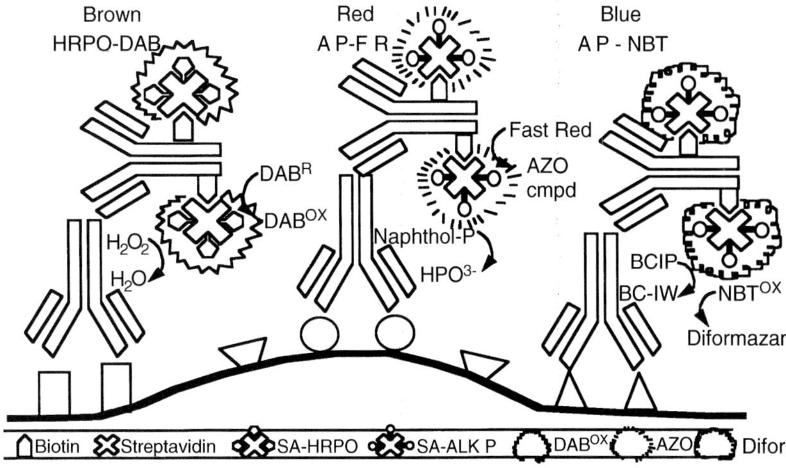

Figure 8–1. Diagrammatic representation of multichromogen immunohistochemical detection system that uses biotin-streptavidin and streptavidin-enzyme links to react with chromogens. HRPO, horseradish peroxidase; DAB, diaminobenzidine; AP, alkaline phosphatase; FR, fast red; AZO cmpd, diazonium compound; NBT, nitroblue tetrazolium; BCIP, 5-bromo-4-chloro-3-indolyl phosphate; BC-IW, BC-indigo white; SA, streptavidin.

The second step in our laboratory entails the use of a cocktail of secondary biotinylated (biotin, or vitamin-B–labeled) antibodies. This cocktail includes two goat anti-mouse antibodies (anti-IgG and anti-IgM) and a goat antirabbit IgG.[5] This universal cocktail ensures a broad spectrum of primary antibody detection. It allows detection of monoclonal or polyclonal primary antibodies in a single run. This universal detection also allows frozen sections, paraffin sections, and cytospin preparations to be run simultaneously; not frozen assays one day and paraffin runs the next. Thus, in evaluating a lymphoma biopsy specimen (see Fig. 8–11), the pathologist may consider at once the findings related to monoclonal mouse antihuman IgG antibodies (pan B and pan T) and IgM antibodies (CD15) as well as polyclonal rabbit antihuman antibodies (CD3).

The third step entails a large streptavidin molecule linked to an enzyme, either horseradish peroxidase (HRPO) or alkaline phosphatase (AP). The avidin provides two attributes: (1) a large molecular platform for further reactivity and (2) a tight lock-and-key fit with vitamin B (biotin) on the secondary antibody. The high affinity of the biotin-avidin (egg white) complex ensures that the IHC detection signal remains bound and does not diffuse. Incidentally, the strength of the vitamin B–egg white link was first realized from a pathologic circumstance: feeding egg whites back to chickens resulted in beri beri due to bound vitamin B.[1]

The fourth step involves reactivity of the linked enzyme with a chromogen to produce a colored precipitated compound or dye that decorates the site of localization (e.g., cell surface). A chromogen is a colorless compound that becomes a colored compound or dye when oxidized or reduced by another.[5] The oxidizing-reducing substance in this case is acted on by the linked enzyme that serves as the catalyst and the physical site of the oxidative:reductive process, as shown in Figure 8–1. To produce a brown precipitate, we use a diaminobenzidine (DAB) hydrogen peroxide (H_2O_2) solution. The H_2O_2 serves as the initial oxidizing substrate acted on by HRPO. To produce a red precipitate, naphthol solution serves as the substrate for the AP enzyme, which acts on the fast red chromogen to produce a stable diazonium compound. To produce a blue precipitate, the nitroblue tetrazolium chromogen is reduced by AP acting on the 5-bromo-4-chloro-3-indolyl phosphate (BCIP) substrate.[5]

The value of multiple chromogens is the ability to colocalize antigens. This reduces inferences from single-antigen analyses and allows the study of interactive molecules (e.g., p53 and *BCL2*; see Fig. 8–13) or differentiation of lymphoid subpopulations (e.g., T-TIL versus Ki67, see Fig. 8–21). The value of multiple enzyme systems lies partly in the ability to avoid the periodic pitfall of confounding endogenous enzymes (neutrophilic peroxidase) or pigments (e.g., melanin) or pseudoperoxidase (e.g., red blood cells).[5]

Finally, we use a kinetic-mode method that mixes and heats the IHC reactants in an automated manner. This instrument-controlled process ensures a rapid reaction driven to equilibrium to ensure uniform, clinically timely results. The gain in time and reduction in labor, aided by a multichromogen-compatible system, greatly facilitates double labeling.[5]

IMMUNOPHENOTYPING PROFILES ASSOCIATED WITH LYMPHOID MALIGNANCY

CONCEPT OF A MALIGNANT PHENOTYPE-GENOTYPE

Over the past 20 years, batteries of antibodies have generated immunophenotypic profiles or patterns of antigenic expression that distinguish lymphoma from normal variations in lymphoid tissue. In many instances, a characteristic phenotypic "fingerprint" is associated with a specific lymphoma entity.[1–3] A case in point would be the unique combination of activation antigens (CD30), myelomonocytic antigen (CD15), and absent universal lymphoid antigen (CD45) found in typical Hodgkin's disease–related Reed-Sternberg cells (see Fig. 8–8). On this basis immunotyping is beginning to achieve status as a useful adjunct to lymphoma diagnosis. These IHC phenotypic profiles are now being codified as in the 1994 REAL classification.[3]

A burgeoning literature details the usefulness of IHC phenotypes in distinguishing Hodgkin's disease and B-cell and T-cell lymphomas from reactive lymphoid lesion tissues.[3] From this literature, it emerges that Hodgkin's disease and B-cell and T-cell lymphomas are typically an amalgam of neoplastic and normal traits.[3, 6] Neoplastic lymphoid cells differ from normal lymphoid cells by a wide array of changes. These genotypic and phenotypic changes lead to a single immortalized clone. This singular clone has admixed abnormal and normal features. Although the abnormal genetic tracts may confer immortality, it is sometimes the retained normal attributes that dictate lymphoma cell function or behavior. For example, a neoplastic B cell might express a single light- and heavy-chain Ig and manifest monoclonality but also retain normal homing receptors, allowing the neoplastic cell to follow normal homing patterns and thereby colonize other nodes (germinal center) and extranodal sites (e.g., bone marrow). At other times the neoplastic cell (e.g., B cell) may lose a key functional surface antigen (e.g., LFA-1) and thereby lose capacity for interaction with other cells (CD8+ T cell necessary for immunosurveillance).[6] For this reason, we briefly consider the normal lymphoid traits as a prelude to comprehending the malignant lymphoid cell.

NORMAL LYMPHOID TRAITS RELEVANT TO LYMPHOMA BEHAVIOR

B-Cell and T-Cell Developmental Antigens. Since malignant lymphoid cells mimic normalcy and may be frozen in a state of known B-cell or T-cell development, and finally, since lymphoma cell behavior may be secondary to known developmental stage, it is necessary to place lymphomas in the known scheme of B-cell and T-cell development, as shown in Figures 8–2 and 8–3, respectively.[1, 2, 7] The details of lymphoid ontogeny are given elsewhere in this text; however, these figures should suffice to compare the

phenotypes of B-cell and T-cell malignancies with their normal counterparts. Figures 8–2 and 8–3 may be seen as a "roadmap," suggesting the likely phenotypic profile for a given lymphoma. Thus, as illustrated, the follicular lymphomas (FLs) as a mid-phase B-cell lymphoma of germinal center origin expectedly coexpress surface Ig, CD10, CD21, and certain other pan-B antigens. In the T-cell scheme, for example, the precursor T-LBL expectedly coexpresses the immature nuclear enzyme (terminal deoxynucleotidyl transferase [Tdt]) and the cortical thymic antigen CD1. It also commonly presents as an anterior mediastinal mass consistent with its immature cortical thymic phenotype and origin.[1, 2, 7] In a subsequent section, each of the common lymphomas is placed in the illustrated scheme, except for Hodgkin's disease, the position of which in normal lymphoid ontogeny is uncertain. The illustrated scheme facilitates an understanding of the expected array of markers associated with a given lymphoma and reveals the differential phenotypic features separating morphologically similar entities (e.g., the small lymphoid cell lymphomas, small lymphocytic leukemia [SLL], marginal zone lymphoma [MZL], and mantle cell lymphoma [MCL]) In addition to developmental antigens, other antigens are highly relevant to lymphoid cell function. These include surface molecules relevant to B-cell and T-cell interaction; those relevant to sessile versus mobile status; and the oncogenic products relevant to cell proliferation, activation, or resting status. These are briefly considered in turn.

B-Cell and T-Cell Interaction. As illustrated in Figure 8–4, a variety of molecules mediate B-cell and T-cell interactions.[8, 9] They include cell adhesion molecules (CAMs) (e.g., ICAM), integrins (e.g., LFA-1), selectins

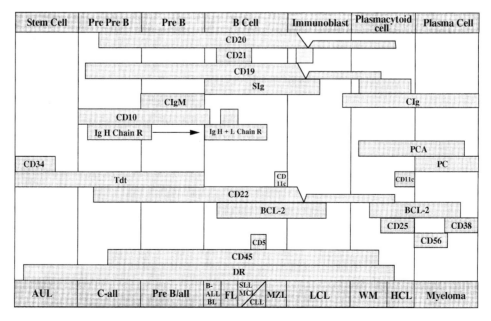

Figure 8–2. B-cell phenotypes. Diagrammatic representation of the range of B-cell antigenic and Ig gene expression both in normal B-cell development (ontogeny) and in the B-cell neoplasms derived from each stage of ontogeny. AUL, acute undifferentiated leukemia; C-all, common acute lymphoblastic leukemia; pre B/all, pre-B-cell acute lymphoblastic leukemia; B-ALL, B-cell acute lymphoblastic leukemia; BL, Burkitt's/Burkitt's-like leukemia/lymphoma; FL, follicular lymphoma; SLL, small lymphocytic lymphoma; MCL, mantle cell lymphoma; CLL, chronic lymphocytic leukemia; MZL, mantle zone lymphoma; LCL, large cell lymphoma; WM, Waldenström's macroglobulinemia; HCL, hairy cell leukemia; myeloma, multiple myeloma. See Table 8–1 for descriptions of antibodies and CD abbreviations.

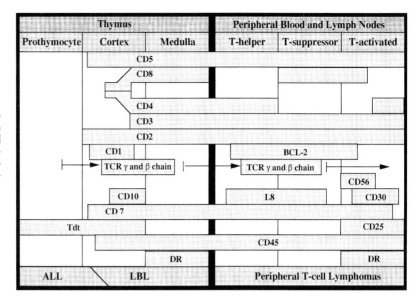

Figure 8–3. T-cell phenotypes. Diagrammatic representation of the range of T-cell antigenic and T antigen receptor (TCR) gene expression in both normal T-cell ontogeny and T-cell neoplasms derived from the developmental phases. See Table 8–1 for descriptions of antibodies. ALL, acute lymphoblastic leukemia; LBL, lymphoblastic lymphoma.

(e.g., LAM-1), histocompatibility antigens (e.g., human leukocyte antigens [HLAs]), and Ig superfamily molecules (e.g., CD22).[8–10] Differential expression of these molecules is relevant to cell behavior. The LFA-1–ICAM interaction shown in Figure 8–4 is a prime example. This molecular pairing is a critical factor for (1) B-cell homotypic adhesion; (2) T-cell adhesion for cytotoxic T-lymphocyte (CTL) recognition and T-cell immunosurveillance; and (3) lymphocyte–endothelial cell interaction.[9, 10] T-cell immunosurveillance, as shown in Figure 8–4, is a complex interaction that has an initial antigen-independent phase mediated by large docking molecules such as CD22, LFA-1, and ICAM-1.[8] The subsequent antigen-dependent phase, giving

a tighter, more antigen-specific fit, entails cross-linking the T-cell antigen receptor through binding to HLA antigens and associated foreign antigens on the opposing B cells, as shown.[8] The HLA-1 surface antigens (A, B, and C) are major determinants of graft rejection and serve as self-recognition elements for CTLs (CD8+) in foreign body or tumor rejection.[11] A second family, known as HLA class II or Ia (immune-associated gene), is subdivided into DP, DR, and DQ subunits that function in antigen presentation and in self-recognition by helper T cells (CD4+), which are also relevant to tumor containment via secondary stimulation of T-cell cytotoxicity.[12] In the end, there are multiple adhesion and recognition molecules that participate in cell adhesion

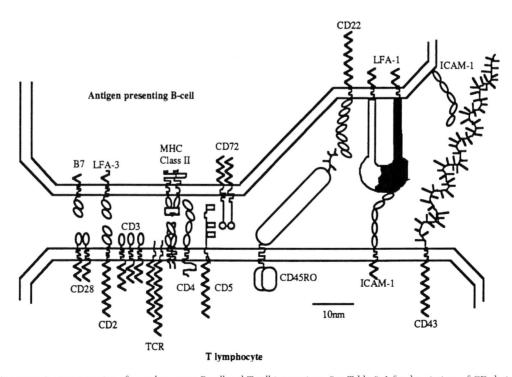

Figure 8–4. Diagrammatic representation of complementary B-cell and T-cell interactions. See Table 8–1 for descriptions of CD designation. (Adapted from Barclay N: Leucocyte Antigen Facts Book. London, Academic Press, 1993, p. 34.)

and aid in effective T-cell surveillance, which serves to eliminate aberrant, neoplastic cells.[12]

Sessile Versus Mobile Phenotype. Critical to lymphoid cell development and function is the cells' regulated ability to either stay put or migrate "home" and traffic through target organs. Specific phenotypes are associated with either sessile or mobile phenotypes. Regarding the sessile phenotype, the very late activation (VLA) molecules, including VLA-4, VLA-5, and VLA-6, are important for cell attachment of the extracellular matrix (ECM) (see Table 8–1).[10] In particular, it is the B1 chain of VLA that mediates interaction with fibronectin (FN) and laminin (LN), giving lymphoid cells an anchoring effect in the ECM. This VLA-FN-LN bond is the essential sessile phenotype dictating lymphocyte anchoring at sites of inflammation and in lymphoid organs.[13, 14]

In contrast, the mobile phenotype is associated with lymphoid cell migration, homing, and organ specificity. In particular, the lymphocyte homing receptor (LHR), (CD44, Hermes 3) is known to play a role in lymphocyte trafficking.[15] LHR interacts with a vascular endothelium receptor (addressin) on the postcapillary venules of the lymph nodes. This addressin and its CD44 ligand facilitate recruitment of circulating memory B cells and T cells into the lymph nodes. Thus, circulating peripheral blood memory cells have high-level LHR or CD44, whereas anchored, sessile lymphoid cells express very-low-level LHR.[15] In some instances lymphoid traffic may be organ specific. This organ specificity may be mediated by surface markers such as CD103+ mucosal lymphocyte antigen (MLA), which is found on some gut mucosal-associated T cells.[16]

Ultimately, multifactorial phenotypic analysis defines the complete mobile versus sessile phenotype. As described by Springer in his "area code" hypothesis, the transition from mobile to sessile may involve a specific sequential expression of a specific selection, integrin, and CAM so that a complete phenotype, not a single marker, is needed to predict lymphocyte behavior.[17, 18]

Proliferative Versus Resting Memory Status. When a given foreign antigen is presented, some lymphoid cells are specifically stimulated to activation and proliferation, whereas immediately adjacent clones are not stimulated. In germinal centers, there is either initial clonal expansion and prolonged survival of high-affinity clones or loss or culling of clones with low affinity for antigen. This balance between clone expansion or demise, between clonal proliferation or resting status, is largely regulated by the products of protooncogenes and tumor suppressor genes.[19] The products of these genes control lymphoid cell proliferation, differentiation, and survival.[19] These protein products are readily detected by IHC assay.

In lymphoid ontogeny, three categories of genes are commonly involved: (1) growth-promoting genes (e.g., C-*MYC*); (2) tumor suppressor genes (e.g., *p53*); and (3) death-sparing, survival genes (e.g., *BCL 2*).[19] C-*MYC* is a mitogenic nuclear transcription factor that results in increased unbridled growth, if amplified.[20] The counterbalancing category II gene *p53* inhibits growth in its wild form.[21] In reactive lymphoid tissues, little wild-type *p53* or C-*MYC* is found, suggesting that small amounts of these short-lived molecules are needed for normal physiologic function.[19–21] In certain lymphomas, these genes may be altered by mutation or translocation and upregulated. The upregulated forms are more abundant owing to constitutive synthesis or increased stability, leading to unbridled growth and consequent loss of proliferative control.[21] They are also more readily detected by IHC. The category III, death-sparing *BCL 2*, blocks cell death and confers resting status, thereby creating the long-lived physiologic trait of memory B cells and T cells.[19, 22] This resting status is subsequently overcome by antigen activation with proliferative escape, resulting in a "rebirth" of memory B-cell and T-cell clones.[17, 20]

MALIGNANT LYMPHOID PROFILES

The collective "malignant" aberrancies of neoplastic lymphoid cells are shown in Table 8–2. The listed malignant properties and their associated markers allow speculation as to the biologic principles at play in lymphoma tumorigenicity.[6] In some instances, there is abnormal expression of an oncogene or tumor suppressor gene (e.g., C-*MYC* or *p53*), leading to loss of growth control. In other instances, there is loss of a normal antigen with consequent loss of normal B-cell and T-cell interaction, resulting in a loss of cell cohesion or a loss of immunosurveillance. In some instances, there are aberrant, inappropriate lineage markers (such as CD15 myeloid antigen in a B-cell neoplasm). Collectively, the aberrancies lead to a single immortalized clone; individually, they may be used as diagnostic markers to herald malignancy.[6] These malignant properties relevant to tissue IHC diagnosis are discussed in turn.

Table 8–2. Malignant Properties of Lymphoma

Malignant Phenotypes	Markers	Biologic Principles
High proliferative rate	Ki67, p53, C-*MYC*	Loss of growth control
Low proliferative rate	BCL2	Resting status conferred
Loss of CAM	LFA-1, CD54, CD22	Loss of cell cohesion
Gain of CAM	CD56	Extranodal localization
Loss of lineage Ag (pan-B and T)	CD2, 5, 22, 23	Loss of cell cohesion
Loss of HLA	HLA I, II	Loss of immunosurveillance
Loss of T-TIL	CD3, 4, 8	Loss of immunosurveillance
Drug resistance protein	P-glycoprotein	Gain of efflux pump
Homing receptor expression	CD44	Gain of mobile phenotype
Collagenase expression	Collagenase IV	Gain in invasiveness

See text for abbreviations.

FOLLICULAR LYMPHOMA

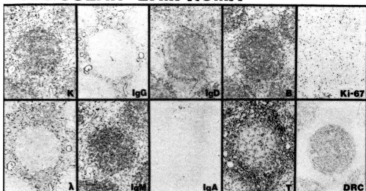

Figure 8–5. Comparison of monoclonal follicular lymphoma and polyclonal reactive lymph node tissue section phenotypes. DRC, dendritic reticulum cell (detected with anti-CD21). Ki67, anti-proliferation antibody directed at nuclear proliferation protein.

REACTIVE LYMPH NODE

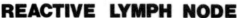

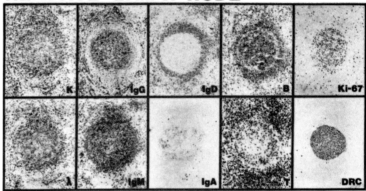

Monoclonality. Fundamentally, lymphoma represents a single immortalized clone, and as such it is a paradigm of monoclonality.[23, 24] In neoplastic B-cell lymphomas of mid and late phase, there is generally light- and heavy-chain Ig restriction, indicating a monoclonal B-cell proliferation.[23, 24] Figure 8–5 demonstrates this light- and heavy-chain restriction in a follicular lymphoma, in contrast with the polyclonal pattern of a reactive lymph node. This figure illustrates the importance of the microanatomic context. That is, the monoclonality is evident within follicles, and yet it may be polyclonal in adjacent normal tissues; therefore, monoclonality is defined contextually.[1] Additional genetic evidence of clonality comes from demonstrating clonal rearrangement of Ig heavy- and light-chain genes in B-cell tumors.

Although T-cell lymphomas typically also derive from a single clone, monoclonality may be difficult to judge on a phenotypic basis. Normally, T-helper and T-cytotoxic-suppressor cells are admixed in a 3 to 4 : 1 ratio.[1, 25] In mature T-cell neoplasia, one subset may be present to the near exclusion of the other, as shown in Figure 8–6. The difficulty is that some benign reactive T-cell proliferations may show a remarkable predominance of one subset without neoplastic transformation.[26] In this circumstance, judgment of T-cell monoclonality is greatly aided by assessment of T antigen receptor genes to establish clonal rearrangements. However, even molecular assay of clonality may prove problematic unless both α/β and γ/δ assays are performed.[27] Furthermore, phenotypically proven mature T-cell lymphomas without T-cell receptor rearrangements have been de-

scribed.[28] Finally, the issue of clonality is clouded with immature T-cell neoplasms. These immature tumors may have both T subset antigens, or they may have neither (see Fig. 8–12).[29] Nonetheless, the unique presence of Tdt and CD1 usually ensures proper lineage identification.[29]

In certain etiologic and clinical circumstances, notably human immunodeficiency virus (HIV)-related lymphomas and posttransplantation lymphomas, judgment of monoclonality may be highly ambiguous. In these circumstances, lymphoid tumors that appear morphologically neoplastic have proved to be variously monoclonal, oligoclonal, or polyclonal by genotyping.[30] Some of the latter were self-limiting when immunosuppressive therapy ceased, suggesting that clonality does not always equate precisely with true malignancy.[30]

Lineage Aberrancies. Although monoclonality is a powerful indicator of likely lymphoid neoplasia, it is not the sole determinant, since other notable phenotypic aberrancies herald the neoplastic condition. In particular, two lineage-related phenomena are associated with lymphoid neoplasia: (1) loss of pan-B- and pan-T-cell antigens and (2) unusual cross-lineage coexpressions.[31–33] In the first instance, either B-cell or T-cell lymphomas may fail to express or may lose expression of some pan-B- or pan-T-cell antigens, indicating a novel, aberrant phenotype that has no normal counterpart (see Fig. 8–6).[31–33] A case in point is that certain mature B-cell lymphomas may fail to express either a heavy- or light-chain Ig, presenting an Ig-negative phenotype with no normal counterpart (see Fig. 8–2). The phenomenon of idiosyncratic phenotypes indicates that lymphomas are not invariant mimics of normalcy.[31–33] Regarding unusual cross-lineage coexpressions, these include (1) CD5, T antigen, coexpression in B-cell small lymphocytic lymphoma; (2) CD11c, histiocytic antigen, in B-cell monocytoid B-cell, SLL, or hairy cell leukemias; (3) CD15, myeloid antigen, in some non-Hodgkin's lymphoma (NHL); (4) CD20, pan-B antigen, in some T-cell lymphomas; and (5) CD43, pan-T antigen, in some B-cell lymphomas.[31–33] These cross-lineage expressions may have a normal counterpart in the form of a rare clone (less than 1% of the population). In the neoplastic process, the emergence of this rare clone to predominance is heralded by the unexpected cross-lineage pattern of markers. In a battery of antibodies, this unusual IHC pattern is useful diagnostically. Caution is necessary, even with aberrant coexpressions such as CD20/43, since this coexpression may occur in cases of infectious mononucleosis.[34]

Oncogenic Changes Leading to a Loss of Proliferative Control. In general, the alterations in oncogenes and tumor suppressor genes that occur in lymphoma result in deregulated lymphoid cell growth.[6, 35] The loss of proliferative control may occur at two extremes of high and low proliferation. In general, upregulated or overexpressed category I and II genes (e.g., C-MYC and p53) result in high proliferation, whereas upregulated category III genes (e.g., BCL2) lead to a hypoproliferative state that immortalizes the neoplastic cell in the resting state

locked in perpetual "memory" status incapable of programmed cell death.[6, 19]

These overexpressed gene products are especially useful in IHC assessment of malignancy, since in normal, physiologic lymph nodes their expression is low (C-MYC or p53) or restricted to certain microanatomic compartments (e.g., BCL2 abundant in mantle zones, but nearly absent in germinal centers). In tissue sections of lymphoid tissues, the mere detection of C-MYC or p53 connotes malignancy (see Fig. 8–13). With BCL2, the presence of this oncogene product in follicles (see Fig. 8–14) heralds malignancy.[36] Thus, the microanatomic context is pivotal, and the use of tissue section IHC is critical because a suspension method would not distinguish the *site* or context of expression.

Another IHC feature secondarily related to altered oncogene status may be of diagnostic usefulness: altered microanatomic patterns of cell proliferation as measured by Ki67. The Ki67 monoclonal antibody detects a nuclear proliferation antigen.[37] In Burkitt's lymphoma, which commonly overexpresses C-MYC, assay with Ki67 reveals a very high proliferative rate (>80%) representing a "pathologically" high proliferative rate with no physiologic equivalent (see Fig. 8–18).[38, 39] In follicular lymphoma, with overexpression of BCL2 related to the (14,18) translocation, assay by Ki67 reveals a pathologically low proliferative rate (<5%), far lower than the normal physiologic germinal center proliferative rate (see Fig. 8–5).[1] In the Burkitt's instance, it

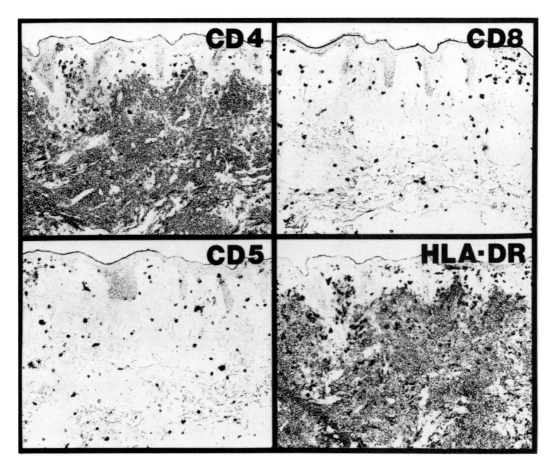

Figure 8–6. Peripheral T-cell lymphoma of skin with a novel T-cell phenotype (absent CD5 and CD8), T-helper predominance (CD4), and activated status (Ia+ [HLA-DR]).

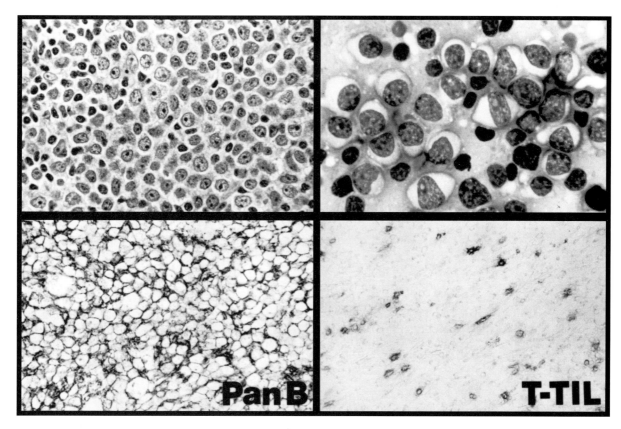

Figure 8–7. T-cell tumor-infiltrating lymphocytes (T-TILs). The large blastic cells are of B-cell phenotype (pan B, CD20+), whereas the smaller cells are of T-cell phenotype (CD8+), representing CD8+ cytotoxic T-TIL infiltrating the tumor.

is the diffuse sheet of Ki67-positive blastic cells that is pathologically distinctive; in the follicular instance it is the sometime near-absence of Ki67-positive cells in the neoplastic nodules that is distinctive. Once again, the pattern or context of the IHC finding is pivotal.[33]

Among FLs, both C-*MYC* and *p53* may also have prognostic value because the overexpression of both or either is associated with transition from indolent to high-grade status. Indeed, overexpression of either one in FL is an IHC finding heralding clinical progression.[40]

Regarding altered *p53*, it is most commonly found by IHC in high-grade Burkitt's-like lymphoma and large cell immunoblastic lymphomas, especially in HIV-associated cases (31%).[21] In contrast, *p53* overexpression is rare in low-grade lymphoma except in scattered large cells, which might herald progression to high grade. Within Hodgkin's disease mutated, overexpressed *p53* is most common (30%) among the nodular sclerosis subtype and not other subtypes.[21]

Regarding *BCL2* overexpression, most FLs manifest aberrant overexpression related to the translocation of the gene on chromosome 18. This leads to "pathologic" deregulated *BCL2* expression by fusing the *BCL2* gene to the IgH locus, leading to production of a chimeric transcript.[19] Some diffuse lymphomas overexpress *BCL2* independent of this translocation, suggesting that other more physiologic factors lead to *BCL2* expression.[19]

Altered B-Cell Versus T-Cell Interactions. Loss or lack of expression of adhesion-recognition molecules (e.g., HLA, ICAM, and LFA-1) is a broad phenomenon of biologic and clinical prognostic importance, as discussed in detail later. For now, the lack of these normal surface molecules on lymphomas has IHC diagnostic utility.[6] For example, the absence of LFA-1 or ICAM in a lymphoid proliferation is decidedly nonphysiologic. The absence of the CAM CD22 or HLA I or II in a B-cell proliferation is decidedly pathologic.[6] The absence of these key mediators of B-cell and T-cell interaction has another secondary consequence also detectable by IHC: a deficiency of tumor-infiltrating CTLs (CD8) (Fig. 8–7; see also Fig. 8–22).[41]

Effect of Sessile Versus Mobile Phenotype. The expression of LHRs appears relevant to lymphoma dissemination and has prognostic import, as discussed later. [15] For now, regarding IHC usefulness in diagnosis, high-level LHR expression correlates with more extensive lymphoma dissemination and higher stage.[15] Molecules other than LHR may account for organ-specific dissemination of lymphoma.[16] For example, CD103+, found on some gut-associated T-cells, is highly expressed on the neoplastic cells of intestinal T-cell lymphoma associated with gluten-sensitive enteropathy.[16] The localization of this rare lymphoma is probably largely dictated by this organ-specific homing receptor.

PHENOTYPIC PROPERTIES OF HODGKIN'S DISEASE

THE CLASSIC PHENOTYPE

Most Hodgkin's disease subtypes, including nodular sclerosis, mixed cellularity, and lymphocyte depleted, have a distinctive phenotype comprising a unique combination of a lymphoid activation antigen (CD30+, Kil, Ber-H2) and a myelomonocytic antigen (CD15, LM1), with absence of the "universal" leukocyte common antigen (LCA) (CD45 RB) and absence of lineage markers (B and T cell) (Fig. 8–8; see also color section).[42–44] This characteristic "classic" Hodgkin's disease phenotype, found in 85% of clinical cases using paraffin-active antibodies, has no normal counterpart among lymph node–derived cells.[42–44] Perhaps the neoplastic Hodgkin's cells (Reed-Sternberg cells) is the unique consequence of "aberrant gene expression."[45] The neoplastic Reed-Sternberg cell may be a phenotypic "platypus," suggesting that lymphoid and myeloid ontogeny may be linked in early embryogenesis.[46] Alternatively, perhaps the neoplastic cell is a phenotypic hybrid owing to fusion or syncytial formation of separate lymphoid-myelomonocytic cells.[47, 48] The absent LCA (CD45, RB) suggests a mutational or deletional event in Hodgkin's pathogenesis.[45]

The uniqueness of the classic Hodgkin's disease phenotype is compounded by an equally unique pattern of cellular localization. In particular, CD15 and CD30 characteristically localize in both the Golgi complex and on the surface of Reed-Sternberg cells and variants. The combined Golgi and surface activity gives a "targetlike" pattern (Fig. 8–9).[49]

Furthermore, beyond the unique phenotype and cellular localization, the classic Hodgkin's disease may have a distinctive microanatomic pattern, particularly in the nodular sclerosis subtype. In this subtype, the neoplastic variants known as lacunar cells occur in groups or clusters, suggesting a cohesive syncytium of cells.[49] Thus a syncytial sheet of CD15+, 30+, 45– "targets" is characteristic of nodular sclerosis Hodgkin's disease (NSHD) (see Fig. 8–9).[45, 49] In the end, it is not simply whether a marker is present or absent but the microanatomic context or immunoarchitecture of the lesional tissue that is pathognomonic and the best guide to Hodgkin's disease. It is the unique hybrid (lymphoid-myeloid–absent LCA) phenotype, unique cellular localization of CD15 and CD30, compounded with the unique immunoarchitecture (grouped sheets of CD15–30 targets), that is definitive.[42–45]

In addition to unique tumor cell characteristics, classic Hodgkin's disease may also manifest unique surrounding host cell attributes reflecting paracrine effects. In particular, the neoplastic cells may constitutively express cytokines that alter the surrounding stroma and immune response.[50] A case in point is the nodular sclerosis subtype in which the neoplastic cells secrete transforming growth factor-β (TFG-β), accounting for the distinct histologic constellation of NSHD and some of the clinical symptoms.[50] TFG-β from

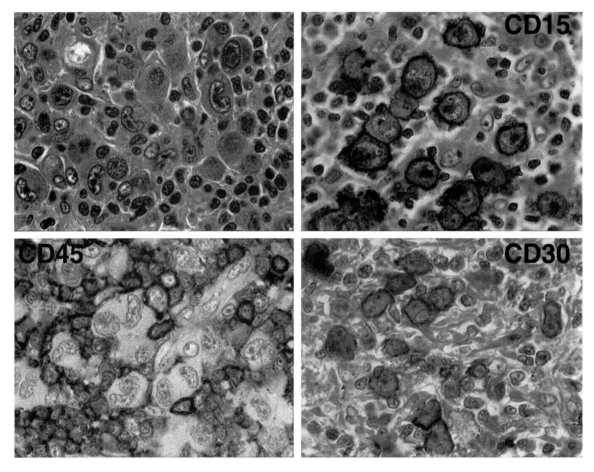

Figure 8–8. Classic Hodgkin's disease phenotype *(upper left)* with neoplastic Reed-Sternberg cells coexpressing CD15 *(upper right)* and CD30 *(lower right)* with absent CD45 *(lower left)*. Note that the CD15 occurs in both the Golgi complex and cell surface, creating a "target." CD45 expression is found in adjacent normal leukocytes, but the polylobated cells are negative. (See also color section.)

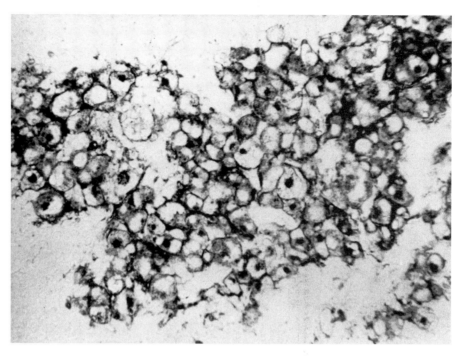

Figure 8–9. Hodgkin's disease cluster of CD15+ targets with both Golgi complex and surface staining. This is the characteristic immunotopographic feature of the "classic" Hodgkin's disease phenotype.

Reed-Sternberg cells is believed to promote the "C" bands of collagenosis, zones of necrosis, and syncytial formation among lacunar cells.[50] TFG-β is known to suppress proliferation of activated lymphocytes, and its expression by Reed-Sternberg cells may explain the loss of cell-mediated immunity among Hodgkin's disease patients. Although Reed-Sternberg cells secrete TFG-β, they lack TFG-β receptors, suggesting a loss of TFG-β regulation, thus contributing to the malignant behavior of Hodgkin's cells.[51] It is also possible that this growth factor confers a growth advantage on Reed-Sternberg cells that is reflected in their high growth fraction as measured by Ki67 or Mib1. In addition to TFG-β, Reed-Sternberg cells and variants may express interferon-γ (IFN-γ),[51] interleukin-1 (IL-1),[52] colony-simulating factor,[53] IL-5,[54] and eosinophilic chemotactic factors (ECFs).[55] The IFN-γ could account for the known enhanced HLA expression on Reed-Sternberg cells, which in turn could favor the E-rosetting phenomenon described around Reed-Sternberg cells.[51] The IFN-γ could explain the fever and chills or some of the B symptoms in patients with Hodgkin's disease. In addition, IL-5 and ECF could explain clinical instances of extreme granulocytopoiesis and the frequent eosinophilia in distant sites, such as the marrow, that are uninvolved by Hodgkin's disease.[54, 55]

THE HODGKIN'S B-CELL PHENOTYPE

The second major paraffin-associated phenotype, a unique B-cell phenotype, is common (almost 100%) in nodular lymphocyte-predominant Hodgkin's disease (NL-PHD) and in some cases of diffuse lymphocyte-predominant Hodgkin's disease but is uncommon (<15%) in mixed cellularity or NSHD.[56, 57] This phenotype features coexpression of a pan-B antigen (e.g., CD20/L26) with CD45 coexpression and absent CD15 (Fig. 8–10; see also color section).

Like the aberrant myeloid antigen coexpression (CD15) in the classic Hodgkin's phenotype discussed earlier, this B-cell entity demonstrates a unique lineage aberrancy: coexpression of epithelial membrane antigen (EMA).[56] Like the classic phenotype, it also manifests distinctive immunoarchitecture features: (1) the scattered neoplastic B cells are surrounded by T-cell rosettes composed of CD57+ natural killer (NK)-like T cells (see Fig. 8–10)[58]; (2) within the vague nodules of the neoplasm there is a well-defined meshwork of CD21+ (C3dr) expressive follicular dendritic cells that, unlike the dendritic cells of reactive germinal centers, do not react with antiimmunoglobulin antibodies.[59] Once again, the microanatomy (nodular growth pattern) is strongly related to the immunologic detail (derivation from germinal centers as evidenced by B-cell lineage and associated mesh of follicular dendritic and CD57-associated cells).[58] In physiologic lymph nodes, CD57+ NK-like T cells occur preferentially as scattered single cells within germinal centers; in NLPHD, these CD57 cells occur in clusters surrounding neoplastic B cells, within polyclonal B-cell nodules, as an immunoarchitectural feature that heralds a specific diagnosis (see Figs. 8–10 and 8–11).[58] The germinal center–related properties of the NLPHD neoplasm may also account for some of the clinical features of this entity. As reported by Regula and associates,[60] NLPHD may clinically be an ever-relapsing disease, highly analogous to follicular small cell lymphoma, also of germinal center origin.

Studies using frozen section IHC have added to the detailed definition of this entity.[56] Regarding the neoplastic cells, which include scattered, polylobated Reed-Sternberg variants called "L & H" or "popcorn" cells, these may express

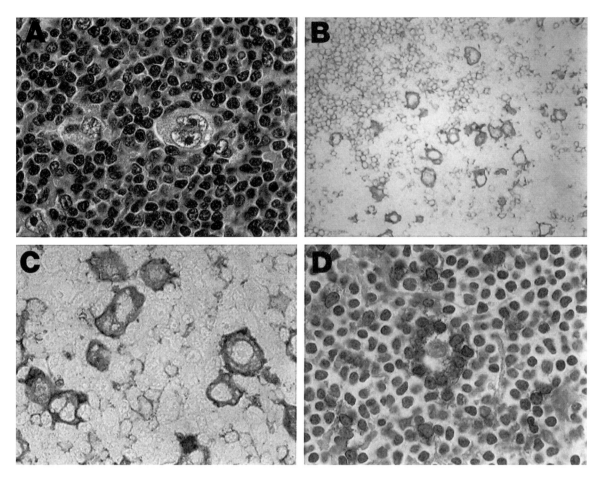

Figure 8–10. *A*, B-cell phenotype in lymphocyte-predominant Hodgkin's disease (LPHD). The large neoplastic cells are CD20+ (*B* and *C*). Immediately surrounding the CD20+ neoplastic cells is a wreath or rosette of CD57+ and positive-like T natural killer cells representing the characteristic immunotopographic feature of LPHD (*D*). (See also color section.)

Ig J chains or light chains and pan-B antigens such as CD19, 20, and 22 (see Fig. 8–10). In some studies, the L & H variants have had monoclonal light-chain expression.[61–64] The L & H cells may also express activation antigens (CD25, 38, and 71) and, in contrast with less-sensitive paraffin-embedded tissue, may show expression of CD30 and CD15.[44, 65] Thus, the curiosity of aberrant myelomonocytic (CD15) and neural growth factor receptor (CD30) coexpression is not restricted to the classic phenotype. Sensitive frozen cell typing also reveals altered CAM expression (upregulated LFA-3 and ICAM-1) related to malignant transformation of Hodgkin's cells.[66, 67] This exaggerated CAM expression is believed to enhance normal T-cell adhesion, resulting in the spontaneous rosetting of T cells to Reed-Sternberg cells, as described earlier. T-rosetting of Reed-Sternberg cells suggests effective T-cell immunosurveillance or T-cell containment of neoplasia.[66, 67] The operative word is "containment," not elimination, of Hodgkin's neoplasia, suggesting an element of aberrant neoplastic B–T-cell symbiosis.

Immunosurveillance aside, the large, scattered, polylobated L & H B cells surrounded by CD57+ T-cell rosettes present a pathognomonic IHC phenotypic pattern.[58] This pattern differs conspicuously from the usual continuous sheet of neoplastic cells in B-cell NHLs.[33] Again, it is

phenotype merged with microanatomy (immunoarchitectural pattern) that is diagnostic.

Outside the T-cell rosettes, the remaining small lymphoid cells in the vague nodules of NLPHD are predominantly B cells with a mantle zone phenotype (e.g., IgM+ and IgD+) with admixed T-helper cells.[56–58]

The relationship between NLPHD and other lymphocyte-rich subtypes remains uncertain. In general, the lymphocyte-rich entities (diffuse lymphocyte-predominant Hodgkin's disease and some cases of mixed cellularity and nodular sclerosis) have the classic, non–B-cell phenotype, suggesting they are different from NLPHD from the onset.[45] Indeed, on this basis, the lymphocyte-rich categories are given a separate category in the 1994 REAL classification.[3] Nonetheless, exceptional cases, as described in the following section, indicate some ambiguity in these characterizations.

NODULAR LYMPHOCYTE-PREDOMINANT HODGKIN'S DISEASE WITH COEXISTING LARGE CELL LYMPHOMA OF B-CELL TYPE

Several reports now detail sporadic cases (2%) of either coexisting NLPHD and large cell lymphoma (LCL) or cases of NLPHD with subsequent transition to LCL, typically of B-cell type.[68–70] In the coexisting or composite cases, L & H cells cluster into large confluent sheets resembling LCL with features of large, noncleaved follicular center cells. This variant of NLPHD with LCL progression surprisingly follows a benign course, showing radiotherapeutic sensitivity and prolonged survival comparable with that expected for the usual NLPHD.[68–70] Thus, this morphologic variant does not have special clinical significance except that its appearance could falsely lead to overaggressive high-grade therapy for LCL of NHL type.

Phenotyping and genotyping of coexisting cases reveals identical B-cell phenotype in both the NLPHD and LCL.[68] As with the usual NLPHD, most related LCLs have expressed pan-B antigens, CD45, and absent CD15 and CD30. Nonetheless, there are combined NLPHD and LCL cases with classic Hodgkin's phenotype (CD15+ 30+ 20– 45–) in both components.[68, 70]

Prior to phenotyping and genotyping, Hodgkin's disease and LCL were considered entirely separate on the basis of clinical behavior and morphology. However, an entity like NLPHD with B-cell LCL (B-LCL) progression suggests that the distinction may be less absolute and more problematic—an observation only strengthened by genotyping. Finally, this entity suggests that some LCLs (those derived from NLPHD), have a favorable prognosis worthy of clinical recognition, given its inherent radiosensitivity.[38]

ATYPICAL PHENOTYPES OF HODGKIN'S DISEASE

The two major phenotypes of Hodgkin's disease are so well defined that exceptional phenotypic variants may seem to preclude the diagnosis of Hodgkin's disease. Nonetheless, exceptional phenotypes occur and are truly Hodgkin's related. A case in point is illustrated in Figure 8–11 (see also color section), wherein a case of NLPHD is shown to have a crossover phenotype with combined elements of the classic and B-cell phenotypes. There is coexpression of CD15 (myelomonocytic antigens), activation antigens (CD30), and pan-B antigens CD20 in the context of CD57+ CD3+ T-cell rosettes. This hybrid phenotype is a rarity but an indication that atypical phenotypes may occur. The detection of the CD15+ in NLPHD may increase based on a maneuver known as "antigen unmasking."[4] With this method, a specific neuraminidase may be employed to unmask CD15 glycosylation, allowing more sensitive CD15 detection.[71]

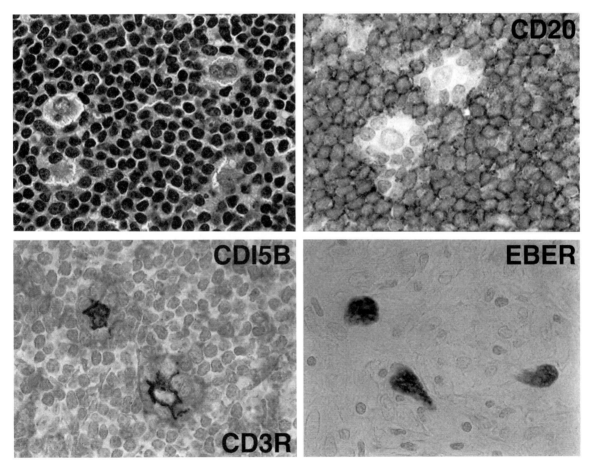

Figure 8–11. Atypical Hodgkin's disease phenotype. This lymphocyte-predominant Hodgkin's disease *(upper left)* has CD20+ B-cell nodules *(upper right)* with CD57+/CD3+ rosettes surrounding CD15+ Reed-Sternberg and Hodgkin's cell variants *(lower left)*. Some of the Reed-Sternberg variants also coexpressed CD20 (not shown.) The Reed-Sternberg cells also demonstrated Epstein-Barr virus transcripts (EBER) by in situ hybridization *(lower right)*. (See also color section.)

EPSTEIN-BARR VIRUS–ASSOCIATED HODGKIN'S PHENOTYPES

Historically, epidemiologic and serologic findings have linked Hodgkin's disease and Epstein-Barr virus (EBV).[72] Patients with EBV-associated infectious mononucleosis have a fourfold increased risk of Hodgkin's disease, and patients with Hodgkin's disease have higher titers of EBV antibodies (e.g., early antigen[EA] and viral capsid antigen [VCA]). In some instances, the higher EA/VCA titers preceded overt Hodgkin's disease by several years.[72] Although EBV genomes were identified in most cases by blotting methods, it was uncertain whether these foreign genomes were in neoplastic cells or nearby nonneoplastic lymphoid cells.[73] In situ hybridization with DNA probes established cellular localization with Reed-Sternberg cells and variants.[74] Furthermore, probes to the terminal region of EBV genomes established the presence of episomal EBV DNA in a monoclonal form consistent with a single-cell origin of neoplasia.[75] Even so, the possibility remained that EBV could be a silent passenger in Hodgkin's disease as a remnant of universal latent EBV infection in nearly all adult human lymph nodes.[76] Subsequently, the demonstration of EBV RNA transcripts (EBER, EB early region)[77–79] and gene products such as latent membrane protein (LMP-1 and LMP-2)[80] specifically within tumor cells established that EBV likely contributed directly to the immortalization of Reed-Sternberg cells and was not a silent passenger (see Fig. 8–11).

The IHC demonstration of LMP in the neoplastic cells of Hodgkin's disease[80, 81] has particular pathogenic implications, since LMP-1 has known oncogenic and immunogenic properties, including (1) potent growth-transforming activity[82]; (2) upregulation of proliferation antigens; (3) upregulation of the cellular oncogene *BCL2*, which promotes enhanced cell survival by blocking programmed cell death[83]; (4) upregulation of cell adhesion molecules (ICAM-1, LFA-1, and LFA-3)[84, 85]; and (5) high immunogenicity for EBV-specific cytotoxic cells relevant to curtailment of latently infected cells.[86, 87]

LMP and EBER are highly associated in clinical Hodgkin's disease, occurring in tandem in as many as 50% of Hodgkin's disease cases.[81, 88, 89] The LMP is found exclusively in the cytoplasm and on the surface neoplastic cells and not in nearby "normal" lymphocytes, in contrast with EBER, which may also be in normal lymphocytes.[81, 88, 89] This LMP/EBER tandem shows histologic specificity, with LMP in most (60% to 70%) mixed cellularity and lymphocyte-depleted cases and only a small proportion (10%) of nodular sclerosis cases (10%) or lymphocyte-predominant cases (<5%).[81, 88, 89] The low incidence of EBV-associated LMP/EBER in lymphocyte-predominant Hodgkin's disease (LPHD) is odd given the typical B-cell phenotype of LPHD and the known proclivity of EBV to infect B cells. Furthermore, the EBV receptor on lymphocytes (C3Dr, CD21) is found on germinal center B cells and some neoplastic LPHD cells, yet, again enigmatically, LPHDs are only rarely EBER or LMP positive.[90] Outside mixed-cell Hodgkin's disease (MCHD) and LDHD, EBV-associated LMP and EBER also have a high incidence in HIV-positive Hodgkin's disease,[91] childhood Hodgkin's disease,[92] and Hodgkin's disease occurring in underdeveloped

countries.[93] Two types (A and B) of EBV that differ at the EBV nuclear antigen gene loci have been described.[91, 94] The type A virus, most common in healthy adults, is the predominant type in usual Hodgkin's disease,[94] whereas type B EBV is most common in Hodgkin's disease occurring in immunocompromised patients with HIV or cardiac transplant recipients.[91]

In addition to immunoreactivity for LMP, other EBV gene products are relevant to the EBV phenotype. In particular, the EBV nuclear antigens (1, 2, 3a, 3b, 3c, –LP) are negative in Hodgkin's disease as are the membrane antigen and the VCA.[89] This phenotype (EBNA negative, LMP positive, EA negative, VCA negative, EBER positive) generally confirms that the virus remains in latency. However, rare cells (<1%) of LMP1-positive Hodgkin's disease cells may have an EBV replication protein known as ZEBRA (BZLFI) protein.[95–97] This protein is known to be involved in the switch of EBV from a latent to lytic or productive cycle. Thus, EBV replication in Reed-Sternberg cells is an exceptional event but probably necessary for sustained EBV persistence and may be detected by IHC analysis.[95]

In general, the immunoreactivity pattern observed in Hodgkin's disease is similar to that in nasopharyngeal carcinoma (EBNA-2 negative, LMP1 positive) and contrasts with the EBNA-2-positive, LMP-1-positive phenotype observed in infectious mononucleosis, lymphoblastoid lines, and EBV-associated transplant lymphomas. It also differs from Burkitt's lymphoma cells, which are EBNA-2 negative, LMP negative, EBNA-1 positive.[81, 88]

The role of LMP in Hodgkin's disease immunosurveillence remains unresolved. On the one hand, LMP-1 is highly immunogenic and a known target for EBV-stain–specific T-cell cytotoxicity and probably limits physiologic EBV spread.[86, 87] On the other hand, why does LMP not favor T cell removal of Hodgkin's cells? Certainly the enhanced LMP-1–related upmodulation of LFA-1, ICAM, and LFA-3 favors the T-rosetting phenomenon surrounding Hodgkin's and Reed-Sternberg cells.[84, 85] Yet T-rosettes in Hodgkin's disease and increased LMP in Hodgkin's disease are not associated with disease elimination. Possibly it is because LMP may occur in truncated or mutated form, which is less immunogenic.[86, 98] Second, the absence of EBNA-2 may be a factor, as both EBNA-2 and LMP are targets for effective T-cell immunosurveillance.[81, 88, 99] Third, the EBV itself may directly involve T cells, precluding their subsequent function in T cytotoxicity. Additionally, certain HLA antigens may be downregulated in Reed-Sternberg cells, precluding an HLA-related EBV-specific T-cytotoxicity response.[100]

Other than overt Hodgkin's disease, there are other conditions, both benign and malignant, in which Reed-Sternberg–like cells are described. These conditions include infectious mononucleosis[101, 102] and chronic lymphocytic leukemia (CLL) or SLL.[102] In each of these conditions the widely scattered Reed-Sternberg–like cells may have either LMP protein or EBER RNA transcripts. In infectious mononucleosis, the Reed-Sternberg–like cells adjacent to tonsillar crypts have notably strong LMP expression, suggesting that the portal of entry of EBV may be the tonsillar crypt epithelium known to be rich in C3Dr EBV receptors.[101] Adding to the difficulty of IHC diagnosis, the LMP-positive infectious mononucleosis Reed-Sternberg–

like cells typically are also CD30+ and may lack CD45 and lineage markers (e.g., CD20) like true Reed-Sternberg cells, although CD15 is noticeably lacking.[101] The oncogenic potential of LMP raises the prospect that these LMP-positive Reed-Sternberg–like cells would be progenitors of Hodgkin's disease Reed-Sternberg cells.[101] In the case of CLL/SLL, the EBV-associated phenotype of the large Reed-Sternberg–like cells may be incidental.[102] However, in one study of 13 cases of EBV-positive Reed-Sternberg–like cells in CLL, three cases progressed to disseminated Hodgkin's disease, suggesting these EBV-positive Reed-Sternberg–like cells may rarely convert to overt Hodgkin's disease.[102] The latter circumstance is another phenotypic example of the sometimes blurred boundary between Hodgkin's lymphomas and NHLs.

IMMUNOPHENOTYPES OF THE NON-HODGKIN'S LYMPHOMA

As emphasized by the 1994 REAL classification of NHLs, there is now a broad range of NHL which has characteristic immunophenotypic microanatomic and cytogenetic features. The following discussion emphasizes some of the salient IHC and microanatomic features for most, but not all, of the REAL B-cell and T-cell lymphomas.[3]

B-CELL LYMPHOMAS

As shown in Figure 8–2, the immunotypes of the B-cell neoplasms reflect stages of normal B-cell development. In general, there are precursor B-cell neoplasms that derive from B cells before antigen experience and mature or peripheral B-cell neoplasms that derive after antigen or bone marrow stage development. The general category of B-cell lymphomas includes the small lymphoid B-cell entities, which are typically indolent or low grade, and the B-cell lymphoma with a large or blastic cell component, which are typically intermediate- or high-grade lymphomas.

Precursor B-Lymphoblastic Leukemia/Lymphoma

Although most lymphoblastic lymphomas (LBLs) are an immature T-cell phenotype, a few (15%) are an immature pre-pre-B or pre-B-cell phenotype (Fig. 8–12).[29, 104, 105] These immature B-cell and T-cell LBLs are morphologically indistinguishable. The lymphoblastic cells within these tumors express the nuclear enzyme Tdt and lack Ig, although the pre-B-cell forms may express cytoplasmic μ and not surface Ig.[29, 104, 105] A rare pre-B-LBL with primary hepatic involvement is described recapitulating embryonic pre-B-cell origin in the liver.[106] Some also express CD10 (CALLA), CD34 (PCNA), and other early B-cell antigens (e.g., CD19), further indicating immaturity. Later B antigens (CD20, 22) and universal antigens (e.g., CD45) may be lacking (see Fig. 8–2).

Both precursor acute lymphoblastic leukemia (ALL) and B-LBL may present with leukemia-like marrow and peripheral blood involvement; however, B-LBL also has a high incidence of cutaneous and osteolytic bone lesions, although it may be without the usual mediastinal involvement of T-LBL.[104, 107]

Low-Grade or Indolent B-Cell Lymphomas

The comparative microanatomic and immunophenotypic features for the low-grade or indolent B-cell lymphomas are listed in Table 8–3. Each has distinctive immunoarchitectural features. They generally have in common a predominance of small lymphoid cells and mature B-cell phenotype.

Follicular Lymphomas

FLs are mature B-cell neoplasms (Fig. 8–13; see also color section; also see Fig. 8–5) with phenotypic and microanatomic features that mimic the germinal centers from which they are derived. Reflecting their germinal center origin, these FL cells typically express Ig, pan-B markers (CD19, 20, 22), and CD10.[1–3, 108] FLs characteristically preserve the germinal center microanatomic environment of dendritic reticulum cells (DRCs), complement receptors (C3Dr), and CD57+ T cells. As shown in Figure 8–5, a tightly organized mesh work of DRC and C3Dr is typically present in follicular areas.[1–3, 108] Regarding T cells, these are characteristically found as single scattered admixed cells, including the CD57+ NK-like T cells and T-helper-cytotoxic cells. This is the single-cell pattern of the physiologic germinal center, not the rosetted CD57+ cells of Hodgkin's disease.[58, 109] FL cells also retain normal homing properties (e.g., CD44 expression) and trafficking abilities (e.g., traffic to bone marrow paratrabeculum). This retained aspect of normalcy accounts for frequent simultaneous involvement of the marrow, spleen, and liver by FL cells.[1, 6]

In contrast with normal germinal centers, FL nodules have some neoplastic aberrancies: Ig monotypia, altered growth-related genes (e.g., *BCL2* and *p53*) and altered proliferative status (see Fig. 8–13).[36, 40] Figure 8–5 illustrates the conspicuous immunologic aberrancies of FL compared with normal lymph nodes. Regarding Ig, there is typically light- and heavy-chain restriction, indicating a monoclonal phenotype (e.g., IgM and κ) in contrast with the usual polyclonal circumstance. Occasionally, the monoclonal Ig is also aberrant on a microanatomic basis: IgD expression on some FL nodules contrasts with the usual physiologic IgD-negative germinal center expression (see Fig. 8–5). This "out-of-place" IgD expression suggests that the usual microanatomic basis of heavy-chain switching may be altered in FL.[1]

Regarding altered oncogene status, in contrast with normal germinal centers, FL nodules constitutively overexpress the *BCL2* gene, a useful diagnostic finding distinguishing neoplastic from reactive follicles (Fig. 8–14; see also color section).[36] This altered oncogene status relates to a specific chromosome translocation t(14;18), as discussed earlier.[110] The *BCL2* overexpression induces a hypoproliferative state, as illustrated in Figure 8–5).[37] Note that the FL neoplasm has a conspicuously lower proliferative rate than the reactive lymph node. However, not all FLs are in a hypoproliferative state. As shown in Figure 8–15, the FL with a large cell component known as follicular mixed and LCL have a progressively increasing proliferative rate reflected in their respectively more aggressive clinical course.[1]

As shown in Table 8–3, FLs differ from the other indolent lymphomas in growth pattern (nodular growth) and phenotypic specifics. In contrast with SLL, FLs typically express

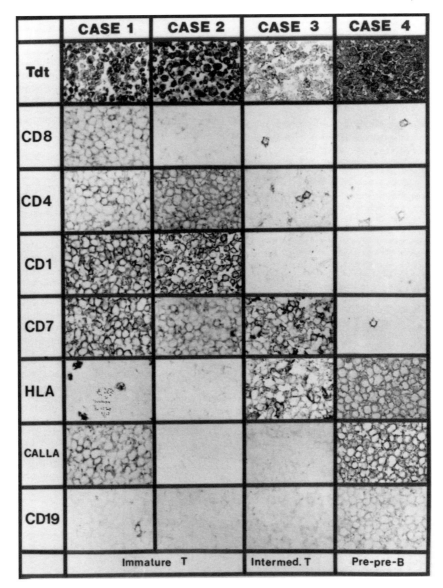

Figure 8–12. Comparative immunotypes of lymphoblastic lymphoma, as illustrated by four examples. Abbreviations: Tdt = terminal deoxynucleotidyl transferase; otherwise, see Table 8–1.

Table 8–3. Low-Grade Non-Hodgkin's Lymphomas: Comparative Morphologic and Immunophenotypic Features

Entity	Characteristic Morphology	Phenotypic and Genotypic Features
FL	Small cleaved and large lymphs in nodules	Strong Ig, pan B+ (CD20 > 19), CD5– 10+, 11c–, 23±, 43–, **BCL2+, t(14;18)**
MALT	Small slightly irregular lymphs, lymphoepithelial lesion, marginal zone growth	Strong Ig, pan B+, CD5–, 10–, 11c±, 23–, 43±, t(1;14); trisomy 3, 7, 12
Monocytoid B-cell	Small lymphs with abundant clear cytoplasm; confluent sinusoidal growth	Moderate Ig, pan B+, CD5–, 10–, 11c+, 23–, 43±,
Mantle cell	Small, slightly irregular lymphs in mantle zone (no large cells)	Strong Ig, pan B+, CD5+, 10–, 11c 23–, 43+, *BCL1+*, t(11;14)
SLL	Small, round lymphocytes ±proliferation centers	Faint Ig (IgM+D+), CD19>20, CD5+, 10–, 11c±, 23+, 43+, BCL–3+, t(14;19); trisomy 12
HCL	Sinusoidal small cells with abundant cytoplasm	Strong Ig (IgM+D–), pan B+, CD5–, 10–, 11c+ (strong), 25+ (strong), 103+, TRAP+

HCL, hairy cell leukemia. See text for other abbreviations.

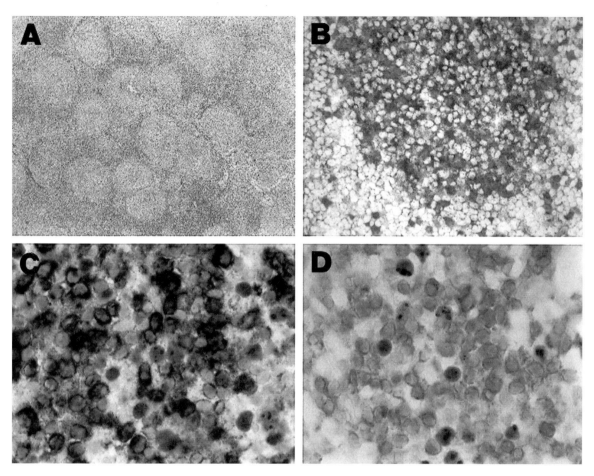

Figure 8–13. Follicular lymphoma *(A)* oncogene and proliferative status. As shown in *B,* the neoplastic cells strongly express CD10 *(Calla)* (blue), and a minority of the cells coexpress the nuclear proliferative antigen Ki67 (brown). As shown in *C,* a minority of the follicular lymphoma cells express nuclear p53 (brown), whereas most express surface *BCL2* (blue). This p53 overexpression heralds clinical progression. As shown in *D,* a few lymphoma cells are proliferating, as evidenced by nuclear Ki67 expression (brown), whereas most of the resting cells (Ki67 negative) are *BCL2* positive (red). This mutually exclusive pattern of Ki67 and *BCL2,* shown in *D,* is common in follicular lymphoma. (See also color section.)

CD20 more intensely than CD19, express surface Ig strongly (rare Ig-negative FLs are described), and do not express CD5.[3] In contrast with MCL, FL expresses CD10 and not CD43 or CD5. The FL overexpression of *BCL2* is not a point of differentiation since most indolent lymphomas express *BCL2,* although typically unrelated to the t(14,18).[3]

Marginal Zone B-Cell Lymphoma

Marginal zone B-cell neoplasms have distinctive histologic, immunologic, and clinical features. They include extranodal low-grade mucosa-associated lymphoid tissue lymphoma (MALToma), splenic MZL, and a monocytoid B-cell lymphoma.[3] These entities have sufficient morphologic and immunophenotypic similarities to suggest relatedness. In particular, they have common tissue-specific homing patterns involving the lymphoid tissues in a patchy or circular pattern just outside the follicular mantle zones in the region known as the marginal zone.[3, 111] Two of these entities are considered in more detail in the following sections.

MALToma. This mature B-cell lymphoma (Fig. 8–16; see also color section) characteristically involves epithelial-lined organs, especially the gastrointestinal tract, salivary glands, orbit, breasts, conjunctiva, and skin.[112, 113] The characteristic

pathologic lesion is the lymphoepithelial lesion representing invasion of the epithelial mucosa by a cluster on monoclonal B cells.[112, 113] These epithelial clusters of lymphocytes represent epithelial invasion highly analogous to the clustered cutaneous T cells (Pautrier's microabscesses) found in mycosis fungoides (see Figs. 8–16 and 8–20). With MALTomas the adjacent submucosa typically shows a lymphocyte infiltrate in the marginal zone of adjacent lymphoid follicles. The neoplastic lymphoid cells are typically small and vary from round to cleaved. Typically, there are admixed small lymphoid cells with abundant clear cytoplasm known as monocytoid B cells. Plasmacytic differentiation is common.[112, 113]

Phenotyping reveals that tumor cells express monoclonal Ig (IgM, G, or A and not D). Typically, this is surface Ig, although the plasmacytic component is monoclonal in 40%.[3, 114] Pan-B-cell antigens are expressed without CD5, CD10, or CD23 coexpression, as found in other indolent lymphocytic lymphomas (see Table 8–3).[3, 114] The monocytoid component may coexpress the monocytoid histiocytic antigen CD11c.[115] Normal epithelial or glandular structures are focally disrupted, an observation made more obvious by cytokeratin stains (see Fig. 8–16). Nearby normal germinal centers may be colonized secondarily, leading to confusion

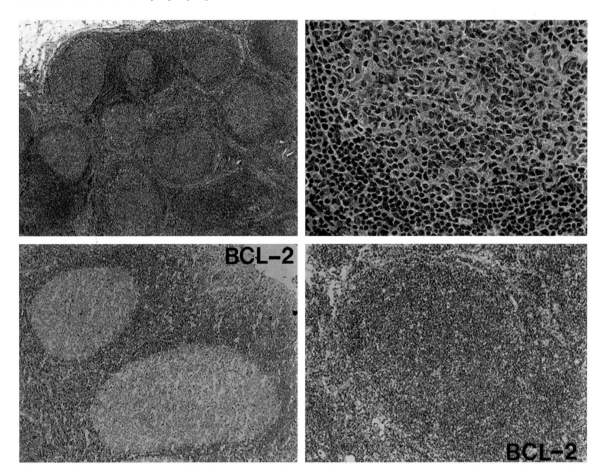

Figure 8–14. Follicular lymphoma with *BCL2* overexpression. This follicular lymphoma manifests follicular overexpression of the *BCL2* oncogene product *(lower right)*, which contrasts with the usual *BCL2* near-absence in a normal physiologic germinal center *(lower left)*. (See also color section.)

with FL.[3] However, MALToma cells lack CD10 expression, and *BCL2* expression occurs unrelated to chromosome translocation.[3]

The disease is typically localized, and it may be cured by local therapy.[116] Recent studies suggest that proliferation in some MALTomas may be antigen driven and

that therapy directed at the antigen may result in regression. Specifically, triple-antibiotic therapy may result in elimination of *Helicobacter pylori* and, in turn, gastric MALToma.[117] More recently, studies by the Southwest Oncology Group (SWOG) and other groups suggest that dissemination and conversion to high-grade lymphoma may

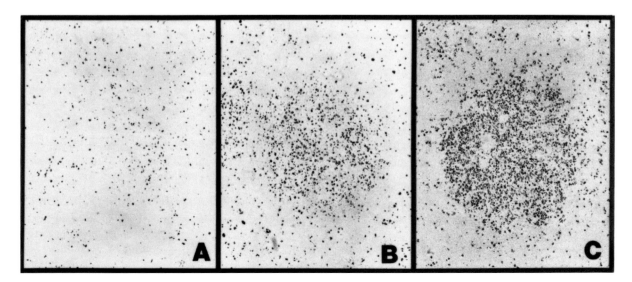

Figure 8–15. The range of cell proliferation among follicular lymphomas as revealed by Ki67: *A*, follicular small cleaved; *B*, follicular mixed; *C*, follicular large cell.

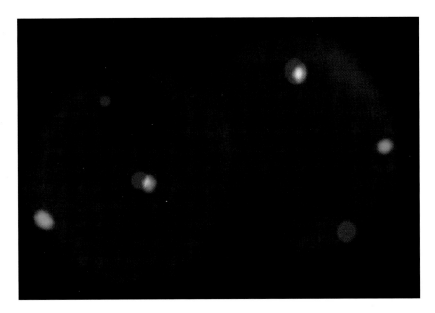

Figure 7–7. Detection of chromosome translocations by interphase fluorescence in situ hybridization (FISH). The figure shows a digitized image of two nuclei that were isolated from a paraffin section of a gastric lymphoma of mucosa-associated lymphoid tissue (MALT) and then analyzed for the presence of the t(11;18)(q21;q21), a translocation found in about 20% of MALT lymphomas. Two bacterial artificial chromosomes (BACs) that flank the chromosome 11 breakpoint on either side were used as hybridization probes and appear as red or green dots. The normal chromosome 11q21 region is identified by closely lying or superimposed red and green dots. The discrete green and red dots identify the two translocation derivatives and demonstrate that the translocation breakpoint in chromosome 11 occurred between the sequences contained within the two BACs.

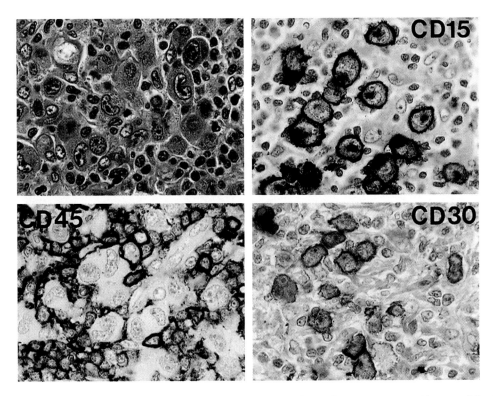

Figure 8–8. Classic Hodgkin's disease phenotype *(upper left)* with neoplastic Reed-Sternberg cells coexpressing CD15 *(upper right)* and CD30 *(lower right)* with absent CD45 *(lower left)*. Note that the CD15 occurs in both the Golgi complex and cell surface, creating a "target." CD45 expression is found in adjacent normal leukocytes, but the polylobated cells are negative.

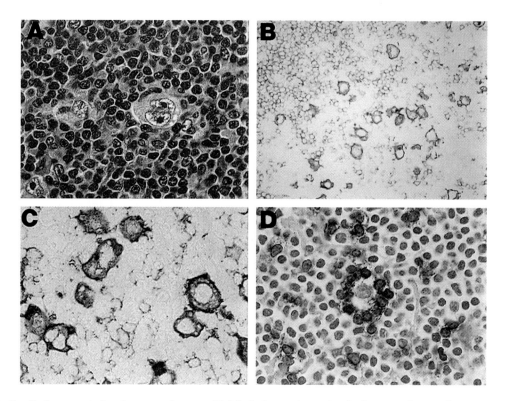

Figure 8–10. *A,* B-cell phenotype in lymphocyte-predominant Hodgkin's disease (LPHD). The large neoplastic cells are CD20+ *(B* and *C).* Immediately surrounding the CD20+ neoplastic cells is a wreath or rosette of CD57+ and positive-like T natural killer cells representing the characteristic immunotopographic feature of LPHD *(D).*

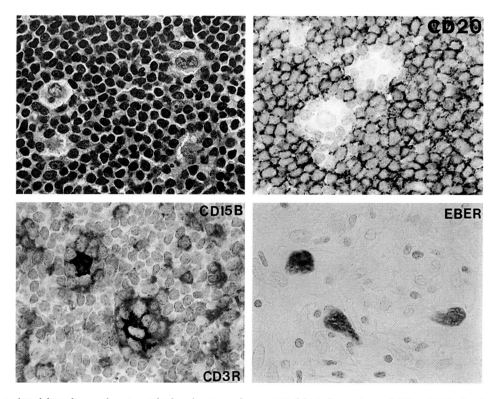

Figure 8–11. Atypical Hodgkin's disease phenotype. This lymphocyte-predominant Hodgkin's disease *(upper left)* has CD20+ B-cell nodules *(upper right)* with CD57+/CD3+ rosettes surrounding CD15+ Reed-Sternberg and Hodgkin's cell variants *(lower left).* Some of the Reed-Sternberg variants also coexpressed CD20 (not shown.) The Reed-Sternberg cells also demonstrated Epstein-Barr virus transcripts (EBER) by in situ hybridization *(lower right).*

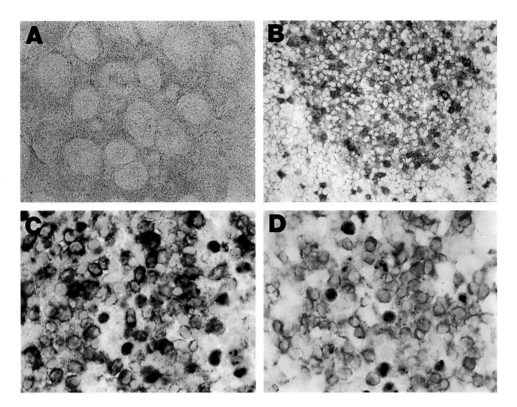

Figure 8–13. Follicular lymphoma *(A)* oncogene and proliferative status. As shown in *B,* the neoplastic cells strongly express CD10 *(Calla)* (blue), and a minority of the cells coexpress the nuclear proliferative antigen Ki67 (brown). As shown in *C,* a minority of the follicular lymphoma cells express nuclear p53 (brown), whereas most express surface *BCL2* (blue). This p53 overexpression heralds clinical progression. As shown in *D,* a few lymphoma cells are proliferating, as evidenced by nuclear Ki67 expression (brown), whereas most of the resting cells (Ki67 negative) are *BCL2* positive (red). This mutually exclusive pattern of Ki67 and *BCL2,* shown in *D,* is common in follicular lymphoma.

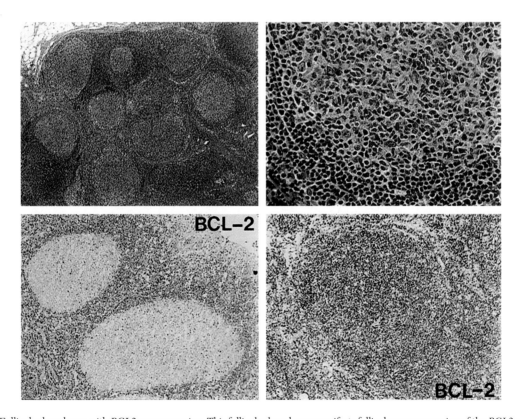

Figure 8–14. Follicular lymphoma with *BCL2* overexpression. This follicular lymphoma manifests follicular overexpression of the *BCL2* oncogene product *(lower right),* which contrasts with the usual *BCL2* near-absence in a normal physiologic germinal center *(lower left).*

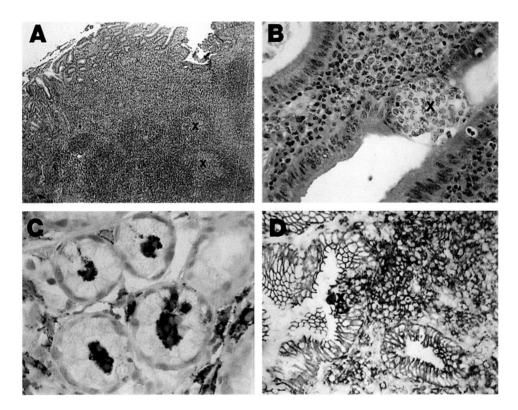

Figure 8–16. Phenotype of mucosa-associated lymphoma (MALToma). As shown in *A*, this gut-associated lymphoid proliferation occurs in the submucosa in a complex pattern: surrounding intact germinal centers (marked "x") with mantle zones. As shown in *B*, the mucosa shows focal, clustered invasion by small lymphoid cells producing a lesion known as a lymphoepithelial lesion (marked "x"). As shown in *C*, the lymphoepithelial lesion is composed of a cluster of B cells (brown, CD20+). As shown in *D*, the neoplastic B cells (blue, CD20+) focally invade (marked "x") and displace normal mucosa (brown, keratin).

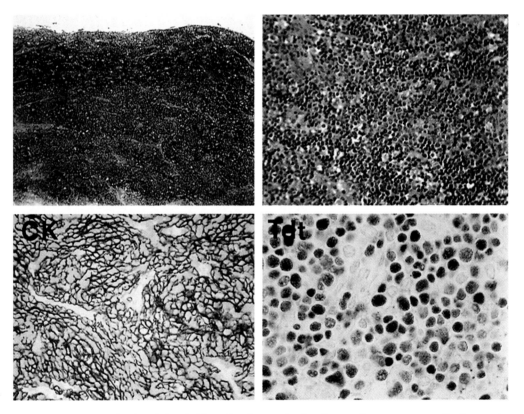

Figure 8–19. Lymphocytic thymoma confused with lymphoblastic lymphoma. This lymphocytic thymoma was initially diagnosed as a lymphoblastic lymphoma based on the morphology and nuclear Tdt finding *(lower right)*. Subsequently, a keratin stain *(lower left)* showed an extensive epithelial network in the tumor, favoring thymoma in agreement with radiographic findings.

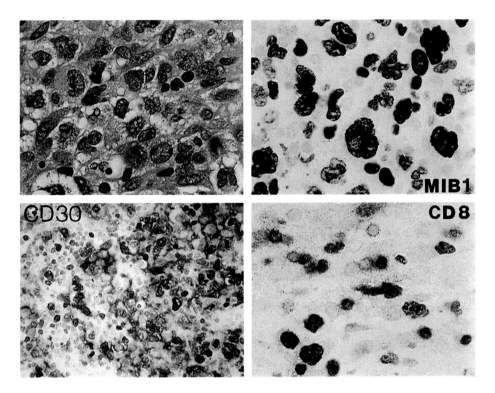

Figure 8–21. Anaplastic large cell lymphoma. The large blastic cells *(upper left)* have a high proliferative rate, as evidenced by nuclear Ki67 reactivity (brown, Ki67) *(upper right).* As shown in the lower left, the large neoplastic cells are mostly CD30+ (blue, Ki1 antigen), with Ki67-positive (brown) nuclei indicating a high proliferation rate. As shown in the lower right, the smaller nonneoplastic CD8+ T-cytotoxic cells (blue), representing T-TIL, are admixed with the larger tumor cells, and in this double-labeled assay, some CD8+ are proliferative (brown, Ki67 positive) and others are Ki67 negative. This indicates that a proliferative CD8+ T-TIL response is active in this high-grade lymphoma.

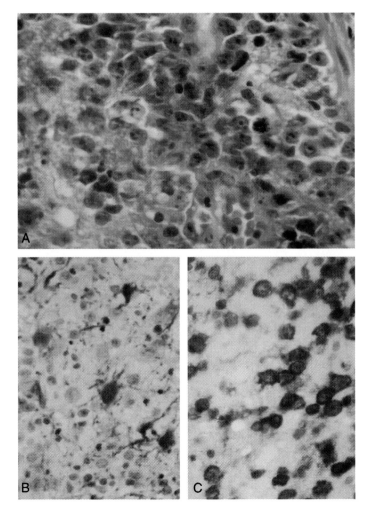

Figure 26–2. Histologic sections of a large cell primary central nervous system lymphoma. *A,* The tumor is characterized by angiocentricity (tendency to aggregate around small blood vessels), as well as clumped, peripherally located nuclear chromatin, and prominent nucleoli (hematoxylin and eosin, ×400). *B,* Glial fibrillary acidic protein (GFAP) immunoperoxidase staining of the tumor. GFAP is a known intermediate filament found exclusively in cells of astrocytic origin. The darkly staining cells with the elongated processes are reactive astrocytes, often found in areas of abnormality within the cerebrum (tumor, infection, ischemia). *C,* Leukocyte common antigen (LCA) immunoperoxidase staining of the tumor. LCA is a protein found on the surface of almost all cells of lymphocytic origin. The darkly staining cells are the tumor cells, proving the lymphocytic nature of this neoplasm.

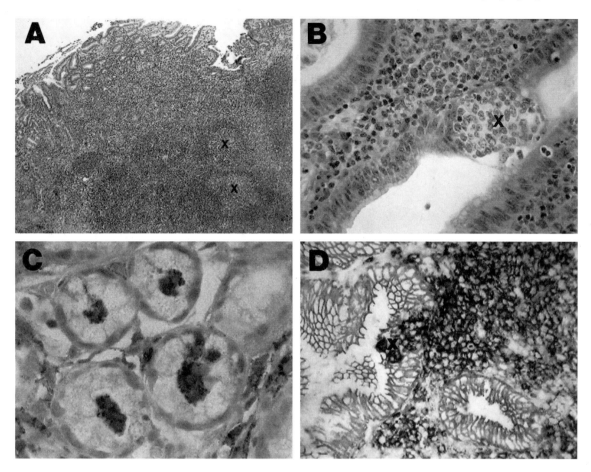

Figure 8–16. Phenotype of mucosa-associated lymphoma (MALToma). As shown in *A*, this gut-associated lymphoid proliferation occurs in the submucosa in a complex pattern: surrounding intact germinal centers (marked "x") with mantle zones. As shown in *B*, the mucosa shows focal, clustered invasion by small lymphoid cells producing a lesion known as a lymphoepithelial lesion (marked "x"). As shown in *C*, the lymphoepithelial lesion is composed of a cluster of B cells (brown, CD20+). As shown in *D*, the neoplastic B cells (blue, CD20+) focally invade (marked "x") and displace normal mucosa (brown, keratin). (See also color section.)

be more common than previously reported. When disseminated, MALTomas appear to be incurable even with curative-intent therapy.[111] When MALToma spreads to distant sites, such as the lymph nodes, or the spleen, the monocytoid cells may predominate, occurring in a marginal zone pattern.[112, 113]

Monocytoid B-Cell Lymphoma. In contrast with extranodal epithelial-based MALToma, monocytoid B-cell lymphomas are typically node based.[111, 115, 118–121] Node-based monocytoid B-cell lymphomas occur in a disseminated pattern and follow an indolent disease course similar to FLs.[111, 120] The neoplastic cells are small lymphoid cells with abundant cytoplasm, suggesting monocytes. These neoplastic cells have a hybrid phenotype with monotypic Ig, pan-B, and monocytic/histiocytic (CD11c) antigen coexpression.[119] The distinctive microanatomic features include a sinusoidal pattern of spread with characteristic confluent sinuses filled with monocytoid cells showing secondary follicle invasion. Distinction from physiologic monocytoid B-cell responses is based on the greater pleomorphism and monotypic Ig found in the neoplastic state.[121] Confusion with hairy cell leukemia is possible based on similar morphology and similar phenotypic features (pan-B/CD11c) coexpression. However, hairy cell leukemia cells are characteristically positive for CD25, PCA-1, and tartrate-resistant acid phosphatase (TRAP),

whereas monocytoid B-cell lymphomas are not.[3] There is a high occurrence of composite lymphoma, suggesting the monocytoid B-cell population may involve a range of morphologic and differentiation expressions.[111, 121] Like MALToma, monocytoid B lymphoma is associated with Sjögren's syndrome, and it may secondarily involve the gut in a few cases, suggesting considerable overlap with the two entities.[118–120]

Mantle Cell Lymphoma

MCL was initially defined as centrocytic lymphoma by Tolksdorf and associates,[122] intermediately differentiated lymphocytic lymphoma by Berard and Dorfman,[123] and MZL by Weisenburger and colleagues.[124] It is derived from cells of the follicular mantle zone. There are two histologic patterns, including the nodular variant and the diffuse variant.[124] In the American literature, the nodular variant is typically referred to as the MZL, whereas the diffuse variant is typically referred to as the diffuse intermediate differentiated lymphocytic lymphoma (DILL).[123, 124] The tumor cells are small, slightly irregular, oval to round lymphocytes with moderate chromatin condensation. Larger transformed cells are rare. Rarely, histologic transformation to a lymphoblastic large cell or highly proliferative form may occur.[125]

Many cases have scattered epithelial histiocytes, creating a "starry-sky" pattern. The tumor cells express monotypic surface Ig and coexpress CD5 with typical absence of CD10, 11c, and 23 (Fig. 8–17). By IHC analysis, a prominent disorganized meshwork of follicular dendritic cells (FDCs) is present, in contrast with the tight-knit FDC of FL.[3] Absence of CD23 is useful in distinguishing from B-cell chronic lymphocytic leukemia (B-CLL); CD5 is useful in distinguishing from FL or MZL.[126] There is a chromosome translocation t(11;14), which involves the *BCL1* locus on 11 and the IgH locus on 14. This translocation results in overexpression of the *PRAD-1* protooncogene, which encodes the cell cycle D1, not normally detectable in physiologic lymphoid cells.[127] The occurrence of *PRAD-1*-positive lymphoid cells in a mantle zone configuration is the characteristic tissue section IHC pattern for MCL.

Clinically, the tumor is prevalent in older men, who usually present with stage III or IV disease.[111] Sites involved include lymph nodes, spleen, peripheral blood, marrow, Waldeyer's rings, and gastrointestinal tract in the form of multifocal lymphomatous polyps. The latter involvement is submucosal in association with polyps, without evident lymphoepithelial lesions, as found in MALToma.[3] The disease course is aggressive, without evidence of curability, since the survival curves do not show evidence of a plateau effect.[111, 114]

Small Lymphocytic Lymphoma

This tissue counterpart of CLL is composed of small, round, monotonous lymphoid cells with clumped "tortoise shell–like" chromatin and inapparent nucleoli growing in a diffuse pattern.[128] Larger prolymphocytes and immunoblasts occur clustered in pseudofollicles or proliferation centers.[129] The immunophenotype is typically (>95%) of B-cell type with a characteristic amalgam of findings: faint monoclonal Ig expression with frequent IgM and IgD coexpression, general pan-B antigen (CD19,20,22,23) expression with aberrant CD5, and CD43 pan-T antigen coexpression.[114, 130, 131] Characteristically, CD22 and 20 expression is weaker than CD19, with the former sometimes undetectable.[114, 130, 131] The CD23 expression is useful in distinguishing B-SLL/CLL from CD23– MCL.[3] Expression of IgD and CD5 in SLL has a high association with eventual lymphocytosis, further blurring the distinction from CLL (see Table 8–3).[114, 131] The lack of CD5 and IgD in nonleukemic SLL suggests that these molecules are relevant to SLL cell spread and localization.[114, 131] The normal cellular equivalent of SLL is the CD5+ autoantibody-

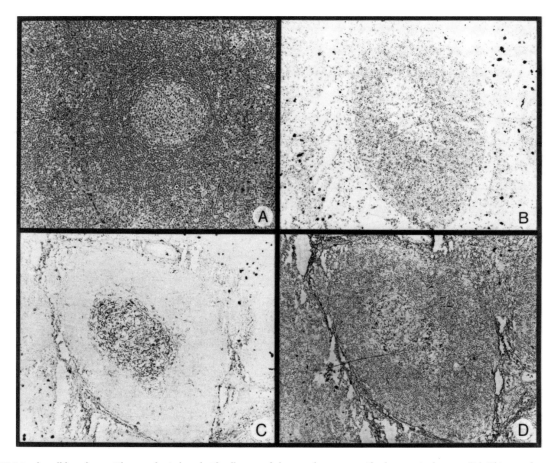

Figure 8–17. Mantle cell lymphoma. The neoplastic lymphoid cells expand the mantle zone outside the germinal center (*A*). This mantle zone expansion manifests immunoglobulin monoclonality with the presence of κ (*D*) and absence of λ (*C*) in the mantle zone, whereas the centrally located normal germinal centers express both light chains and manifest polyclonality (*C* and *D*). An additional characteristic phenotypic feature is the coexpression of CD5 (*B*).

producing B cell at the edge of germinal centers[132] and in primary fetal follicles.[133] Cytogenetics reveal trisomy 12 (one third of cases)[10] translocations of chromosomes 11 and 14 in a minority of cases,[11] and *BCL3* rearrangements are reported[12] relative to the translocation of chromosomes 14 and 19 (t14;19) in scattered patients. Using IHC, transition to aggressive disease is also heralded by high mitotic rate[17] (>30/20 hpf) and a high proliferative rate (>20%) as measured by Ki67.[134]

SLL Plasmacytoid Variant (Immunocytoma)

Twenty-five percent of SLLs have either plasma cells or lymphoid-plasma cell hybrids or plasmacytoid cells.[128] Morphologically, intranuclear (Dutcher bodies) and intracytoplasmic (Russell bodies) inclusions are common, as is associated gammopathy due to monoclonal Ig secretion.[128] These tumors usually lack CD5 and commonly have surface and cytoplasmic Ig, usually of IgM type without IgD. Many cases represent Waldenström's macroglobulinemia with monoclonal IgM secretion and hyperviscosity syndromes.[114, 131]

Hairy Cell Leukemia

Hairy cell leukemia, a leukemic form of mature B-cell neoplasia, causes morphologic confusion with other tissue-based small cell lymphocytic lymphomas. The distinctive cytology of hairy cell leukemia usually suffices for diagnostic identification. However, sometimes hepatic, nodal, or splenic involvement can be problematic. Using IHC criteria, hairy cell leukemia is readily distinguished from other indolent lymphocytic lymphoma/leukemia by a unique pattern of coexpression: pan-B antigens with monocytic (CD11c) and IL-2 growth receptors (CD25) along with TRAP.[3, 16] Although IgM is usually present, IgD is not, and CD5, CD23, CD43, and LFA-1 are usually absent. Hairy cell leukemia also coexpresses CD103+ and is useful in differential IHC diagnosis.[16]

Diffuse Aggressive B-Cell Lymphomas

The diffuse aggressive B-cell neoplasms have a B-cell phenotype with a high proliferative rate. In particular, although the low-grade lymphomas may have an average Ki67 proliferative rate below 20%, the aggressive B-cell lymphomas have an average proliferative rate exceeding 40% to 50%.[6, 37] They also typically express activation markers (e.g., HLA-DR and CD38) more strongly than indolent B-cell lymphomas.[3] They show a higher incidence of aberrant phenotypes with more frequent loss of pan-B, Ig, and CAM markers than low-grade B-cell lymphomas.[6] These lymphomas in the Working Formulation (WF) include cases of diffuse mixed large cell type and small, noncleaved Burkitt's and Burkitt's-like lymphoma.

Diffuse Large Cell Lymphomas

Immunotyping reveals that 80% of large cell lymphomas are B cell, 15% are T cell, 4% are null, and 1% are biphenotypic.[135, 136] The B-cell diffuse large cell lymphomas (DLCL) typically express at least one of several pan-B antigens, including CD19, 20, 22, and 79a.[3, 135, 136] Surface Ig is found in many but not all B-cell DLCLs, and cyto-

plasmic Ig may occur in a minority, particularly in plasmacytoid variants. The latter may prove difficult for IHC diagnosis because they commonly lack pan-B antigens (see Fig. 8–2). They typically express various activation antigens (e.g., CD25 and HLA-DR).[136] DLCL may present challenges because loss of pan-B antigens and pan-T antigens may accompany their transformed status.[136] Some B-cell DLCLs are anaplastic LCL with CD30 coexpression and may show cohesive cell growth and lack CD45, making certain distinction from carcinoma difficult.[3] In some cases, the extranodal DLCL may be accompanied by compartmentalizing fibrosis, giving a nesting appearance and suggesting carcinoma.[3] IHC phenotyping is critical to proper diagnosis in these instances. DLCL phenotyping may identify prognostic differences, as described later.

Burkitt's and Burkitt's-Like Lymphomas

Burkitt's lymphomas are high-grade lymphomas that are monomorphic proliferations of intermediate-sized cells with round blastic nuclei and multiple (two to five) basophilic nucleoli.[137, 138] There is a high mitotic rate and a starry-sky pattern reflecting ingested apoptotic tumor cells within macrophages.[137, 139] The usual pattern of growth is diffuse, although involved germinal centers suggest follicular derivation.[140] There is a morphologic variation known as Burkitt's-like lymphoma that shows greater nuclear viability (pleomorphism). Burkitt's-like lymphoma typically has nuclei containing one or two eosinophilic nuclei with basophilic vacuolated cytoplasm.[138] The latter appearance is intermediate between Burkitt's and large cell (immunoblastic) lymphomas. The Burkitt's-like lymphoma is the most common lymphoma, complicating HIV,[141] treated Hodgkin's disease,[142] and the immunosuppressive posttransplantation state.[143]

Immunologic findings reflect the likely germinal center origin with pan-B antigen expression, including CD10 and monoclonal Ig expression ($\lambda > \kappa$, M > G) (Fig. 8–18).[38, 39] Burkitt's lymphomas typically have absent expression of both LFA-1 (CD18) and ICAM (CD54).[144, 145] The loss of these CAMs relevant to B–T-cell interaction has been shown to result in poor T-cell immunosurveillance of Burkitt's cells and may also account for loss of B-cell cohesion and ready extranodal spread.[145] Occasional Burkitt's-like tumors are described of more immature pre-B-cell (Tdt-positive, CIgM-positive) phenotype.[106] Rare examples of Burkitt's-like lymphoma of T-cell phenotype are described.[146] Typically, translocation of C-*MYC* results in overexpression of this gene and a consequent markedly elevated Ki67 proliferative rate exceeding 80%.[38, 39] IHC analysis reveals a diffuse sheet of Ki67-positive blastic lymphoid cells with a proliferative rate higher than that of any other lymphoma (see Fig. 8–18).

T-CELL LYMPHOMAS

Precursor T-Lymphoblastic Lymphoma/Leukemia

LBLs of immature T-cell type, indistinguishable from immature B-LBL, have blastic nuclei with fine dusky chromatin, inconspicuous nucleoli, and scant cytoplasm. Most LBLs (85%) (see Fig. 8–12) have an immature T-cell

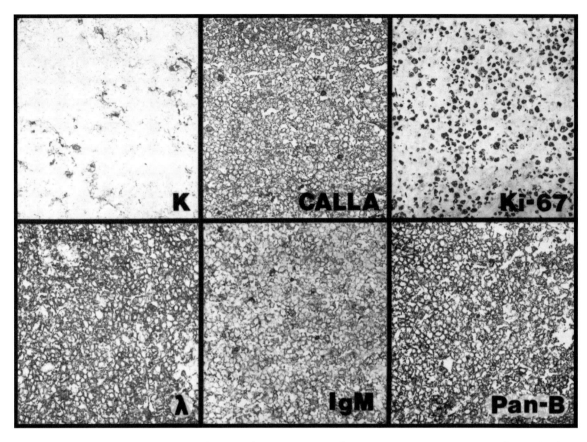

Figure 8–18. Burkitt's lymphoma. The characteristic phenotype shows coexpression of pan-B antigens, CD10 (CALLA), and monoclonal Ig with a very high Ki67 proliferative rate (>80%).

phenotype that mimics the cortex of the thymus.[29, 104, 105] As shown in Figure 8–12, this immaturity is manifested by coexpression of T-helper (CD4) and T-cytotoxic antigens (CD8) with strong nuclear coexpression of the thymic-derived nuclear enzyme Tdt. The more immature forms coexpress CD10 (CALLA) and lack HLA-DR, as shown in Figs. 8–3 and 8–12). More mature T-LBLs have a single functional subset (e.g., CD4) and lack CALLA. Rarely, as shown in Figure 8–12 (case 3), even more mature forms occur with faint Tdt and aberrant T antigens (e.g., CD7+, CD1–, 4–, 8–). In the latter instance of more mature T-LBL, the patients nonetheless fit the clinicopathologic profile of LBL, with mediastinal presentation in young males, subsequent leukemic involvement, and classic convoluted LBL morphology.[29] There is considerable overlap with T-cell acute lymphoblastic leukemia (T-ALL) with peripheral blood and marrow involvement in one third of LBL cases. Sanctuary sites such as the gonads and central nervous system (CNS) are commonly involved. This similarity to T-ALL (i.e., involvement of sanctuary sites and similar phenotype) prompts treatment of LBL similar to ALL. Rarely, T-LBL may express NK cell antigens (CD16+, 57+); these patients follow an aggressive course, and females predominate in contrast with the usual T-LBL male predominance.[147]

A serious error in diagnosis may result when lymphocytic thymoma is confused with LBL.[1] Since lymphocytic thymoma has a mediastinal presentation and a predominance of

immature T cells with coexpression of Tdt/CD10/CD1, 2, 3, 4, 5, 7, 9, this mistake is not unreasonable on clinical and immunologic levels. Since LBL requires elaborate multidrug chemotherapy with CNS prophylaxis and thymoma requires simple surgery, the clinical stakes are high.[1]

As illustrated in Figure 8–19 (see also color section), the key to deciphering this difference is histologic and immunologic detection of the epithelial cell component. Figure 8–19 demonstrates the simultaneous Tdt and cytokeratin expression in a lymphocytic thymoma. This 35-year-old man presented with a large anterior mediastinal mass. The biopsy specimen obtained from mediastinoscopy was interpreted as a lymphoblastic lymphoma. A consulting hematopathologist concurred with this diagnosis but only after confirming that the cytokeratin antibody on formalin-fixed material was negative. Chemotherapy was initiated. However, since a thymoma was strongly suspected on radiologic grounds, an antikeratin antibody test on frozen tissue was performed, revealing the striking epithelial framework. Frozen tissue assessment indicated both an immature T-cell lymphoid component (pan T+, CD1a+, CD10+, Tdt+) and epithelial components, mirroring the phenotype of normal thymus and supporting the diagnosis of a thymoma with a predominance of lymphocytes.[1]

This case emphasizes several important rules in phenotyping: (1) immunotyping should not be performed in a clinical vacuum (the radiologist strongly suspected a thymoma); (2) avoid "tunnel vision" (lymphoid phenotyping should be counterbalanced with other findings [e.g., histologic evidence of lobation]); (3) beware of false negatives, in general, and in formalin-fixed material, in particular; (4) freezing generally results in fewer antigenic false-negative results; and (5) cell suspension studies, without cytoplasmic fixatives and without methods to free epithelial cells from stroma, may be misleading.[1]

Peripheral T-Cell Lymphomas

Peripheral T-cell lymphomas (PTLs) are a morphologically heterogeneous group of lymphomas with a mature, activated postthymic phenotype.[31, 32, 148] The PTL neoplastic cells typically express HLA-DR and other activation antigens (e.g., CD38). Characteristically, PTLs show aberrant pan-T antigen expression with loss or absence of some expected pan-T antigens (see Fig. 8–6).[31, 32, 148] This frequent idiosyncratic pan-T antigen loss in PTL is not usual in inflammation and greatly helps to identify true T-cell neoplasia.[31, 32, 149] Morphologically, most PTL would be classified in the WF as mixed cell or large cell lymphomas, with a few CLL-like lymphocytic lymphomas. Histologically, PTLs are characterized by their pleomorphism and polymorphism.[31, 149] The pleomorphism may take the form of large polylobated Reed-Sternberg–like cells that require the

distinction of PTL from Hodgkin's disease.[31, 49] The polymorphism, representing admixed eosinophils, plasma cells, fibroblasts, histiocytes, and vascular elements, is largely the result of the functional cytokines produced by PTL cells.[150] Commonly in PTL, these admixed reactive elements may outnumber neoplastic elements, leading to great diagnostic difficulty and confusion with IHC interpretation. In any event, there has emerged an understanding that under the rubric of PTL there are a number of distinct clinical, etiologic, and cytogenetic syndromes not accounted for in the WF. These entities, as listed in the REAL classification[3] and elsewhere, include (1) angiocentric PTL (e.g., lethal midline granuloma); (2) virus-associated PTL (e.g., adult Japanese T-lymphoma/leukemia); (3) cytogenetic-specific PTL (e.g., anaplastic large cell lymphoma); (4) lymphokine-related PTL (e.g., Lennert's lymphoma); and (5) organ-specific PTL (e.g., skin: mycosis fungoides; CNS: CD56+ PTL). The emergence of PTL as an entity, in spite of such diversity, reflects several factors: (1) its immunologic specificity (mature activated T-cell status with a novel pan-T antigen pattern)[31, 32]; (2) the occurrence of distinctive clinical syndromes (e.g., gluten-enteropathy associated)[151]; (3) distinctive etiologic definition (human T-cell lymphotropic virus, type I–related PTL)[152–154]; and (4) specific genetic definition (e.g., the t[2;5] in anaplastic LCL-PTL).[155]

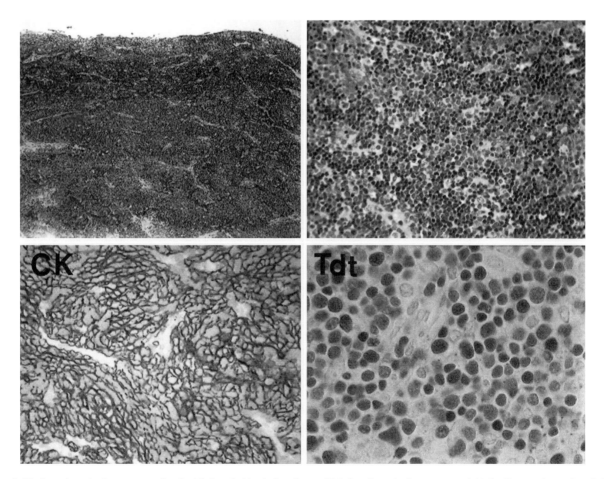

Figure 8–19. Lymphocytic thymoma confused with lymphoblastic lymphoma. This lymphocytic thymoma was initially diagnosed as a lymphoblastic lymphoma based on the morphology and nuclear Tdt finding (*lower right*). Subsequently, a keratin stain (*lower left*) showed an extensive epithelial network in the tumor, favoring thymoma in agreement with radiographic findings. (See also color section.)

Several of these PTL variants are discussed because they are of particular interest in IHC assay or diagnosis.

PTL Variants

Mycosis Fungoides. Mycosis fungoides is a cutaneous T-cell lymphoma characterized by a distinctive immunotopographic lesion: a cutaneous cluster of aberrant mature T cells (Fig. 8–20). The clustered epidermal invasion results in a histologic lesion referred to as a Pautrier's microabscess. This cutaneous lesion is highly analogous to the clustered mucosal invasion (e.g., lymphoepithelial lesion) described in the section on MALTomas (see Fig. 8–16). An additional microanatomic feature of note is the presence of S100+, CD1a+ interdigitating reticulum cells (IDCs), and Langerhans' cells (LCs) within the Pautrier's microabscess (see Fig. 8–20).[1, 3] It appears that the IDC/LCs are the nidus of neoplastic T-cell localization, suggesting that these antigen-presenting cells are part of the pathogenesis of mycosis fungoides. Perhaps a carcinogenic agent in LC or IDC (e.g., viral or petrochemical) leads to aberrant T-cell pathogenesis.

The neoplastic helper T cells typically have aberrant T-cell phenotype with an absence of CD7 and Leu-8.[31, 156, 157] Although CD7 and Leu-8 antigen are occasionally separately absent in cutaneous inflammation, the absence of both speaks decidedly for true T-cell neoplasia.[31, 157] Occasional cases of mycosis fungoides with T-cytotoxic antigens or no subset antigens are described; the latter are more commonly associated with the tumor phase and progression of disease.[156] In the final disseminated phase of mycosis fungoides, large pleomorphic cells may be found that coexpress CD15, leading to difficulty in distinction from Hodgkin's disease morphologically and immunologically.[156]

Lennert's Lymphoma. This PTL variant is noteworthy because of its frequent misdiagnosis.[158] These older patients typically present with fever and generalized lymphadenopathy, suggesting an infectious process.[158] On biopsy, this PTL variant characteristically is found to have clusters of epithelioid histiocytes, further suggesting an inflammatory or infectious process.[158, 159] In particular, the reactive histiocytes, eosinophils, and plasma cells may greatly outnumber the rare Reed-Sternberg–like cells. Eventually the entire reticuloendothelial system is involved, with bone marrow and liver involvement the rule.[158] Diagnosis relies on the cytologic atypia of the smaller and intermediate cells' giving the appearance of a diffuse mixed cell lymphoma. The presence of a novel aberrant pan-T antigen coexpression on IHC analysis is also characteristic.[158, 159] A further aid to IHC diagnosis is the pattern of tissue involvement with prominent bone marrow and liver involvement relative to nodal involvement. The disease course is fulminant without therapy, with progression to large cell PTL and loss of histiocytic reaction.[158, 159] Rarely, NHL with excess histiocytes may be of B-cell phenotype and may portend a better prognosis unless of a high-grade histology.[159]

Anaplastic Large Cell Lymphoma (CD30+). This PTL variant composed of large, pleomorphic horseshoe-shaped multinuclear cells was first recognized by its expression of the CD30 activation antigen in the context of other mature T-cell antigens (Fig. 8–21; see also color section).[160]

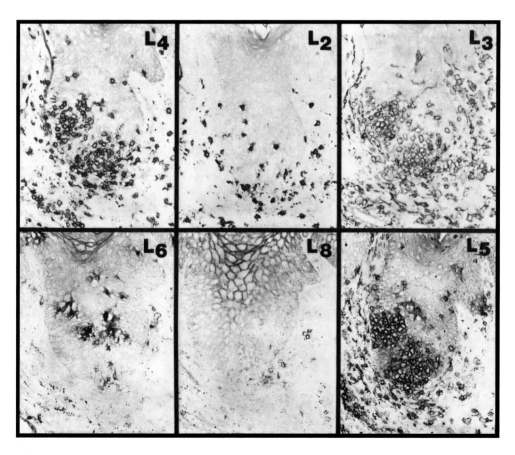

Figure 8–20. Mycosis fungoides. The clustered invasion of the epidermis typically shows an aberrant T-helper phenotype with CD2 (L_5), CD3 (L_4), CD4 (L_3) coexpression and unexpected absence of Leu-8 (L_8 shown) and CD7 (L_9, not shown). The aberrant T cells are associated with CD1a (L_6)-positive Langerhans' cells. CD8 (L_2) cells are sparse.

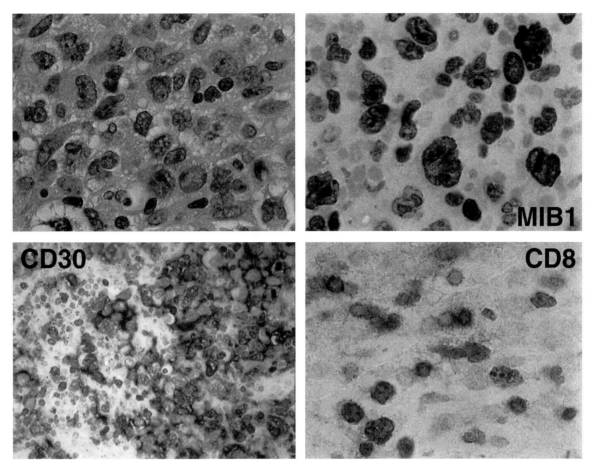

Figure 8–21. Anaplastic large cell lymphoma. The large blastic cells *(upper left)* have a high proliferative rate, as evidenced by nuclear Ki67 reactivity (brown, Ki67) *(upper right)*. As shown in the lower left, the large neoplastic cells are mostly CD30+ (blue, Ki1 antigen), with Ki67-positive (brown) nuclei indicating a high proliferative rate. As shown in the lower right, the smaller nonneoplastic CD8+ T-cytotoxic cells (blue), representing T-TIL, are admixed with the larger tumor cells, and in this double-labeled assay, some CD8+ are proliferative (brown, Ki67 positive) and others are Ki67 negative. This indicates that a proliferative CD8+ T-TIL response is active in this high-grade lymphoma. (See also color section.)

Occasionally, null type and B-cell phenotypes are found.[160, 161] Nonetheless, CD30+ anaplastic LCL is believed to be a distinct clinicopathologic entity.[160] Histologically, it characteristically involves the perifollicular and sinus regions of the node with a sheetlike infiltration of cells.[160] In particular, the cohesive property (sheetlike growth pattern) has caused historical confusion with metastatic carcinoma—an error that may be compounded in IHC analyses because some ALCLs may coexpress the EMA and may lack CD45 expression.[162] Cytogenetic analysis characteristically reveals a translocation t(2;5) in the systemic form of ALCL, while not in the primary cutaneous form.[155] ALCL may occur as a primary disease or secondary to disorders such as mycosis fungoides and Hodgkin's disease.[3] Clinically, two forms are described: (1) a systemic form that follows an aggressive course but, like other LCLs, may be curable; and (2) a primary cutaneous form that either may spontaneously regress or persist as an indolent incurable entity.[163]

In the REAL classification, a Hodgkin's-like variant with some features (e.g., bands of sclerosis) similar to NSHD is described.[3] The latter patients typically are young adults with aggressive nodal disease and often with bulky mediastinal masses. IHC assay typically reveals a non-Hodgkin's phenotype with either pan-B or pan-T lineage markers without CD15 coexpression, except as a minority component. Conventional therapy for HD is said to be insufficient, but good response to third-generation chemotherapy for high-grade NHL is described.[164]

CD56+ Lymphoma. Some PTL may coexpress the CD56 antigen and neuronal cell adhesion molecule (NCAM) and manifest unusual sites of disease involvement (e.g., CNS), as described in the following sections.[165–167]

PHENOTYPIC MARKERS OF PROGNOSIS

IHC has been used to detect cell surface, cytoplasmic, and nuclear antigens that correlate with prognosis, and this body of literature has recently been reviewed in detail.[6] The IHC study of prognostic significance to date has been largely developmental, since most of the published studies are retrospective analyses of small patient groups with heterogenous clinical features, variable treatments, variable assay conditions, and variable statistical cutpoints. More recently, larger prospective IHC trials among uniformly staged and treated, unselected populations have been published and suggest that some IHC markers may have independent clinical significance.[168, 169] Although more time and studies are needed to give ultimate clinical proof of usefulness, even the initial studies have value, since they reveal the biologic features and principles that underlie the failure of lymphoma therapy.[6] Furthermore, the specific antigens identified as factors in lymphoma tumorigenicity present new targets for therapy and new testable treatment hypotheses.

SINGLE-INSTITUTION, RETROSPECTIVE STUDY

A case in point regarding these factors is illustrated in Figure 8–22. This figure illustrates several immunopheno-typic features that are predictive of poor outcome in a consecutive series of 105 patients with DLCL at the University of Arizona. This figure, a composite of the six published papers[37, 41, 136, 170–172] from the single study, reveals that poor outcome relates to (1) loss or absence of HLA-DR antigen; (2) a high proliferative rate, with Ki67 higher than 60%; (3) presence of T-cell lineage; (4) loss of a pan-B antigen (CD22); and (5) a deficiency of tumor-infiltrating T cells (T-TIL, CD8). Finally, as shown in the illustrated model, these immunologic parameters were important independent predictors of outcome among these patients with LCL and have value in identifying patients who will not respond to currently available therapy.[173] These findings suggest at least four factors relevant to prognosis: proliferative status, B-cell versus T-cell lineage, CAMs or recognition molecule status, and host cell response (immunosurveillance).

Beyond this Arizona experience, the literature, focused on these same four areas, indicates mixed results. Studies from several groups have found that loss of class I or II antigens predict a poor prognosis[170, 174–177]; other studies have not.[178, 179] Regarding cell lineage, the prognostic significance of determining B-cell versus T-cell lineage is well established among certain subtypes of lymphoma, specifically lymphoblastic T-cell lymphoma and mature T-cell subtypes of DSCL.[180] However, the usefulness of determining B-cell versus T-cell phenotype among other diffuse intermediate- and high-grade lymphomas is more controversial, with some studies showing no difference[181, 182] and others showing a clear survival difference, with T-cell phenotype always inferior to B-cell phenotype.[168, 172, 183, 184] Regarding proliferation, two studies of LCL have found that poor survival correlates with elevated Ki67 higher than 60%.[37, 185] In contrast, other studies have shown the opposite, with poor outcome related to a low Ki67 value.[186] However, the latter study in particular did not account for, or balance, all known prognostic or treatment factors, as in the Arizona study discussed earlier. Therefore, a comparison among studies cannot be made, and the issue of Ki67 value might be considered moot based on results of single-institution studies, with a clear need for future prospective studies.

MULTIINSTITUTIONAL, PROSPECTIVE STUDIES

More recent studies seeking to answer this call have focused on multiinstitutional, prospective design with predetermined cutpoints looking at uniformly staged and treated patients.[168, 169] These studies balance known clinical prognostic factors (e.g., age, sex, stage, and lactic dehydro-

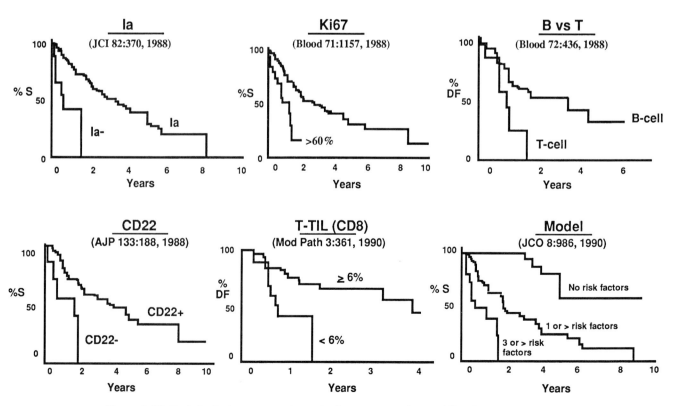

Figure 8–22. Single-institution, retrospective study of prognostic markers in diffuse large cell lymphoma.

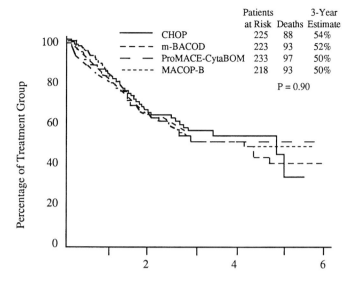
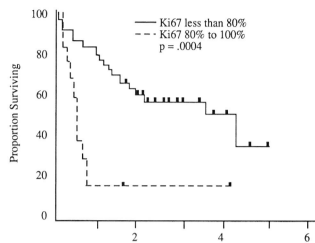

Figure 8–23. Multiinstitutional, prospective trial of Ki67. *Left,* Data are from Fisher R, Gaynor E, Dahlberg S, et al: A phase III comparison of CHOP vs. m-BACOD vs. ProMACE-cytaBOM vs. MACOP-B in patients with intermediate- or high-grade non-Hodgkin's lymphoma: Results of SWOG 8516—The National High-Priority Lymphoma Study. N Engl J Med 1993; 328:1002. *Right,* The same SWOG-8516 patients studied for the proliferative index by Ki67 assay. Data are from Miller T, Grogan T, Dahlberg S, et al: Prognostic significance of the Ki67-associated proliferation antigen in aggressive non-Hodgkin's lymphomas: A prospective Southwest Oncology Group Trial. Blood 1994; 83:1460.

genase [LDH] status). One of these studies, a prospective test of Ki67 in SWOG, is illustrated in Figure 8–23.[169] In this study, a high Ki67 level was found to be useful in identifying a group of intermediate- and high-grade patients with rapidly progressive and fatal disease. The patients with high Ki67 levels experienced 1-year survival of 18% versus 82% for those with a low proliferative rate. A multivariant regression comparing the effect of Ki67 level to performance status, age, stage, extranodal sites of disease, and serum LDH level confirmed the independent effect of proliferation and survival.[169]

In this study incorporating the Ki67 proliferative index, stage (tumor burden), and LDH, the relative risk assigned to each factor (relative risk 5.9, 1.3, and 0.8, respectively) suggests that a direct IHC measure of the growth rate with Ki67 is a more powerful prognostic tool than serum LDH levels and largely displaces LDH as a significant variable. Further evidence of the usefulness of the Ki67 index is the finding that 5 (45%) of 11 patients with high values were identified among the two lowest risk groups as defined by the new International Prognostic Index.[169] The usefulness of Ki67 has also been tested among patients with lower grades of NHL and may prove valuable in selecting patients for more aggressive therapy.[180]

Regarding lineage, a recent large multiinstitutional test by Groupe d'Etudes des Lymphomes des L'Adulte (GELA), which involved a consecutive series of 361 French and Belgian patients with aggressive lymphoma, showed that peripheral T-cell phenotype was associated with a poor prognosis and that the T-cell phenotype is independent of other adverse clinical prognostic factors.[168] Multivariate analysis established four adverse factors: T-cell phenotype, LDH level, serum albumin level, and number of extranodal sites. The French, Arizona, and Nebraska studies of lineage reveal a high level of relapse, suggesting that peripheral T-cell lymphomas may be an incurable subset of intermediate and LCL.[168, 172, 184]

As evidenced by the SWOG[169] and GELA[168] studies, immunophenotypic markers are showing promise for clinical usefulness in multigroup lymphoma trials. In particular, IHC as cited might aid patients who are highly likely to fail conventional therapy and require alternative therapy. Markers such as Ki67 may serve in judging the comparability of lymphoma groups studied. However, more important than any of these uses, IHC markers might give specific insight into why certain patients fail therapy.[6]

MALIGNANT PHENOTYPES SUGGEST BIOLOGIC PRINCIPLES

The "malignant" phenotypes and the related biologic principles are shown in Table 8–2. As shown, each altered phenotypic property suggests a principle (e.g., absent LFA-1) reflecting loss of cell adhesion or loss of immunosurveillance. Many of the listed malignant phenotypes entail a loss or deficiency of marker expression. This suggests that loss of pivotal physiologic surface molecules is commonly adversely related to prognosis. Relevant to this hypothesis, loss of multiple recognition molecules has been shown to result in progressively worse prognosis, whereby a patient with three lost antigens has a worse rate of survival than a patient with one loss (median survival of 4 versus 12 months).[136] This suggests a series or progression of deletional events in lymphoma similar to the allelotypic deletional events described in colon carcinoma progression.[187]

Altered B-Cell Versus T-Cell Interactions

Loss or lack of expression of these adhesion/recognition molecules (e.g., HLA, ICAM, and LFA-1) is a broad phenomenon of biologic importance to IHC diagnosis, as mentioned earlier, and of prognostic import (as discussed in this section) among lymphomas.[6] This is not surprising, given that normal B-cell and T-cell interactions, cohesion, and immunosurveillance are highly dependent on expression of surface recognition molecules (see Fig. 8–4). In general, two factors may be at play: loss of lymphoid cell cohesion and loss of the adhesion molecules relevant to immunosurveillance.[145]

Regarding loss of cohesion, this observation as a factor in lymphoma tumorigenicity fits well with the general observation among solid tumors that lack or loss of CAM expression facilitates tumor progression in the metastatic cascade hypothesized by Liotta and Stetler-Stevenson.[188] Three relevant lymphoma examples may be cited: (1) loss of ICAM-1, normally found on mature B cells, has been correlated with leukemic behavior among NHLs[189]; (2) CD22 loss among B-cell LCL is associated with poor prognosis[136]; and (3) LFA-1-deficient mutants have shown greater invasiveness.[190]

Regarding loss of T-cell immunosurveillance, several examples may be cited. First, loss of LFA-1, necessary for initial T-cell blocking, is more commonly lost in higher-grade lymphomas, suggesting that LFA loss is an inherent part of greater tumorigenicity in lymphoma.[145] More specifically, lymphomas lacking LFA-1 are known as poor stimulators of a CTL response, and it is believed that loss of LFA precludes T-cell adhesion to B cells and thereby obviates immunosurveillance.[145] Second, because HLA antigens are required in the presentation of new antigens on tumor cells to CTLs, absence of HLA in lymphoma may lead to escape from immunosurveillance owing to a lack of tumor immunogenicity. Studies from several groups[170, 174–177] have indeed found that loss of class I or II antigens predict a poor prognosis (see Fig. 8–22). As with LFA, HLA loss increases with lymphoma grade, again suggesting that HLA loss is an inherent part of increased tumorigenicity in lymphoma.[191]

The importance of T-cell immunosurveillance in B-cell neoplasia has been underscored in a number of studies.[42, 134, 192, 193] In particular, in these studies, lymphoma relapse and patient survival have been related to the type and number of specific T-cell subsets, known as T-TIL, that infiltrate B-cell lymph. In one study of BLCL, the finding of CTLs below the 6% level was invariably associated with patient relapse (see Fig. 8–22).[42] In the latter study, the relapsing patients with low T-TIL frequently demonstrated either HLA or LFA-1 loss in 85% of patients.[171] This loss of recognition/adhesion molecule status correlates with loss of immunosurveillance, tumor escape, and prompt relapse. Other studies emphasize a decreased frequency of memory T cells in high-grade relative to low-grade lymphoma, implying that a memory T-TIL response, rather than a naive T-cell response, is active in maintaining less-aggressive NHL status.[192, 193] Although the loss of immunosurveillance is emerging as an adverse factor, the obverse—a gain of immunosurveillance—is a less-documented phenomenon. Perhaps demonstration of a highly proliferative T-TIL–cytotoxic (CD8) component by double labeling, as shown in Figure 8–21, will prove a useful indicator of favorable outcome. The patient illustrated remains alive 7 years after diagnosis in spite of a high proliferative rate, suggesting that a strong, CD8 proliferative rate may be a favorable survival factor.

Not all lymphoma tumorigenicity relates to CAM loss. In other instances, a gain of CAM status may effect tumorigenicity. A case in point would be the T-cell-associated expression of NCAM (CD56).[165–167] This oncofetal adhesion molecule, which is highly analogous to carcinoembryonic antigen, is expressed in 25% of peripheral T-cell or NK-like T-cell lymphomas. Recently, NCAM studies by both the SWOG repository[165, 167] and Wong and colleagues[194] have found that these NCAM-positive lymphomas showed a striking predilection for unusual sites of involvement, including the nasopharynx, CNS, skeletal muscle, and gastrointestinal tract. These anatomic sites naturally express high levels of NCAM, and the known "like-like" homophilic attraction of NCAM molecules could account for the preferential homing of NCAM-positive lymphomas to these sites.[165] Lymphoma involving either the CNS or the nasopharynx is known to portend a poor outcome. The median survival of NCAM-positive lymphomas is less than 50% of the median survival of NCAM-negative lymphomas.[165–167]

The recent observation that NCAM-positive lymphomas with CNS involvement have a high $\alpha2,8$-linked polysialic acid content is intriguing, since similar $\alpha2,8$-linked polysialic acid expression dictates entry of neuroinvasive bacteria into the meninges.[195] This suggests that glycosylation of surface receptors may sometimes be the pivotal factor in site-specific lymphoma spread.

Effect of Sessile Versus Mobile Phenotype

Expression of the LHR (CD44 and Hermes 3) may exert an unfavorable prognostic influence.[15, 196, 197] NHL with a putative derivation from mobile, recirculating, or mature memory T and mature B lymphocytes almost invariably expresses high levels of the LHR, whereas NHLs of sessile derivation (e.g., germinal centers) express lower levels. This gives further credence to the notion that a sessile-mobile phenotype may be relevant to lymphoma dissemination.[6]

In a survey, high-level LHR expression occurred in 85% of patients with stages III and IV LCL, whereas it occurred in only 12% of patients with stages I and II disease.[15] This correlation between LHR expression and disease stage suggests there could ultimately be a "stage-specific" phenotype. A similar trend was found in one study[198] and statistically confirmed in another.[183] In any event, the correlation in the study by Pals and associates is not absolute, because approximately 15% of patients with stages III and IV LCL had low-level LHR and 12% of patients with stages I and III LCL had high levels.[15] This suggests that molecules other than LHR are relevant to dissemination. Indeed, LFA-1 is also involved in lymphocyte migration through high endothelial venules. In a study of LHR-negative lymphomas, lack of LFA-1B expression correlated with dissemination and poor outcome, whereas LHR-negative LFA-1B-positive lymphomas did not disseminate and had favorable outcome.[197]

Several studies now suggest that LHR staining intensity is an independent prognostic factor in multivariant analysis of lymphoma. In one study, the actuarial survival rate at 2 years among patients with high CD44 was 47% versus 91% among patients with low CD44.[15] Similarly, poor response to treatment correlates with a high level of CD44. In the study by Jalkanen and colleagues, the actuarial survival rate at 5 years among patients with high LHR was 45% versus 74% among patients with low or no LHR.[197] From a clinical perspective, CD44 not only identifies lymphomas with high metastatic potential and poor prognosis but also identifies and defines a new entity among lymphomas. This new entity is a subgroup characterized by high histologic grade and large S-phase fraction (high proliferative index) with LHR negativity, showing a decreased tendency for dissemination and generally favorable prognosis.[197] Because morphologic high-grade malignant lymphomas receive aggressive combination chemotherapy with toxicity that might be life threatening, identification of a subgroup with less serious prognosis and a tendency to remain localized may be of therapeutic importance.[197]

Drug Resistance Phenotype

P-glycoprotein is a transmembrane protein believed to function as an efflux pump, removing cytotoxic or xenobiotic agents from cells, thereby protecting them from toxic effects.[199] P-glycoprotein expression is described in normal hematopoietic elements (e.g., CD34+ stem cells and CD56+ T cells) and in hematopoietic neoplasms.[200, 201] Among lymphomas, detectable levels of P-glycoprotein are uncommon (2%) in untreated patients and frequent (64%) in those with clinically drug-resistant disease.[199] Several reports [202, 203] indicate that the presence of P-glycoprotein in malignant lymphomas is associated with poor response to therapy, although other studies do not find this association.[204] Recent clinical data suggest that patients with P-glycoprotein–positive lymphoma benefit from alternative supplemental therapy with chemosensitizers (e.g., verapamil, quinine, and cyclosporine) that may competitively combine with P-glycoprotein and reverse the efflux pump effect.[199] In particular, among 18 patients with drug-refractory lymphoma, 72% responded to standard chemotherapy plus the added P-glycoprotein–binding chemosensitizers, suggesting that carefully selected lymphoma patients with clinical evidence of multidrug resistance and detectable P-glycoprotein benefit from this alternative therapy.[199] This suggests that P-glycoprotein is an important object of clinical immunophenotypic assay among patients with lymphoma. As described earlier, the high frequency of physiologic P-glycoprotein expression among CD56+ T cells may explain the relatively poor survival among patients with CD56+ lymphomas.[165–167]

THE MALIGNANT PHENOTYPE AS A THERAPEUTIC TARGET

As evidenced by P-glycoprotein treatment with a chemosensitizer, the malignant phenotypes may serve as new therapeutic targets. The changes in therapy would involve the use of adjuvant cytokine therapy. For example, they might include (1) upmodulation of LFA-1 with interferon-α; (2) restoration of HLA deficiency with IFN-γ; or (3) restoration of TIL with IL-2.[6] These new supplemental cytokine treatments would have to be phenotype specific (e.g., use of IFNα directed at LFA-1 deficiency). In another

example, loss of proliferative control, therapy could be risk adapted. That is, the high-risk patients, with a high Ki67 (>80%) and a high probability of failing conventional therapy, might receive high-dose infusional chemotherapy with autologous marrow rescue as currently instituted in SWOG. This would constitute a high-risk therapeutic choice tailored to the patient's high-risk status. Although the outcome is unproven, the phenotype-adapted, risk-adapted therapies seem compelling as progress in the development of conventional chemotherapy in multiple combinations has seemingly plateaued.[205]

Phenotype-adapted therapy holds considerable promise, provided that an important factor is not underestimated: genetic alteration. If genetic loss underlies HLA or LFA loss, then cytokine therapy would be of no consequence. In this regard, a recent study of HLA deficiency in lymphoma suggests that nongenetic causes are common, whereas specific HLA gene change is rare, suggesting that cytokine therapy is rational with this biologic entity.[206] In contrast, a recent combined phenotypic and genotypic study of DLCL found that double-positive status with both *BCL2* phenotypic expression and *BCL2* translocation t(14;18) identified an incurable subset of B-cell LCL with low proliferative rate and late relapse.[207] These features were not found in the patients with *BCL2* expression independent of the translocation, suggesting that a constitutive genetic overexpression of *BCL2* is necessary to confer ever-relapsing status on B-LCL. In the end, there is an incomplete prediction of outcome unless both phenotype and genotype of *BCL2* are known.[207] With this example in mind, we await future prospective trials of combined lymphoma phenotypic and genotypic traits as possible indicators for alternative therapy.

REFERENCES

1. Grogan TM, Spier CM, Richter LC, et al: Immunologic approaches to the classification of non-Hodgkin's lymphomas. *In* Bennett JM, Foon KA (eds): Immunologic Approaches to the Classification and Management of Lymphomas and Leukemias. Norwell, MA, Kluwer, 1988, pp 31–148.
2. Jaffe ES: The role of immunophenotypic markers in the classification of non-Hodgkin's lymphomas. Semin Oncol 1990; 17:11.
3. Harris NL, Jaffe ES, Stein H, et al: A revised European-American classification of lymphoid neoplasms: A proposal from the International Lymphoma Study Group. Blood 1994; 84:1361.
4. Cattoretti G, Svurmeijer A: Antigen unmasking on formalin-fixed paraffin-embedded tissues using microwaves: A review. Adv Anatom Pathol 1995; 2:2.
5. Grogan TM, Casey T, Miller P, et al: Automation of immunohistochemistry. Adv Pathol Lab Med 1993; 6:253.
6. Grogan TM, Miller P: Immunobiologic correlates of prognosis in lymphoma. Semin Oncol 1993; 20:58.
7. Foon KA, Todd RF: Immunologic classification of leukemia and lymphoma. Blood 1986; 68:1.
8. Barclay N: Leucocyte Antigen Facts Book, London, Academic Press, 1993, p 34.
9. Rothlein R, Springer T: The requirement for lymphocyte function–associated antigen 1 in homotypic leukocyte adhesion stimulated by phorbol ester. J Exp Med 1986; 163:1132.
10. Shimizu Y, Van Seventer GA, Horgan KJ, et al: Roles of adhesion molecules in T -cell recognition: Fundamental similarities between four integrins on resting human T-cells (LFA-1, VLA-4, VLA-5, VLA-6) in expression, binding, and co-stimulation. Immunol Rev 1990; 114:109.

11. Tanaka K, Yoshioka T, Bieberich C, et al: Role of the major histocompatibility complex class I antigens in tumor growth and metastasis. Annu Rev Immunol 1988; 6:359.

12. Hämmerling GJ, Klar D, Pulm W, et al: The influence of major histocompatibility complex class I antigens on tumor growth and metastasis. Biochim Biophys Acta 1987; 907:245.

13. Buck CA, Horwitz AF: Cell surface receptors for extracellular matrix molecules. Annu Rev Cell Biol 1987; 3:179.

14. Hemler ME: Adhesion protein receptors on hematopoietic cells. Immunol Today 1988; 9:109.

15. Pals ST, Host E, Ossekoppele GJ, et al: Expression of lymphocyte homing receptor as a mechanism of dissemination in non-Hodgkin's lymphoma. Blood 1989; 73:885.

16. Moller P, Mielke B, Moldenhauer G: Monoclonal antibody HML-1, a marker for intraepithelial T cells and lymphomas derived thereof, also recognizes hairy cell leukemia and some B-cell lymphomas. Am J Pathol 1990; 136:509.

17. Ezzell C: Sticky situations: Picking apart the molecules that glue cells together. Sci News 1992; 141:392.

18. Dustin ML, Springer TA: Role of lymphocyte adhesion receptors in transient interactions and cell locomotion. Annu Rev Immunol 1991; 9:27.

19. Korsmeyer SJ: Bcl-2 initiates a new category of oncogenes: Regulators of cell death. Blood 1992; 80:879.

20. Klein G: The role of gene dosage and genetic transpositions in carcinogenesis. Nature 1981; 294:313.

21. Said JW, Barrera R, Shintaku IP, et al: Immunohistochemical analysis of p53 expression in malignant lymphomas. Am J Pathol 1992; 141:1343.

22. Nunez G, London L, Hockenbery D, et al: Deregulation bcl-2 gene expression selectively prolongs survival of growth factor–deprived hemopoietic cell lines. J Immunol 1990; 144:3602.

23. Leder P: The genetics of antibody diversity. Sci Am 1982;246:102.

24. Tonegawa S: Somatic generation of antibody diversity. Nature 1983; 302:575.

25. Stein H, Bonk A, Tolksdorf G: Immunohistologic analysis of the organization of normal lymphoid tissue and non-Hodgkin's lymphomas. J Histochem Cytochem 1980; 28:746.

26. Grogan TM, Payne CM, Payne TB, et al: Cutaneous myiasis: Immunohistologic and ultrastructural morphometric features of a human botfly lesion. Am J Dermatopathol 1987; 9:232.

27. Waldman TA, Davis MM, Bongiovanni KF: Rearrangements of genes for the antigen receptor on T cells as markers of lineage and clonality in human lymphoid neoplasms. N Engl J Med 1985; 313:776.

28. Weiss LM, Picker LJ, Grogan TM, et al: Absence of clonal beta and gamma T-cell receptor gene rearrangements in a subset of peripheral T-cell lymphomas. Am J Pathol 1988; 130:436.

29. Grogan T, Spier C, Wirt DP, et al: The immunologic complexity of lymphoblastic lymphoma. Diagn Immunol 1986; 4:81.

30. Lippman SM, Volk JR, Spier CM, et al: Human immunodeficiency virus (HIV)-associated lymphomas with initial clonal ambiguity and their similarity to post-transplantation lymphomas. Arch Pathol Lab Med 1988; 112:128.

31. Picker L, Weiss LM, Medeiros LJ: Immunophenotypic criteria for the diagnosis of non-Hodgkin's lymphoma. Am J Pathol 1987; 128:181.

32. Grogan TM, Fielder K, Rangel C, et al: Peripheral T-cell lymphoma: Aggressive disease with heterogeneous immunotypes. Am J Clin Pathol 1985; 83:279.

33. Gelb AB, Rouse RV, Dorfman RF: Detection of immunophenotypic abnormalities in paraffin-embedded B-lineage non-Hodgkin's lymphomas. Am J Clin Pathol 1994; 102:825.

34. Shin SS, Berry GJ, Weiss LM: Infectious mononucleosis diagnosis by in situ hybridization in two cases with atypical features. Am J Surg Pathol 1991; 15:625.

35. Gaidano G, Ballerini P, Gong JZ, et al: P53 mutations in human lymphoid malignancies: Association with Burkitt lymphoma and chronic lymphocytic leukemia. Proc Natl Acad Sci U S A 1991; 88:5413.

36. Ngan BY, Chen-Levy Z, Weiss LM, et al: Expression in non-Hodgkin's lymphoma of the bcl-2 protein associated with the t(14;18) chromosomal translocation. N Engl J Med 1988; 318:1638.

37. Grogan TM, Lippman SM, Spier CM, et al: Independent prognostic significance of a nuclear proliferation antigen in diffuse large cell lymphomas as determined by the monoclonal antibody Ki67. Blood 1989; 71:1157.

38. Garcia CF, Weiss LM, Warnke RA: Small noncleaved cell lymphoma: An immunophenotypic study of 18 cases and comparison with large cell lymphoma. Hum Pathol 1986; 17:454.

39. Payne CM, Grogan TM, Cromey DW, et al: An ultrastructural morphometric and immunophenotypic evaluation of Burkitt's and Burkitt's-like lymphomas. Lab Invest 1987; 57:200.

40. Sander C, Yano T, Clark HM: P53 mutation is associated with progression in follicular lymphomas. Blood 1993; 82:1994.

41. Lippman SM, Spier CM, Miller TP, et al: Tumor-infiltrating T-lymphocytes in B-cell diffuse large cell lymphoma related to disease course. Mod Pathol 1990; 3:361.

42. Kadin ME, Muramoto L, Said J: Expression of T-cell antigens on Reed-Sternberg cells in a subset of patients with nodular sclerosing and mixed cellularity Hodgkin's disease. Am J Pathol 1988; 130:345.

43. Stein H, Uchanska-Ziegler B, Gerdes J, et al: Hodgkin and Sternberg-Reed cells contain antigens specific to late cells of granulopoiesis. Int J Cancer 1982; 29:283.

44. Falini B, Stein H, Pileri S, et al: Expression of lymphoid-associated antigens on Hodgkin's and Reed-Sternberg cells of Hodgkin's disease: An immunocytochemical study on lymph node cytospins using monoclonal antibodies. Histopathology 1987; 11:1229.

45. Grogan T: Hodgkin's disease. In Jaffe E (ed): Surgical Pathology of the Lymph Nodes and Related Organs, 2nd ed., Philadelphia, WB Saunders, 1995, p 136.

46. Brown G, Bunce CM, Howie AJ, Lord JM: Stochastic or ordered lineage commitment during hemopoiesis. Leukemia 1987; 1:150.

47. Larizza L, Schirrmacher. V: Somatic cell fusion as a source of genetic rearrangement leading to metastatic variants. Cancer Metastasis Rev 1984; 3:193.

48. Munzarova M, Kovarik J: Is cancer a macrophage-mediated autoaggressive disease? Lancet 1987; 1:952.

49. Strickler JG, Michie SA, Warnke RA, Dorfman RF: The syncytial variant of nodular sclerosing Hodgkin's disease. Am J Surg Pathol 1986; 10:470.

50. Kadin ME, Agnarsson BA, Ellingsworth LR, Newcom SR: Immunohistochemical evidence of a role for transforming growth factor beta in the pathogenesis of nodular sclerosing Hodgkin's disease. Am J Pathol 1990; 136:1209.

51. Naumovski L, Utz RJ, Bergstrom SK, et al: SUP-HD1: A new Hodgkin's disease–derived cell line with lymphoid features produces interferon-gamma. Blood 1989; 74:2733.

52. Kortmann C, Burrichter H, Monner D, et al: Interleukin-1–like activity constitutively generated by Hodgkin-derived cell lines: Measurement in a human lymphocyte co-stimulator assay. Immunobiology 1984; 166:318.

53. Burrichter H, Heit W, Schaadt M, et al: Production of colony-stimulating factors by Hodgkin cell lines. Int J Cancer 1983; 31:269.

54. Samoszuk M, Nansen L: Detection of interleukin-5 messenger RNA in Reed-Sternberg cells of Hodgkin's disease with eosinophilia. Blood 1990; 75:13.

55. Ben-Ezra J, Sheibani K, Swartz W, et al: Relationship between eosinophil density and T-cell activation markers in lymph nodes of patients with Hodgkin's disease. Hum Pathol 1989; 20:1181.

56. Nicholas DS, Harris S, Wright DH: Lymphocyte predominance Hodgkin's disease—an immunohistochemical study. Histopathology 1990; 16:157.

57. Agnarsson BA, Kadin ME: The immunophenotype of Reed-Sternberg cells: A study of 50 cases of Hodgkin's disease using fixed frozen tissues. Cancer 1989; 63:2083.

58. Kamel OW, Gelb AB, Shibuya RB: Leu 7 (CD57) reactivity distinguishes nodular lymphocyte predominance Hodgkin's disease from nodular sclerosing Hodgkin's disease, T-cell–rich B-cell lymphoma, and follicular lymphoma. Am J Pathol 1993; 142(2):541.

59. Hansmann ML, Stein H, Dallenbach F, et al: (Diffuse lymphocyte-predominant Hodgkin's disease (diffuse paragranuloma): A variant of the B-cell–derived nodular type. Am J Pathol 1991; 138:29.

60. Regula D, Hoppe R, Weiss L: Nodular and diffuse types of lymphocytic predominance Hodgkin's disease. N Engl J Med 1988; 318:214.

61. Stein JH, Hansmann MI, Lennert K, et al: Reed-Sternberg and Hodgkin cells in lymphocyte-predominant Hodgkin's disease of nodular subtype contain J chain. Am J Clin Pathol 1986; 86:292.

62. Regula DP, Weiss LM, Warnke RA, et al: Lymphocyte-predominance Hodgkin's disease: A reappraisal based upon histological and immu-

nophenotypical findings in relapsing cases. Histopathology 1987; 11:1107.

63. Coles FB, Cartun RW, Pastuszak WT: Hodgkin's disease, lymphocyte-predominant type: Immunoreactivity with B-cell antibodies. Mod Pathol 1988; 1:274.

64. Pinkus GS, Said JW: Hodgkin's disease, lymphocyte predominance type, nodular—further evidence for a B-cell derivation. Am J Pathol 1988; 133:211.

65. Abdulaziz Z, Mason DY, Stein H, et al: An immunohistological study of the cellular constituents of Hodgkin's disease using a monoclonal antibody panel. Histopathology 1984; 8:1.

66. Sanders ME, Makgoba MW, Sussman EH, et al: Molecular pathways of adhesion in spontaneous rosetting of T-lymphocytes of Hodgkin's line L428. Cancer Res 1988; 48:37.

67. McGuire R, Pretlow T, Wareing T, Bradley E: Hodgkin's cells and attached lymphocytes: A possible prognostic indicator in splenic tumor. Cancer 1979; 44:183.

68. Sundeen JT, Cossman J, Jaffe ES: Lymphocyte predominant Hodgkin's disease nodular subtype with coexistent large cell lymphoma: Histological progression or composite malignancy? Am J Surg Pathol 1988; 12:599.

69. Miettinen M, Franssila KO, Sanen E: Hodgkin's disease, lymphocytic predominance nodular—increased risk for subsequent non-Hodgkin's lymphomas. Cancer 1983; 54:2293.

70. Hansmann ML, Stein H, Fellbaum C, et al: Nodular paragranuloma can transform into high-grade malignant lymphoma of B-type. Hum Pathol 1989; 20:1169.

71. Hsu S, Ho Y, Li PJ, et al: L&H variants of Reed-Sternberg cells express sialylated Leu M1 antigen. Am J Pathol 1986; 122:199.

72. Mueller N, Evans A, Harris NL, et al: Hodgkin's disease and Epstein-Barr virus: Altered antibody patterns before diagnosis. N Engl J Med 1989; 320:689.

73. Weiss LM, Strickler JG, Warnke RA, et al: Epstein-Barr viral DNA in tissues of Hodgkin's disease. Am J Pathol 1987; 129:86.

74. Weiss LM, Movahed AM, Warnke RA, et al: Detection of Epstein-Barr viral genomes in Reed-Sternberg cells of Hodgkin's disease. N Engl J Med 1989; 320:502.

75. Anagnostopoulos I, Herbst H, Niedobitek G, et al: Demonstration of monoclonal EBV genomes in Hodgkin's disease and Ki-1 positive anaplastic large cell lymphoma by combined Southern blot and in situ hybridization. Blood 1989; 74:810.

76. Masih A, Weisenburger D, Duggan M, et al: Epstein-Barr viral genome in lymph nodes from patients with Hodgkin's disease may not be specific to Reed-Sternberg cells. Am J Pathol 1991; 139:37.

77. Lerner MR, Andrews NC, Miller G, et al: Two small RNAs encoded by Epstein-Barr virus and complexed with protein are precipitated by antibodies from patients with systemic lupus erythematosus. Proc Nat Acad Sci U S A 1981; 78:805.

78. Howe JG, Steitz JA: Localization of Epstein-Barr virus encodes small RNAs by in situ hybridization. Proc Nat Acad Sci U S A 1986; 83:9006.

79. Weiss LM, Chen YY, Liu XF, et al: Epstein-Barr virus in Hodgkin's disease: A correlative in situ hybridization and polymerase chain reaction study. Am J Pathol 1991; 139:1259.

80. Pallesen G, Hamilton-Dutoit SJ, Rowe M, et al: Expression of Epstein-Barr virus latent gene products in tumour cells of Hodgkin's disease. Lancet 1991; 337:320.

81. Pinkus GS, Lones M, Shintaku P, et al: Immunohistochemical detection of Epstein-Barr virus–encoded latent membrane protein in Reed-Sternberg cells and variants of Hodgkin's disease. Mod Pathol 1994; 7:454.

82. Wang D, Liebowitz D, Kieff E: An EBV membrane protein expressed in immortalized lymphocytes transforms established rodent cells. Cell 1985; 43:831.

83. Henderson S, Rowe M, Gregory C, et al: Induction of *BCL-2* expression by Epstein-Barr virus latent membrane protein 1 protects infected B-cells from programmed cell death. Cell 1991; 65:1107.

84. Young L, Alfieri C, Hennessy K, et al: Expression of Epstein-Barr virus transformation–associated genes in tissues of patients with EBV lymphoproliferative disease. N Engl J Med 1989; 321:1080.

85. Wang F, Gregory C, Sample C, et al: Epstein-Barr virus latent membrane protein (LMP1) and nuclear proteins 2 and 3C are effectors of phenotypic changes in B lymphocytes: EBN?A-2 and LMP1 cooperatively induced CD23. J Virol 1990; 64:2309.

86. Moss DJ, Misko IS, Burrows SR, et al: Cytotoxic T-cell clones discriminate between A- and B-type Epstein-Barr virus transformants. Nature 1988; 331:719.

87. Murray RJ, Wang D, Young LS, et al: Epstein-Barr virus–specific cytotoxic T-cell recognition of transfectants expressing the virus-encoded latent membrane protein LMP. J Virol 1988; 62:3747.

88. Hummel M, Anagnostopoulos I, Dallenbach F, et al: EBV infection patterns in Hodgkin's disease and normal lymphoid tissue: Expression and cellular localization of EBV gene products. Br J Haematol 1992; 82:689.

89. Delsol G, Brousset P, Chittal S, et al: Correlation of the expression of Epstein-Barr virus latent membrane protein and in situ hybridization with biotinylated BamHI-W probes in Hodgkin's disease. Am J Pathol 1992; 140:247.

90. Fingeroth JD, Weis JJ, Tedder TF, et al: Epstein-Barr virus receptor of human B lymphocytes is the C3d receptor CR2. Proc Natl Acad Sci U S A 1984; 81:4510.

91. Boyle MJ, Vasak E, Tschuchnigg M, et al: Subtypes of Epstein-Barr virus (EBV) in Hodgkin's disease: Association between B-type EBV and immunocompromise. Blood 1993; 81 :468.

92. Ambinder RF, Browning PJ, Lorenzana I, et al: Epstein-Barr virus and childhood Hodgkin's disease in Honduras and the United States. Blood 1993; 81:462.

93. Chang KL, Albujar PF, Chen YY, et al: High prevalence of Epstein-Barr virus in the Reed-Sternberg cells of Hodgkin's disease occurring in Peru. Blood 1993; 81:496.

94. Lin JC, Lin SC, De BK, et al: Precision of genotyping of Epstein-Barr virus by polymerase chain reaction using three gene loci (EBNA-2, EBNA-3C, and EBER): Predominance of type A virus associated with Hodgkin's disease. Blood 1993; 81:3372.

95. Brousset P, Knecht H, Rubin B, et al: Demonstration of Epstein-Barr virus replication in Reed-Sternberg cells of Hodgkin's disease. Blood 1993; 82:872.

96. Joske DJ, Emery-Goodman A, Bachmann E, et al: Epstein-Barr virus burden in Hodgkin's disease is related to latent membrane protein gene expression but not to active viral replication. Blood 1992; 80:2610.

97. Pallesen G, Sandvy K, Hamilton-Dutoit SJ, et al: Activation of Epstein-Barr virus replication in Hodgkin's and Reed-Sternberg cells. Blood 1991; 78:1162.

98. Rowe M, Evans HS, Young LS, et al: Monoclonal antibodies to the latent membrane protein of Epstein-Barr virus reveal heterogeneity of the protein and inducible expression in virus-transformed cells. J Gen Virol 1987; 68:1575.

99. Herbst H, Dallenbach F, Hummel M, et al: Epstein-Barr virus latent membrane protein expression in Hodgkin and Reed-Sternberg cells. Proc Natl Acad Sci U S A 1991; 88:4766.

100. Pileri S, Sabattini E, Tazzari PL, et al: Hodgkin's disease: Update of findings. Haematologica 1991; 76:175.

101. Isaacson PG, Schmid C, Pan L, et al: Epstein and Hodgkin's virus latent membrane protein expression by Hodgkin and Reed-Sternberg–like cells in acute infectious mononucleosis. J Pathol 1992; 167:267.

102. Momose H, Jaffe ES, Shin SS, et al: Chronic lymphocytic leukemia/small lymphocytic lymphoma with Reed-Sternberg–like cells and possible transformation to Hodgkin's disease. Am J Surg Pathol 1992; 16:859.

103. Jaffe ES, Berard CW: Lymphoblastic lymphoma: A term rekindled with new precision. Ann Intern Med 1978; 89:415.

104. Cossman J, Chused TM, Fisher RI, et al: Diversity of immunological phenotypes of lymphoblastic lymphoma. Cancer Res 1983; 43:4486.

105. Weiss LM, Bindl JM, Picozzi VJ, et al: Lymphoblastic lymphoma: An immunophenotype study of 26 cases with comparison to T-cell acute lymphoblastic leukemia. Blood 1986; 67:474.

106. Verdi CJ, Grogan TM, Protell R, et al: Liver biopsy immunotyping to characterize lymphoid malignancies. Hepatology 1986; 6:6.

107. Sander C, Medeiros L, Abruzzo L, et al: Lymphoblastic lymphoma presenting in cutaneous sites: A clinicopathologic analysis of six cases. J Am Acad Dermatol 1991; 25:1023.

108. Stein H, Berdes J, Mason DY: The normal and malignant germinal centre. Clin Haematol 1982; 11:531.

109. Grogan T, Jolly C, Rangel C: Immunoarchitecture of the human spleen. Lymphology 1983; 16:72.

110. Hockenberry DM, Zutter M, Hickey W, et al: *BCL2* protein is topographically restricted in tissues characterized by apoptotic cell death. Proc Natl Acad Sci U S A 1991; 88:6961.

111. Fisher R, Dahlber S, Banks P, et al: A clinical analysis of two indolent lymphoma entities: Mantle cell lymphoma and marginal zone lymphoma, including MALT and monocytoid B subcategories. Blood 1995; 85:1075.

112. Isaacson P, Wright D: Malignant lymphoma of mucosa-associated lymphoid tissue: A distinctive B cell lymphoma. Cancer 1983; 52:1410.

113. Isaacson P, Spencer J: Malignant lymphoma of mucosa-associated lymphoid tissue. Histopathology 1987; 11:445.

114. Zukerberg L, Medeiros L, Ferry L, et al: Diffuse low grade B-cell lymphomas: Four clinically distinct subtypes defined by a combination of morphologic and immunophenotypic features. Am J Clin Pathol 1993; 100:373.

115. Piris M, Rivas C, Morente M: Monocytoid B-cell lymphoma, a tumour related to the marginal zone. Histopathology 1988; 12:383.

116. Cogliatti S, Schmid U, Schumaeher U, et al: Primary B-cell gastric lymphoma: A clinicopathological study of 145 patients. Gastroenterology 1991; 101:1159.

117. Wotherspoon A, Doglioni C, Diss T, et al: Regression of primary low-grade B-cell gastric lymphoma of mucosa-associated lymphoid tissue type after irradiation of *Heliobacter pylori*. Lancet 1993; 342:575.

118. Sheibani K, Burke J, Swartz W, et al: Monocytoid B-cell lymphoma: Clinicopathologic study of 21 cases of a unique type of low-grade lymphoma. Cancer 1988; 62:1531.

119. Ngan B-Y, Warnke R, Wilson M, et al: Monocytoid B-cell lymphoma: A study of 36 cases. Hum Pathol 1991; 22:409.

120. Nizze H, Cogliatti S, von Schilling C, et al: Monocytoid B-cell lymphoma: Morphologic variants and relationship to low-grade B-cell lymphoma of the mucosa-associated lymphoid tissue. Histopathology 1991; 18:403.

121. Nathwani BN, Mohrmann RL, Brynes RK, et al: Monocytoid B-cell lymphomas: An assessment of diagnostic criteria and a perspective on histogenesis. Hum Pathol 1992; 23:1061.

122. Tolksdorf G, Stein H, Lennert K: Morphological and immunological definition of a malignant lymphoma derived from germinal centre cells with cleaved nuclei (centrocytes). Br J Cancer 1980; 41:168.

123. Berard CW, Dorfman RF: Histopathology of malignant lymphomas. Clin Haematol 1974; 3:39.

124. Weisenburger DD, Kim H, Rappaport H: Mantle-zone lymphoma: A follicular variant of intermediate lymphocytic lymphoma. Cancer 1982; 49:1429.

125. Lardelli P, Bookman M, Sundeen L, et al: Lymphocytic lymphoma of intermediate differentiation: Morphologic and immunophenotypic spectrum and clinical correlations. Am J Surg Pathol 1990; 14:752.

126. Banks P, Chan J, Cleary M, et al: Mantle cell lymphoma: A proposal for unification of morphologic, immunologic, and molecular data. Am J Surg Pathol 1992; 16:637.

127. Rosenberg C, Wong E, Petty E, et al: Overexpression of *PRAD1*, a candidate *BCL1* breakpoint region oncogene, in centrocytic lymphomas. Proc Natl Acad Sci U S A 1991; 88:9638.

128. Pangalis GA, Nathwani BN, Rappaport H: Malignant lymphoma, well-differentiated lymphocytic: Its relationship with chronic lymphocytic leukemia and macroglobulinemia of Waldenström. Cancer 1977; 39:999.

129. Dick FR, Maca RD: The lymph node in chronic lymphocytic leukemia. Cancer 1978; 41:283.

130. Spier CM, Grogan TM, Fielder K, et al: Immunophenotypes in well-differentiated lymphoproliferative disorders, with emphasis on small lymphocytic lymphoma. Hum Pathol 1986; 17:1126.

131. Harris NL, Bhan AK: B-cell neoplasms of the lymphocytic, lymphoplasmacytoid, and plasma cell types: Immunohistologic analysis and clinical correlation. Hum Pathol 1985; 16:829.

132. Bofill M, Janossy G, Jannosa M, et al: Human B-cell development: II. Subpopulations in the human fetus. J Immunol 1985; 134:1531.

133. Antin JH, Emerson SG, Martin P, et al: Leu–1+ (CD5+) B cells: A major lymphoid subpopulation in human fetal spleen–phenotypic and functional studies. J Immunol 1986; 136:505.

134. Medeiros JL, Picker LJ, Gelf AB, et al: Numbers of host "helper" T-cell and proliferating cells predict survival in diffuse small cell lymphomas. J Clin Oncol 1989; 7:1009.

135. Doggett RS, Wood GS, Horning S, et al: The immunological characterizations of 95 nodal and extranodal diffuse large cell lymphomas in 89 patients. Am J Pathol 1984; 115:245.

136. Spier CM, Grogan TM, Lippman SM, et al: The aberrancy of immunophenotype and immunoglobulin status as indicators of prognosis in B-cell diffuse large cell lymphoma. Am J Pathol 1988; 133:118.

137. Berard C, O'Conner GT, Thomas LB, et al: Histopathological definition of Burkitt's tumor. Bull WHO 1969; 40:601.

138. Grogan TM, Warnke R, Kaplan HS: A comparative study of Burkitt's and non-Burkitt's types of "undifferentiated malignant lymphoma": Histopathologic, cytochemical, ultrastructural, immunologic, clinical and tissue culture features. Cancer 1982; 49:1817.

139. Miliauskas MB, Berard CW, Young RC, et al: Undifferentiated non-Hodgkin's lymphomas (Burkitt's and non-Burkitt's types): The relevance of making this histologic distinction. Cancer 1982; 50:2115.

140. Mann RB, Jaffe ES, Braylan RC, et al: Non-endemic Burkitt's lymphoma: A B-cell tumor related to germinal centers. N Engl J Med 1976; 295:685.

141. Ziegler JL, Beckstead JA, Volberding PA, et al: Non-Hodgkin's lymphoma in 90 homosexual men: Relation to generalized lymphadenopathy and the acquired immunodeficiency syndrome. N Engl J Med 1984; 311:565.

142. Krikorian JG, Burke JS, Rosenberg SA, et al: Occurrence of non-Hodgkin's lymphoma after therapy for Hodgkin's disease. N Engl J Med 1979; 300:452.

143. Swinin LJ, Costanzo-Nordin MR, Fisher SG, et al: Increased incidence of lymphoproliferative disorder after immunosuppression with the monoclonal antibody OKT3 in cardiac transplant recipients. N Engl J Med 1990; 323:1723.

144. Aiello A, Delia D, Fontanella E, et al: Expression of differentiation and adhesion molecules in sporadic Burkitt's lymphoma. Hematol Oncol 1990; 8:229.

145. Clayberger C, Wright A, Medeiros LJ, et al: Absence of cell surface LFA-1 as a mechanism of escape from immunosurveillance. Lancet 1987; 2:533.

146. Oliver JD, Grogan TM, Payne CM, et al: Burkitt's-like lymphoma of T-cell type. Mod Pathol 1988; 1:15.

147. Shebani K, Winberg CD, Burke JS, et al: Lymphoblastic lymphoma expressing natural killer cell–associated antigens: A clinicopathologic study of six cases. Leuk Res 1987; 11:371.

148. Weiss LM, Crabtree GS, Rouse RV, et al: Morphologic and immunologic characterization of 50 peripheral T-cell lymphomas. Am J Pathol 1985; 118:316.

149. Jaffe ES: Pathologic and clinical spectrum of post-thymic T-cell malignancies. Cancer Invest 1984; 2:413.

150. Wright DH: T-cell Lymphomas. Histopathology 1986; 10:321.

151. Isaacson PG, Spencer J, Connolly CE, et al: Malignant histiocytosis of the intestine: A T-cell lymphoma. Lancet 1985; 2:688.

152. Uchiyama T, Yodoi J, Sagawa K, et al: Adult T-cell leukemia: Clinical and hematologic features of 16 cases. Blood 1977; 50:481.

153. Jaffe ES, Blattner EA, Blaynew DW, et al: The pathologic spectrum of adult T-cell leukemia/lymphoma in the United States: Human T-cell leukemia/lymphoma virus–associated lymphoid malignancies. Am J Surg Pathol 1984; 8:263.

154. Blattner WA, Kalyanaraman VS, Robert-Guroff M, et al: The human type-C retrovirus, HTLV, in blacks from the Carribean region and relationship to adult T-cell leukemia/lymphoma. Int J Cancer 1982; 30:2457.

155. Mason D, Bastard C, Rimokh R, et al: CD30-positive large cell lymphomas ("Ki-1 lymphoma") are associated with a chromosomal translocation involving 5q35. Br J Haematol 1990; 74:161.

156. Ralfkiaer E, Wantzin GL, Mason DY, et al: Phenotypic characterization of lymphocyte subsets in mycosis fungoides: Comparison with large-plaque parapsoriasis and benign chronic dermatoses. Am J Clin Pathol 1985; 84:610.

157. Wood GS, Abel EA, Hoppe RT, et al: Leu 8 and Leu 9 antigen phenotypes: Immunologic criteria for the distinction of mycosis fungoides from cutaneous inflammation. J Am Acad Dermatol 1986; 14:1006.

158. Kim H, Jacobs C, Warnke RA, et al: Malignant lymphoma with a high content of epithelioid histiocytes: A distinct clinicopathologic entity and a form of so-called "Lennert's lymphoma." Cancer 1978; 41:620.

159. Spier CM, Lippman SM, Miller TP, et al: Lennert's lymphoma: A clinicopathologic study, with emphasis on phenotype and its relationship to survival. Cancer 1988; 61:517.

160. Stein H, Mason D, Gerdes J, et al: The expression of the Hodgkin's disease–associated antigen Ki-1 in reactive and neoplastic lymphoid tissue: Evidence that Reed-Sternberg cells and histiocytic malignancies are derived from activated lymphoid cells. Blood 1985; 66:848.

161. Piris M, Brown D, Gatter K, et al: CD30 expression in non-Hodgkin's lymphoma. Histopathology 1990; 17:211.

162. Delsol G, Al Saati T, Gatter K, et al: Coexpression of epithelial membrane antigen (EMA), Ki-1, and interleukin-2 receptor by anaplastic large cell lymphomas: Diagnostic value in so-called malignant histiocytosis. Am J Pathol 1988; 130:59.

163. de Bruin P, Beljaards R, van Heerde P, et al: Differences in clinical behavior and immunophenotype between primary cutaneous and primary nodal anaplastic large cell lymphoma of T-cell or null cell phenotype. Histopathology 1993; 23:127.

164. Pileri S, Bocchia M, Baroni C, et al: Anaplastic large cell lymphoma (CD30; pl/Ki−1+): Results of a prospective clinicopathologic study of 69 cases. Br J Haematol 1994; 86:513.

165. Kern WF, Spier CM, Grogan TM: N-CAM-positive peripheral T-cell lymphomas: A rare variant with a propensity for unusual sites of involvement. Blood 1992; 79:2432.

166. Wong KF, Chan JKC, Ng CS, et al: CD56 (NKH-1)-positive hematolymphoid malignancies: An aggressive neoplasm featuring frequent cutaneous mucosal involvement, cytoplasmic azurophilic granules, and angiocentricity. Hum Pathol 1992; 23:798.

167. Kern WF, Spier CM, Miller TP, et al: NCAM(CD56)-positive malignant lymphoma. Leuk Lymphoma 1993; 12:1.

168. Coiffier B, Brousse N, Peuchmaur M, et al: Peripheral T-cell lymphomas have a worse prognosis than B-cell lymphomas: A prospective study of 361 immunophenotyped patients treated with the LNH-84 regimen. Ann Oncol 1990; 1:45.

169. Miller T, Grogan T, Dahlberg S, et al: Prognostic significance of the Ki67–associated proliferation antigen in aggressive non-Hodgkin's lymphomas: A prospective Southwest Oncology Group Trial. Blood 1994; 83:1460.

170. Miller TP, Lippman SM, Spier CM, et al: HLA-DR (Ia) immune phenotype predicts outcome for patients with diffuse large cell lymphomas. J Clin Invest 1988; 82:370.

171. List AF, Spier CM, Miller TP, et al: Deficient tumor-infiltrating T cells in B-cell malignant lymphoma. Leukemia 1993; 7:398.

172. Lippman SM, Miller TP, Spier CM, et al: The prognostic significance of the T-cell phenotype in diffuse large cell lymphoma: A comparative study of the T-cell and B-cell phenotype. Blood 1988; 72:436.

173. Slymen DJ, Miller TM, Lippman SM, et al: Immunobiologic factors predictive of clinical outcome in diffuse large cell lymphoma. J Clin Oncol 1990; 8:986.

174. Rybski JA, Spier CM, Miller TP, et al: Prediction of outcome in diffuse large cell lymphoma by the major histocompatibility complex class I (HLA-A, B, C) and class II (HLA-DR, DP, DQ) phenotype. Leuk Lymphoma 1991; 6:31.

175. Hart S, Toghill P, Vaughan-Hudson G, et al: Phenotypic analysis of diffuse large cell lymphoma in paraffin sections: The relationship to prognosis and natural history [Abstract]. Third International Conference of Malignant Lymphomas, Lugano, Switzerland, 1987.

176. Kluin PK, Gromingen KV, Sandt MVD, et al: Histoimmunopathology related to survival in a regional registry of non-Hodgkin's lymphomas [Abstract]. Third International Conference of Malignant Lymphomas, Lugano, Switzerland, 1987.

177. Momburg F, Herrmann B, Moldenhauser G, et al: B-cell lymphomas of high grade malignancy frequently lack HLA-DR, -DP and -DQ antigens and associated invariant chain. Int J Cancer 1987; 40:598.

178. O'Keane JC, Mack C, Lynch E, et al: Prognostic correlation of HLA-DR expressions in large cell lymphoma as determined by LN3 and antibody staining. Cancer 1990; 66:1147.

179. Medeiros LJ, Gelb AB, Wolfson K, et al: Major histocompatibility complex class I and class II antigen expression in diffuse large cell and large cell immunoblastic lymphomas: Absence of a correlation between antigen expression and clinical outcome. Am J Pathol 1993; 143:1086.

180. Leith C, Spier C, Grogan T, et al: Diffuse small cleaved cell lymphoma: A heterogeneous disease with distinct biologic subsets. J Clin Oncol 1992; 10:1259.

181. Cossman J, Jaffe ES, Fisher RI: Immunologic phenotypes of diffuse, aggressive non-Hodgkin's lymphomas: Correlation with clinical features. Cancer 1984; 54:1310.

182. Horning SJ, Doggett RS, Warnke RA, et al: Clinical relevance of immunologic phenotype in diffuse large cell lymphoma. Blood 1986; 63:1209.

183. Jalkanen SH, Joensuu H, Klemi P: Prognostic value of lymphocytic homing heceptor and S-phase fraction in non-Hodgkin's lymphoma. Blood 1990; 75:1549.

184. Armitage JO, Vose JM, Linder J, et al: Clinical significance of immunophenotype in diffuse aggressive non-Hodgkin's lymphoma. J Clin Oncol 1989; 17:1783.

185. Chott A, Augustin I, Wrba F, et al: Peripheral T-cell lymphomas: A clinicopathologic study of 75 cases. Hum Pathol 1990; 21:1117.

186. Gerdes J, Stein H, Pileri S, et al: Prognostic relevance of tumor-cell growth fraction in malignant non-Hodgkin's lymphomas. Lancet 1987 2:448.

187. Fearon ER, Cho KR, Nigro JM, et al: Identification of a chromosome 18q gene that is altered in colorectal cancers. Science 1990; 247:49.

188. Liotta LA, Stetler-Stevenson WG: Principles of molecular cell biology of cancer: Cancer metastasis. *In* Devita VT, Hellman S, Rosenberg S (eds): Cancer: Principles and Practice of Oncology, 3rd ed. Philadelphia, JB Lippincott, 1989, p 98.

189. Stauder R, Greil R, Schulz TF, et al: Expression of leucocyte function–associated antigen-1 and 7F7-antigen, an adhesion molecule related to intercellular adhesion molecule-1 (ICAM-1) in non-Hodgkin lymphomas and leukemias: Possible influence on growth pattern and leukaemic behaviour. Clin Exp Immunol 1989; 77:234.

190. Roossien FF, DeRijk D, Bikker A, et al: Involvement of LFA-1 in lymphoma invasion and metastasis demonstrated with LFA-1–deficient mutants. J Cell Biol 1989; 108:1979.

191. Banks P, Kjeldsberg C, Nathwani B, et al: Refined working formulation (WF) categorization of lymphomas using phenotypic and genotypic analysis: A SWOG Central Repository study. Lab Invest 1991; 64:73A.

192. Jacob MC, Favre M, Lemarc'Hadour F, et al: CD45RA expression by CD44T lymphocytes in tumors invaded by B-cell non-Hodgkin's lymphoma (NHL) or Hodgkin's disease (HD). Am J Hematol 1992; 39:45.

193. Jacob MC, Piccinini MP, Bonnefoix T, et al: T lymphocytes from invaded lymph nodes in patients with B-cell–derived non-Hodgkin's lymphoma: Reactivity toward the malignant clone. Blood 1990; 75:1154.

194. Wong KF, Chan JKC, Ng CS: CD56 (NCAM)-positive malignant lymphoma. Leuk Lymphoma 1994; 14:29.

195. Grogan T, Guptill V, Mullen J, et al: Polysialated NCAM as a neurodeterminant in malignant lymphoma. Lab Invest 1994; 70: 110A(637).

196. Horst E, Meijer CJLM, Radaszkiewicz T, et al: Adhesion molecules in the prognosis of diffuse large-cell lymphoma: Expression of a lymphocyte homing receptor (CD44), LFA-1 (CD11a/18), and ICAM-1 (CD54). Leukemia 1990; 4:595.

197. Jalkanen S, Joensuu H, Söderstrom KO, et al: Lymphocyte homing and clinical behavior of non-Hodgkin's lymphoma. J Clin Invest 1991; 87:1835.

198. Picker L, Meideros J, Weiss L, et al: Expression of lymphocyte homing receptor antigen in non-Hodgkin's lymphoma. Am J Pathol 1988; 130:496.

199. Miller TP, Grogan TM, Dalton WS, et al: P-glycoprotein expression in malignant lymphoma and reversal of clinical drug resistance with chemotherapy plus high-dose verapamil. J Clin Oncol 1991; 9:17.

200. Chaudhary PM, Mechetner EB, Roninson IP: Expression and activity of the multidrug resistance P-glycoprotein in human peripheral blood lymphocytes. Blood 1992, 80:2735.

201. Drach D, Zhao S, Drach J, et al: Subpopulations of normal peripheral blood and bone marrow cells express a functional multidrug resistant phenotype. Blood 1992; 80:2729.

202. Dan S, Esumi M, Sawada U, et al: Expression of a multidrug resistance gene in human malignant lymphoma and related disorders. Leuk Res 1991; 15:1139.

203. Pileri SA, Sabattini E, Falini B, et al: Immunohistochemical detection of the multidrug transport protein P170 in human normal tissues and malignant lymphomas. Histopathology 1991; 19:131.

204. Niehans GA, Jaszez W, Brunetto V, et al: Immunohistochemical identification of P-glycoprotein in previously untreated diffuse large cell and immunoblastic lymphomas. Cancer Res 1992; 52:3768.

205. Fisher R, Gaynor E, Dahlberg S, et al: A phase III comparison of CHOP vs. m-BACOD vs. ProMACE-cytaBOM vs. MACOP-B in patients with intermediate- or high-grade non-Hodgkin's lymphoma: Result of SWOG 8516—the National High-Priority Lymphoma Study. N Engl J Med 1993; 328:1002.

206. Kadin ME: HLA modulation in lymphomas. Am J Pathol 1990; 136:342.

207. Miller TP, Levy N, Bailey NP, et al: The *BCL2* gene translocation (T14;18) identifies a subgroup of patients with diffuse large cell lymphoma (DLCL) having an indolent clinical course with late relapse. Proc Am Soc Clin Oncol 1994; 13:1249(370).

INVESTIGATION

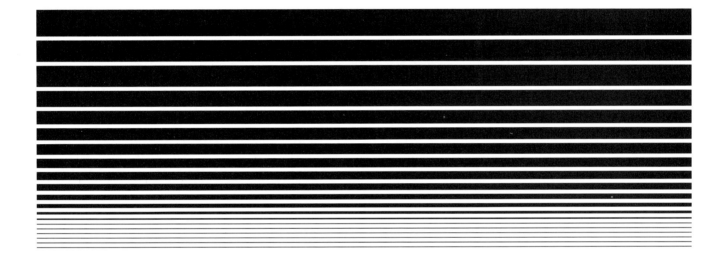

Diagnostic Radiology

Ronald A. Castellino

When determining which imaging study, or studies, should be performed on patients with Hodgkin's disease and the non-Hodgkin's lymphomas, one should consider several interrelated factors. Although Hodgkin's disease and the disorders included in the non-Hodgkin's lymphoma classification are similar in many respects, their important differences in pathologic findings, methods of presentation, response to therapy, and prognosis are, to some extent, mirrored in the utility of diagnostic imaging studies in their management. It is therefore important for the oncologist to be mindful of the following when ordering diagnostic imaging tests:

1. What specific information is being sought from the imaging study? Is the intent to *detect* whether disease is present at a certain site, or is it also important to *delineate* the anatomic extent of disease at a specific site? The former is usually sufficient to determine stage, whereas the latter may be needed for therapeutic management, for example, to precisely define radiation therapy portals, to determine specific anatomic boundaries, to provide measurements for "bulky" disease, and so forth.

2. Will the results of the imaging study, either positive or negative, influence patient management? In large part, this is based on the known patterns of disease at presentation. Imaging studies (as well as other tests) are generally directed at sites that have a high probability of involvement or, if there is a low probability of involvement, at sites where the results will have a major impact on therapy.

3. What is the value of a "baseline" imaging study? Having a reference study is often useful for comparison purposes to determine if an observed finding was previously present. Are there different requirements for a baseline examination before therapy, compared with an examination after therapy?

4. What is known about the diagnostic accuracy of the imaging test to evaluate a specific site? Accuracy of imaging tests (as well as other diagnostic tests) is generally defined in terms of the following (Fig. 9–1)[1]:
   a. Sensitivity—the ability of a test to correctly identify disease when present
   b. Specificity—the ability of a test to correctly identify the absence of disease when no disease is present
   c. Positive predictive value—how often the test is correct when interpreted as positive
   d. Negative predictive value—how often the test is correct when interpreted as negative
   e. Overall accuracy—the proportion of correct test results in the total number of tests

5. Since most imaging studies are subjectively interpreted, they often do not have clear-cut positive or negative results, but instead results that are properly stated as negative, probably negative, indeterminate, probably positive, or positive. These results cannot be readily analyzed by the earlier terminology, and for this reason receiver operating characteristic (ROC) curves are used for comparing imaging tests.[1] These ROC curves plot sensitivity and specificity pairs; an accurate test is one in which the sensitivity is high and the false-positive ratio is low (Fig. 9–2).

6. What is the access to advanced imaging technology, and what is the local expertise of the diagnostic radiology group? Although certain imaging studies may be judged optimal for a specific clinical evaluation, perhaps the technology is not readily available (e.g., access to magnetic resonance imaging [MRI], single photon emission computed tomography [SPECT]). Certain technologies, such as computed tomography [CT], MRI, ultrasonography (US), and nuclear medicine cameras, have undergone rapid technologic improvements, so that a study produced on an older unit might well not possess the diagnostic accuracy reported from state-of-the-art units. Local expertise of the diagnostic imaging group is obviously critical, since accuracy is clearly related to the careful supervision, performance, and interpretation of the studies.

7. What is the impact of the newer imaging technologies on oncologic imaging? For example, attempts have been made to use various MRI pulse sequences to explore the tissue composition ("tissue characterization") of masses, information that goes beyond the anatomic detection and delineation of masses with CT. These efforts have been made to try to predict prognostic grades of tumor, the potential size of a residual mediastinal mass after treatment, and the degree of fibrosis in masses before treatment, among others. Such work suggests that MRI can separate

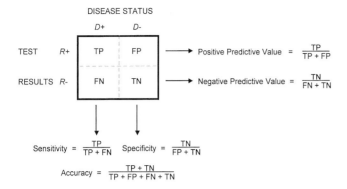

Figure 9–1. Bayesian 2 × 2 classification table of test results compared with a gold standard of diagnosis. TP, true positive; FP, false positive; FN, false negative; TN, true negative; D, disease status; R, test result. (From Castellino RA, DeLaPaz RL, Larson SM: Imaging techniques in cancer. *In* DeVita V, Hellman S, Rosenberg SA [eds]: Cancer: Principles and Practice of Oncology. Philadelphia, JB Lippincott, 1993, pp 507–531.)

high-grade from low-grade non-Hodgkin's lymphoma nodes in many cases, thereby providing prognostic information[2]; can predict the size of the residual mediastinal mass in Hodgkin's disease from the initial size of the tumor mass and its signal intensity ratio[3]; and can help in the evaluation of a persistent mass after treatment (as discussed later in this chapter).[4]

IMAGING STUDIES AT INITIAL STAGING

THORAX

Lymph Nodes. All lymph node stations within the thorax can be involved by both Hodgkin's disease and the non-Hodgkin's lymphomas. At the time of presentation, patients with Hodgkin's disease who have radiographic evidence of intrathoracic involvement almost invariably have involvement of the lymphoid tissue in the superior mediastinum (paratracheal and/or prevascular lymph nodes and/or the thymus) (Fig. 9–3), and in this setting other lymph node sites are frequently involved as well.[5, 6] However, it is highly unusual for these patients to have involvement at other sites, both nodal and extranodal, within the thorax without concomitant involvement of the superior mediastinum. When this is noted, although the observed abnormality in the superior mediastinum may well be due to Hodgkin's disease, other causes should be carefully considered.

In the non-Hodgkin's lymphomas, however, it is not uncommon to find involvement of lymph node sites or extranodal sites within the thorax without apparent involvement of the superior mediastinal lymph nodes.[7, 8] This is particularly true in patients whose major disease is within the abdomen and who demonstrate lower thoracic (paravertebral and cardiophrenic angle lymphadenopathy) disease.

In spite of the frequently bulky lymphadenopathy noted in both Hodgkin's disease and non-Hodgkin's lymphoma, symptomatic evidence of compromise of adjacent organs (e.g., superior vena cava syndrome, phrenic nerve entrapment, dysphagia, airway compromise) is relatively uncommon. As noted on CT scans, this is perhaps related to the tendency for these masses to displace, rather than encase, adjacent mediastinal structures. Evidence of adjacent organ compromise does occur, however, particularly with the large cell non-Hodgkin's lymphomas.

At times, particularly after intravenous contrast media–enhanced CT scans, the nodal masses demonstrate foci of lower attenuation due to necrosis. This finding does not appear to correlate with the subsequent clinical course in patients with Hodgkin's disease, based on a study that found no significant correlation for a number of variables (sex, age, stage, distribution of disease, presence of E disease, cell type, mass diameter, or presence of bulk disease) or on their clinical response to treatment or survival in patients with and without evidence of necrotic nodes.[9]

Lung. Involvement of the lung parenchyma and the bronchial tree can occur as the result of direct invasion from adjacent (usually lymph node) disease or as distinct foci. As mediastinal lymph node masses enlarge, an indistinct interface between the mediastinal mass and adjacent aerated

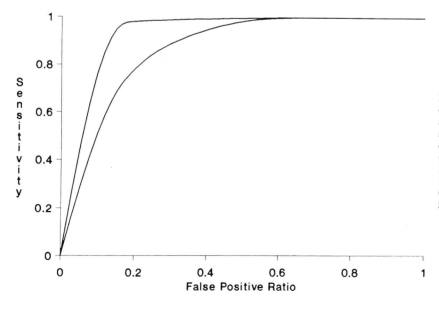

Figure 9–2. Receiver operator characteristic (ROC) curves for comparing two imaging tests. The more accurate test is shown by the curve with the higher sensitivity and lower false-positive ratio (i.e., the curve closest to the left horizontal and upper vertical axes). (From Castellino RA, DeLaPaz RL, Larson SM: Imaging techniques in cancer. *In* DeVita V, Hellman S, Rosenberg SA [eds]: Cancer: Principles and Practice of Oncology. Philadelphia, JB Lippincott, 1993, pp 507–531.)

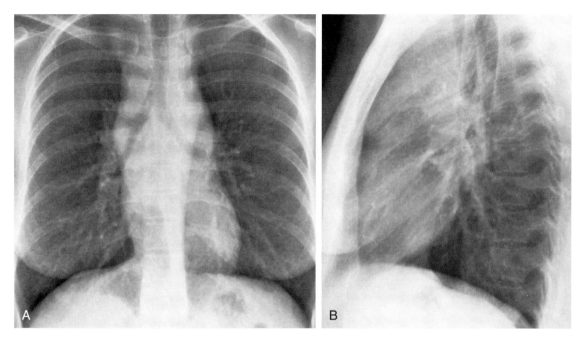

Figure 9–3. Posteroanterior *(A)* and lateral *(B)* chest radiographs in a 34-year-old woman with newly diagnosed Hodgkin's disease. The lobular bilateral superior mediastinal mass, with a prominent anterior component as seen on the lateral projection, is a typical chest radiographic appearance at presentation.

lung at times is seen on chest radiographs and is particularly well demonstrated on chest CT studies (Fig. 9–4). The distinction between local invasion of lung parenchyma versus areas of subsegmental atelectases due to the adjacent mass cannot reliably be made with imaging studies. Since such "local invasion" would represent an E lesion in the Ann Arbor classification, which does not change stage and infrequently affects treatment, such distinction is often not that critical for patient management.

Infiltration of the rich lymphatic network along the bronchovascular bundle, both external to the bronchi and endobronchially in a submucosal location, can often be inferred on chest radiographs by evidence of thickening and/or indistinctness of the bronchial wall. This is better demonstrated on CT scanning, particularly with high-resolution imaging.

Parenchymal deposits of malignant lymphoma often have somewhat ill defined margins compared with the more

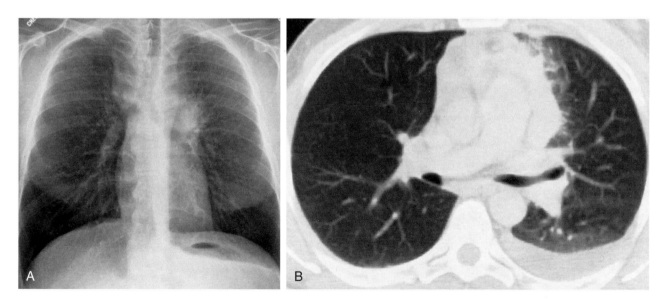

Figure 9–4. A 45-year-old man with newly diagnosed diffuse large cell lymphoma. *A,* Posteroanterior chest radiograph demonstrates bilateral superior mediastinal lymphadenopathy and a left pleural effusion. Note the indistinct margin of the left mediastinal mass, compared with the sharply demarcated margin to the right-sided component. (Also compare with Fig. 9–3*A,* which demonstrates sharply marginated contours.) *B,* Lung windows of a computed tomographic (CT) scan at the level of the right pulmonary artery show a sharply demarcated right anterior mediastinal contour compared with the poorly marginated left mediastinal contour, as well as patchy areas of relatively higher attenuation within the adjacent left lung field. These appearances are worrisome for local infiltration of lung parenchyma by the adjacent mediastinal adenopathy, although a similar appearance could be caused by subsegmental atelectasis due to the adjacent mediastinal mass.

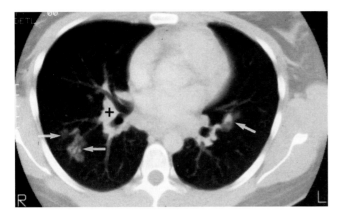

Figure 9–5. CT scan, lung windows, shows bilateral poorly defined pulmonary parenchymal lesions *(arrows)*, with associated right hilar (+) and superior mediastinal (not shown) adenopathy. Note the air bronchograms in the right lung lesion.

sharply demarcated masses typically seen with metastasis from carcinomas and sarcomas. In addition, lymphomatous masses may demonstrate air bronchograms, also unusual in other types of metastasis (Fig. 9–5). Other causes of such masses, such as infectious and/or inflammatory lesions, should always be considered. Comparison with prior studies, if available, is useful to determine the chronicity of such findings.

In patients with newly diagnosed Hodgkin's disease, the lung parenchyma is almost never involved without concomitant involvement of mediastinal lymph nodes (see earlier) and, almost invariably, involvement of the ipsilateral hilar lymph nodes.[5] This is different from non-Hodgkin's lymphoma, when pulmonary lesions can be seen as the only manifestation of intrathoracic disease, or without evidence of superior mediastinal or hilar lymphadenopathy.

Pleura and Pericardium. The presence of fluid in the pleural space is well evaluated by chest radiography, whereas only moderate to large pericardial effusions are seen with this technique. CT, on the other hand, readily depicts relatively small amounts of pericardial fluid and/or thickening. When pleural fluid is noted in association with mediastinal lymphadenopathy, such effusions may simply be the result of lymphatic and/or vascular compromise (since the effusion may resolve after radiation therapy directed only to the mediastinum). Pericardial fluid (or at times "thickening," since the area of pericardial widening noted on CT scans is often too small to accurately categorize as representing fluid versus soft tissue) is usually noted with adjacent mediastinal adenopathy (Fig. 9–6), raising the possibility of local invasion as its cause (although compromise of lymphatic drainage could play a similar role as it does with pleural effusions).

At times, focal pericardial or pleural (Figs. 9–6 and 9–7) soft tissue foci are noted in association with the fluid accumulations. When this occurs, such soft tissue masses are reasonably attributed to discrete tumor deposits (and frequently resolve after therapy). When necessary, histologic confirmation of pleural masses can be obtained with CT-guided fine-needle biopsy.[10]

Chest Wall. Although bulky intrathoracic masses are often contiguous with the chest wall, it is only when CT scans show that the intervening fascial planes are disrupted, or that there is convincing evidence of anatomic extension into the chest wall (Fig. 9–8A), that local invasion can be suggested with confidence.[11] MRI has particular potential in this evaluation, as described later.[12]

Enlarged axillary lymph nodes are frequently noted on chest CT scans, and this usually correlates with the physical examination findings. At times, enlarged axillary nodes noted on CT scans are not palpable, but how often this added information affects stage or treatment is unknown. Extension of nodal disease into the subpectoral region (Fig. 9–8B) is generally not noted on physical examination, and CT demonstration of this process may be valuable in radiation therapy treatment planning.

Comment. Well-performed and carefully interpreted frontal and lateral radiographs of the chest detect the majority of abnormalities affecting mediastinal and hilar lymph nodes, lung parenchyma, and pleura, and such information is generally sufficient to determine the stage of diseases. However, compared with cross-sectional imaging techniques, chest radiographs often underestimate the extent of disease at these and other sites. Furthermore, chest radiographs often cannot demonstrate even modest involvement in "blind" areas, such as enlarged lymph nodes in the subcarinal and cardiophrenic spaces and modest pericardial fluid and/or thickening. Cross-sectional imaging techniques clearly provide unique information regarding invasion into adjacent structures, such as the adjacent soft tissue and bony structures of the chest wall, including the spine and spinal canal. Furthermore, subtle pulmonary and pleural masses, as well as only modestly enlarged mediastinal lymph nodes, can often be detected on CT scans when even on retrospective review the chest radiograph is unremarkable at these specific sites. For these reasons, chest CT studies are frequently routinely employed in the initial staging evaluation, as well as periodically as a surveillance technique after treatment, in

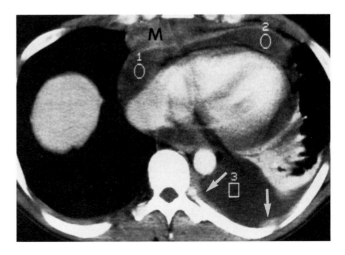

Figure 9–6. A 36-year-old man with newly diagnosed diffuse large cell lymphoma. The CT scan shows a pleural effusion (number 3) associated with focal pleural soft tissue densities *(arrows)*. A pericardial effusion (numbers 1 and 2) and a paracardiac mass (M) are also present, not noted on the concomitant chest radiograph.

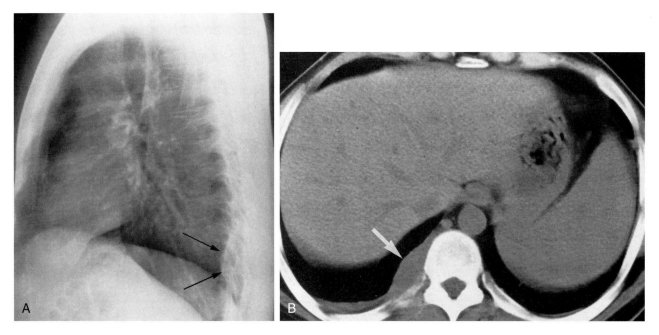

Figure 9–7. A 25-year-old man with recurrent diffuse large cell lymphoma. *A,* Lateral chest radiograph demonstrates focal pleural thickening in the lower posterior right thorax *(arrows),* without other evidence of intrathoracic disease. *B,* Chest CT scan confirms a right paravertebral mass *(arrow)* with adjacent rib involvement, without further evidence of intrathoracic disease.

Figure 9–8. *A,* A 40-year-old human immunodeficiency virus–positive man with Burkitt's lymphoma. A CT scan demonstrates a large mediastinal mass that involves the right, as well as left, anterior chest wall. (*A* From Caravella BA, DeLaPaz RL, Castellino RA: Malignant lymphoma in AIDS. Postgrad Radiol 1993; 13:151.) *B,* A 60-year-old man with newly diagnosed non-Hodgkin's lymphoma. A CT scan demonstrates bilateral axillary lymphadenopathy, left greater than right, with extension of enlarged lymph nodes medially in a subpectoral location *(arrows).* Also noted is superior mediastinal lymphadenopathy and a left pleural effusion.

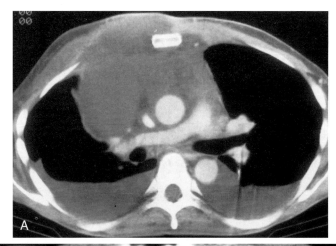

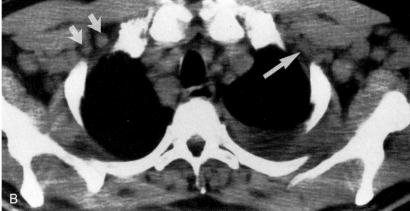

patients with Hodgkin's disease and the non-Hodgkin's lymphomas.

Although chest CT studies clearly provide information incremental to that derived from conventional chest radiographs, it is important to determine how often such incremental information will change the stage of the disease and, most important, alter patient management. When patients with newly diagnosed Hodgkin's disease are staged, there is general agreement that routinely performed chest CT studies provide sufficient incremental information that affects stage and/or management to justify its routine use. In a study of 203 such patients at Stanford Medical Center,[5] routinely performed chest CT studies detected disease not shown on chest radiographs at specific anatomic sites (various lymph node stations, lung, pleura, pericardium, chest wall) in as many as 15% of cases (Table 9–1). Based on this incremental information, patient management was modified in 9.4% of all patients (13.8% of those receiving radiation therapy alone and 8.2% of those receiving combined radiation therapy and chemotherapy). A similar analysis by Hopper and colleagues of their own case material, which they then applied in a theoretical model to other treatment protocols in place at other medical centers, demonstrated an impact on management in 6.5% to 62.7% of cases.[13]

Similar analysis in newly diagnosed patients with non-Hodgkin's lymphoma is limited. Some authors suggest that routinely performed CT, at the time of initial staging of patients with non-Hodgkin's lymphoma, provides important information regarding changes in stage, although the impact on patient management is less clear. Our recently completed study at Memorial Sloan-Kettering Cancer Center, on 181 consecutive patients with newly diagnosed non-Hodgkin's lymphoma who had concomitant chest radiographs and chest CT studies, demonstrated that incremental information derived from CT scans affected the stage in 8.8% of patients. However, this change in stage had no impact on patient management (0%), suggesting that routine chest CT is not indicated in all such patients.[8] This experience requires validation from other centers.

There is little published information regarding the role

that routine chest MRI might have in contributing to patient management at the time of initial staging of Hodgkin's disease and non-Hodgkin's lymphoma.[14, 15] Since MRI interpretation relies on demonstration of masses and size criteria for lymph nodes similar to those of CT, the decreased spatial resolution with current MRI technology compared with CT suggests that MRI would not have a major role in the initial staging of these diseases. This is particularly true in the evaluation of the lung parenchyma for pulmonary involvement, a particularly difficult site for MRI. However, various MRI pulse sequences can enhance contrast resolution, a significant advantage over x-ray CT. Preliminary experience suggests, for example, that MRI is superior to CT in evaluating chest wall involvement in newly diagnosed, as well as in previously treated, patients with the malignant lymphomas, with subsequent impact on patient management.[12] In addition, preliminary experience with MRI and two-dimensional echocardiography suggests that paracardiac and cardiac involvement with lymphoma can be detected with these modalities with greater frequency than with CT.[16] MRI technology is rapidly changing, with continued improvement in spatial and contrast resolution as well as decreased acquisition times, and, in many areas MRI units are becoming more widely available and charge-competitive compared with CT. Studies need to be done to compare MRI and CT results in this assessment.

ABDOMEN AND PELVIS

Lymph Nodes. Lymphography (LAG) was the method of choice for evaluating the retroperitoneal and pelvic lymph nodes during the 1960s and 1970s. Improved CT technology, particularly markedly increased spatial resolution and decreased scan acquisition times, has clearly challenged the utilization of LAG since the early 1980s, so that CT has supplanted LAG in many oncology practices, including many major medical centers.

The advantages of LAG are that subtle alterations in internal architecture of the opacified lymph nodes can demonstrate manifestations of metastasis before significant lymph node enlargement (Fig. 9–9), whereas CT (and other

Table 9–1. Location of Thoracic Hodgkin's Disease at Initial Presentation (%) (n = 203)

	CX− CT−	CX+ CT+	CX− CT+	Change in Treatment*
Lymph nodes				
Superior mediastinal	16	77	7	0.5
Hilar	72	21	7	1.0
Subcarinal	78	7	15	3.5
Internal mammary	95	1	4	0
Posterior mediastinal	95	2	3	1.0
Cardiophrenic angle	92	1	7	1.5
Lung parenchyma	92	8	0	0
Pleura	87	10	3	0
Pericardium	94	2	4	1.0
Chest wall	94	1	6	2.5
Any site	13	78	8	9.4

*Incidence of treatment modification based on incremental CT data in total patient study (n = 203).
CT, computed tomography; CX, chest radiography; − = negative findings; + = positive findings.
From Castellino RA, Blank N, Hoppe RT, Cho C: Hodgkin's disease: Contributions of chest CT in the initial staging evaluation. Radiology 1986; 106:603.

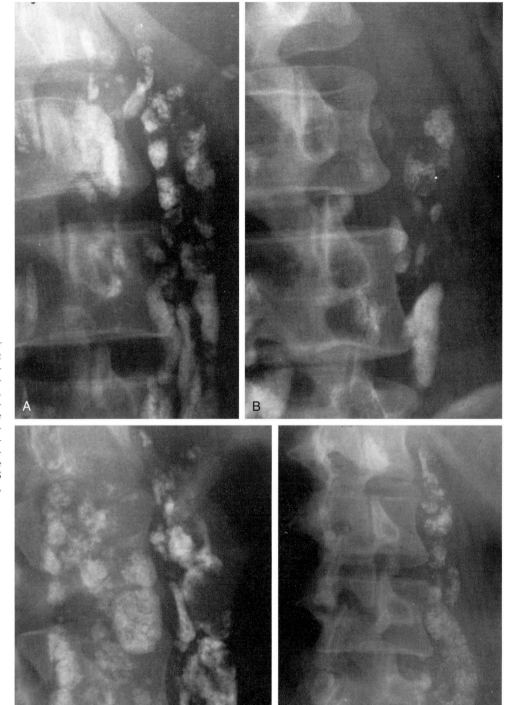

Figure 9–9. Coned left posterior oblique projections of the left paraaortic lymph nodes in four different patients with newly diagnosed malignant lymphoma (*A, C,* and *D,* Hodgkin's disease; *B,* non-Hodgkin's lymphoma). Note the compelling architectural abnormalities in normal-sized to slightly enlarged lymph nodes. (From Castellino RA: Lymphography of the malignant lymphomas. *In* Baum S [ed]: Angiography, 4th ed. Boston, Little, Brown, in press.)

Table 9–2. Accuracy of Lymphography in 632 Patients with Newly Diagnosed Malignant Lymphoma, Based on Staging Laparotomy Findings

	Hodgkin's Disease (n = 416)		Non-Hodgkin's Lymphoma (n = 216)	
	Percentage	*No.*	*Percentage*	*No.*
Sensitivity	93	100/107	89	101/114
Specificity	92	284/309	86	88/102
Overall accuracy	92	384/416	88	189/216
Positive predictive value	80	100/125	88	101/115
Negative predictive value	98	284/291	87	88/101

Modified from Marglin S, Castellino RA: Lymphographic accuracy in 623 consecutive, previously untreated cases of Hodgkin's disease and non-Hodgkin's lymphoma. Radiology 1981; 140:351.

cross-sectional imaging studies) requires lymph nodes to become enlarged beyond established size criteria to be considered abnormal. Also, at times LAG can correctly identify generalized lymph node enlargement due to reactive follicular hyperplasia, which would be mistaken for tumor involvement on CT studies. However, abnormalities of internal architecture caused by benign processes, such as sinus histiocytosis or fatty and fibrous infiltration, can lead to false-positive LAG diagnosis, whereas the CT study would not recognize such alterations and thus would be considered a correct true-negative diagnosis. LAG requires experience with lymphatic cannulation and does not opacify the upper retroperitoneal lymph nodes (those above the renal vascular pedicle) consistently, nor nodes in the porta hepatis, peripancreatic region, and mesentery.

There are good data on the accuracy of LAG in newly diagnosed patients with Hodgkin's disease and non-Hodgkin's lymphoma,[17] gathered when routine staging laparotomies were performed, which provided an excellent opportunity for careful lymphangiographic-histopathologic correlation (Table 9–2). In experienced hands, LAG has a high level of accuracy. In two comparative studies with CT in patients with Hodgkin's disease, also based on staging laparotomy data, LAG was superior to CT (Tables 9–3 and 9–4).[18, 19] Only limited information is available for the non-Hodgkin's lymphomas,[20] since routine staging laparotomies in this group of patients were no longer performed when relatively current CT technology was available (Table 9–5).

Mesenteric lymph nodes are infrequently involved by Hodgkin's disease at the time of initial presentation (<5%);

and, when involved, these nodes are almost always normal in size. Further, when Hodgkin's disease involves the highest abdominal lymph node groups (celiac axis, porta hepatis, splenic hilar) before involvement of the mid and lower retroperitoneal lymph nodes, these upper abdominal nodes are frequently normal in size. (When these nodes become large enough to be detected by CT because of more extensive disease, the mid and lower retroperitoneal nodes are usually also involved.) Therefore, to decide to use CT rather than LAG (the latter being a more accurate test) because CT can also evaluate these specific lymph node sites does not necessarily follow.

In non-Hodgkin's lymphoma, the situation is quite different. Many of these patients (particularly those with follicular histologic subtype) have bulky lymphadenopathy at multiple lymph node sites within the abdomen and pelvis, a situation readily detected by CT (Fig. 9–10A). Based on staging laparotomy data, more than 50% of these patients have biopsy-proven mesenteric lymph node disease, and these nodes are frequently bulky. Although LAG can readily detect the involved retroperitoneal and pelvic lymph nodes, it will not identify multiple other lymph node sites that may be enlarged and readily seen on CT studies (Figs. 9–11 and 9–12B). However, detecting additional sites of lymph node involvement does not necessarily change the stage and/or patient management.

With newer CT technology, there is increasing evidence that LAG in a patient with newly diagnosed Hodgkin's disease whose abdominal and pelvic CT study is unequivocally negative for enlarged (>10 mm) lymph nodes has a low yield of relevant incremental information (Table 9–6).[21, 22]

Table 9–3. Histopathologic Correlations of Computed Tomography (CT) and Lymphography (LAG) in Newly Diagnosed, Previously Untreated Patients with Hodgkin's Disease Based on Staging Laparotomy Findings (n = 121)

	Paraaortic Nodes, LAG		Paraaortic Nodes, CT°		Mesenteric Nodes, CT		Spleen, CT		Liver, CT	
	No.	*(%)*	*No.*	*(%)*	*No.*	*(%)*	*No.*	*(%)*	*No.*	*(%)*
Sensitivity	17/20	(85)	13/20	(65)	0/1	(0)	17/51	(33)	1/4	(25)
Specificity	85/87	(98)	80/87	(92)	90/91	(99)	53/70	(76)	117/117	(100)
Accuracy										
Overall	102/107	(95)	93/107	(87)	90/92	(98)	70/121	(58)	118/121	(98)
Positive report	17/19	(89)	13/20	(65)	0/1	(0)	17/34	(50)	1/1	(100)
Negative report	85/88	(97)	80/87	(92)	90/91	(99)	53/87	(61)	117/120	(98)

°In seven patients, no retroperitoneal node biopsies were performed and in an additional seven patients, the lymphangiographically positive node biopsy specimens were not obtained, leaving 107 cases for analysis.

From Castellino RA, Hoppe RT, Blenk N, et al: Computed tomography, lymphography, and staging laparotomy: Correlations in initial staging of Hodgkin's disease. AJR Am J Roentgenol 1984; 143:37.

Table 9–4. Histopathologic Correlation of Computed Tomography (CT) and Lymphography (LAG) in Newly Diagnosed Children (<17 Years of Age) with Hodgkin's Disease, Based on Staging Laparotomy Findings*

	Sensitivity		Specificity		Accuracy	
Organ	No.	(%)	No.	(%)	No.	(%)
Lymph nodes						
Retroperitoneal						
Lymphangiography	4/5	(80)	41/41	(100)	45/46	(98)
Computed tomography (CT)	2/5	(40)	39/41	(95)	41/46	(89)
Splenic hilar (CT)	0/10	(0)	26/26	(100)	26/36	(72)
Mesenteric (CT)	0/0		35/35	(100)	35/35	(100)
Celiac (CT)	0/0		11/11	(100)	11/11	(100)
Porta hepatis (CT)	0/1		11/11	(100)	11/12	(92)
Spleen (CT)	3/16	(19)	25/30	(83)	28/46	(61)
Liver (CT)	—		—		—	

*No patient had biopsy-proven hepatic involvement.
From Baker LL, Parker BR, Donaldson SS, Castellino RA: Staging of Hodgkin disease in children: Comparison of CT and lymphography with laparotomy. AJR Am J Roentgenol 1990; 154:1251.

Table 9–5. Histopathologic Correlations of Computed Tomography (CT) and Lymphography (LAG) in Newly Diagnosed, Previously Untreated Patients with Non-Hodgkin's Lymphoma Based on Staging Laparotomy Findings (n = 23)

	Retroperitoneal Nodes, LAG		Retroperitoneal Nodes, CT		Mesenteric Nodes, CT		Spleen, CT	
	Percentage	No.	Percentage	No.	Percentage	No.	Percentage	No.
Sensitivity	100	14/14	86	12/14	67	10/15	45	5/11
Specificity	75	6/8	75	6/8	75	6/8	83	10/12
Accuracy	91	20/22	82	18/22	70	16/23	65	15/23

Modified from Castellino RA: Imaging techniques for extent determination of Hodgkin's disease and non-Hodgkin's lymphoma. *In* Progress in Clinical and Biological Research, Vol 132 D. Proceedings of the 13th International Cancer Congress. Seattle, 1982. New York, Alan R Liss, 1983, pp 365–372.

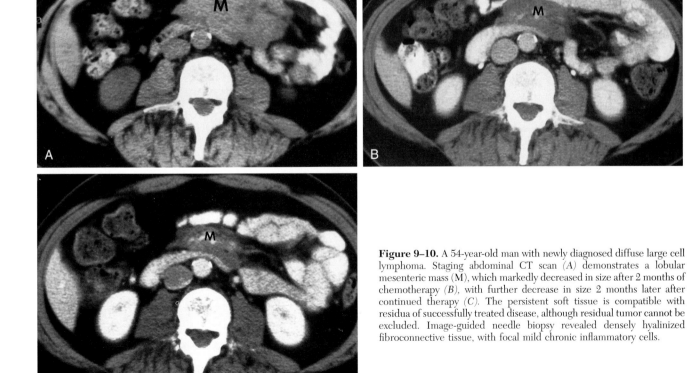

Figure 9–10. A 54-year-old man with newly diagnosed diffuse large cell lymphoma. Staging abdominal CT scan (*A*) demonstrates a lobular mesenteric mass (M), which markedly decreased in size after 2 months of chemotherapy (*B*), with further decrease in size 2 months later after continued therapy (*C*). The persistent soft tissue is compatible with residua of successfully treated disease, although residual tumor cannot be excluded. Image-guided needle biopsy revealed densely hyalinized fibroconnective tissue, with focal mild chronic inflammatory cells.

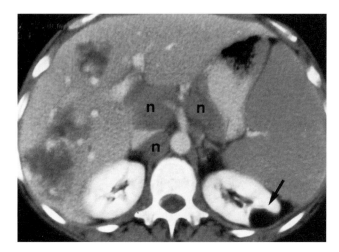

Figure 9–11. A 52-year-old woman with newly diagnosed diffuse mantle zone lymphoma. Multiple abnormalities are noted on this CT scan of the upper abdomen, including lymphadenopathy (n) in the celiac, porta hepatis, and retrocaval regions. In addition, the homogeneous lower attenuation within the enlarged spleen is compatible with diffuse infiltration by lymphoma. These findings resolved after treatment. Also noted are poorly defined lower-attenuation masses within the liver, with foci of contrast accumulation, compatible with cavernous hemangiomas. A focal, low-attenuation lesion in the posterior lateral left kidney *(arrow),* with measurements indicative of fat, is diagnostic of an incidental angiomyelolipoma (renal hamartoma). These latter findings were unchanged after therapy, indirectly confirming their nonlymphomatous cause.

No imaging modality successfully evaluates the spleen, which is the most common site of subdiaphragmatic disease in patients presenting with cervical or mediastinal disease with negative abdominal CT scans.

There is limited staging laparotomy data from which to evaluate the accuracy of imaging studies in newly diagnosed patients with non-Hodgkin's lymphoma (see Table 9–5). One study evaluated the contributions of LAG, abdominal and pelvic CT, and bone marrow biopsy and cytologic examination to the staging and management of 168 patients with newly diagnosed non-Hodgkin's lymphoma (Tables 9–7 and

9–8).[23] LAG and/or CT detected clinically inapparent retroperitoneal adenopathy and/or extranodal disease, which influenced clinical stage in 23% (39 of 168) and pathologic stage in 14% (13 of 168) of patients. Although bone marrow biopsy and cytologic examination influenced staging in 32% (53 of 168), 42 of these 53 patients already had advanced disease (clinical stage III) based on LAG and/or CT data. Thus, of the 16% (27 of 168) of patients whose management was changed by CT, LAG, or bone marrow results, the LAG and/or CT results influenced management more frequently (20 cases) compared with bone marrow results (7 cases).

The role of MRI in staging lymph nodes in the abdomen and pelvis is currently being evaluated.[14, 24] Since MRI relies on similar size criteria as CT for distinguishing normal from abnormal nodes, one would not expect MRI to have significant benefit over CT in this assessment. However, certain pulse sequences can increase contrast resolution between nodes and surrounding tissues, enhancing lymph node detection. Since staging laparotomies are done infrequently, studies evaluating MRI in this assessment will suffer from lack of histologic verification.

Liver and Spleen. Detection of lymphomatous deposits within the liver and spleen by cross-sectional imaging techniques is dependent on the size of the tumor deposit. Size criteria for these organs as predictors of involvement by tumor have repeatedly been shown to be inaccurate (unless there is massive enlargement, a situation readily detected by the physical examination). Although lesions 1.0 cm or larger can be detected with a high degree of confidence (Fig. 9–13; see also Fig. 9–12), at the time of initial presentation involvement of the spleen (as demonstrated by splenectomy) and liver (as evaluated by multiple needle and wedge biopsies) often occurs as several subcentimeter deposits of tumor in the former, and periportal infiltration of malignant cells in the latter. Such lesions cannot be identified even in retrospect on imaging studies (see Tables 9–3 to 9–5). Larger lesions are readily detected by CT, US, or MRI.[25, 26] When lesions are detected, and other causes confidently excluded (such as the relatively common occurring small hepatic cysts

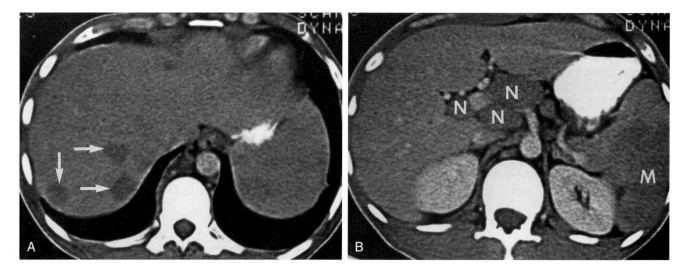

Figure 9–12. A 22-year-old man with newly diagnosed Hodgkin's disease. CT scans through the upper abdomen (*A* and *B*) demonstrate bulky lymphadenopathy in the celiac axis and porta hepatis (N), a large mass occupying a large portion of the spleen (M), and discrete intrahepatic masses *(arrows).* These abnormalities resolved after treatment, indirectly confirming their Hodgkin's etiology.

Table 9–6. Analysis of Computed Tomography (CT), Lymphography (LAG), and Gallium Scanning for Detection of Abdominal Lymph Node Involvement in Hodgkin's Disease Staging

| | Detection with CT, by Lymph Node Size° | | | | | | Detection with LAG° | | Detection with Gallium Scanning† | |
| | ≥ 10 mm | | ≥ 15 mm | | ≥ 20 mm | | | | | |
	No.	(%)	No.	(%)	No.	(%)	No.	(%)	No.	(%)
Sensitivity	6/12	(50)	4/12	(33)	3/12	(25)	5/12	(42)	3/11	(27)
Specificity	30/39	(77)	36/39	(92)	39/39	(100)	32/39	(82)	29/30	(97)
Accuracy	36/51	(71)	40/51	(78)	42/51	(82)	37/51	(73)	32/41	(78)
Positive predictive value	6/15	(40)	4/7	(57)	3/3	(100)	5/12	(42)	3/4	(75)
Negative predictive value	30/36	(83)	36/44	(82)	39/47	(83)	32/39	(82)	29/37	(78)

Data include involvement in the celiac axis and/or retroperitoneal lymph nodes.
°n = 51.
†n = 41.
From Stomper PC, Cholewinski SP, Park J, et al: Abdominal staging of thoracic Hodgkin disease: CT–lympangiography–Ga-67 scanning correlation. Radiology 1993; 187:381.

Table 9–7. Influence of Lymphography and/or Computed Tomography Findings on Pathologic Stage (Including Bone Marrow Biopsy and/or Cytologic Examination Results) and on Case Management in 168 Patients with Newly Diagnosed Non-Hodgkin's Lymphoma

| NHL Grade | No. of Patients | Stage Change | | Management Stage | |
		No.	(%)	No.	(%)
Low	57	11	(19)	11	(19)
Intermediate	78	12	(15)	9	(12)
High	33	0	(0)	0	(0)
Total	**168**	**23**	**(14)**	**20**	**(12)**

NHL, non-Hodgkin's lymphoma.
From Pond GD, Castellino RA, Horning S, Hoppe RT: Non-Hodgkin's lymphoma: Influence of lymphography, CT, and bone marrow biopsy on staging and management. Radiology 1984; 170:159.

or hepatic hemangiomas [Fig. 9–14; see also Fig. 9–11]), then such information is useful in determining if these organs are involved by lymphoma and can be confirmed by image-guided percutaneous needle biopsy[27] or laparoscopy.

Diffuse infiltration of the spleen, rather than focal tumor deposits, may go unrecognized by conventional cross-sectional imaging studies since no focal "masses" are identified. MRI after intravenous administration of super-paramagnetic contrast agents might have a role in this clinical setting, if such information would affect manage-

ment.[28] Since this situation occurs most commonly in the non-Hodgkin's lymphomas and is usually accompanied by obvious subdiaphragmatic lymphadenopathy, stage and management would infrequently be affected by such information.

Genitourinary Tract. Invasion of the genitourinary organs by adjacent lymph node masses in Hodgkin's disease can occur and is readily demonstrated on cross-sectional imaging studies. Intrinsic involvement of these organs by Hodgkin's disease, however, rarely occurs.

Table 9–8. Influence of Positive Bone Marrow Biopsy and/or Cytologic Examination Results on Management of Clinical Stage (Including Lymphography and Computed Tomography Results) I and II Cases° of Newly Diagnosed Non-Hodgkin's Lymphoma

NHL Grade	No. of CS I and CS II Patients	No. of Patients with Positive Biopsy and Cytologic Results	No. of Cases with Management Change
Low	9	1	1
Intermediate	34	4	4
High	18	6	2
Total	**61**	**11**	**7**

°No case of CS III or CS IV disease had a management change as a consequence of positive findings from bone marrow biopsy and cytologic examination.
NHL, non-Hodgkin's lymphoma; CS, clinical stage.
From Pond GD, Castellino RA, Horning S, Hoppe KT: Non-Hodgkin's lymphoma: Influence of lymphography, CT, and bone marrow biopsy on staging and management. Radiology 1984; 170:159.

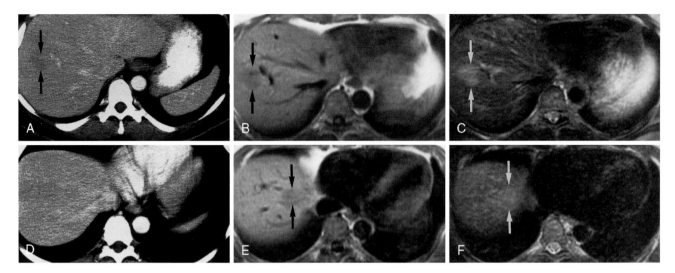

Figure 9–13. A 41-year-old man with follicular small cell lymphoma. CT scan *(A)* demonstrated a low-attenuation liver lesion *(arrows)* for which magnetic resonance imaging (MRI) was done for further evaluation (i.e., to exclude focal fatty infiltration, cavernous hemangioma). The MRI findings are compatible with metastasis, that is, a low signal on a T_1-weighted image *(B)* and higher signal on fat-suppressed T_2-weighted image *(C)*. Unexpectedly, a second similar lesion was seen on the MRI study *(arrows, E and F,* same pulse sequences as B and C) near the dome of the liver, which could not be seen in retrospect on the CT study *(D)*.

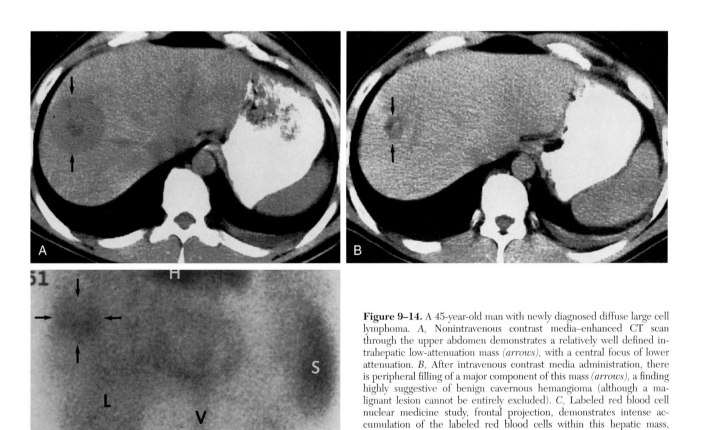

Figure 9–14. A 45-year-old man with newly diagnosed diffuse large cell lymphoma. *A,* Nonintravenous contrast media–enhanced CT scan through the upper abdomen demonstrates a relatively well defined intrahepatic low-attenuation mass *(arrows)*, with a central focus of lower attenuation. *B,* After intravenous contrast media administration, there is peripheral filling of a major component of this mass *(arrows)*, a finding highly suggestive of benign cavernous hemangioma (although a malignant lesion cannot be entirely excluded). *C,* Labeled red blood cell nuclear medicine study, frontal projection, demonstrates intense accumulation of the labeled red blood cells within this hepatic mass, confirming its etiology as a cavernous hemangioma *(arrows)*. Activity is also noted in the base of the heart (H), spleen (S), liver (L), and retroperitoneal vessels (V).

Table 9–9. Computed Tomographic Evidence of Intrinsic Genitourinary Tract Disease in 170 Newly Diagnosed Cases of Non-Hodgkin's Lymphoma

Findings	No. of Patients	Kidney	Other Sites
Nodular lymphocytic, well differentiated	0	0	0
Nodular lymphocytic, poorly differentiated	36	1	0
Nodular mixed	17	0	0
Nodular histiocytic	6	0	0
Diffuse lymphocytic, well differentiated	5	0	0
Diffuse lymphocytic, poorly differentiated	9	1	0
Diffuse mixed	11	0	0
Diffuse histiocytic	53	5	4°
Immunoblastic	8	0	2†
Lymphoblastic	10	3	0
Diffuse undifferentiated	10	0	1‡
Unclassified	5	0	0
Total	**170**	**10**	**7**

°Testis was involved in two patients and the uterus/cervix and ovaries in one patient each.
†Ovaries were involved in both patients.
‡Uterus/cervix was involved.
From Gilbert TJ, Castellino KA: Linfomi maligni dell'apparato genito-urinario. *In* Dalla Palma L (ed): Progressi in Radiologia 2: Radiourologia 1986. Trieste, Edizioni Lint, 1986, pp 265–280.

In non-Hodgkin's lymphoma, the prevalence of intrinsic involvement of these organs at the time of initial presentation has clearly been revised upward, based on information from CT studies (Table 9–9).[29] Not surprisingly, these organs are more frequently involved in the intermediate and high-grade histologic types. The kidney is most frequently involved, usually by one or more discrete masses that affect one or both kidneys, or by diffuse renal enlargement. Diffuse infiltration with thickening of the wall of the bladder (Fig. 9–15) and the ureter, as well as mass lesions within the uterus and/or cervix and prostate and/or seminal vesicles, are also readily detected by CT, as well as other cross-sectional

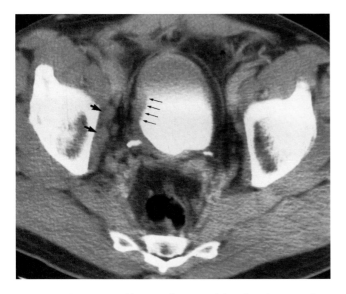

Figure 9–15. A 60-year-old man with non-Hodgkin's lymphoma involving the orbits, treated with radiation therapy 8 and 3 years ago. The patient developed incontinence for which a CT scan of the pelvis was done. Irregular soft tissue thickening was noted along the right posterolateral wall of the bladder *(narrow arrows)*, with enlarged lymph nodes adjacent to the obturator internus muscle *(broad arrows)*. Endoscopic biopsy revealed diffuse mixed lymphoma.

imaging studies.[30, 31] US is the preferred modality for evaluating the testes for involvement for lymphoma, although MRI can provide similar information.

Gastrointestinal Tract. Invasion of the gastrointestinal tract by adjacent lymph node masses in Hodgkin's disease does occur and can readily be noted on cross-sectional imaging studies. Intrinsic involvement of these organs by Hodgkin's disease, however, rarely occurs.

In the non-Hodgkin's lymphomas, intrinsic involvement of this organ system does occur, particularly with the higher-grade histologic types.[32] Barium contrast gastrointestinal tract studies provide excellent evaluation of the mucosal surface of these organs, as well as assessment of pliability, which reflects involvement of the gastrointestinal tract wall. Cross-sectional imaging techniques can also identify such involvement (with the exception of minimal mucosal abnormalities in early disease), and they have the added advantage of displaying the extraluminal extent of tumor, which is frequently considerable. Whether such information affects patient management, however, is unclear. Obviously, such techniques also provide information about the relationship of such lesions to adjacent structures, as well as whether regional lymph nodes are involved (Figs. 9–16 and 9–17).

In that subset of patients who have a high prevalence of concomitant gastrointestinal tract involvement (the so-called Mediterranean lymphomas or mucosal-associated lymphoid tissue lymphomas), screening barium contrast studies are frequently used to detect possible unsuspected involvement. If the staging abdominal and/or pelvic CT demonstrates such involvement, then barium studies are probably redundant. It is not known, however, if barium studies will detect gastrointestinal tract involvement in patients whose CT scan is negative, and if this does occur, if it occurs frequently enough to make it worthwhile to pursue.

OTHER SITES

Central Nervous System. In general, MRI is the imaging modality of choice for evaluating the cerebral spinal

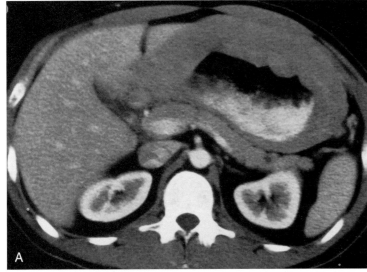

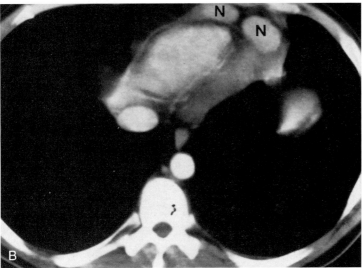

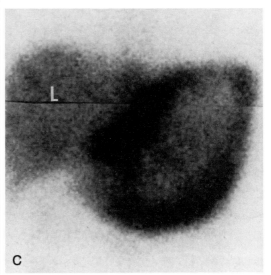

Figure 9–16. A 40-year-old man with newly diagnosed diffuse small cell gastric lymphoma. *A*, CT scan demonstrates concentric lobular soft tissue thickening of the gastric wall, without evidence of additional subdiaphragmatic disease. *B*, CT scan of the lower thorax demonstrates unsuspected bulky cardiophrenic angle lymphadenopathy (N). *C*, Gallium scan, frontal view, demonstrates intense circumferential uptake around the stomach, correlating with the CT findings (*A*). The bulky cardiophrenic angle lymphadenopathy was not identified, perhaps because of the adjacent high radioactivity in the gastric wall. L, liver.

axis.[33] Intrinsic involvement of the brain and spinal cord is rare in Hodgkin's disease but occurs with some frequency in the non-Hodgkin's lymphomas, particularly in those lymphomas occurring in immunocompromised patients. A more common manifestation of central nervous system disease is infiltration of the leptomeninges by tumor, as well as extradural masses that produce symptoms by compression (Fig. 9–18).[34] Such involvement is readily detected by MRI, with or without contrast enhancement. In those patients with an underlying likelihood of central nervous system involvement, that is, those with immunocompromise or with certain histologic subtypes, appropriate signs or symptoms, or worrisome cerebrospinal fluid results, screening of the central nervous system with MRI is appropriate.

Musculoskeletal System. Involvement of bone by direct invasion from adjacent lymph node masses occurs in both Hodgkin's disease and non-Hodgkin's lymphoma. Although frequently recognized on conventional skeletal radiographs or on the "bone windows" obtained during performance of staging CT studies, radionuclide bone scanning is a more sensitive imaging study. However, radionuclide bone scans

lack specificity, and if detailed bone radiographs fail to elucidate the cause of the increased activity on radionuclide bone scans, MRI has been found to be useful to demonstrate previously unrecognized cortical, as well as marrow, involvement, and relationships with adjacent soft tissue masses (Fig. 9–19).

Involvement of muscle, as well as adjacent soft tissues such as fat and fascial planes, usually is seen when lymph node masses enlarge and infiltrate adjacent structures.[35] On cross-sectional imaging studies, the maintenance of a distinct fat plane between a large mass and adjacent structures is a reliable indicator of lack of invasion. However, at times the mass obliterates the intervening soft tissue fat plane, in which instance direct invasion of adjacent structures cannot be reliably determined. Such invasion can be strongly suggested, however, when there is distortion of the normal texture or contour of the adjacent structures. Isolated nodules of tumor, distant from adjacent lymph node masses, can also be noted, more frequently in the non-Hodgkin's lymphomas. Apparent isolated involvement of muscles, with or without adjacent lymph node enlargement, is more common in non-Hodgkin's lymphoma. Extensive, often uniform, involvement of a muscle or muscle group is readily depicted on cross-sectional imaging studies (Fig. 9–20).

Intrinsic involvement of bone, that is, without an adjacent lymph node mass infiltrating bone, is seen in the non-Hodgkin's lymphomas, particularly those of diffuse histologic type. The entity "primary lymphoma of bone" (previously called "reticulum cell sarcoma" or "histiocytic lymphoma of bone"), in which there is no evidence of other sites of involvement, is less common than it used to be, probably because improved imaging techniques are able to demonstrate disease at sites that could not be evaluated as recently as several decades ago.

Bone Marrow. MRI can readily distinguish bone marrow that has undergone the normal fatty replacement (yellow marrow) from that which maintains active hematopoieses (red marrow). When tumor is present within the fat-containing marrow, it can be identified on conventional MRI, and there is increasing evidence to suggest that tumor deposits can often be identified within the cellular (red) marrow. Spotty, focal involvement of marrow (such as is typically seen with Hodgkin's disease) is probably more

readily identified than when the marrow is diffusely infiltrated by tumor, such as is seen in the low-grade lymphomas. Preliminary experience suggests that in patients who have normal posterior iliac crest bone marrow sampling, MRI can demonstrate areas of abnormal marrow signal at other sites that, when biopsied, are positive for tumor.[36, 37] MRI of the bone marrow, therefore, appears to have great promise in evaluating large portions of the bone marrow (compared with the minute sample obtained with aspiration techniques) and serves as a guide for directed marrow sampling, when indicated for patient management (Fig. 9–21). This application of MRI needs to be further evaluated to determine accuracy as well as impact on patient management.

IMAGING STUDIES AFTER TREATMENT

Surveillance Imaging Studies. Although different groups might prefer one imaging modality over another in

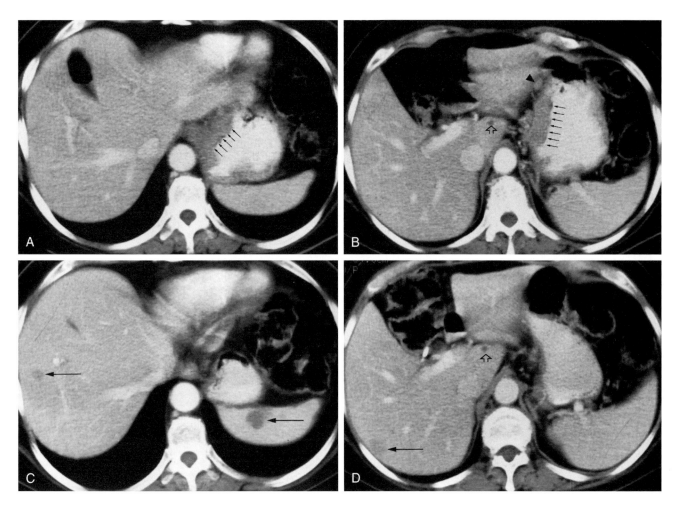

Figure 9–17. A 63-year-old woman with newly diagnosed gastric diffuse large cell lymphoma. *A* and *B*, CT scans demonstrate irregular thickening of portions of the gastric wall *(arrows)* due to gastric lymphoma. In addition, several enlarged perigastric lymph nodes are seen *(arrowhead)*. A sharply demarcated low-attenuation lesion in the caudate lobe of the liver *(open arrow)* is compatible with a hepatic cyst. *C* and *D,* Seven months later, after chemotherapy, CT scans at similar levels demonstrate resolution of the gastric wall thickening and perigastric lymphadenopathy. However, there has been interval appearance of poorly defined, low-attenuation lesions *(arrows)* within the spleen and liver because of unsuspected disease progression.

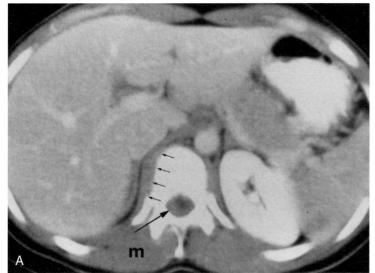

Figure 9–18. A 27-year-old woman with newly diagnosed Hodgkin's disease. *A,* CT scan demonstrates modest thickening of the paravertebral soft tissues *(short arrows),* minimal asymmetric fullness of the right paravertebral musculature (m), and soft tissue infiltration into the right spinal canal *(long arrow).* T_1 *(B)* and T_2 *(C)* weighted MRI scans confirm the infiltration into the spinal canal *(arrow),* with displacement of the spinal cord (c) to the left. Note the improved tumor delineation within the posterior musculature on the T_2-weighted image *(arrows).*

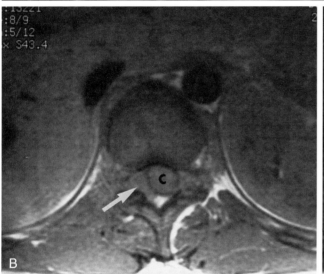

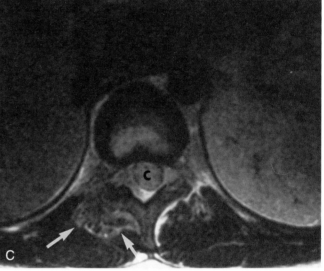

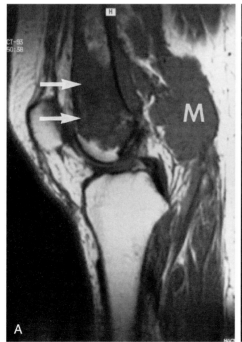

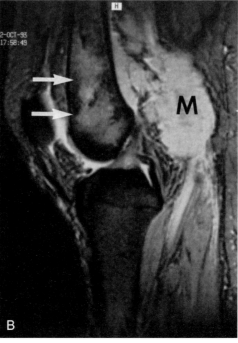

Figure 9–19. A 56-year-old woman with diffuse large cell lymphoma presented with knee pain, for which an MRI scan was done. *A,* Sagittal views of the knee show an irregular low signal within the marrow cavity of the distal left femur *(arrows)* on the T_1-weighted image, which normally should demonstrate a uniform bright signal owing to fat within the marrow space (as is present in the proximal tibia and patella). *B,* This area develops a brighter signal on the T_2-weighted image, a pulse sequence that enhances signal from water-containing (in this case, tumor) tissue and decreases signal from fat. Also noted is a large, irregular soft tissue mass (M) in the popliteal space, as well as a joint effusion. Other images demonstrated partial destruction of cortical bone in the distal femur.

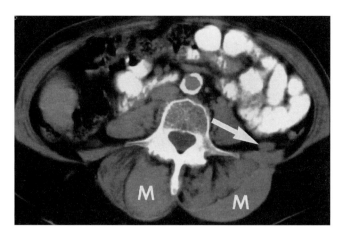

Figure 9–20. A 72-year-old woman with diffuse large cell lymphoma. CT scan shows diffuse, homogeneous increase in size of the posterior back muscles (M), which extended uniformly over multiple levels. Note enlargement of a lymph node anterior to the quadratus lumborum muscle *(arrow)*.

the initial staging evaluation of Hodgkin's disease and non-Hodgkin's lymphoma, there is general agreement on the imaging workup of these patients during initial staging, as noted in the prior section. Considerably less attention has been paid to assessing imaging studies in the subsequent management and followup of these patients, both as a monitor of treatment response and for periodic surveillance for disease relapse in the posttreatment period (see Fig. 9–17).[38] For example, how frequently should patients be reevaluated during treatment to verify that their disease is

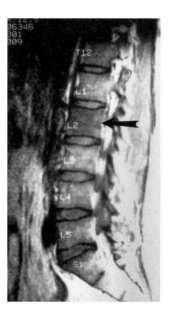

Figure 9–21. A 28-year-old man with newly diagnosed Hodgkin's disease with complaints of back pain. Conventional spine radiographs and radionuclide studies were negative. MRI demonstrated abnormally low signal at T12 and L2 on T_1-weighted images, suggesting infiltration of the marrow. Conventional iliac crest bone marrow biopsy results were negative; however, image-guided percutaneous biopsy of L2 *(arrow)* was positive for marrow involvement by Hodgkin's disease. (From Castellino RA: Malignant lymphoma in adults. *In* Bragg DG, Thompson WM [eds]: Categorical Course on Imaging of Cancers: Diagnosis, Staging and Follow-up Challenges. American College of Radiology, 1992, pp 127–136.)

Table 9–10. Results of Transthoracic Fine-Needle Biopsy in 54 Patients with a History of Lymphoma

Final Diagnosis	No. of Cases	Biopsy Results	
		No.	*(%)*
Lymphoma	21		
Initial biopsy		17/21	(81)
Repeat biopsy		20/21	(95)
Other malignancy	14	14/14	(100)
Infection	19	11/19	(58)

Modified from Wittich GR, Nowels KW, Korn RL, et al: Coaxial transthoracic fine-needle biopsy in patients with a history of malignant lymphoma. Radiology 1992; 183:175.

responding as anticipated? Although most would agree that only those sites positive for disease at the time of staging need to be reevaluated to determine response to treatment, the frequency during treatment at which this should occur is unclear. After completion of treatment, most would agree that a set of "baseline" studies is warranted on which subsequent studies can be compared. However, the frequency of performing surveillance studies on a routine basis (compared with when a patient develops symptoms or signs that initiate a directed reevaluation) is not clearly established for these diseases (nor for many other oncologic diseases as well). This can be addressed, to some extent, by dynamic probabilistic modeling that requires that several important assumptions be made by the clinical oncologist.[39] In such analysis, the frequency of periodic monitoring may differ for subsets of different biologic behavior within these diseases.

The Posttreatment "Residual Mass." With improved imaging techniques, the demonstration of a residual mass after therapy frequently occurs. Whether such masses represent persistent viable tumor or simply residual fibrosis of successfully treated disease is an important clinical distinction. Stability over time after completion of therapy provides increasing reassurance that the residual mass in fact does not represent viable tumor. However, since additional therapy is often available for patients in which the residual mass represents tumor, there is often need to make this determination in a timely fashion. Tissue sampling of such masses can be readily accomplished with image-guided percutaneous needle biopsy techniques (see Fig. 9–10). Such samples are adequate for relatively extensive evaluation by experienced pathologists.[40] A positive biopsy provides meaningful information; with a negative result, however, one must always consider that the limited sampling of the mass might have "missed" areas of viable tumor, or other pathologic lesions (Table 9–10).

Analysis of the morphology of these residual masses does not provide such information. However, some information can be obtained from the MRI signal characteristics of these masses, and from nuclear medicine studies that directly evaluate the avidity of some tumors for specific agents (such as gallium) or tissue metabolism (such as thallium and fluorodeoxyglucose positron emission tomographic scanning) (Fig. 9–22). CT cannot provide reliable information about the viability of tissue in this setting, except in the rare instance in which there is convincing evidence of lack of any contrast enhancement after intravenous bolus injection of

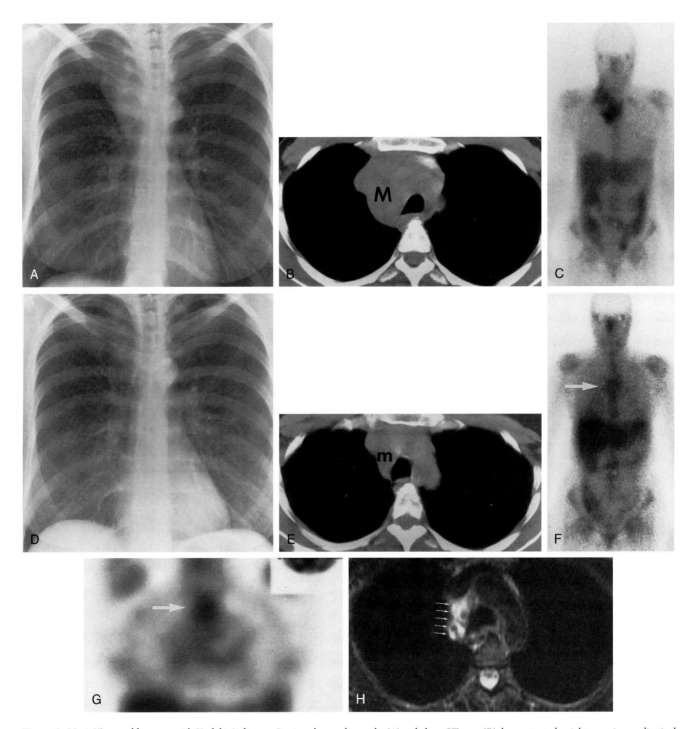

Figure 9–22. A 37-year-old woman with Hodgkin's disease. Staging chest radiographs (*A*) and chest CT scan (*B*) demonstrated a right superior mediastinal mass (M). The staging gallium scan (*C*) demonstrated right supraclavicular lymphadenopathy in addition to the right superior mediastinal mass. Approximately 6 months later, after treatment, a repeat chest radiograph (*D*) demonstrated complete resolution of the mass. However, chest CT at that time (*E*) demonstrated a markedly smaller, but persistent, soft tissue mass (m) in the right superior mediastinum. Gallium study with planar (*F*) and single photon emission computed tomography (*G*) coronal imaging showed persistent, although decreased, activity in the right superior mediastinum (*arrow*). MRI scan (*H*), performed with a pulse sequence designed to suppress signal from fat and increase the conspicuity of tissues containing water, demonstrated a bright signal in the right superior mediastinum (*arrows*). Although highly suspicious for persistent viable tumor, such findings can be seen on MRI scans 6 to 9 months after cessation of treatment. (From Castellino RA, DeLaPaz RL, Larson SM: Imaging techniques in cancer. *In* DeVita V, Hellman S, Rosenberg SA [eds]: Cancer: Principles and Practice of Oncology. Philadelphia, JB Lippincott, 1993, pp 507–531.)

contrast media of a structure that does not contain a thickened, irregular wall. MRI has significantly greater promise in this evaluation, since choosing specific pulse sequences can provide important information regarding the cellular content of such masses.[4, 41] In general, masses that demonstrate a brighter signal than muscle on T_2-weighted images have sufficient mobile water content to suggest viable tumor cells, whereas those of low signal intensity on T_2-weighted images frequently represent relatively acellular tissue, such as "mature" fibrosis.[42] Correlating changes in tumor or mass size with patterns of MRI signal intensity shows promise, particularly after the first 6 months following therapy. A mass decreasing or stable in size with homogeneously low signal intensity on T_2-weighted images is reassuring for "sterilized" tumor; whereas, areas of high signal intensity on T_2-weighted images in any residual mass, whether stable in size or larger, are worrisome for persistent active tumor. However, this assessment is made most confidently from 6 to 9 months after treatment, since there is frequently "cellular" fibrosis and associated inflammation in the early months following therapy that can mimic persistent viable tumor. And it is during this period when it is important to determine if the residual mass requires further treatment. Clearly, more experience is needed with MRI in this evaluation, as well as comparative studies with radionuclide scans,[43] which have a demonstrated usefulness in this clinical setting.

Several reports from Europe suggest that US can be useful in this assessment, based not on the morphology of the persistent residual mass but instead on the "echo texture" of the lesion.[44] This work requires corroboration from other institutions, but there appears to be little interest at this time from other groups, perhaps because it appears to be a highly operator-dependent examination requiring considerable technical skill.

Nuclear medicine studies, particularly for those tumors that are known to be gallium avid at the outset, are perhaps the most useful at this time. Persistence of gallium avidity certainly suggests persistent viable tumor, and the conversion from a positive to a negative gallium study would support tumor eradication. Such information is often used in patient management, particularly when it reaffirms the overall clinical evaluation.

REFERENCES

1. Begg CB, McNeil BJ: Assessment of radiologic tests: Control of bias and other design considerations. Radiology 1988; 167:565.
2. Rehn SM, Nyman RS, Glimelius BLG, et al: Non-Hodgkin's lymphoma: Predicting prognostic grade with MR imaging. Radiology 1990; 176:249.
3. Nyman RS, Rehn SM, Glimelius BLG, et al: Residual mediastinal masses in Hodgkin's disease: Prediction of size with MR imaging. Radiology 1989; 170:435.
4. Rahmouni A, Tempany C, Jones R, et al: Lymphoma: Monitoring tumor size and signal intensity with MR imaging. Radiology 1993; 188:445.
5. Castellino RA, Blank N, Hoppe RT, Cho C: Hodgkin's disease: Contributions of chest CT in the initial staging evaluation. Radiology 1986; 106:603.
6. Wernecke K, Vassallo P, Rutsch F, et al: Thymic involvement in Hodgkin's disease: CT and sonographic findings. Radiology 1991; 181:375.
7. Castellino RA, Goffinet DR, Blank N, et al: The role of radiography in the staging of non-Hodgkin's lymphoma with laparotomy correlation. Radiology 1973; 110:329.
8. Castellino RA, Hilton S, O'Brien JP, Portlock CS: Non-Hodgkin's lymphoma: Contribution of chest CT in the initial staging evaluation. Radiology 1996; 199:129.
9. Hopper KD, Diehl LF, Cole BA, et al: The significance of necrotic mediastinal lymph nodes on CT in patients with newly diagnosed Hodgkin disease. AJR Am J Roentgenol 1990; 155:267.
10. Celicoglu F, Trerstein AS, Krellenstein DJ, Strauchen JA: Pleural effusion in non-Hodgkin's lymphoma. Chest 1992; 101:1137.
11. Cho CS, Blank N, Castellino RA: Computerized tomography evaluation of chest wall involvement in lymphoma. Cancer 1985; 55:1892.
12. Carlsen SE, Bergin CJ, Hoppe RT: MR imaging to detect chest wall and pleural involvement in patients with lymphoma: Effect on radiation therapy planning. AJR Am J Roentgenol 1993; 160:1191.
13. Hopper KD, Diehl LF, Lesar M, et al: Hodgkin's disease: Clinical utility of CT in initial staging and treatment. Radiology 1988; 169:17.
14. Tesoro-Tess JD, Balzarini L, Ceglia E, et al: Magnetic resonance imaging in the initial staging of Hodgkin's disease and non-Hodgkin's lymphoma. Eur J Radiol 1991; 12:81.
15. Greco A, Jelliffe AM, Maher EJ, Leung AWL: MR imaging of lymphomas: Impact on therapy. J Comput Assist Tomogr 1988; 12(5):785.
16. Tesoro-Tess JD, Biasi S, Balzarini L, et al: Heart involvement in lymphomas: The value of magnetic resonance imaging and two-dimensional echocardiography at disease presentation. Cancer 1993; 72:2484.
17. Marglin S, Castellino RA: Lymphographic accuracy in 623 consecutive, previously untreated cases of Hodgkin's disease and non-Hodgkin's lymphoma. Radiology 1981; 140:351.
18. Castellino RA, Hoppe RT, Blank N, et al: Computed tomography, lymphography, and staging laparotomy: Correlations in initial staging of Hodgkin's disease. AJR Am J Roentgenol 1984; 143:37.
19. Baker LL, Parker BR, Donaldson SS, Castellino RA: Staging of Hodgkin disease in children: Comparison of CT and lymphography with laparotomy. AJR Am J Roentgenol 1990; 154:1251.
20. Castellino RA: Imaging techniques for extent determination of Hodgkin's disease and non-Hodgkin's lymphoma. In Progress in Clinical and Biological Research. Vol 132D. Proceedings of the 13th International Cancer Congress. Seattle, 1982. New York, Alan R Liss, 1983, pp 365–372.
21. Stomper PC, Cholewinski SP, Park J, et al: Abdominal staging of thoracic Hodgkin disease: CT–lymphangiography–Ga-67 scanning correlation. Radiology 1993; 187:381.
22. North LB, Wallace S, Lindell MM, et al: Lymphography for staging lymphomas: Is it still a useful procedure? AJR Am J Roentgenol 1993; 161:867.
23. Pond GD, Castellino RA, Horning S, Hoppe RT: Non-Hodgkin's lymphoma: Influence of lymphography, CT, and bone marrow biopsy on staging and management. Radiology 1984; 170:159.
24. Hanna SL, Fletcher BD, Boulden TF, et al: MR imaging of infradiaphragmatic lymphadenopathy in children and adolescents with Hodgkin's disease: Comparison with lymphography and CT. J Magn Reson Imaging 1993; 3:461.
25. Sanders LM, Botet JF, Straus DJ, et al: CT of primary lymphoma of the liver. AJR Am J Roentgenol 1989; 152:973.
26. Soyer P, Van Beers B, Teillet-Thiébaud F, et al: Hodgkin's and non-Hodgkin's hepatic lymphoma: Sonographic findings. Abdom Imaging 1993; 18:339.
27. Cavanna L, Civardi G, Fornari F, et al: Ultrasonically guided percutaneous splenic tissue core biopsy in patients with malignant lymphomas [Abstract] Radiology 1993; 186:584.
28. Weissleder R, Elizondo G, Stark DD, et al: The diagnosis of splenic lymphoma by MR imaging. AJR Am J Roentgenol 1989; 152:175.
29. Gilbert TJ, Castellino RA: Linfomi maligni dell'apparato genito-urinario. In Dalla Palma L (ed): Progressi in Radiologia 2: Radiourologia 1986. Trieste, Italy, Edizioni Lint, 1986, pp 265–280.
30. Yeoman LJ, Mason MD, Olliff JFC: Non-Hodgkin's lymphoma of the bladder—CT and MRI appearances. Clin Radiol 1991; 44:389.
31. Buck DS, Peterson MS, Borochovitz D, Bloom EJ: Non-Hodgkin lymphoma of the ureter: CT demonstration with pathologic correlation. Urol Radiol 1992; 14:183.
32. Rubesin SE, Gilchrist AM, Bronner M, et al: Non-Hodgkin lymphoma of the small intestine. Radiographics 1990; 10:985.

33. Zimmerman RA: Central nervous system lymphoma. Radiol Clin North Am 1990; 28:697.
34. Li MH, Holtåas S, Larsson EM: MR imaging of spinal lymphoma. Acta Radiol 1991; 33:338.
35. Malloy PC, Fishman EK, Magid D: Lymphoma of bone, muscle, and skin: CT findings. AJR Am J Roentgenol 1992; 159:805.
36. Hoane BR, Shields AF, Porter BA, Shulman HK: Detection of lymphomatous bone marrow involvement with magnetic resonance imaging. Blood 1991; 78:728.
37. Linden A, Zankovich R, Theissen P, et al: Malignant lymphoma: Bone marrow imaging versus biopsy. Radiology 1989; 173:335.
38. Heron CW, Husband JE, Williams MP, Cherryman GR: The value of thoracic computed tomography in the detection of recurrent Hodgkin's disease. Br J Radiol 1988; 61:567.
39. Chang PJ, Parker BR, Donaldson SS, Thompson EI: Dynamic probabilistic model for determination of optimal timing of surveillance chest radiography in pediatric Hodgkin disease. Radiology 1989; 173:71.
40. Wittich GR, Nowels KW, Korn RL, et al: Coaxial transthoracic fine-needle biopsy in patients with a history of malignant lymphoma. Radiology 1992; 183:175.
41. Webb R: MR imaging of treated mediastinal Hodgkin disease. Radiology 1989; 170:315.
42. Lee JKT, Glazer HS: Controversy in the MR imaging appearance of fibrosis. Radiology 1990; 177:21.
43. Gasparini MD, Balzarini L, Castellani MR, et al: Current role of gallium scan and magnetic resonance imaging in the management of mediastinal Hodgkin lymphoma. Cancer 1993; 72:577.
44. Wernecke K, Vassallo P, Hoffmann G, et al: Value of sonography in monitoring the therapeutic response of mediastinal lymphoma: Comparison with chest radiography and CT. AJR Am J Roentgenol 1991; 156:265.

GENERAL REFERENCES

Castellino RA: Hodgkin disease: Practical concepts for the diagnostic radiologist. Radiology 1986; 159:305.
Castellino RA: The non-Hodgkin lymphomas: Practical concepts for the diagnostic radiologist. Radiology 1991; 178:315.
Castellino RA: Malignant lymphoma in adults. In Bragg DG, Thompson WM (eds): Categorical course on imaging of cancers: Diagnosis, staging and follow-up challenges. American College of Radiology, 1992, pp 127–136.
Libshitz HJ (ed): Imaging the lymphomas. Radiol Clin North Am July 1990, vol 28.
Musumeci R, Tesoro-Tess JD: New imaging techniques in staging lymphomas. Curr Opin Oncol 1994; 6:464.

Chapter Ten

Approach to the Patient with Suspected Lymphoma

Arthur T. Skarin

Although lymphomas are relatively common, there are a number of other conditions characterized by lymphadenopathy, with or without hepatosplenomegaly, that may mimic an underlying lymphoma. These conditions include numerous benign diseases as well as other malignancies, both primary and metastatic (Table 10–1). Seemingly healthy adults may have palpable lymph nodes, particularly in the cervical area. In one study, as many as 56% of patients examined for other reasons were found to have cervical adenopathy.[1] Likewise, it is not uncommon to discover slight adenopathy and even splenomegaly, findings reported in the past in otherwise healthy college students.[2] In these circumstances followup evaluation is important, since pathologic or progressive enlargement of lymph nodes or spleen requires investigation and a histologic diagnosis.

In the differential diagnosis of adenopathy, infections are usually associated with tender or painful nodes; allergic or autoimmune processes with soft, rubbery nodes; lymphomas with firm, occasionally rubbery nodes that may be matted together; and carcinoma with hard nodes, sometimes matted or fixed to the underlying tissues. Sarcomas rarely spread to lymph nodes, but adenopathy is occasionally seen in metastatic rhabdomyosarcoma, malignant fibrous histiocytoma, and Ewing's sarcoma. Metastatic Kaposi's sarcoma may also be found in enlarged nodes of acquired immunodeficiency syndrome (AIDS) patients, particularly with associated skin lesions, but even in those without typical skin involvement. Tenderness of a lymph node can occur when rapid enlargement develops, resulting in expansion of the capsule, or when hemorrhage occurs into the necrotic center of a neoplastic node, also resulting in sudden enlargement.[3]

Acute nonspecific lymphadenitis is most often the result of acute bacterial infection. Foreign material introduced into the circulation via injury or intravenous drug abuse also results in regional acute adenitis. These conditions are usually not confused with lymphoma due to the classic signs and symptoms of infection and inflammation. Chronic lymphadenitis may be due to nonspecific reactions induced by a variety of antigens (e.g., drugs), resulting in follicular hyperplasia (B-cell proliferation), paracortical lymphoid hyperplasia (T-cell expansion), or sinus histiocytosis (usually in nodes draining malignancies). These conditions are discussed in more detail in the following section.

PATTERNS OF ADENOPATHY

Adenopathy may be localized or solitary (restricted to one lymph node area), limited to several adjacent sites, or generalized. The last pattern more often signifies a lymphoma, since carcinomas tend to spread to regional or contiguous lymph node sites (e.g., head and neck cancer). This tendency, however, is also characteristic of Hodgkin's disease. A haphazard nodal enlargement may be seen in malignant melanoma, because of extensive spread though subcutaneous lymphatics and the unpredictable biologic behavior of melanoma.

The probability of various etiologies (nonspecific, specific, or malignant) related to the extent of lymphadenopathy (localized, limited or regional, and generalized) have been reviewed.[4] The three most common causes in localized disease were lymphomas, tuberculosis, and toxoplasmosis; in limited disease, toxoplasmosis, infectious mononucleosis, and Hodgkin's disease; and in generalized disease, infectious mononucleosis and lymphoma (same rate), and toxoplasmosis. The frequency of these categories, however, may be biased by referral patterns.

Lymph node size varies considerably, mainly related to the patient's awareness of adenopathy and eagerness in obtaining medical evaluation. In one series, most patients with lymph nodes larger than 1 cm² had nonspecific adenopathy, with only a few cases of infections mononucleosis or toxoplasmosis found.[5] It was concluded that patients with adenopathy smaller than 1 cm could be observed as long as infectious mononucleosis, toxoplasmosis, or an underlying systemic disease had been ruled out. Classic B symptoms suggest that underlying Hodgkin's disease can occur in about 20% of cases or in 20% to 30% of patients with non-Hodgkin's lymphoma. The lymphoma may be difficult to locate, although it is occasionally initially restricted to pelvic nodes. Unusual symptoms such as generalized pruritus or pain in enlarged lymph nodes after ingesting alcohol are

Table 10–1. Causes of Lymphadenopathy°

Infections

Viral: infectious mononucleosis (EBV), cytomegalovirus, infectious hepatitis, postvaccinial lymphadenitis, adenovirus, herpes zoster, HIV, (AIDS), HTLV-I
Bacterial: *Staphylococcus, Streptococcus,* cat scratch disease, chancroid, melioidosis, tuberculosis, atypical mycobacteria, primary and secondary syphilis
Chlamydial: lymphogranuloma venereum
Protozoan: toxoplasmosis
Mycotic: histoplasmosis, coccidiomycosis
Rickettsial: scrub typhus
Helminthic: filariasis

Autoimmune Disorders

Rheumatoid arthritis, systemic lupus erythematosus, dermatomyositis, mixed connective tissue disease, Sjögren's syndrome

Hypersensitivity (iatrogenic)

Serum sickness
Drug hypersensitivity: diphenylhydantoin, carbamazepine, primidone, gold, allopurinol, indomethacin, sulfonamides, others
Silicone reaction
Vaccination related
Graft vs. host disease

Atypical Lymphoproliferative Disorders (potentially malignant)

Angiofollicular (giant) lymph node hyperplasia (Castleman's disease)
Angioimmunoblastic lymphadenopathy with dysproteinemia
Angiocentric immunoproliferative disorders
  Lymphomatoid granulomatosis
  Wegener's granulomatosis

Unusual Causes of Lymphadenopathy

Inflammatory pseudotumor of lymph nodes
Histiocytic necrotizing lymphadenitis (Kikuchi's lymphadenitis)
Sinus histiocytosis with massive lymphadenopathy (Rosai-Dorfman disease)
Vascular transformation of sinuses
Progressive transformation of germinal centers

Miscellaneous Benign Disorders

Hyperthyroidism, sarcoidosis, amyloidosis, dermatopathic lymphadenopathy, mucocutaneous lymph node syndrome (Kawasaki disease), storage diseases (Gaucher's, Niemann-Pick, Letterer-Siwe disease), Whipple's disease, hypertriglyceridemia, extramedullary hematopoiesis

Malignant Diseases

Hematologic: lymphoma, acute and chronic leukemia, Waldenström's macroglobulinemia, multiple myeloma (uncommon), systemic mastocytosis
Metastatic: breast, lung, renal cell, prostate, other cancers

°The listings are by no means all inclusive.
EBV, Epstein-Barr virus; AIDS, acquired immunodeficiency syndrome; HIV, human immunodeficiency virus; HTLV-I, human T-cell lymphotropic virus, type I.
Modified from Pangalis GA, Vassilakopoulos TP, Boussiotis VA, et al: Clinical approach to lymphadenopathy. Semin Oncol 1993; 20:570.

associated with Hodgkin's disease. Systemic B symptoms, however, may also be seen in infections, connective tissue disease, and angioimmunoblastic lymphadenopathy. Intermittent fevers may also be seen in metastatic carcinomas, especially if liver involvement is present. Recurrent fevers

may also be a hallmark of underlying renal cell carcinoma, which may be still restricted to the kidney. A complex of fever, splenomegaly, and anemia (especially in the presence of a heart murmur) is the hallmark of subacute bacterial endocarditis, a diagnosis that appears to be decreasing in incidence but one that must not be missed. A complex of fever, malaise, and migratory arthritis, along with persistent inflammatory nasal and sinus disease, strongly suggests Wegener's granulomatosis.[6]

Anatomic locations often predict the type of underlying disorder. Cervical nodes are the most often enlarged but are also the least likely to reveal a specific diagnosis at the time of biopsy. Malignancies involving upper cervical nodes most often arise from the oral pharynx, larynx, and nasal and paranasal sinuses, whereas in the lower neck numerous sites must be considered, including the lung, breast, and abdominal organs. Enlarged epitrochlear nodes are most often due to non-Hodgkin's lymphoma and, rarely, Hodgkin's disease. Supraclavicular adenopathy, especially on the left side (Virchow's node), is a classic clue to underlying lung or gastrointestinal cancer. Axillary adenopathy is often nondiagnostic but may be due to cat scratch disease, lymphoma, or metastatic breast cancer. Enlarged inguinal nodes 1 cm in diameter or smaller may occur in normal adults related to minor infections in the lower extremities or unknown factors. Malignancies of the lower extremities, tumors of the anal or urogenital area, or lymphomas must also be considered.

Mediastinal adenopathy may be due to a number of entities, some of which are benign, including neurogenic tumors and benign cysts. Consideration of the anatomic location within the mediastinum is helpful in the differential diagnosis.[7] In the anterior mediastinum, most tumors are lymphomas, thymomas, germ cell tumors, or lipomas, whereas the posterior mediastinum is the location for neurogenic tumors, esophageal cysts and tumors, spinal column tumors, and paragangliomas. Common tumors in the middle mediastinum include lymphomas, bronchogenic and pericardial cysts, sarcoidosis, and metastatic malignancies. The superior mediastinum is often a site for parathyroid adenomas, thyroid tumors, lymphomas, and thymic tumors and cysts. With advanced disease, and especially lung cancer, the tumor may involve contiguous or multiple mediastinal compartments. Of note, hilar adenopathy suggests sarcoidosis (particularly if bilateral), lymphoma, or underlying lung cancer.

Although some patients with lymphoma may present with splenomegaly, with the lymphoma restricted to the spleen (especially non-Hodgkin's lymphomas), a variety of other benign and malignant processes may be characterized by initial isolated splenomegaly.[8] In this situation, a specific diagnosis may be difficult to make by standard studies, and splenectomy may be indicated, which is occasionally therapeutic.

Lymphomas may also arise within the bone marrow, resulting in pancytopenia.[9] The differential diagnosis of pancytopenia is extensive, including benign hematologic as well as malignant disorders, but occasional benign processes such as drug reactions or sepsis must be ruled out.

Finally, lymphomas may arise primarily in extranodal sites such as the central nervous system,[10] head and neck,[11] thyroid,[12] lungs,[13] heart,[14] liver,[15] pancreas,[16] gastrointestinal tract,[17] adrenal glands,[18] kidneys,[19] testes,[20] ovaries,[21] subcutaneous tissues,[22] and skin.[23] In these circumstances, other malignancies, either primary or metastatic, enter into the differential diagnosis.

Skin involvement occurs in lymphomas, particulary T-cell types, but may also be seen in B-cell lymphomas.[24, 25] The lesions may be primary[23] or develop as part of disseminated disease. Primary cutaneous T-cell lymphomas (CTCLs) such as mycosis fungoides (see Chapter 26) often spread into regional lymph nodes as the disease progresses. Cutaneous lesions that simulate lymphoma include erythema nodosum (related to underlying sarcoidosis, tuberculosis, streptococcal infection, or drug reaction), sarcoidosis, and a variety of chronic dermatoses that may result in regional adenopathy. In the last condition, lymph node biopsy often reveals dermatopathic lymphadenopathy.[26]

An unusual and uncommon chronic skin disorder, lymphomatoid papulosis, is characterized by intermittent, self-healing papular skin lesions that histologically may resemble a malignant lymphoma.[27] Epidemiologic studies of patients with lymphomatoid papulosis show a significantly increased frequency of prior or coexisting Hodgkin's disease or CTCL, an increased frequency of nonlymphoid malignancies, and exposure to radiation therapy but not human T-cell leukemia/lymphoma virus, type I infections.[27] A recent report reveals an increased risk of subsequent Hodgkin's disease as well as non-Hodgkin's lymphomas occuring in 5 (24%) of 21 patients over a 15-year interval.[28] Anaplastic large cell lymphoma (Ki1+) involving skin and nodes has been documented in two patients with previous lymphomatoid papulosis.[29] The association of the earlier mentioned disorders remains unknown but suggests an underlying immunoregulatory defect of T lymphocytes.

INITIAL EVALUATION OF ADENOPATHY

The initial studies after a detailed history and physical examination should include a complete blood count, platelet count, erythrocyte sedimentation rate, and examination of the peripheral blood smear. Infectious mononucleosis can often be diagnosed by the presence of abnormal or atypical monocytes and lymphocytes, often before the leukocyte level becomes elevated. The blood smear shows a heterogenous or pleomorphic population of mononuclear cells compared with leukemia or lymphoma, wherein the abnormal cells are homogenous in appearance. The presence of a left shift in the myeloid series with toxic vacuoles and coarse granules (especially in polymorphonuclear leukocytes) suggests an underlying infection.

When indicated, blood cultures for infection and serologic studies for infectious mononucleosis, cytomegalovirus, human immunodeficiency virus, and other viruses and also autoimmune diseases should be obtained. The heterophile antibody test results may be negative in early infectious mononucleosis, but a repeated test is required and is positive in 40%, 60%, and 90% of patients by the end of the first, second, and third weeks of illness, respectively.[4] Blood chemistries are also helpful, especially lactate dehydrogenase levels, which can be elevated in leukemia and advanced non-Hodgkin's lymphoma. Other tumor markers such as

C-reactive protein, Ca125, and carcinoembryonic antigen are nonspecific and more valuable in following the course of an established diagnosis than as a screening test. Serum calcium and angiotensin-converting enzyme levels may be increased in active sarcoidosis in 2% to 10% and 50% to 80% of cases, respectively.[4]

Initial radiographic studies should be limited to a chest radiographic examination for adenopathy above the diaphragm. Other than sarcoidosis, tuberculosis, toxoplasmosis, histoplasmosis, and infectious mononucleosis, few benign diseases result in mediastinal or hilar adenopathy or parenchymal lesions. Computed tomographic (CT) scan of involved lymph node sites is not often helpful, except in head and neck adenopathy when extension to bone or other soft tissue may be diagnosed, which is a part of staging evaluation in diagnosed cases.

WHEN TO PERFORM LYMPH NODE BIOPSIES

The lymphatic system grows during childhood and achieves twice its adult size by early adolescence. During mid-adolescence lymphoid tissue begins to regress, reaching stable adult size by age 20 to 25 years.[30] Peripheral lymphadenopathy is commonly seen in children and young adults and is mostly related to benign causes.[31] The probability of malignancy rises with increasing age. Mathematical models have been developed for predicting the need to carry out a lymph node biopsy. In a study of adults, a discriminate analysis was carried out based on assessment of patient age, lymph node size, texture, tenderness, and location.[4] Of patients in whom biopsy was finally proven unnecessary, 88% were correctly classified. Of those whose mathematical score indicated a need for biopsy, 91% were correctly classified by the model. A similar study was performed in young patients aged 9 to 25 years in an attempt to differentiate "no treatment" categories (normal lymph nodes, reactive follicular hyperplasia, miscellaneous viral infections, or autoimmune disorders) from "treatment" categories (granulomatous reactions to tuberculosis, sarcoidosis and cat-scratch disease, lymphomas, and metastatic cancers) by another group.[26] Based on lymph node size, the presence of upper respiratory symptoms, and chest radiographic abnormalities, they managed to classify correctly 95% and 96% of their patients who were or were not in need of lymph node biopsy, respectively.[26, 32]

Although the multivariate models are of interest in determining whether a lymph node biopsy is indicated, the final decision should be based on clinical judgment. A high index of suspicion may result in many nondiagnostic biopsies, however, as noted by a 63% rate of benign adenopathies in the European study.[4] In the Philadelphia study of young patients, 9.8% of all biopsies showed normal lymph nodes, 31.7% reactive follicular hyperplasia, and 17% miscellaneous conditions.[26] Careful followup of the latter categories is important, however, since 17% to 24% of patients have specific diseases diagnosed on a later biopsy, with 90% of subsequent lymphomas diagnosed within 8 months.[4] Use of modern polymerase chain reaction techiques allows for earlier diagnosis of lymphomas compared with traditional histopathologic and immunologic methods (see Chapter 5). In one report, a 35-year-old woman had lymphadenopathy for 9 years, with serial lymph node biopsies showing benign reactive changes before Hodgkin's disease eventually developed.[33]

One type of "prelymphoma" is progressive transformation of germinal centers (PTGCs).[34] In this entity there is a high tendency for subsequent development of nodular lymphocyte predominance Hodgkin's disease (see later). However, in a recent report, a syndrome of lymphoid hyperplasia and florid PTGC occurred in adolescent boys and young men, with no progression to Hodgkin's disease in as long as 10 years of followup.[35] The availability of molecular probes may allow for early diagnosis of a lymphoma.

What are the indications for biopsy of enlarged lymph nodes? As noted earlier, clinical judgment based on clinical and laboratory features is a major factor in the decision. Table 10–2 outlines several aspects that should be considered. An abdominal and pelvic CT scan may be indicated, particularly in patients with abdominal complaints or abnormal liver function studies. Careful observation of lymphadenopathy for a few weeks is not unreasonable in otherwise asymptomatic patients since regression may occur in benign diseases. However, spontaneous regression has been reported in 23% of patients with early non-Hodgkin's lymphoma, particularly those with low-grade or nodular histology.[36] Lymph node enlargement in Hodgkin's disease may also wax and wane, sometimes for several months, before progressive enlargement occurs.

LYMPH NODE BIOPSY

A specific tissue diagnosis may be made by fine-needle aspiration (FNA), Tru-Cut needle biopsy, or lymph node excisional biopsy. Indications are listed in Table 10–2. Although FNA has many advantages, particularly minimal morbidity, the size of the specimen may limit its usefulness in accurately classifying a malignant lymphoma. In patients with cervical lymphadenopathy, however, FNA has been preferred by some investigators since, if occult head and neck cancer is present, biopsy of an involved node may lead to regional spread of disease.[37] This concept, however, is not universally accepted.

In patients with suspected lymphoma or those with an "unknown" primary malignancy, excisional lymph node biosy offers ample tissue for detailed study using a variety of diagnostic immunoperoxidase reactions (see Chapter 5). In addition, tissue can be obtained or stored for special studies, including electron microscopy, cytogenetics, biologic (oncogene) assay, immunophenotyping, and immunogenotyping.[38]

The percentage of patients with adenopathy who eventually require a lymph node biopsy for diagnosis varies from 33% to 66%, depending on the results of noninvasive studies, patient referral patterns, and age of the patient. In a patient with suspected infectious mononucleosis or other viral syndrome, lymph node biopsy should not be carried out because the histologic features may be confused with a malignant lymphoma.[39] For the same reason, biopsy of enlarged nodes should be avoided in patients suspected of phenytoin or other drug-related hypersensitivity adenopathy.

In selection of the node for biopsy, the largest and thus most pathologic lymph node should be removed. Inguinal nodes should be avoided if at all possible, owing to the high frequency of nonspecific adenitis that can occur in this region. The surgeon must carefully resect the node intact, and not in fragments, to allow for careful examination by an experienced hematopathologist. It is also important to notify the pathology laboratory before the lymph node biopsy is scheduled so that special studies can be discussed and planned.

REFERENCES

1. Linet OI, Metzler C: Incidence of palpable cervical nodes in adults. Postgrad Med 1977; 62:210.
2. Hoagland, RJ: Infectious Mononucleosis. New York, Grune & Stratton, 1967.
3. Kubotta TT: The evaluation of peripheral lymphadenopathy. Prim Care 1980; 7:461.
4. Pangalis GA, Vassilakopoulos TP, Boussiotis VA, et al: Clinical approach to lymphadenopathy. Semin Oncol 1993; 20:570.
5. Fessas PH, Panglais GA: Non-malignant lymphadenopathies: Reactive non-specific and reactive specific. In Panglais GA, Polliack A (eds): Benign and Malignant Lymphadenopathies: Clinical and Laboratory Diagnosis. London, Harwood, 1993, pp 31–45.
6. Sneller MC: Wegener's granulomatosis. JAMA 1995; 273(16):1288.
7. Skarin AT: Atlas of Diagnostic Oncology, 2nd ed. London, Mosby-Year Book Europe, 1996.
8. Salgia R, Skarin AT, Kraus M, et al: The spleen: An oncopathologic approach. Contemp Surg 1994; Oct:197.
9. Rathmell AJ, Gospodarowicz MK, Sutcliffe SB, et al: Localized lymphoma of bone: Prognostic factors and treatment recommendations—The Princess Margaret Hospital Lymphoma Group. Br J Cancer 1992; 66:603.
10. Fine H, Mayer R: Primary CNS lymphoma. Ann Intern Med 1993; 119:1093.
11. Economopoulos T, Asprou N, Stathakis N, et al: Primary extranodal non-Hodgkin's lymphoma of the head and neck. Oncology 1992; 49:484.
12. Doria R, Jekel JF, Cooper DL: Thyroid lymphoma. Cancer 1994; 73:200.
13. Mentzer SJ, Reilly JJ, Skarin AT, et al: Patterns of lung involvement by malignant lymphoma. Surgery 1993; 113:507.
14. Nand S, Mullen GM, Lonchyna VA, et al: Primary lymphoma of the heart. Cancer 1991; 62:2289.
15. Harris AC, Kornstein MJ: Malignant lymphoma imitating hepatitis. Cancer 1993; 71:2639.
16. Webb TH, Lillemoe KD, Pitt HA, et al: Pancreatic lymphoma. Ann Surg 1989; 209:25.
17. Hall PA, Levinson DA: Malignant lymphoma in the gastrointestinal tract. Semin Diagn Pathol 1991; 8:163.
18. Gamelin E, Beldent V, Rousselet MC, et al: Non-Hodgkin's lymphoma presenting with primary adrenal insufficiency. Cancer 1992; 69:2333.
19. Mills NE, Goldenberg AS, Liu D, et al: B-cell lymphoma presenting as infiltrative renal disease. Am J Kidney Dis 1992; 19:181.

Table 10–2. Indications for Lymph Node Biopsy

Constitutional symptoms (weight loss, fever, and night sweats) that are otherwise unexplained

Persistent adenopathy (>2–3 weeks)

Increasing size of lymph nodes over several weeks

Appearance of additional enlarged lymph nodes

High risk for AIDS or HIV-positive patient (to rule out early lymphoma or other malignancy)

Abnormal blood test results (anemia, elevated sedimentation rate, LDH, or liver chemistries) otherwise unexplained

Abnormal chest radiograph (e.g., mediastinal adenopathy)

LDH, lactate dehydrogenase.

20. Connors JM, Klimo P, Voss N, et al: Testicular lymphoma: Improved outcome with early brief chemotherapy. J Clin Oncol 1988; 6:776.
21. Monterroso V, Jaffe ES, Merino MJ, et al: Malignant lymphomas involving the ovary: A clinicopathologic analysis of 39 cases. Am J Surg Pathol 1993; 17:154.
22. Jeon HJ, Akagi T, Hoshida Y, et al: Primary non-Hodgkin malignant lymphoma of the breast. Cancer 1992; 70:2451.
23. Joly P, Charlotte F, Leibowitch M, et al: Cutaneous lymphomas other than mycosis fungoides: Follow-up study of 52 patients. J Clin Oncol 1991; 9:1994.
24. Watsky KL, Longley BJ, Dvoretzky I: Primary cutaneous B-cell lymphoma. J Dermatol Surg Oncol 1992; 18:951.
25. Vonderheid EC, Diamond LW, van Vloten WA, et al: Lymph node classification systems in cutaneous T-cell lymphoma. Cancer 1994; 73:207.
26. Slap GB, Brooks JSJ, Schwartz JS: When to perform biopsies of enlarged peripheral lymph nodes in young patients. JAMA 1984; 252:1321.
27. Wang HH, Lach L, Kadin ME: Epidemiology of lymphomatoid papulosis. Cancer 1992; 70:2951.
28. Cabanillas F, Armitage J, Pugh W et al: Lymphomatoid papulosis: A T-cell dyscrasia with a propensity to transform into malignant lymphoma. Ann Intern Med 1995; 122:210.
29. McCarty MJ, Vukelja SJ, Sausville EA et al: Lymphomatoid papulosis associated with Ki-1–positive anaplastic large cell lymphoma. Cancer 1994; 74:3051.
30. Boyd E: Weight of the thymus and its component parts and number of Hassall corpuscles in health and disease. Am J Dis Child 1936; 51:313.
31. Zuelzer WW, Kaplan J: The child with lymphadenopathy. Semin Hematol 1975; 12:323.
32. Slap GB, Connor JL, Wigton RS, et al: Validation of a model to identify young patients for lymph node biopsy. JAMA 1986; 255:2768.
33. Hyland CH, Murad TM, Dismukes WE: Evolution of reactive lymphadenopathy into lymphoma over a nine-year period. Am J Clin Pathol 1977; 68:606.
34. Lennert K, Hansmann ML: Progressive transformation of germinal centers: Clinical significance and lymphocytic predominance of Hodgkin's disease—the Kiel experience. Am J Surg Pathol 1987; 11:149.
35. Ferry JA, Zukerberg LR, Harris NL: Florid progressive transformation of germinal centers. Am Surg Pathol 1992; 16:252.
36. Horning SJ: Natural history of and therapy for the indolent non-Hodgkin's lymphomas. Semin Oncol 1993; 20(5, Suppl 5):75.
37. Browder JP: Biopsy of cervical node [Letter]. JAMA 1979; 241:565.
38. Knowles DM: Immunophenotypic and immunogenotypic approaches useful in distinguishing benign and malignant lymphoid proliferations. Semin Oncol 1993; 20:583.
39. Tindle BH, Parker JW, Lukes RJ: "Reed-Sternberg cells" in infectious mononucleosis? Am J Clin Pathol 1972; 58:607.

FOUR

PRINCIPLES OF THERAPY

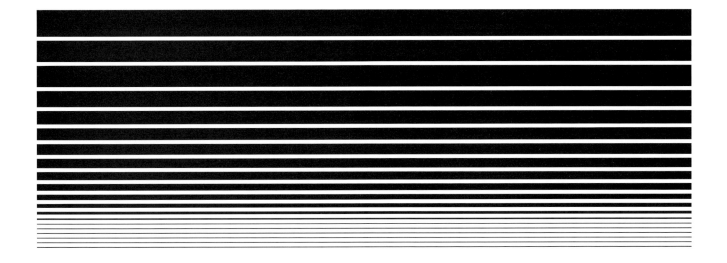

Chapter Eleven

—Principles of Radiation Therapy— for Lymphomas

Karen C. Marcus
Beverly Buck
Peter M. Mauch

HODGKIN'S DISEASE

From 1832, when Thomas Hodgkin first described seven patients with massive enlargement of the lymph nodes and spleen, until 1902, there was no effective treatment for the disease that now bears Hodgkin's name. A major breakthrough in treatment came in the early 1900s after the recognition of the responsiveness of Hodgkin's disease (HD) to ionizing radiation.[1, 2] Unfortunately, only crude radiation therapy techniques were available, limiting the dose that could be delivered to involved nodal regions. Techniques administering small weekly doses to the entire trunk for several weeks or high single doses to the area of clinical disease were associated with high complication rates and frequent recurrences. Using some of the principles advocated by Dr. Rene Gilbert, Drs. Vera Peters and Gordon Richards at Toronto General Hospital treated patients with early HD with higher total doses to primary sites of involvement than those used by Gilbert.[3] In 1950, Peters reported on a series of 113 patients with HD treated between 1924 and 1942; patients with stage I disease had 5-year and 10-year survivals of approximately 80%.[4] Peters was one of the first physicians to demonstrate that early HD treated with adequate doses of radiation therapy was highly curable. Similar results were published in 1963 by Easson and Russell in an article describing the cure of HD with radiation therapy.[5]

Many of the modern concepts of the importance of radiation therapy in the treatment of stage I–II HD come from the work of Dr. Henry Kaplan at Stanford University. Kaplan helped define the concept of a dose response in the permanent eradication of disease.[6] He helped pioneer the use of the linear accelerator and delivery of higher doses in the treatment of adjacent prophylactic lymph node regions. He was a strong advocate of randomized trials to answer questions concerning the treatment of HD. He also made major contributions in arguing for techniques that would improve the accuracy of staging. These techniques included pioneering the use of bipedal lymphangiography and staging laparotomy.

Radiation therapy continues to be the primary treatment of early HD and is used as an adjuvant treatment of patients with more advanced HD.[7] Patients with early disease (stages I and II) treated with radiation therapy alone have only a 20% actuarial risk of relapse 15 to 20 years after treatment. In addition, radiation therapy improves the relapse-free survival when used as an adjuvant to chemotherapy in selected stage I–II patients who have a higher risk of relapse after radiation therapy alone (i.e., those with multiple B symptoms and large mediastinal adenopathy [LMA]). The success of radiation therapy in the treatment of stage I–II HD results from the current practices of thorough staging and the employment of modern radiation therapy techniques detailed in this chapter.

STAGING AND TREATMENT DECISIONS

The successful treatment of patients with HD includes maintaining a high probability of cure and a low risk of complications. Attaining these goals requires a careful assessment of the extent of disease to determine which patients are best suited for radiation therapy alone and to minimize treatment fields and doses whenever possible. A careful history and physical examination, blood studies (including the erythrocyte sedimentation rate and liver function tests), and radiographic evaluation should be performed in all patients. Most patients need a bone marrow biopsy, and staging laparotomy and splenectomy should be considered in early-stage patients when a negative laparotomy would result in reduction of treatment.

Radiographic studies commonly performed in evaluating patients with HD include a chest radiograph; computed tomography (CT) of the thorax, abdomen, and pelvis; and gallium 67 scanning. CT scans of the thorax are required to determine the extent of disease in patients with a positive chest radiograph. Because of the high percentage of mediastinal involvement with HD, most patients should undergo this staging procedure. The role of gallium scanning is still controversial, but the procedure may be particularly valuable as a means to monitor patients after completion of treatment. The results of these studies dramatically affect treatment decisions and outcome.

Thoracic Staging. Many patients who are candidates for primary radiation therapy may have more extensive disease on thoracic CT scanning than is evident from the plain chest radiograph. CT scanning is especially apt at detecting pulmonary parenchymal disease, pleural involvement, pericardial involvement, paracardiac nodal enlargement, extension into the chest wall, and hilar adenopathy and in defining the extent of involved axillary lymph nodes. An example of a thoracic CT scan is shown in Figure 11–1, demonstrating extensive axillary and pleural disease that would not be apparent on plain chest radiograph. The presence of multiple pulmonary nodules or gross pericardial or cardiophrenic angle nodal disease renders most patients ineligible for treatment with radiation therapy alone. Extension into the lung, involvement of the hilar nodes or chest wall, or the presence of a pericardial effusion may still allow the patient to be treated with radiation therapy alone, but with modification of the treatment field size and block placement. For example, prophylactic low-dose whole-heart irradiation may be indicated when pericardial fluid is present. Most patients who have significant subcarinal, hilar, or pericardial disease should be treated with a combination of chemotherapy and radiation therapy so as to lower the risk of relapse, eliminate the need for staging laparotomy, and reduce the dose and volume of normal tissue irradiated.[8–10]

Patients with LMA, defined as a mass greater than one third the maximum thoracic diameter on an upright chest radiograph, have an increased risk of relapsing in nodal and extranodal sites above the diaphragm following radiation therapy alone.[8, 11–17] The upright chest radiograph from a patient with LMA is shown in Figure 11–2; the mediastinal mass ratio is the ratio of the width of the mass divided by the width of the greatest intrathoracic chest diameter. Patients with bulky mediastinal disease are the most likely to have a large number of anatomic nodal regions involved above the diaphragm.[13, 18] This may partly explain the high thoracic nodal failure rate with radiation therapy alone. The use of careful staging with thoracic CT and gallium scanning can identify more precisely sites of initial involvement.[19] This information, coupled with the use of combined chemotherapy and radiation therapy in most patients (since the location of disease would often require irradiation of large volumes of heart and lungs when using radiation therapy alone), has greatly reduced the risk of relapse.[12]

Abdominal Staging. CT scanning, lymphangiography, magnetic resonance imaging (MRI), and gallium scanning all

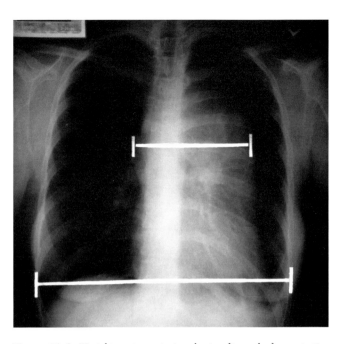

Figure 11–2. Upright posteroanterior chest radiograph demonstrating mediastinal adenopathy greater than one third of the largest intra-thoracic chest diameter (large mediastinal adenopathy). Mediastinal mass ratio (MMR) is defined as the ratio of the width of the mass divided by the greatest intrathoracic diameter. In this example, the MMR is 0.5.

have limitations in the radiologic evaluation of the abdominal nodes. No single study is reliable for detecting HD in normal-sized nodes, and all studies have a 20% to 25% false-negative rate owing to the inability to detect occult HD in the spleen. Ninety percent of patients who are upstaged have splenic involvement either alone or in addition to other infradiaphragmatic nodal sites. Lymphangiography continues to be an important study for treatment planning for patients who present with infradiaphragmatic HD.

Surgical staging with laparotomy and splenectomy remains the most precise method of determining abdominal involvement in patients who present with supradiaphragmatic HD who are candidates for radiation therapy alone. Surgical staging includes removal of the spleen; inspection, palpation, and biopsy of nodes in the abdomen and pelvis; wedge and needle biopsies of the liver; and placement of splenic pedicle clips. Twenty to 30% of clinical stage (CS) IA–IIA patients and 35% of CS IB–IIB patients have occult splenic or upper abdominal HD identified at staging laparotomy that was not detected on presurgical clinical staging studies. Clinical factors predictive of abdominal involvement have been identified and include male sex, stage II disease, and B symptoms.[20, 21] Selected subgroups of patients can be identified whose risk of occult abdominal disease is less than 10%. These subgroups include all CS IA females and CS IA males with lymphocyte predominant histology. However, most patients with CS I–II HD have a substantial risk (24% to 36%) of abdominal involvement that cannot be detected on clinical staging.[20, 21]

Two different philosophies have emerged for the treatment of early-stage HD. The first philosophy reflects the continued use of staging laparotomy and splenectomy for selected CS I–II patients in the United States. This philosophy of more extensive staging enables treatment to be

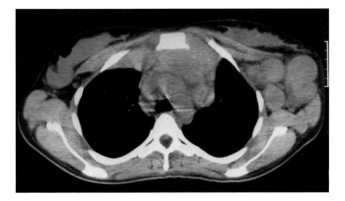

Figure 11–1. CT scan demonstrating extensive left-sided axillary disease and bilateral anterior pleural disease that would not be apparent on plain chest radiograph.

tailored to the extent of disease and reduces potential overtreatment with both radiation therapy and chemotherapy. Surgical staging selects patients who can be treated with radiation therapy alone. Removal of the spleen in those patients who are to receive abdominal irradiation substantially reduces the abdominal tissue in the treatment field and allows some patients with early HD to avoid abdominal irradiation entirely. For most CS I–II patients, treatment with mantle and paraaortic (MPA) irradiation following a negative laparotomy is associated with a low rate of recurrence, a low probability of needing chemotherapy, and excellent long-term survival.[8, 9, 17, 22] Staging laparotomy and splenectomy are indicated when the results will influence treatment recommendations. Patients who have extensive mediastinal disease, multiple B symptoms, or CS III disease require chemotherapy as part of their management and should not undergo staging laparotomy.

Staging laparotomy is associated with potential morbidity and mortality, but these should be minimal at large centers that routinely perform this surgical procedure. Among the 692 patients in the Harvard University series, there were no surgical deaths in the immediate postoperative period.[20] However, complications at laparotomy eventually resulted in death in two patients (0.3%). Major morbidity included a small bowel obstruction in nine patients (1.3%), development of wound or subdiaphragmatic abscess in nine patients (1.3%), and postoperative bleeding in three patients (0.4%). Following splenectomy, patients are also at increased risk for infection with encapsulated bacteria.[23] Vaccinations against *Pneumococcus* and *Meningococcus* or prophylactic antibiotics probably decrease this risk.[24] An increased (approximately twofold) risk of leukemia following splenectomy has been reported in some studies, although mechanisms are poorly understood, and the increase is not recognized by all observers.

The alternative approach for CS I–II patients, based on clinical trials done in Europe, Canada, and South America, uses prognostic factors in clinically staged patients. Treatment is determined based on the presence of adverse factors. These factors predict in part for the likelihood of occult abdominal disease. Treatments are tailored according to the number of adverse prognostic factors. The following have been identified as adverse factors in CS I–II patients: age older than 40 years, mixed cellularity/lymphocyte depleted (MC/LD) histology, number of sites of involvement, B symptoms, and high erythrocyte sedimentation rate.[25, 26] The most favorable patients receive radiation therapy alone either to a mantle field or to MPA lymph nodes, and to the spleen. Patients with a less favorable prognosis receive chemotherapy and involved-field (IF) or regional field irradiation.[26–28] Overall, this approach requires more treatment for early-stage patients than would be required following a staging laparotomy.

TECHNIQUES OF IRRADIATION

Long-term studies from single institutions of patients with pathologic stage I–IIA HD treated with MPA irradiation report freedom from relapse (FFR) rates higher than 80% at 10 to 15 years. These excellent results have been achieved through careful delineation of disease (including staging laparotomy and splenectomy) and meticulous attention to technique (including treatment simulation, individually contoured divergent blocks, equally weighted treatment from the anterior and posterior fields, and machine-generated verification films). The techniques are detailed in this section.

The Patterns of Care Study[29] for HD correlated relapse rates with accuracy of treatment delivery and helped define the standards of practice for the treatment of HD with radiation therapy. It demonstrated that attention to treatment detail minimized the risk of relapse. This study examined 407 records from 101 institutions and separately collected 50 cases from each of the five institutions seeing the largest number of patients. The relative rate of recurrence from these five institutions was 0.75 as compared with 1.17 for the regular survey ($P \leq 0.01$). This suggested that treatment with radiation therapy alone yielded better results when administered in institutions treating large numbers of HD patients compared with centers seeing fewer patients, perhaps because of better quality control at larger centers.

Portal films examined in the Patterns of Care Study demonstrated that when there were inadequate margins between the protective lung and cardiac blocks and the tumor, both the overall recurrence rate (54% versus 14%, $P \leq 0.0001$) and the infield or marginal recurrence rate increased dramatically (33% versus 7%, $P \leq 0.001$) as compared with patients treated with adequate margins. Treatment with involved or small radiation fields, cobalt 60 machines with source-to-skin distance (SSD) less than 80 cm, or the absence of treatment simulation were also associated with a significantly increased risk of relapse.

Careful treatment planning and delivery are essential for preventing relapse and minimizing complications in patients with HD. Results from the Southwest Oncology Group (SWOG) 781 trial and the Stanford S1 trial illustrate how variations in treatment technique and uniform application can result in significant outcome differences.[30, 31] Both trials studied the use of MPA irradiation compared with IF irradiation plus MOPP (mechlorethamine, Oncovin, procarbazine, prednisone) chemotherapy in IA–IIA patients. In both studies, MOPP chemotherapy and IF irradiation resulted in FFR rates higher than 80% and overall survival rates higher than 90%. However, the FFR after MPA irradiation in the SWOG trial was 30% at 5 years in contrast with 83% in the Stanford study. The SWOG 781 study used radiation therapy techniques no longer employed that were more likely to have resulted, in retrospect, to the poor FFR. "Patchwork" nodal instead of continuous nodal irradiation was used, and the hilar lymph nodes were not treated. This study also involved multiple institutions, perhaps making quality control more difficult. The single-institution Stanford study, in contrast, used doses given equally from front and back to all nodal regions. Surgical staging and careful radiation techniques used at Stanford allowed most patients treated with initial radiation therapy alone to remain in remission without the need for subsequent chemotherapy.

The European Organization for the Research and Treatment of Cancer (EORTC) performed a series of randomized trials to determine the need for abdominal irradiation in patients with disease limited to supradiaphragmatic sites.[26] The EORTC H-5 trial randomized favorable patients to mantle field alone or to mantle plus paraaortic–splenic pedicle irradiation. Patients had to have nodular sclerosing (NS) or lymphocyte predominant (LP) histology, pathologic stage I or II without mediastinal involvement, and an erythrocyte sedimentation rate of less than 70 and had to be 40 years of age or younger. Patients treated with mantle irradiation alone had an 11% risk of relapsing below the diaphragm.

Specific technical recommendations for radiation therapy employed at the Joint Center for Radiation Therapy in Boston are as follows. Routine treatment machine–generated verification films should be used to ensure proper alignment. A mantle simulation film and the corresponding portal film are shown in Figure 11–3. Equal dose delivery from anterior and posterior fields and treatment of both fields daily minimize the anterior cardiac dose and reduce the risk to the heart. Similar blocks are used for both anterior and posterior fields, in contrast with other centers that employ larger posterior blocks and therefore treat the infraclavicular nodes only from the anterior. Daily doses of 180 to 200 cGy per day are recommended unless the treatment field includes the entire heart or entire lung, in which case the dose should be limited to 150 cGy or less per day. Off-central-axis dose calculations should be obtained and adjustments made to improve the dose inhomogeneity that occurs from differences in patient separation within the large mantle field. For example, nodes in the axilla and neck receive a higher effective dose owing to decreased patient thickness in those regions as compared with the dose received to the upper mediastinum. The subcarinal (low cardiac) region receives a lower effective dose owing to the loss of scatter from within the tissue protected by the lung

blocks. Adjustment of the total dose to these regions can be made through a few cone-down treatments at the end of the radiation course.

Inhomogeneities in the mantle field can also be reduced by using an extended SSD of 110 cm or greater rather than an SSD of 100 cm. For example, by using a 130-cm SSD on a 6-megavolt (MV) linear accelerator, the increased dose to the neck and axilla can be kept to less than 110% of the central axis dose (as opposed to nearly 120%). Because of the increased dose to the neck, the cervical spinal cord receives more than the prescribed central axis dose. To decrease the dose to the upper spinal cord, a posterior cervical spine block extending from the top of the field down to the level of C7 is added at 3000 cGy. Blocking the thoracic spine is not necessary, and, in fact, the use of a thoracic cord block risks underdosing mediastinal nodes. At our center adult patients are treated in the arms-over-the-head position as shown schematically in Figure 11–4*A* and *C*. This arm position pulls the axillary nodes laterally and allows more lung tissue to be shielded. When prepubertal children are treated, the arms are positioned at the sides to allow blocking of the humeral heads (Fig. 11–4*B* and *D*). Some centers advocate the arms-down position for all patients to block the humeral heads; however, in this position the axillary nodes overlie more lung, and to adequately treat these nodes, more lung is within the radiation field. The position of the axillary nodes relative to the arm position is illustrated in Figure 11–5. In addition, there can be increased skin reaction in the folds of the axillary region with the arms-down position.

Patients with unilateral high cervical or preauricular involvement should receive a modified mantle technique to

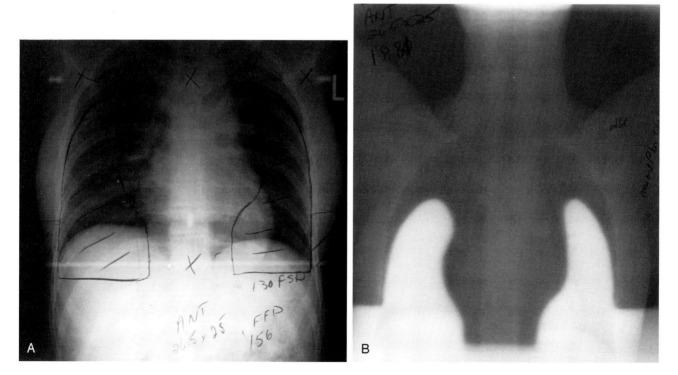

Figure 11–3. Examples of mantle simulation film (*A*) and representative portal film (*B*). Lung blocks are shaped to treat the hilar and subcarinal nodes; blocks shield the cardiac apex. A subcarinal block positioned 5 cm below the carina can be added if there is no subcarinal nodal involvement and the prescribed mantle dose is higher than 3600 cGy.

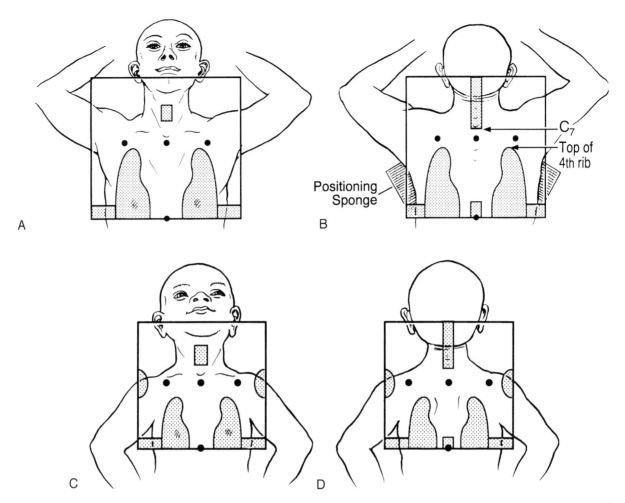

Figure 11–4. Placement on the anterior (*A* and *C*) and posterior (*B* and *D*) mantle fields of the lung, iliac wing, and larynx, and cervical spine blocks in the arms-up position (*A* and *B*) and placement of the humeral head blocks in the arms-akimbo position (*C* and *D*), with tattoos shown as a solid circle. Note the positioning sponges placed under the shoulders on the posterior projection (*B*) to prevent medial rotation of the shoulders and axillary lymph nodes.

include the ipsilateral preauricular nodes without coverage of Waldeyer's ring. This is done either through a matched-on electron field or by extending the top border of the mantle field and blocking out the mouth and contralateral parotid region. The "high mantle" technique is demonstrated in Figure 11–6. The advantages of photon beam include avoidance of matching electron to photon fields and coverage of the lateral tonsillar area. Involvement of tonsils, nasopharynx, or bilateral preauricular nodes requires treatment of Waldeyer's ring. In this setting our policy is to use large opposed lateral fields to cover Waldeyer's ring and match this to the mantle field.

A characteristic of megavoltage irradiation is the dose sparing of skin and subcutaneous tissue. Proper use of megavoltage energies ensures that superficial nodes are not underdosed in the "buildup region." A 4- to 6-MV linear accelerator should be used for mantle and pelvic fields, whereas higher energies (10 to 15 MV) can be used for treating paraaortic nodes. If a higher-energy linear accelerator is used for the mantle field, the use of a beam spoiler is suggested to ensure delivery of a sufficient dose to the superficial cervical lymph nodes.

A total dose of 3600 cGy to the entire mantle field is sufficient for patients with supradiaphragmatic HD. Areas of gross involvement should receive a total of 4000 to 4400 cGy through the addition of a cone-down field. The total doses and daily doses currently used are reduced over the early days of radiation therapy for HD developed at Stanford by Henry Kaplan.[32] In 1966 Kaplan compiled data on the recurrence rate of HD as a function of dose.[6] He demonstrated that the rate of recurrence was inversely proportional to dose, with a recurrence rate of 4.4% for doses of 3500 to 4000 cGy delivered over 4 weeks. Based on the Stanford experience of a true recurrence rate of 1.3% following 4400 cGy in 4 to 5 weeks, Kaplan recommended 4000 to 4400 cGy for gross disease treated with radiation therapy alone. Reduction of the radiation dose to 3000 to 3600 cGy to uninvolved regions and 3600 to 4000 cGy to areas of residual disease is recommended for patients receiving combined-modality therapy (CMT). Further reduction to 1500 to 2500 cGy may be desirable in prepubertal patients receiving CMT or occasionally in patients with extensive nodal involvement receiving large radiation fields after chemotherapy. The dose to the entire heart should not exceed 3000 cGy and should be kept at 2500 cGy or lower in patients treated with doxorubicin. With a prescribed dose of 3600 cGy to the

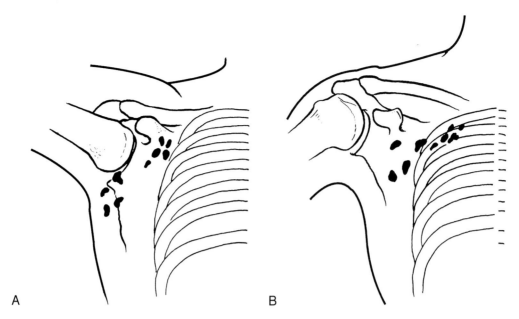

Figure 11–5. Positioning the arms above the head pulls the axillary nodes away from the chest wall (*A*) and allows tighter lung blocks. With the arms akimbo (*B*), the axillary nodes overlie more of the lungs. Lung blocks must be shaped to include these nodes.

central axis, the dose to the lower central cardiac region is 3200 to 3300 cGy. Provided a left ventricular block has been used, this dose is within the tolerance limits of the heart. If the prescribed mantle dose is higher than 3600 cGy, a subcarinal block should be added to limit the dose to the low central cardiac region to 3000 cGy. The use of lower doses will likely contribute to a lower complication rate to heart and lung tissue.

The paraaortic field encompasses the paraaortic nodes as well as the splenic pedicle. Treatment of the splenic pedicle is optional in patients who have a negative staging laparotomy. Although once routinely recommended, the development of gastric cancers many years after treatment has caused a reconsideration of this policy.[33] At splenectomy, surgical clips should be placed to mark the splenic pedicle. The splenic tag portion of the paraaortic field should have a 2.5- to 3-cm margin around the clips. The paraaortic field is

shown in Figure 11–7. If a splenectomy has not been done, the entire spleen needs to be irradiated. A CT scan should be used to localize the position of the spleen and enable blocking of as much of the left kidney as possible. An intravenous pyelogram at treatment simulation may also help with optimum placement of the kidney block. The paraaortic field is positioned to encompass the lateral transverse processes of the lumbar vertebrae, unless the lymphangiogram (LAG), CT scan, or laparotomy demonstrates more extensive disease. The inferior border is positioned at L4–L5. The dose to the paraaortic lymph nodes should be 3000 to 3600 cGy when there is no gross disease and radiation therapy alone is used. The dose can be limited to 3000 cGy if CMT is used.

Beam divergence from the mantle and paraaortic fields creates the potential for an overdose at the spinal cord. A number of different matching techniques have been pub-

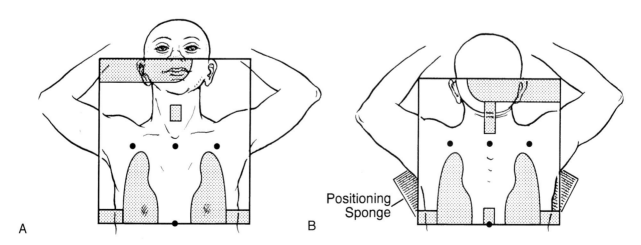

Figure 11–6. Placement on the anterior (*A*) and posterior (*B*) "high mantle" of the superior border and mouth block when treating a patient with high neck disease (tattoos shown as a solid circle).

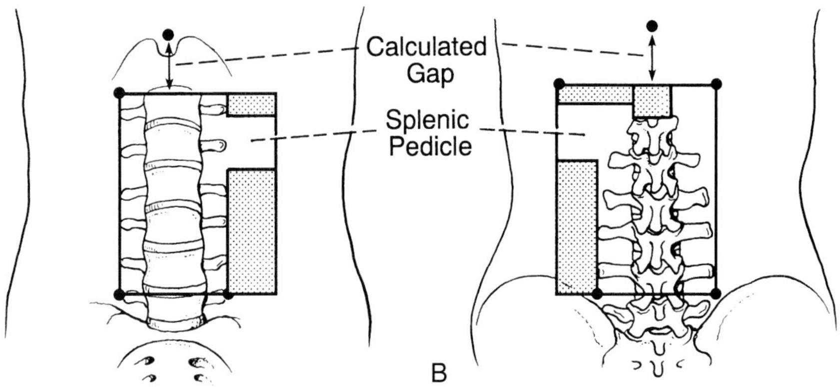

Figure 11–7. Position of the anterior (A) and posterior (B) paraaortic field from the calculated gap down to the inferior border of L4. The left lateral border is extended to encompass the splenic pedicle or the entire spleen (tattoos shown as a solid circle).

lished.[34, 35] Figure 11–8 shows the technique developed at the Joint Center for Radiation Therapy, which is briefly described as in the following paragraphs.

To determine the match position on the anterior skin surface (point P), the anterior mantle is set up using clinical

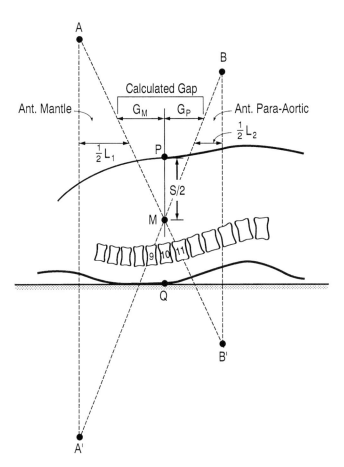

Figure 11–8. Schematic of the gap localization and calculation technique, where A = source-surface distance (SSD) and beam divergence of the inferior half (½ L1) of the anterior mantle and A′ = the same dimensions for the posterior mantle; B = SSD and beam divergence of the superior half (½ L2) of the anterior paraaortic field and B′ = the same dimension for the posterior paraaortic field; P = match position on the anterior skin surface; Q = match position on the posterior skin surface; S/2 = one half the measured separation from point P to point Q; M = the midline match point of all four fields; G_M = the calculated gap using the mantle parameters; and G_P = the calculated gap using the paraaortic parameters. (Adapted from Int J Radiat Oncol Biol Phys, vol 9. Lutz W, Larsen R: Technique to match mantle and paraaortic fields, p 1753, 1983, with permission from Elsevier Science.)

considerations. The mantle gap calculation (Gm) is done using the length of the mantle (Lm) and the separation (S) taken at approximately 1 cm below the inferior border of the mantle field (the approximate position of point P).

The following gap formula is used:

$$G = \frac{S}{2} \times \frac{L/2}{(FID)} = \frac{S \times L}{4(FID)}$$

where FID = focus-isocenter distance.

The calculated distance is measured down from the inferior border of the anterior mantle and marked on the patient's skin. The central axis of the beam is moved to this point, the collimator size adjusted to encompass the spine, and a spine-technique diagnostic radiograph taken. Using the nondivergent central axis, the exact location of the match point (M) on a specific vertebral body can be determined by careful measurements on film. The location is documented on the Hodgkin's Match Summary form (not shown) along with the divergence points of the anterior mantle field on the vertebral bodies. The patient is then turned over and positioned for the posterior mantle.

To determine the position of the posterior match point (point Q) with the patient in the prone position, fluoroscopy is used to place the central axis at the same point on the same vertebral body as point P. A spine-technique diagnostic radiograph is once again taken, measurements made on the film, and any necessary adjustments made to position point Q. The calculated gap, Gm, is measured superiorly to point Q to position the inferior border of the posterior mantle. The remaining borders of the posterior mantle are determined clinically, and a film is taken. The divergence points on the vertebral bodies are documented on the Hodgkin's Match Summary form. A 1-half-value layer (HVL) thickness block measuring 3 cm wide and 1.5 cm long on skin is placed over the spinal cord at the inferior border of the posterior mantle to decrease any potential overlap due to variations in the day-to-day setup.

At the time of simulation of the paraaortic fields, the patient is positioned supine, Gm is measured down from the inferior mantle tattoo, and the spine-technique film of the match point is repeated to determine whether the tattoos have changed position due to weight loss or gain. If necessary, the central axis is shifted until the original match point (M) is localized on the vertebral body. An approximate field length (Lp) and the separation (S) taken at point P are entered on the same Hodgkin's Gap Calculation form as for the mantle and are used to calculate the gap from point P down to the superior border of the anterior paraaortic field (Gp) using the following formula:

$$G = \frac{S}{2} \times \frac{L/2}{(FID)} = \frac{S \times L}{4(FID)}$$

The gap is measured and marked on the patient's skin, and the remaining borders of the field are set up using clinical considerations. The simulation film of the anterior paraaortic field is compared with the simulation film of the posterior mantle to verify the match. Beam divergence of the paraaortic field is documented on the same Hodgkin's Match Summary form as the mantle. If there is misalignment of the fields, the superior border of the paraaortic field should be adjusted.

The patient is then placed in the prone position, and the procedure is repeated to localize and document the position of point Q and the posterior paraaortic field. The posterior simulation film is compared with the anterior mantle simulation film to verify the match. A 1 HVL block (3 cm wide and 1.5 cm long on skin) is placed over the spinal cord at the superior border of the posterior paraaortic field as discussed previously.

The match technique described earlier delivers 15% to 20% less dosage to the anterior pericardial nodes, but recurrences in the gap region are rare as long as care is taken to not place the match over areas of known disease. Some have reported the use of an extended mantle technique designed to treat both the mantle and paraaortic nodes in one field to avoid problems in the match area.[36] Although toxicity is only minimally increased with this technique, accurate placement of blocks is more difficult, and the full paraaortic nodal region cannot be treated in taller patients. The availability of new extended travel distance treatment couches may obviate the need for patients to change position for the opposed-field treatments. The use of a pelvic field as part of total-nodal irradiation (infrequently used in current practice) includes a calculated gap for matching with the paraaortic field. The superior border of the pelvic field is usually located on L5, and the inferior border should include the iliac and inguinal nodes. Figure 11-9 is an example of the pelvic field treated as part of total-nodal irradiation. The total dose should be 3000 to 3600 cGy if the pelvic nodes are not involved with gross disease and radiation therapy alone is used. The total dose can be reduced to 3000 cGy if CMT is used. For patients with infradiaphragmatic HD, treatment with radiation therapy alone should include a boost to the involved nodes to a total dose of 4000 to 4400 cGy. Iliac wing blocks to spare bone marrow and a pelvic block to shield the bladder and central pelvic organs should be part of the treatment technique (which includes irradiation of inguinal nodes). It is possible to spare fertility in both men and women with conventional pelvic nodal treatment. Irradiation of the ovaries to 3500 cGy causes sterility and amenorrhea in 100% of women. Oophoropexy, a technique to move the ovaries into the midline, allows their shielding with a full-thickness block. With this technique, the dose to the ovaries is usually kept under 300 to 600 cGy, allowing 60% of women to maintain menstrual function. Normal pregnancies have been reported.[37] The probability of retaining normal menses decreases with increasing age. In

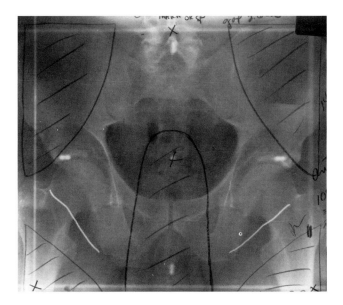

Figure 11–9. Simulation film of a pelvic field for a male patient. Wires are on the inguinal nodes. The central block shields the bladder, bowel, and scrotum. Blocks over the iliac wings protect the pelvic bone marrow.

men, blocking of central pelvic structures and careful placement of a scrotal shield can limit the dose to the testicles to 2% to 3% of the total prescribed dose (approximately 75 to 105 cGy). Initial oligospermia is seen in this dose range, but long-term return to normal counts and fertility is possible.[38] Radiation dose to the testes results from scatter from the pelvic field and depends on the field size, field shape, and distance from the field edge to the testes.

Patients with early-stage subdiaphragmatic HD with primary inguinal or iliac involvement should also have the femoral nodes treated. Generous central blocking of the pelvis is usually not feasible when the inguinal or pelvic nodes are involved. However, an LAG may help limit the amount of normal tissue treated. Most patients do not retain fertility following radiation therapy for HD presenting in inguinal or iliac nodes owing to the increased internal scatter to the ovaries in women under the smaller-than-usual blocks (even after oophoropexy) and to the testes in men owing to the lower than usual inferior border needed to treat femoral nodes. Even with a carefully placed scrotal shield, the estimated dose to the testes is 8% of the total dose (approximately 300 cGy) if the femoral nodes are treated. This dosage results in loss of fertility in most patients.

SHORT-TERM TOXICITY

The acute toxicities associated with mantle irradiation include mild pharyngitis; low posterior scalp epilation; loss of or change in taste; mouth dryness and thickening of saliva; mild skin erythema on the shoulders, axillae, and neck; generalized fatigue; and nausea. Patients may lose 5 to 10 pounds during treatment owing to salivary and taste changes. Mouth dryness and taste changes occur 1 to 2 weeks into treatment; pharyngitis and epilation occur after 2 to 3 weeks. These acute symptoms are transitory. Pharyngitis lasts approximately 1 to 2 weeks after completion of treatment; taste gradually returns in 1 to 2 months; hair starts to regrow after 3 months; fatigue and weight loss diminish after 2 to 4 weeks; and, in patients younger than 40 years of age, saliva returns to normal after 6 months. For patients older than 40, the recovery may be prolonged, with xerostomia lasting as long as 1 year or more. Patients should be treated with daily fluoride prophylaxis during and after radiation to help prevent an increase in dental caries from the radiation-induced chemical changes in the saliva. During the first 2 years following mantle irradiation, patients are encouraged to see their dentist three or four times per year. Fluoride applications are continued for at least 1 year or longer if the patient's salivary function has not returned to normal.

The common acute reactions of treatment of the paraaortic field are nausea and vomiting associated with treating part of the stomach. These toxicities can be ameliorated by prophylactic treatment with an antiemetic medication. The acute effects of pelvic irradiation include transient diarrhea and urinary frequency; however, these effects occur in fewer than 10% of patients undergoing treatment.

LONG-TERM COMPLICATIONS

Long-term complications of mantle irradiation include lung, heart, and thyroid dysfunction; second primary cancers; and Lhermette's syndrome. Complications such as transverse myelitis and constrictive pericarditis are totally avoidable with modern radiation therapy techniques. Other long-term toxicities are not totally avoidable but can be reduced in severity or frequency.

Radiation pneumonitis, which typically occurs 1 to 6 months after completion of mantle irradiation, is characterized by a mild, nonproductive cough, low-grade fever, and dyspnea on exertion. Infection and recurrent HD must also be considered in the diagnosis. The overall incidence of symptomatic pneumonitis is less than 5% after mantle

irradiation; patients with LMA or who receive CMT are at increased risk.[16, 39] Radiographically, pneumonitis is characterized by the formation of infiltrates confined to the original radiation fields. The chest radiograph and CT scan from a patient with radiation pneumonitis is shown in Figure 11–10A and B. Infection rather than pneumonitis is a more likely diagnosis if the infiltrates extend into areas of the lung initially protected from radiation. Severe pneumonitis may require treatment with steroids. If the symptoms do not respond to steroid treatment, the presence of a superimposed infection, such as *Pneumocystis carinii*, should be considered. Patients who develop pneumonitis generally do not have long-term pulmonary sequelae. Perihilar and perimediastinal pulmonary fibrosis, a separate subacute-to-chronic pulmonary process from acute pneumonitis, can be seen as soon as 6 months following irradiation and, if severe, may be associated with a mild decrease in lung capacity.

Radiation therapy can damage the pericardium, the myocardium, or the cardiac vessels, although with modern radiation therapy techniques symptomatic pericardial and myocardial damage are rare. Clinical pericarditis occurs in about 1% of cases, and constrictive pericarditis is almost never seen. The relative risk (RR) of coronary artery disease and myocardial infarction is modestly increased following mantle irradiation.[40] The total dose, the radiation technique used, the size of the left ventricular block, and the fraction size all are factors that can modify the risk of myocardial damage. Boivin and colleagues followed 4665 patients treated for HD between 1940 and 1985, with median followup of 7 years.[40] Patients had received either chemotherapy or radiation therapy, or both. They reported an increased risk of death from myocardial infarction after mediastinal irradiation (RR, 2.56) but not after chemotherapy (RR, 0.97). The RR was 1.97 in patients treated between 1967 and 1985 compared with an RR of 6.33 in

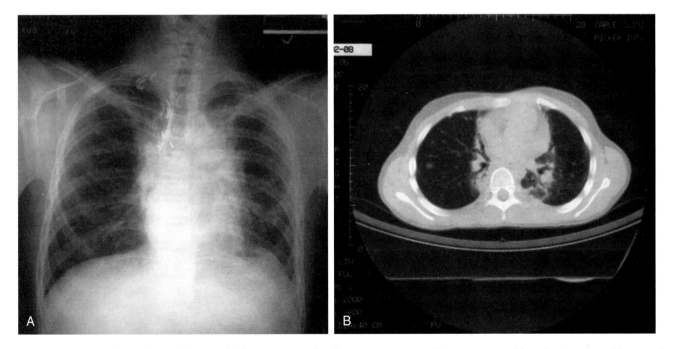

Figure 11–10. Chest radiograph (A) and CT scan (B) from a patient with radiation pneumonitis. Infiltrates are paramediastinal in the region of the original radiation fields. This patient had also relapsed in the pulmonary parenchyma.

patients treated from 1940 to 1966. This decrease in risk is consistent with the changes in treatment technique that have occurred in the 1970s and 1980s. Although their impact on radiation-induced cardiac damage is unknown, blood pressure and cholesterol screening should be routinely performed on patients treated for HD to try to modify risk factors.

Awareness of the potential development of thyroid dysfunction following radiation therapy can ameliorate clinical symptoms. The degree and frequency of thyroid abnormalities depend on the thoroughness of followup and the routine use of thyroxine for patients with elevated thyroid-stimulating hormone (TSH) levels. Although elevation of TSH is common and occurs in nearly 30% of adult patients and two thirds of pediatric patients,[16] clinical hypothyroidism occurs less than 5% of the time and reflects the practice of placing patients on supplemental therapy prior to development of clinical symptoms. The most common abnormality is the elevation of TSH levels sometimes associated with low serum levels of thyroxine. Although radiation-induced hypothyroidism is believed to result from direct cellular injury, the presence of thyroiditis in some patients suggests that injury may also develop from autoantibodies. Some patients, in rare instances, have developed palpable thyroid nodules, lymphocytic infiltration, and Hürthle cell nodules. Graves' disease with exophthalmos has also been described in some patients receiving high-dose thyroid irradiation.[41, 42]

Lhermette's syndrome, a form of mild radiation myelitis, occurs in approximately 15% of patients receiving mantle irradiation. It is characterized by an "electric shock sensation" radiating down the back of both legs on flexion of the head. The symptoms are mild, do not require treatment, and last anywhere from 3 months to several years (unusual). The symptoms eventually resolve spontaneously, and there are no long-term sequelae.

One of the more devastating long-term complications associated with treatment for HD (in addition to HD recurrence) is the development of second primary cancers following treatment. Patients treated with chemotherapy, radiation therapy, or both modalities, have an increased risk of developing acute leukemia, NHL, and solid tumors.[43–46] The development of leukemia is primarily associated with the use of alkylating agent regimens, and most cases occur within 10 years of treatment. Following chemotherapy or CMT, the observed-to-expected ratio (RR) for developing leukemia was greater than 100 to 1.[46] In large reported series the RR of developing NHL after HD varies between 8 to 1 and 31 to 1. These ratios appear to be the same for patients receiving radiation therapy alone compared with CMT in some studies,[46, 47] but they were lower following radiation therapy alone than after CMT in other reports.[44] The increased risk of developing NHL continues beyond 10 years of treatment.[44, 46, 47] Most cases of secondary NHL are of intermediate-grade or high-grade histology.[44, 48–50] Similar histologic subtypes occur with immunodeficiency diseases or in association with chronic immunosuppressive therapy in patients who are also at increased risk to develop NHL.

The RR of developing a solid tumor following treatment for HD is considerably less than the RR of developing leukemia or NHL (2.8:1 versus 22:1 versus 120:1, respectively). However, because the overall background risk of developing a solid tumor in the general population is much higher than for the development of leukemia or NHL, the absolute excess risk (per 10,000 person-years, AR) of solid tumors is greater than the AR for NHL or leukemia. The increased RR for developing solid tumors continues beyond 10 years after treatment for HD. Tucker and associates reported an observed-to-expected ratio of 1.9 to 1 for the development of a second solid tumor within the first 5 years after treatment.[46] During the second followup interval of 5 to 10 years, this ratio increased to 4.9 to 1, and for patients followed longer than 10 years this risk ratio was 6.3 to 1. The most frequently observed second solid tumors have been lung, stomach, melanoma, connective tissue, and bone tumors. An age-related increased risk of breast cancer has also been reported, with the highest risk period being patients treated between the ages of 10 and 20 years.[33, 51] Risk factors for the development of second tumors include the use of combined radiation therapy and chemotherapy compared with radiation therapy alone.[46, 52] Age older than 40 at treatment is associated with an absolute excess rates similar to that of younger patients. The extent of the radiation therapy field is a likely factor in the development of solid tumors, but little data exist to confirm this. There is little information on the risk of second solid tumors after chemotherapy alone.

FOLLOWUP

Patterns of recurrence and risks of second tumors should be reflected in the followup studies obtained. Patients with lymphocyte-predominant histology have experienced recurrences at later times than other histologies. Patients with bulky disease relapse earlier than those without bulky disease. Patients should be seen in followup every 3 months for the first 2 years following treatment, every 4 months during the third year, twice yearly for the fourth and fifth years, and then once or twice yearly after 5 years. Thyroid functions should be monitored at least twice yearly in addition to complete blood counts and erythrocyte sedimentation rate. Chest radiographs should be obtained at each visit. Abdominopelvic CT or gallium scans are recommended every 6 to 12 months for the first 5 years for patients at increased risk of infradiaphragmatic recurrence. This would include pathologically staged patients with mixed-cellularity histology treated with MPA irradiation and pathologically staged patients treated with mantle alone. Patients with LMA should undergo chest CT and gallium scanning every 6 to 12 months for the first 3 to 4 years. Other patients should undergo abdominal CT, gallium scanning, or both at 2.5 years and 5 years after treatment. Initiation of annual screening mammography should be considered before 30 years of age in women treated with radiation therapy during puberty.

Great advances have been made in the treatment of HD during the last 25 years. Long-term studies have shown that patients with HD who are carefully staged and who undergo treatment at experienced institutions can enjoy an FFR rate of greater than 80% with 15 to 20 years of followup. Analysis of causes of death in these patients suggests that HD is still the major cause of death, especially in patients with advanced-stage disease, although the risk for recurrence and death from HD becomes small beyond 10 years. Death from other causes such as cardiac disease and second tumors increases with time off treatment. Routine patient followup intervals and testing should reflect these differences in events with time.

NON-HODGKIN'S LYMPHOMA

As more sophisticated molecular biologic techniques have become available, the pathologic classification for NHLs has changed. Many new classifications have been developed, and a recent consensus conference has proposed restructuring of the Working Formulation. However, for the purposes of this review, treatment discussions are made according to the Working Formulation.[53, 54] The role of radiation therapy in the treatment in NHL is dependent on the histology, disease stage, and physiologic status of the patient. With more effective chemotherapy, the techniques of radiation therapy have been modified or even eliminated under some circumstances. Often, field sizes can be reduced and doses modified when used in conjunction with chemotherapy. Radiation therapy continues to play a major role in specific clinical situations. For example, patients with early-stage low-grade lymphomas can often be managed with radiation therapy alone. Patients with lymphomatous involvement of organs such as the eye, even when disease is advanced, are often treated with IF radiation therapy with excellent control of symptoms.

STAGING STUDIES

With the increasing use of chemotherapy, radiographic studies have become the predominant form of staging, virtually replacing staging laparotomy in lymphocytic lymphomas. The choice of treatment and, in patients with low-grade lymphoma, even the decision to institute treatment are influenced by the stage of disease. Although the Ann Arbor staging system has shown prognostic value for HD, its prognostic usefulness in lymphocytic lymphomas is diminished because it fails to include other parameters that have more influence on prognosis. For the aggressive lymphomas several parameters have been identified that are not accounted for by the Ann Arbor system; these parameters allow placement of patients into prognostic groups. Of the many factors analyzed, age, lactate dehydrogenase (LDH) level, stage, tumor bulk, and number of extranodal sites have been used to construct a prognostic index to identify patients in need of more intensive treatment.[55, 56]

CT and gallium scanning have become standard practice in the staging of patients with lymphocytic lymphoma. Bipedal lymphangiography has been largely replaced by the use of the CT scan, with its improved visualization of abdominal structures.[57] The LAG continues to be a useful study in those patients who present with femoral, inguinal, or pelvic disease. In these patients, the LAG can assist in determining the extent of disease and can improve the definition of radiation therapy fields for treating limited disease. The abdominopelvic CT scan can identify mesenteric, porta hepatic, retrocrural, and splenic hilar lymph nodes; the presence of bulky splenic disease; and extranodal involvement of liver, bone, and kidney. These radiographic studies are particularly important in patients who are to receive radiation therapy. These tests not only allow precise localization of nodes and protection of normal tissue but can influence treatment decisions, particularly when bulky disease or parenchymal organ involvement is detected. Other routine staging studies performed include bone marrow biopsies and blood counts and chemistries.

Gallium 67 scanning has been used to identify sites of initial disease, to detect early recurrences, and to measure response to chemotherapy.[58–60] The use of high-dose gallium 67 (8 to 11 mCi), spot imaging, double or triple peak angle cameras, single-photon emission CT, and delayed views of the abdomen all increase the sensitivity of the study. The gallium scan is most useful in the large cell lymphomas, in which it appears to have prognostic importance.[59] Patients who are gallium positive at mid-course of chemotherapy have a significantly worse survival compared with patients whose gallium scan results are normal. These findings suggest that patients who remain gallium positive should be considered for more aggressive treatment, such as autologous bone marrow transplantation (BMT).

Low-Grade Lymphomas

Stage I–II. Many published studies have demonstrated the efficacy of radiation therapy in the treatment of clinically staged patients with localized low-grade lymphoma.[61–66] Although the 10-year survival of patients treated with radiation therapy alone is very good, late recurrences beyond 10 years are seen. The curative potential of localized radiation therapy is best demonstrated by a plateau in the disease-free survival curve in patients followed for 10 years or longer. Several different studies have demonstrated such a plateau, suggesting various subgroups of patients for whom a cure might be achieved.[63–65] In the Stanford series,[63] 80% of patients with CS I or II follicular lymphoma (including some patients with the aggressive follicular large cell lymphoma) who were 40 years of age or younger appeared to be cured with IF, extended-field, or total-nodal radiation therapy. There were no recurrences in this subgroup of patients after 4 years. In contrast, there was no plateau on the survival curve for patients older than 40 years of age, and the survival for this subgroup of patients was significantly less than for the younger patients. At the National Cancer Institute (NCI), patients with stage I disease appeared to have a plateau in the disease-free survival curve with no relapses after 7 years, whereas for stage II patients no such plateau was observed, with relapses occurring past 18 years.[65] Survival rates for patients with low-grade lymphoma are difficult to evaluate because the 10-year survival is good and does not reflect the consequences of late relapses.

The techniques of radiation therapy in the treatment of NHLs depend not only on the histologic subtype and stage of disease but on the patterns of failure. Early-stage indolent lymphomas treated with radiation therapy alone have been shown to relapse in extranodal sites or in nodal sites distant from the radiation therapy fields when less than total-lymphoid irradiation has been used.[63] This observation has led some to recommend the use of total-lymphoid irradiation. Several factors, however, argue against the use of such extensive radiation therapy in patients with early-stage indolent lymphomas. These factors include (1) the lack of evidence that patients with stage I–II presentations have benefited from the use of extended-field when compared with IF or regional irradiation; (2) the lack of a survival advantage for patients receiving total-body irradiation (TBI); (3) late recurrences of 50% in patients with indolent lymphoma; and (4) the eventual high conversion rate of these lymphomas to a more aggressive histology requiring treatment with chemotherapy. In addition, there is an increasing role for high-dose chemotherapy (often with autologous marrow rescue) in the management of recurrent disease. Such treatment would be difficult to deliver after total lymphoid irradiation (TLI). All these considerations make the use of TLI unattractive as an initial therapy for early-stage indolent lymphoma.

For patients with stage I–II indolent lymphomas the current recommendation is the use of regional radiation therapy fields. This consists of irradiating the involved nodal region plus one additional uninvolved region on each side of the involved nodes. For example, the treatment field for lymphoma of the left inguinal nodes would include the ipsilateral femoral, inguinal, and iliac nodes. The treatment of stage I lymphoma of the right supraclavicular nodes would include the ipsilateral axilla, bilateral supraclavicular regions, and bilateral cervical nodes. The cervical, supraclavicular, oropharyngeal, and nasopharyngeal nodes would be irradiated in patients with involvement of Waldeyer's ring.

The recommended doses for patients with low-grade lymphoma are 3000 to 3600 cGy with a boost to areas of initial involvement to 3600 to 4000 cGy. These doses have been reported to control disease in most patients with low-grade lymphoma.[67] When there is a possibility of significant morbidity from the treatment, such as the inclusion of the salivary glands or in the treatment of orbital lymphoma, the lower doses to the uninvolved nodal areas are recommended (i.e., 3000 cGy).

Stage III–IV. The management of stage III–IV lymphomas remains more controversial. There are four approaches to patients with advanced NHL low-grade lymphomas: (1) no initial therapy with palliative treatment using chemotherapy or IF radiation therapy as needed to control symptoms; (2) single-agent chemotherapy; (3) aggressive multiagent chemotherapy with or without TLI for stage III and multiagent chemotherapy for stage IV disease; and (4) autologous BMT. Although these approaches are quite diverse, there is no convincing evidence that initial aggressive or intensive therapy improves survival.[30] Advanced-stage low-grade lymphomas are responsive to single-agent and combination chemotherapy as well as radiation therapy; however, responses last a median of 2 years in many studies, and 10% or less of patients with low-grade lymphomas remain in remission beyond 5 years.

The "watch-and-wait" approach to patients with advanced-stage disease was suggested by Rosenberg and Kaplan, who withheld treatment from selected asymptomatic patients with advanced-stage disease.[30] Patients with bulky peripheral or massive retroperitoneal adenopathy, B symptoms, or splenomegaly causing cytopenia were excluded from the observation arm. No survival differences were observed between the group of patients selected for no initial therapy compared with those treated immediately.[30, 68] Despite the lack of survival advantage to initial treatment, not all patients are appropriate for a watch-and-

wait approach. Not only do the patients' clinical findings often indicate the need for immediate intervention, but many patients are reluctant to be followed without therapy. A second approach, used at the St. Bartholomew's Hospital and other institutions, has been the use of single-agent chemotherapy.[69] This approach leads to a lower rate of complete response than multiagent chemotherapy; however, when single-agent chemotherapy is given for 1 year or longer, there is no difference in the complete response rate, disease-free survival, or overall survival compared with combination chemotherapy such as CVP (cyclophosphamide, vincristine, prednisone).[30]

The third approach of using TLI or aggressive multiagent chemotherapy with or without TLI has been studied, with improvements in complete remission rates but without a benefit in overall survival. TLI is extremely toxic treatment, and it limits the delivery of subsequent chemotherapy. The Stanford trial that administered TLI demonstrated continuous relapse rates in patients treated with TLI, with the exception of a cohort of eight patients with more limited disease for whom there appeared to be a plateau in the disease-free survival curve.[70] Two institutions used TLI plus chemotherapy in patients with stage III low-grade NHL. The M. D. Anderson Cancer Center evaluated the use of TLI plus CHOP (cyclophosphamide, hydroxydaunomycin, Oncovin, prednisone) chemotherapy in patients with stage III low-grade lymphomas.[71] The relapse-free survival at 5 years was 52%; however, the followup period of 6 years was not sufficiently long to show that patients with small cleaved NHL were being cured. A prospective, randomized trial comparing no initial therapy with aggressive CMT using ProMACE/MOPP (prednisone, methotrexate [with leucovorin rescue], Adriamycin, cyclophosphamide, etoposide/mechlorethamine, Oncovin, procarbazine, prednisone) chemotherapy followed by low-dose TLI (2400 cGy) was undertaken by the NCI.[72] Eighty-nine patients were randomized. The disease-free survival at 4 years was significantly higher for the patients receiving CMT (51% versus 12%); however, no differences in overall survival were observed. None of these studies has shown a survival advantage using initial aggressive therapy in the management of patients with advanced-stage low-grade lymphoma compared with less aggressive initial therapy.

High-dose chemotherapy followed by autologous bone marrow rescue has been used at a number of institutions to treat selected patients with recurrent low-grade lymphoma.[73–76] Investigators at the Dana-Farber Cancer Institute have employed cyclophosphamide 60 mg/kg on two successive days followed by 1200 cGy of TBI and autologous bone marrow purged of malignant cells using monoclonal antibodies. Patients were either in a complete remission or minimal disease state before marrow harvest. Fifty-one patients with relapsed low-grade lymphoma and 18 patients with histologic transformation of low-grade lymphoma were treated. The 5-year disease-free survival of the patients without transformation who were in complete remission at the time of transplant was higher than 80% and 20% for the patients in partial remission.[73]

The Dana-Farber Cancer Institute initiated a trial of up-front autologous BMT for advanced-stage patients with indolent lymphomas in first remission.[77] Patients were given six to eight cycles of CHOP chemotherapy and, if not in a minimal disease state (as previously defined), IF pretransplant radiation therapy. Marrow was harvested once patients were in a minimal disease state (<10% bone marrow involvement as determined by histologic examination of iliac crest biopsy). They were then given high-dose cyclophosphamide and 1200 cGy of TBI followed by antibody-purged marrow. The 2-year disease-free survival is 65%, and overall survival is 95%. The followup period is too short to determine the impact on curability that autologous BMT will have on low-grade lymphoma.

Intermediate-Grade Lymphomas

Stage I–II. Prior to 1980, radiation therapy was the primary treatment for patients with localized diffuse large cell lymphomas. With the development of effective multi-agent chemotherapy, the treatment of localized large cell lymphoma has changed dramatically. Randomized trials comparing radiation therapy alone with radiation therapy followed by chemotherapy demonstrated significant advantages for the inclusion of chemotherapy.[78–80] Staging laparotomy and large-field radiation therapy became obsolete as combination chemotherapy with or without radiation therapy produced disease-free and overall survival rates better than those seen even in the most selected studies reporting results with radiation therapy alone.

With effective multiagent chemotherapy, there is controversy regarding the benefit of radiation therapy in early-stage diffuse large cell lymphomas. Limited data on the use of multiagent chemotherapy alone has yielded 65% to 83% 10-year disease-free survival for stage I–II patients and 68% to 80% 10-year survival for stage I–II patients.[81, 82] In some series, patients were given radiation therapy when disease was slow to respond to initial chemotherapy.[82] Retrospective studies suggest that the addition of radiation therapy to chemotherapy yields a moderately improved freedom from recurrence compared with chemotherapy alone.[83–86] At the NCI, four cycles of modified dose ProMACE-MOPP chemotherapy followed by 4000 cGy to involved sites in patients with stage I–II aggressive lymphomas resulted in complete responses in 47 of 49 patients in the stage I–IE patients, all of whom remained in continuous remission with median followup of 4 years.[84] Adjuvant IF radiation therapy in this setting does appear to permit the delivery of fewer cycles and lower doses of chemotherapy than those used for more advanced disease.[84, 87]

The prognosis of patients with stage I–II large cell lymphomas varies greatly. At our institution, a subgroup of early-stage patients with bulky thoracic or abdominal disease or with three or more sites of involvement had a significantly worse survival independent of treatment than patients with only one or two contiguous sites that were nonbulky.[85] Further analysis of 57 patients with stage I–II bulky large cell lymphoma of the mediastinum (all treated with intensive chemotherapy) experienced disease-free survival of only 44% and overall survival of 50%.[56] Prognostic factors associated with a poor outcome identified in this retrospective study included presentation with multiple extranodal sites, pleural effusion, high LDH level, and a positive gallium scan following chemotherapy. More recently, the International Non-Hodgkin's Lymphoma Prognostic Factors Project developed a model to identify patients with intermediate-grade and high-grade lymphomas who appear to have a worse survival with conventional treatment.[56] The model was based on age, tumor stage, serum LDH level, performance status, and number of extranodal sites. The international index and the age-adjusted international index are significantly more accurate in predicting long-term survival than the Ann Arbor classification and may help to identify early-stage patients who may require more intensive treatment.

Higher doses of radiation therapy are required for patients with large cell lymphomas compared with small cell lymphomas when radiation therapy is used as a single modality. In experiences from both the Stanford University Medical Center and the Princess Margaret Hospital, approximately 20% of patients with large cell lymphomas developed in-field recurrences with total doses of 5000 cGy or greater compared with 3500 cGy or less for low-grade lymphomas.[67, 88] Following multiagent chemotherapy, it may be feasible to reduce the total dose of radiation. We currently recommend doses of approximately 4000 cGy for patients with diffuse large cell lymphoma who have had a complete response to chemotherapy. Patients with persistent disease require higher doses. Treatment volumes are generally designed to include the initial extent of the tumor but not necessarily the initial volume of tumor. For example, in a mediastinal lymphoma, the initial superior to inferior extent would be need to be treated; however, following the response to chemotherapy, a large nodal mass without extension into the chest wall would have shrunk such that a larger volume of normal lung can be blocked.

In summary, the best treatment for patients with early-stage large cell lymphomas is still controversial. We recommend that clinically staged patients with fewer than three sites of disease and no bulky (>10 cm) masses receive CHOP chemotherapy for four to six cycles followed by IF radiation therapy.[84, 87] Patients with bulky masses or other factors associated with poorer outcome should be managed similarly to patients with advanced-stage disease.

Stage III–IV. The treatment of advanced-stage large cell lymphoma is combination chemotherapy. Patients who are considered high risk because of masses larger than 10 cm in diameter (particularly involving the mediastinum or gastrointestinal tract), involvement of multiple extranodal sites, presence of B symptoms, or elevated serum LDH level should be considered for treatment with more aggressive regimens that provide more dose intensification.[55, 56, 89–93] As an alternative, myeloablative therapy and hematopoietic stem cell rescue has been used at several centers. Freedman and colleagues at the Dana-Farber Cancer Institute recently reported results of purged-marrow autologous transplantation including TBI as part of upfront treatment of poor-prognosis patients with intermediate- and high-grade B-cell lymphomas.[77] The 3-year disease-free survival was 85%. TBI is delivered using a fractionated low-dose rate (5 to 10 cGy/minute) treatment technique delivering 1200 cGy total dose in 200 cGy fractions, two fractions per day 6 hours apart. Thin lung shields are also placed on the patient during treatment delivery to decrease the lung dose by 10% to 15%, which compensates for the excess dose deposited in the air-filled lungs. With the use of these techniques the risk of acute radiation pneumonitis is less than 10%.[94]

High-Grade Lymphomas

The management of patients with large cell immunoblastic NHL follows the same approach as that used with similarly staged diffuse large cell lymphoma of intermediate grade. High-grade diffuse small noncleaved cell subtypes (Burkitt's and non-Burkitt's), and lymphoblastic lymphomas behave like leukemias of similar histology and are treated as their systemic counterparts. Human T-cell leukemia/lymphoma virus, type I (HTLV-I)-related adult T-cell lymphomas (ATLs) are observed most often in HTLV-I endemic regions. For example, the cumulative lifetime risk of developing ATL in Japan is 4.5% for HTLV-I infected males and 2.5% for infected females. ATL is highly aggressive and most often disseminated at diagnosis. Diffuse small noncleaved cell lymphomas (non-Burkitt's) account for less than 10% of diffuse lymphomas. These lymphomas are treated with aggressive multiagent chemotherapy regimens. Aside from prophylactic cranial irradiation in patients with lymphoblastic lymphoma, there is no role for radiation therapy in the primary treatment of patients with high-grade NHL.

RADIATION THERAPY TECHNIQUES

Recommended Fields for Nodal Sites Treated with Radiation Therapy Alone

Nodal disease involving one side of the neck is generally treated to both neck and supraclavicular regions, with a boost to the involved side of the neck. Involvement limited to the supraclavicular nodes would include the supraclavicular, infraclavicular, axillary, and cervical nodes. Disease limited to the mediastinum would be treated to a field including the mediastinal, bilateral hilar, and supraclavicular nodes. Ipsilateral inguinal nodal disease would be treated to the ipsilateral external iliac, inguinal, and femoral nodes. Recommended doses for low-grade lymphoma are 3000 to 3500 cGy, with boost to 4000 cGy if bulky disease is present.

Specific Extranodal Sites

Patients with early-stage lymphoma presenting in an extranodal site have a prognosis similar to those with similar stage and histology involving purely nodal sites.[95] Radiation therapy guidelines and doses are similar to those for nodal presentations. Specific sites of extranodal involvement do require special consideration and are discussed in the following sections.

Conjunctiva and Orbit. Lymphomatous involvement occurs in the orbit and in the conjunctiva with about equal frequency, accounting for between 5% and 14% of all extranodal presentations. These locations should be considered individually because they are often histologically distinct and have distinct natural histories. Conjunctival lymphoma tends to be localized but may be associated with advanced disease. Owing to its infiltrative nature, conjunctival lymphoma recurs with a high frequency following surgical excision alone. Surgery is used for diagnosis, but local radiation therapy to the entire conjunctiva is the definitive treatment of choice for local control. Treatment of

conjunctival lymphoma can be accomplished with either electrons or photons.[96] Dunbar and colleagues from the Massachusetts General Hospital have recommended doses of 2400 to 3000 cGy for conjunctival lymphoma without local recurrence in a series of 12 patients treated with electron-beam radiation therapy.[96] Alternatively, a simple anterior photon field can be used; a bolus may be required to increase the dose to the conjunctiva. The lens can be blocked, but care must be taken not to shield disease.

CT scanning is useful in the evaluation of the extent of disease and radiation therapy treatment planning, especially when the orbit is involved. Various treatment field arrangements can be employed, depending on the location of the disease, that is, disease limited to the anterior portion of the orbit, involving both eyes, or involving the lacrimal glands. When disease is unilateral, a single anterior photon field can be used to avoid dose to the contralateral eye; however, this field can produce "hot spots" that may be in the lacrimal gland, resulting in eye dryness. Dry eye can be more problematic than the development of a cataract from treatment of the lens. An anterior and a lateral field can be used or opposed lateral fields, although using this treatment plan, there is dose to the contralateral eye. Figure 11–11 is an orbital CT scan demonstrating involvement of both the lateral orbits. The patient also had involvement of both lacrimal glands. An example of the treatment field arrangement for this patient is shown in Figure 11–12A, where an en face (anterior) photon field was used up to a dose of 2000 cGy followed by the use of two separate anterior fields. This allowed the use of the hanging eye block to protect each lens (Fig. 11–12B). The hanging eye block can only protect one lens at a time because it is positioned clinically with the patient looking up at the block. The dose was limited to 3500 cGy, which produced neither retinal damage nor a permanent dry eye. The location of the orbital disease prevents the use of the hanging eye block in most patients, and even with the lateral location of the orbital lymphoma in this patient, its use was restricted to after 2000 cGy.

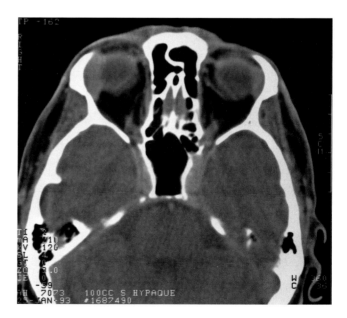

Figure 11–11. CT scan of orbital lymphoma with bilateral involvement in the lateral aspect of each orbit.

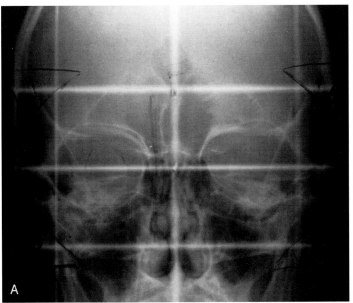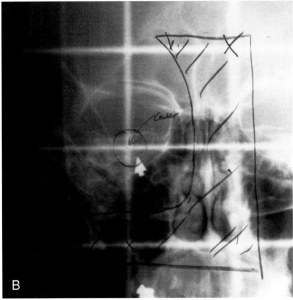

Figure 11–12. The initial anterior treatment field (*A*) covers both orbits and is used to deliver 2000 cGy, after which the fields are modified and each eye is treated separately (*B*) and a hanging eye block (labeled "center") is used to protect the lens. The dose is increased to 3500 cGy.

Lymphocytic lymphoma can also involve the orbit or the globe itself. Patients with diffuse large cell lymphoma of the orbit usually receive chemotherapy and radiation therapy. Again, the orbital CT scan is useful for determining the extent of disease and planning the treatment for these patients. Those patients with DHL of the globe have a high risk of relapsing in the central nervous system (CNS). Patients with extension into the CNS should be treated as though there is primary CNS disease.

Gastric Lymphoma. The treatment of patients with extranodal lymphoma presenting in the gastrointestinal tract follow similar guidelines to that of localized nodal disease of the same histologic subtype. The stomach is the most common site of primary extranodal lymphoma, but it is more often secondarily involved in the dissemination of nodal lymphomas. Gastric lymphomas spread submucosally, often leading to an underestimate of disease. Local/regional failure is frequent and is a common cause of death. The diagnosis can be made by endoscopic biopsy, reserving surgery for those patients in whom diagnosis is not obtained by endoscopy.

Most primary gastric lymphomas are of B-cell lineage and are a large cell histologic subtype. The role of surgery in diffuse large cell lymphoma is controversial owing to historical concerns of life-threatening perforation associated with the use of chemotherapy. These risks have been overstated so that surgical resection is reserved for large or ulcerating lesions. With the use of CMT, total gastrectomy is rarely warranted. Partial gastrectomy does remain an option for the local treatment of localized large cell lymphoma. There are no prospective, randomized trials on the optimal treatment for primary localized gastric lymphoma; however, patients with positive margins following resection or with tumor beyond the submucosa may have an improved disease-free survival with the addition of radiation therapy after chemotherapy. Otherwise, chemotherapy alone should be used.[97]

Local/regional radiation therapy is recommended in the treatment of low-grade gastric lymphoma owing to their infiltrative nature; however, a total gastrectomy need not be performed. The radiation therapy fields include the perigastric lymph nodes, with the total dose being 3500 cGy for low-grade lymphomas, followed by a boost to gross disease of 500 cGy. CT planning minimizes the dose to the small bowel and kidneys.

MALT Lymphoma of the Stomach. Low-grade B-cell lymphoma of mucosal-associated lymphoid tissue (MALT) occurs in the stomach, small intestine, salivary gland, lung, and thyroid.[98] These lymphomas are characterized by prolonged clinical course, localized but persistent disease, and when dissemination occurs, involvement of other mucosal sites. They may progress to high-grade lesions through blastic transformation of the low-grade component.[99] *Helicobacter pylori* infection has been recognized as a risk factor for gastric adenocarcinoma and has been reported in association with the development of gastric lymphoma.[100, 101] In a case-control study of more than 230,000 participants, patients with previous *H. pylori* infection were significantly more likely to develop gastric lymphoma than those without prior infection (odds ratio of 6.3). Other studies have also linked *H. pylori* infection and lymphoma, in particular those arising in MALT.[101, 102] Eradication of the *H. pylori* infection with antibiotics in one study led to tumor remission in five of six patients with biopsy-proven low-grade MALT lymphoma.[102] However, in our experience, patients whose lymphoma regresses with *H. pylori* treatment eventually develop recurrent gastric lymphoma. We have had excellent local control of gastric MALT lymphomas with the use of 3500 cGy of gastric irradiation.

Testicular Lymphoma. Primary NHL of the testis is rare, although it is the most common testicular neoplasm in men older than 60 years of age. These lymphomas are most often of intermediate-grade histology, although some patients had areas with features similar to those seen in MALT lymphomas. Most patients have early-stage disease; bilateral involvement either synchronously or metachronously is reported in 0 to 30% of reported series.[103–105] CNS involvement is reported in 8% of patients in various series but is influenced by the histologic subtype, with lymphoblastic and diffuse undifferentiated lymphoma having the highest incidence.[104] Involvement of Waldeyer's ring and adjacent structures is another feature associated with testicular lymphoma. Diagnosis of testicular lymphoma is established by orchiectomy. Staging studies that include an evaluation of abdominal and pelvic lymph nodes, bone marrow, and cerebrospinal fluid should be considered. Systemic chemotherapy is the primary modality. The role of irradiation of the contralateral testicle is recommended by some authors, but it remains controversial.[103–106] Patients who cannot tolerate chemotherapy can be treated with radiation therapy to the inguinal, pelvic, and paraaortic lymph nodes with a low expectation of cure. Radiation therapy should also be considered for patients with diffuse, poorly differentiated small cleaved cell histology because the efficacy of chemotherapy in this subtype is limited.

Lymphoma of the Head and Neck. The most common sites of presentation in the head and neck regions are the cervical lymph nodes and Waldeyer's ring. Waldeyer's ring consists of nasopharyngeal, palatine, and lingual tonsils. There is an association between involvement of Waldeyer's ring and involvement of the gastrointestinal tract, which may be part of the aforementioned MALT lymphoma. Selection of treatment of head and neck lymphoma is based on the stage, histology, and patient characteristics. Patients with early-stage low-grade lymphomas limited to the head and neck are treated with radiation therapy alone. Patients with early-stage large cell lymphoma are given chemotherapy, with consolidation with radiation therapy as an option.[83, 84]

Treatment technique depends on the site of involvement as well as whether radiation therapy alone is being used. Patients with stage I and localized stage II extranodal low-grade lymphoma of the head and neck are treated with fields covering the next-echelon lymph node group. Sites such as the orbit are less likely to have nodal involvement and treatment fields cover involved areas unless clinically involved nodes are present. Patients with low-grade lymphoma involving Waldeyer's ring who are to receive radiation therapy alone are generally treated with comprehensive fields covering the nasopharynx, the base of the tongue, the tonsillar fossae, the cervical lymph nodes, and the preauricular, postauricular, and occipital lymph nodes. Opposed lateral fields are used with an anterior low neck field junctioned to the lateral fields. The treatment fields must be individualized for each patient. Patients with large cell lymphoma of Waldeyer's ring are treated to more limited fields covering originally involved sites and nodes following chemotherapy. The dose required for local control in low-grade NHL is 3000 to 3600 cGy with radiation therapy alone. Patients with large cell NHL are treated with 4000 to 4500 cGy following chemotherapy.

Radiation therapy to the head and neck produces transient mucositis and xerostomia. Following total doses of 3000 cGy, most patients recover adequate salivary function. Doses higher than 4500 to 5000 cGy can result in permanent xerostomia of moderate to severe in most adults, with older patients more susceptible to permanent xerostomia at doses above 3500 cGy. Hypothyroidism can result from irradiation of the neck. Patients are managed with thyroid examination and thyroid function analysis on a regular basis to detect hypothyroidism before it becomes clinically evident. Treatment is with hormone replacement and continued monitoring of TSH levels.

Primary Central Nervous System Lymphoma. Primary CNS lymphoma is increasing in both the immunocompetent and immunocompromised patient population. These two conditions are different diseases with respect to presentation and prognosis as well as patient characteristics.[107] Despite these differences, radiation therapy remains part of the standard treatment in both patient groups. Using whole-brain doses of 4000 to 5000 cGy, complete responses occur in most patients, although long-term survival is rare.[108, 109] The Radiation Therapy Oncology Group (RTOG) examined the use of higher doses to the involved areas (4000 cGy to the whole brain with 2000 cGy boost) and found that the median survival was 11.6 months and that 92% of patients recurred in the initially involved region.[109] Radiation therapy alone has not been curative for most patients with non–human immunodeficiency virus (HIV) primary CNS lymphoma. These disappointing results have prompted the initiation of CMT approaches in immunocompetent patients, including regimens designed to disrupt the blood-brain barrier. (Primary CNS lymphoma is discussed in detail in Chapter 25.)

Lymphoma in Acquired Immunodeficiency Syndrome. Patients with HIV infection are at risk for the development of NHL. The case definition of the acquired immunodeficiency syndrome (AIDS) includes primary CNS lymphoma as well as intermediate- or high-grade lymphoma of B-cell origin in patients with HIV infection.[110] Most patients have widely disseminated disease at diagnosis, and 65% to 98% have extranodal involvement. The sites of involvement are unusual and include the myocardium, rectum, popliteal fossa, earlobe, orbit, and gallbladder. Involvement of the bone marrow, CNS, and gastrointestinal tract occurs in one third of patients. Most patients with AIDS and NHL die from opportunistic infections, although lymphoma was present in 100% at the time of death in one series and was the cause of death in 35% to 50% in another series.[111] In the HIV-infected patients with primary CNS lymphoma (this is now considered to fulfill the criteria for the diagnosis of AIDS) radiation therapy alone may still be appropriate for those patients unable to receive more aggressive chemotherapy. Without radiation therapy, all these patients develop progressive lymphoma.[112] Whole-brain treatment using doses of 3000 to 4000 cGy are recommended for these patients.

Optimal treatment of AIDS lymphoma is not established. Aggressive chemotherapy as well as protocols using less intensive regimens have been used; however, few patients are expected to experience long-term survival. Patients with a better performance status, without prior history of opportunistic infections, and with lower stages of NHL may tolerate more aggressive treatment. Radiation therapy is a reasonable option and can provide good short-term palliation for AIDS patients with NHL.

Lymphoma in the Immunocompromised Host. The incidence of lymphoma occurring in the immunocompromised host has been increasing. This increase is primarily attributed to the increasing number of patients undergoing transplants of solid organ and bone marrow with the resulting immunosuppression to prevent graft rejection. The majority of these lymphomas are of B-cell subtype, usually diffuse large cell lymphoma or diffuse large cell lymphoma-immunoblastic subtypes, and often contain Epstein-Barr virus DNA. An initial approach to treatment involves decreasing the immunosuppression, although this is not always possible (such as in the heart transplant recipient, in whom graft rejection would be fatal). Treatment of diffuse large cell lymphoma subtypes includes initial chemotherapy as tolerated; local radiation therapy can be employed as an adjunct to chemotherapy or for palliation in situations in which chemotherapy would not be tolerated.

Total-Body Irradiation

TBI is often employed as part of the preparative regimen in BMT. The goals of the conditioning regimen in BMT include (1) the creation of space to allow the transplanted marrow space to engraft and expand; (2) the immunosuppression of the recipient to prevent graft rejection; and (3) the elimination of remaining malignant cells. TBI is used in many BMT preparative regimens to help achieve these goals. In addition, because of its ability to penetrate the CNS and testes, TBI is often incorporated into BMT regimens for acute lymphoblastic leukemia. The fractionation, dose rate, and total dose of TBI in the transplant setting has been evolving since it was first employed in Seattle,[113] where the first randomized trial designed to define the optimal method of TBI delivery was carried out. This study used a single fraction (1000 cGy) versus multiple fractions of TBI (200 cGy daily for 6 days) to treat patients with acute non-lymphoblastic leukemia in first remission. The dose rate in both arms was 4 to 7 cGy per minute, considered low dose rate with conventional local-field irradiation delivered at 100 cGy per minute. The survival was significantly better for the patients given single-fraction TBI owing to an increase in mortality from complications.[113] Although there is still some controversy concerning the optimal TBI delivery schedule, most transplant centers use fractionated TBI. Preparative regimens do vary among centers. For example, Memorial Sloane-Kettering Cancer Center administers 120 cGy three times per day for 11 fractions and gives the TBI before cylcophosphamide.[114] Other centers use fractions ranging from 120 to 400 cGy, with dose rates of 2.5 to 20 cGy/min. The chief advantages of fractionated low dose rate TBI are improved normal tissue tolerance and decreased late effects. These normal tissue improvements are of particular advantage in younger patients undergoing BMT.

BMT is associated with significant morbidity and mortality, whether or not TBI is a part of the preparative regimen. The chief causes of morbidity and mortality include infection, idiopathic pneumonitis, graft-versus-host disease, veno-occlusive disease, and relapse of disease. The acute toxicities of TBI include nausea, vomiting, fever, hair loss, mucositis, skin erythema, and veno-occlusive diseases. The subacute and chronic toxicities of TBI, occurring more than 3 months after BMT, are interstitial pneumonitis, veno-occlusive disease, radiation nephritis, and cataract development.

Interstitial pneumonitis had been associated with a 50% incidence and 70% mortality rate.[115] The cause of interstitial pneumonitis following BMT is often multifactorial, including infection, graft-versus-host disease, and radiation pneumonitis. Radiation factors that are associated with an increased risk of interstitial pneumonitis are the use of high dose rate or single-fraction TBI. Greater degrees of histoincompatibility, which require extensive use of immunosuppressive agents and result in more graft-versus-host disease, are also associated with an increased risk of interstitial pneumonitis. At experienced transplant centers the risk of interstitial pneumonitis is approximately 10% in allogeneic BMT and 5% in autologous BMT.

Complications of Radiation Therapy

Toxicities of radiation therapy in the treatment of lymphomas are related to the dose and volume of tissue treated. Treatment of the head and neck region results in temporary xerostomia, taste change, and mucositis. Recovery of salivary function may be incomplete with doses higher than 3500 cGy and particularly in patients 40 years of age and older. Radiation therapy to lymphomas involving the mediastinum requires careful attention to the lung volumes irradiated to decrease the risk of significant radiation pneumonitis. Patients who have received prior thoracic irradiation are at increased risk of developing pneumonitis after BMT. Treatment of pelvic nodes requires shielding of the iliac crests (if possible) to avoid excessive bone marrow toxicity. This is of particular importance for patients who may be likely to undergo a BMT and need to have bone marrow harvested from the iliac crests. Although bowel complications are rare with the doses generally used in lymphomas, treatment of the upper abdomen requires careful attention to the dose to the kidneys. Total dose to the spinal cord should also be kept as low as possible to allow for additional dose if a BMT with TBI is ever to be considered.

Palliation

External-beam radiation therapy is a useful palliative treatment owing to the responsiveness of HD and NHLs to low doses of irradiation. Patients treated for palliation can be given relatively low doses (2500 to 3000 cGy) using a variety of fractionation schemes, depending on the clinical situation. Generally, 150 to 180 cGy/fraction provides less long-term toxicity without comprising efficacy. Larger fractions can be used but usually are not necessary owing to the sensitivity of lymphomas. For very rapidly growing lymphomas, twice daily fractionation should be considered. For some selected sites such as the eye, doses closer to the upper range (3000 cGy) may be more likely to provide long-term local control.

RECOMMENDATIONS

Chemotherapy has assumed a greater role in the treatment of the NHL, in particular for the aggressive lymphomas. Chemotherapy for the low-grade lymphomas is not as successful. Patients with low-stage indolent lymphomas are still often best treated by local radiation therapy. The use of low doses and small fields can provide good local control with a minimum of morbidity and still not jeopardize a more aggressive approach should such be required for relapse. In the localized large cell lymphoma with very bulky disease, IF radiation therapy may prevent local relapse, because such patients have tended to experience recurrence in sites of bulk disease. Despite promising advances in the treatment of lymphoma, including newer approaches with myeloablation and hematopoietic stem cell rescue and the use of cytokines with greater dose intensification, radiation therapy continues to play a role in the treatment of lymphoma.

Considerable progress has been achieved in the overall treatment of NHL. Better radiographic studies have improved noninvasive staging and have allowed for better definition of radiation therapy fields. Effective chemotherapy has shifted the role of radiation therapy to the treatment of bulk disease rather than the use of wide-field radiation therapy approaches that have increased morbidity and can compromise the delivery of chemotherapy. Current efforts are focusing on minimizing treatment volumes and, in some situations, decreasing doses so as not to compromise the use of systemic therapy.

REFERENCES

1. Pusey W: Cases of sarcoma and of Hodgkin's disease treated by exposures to x-rays: A preliminary report. JAMA 1902; 38:166.
2. Senn N: Therapeutical value of roentgen ray in treatment of pseudoleukemia. NY Med J 1903; 77:665.
3. Gilbert R: Radiotherapy in Hodgkin's disease (malignant granulomatosis): Anatomic and clinical foundations, governing principles, results. Am J Roentgenol 1939; 41:198.
4. Peters M: A study in survivals in Hodgkin's disease treated radiologically. Am J Roentgenol 1950; 63:299.
5. Easson E, Russell M: The cure of Hodgkin's disease. Br Med J 1963; 1:1704.
6. Kaplan H: Evidence for a tumoricidal dose level in the radiotherapy of Hodgkin's disease. Cancer Res 1966; 26:1221.
7. Mauch P: Controversies in the management of patients with early-stage Hodgkin's disease. Blood 1994; 83:318.
8. Hoppe R, Coleman C, Cox R, et al: The management of stage I–II Hodgkin's disease with irradiation alone or combined modality therapy: The Stanford experience. Blood 1982; 59:455.
9. Mauch P, Tarbell N, Weinstein H, et al: Stage IA and IIA supradiaphragmatic Hodgkin's disease: Prognostic factors in surgically staged patients treated with mantle and paraaortic irradiation. J Clin Oncol 1988; 6:1576.
10. Specht L, Nordentoft A, Cold S, et al: Tumor burden as the most important prognostic factor in early-stage Hodgkin's disease: Relations to other prognostic factors and implications for choice of treatment. Cancer 1988; 61:1719.
11. Leslie N, Mauch P, Hellman S: Stage IA to IIB supradiaphragmatic Hodgkin's disease: Long-term survival and relapse frequency. Cancer 1985; 55:2072.
12. Leopold K, Canellos G, Rosenthal D, et al: Stage IA–IIB Hodgkin's disease: Staging and treatment of patients with large mediastinal adenopathy. J Clin Oncol 1989; 7(8):1059.
13. Mauch P, Goodman R, Hellman S: The significance of mediastinal involvement in early-stage Hodgkin's disease. Cancer 1978; 42:1039.
14. Mauch P, Gorshein D, Cunningham J, Hellman S: Influence of mediastinal adenopathy on site and frequency of relapse in patients with Hodgkin's disease. Cancer Treat Rep 1982; 66:809.
15. Prosnitz L, Curtis A, Knowlton A, et al: Supradiaphragmatic Hodgkin's disease: Significance of large mediastinal masses. Int J Radiat Oncol Biol Phys 1980; 6:809.
16. Tarbell N, Thompson L, Mauch P: Thoracic irradiation in Hodgkin's disease: Disease control and long-term complications. Int J Radiat Oncol Biol Phys 1990; 18:275.
17. Willet C, Linggood R, Stracher M, et al: The effect of the respiratory cycle on mediastinal and lung dimensions in Hodgkin's Disease: Implications for radiotherapy gated to respiration. Cancer 1987; 60:1232.
18. Castellino R, Blank N, Hoppe R, Cho C: Hodgkin's disease: Contributions of chest CT in the initial staging evaluation. Radiology 1986; 160:603.
19. Rostock R, Giangreco A, Wharam M, et al: CT scan modification in the treatment of mediastinal Hodgkin's disease. Cancer 1982; 49:2267.
20. Mauch P, Larson D, Osteen R, et al: Prognostic factors for positive surgical staging in patients with Hodgkin's disease. J Clin Oncol 1990; 8:257.
21. Leibenhaut M, Hoppe R, Efron B, et al: Prognostic indicators of laparotomy findings in clinical stage I–II supradiaphragmatic Hodgkin's disease. J Clin Oncol 1989; 7:81.
22. Tubiana M, Henry-Amar M, Hayat M, et al: Prognostic significance of the number of involved areas in the early stages of Hodgkin's disease. Cancer 1984; 54(5):885.
23. Donaldson S, Glatstein E, Vosti K: Bacterial infections in pediatric Hodgkin's disease. Cancer 1978; 41:1949.
24. Siber G, Gorham C, Martin P, et al: Antibody response to pretreatment immunization and post-treatment boosting with bacterial polysaccharide vaccines in patients with Hodgkin's disease. Ann Intern Med 1986; 104(4):467.
25. Tubiana M, Henry-Amar M, Van Der Werf-Messing B, et al: A multivariate analysis of prognostic factors in early-stage Hodgkin's disease. Int J Radiat Oncol 1985; 11:23.
26. Tubiana M, Henry-Amar M, Carde P, et al: Toward comprehensive management tailored to prognostic factors of patients with clinical stages I and II in Hodgkin's disease: The EORTC Lymphoma Group controlled clinical trials, 1964–1987. Blood 1989; 73:47.
26a. Carde P, Burgers JMV, Henry-Amar M, et al: Clinical stages I and II Hodgkin's disease; A specifically tailored therapy according to prognostic factors. J Clin Oncol 1988; 6:239.
27. Gospodarowicz M, Sutcliffe S, Clark R, et al: Analysis of supradiaphragmatic clinical stage I and II Hodgkin's disease treated with radiation alone. Int J Radiat Oncol Biol Phys 1992; 22:859.
28. Sutcliffe S, Gospodarowicz M, Bergsagel D, et al: Prognostic groups for management of localized Hodgkin's disease. J Clin Oncol 1985; 3:393.
29. Kinzie J, Hanks G, Maclean C, Kramer S: Patterns of Care Study: Hodgkin's disease relapse rates and adequacy of portals. Cancer 1983; 52:2223.
30. Rosenberg S, Kaplan H: The evolution and summary results of the Stanford randomized clinical trials of the management of Hodgkin's disease: 1962–1984. Int J Radiat Oncol Bio Phys 1985; 11:5.
31. Coltman C, Fuller L, Fisher R, Frei E: Extended field radiotherapy versus involved field radiotherapy plus MOPP in stage I and II Hodgkin's disease. *In* Jones S, Salmon S (eds): Adjuvant Therapy of Cancer, 2nd ed. New York, Grune & Stratton, 1979, p 129.
32. Kaplan H: Hodgkin's Disease. Cambridge, MA, Harvard University Press, 1980, p 281.
33. Tarbell NJ, Gelber RD, Weinstein HJ, Mauch P: Sex differences in risk of second malignant tumours after Hodkgin's disease in childhood. Lancet 1993; 34:1428.
34. Lutz W, Larsen R: Technique to match mantle and para-aortic fields. Int J Radiat Oncol Biol Phys 1983; 9:1753.
35. Fraass B, Tepper J, Glatstein E, van de Geijn J: Clinical use of match-line wedge for adjacent megavoltage radiation field matching. Int J Radiat Oncol Biol Phys 1983; 9:209.
36. Farah J, Ultmann J, Griem M, et al: Extended mantle radiation therapy for pathologic stage I and II Hodgkin's disease. J Clin Oncol 1988; 6:1047.
37. Horning S: Female reproductive potential after treatment for Hodgkin's disease. N Engl J Med 1981; 304:1377.
38. Speiser B, Rubin P, Casarett G: Aspermia following lower truncal irradiation in Hodgkin's disease. Cancer 1973; 32:692.
39. Jochelson M, Mauch P, Balikian J, et al: The significance of the residual mediastinal mass in treated Hodgkin's disease. J Clin Oncol 1985; 3:637.
40. Boivin J-F, Hutchison G, Lubin J, Mauch P: Coronary artery disease mortality in patients treated for Hodgkin's disease. Cancer 1992; 69:1241.
41. Loeffler J, Tarbell N, Garber J, Mauch P: The development of Graves' disease following radiation therapy in Hodgkin's disease. Int J Radiat Oncol Biol Phys 1988; 14:175.
42. Wasnich R, Grumet T, Payne R, Kriss J: Graves' ophthalmopathy following external neck irradiation for non-thyroidal neoplastic disease. J Clin Endocrinol Metab 1973; 37:703.

43. Andrieu J-M, Ifrah N, Payen C, Fermanian J, et al: Increased risk of secondary acute nonlymphocytic leukemia after extended-field radiation combined with MOPP chemotherapy for Hodgkin's disease. J Clin Oncol 1990; 8:1148.

44. van Leeuwen F, Somers R, Taal B, et al: Increased risk of lung cancer, non-Hodgkin's lymphoma, and leukemia following Hodgkin's disease. J Clin Oncol 1989; 7:1046.

45. Coleman C, Williams C, Flint A, et al: Hematologic neoplasia in patients treated for Hodgkin's disease. N Engl J Med 1977; 297:1249.

46. Tucker M, Coleman C, Cox R, et al: Risk of second cancers after treatment for Hodgkin's disease. N Engl J Med 1988; 318:76.

47. Abrahamsen J, Andersen A, Hannisdal E, et al: Second malignancies after treatment of Hodgkin's disease: The influence of treatment, follow-up time, and age. J Clin Oncol 1993; 11:255.

48. Tester W, Kinsella T, Waller B, et al: Second malignant neoplasms complicating Hodgkin's disease: The National Cancer Institute experience. J Clin Oncol 1984; 2:762.

49. Krikorian J, Burke J, Rosenberg S, Kaplan H: Occurrence of non-Hodgkin's lymphoma after therapy for Hodgkin's disease. N Engl J Med 1979; 300:452.

50. Jacquillat C, Khayat D, Desprez-Curely J, et al: Non-Hodgkin's lymphoma occurring after Hodgkin's disease. Cancer 1984; 53:459.

51. Hancock S, Tucker M, Hoppe R: Breast cancer after treatment for Hodgkin's disease. J Natl Cancer Inst 1993; 85:25.

52. Biti G, Cellai E, Magrini SM, et al: Second solid tumors and leukemia after treatment for Hodgkin's disease: An analysis of 1121 patients from a single institution. Int J Radiat Oncol Biol Phys 1994: 29:25.

53. Harris N, Jaffe ES, Stein H, Banks PM, et al: Perspective: A Revised European-American classification of lymphoid neoplasms: A proposal from the International Lymphoma Study Group. Blood, 1994; 84:1361.

54. National Cancer Institute–sponsored study of classifications of non-Hodgkin's lymphomas. Summary and description of a working formulation for clinical stage. Cancer 1982; 49:2112.

55. Coiffier B, Gisselbrecht C, Vose J, et al: Prognostic factors in aggressive malignant lymphomas: Description and validation of a prognostic index that could identify patients requiring a more intensive therapy. J Clin Oncol 1991; 9(2):211.

56. Kirn D, Mauch P, Shaffer K, et al: Large cell and immunoblastic lymphoma of the mediastinum: Prognostic features and treatment outcome in 57 patients. J Clin Oncol 1993; 11:1336.

57. Castellino R, Dunnick N, Goffinet D, et al: Predictive value of lymphography for sites of subdiaphragmatic disease encountered at staging laparotomy in newly diagnosed Hodgkin's disease and non-Hodgkin's lymphoma. J Clin Oncol 1983; 1:532.

58. Israel O, Front D, Lam M, et al: Gallium 67 imaging in monitoring lymphoma response to treatment. Cancer 1988; 61:2439.

59. Kaplan W, Jochelson M, Herman T, et al: Gallium 67 imaging: A predictor of residual tumor viability and clinical outcome in patients with diffuse large-cell lymphoma. J Clin Oncol 1990; 8:1966.

60. Weeks J, Yeop B, Canellos G, Shipp M: Value of follow-up procedures in patients with large-cell lymphoma who achieve a complete remission. 1991; 9:1196.

61. Chen M, Prosnitz L, Gonzalez-Serva A, Fischer D: Results of radiotherapy in control of stage I and II non-Hodgkin's lymphoma. Cancer 1979; 43:1245.

62. Gomez G, Barcos M, Krishnamsetty R, et al: Treatment of early-stages I and II-nodular, poorly differentiated lymphocytic lymphoma. Am J Clin Oncol 1986; 9:40.

63. Paryani S, Hoppe R, Cox R, et al: Analysis of non-Hodgkin's lymphomas with nodular and favorable histologies, stages I and II. Cancer 1983a; 52:2300.

64. Bush R, Gospodarowicz M: The place of radiation therapy in the management of patients with localized non-Hodgkin's lymphoma. *In* Rosenberg SA, Kaplan HS (eds): Malignant Lymphomas. London, Academic Press, 1982, p 485.

65. Lawrence T, Urba W, Steinberg S, et al: Retrospective analysis of stage I and II indolent lymphomas at the National Cancer Institute. Int J Radiat Oncol Biol Phys 1988; 14:417.

66. Gallagher C, Gregory W, Jones A, et al: Follicular lymphoma: Prognostic factors for response and survival. J Clin Oncol 1986; 4:1470.

67. Fuks Z, Kaplan H: Recurrence rates following radiation therapy of nodular and diffuse malignant lymphomas. Radiology 1973; 108:675.

68. Horning S, Rosenberg S: The natural history of initially untreated low-grade non-Hodgkin's lymphomas. N Engl J Med 1984; 311(23): 1471.

69. Lister T: The management of follicular lymphoma. Ann Oncol 1991; 2(Suppl 2):131.

70. Paryani S, Hoppe R, Cox R, et al: The role of radiation therapy in the management of stage III follicular lymphomas. J Clin Oncol 1984; 2(7):841.

71. McLaughlin P, Fuller L, Velasquez W, et al: Stage III follicular lymphoma: Durable remissions with a combined chemotherapy-radiotherapy regimen. J Clin Oncol 1987; 5(6):867.

72. Young R, Longo D, Glatstein E, et al: The treatment of indolent lymphomas: Watchful waiting versus aggressive combined modality treatment. Semin Hematol 1988; 25(Suppl 2):11.

73. Freedman A, Ritz J, Neuberg D, et al: Autologous bone marrow transplantation in 69 patients with a history of low-grade B-cell non-Hodgkin's lymphoma. Blood 1991; 77:2524.

74. Rohatiner A, Price C, Arnott S, et al: Myeloablative therapy with autologous bone marrow transplantation as consolidation of remission in patients with follicular lymphoma. Ann Oncol 1991; 2(Suppl 2):147.

75. Schouten L, Bierman P, Vaughan W, et al: Autologous bone marrow transplantation in follicular non-Hodgkin's lymphoma before and after histologic transformation. Blood 1989; 74:2579.

76. Gilewski T, Richards J: Biologic response modifiers in non-Hodgkin's lymphomas. Semin Oncol 1990; 17:74.

77. Freedman A, Takvorian T, Neuberg D, et al: Autologous bone marrow transplantation in poor-prognosis intermediate-grade and high-grade B-cell non-Hodgkin's lymphoma in first remission. J Clin Oncol 1993; 11:931.

78. Monfardini S, Banfi A, Bonadonna G, et al: Improved five-year survival after combined radiotherapy-chemotherapy for stage I–II non-Hodgkin's lymphoma. Int J Radiat Oncol Biol Phys 1980; 6:125.

79. Landberg T, Hakansson L, Moller T, et al: CVP remission maintenance in stage I or II non-Hodgkin's lymphomas: Preliminary results of a randomized study. Cancer 1979; 44:831.

80. Nissen N, Ersboll J, Hansen H, et al: A randomized study of radiotherapy versus radiotherapy plus chemotherapy in stage I–II non-Hodgkin's lymphomas. Cancer 1982; 52:1.

81. Cabanillas F: Chemotherapy as definitive treatment of stage I–II large cell and diffuse mixed lymphomas. Hematol Oncol 1985; 3:25.

82. Miller T, Jones S: Initial chemotherapy for clinically localized lymphomas of unfavorable histology. Blood 1983; 62(2):413.

83. Jones S, Miller T, Connors J: Long-term follow-up and analysis for prognostic factors for patients with limited-stage diffuse large-cell lymphoma treated with initial chemotherapy with or without adjuvant radiotherapy. J Clin Oncol 1989; 7:1186.

84. Longo D, Glatstein E, Duffey P, et al: Treatment of localized aggressive lymphomas with combination chemotherapy followed by involved-field radiation therapy. J Clin Oncol 1989; 7:1295.

85. Mauch P, Leonard R, Skarin A, et al: Improved survival following combined radiation therapy and chemotherapy for unfavorable prognosis stage I–II non-Hodgkin's lymphomas. J Clin Oncol 1985; 3(10):1301.

86. Shafman T, Beard C, Silver B, Mauch P: Prognostic factors in stage I and II diffuse large cell lymphoma patients treated with multiagent chemotherapy or combined with radiation therapy. Int J Radiat Oncol Biol Phys 1992; 24(Suppl 1):228.

87. Connors J, Klimo P, Fairey R, et al: Brief chemotherapy and involved field radiation therapy for limited-stage histologically aggressive lymphoma. Ann Intern Med 1987; 107:25.

88. Bush RS, Gospodarowicz M: The place of radiation therapy in the management of patients with localized non-Hodgkin's lymphoma. *In* Rosenberg SA, Kaplan HS (eds): Malignant Lymphomas. London, London Academic Press, 1982, pp 485–502.

89. Ciampi A, Bush R: An approach to classifying prognostic factors related to survival experience for non-Hodgkin's lymphoma patients: Based on a series of 982 patients: 1967–1975. Cancer 1981; 47:621.

90. Jagannath S, Velasquez W, Tucker S, et al: Tumor burden assessment and its implication for a prognostic model in advanced diffuse large-cell lymphoma. J Clin Oncol 1986; 4(6):859.

91. Vose J, Armitage J, Weisenburger D, et al: The importance of age in survival of patients treated with chemotherapy for aggressive non-Hodgkin's lymphoma. J Clin Oncol 1988; 6(12):1838.

92. Hoskins P, Ng V, Spinelli J, et al: Prognostic variables in patients with diffuse large cell lymphoma treated with MACOP-B. J Clin Oncol 1991; 9(2):220.

93. Litam P, Swan F, Cabanillas F, et al: Prognostic value of serum b$_2$-microglobulin in low-grade lymphoma. Ann Intern Med 1991; 114:855.

94. Jochelson M, Tarbell NJ, Freedman AS, et al: Acute and chronic complications following autologous bone marrow transplantation in non-Hodgkin's lymphoma. Bone Marrow Transpl 1990; 6:329.

95. Paryani S, Hoppe R, Burke J, et al: Extralymphatic involvement in diffuse non-Hodgkin's lymphoma. J Clin Oncol 1983b; 1: 682–688.

96. Dunbar S, Linggood R, Doppke K, et al: Conjunctival lymphoma: Results and treatment with a single anterior electron field—a lens-sparing approach. Int J Radiat Oncol Biol Phys 1990; 19:249.

97. Haber D, Mayer RJ: Primary gastrointestinal lymphoma. Semin Oncol 1988; 15:154.

98. Isaacson P, Spencer J: Malignant lymphoma of mucosa-associated lymphoid tissue (MALT). *In* Lymphoproliferative Diseases. Immunol Med 1990; 15:123.

99. Chan J, Ng C, Isaacson P: Relationship between high-grade lymphoma and low-grade B-cell mucosa-associated lymphoid tissue lymphoma (MALToma) of the stomach. Am J Pathol 1990; 136(5): 1153.

100. Correa P: Is gastric carcinoma an infectious disease? N Engl J Med 1991; 325:1170.

101. Parsonnet J, Hansen S, Rodriguez L: *Helicobacter pylori* infection in gastric lymphoma. N Engl J Med 1994; 330:1267.

102. Wotherspoon A, Doglioni C, Isaacson P: Low-grade gastric B-cell lymphoma of mucosa-associated lymphoid tissue (MALT): A multifocal disease. Histopathology 1992; 20:29.

103. Crellin AM, Hudson BV, Bennett MH, et al: Non-Hodgkin's lymphoma of the testis. Radiother Oncol 1993; 27:99.

104. Doll D, Weiss R: Malignant lymphoma of the testis. Am J Med 1986; 81:515.

105. Martenson J, Buskirk S, Ilstrup D, et al: Patterns of failure in primary testicular non-Hodgkin's lymphoma. J Clin Oncol 1988; 6(2):297.

106. Connors J, Klimo P, Voss N, et al: Testicular lymphoma: Improved outcome with early brief chemotherapy. J Clin Oncol 1988; 6(5):776.

107. Fine HA, Mayer RJ: Primary central nervous system lymphoma. Ann Intern Med 1993; 119:1093.

108. Bush RJ, Gospodarowicz M, Sturgeon J, Alison R: Radiation therapy of localized non-Hodgkin's lymphoma. Cancer Treat Rep 1977; 61: 1129.

109. Murray K, Kun L, Cox J: Primary malignant lymphoma of the central nervous system. J Neurosurg 1986; 65: 600.

110. Centers for Disease Control: Revision of the CDC surveillance definition for acquired immunodeficiency syndrome. MMWR 1987; 36:1S.

111. Levine A: Acquired immunodeficiency syndrome–related lymphoma. Blood 1992; 80:8.

112. Baumgartner J, Rachlin J, Beckstead J, et al: Primary central nervous system lymphomas: Natural history and response to radiation therapy in 55 patients with acquired immunodeficiency syndrome. J Neurosurg 1990; 73:206.

113. Thomas E, Buckner C, Banji M, et al: One hundred patients with acute leukemia treated by chemotherapy, total body irradiation, and allogeneic marrow transplantation. Blood 1977; 49:511.

114. Shank B, Hopfan S, Kim J, et al: Hyperfractionated total body irradiation of bone marrow transplantation: I. Early results in leukemia patients. Int J Radiat Oncol Biol Phys 1981; 7:1109.

115. Buckner C, Meyers J, Springmeyer S, et al: Pulmonary complications of marrow transplantation. Exp Hematol 1984; 12:1.

Twelve

——— Principles of Chemotherapy ——— for Lymphomas

Wyndham H. Wilson
Bruce A. Chabner

It increasingly appears that the fundamental genetic changes leading to neoplasia involve deregulation of cellular proliferation and death, events that are controlled in large measure by cell cycle checkpoints and by the induction and suppression of programmed cell death (PCD). Evidence also suggests that abnormalities in these pathways may determine the sensitivity of tumor cells, compared with normal cells, to the cytotoxic effects of irradiation and chemotherapy.[1–3] Understanding the regulation of these pathways and their impact on the efficacy of treatment with irradiation and chemotherapy lies at the frontier of cancer therapy. However, clinical strategies that take advantage of the abnormalities that occur in the regulation of the cell cycle and PCD have just begun and, as yet, do not have a significant place in the design of therapeutic approaches. Indeed, the classic principles of chemotherapy, including pharmacology, drug resistance, and tumor cell kinetics, continue to be the major guides for the development of chemotherapy approaches. Although these principles are important, our rapidly increasing understanding of the molecular basis of neoplasia has placed them in a new perspective. This chapter discusses the classic principles of chemotherapy within the context of this new tumor biology and attempts to provide the reader with a general understanding of current directions in the development of novel treatment strategies for non-Hodgkin's lymphomas.

KINETIC BASIS OF LYMPHOMA TREATMENT

About 30 years ago, Skipper and associates made a number of fundamental observations regarding the kinetic features of tumor cell growth and the effect of chemotherapy on a rodent leukemia L1210 model system.[4] From these observations, they hypothesized the importance of tumor volume, growth fraction, and the first-order kinetics of chemotherapy cell kill for therapeutic outcome. These concepts have become classic principles of chemotherapy and continue to guide treatment strategies. The clinician must remember, however, that the Skipper model was based on a rapidly proliferating tumor that does not accurately reflect the slower growth and heterogeneity of human tumors. Moreover, recent discoveries in tumor molecular biology clearly demonstrate that malignant cells have numerous abnormalities in cell cycle control that independently affect drug sensitivity.

One of the most basic observations that emerged from this model was that the survival of mice inoculated with L1210 cells was inversely proportional to the tumor cell inoculum. In this model system, a single tumor cell was capable of causing death, and the time interval between inoculation and death was proportional to the inoculum. This interval could be calculated from a knowledge of the tumor doubling time and inoculum size. These observations formed the basis for the concept of tumor cell kinetics. When the effect of chemotherapy was investigated in this system, the fraction of tumor cells undergoing DNA replication, termed the "growth fraction," greatly influenced drug sensitivity, an observation likely the result of the relatively greater sensitivity of tumor cells in the DNA synthetic (S) phase of the cell cycle to many classes of chemotherapeutic agents. As a hypothesis of tumor cell sensitivity, however, the principle of growth fraction was a great oversimplification.

Clinically, tumors are heterogeneous. Tumor masses within the same patient vary owing to diverse factors such as blood flow, tissue hypoxia, and clonal mutational events that determine tumor biology and drug resistance. Moreover, the growth fraction of tumor cells is dynamic, decreasing as tumors grow and increasing as tumor cells are killed by cytoreductive treatment. The growth fraction also does not affect the cytotoxicity of all chemotherapy drugs equally. Although most drugs are more cytotoxic to cells undergoing DNA synthesis, some agents such as BCNU do not show this selectivity. Thus, the growth fraction should be included among those factors that contribute to the sensitivity of tumor cells to therapy but alone is not predictive of a therapeutic response. The low-grade lymphomas are a good example of the limitations of this principle. It has been proposed that the low-growth fraction of indolent (low-grade) lymphomas may explain the incurability of these tumors with chemotherapy. However, most low-grade lymphomas are exquisitely sensitive to chemotherapy, so tumor growth fraction alone cannot explain the low cure rate.[5]

Skipper also observed that the number of tumor cells killed by a cycle of chemotherapy depends on first-order kinetics; that is, in the rapidly growing L1210 leukemia cells, a given drug dose killed a constant fraction of cells, independent of cell number.[1, 6] Of course, the sensitivity of the tumor to the chemotherapy directly affects the fraction of cells killed, and in practice this sensitivity changes over multiple courses of chemotherapy. As previously pointed out, when the number of tumor cells decrease, the growth fraction increases, and this may increase the tumor sensitivity. However, the tendency of chemotherapy to select out a resistant cell population after repeated courses may in fact have the opposite effect, namely the emergence of a population much less susceptible to the drugs. The fraction of cells killed can be affected by other factors that change with chemotherapy, including tumor perfusion and oxygenation, decreased host resistance to drug side effects, and the proliferation of tumor in sanctuary sites such as the central nervous system. When applied clinically, the fractional cell kill concept suggests that surgical resection of tumor, if of sufficient degree, would be beneficial to the therapeutic outcome. Although this may true in selected patients with Burkitt's lymphomas in whom an abdominal tumor can be essentially completely resected, as a general rule, surgical resection of lymphomatous tumors does not increase the cure rate of these tumors.[7]

A corollary of the fractional cell kill hypothesis is the important relationship of drug concentration (or dose) and response (or cell kill). For some but not all drugs, a relatively linear relationship exists between cell kill and dose. This applies particularly to alkylating agents. For other drugs (chiefly the antimetabolites) that depend on cell exposure to drug during vulnerable phases of the cell cycle, the duration of exposure may be more important than drug concentration. Clinically, high-dose therapy with stem cell support takes maximal advantage of the drug concentration-response relationship. Alkylating agents and epipodophyllotoxins are the preferred drugs for this approach because of their relatively linear dose response and favorable therapeutic index.[8]

Although these principles do not adequately explain many features of the tumor cell response to chemotherapy, they have had practical application for the design of chemotherapy regimens. The modulation of drug sensitivity by increasing tumor growth fraction has been tested in the treatment of acute myelogenous leukemia. Clinical trials designed to increase tumor response by administering mitogenic agents such as granulocyte-macrophage colony-stimulating factor (GM-CSF) before and during chemotherapy are currently being tested in acute myelogenous leukemia in cooperative group trials, and similar approaches could be tested in lymphomas once the appropriate growth factors are identified.[9] The concept of fractional cell kill has been exploited by chemotherapy regimens that deliver intensive doses of chemotherapy over multiple cycles. This latter approach still remains an important principle for the development of new chemotherapies for lymphomas and has led to the successful use of high-dose chemotherapy with stem cell rescue in relapsed intermediate-grade lymphomas. However, treatment regimens that incorporate modestly intensified therapy, such as the third-generation regimens, have shown no clear benefit over standard therapy such as

CHOP (cyclophosphamide, hydroxydaunomycin, Oncovin, prednisone) in the low- and intermediate-grade lymphomas.[10] For this reason, novel treatment approaches must be explored.

DOSE INTENSITY

Dose intensity, defined as the dose per unit time, has long been considered to be important for the treatment of lymphomas. Indeed, in animal models, a nonlinear relation between drug dose and tumor cell kill has been demonstrated such that doubling drug doses may increase cell kill by up to 10-fold and reductions of as little as 20% may decrease the cure rate by 50%.[11] Since fractional cell kill is rarely, if ever, 100%, it is not surprising that dose intensity would be important to the clinical outcome. In diffuse aggressive lymphomas, the importance of dose intensity was suggested by an analysis performed by DeVita and colleagues that showed a significant relationship between the average relative dose intensity (RDI) of the major chemotherapy regimens and disease-free survival.[12] A similar analysis performed by Kwak and coworkers of the RDI of the individual drugs in CHOP, M-BACOD (methotrexate, bleomycin, Adriamycin [doxorubicin], cyclophosphamide, Oncovin, dexamethasone), and MACOP-B (methotrexate, cyclophosphamide, Oncovin, prednisone, bleomycin) chemotherapy in 115 previously untreated patients with diffuse large cell lymphomas found a correlation of dose intensity with survival as well.[13] In this latter study, a multivariable analysis of prognostic factors showed that the most important predictor of survival was an actual RDI of doxorubicin greater than 75%, 100% being the full dose of doxorubicin in CHOP.

Although these studies suggested that dose intensity is critical to the clinical outcome, randomized trials comparing regimens that differ in dose intensity are required to answer this question. Such a study was performed by Meyer and coworkers in 238 patients with previously untreated advanced-stage, intermediate- and high-grade non-Hodgkin's lymphoma.[14] Patients were randomized to receive either standard (s)-BACOP (bleomycin, Adriamycin [doxorubicin], cyclophosphamide, Oncovin [vincristine], prednisone) chemotherapy or escalated (esc)-BACOP chemotherapy in which a higher doxorubicin dose was administered; the RDI of doxorubicin delivered in the two groups was 80% and 108%, respectively. However, the 28% difference in RDI of doxorubicin did not affect the response and survival rates. A recently published randomized trial comparing CHOP (first-generation regimen) to m-BACOD, ProMACE/cytaBOM (prednisone, methotrexate [with leucovorin rescue], Adriamycin, cyclophosphamide, etoposide/cytarabin, bleomycin, Oncovin), and MACOP-B (second- and third-generation regimens) reached similar conclusions.[10] Although the drugs in these regimens all were delivered at significantly different RDIs (Table 12–1), all four regimens produced similar response rates and disease-free survival at 3 years. The benefit of high-dose–intense therapy, administered with autologous stem cell rescue, has also been tested in patients with previously untreated aggressive non-Hodgkin's lymphomas. In one trial, patients who were slowly responding to

Table 12–1. Comparative Delivered Dose Intensity (DI) of Selected Chemotherapy Regimens (mg/m²/week)°

Drug	CHOP[15]	m-BACOD[16]	Pro-MACE-CytaBOM[17]	MACOP-B[15]	Range of DI
Cyclophosphamide	221	152.9	173.7	155	1.4
Doxorubicin	14.8	11.2	6.6	22	3.3
Vincristine	0.36†	0.28	0.40	0.54†	1.9
Methotrexate	—	73.6	34.9	93.2	2.7
Bleomycin	—	1.1	1.41	2.08	1.9
Cytarabine	—	—	82.6	—	—
Etoposide	—	—	32.7	—	—

°Delivered dose intensity from three different clinical trials.
†Adjusted to ideal m² of 1.7.
See text for chemotherapy abbreviations.

standard CHOP chemotherapy were randomized either to complete a full course of CHOP or to undergo high-dose therapy, and in another trial, patients who achieved a complete response with standard therapy were randomized either to stop or to receive high-dose consolidation.[18, 19] Although the data need to mature, neither trial has demonstrated a benefit for high-dose therapy.

These trials seriously challenge the concept of dose intensity in the design of treatment strategies for non-Hodgkin's lymphomas. However, they should not be interpreted as suggesting that drug dose is not important. Each drug has an individual dose-response curve that is dependent on the drug type and is obviously influenced by the tumor as well. Although this curve may become relatively flat above a threshold dose, we do not know where that threshold lies for any single drug or tumor, so that the clinician should attempt to administer as close to full doses as possible when using a chemotherapy regimen with proven efficacy.

When applying the concept of dose intensity to the design of new therapies, researchers must understand the implications of these clinical trials. They lead to several preliminary but important conclusions. First, the 1.4- to 3.3-fold variation in dose intensity of individual drugs in the first-through third-generation lymphoma regimens does not appear to affect the clinical outcome (see Table 12–1). Second, the large increases in dose intensity, on the order of 5- to 10-fold, achieved with high-dose therapy and autologous stem cell rescue, also does not obviously affect the clinical outcome when used as consolidation in previously untreated patients, although it does allow the apparent cure of a fraction of patients with relapsed aggressive lymphomas. The concept of dose intensity, however, should not be abandoned because not all aspects of the dose intensity question have been fully addressed, and several approaches, as follows, remain to be tested:

1. Strategies that allow repeated treatment with drugs that have steep dose-response curves should be specifically chosen to take maximal advantage of higher fractional kill that may not be curative in a single dose.
2. Major increases in the dose intensity of selected drugs, on the order of threefold to sevenfold, should be the goal.
3. Alternative schedules of drug administration, such as continuous infusion, may allow more dose-intense administration of the natural products (such as doxorubicin, etoposide, and vincristine) with lower toxic-

ity and may partially overcome multidrug resistance (MDR).[20, 21]

Protocols incorporating these approaches are currently being tested in a number of institutions.

Dose intensity depends on the dose interval as well as the total dose. The randomized trials that have assessed the benefit of dose intensity have generally focused on increased drug doses and not on shorter dosing intervals. However, reducing the interval between treatments may be more beneficial for lymphomas that, by comparison to solid tumors, have high proliferation rates. Delays in drug administration may allow the tumor cells to repair cellular damage and lead to regrowth of surviving tumor in the rest period between cycles. Long delays may ultimately allow the selection and outgrowth of drug-resistant clones. Because the minimal interval between chemotherapy cycles is largely dependent on the rate of hematopoietic recovery, recombinant colony-stimulating factors such as GM-CSF, G-CSF, interleukin-3 (IL-3), and IL-3/GM-CSF fusion protein (Pixy) should allow the more rapid administration of chemotherapy cycles.[22, 23] This concept was applied to the development of the MACOP-B regimen where, unlike other regimens for intermediate-grade lymphomas, chemotherapy was given every week for 12 weeks. However, a randomized trial of untreated patients with intermediate-grade lymphomas comparing MACOP-B and CHOP chemotherapy failed to show any clinical difference, indicating that decreasing the treatment interval alone may not have a demonstrable effect on response.[15]

DRUG RESISTANCE

Because non-Hodgkin's lymphomas typically present with disseminated disease, chemotherapy is the mainstay of treatment, and drug resistance becomes the primary barrier to cure. In 1979, Goldie and Coldman proposed a hypothesis to explain the development of resistance to cytotoxic agents by cancer cells.[24] The hypothesis was based on the observation that resistance of *Escherichia coli* to infection by bacteriophage occurs through the preferential expansion of bacterial clones that have undergone mutation to a resistant phenotype.[25] By extrapolation, Goldie and Coldman predicted that the emergence of drug resistance in human tumors would correlate with the underlying spontaneous mutation rate of specific drug-resistance genes. For example, if the rate of mutation to a drug-resistance phenotype is at least 10^{-6}, there is a reasonable probability that at least one drug-resistant clone would emerge after 10^6 cell divisions, a population size below the limits of clinical detection. The emergence of resistant cells may be further hastened by the genomic instability of tumor cells that, in part, results from mutations in the cell cycle regulatory genes such as the *p53* tumor suppressor oncogene and may be further increased by exposure to mutagens such as chemotherapy and irradiation.[26] Under the selective pressure of chemotherapy treatment, resistant clones eventually predominate in the tumor. The model predicts that drug-resistant cells may emerge within a two-log increase in cell number that, in the case of lymphomas with high proliferation rates, may occur within weeks.

The Goldie-Coldman hypothesis has a number of theoretical implications for the design of chemotherapy protocols and provides a rationale for some of the principles already established through empiric observation. In patients with large tumor burdens, there is a high probability that tumor cells resistant to any single cytotoxic drug already exist at the time of initial treatment, providing an explanation for the inverse relationship between tumor cell number and curability, and for the greater efficacy of combination chemotherapy compared with single agents. Unfortunately, combination chemotherapy has not been able to overcome resistance in most cases of clinical cancer treatment. The reasons for this failure are not clearly identified. One factor is that the probability of the emergence of simultaneous resistance to two different classes of drugs is greater than the simple product of the mutation rate conferring resistance to each drug alone. Although a unique mutation may be responsible for resistance to a specific drug, and that drug alone, this is not always the case. A single mutation leading to overexpression of the *BCL2* or *MDR1* proteins, for example, may induce resistance to more than one class of drugs.[27, 28]

A major barrier to the cure of cancer is the development of simultaneous resistance to multiple classes of anticancer drugs, a phenomenon termed "pleiotropic drug resistance."[29, 30] Evidence suggests that the underlying genetic events occur spontaneously and probably relate to the hypermutability of neoplasms. The best understood mechanism of pleiotropic drug resistance results from the increased expression of the multidrug resistance gene *(MDR1)*.[28, 31] MDR confers resistance to a broad spectrum of cytotoxic agents derived from natural products, including anthracyclines, epipodophyllotoxins, vinca alkaloids, taxanes, and some camptothecin derivatives. The product of this gene, the p-glycoprotein (Pgp), functions as a membrane efflux pump that, when overexpressed, decreases intracellular drug levels. In normal cells, Pgp probably functions to eliminate natural environmental toxins that are encountered.[32]

MDR, the most clinically studied mechanism of drug resistance, serves as a paradigm for the development of drug resistance reversal strategies. The first evidence that MDR may be clinically relevant in lymphomas has come from the analysis of *MDR1* RNA and its product, the Pgp expression, in tumor samples from untreated and relapsed lymphoma patients. In studies of tumor samples from untreated patients, increased *MDR1* RNA was found in 4 (22%) of 18 tumor samples, and increased Pgp immunoreactivity was

found in 28 (49%) of 57 tumor samples.[33, 34] However, in the latter study, no correlation between increased expression of Pgp and either response to chemotherapy or overall survival could be found, casting some doubt on the clinical relevance of MDR. In contrast, another study found increased Pgp immunoreactivity only rarely in untreated patients (1 of 39) but commonly in patients with recurrent tumors (5 of 9), suggesting that MDR possibly plays a role in the emergence of clinical drug resistance.[35]

Despite the evidence of increased expression of MDR in lymphomas, the clinical importance of this efflux system can be answered only by clinical trials that address the efficacy of MDR-reversing agents. Although a number of candidate reversing agents, including verapamil, amiodarone, quinidine, and cyclosporine, all have undergone limited testing in various solid tumors, leukemias, and lymphomas, the trial designs lacked adequate controls.[36–40] In one such trial, Miller and associates added verapamil to a regimen of infusional C-VAD (cyclophosphamide, vincristine, Adriamycin, dexamethasone) chemotherapy in 18 patients with relapsed non-Hodgkin's lymphomas.[35] All patients either had progressed or had an incomplete response to a bolus vincristine/doxorubicin–containing regimen or had relapsed within 3 months of receiving these agents, but it was never established whether the patients were truly resistant to infusional C-VAD. The response rate to C-VAD/verapamil was excellent with 11 (79%) of 14 patients achieving objective responses, although there was no correlation between response and Pgp. These results suggest that the change to an infusional regimen by itself might have been responsible for the high response rate, independent of the inhibition of Pgp by verapamil.

The pitfalls of the trial design used by Miller and associates can be partially overcome by using a crossover strategy in which patients receive the reversing agent plus chemotherapy only after demonstrating resistance (persistent or progressive disease) to the basic chemotherapy regimen by itself. We employed this design in a study of dexverapamil, the dextrorotatory isomer of verapamil, and EPOCH (etoposide, prednisone, Oncovin, cyclophosphamide, Halotestin) chemotherapy in patients with EPOCH-resistant lymphomas.[20, 41] An infusional schedule was chosen for the natural products based on studies in an *MDR1*-expressing colon cell line in which resistance to doxorubicin or vincristine was partially reversed by continuous low-dose exposure, compared with short high-dose exposure.[21] With EPOCH alone, 88 (87%) of 101 patients with non-Hodgkin's lymphoma who had relapsed or become refractory following bolus doxorubicin/vincristine–containing regimens achieved either a complete or partial response.[41] Of these patients, 41 were crossed over to receive dexverapamil at the time they were no longer responding to EPOCH alone and were evaluable for response; the addition of dexverapamil produced three complete (75%), two partial (12%), and five (12%) minor responses.[41] Although the response rate following the addition of dexverapamil was modest, it is important to recognize that the crossover design may have militated against a response by having required a tumor to fail a regimen before addition of a Pgp blocker. Indeed, selection for multiple mechanisms of drug resistance, among them *MDR1*, must occur. Of interest was that *MDR1* expression, determined by quantitative polymerase chain

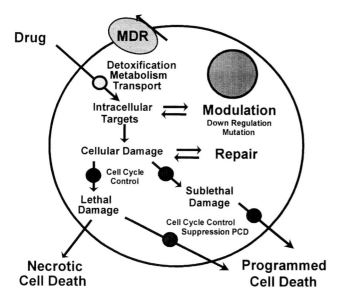

Figure 12–1. Drug resistance mechanisms. MDR, multidrug resistance; PCD, programmed cell death.

reaction, was low in all 17 pretreatment biopsy specimens but was high in 8 of 16 biopsy specimens obtained at the time of crossover to dexverapamil. Furthermore, of six evaluable patients with high *MDR1* levels, three responded to the addition of dexverapamil, whereas only one of eight patients with low *MDR1* levels responded, suggesting that *MDR1* may have played a role in the drug resistance of some patients.

From these preliminary data, a number of conclusions regarding clinical drug resistance in lymphomas can be made. First, *MDR1* is expressed at low levels in untreated patients but may be readily detected at the time of treatment failure. However, other mechanisms of drug resistance must also occur, since most drug-resistant patients do not express high levels of Pgp. Second, the high response rates achieved with EPOCH alone suggest that infusional schedules for the natural products may be more effective than bolus schedules, possibly by partially overcoming drug resistance. Third, the reversal of resistance by dexverapamil in selected cases suggests that MDR is clinically significant in a subset of relapsed or refractory patients. Clearly, further studies are needed to establish the significance of Pgp in clinical drug resistance. Ultimately, reversal strategies for MDR need to be tested in untreated patients to determine if this approach can increase the cure rate of these tumors.

Even if MDR proves to be clinically relevant in lymphomas, its high degree of expression in only a few relapsed patients suggests that the successful reversal of this mechanism alone will not lead to major improvements in therapeutic outcome. As shown in Figure 12–1, multiple mechanisms other than MDR exist by which a cell develops drug resistance. These mechanisms may be drug specific, such as the modulation of a drug target by mutation or altered regulation, or more general, as occurs with increased drug metabolism, transport, or detoxification by glutathione, for example.

Once damage has occurred to vital proteins or DNA, or both, the cell can undergo repair, thereby reversing the cytotoxic effects. The desired effect of cytotoxic therapy, of course, is death of the neoplastic cell, an event accomplished through either cellular necrosis or active cell death.[42] Recent evidence suggests that the cellular apparatus that controls the cell cycle is an essential component of the final common pathways through which cytotoxic agents exert their lethal effects.[1–3, 42] If this proves to be correct, deregulation at any number of steps in this pathway could lead to drug resistance. Among the most common oncogene or tumor suppressor gene mutations found in lymphoid neoplasms are those that occur in cell cycle control genes, further highlighting the central importance of these pathways in the basic biology of neoplasia. Although the clinical significance of these mutations with respect to drug resistance is not established, they are among the most important candidates for investigation.[1–3, 43, 44] The biologic impact of these mutations on tumor cells is discussed in the following section.

PROGRAMMED CELL DEATH AND CELL CYCLE CONTROL IN LYMPHOMAS

Like normal tissues, tumors are composed of mixtures of cells, some of which are undergoing replication while others are resting and still others are undergoing active cell death. The death of malignant cells, like their normal counterparts, may occur by necrosis or by PCD (apoptosis), an active mechanism of cell death characterized by cleavage of cellular DNA into nucleosome-sized fragments (DNA ladder), chromatin condensation, and nuclear fragmentation.[42] The process of PCD can be triggered through multiple pathways, including exposure to chemotherapeutic agents, the loss of essential growth factors, exposure to negative regulators such as tumor necrosis factor (TNF) and transforming growth factor-β (TGF-β), and the loss or induction of specific genes such as c-*myc* and *p53* (Fig. 12–2).[42, 45, 46] Other events suppress PCD, such as the addition of growth factors and the induction or suppression of specific genes and viral proteins.[3, 42, 45, 47] Although pathways leading to PCD are present in many tumor cells, some of the triggering pathways may be disrupted and absent, and experimental evidence

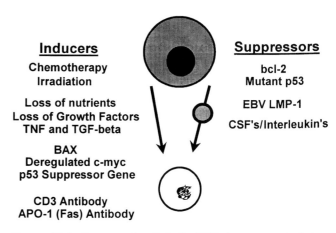

Figure 12–2. Programmed cell death. TNF, tumor necrosis factor; TGF-beta, transforming growth factor-beta; EBV, Epstein-Barr virus; CSF, colony-stimulating factor.

suggests that disruption of these pathways increases the resistance of cancer cells to cytotoxic agents.[1–3, 43, 48, 49]

Abnormalities in the induction of PCD appear to be particularly important in the biology of lymphomas. Indeed, PCD plays a central role in the normal biology of lymphocytes and in the process of clonal deletion.[50] At least two genes (*BCL2* and *p53*) that can affect PCD have been found to be either abnormal or deregulated in lymphomas.[48, 49] Translocations of *BCL2*, located on chromosome 18, to the immunoglobulin (Ig) heavy-chain locus on chromosome 14 (t[14;18]) is present in as many as 85% of follicular lymphomas.[51, 52] This translocation results in elevated levels of the *BCL2* protein product and prolongs cell survival by blocking PCD.[45, 51] Although *BCL2* gene rearrangements are infrequent (approximately 10%) in aggressive lymphomas, significant levels of *BCL2* protein may be detected, suggesting it plays a role in these tumors as well.[53, 54] Viral genes such as Epstein-Barr virus LMP-1, frequently present in Burkitt's lymphomas, can induce expression of *BCL2* and protect cells from PCD. Recently, a second protein, called "BAX," has been identified that blocks the PCD-repressor activity of *BCL2*.[55] The BAX protein, which shares significant homology with *BCL2*, is in equilibrium between homodimerization with itself and heterodimerization with *BCL2*, and it is this ratio that appears to regulate *BCL2* function. When overexpressed, BAX accelerates PCD following a death signal, such as withdrawal of an essential growth factor.

The PCD-repressor activity of *BCL2* affects drug sensitivity. In vitro, cells that express increased levels of *BCL2* are resistant to radiation- and chemotherapy-induced PCD. For example, transfection of *BCL2* into a murine prolymphoid progenitor cell line confers a twofold resistance to the lethal effects of nitrogen mustard and camptothecin by inhibiting PCD.[1] Furthermore, in leukemias, a high level of *BCL2* expression correlated with resistance to several PCD-inducing cytotoxic agents, including doxorubicin, methotrexate, and cytarabine.[56]

The *p53* tumor suppressor gene plays an important role in PCD as well. *P53* controls the cellular responses to DNA damage by arresting cells in G_1 of the cell cycle so that repair of DNA damage may occur before the cell proceeds through DNA synthesis and mitosis; if essential repairs are not possible, *p53* may trigger PCD.[26] For example, *p53* expression increases in cells exposed to DNA-damaging agents and in prostate epithelial cells undergoing PCD following male hormone depletion.[42] Thus, *p53* monitors the fidelity of DNA and reduces the inherent mutability of the genome. The importance of *p53* mutations in the development of the malignant phenotype is suggested by the presence of *p53* mutations in most types of cancers, including chronic lymphocytic leukemias (CLLs) and lymphomas.[1, 48, 57] Mutant *p53* has been detected in tumor biopsy specimens from as many as 15% of CLL patients and 33% of non-Hodgkin's lymphoma patients, and in even higher proportions in biopsy specimens from heavily pretreated patients.[1, 48]

Mutations in the *p53* gene are associated with elevated levels of mutant *p53* protein that inactivate wild-type *p53* and cause profound biologic effects. Because the normal function of wild-type *p53* is to arrest cells in G_1 to allow DNA repair and to promote PCD, inhibition of these activities by

mutant *p53* can lead to genomic instability and a hypermutable state.[26, 56] In vitro, this is reflected by cellular resistance to both radiation therapy and chemotherapy.[1, 2] Moreover, in a drug-resistant human lung cancer cell in which both alleles of *p53* were deleted, chemosensitivity could be restored by transfer of the wild-type *p53* gene into the cells.[58] The hypermutable state that may result from inhibition of normal *p53* theoretically could promote the rapid emergence of resistant clones.

Increased expression of mutant *p53* as well as *BCL2* can also promote the oncogenic potential of c-*myc*. Deregulated c-*myc* by itself has a variety of effects, including enhancement and induction of PCD, induction of cellular proliferation, and inhibition of differentiation.[56, 59] Suppression of the PCD-enhancing effect of deregulated c-*myc* by *BCL2* and/or mutant *p53* allows expression of c-*myc* and an unopposed proliferative signal.

Another molecular abnormality found in a specific lymphoma subtype, called mantle cell, results in the deregulation of the G_1 cell cycle checkpoint.[60] Most mantle cell lymphomas have a reciprocal 11;14 translocation involving chromosome 11q13, which carries the *BCL1* gene, and the Ig heavy-chain locus on chromosome 14q32, resulting in overexpression of *BCL1*. The product of *BCL1*, cyclin D1, belongs to a class of proteins (i.e., cyclins) that initiate mitosis.[61] Although the significance of cyclin D1 in mantle cell lymphomas is not clearly understood, its overexpression would appear to overcome an early G_1 checkpoint.

Although the effect of abnormal cell cycle control on clinical drug resistance is poorly understood, there is reason to believe that their regulation is important for the curability of lymphomas. In follicular lymphomas, for example, the deregulation of *BCL2* inhibits PCD and may increase cellular resistance to chemotherapy and lead to a low probability of cure. A provocative observation is that *BCL2* protein expression is often lower in follicular lymphoma cells that have undergone histologic transformation to a more aggressive lymphoma (Jaffe E, personal communication, 1996). Despite the poorer prognosis associated with histologic transformation, such patients may achieve a long-term complete remission with chemotherapy.[62] Over time, however, tumors may develop mutations in the *p53* gene. In a study of B-cell CLL, *p53* mutations were only detected in the tumor cells from 14% of patients tested; however, compared with CLL patients with normal *p53*, these patients had a low likelihood of responding to chemotherapy and a 13-fold increased risk of death.[1] Furthermore, an increased incidence of *p53* mutations have been found in the tumor cells from patients with Richter's transformation.[48] Similar correlations between *p53* mutations and drug resistance in non-Hodgkin's lymphomas have been described as well.[63] In high-grade Burkitt's lymphomas, the coexpression of deregulated c-*myc* and mutant *p53* may produce a rapidly proliferating and drug-resistant tumor.

Thus, there is sufficient evidence to warrant the development of clinical strategies to overcome the deregulation of PCD and cell cycle control. Drugs and therapeutic peptides could be identified that reverse the deregulation of these pathways. A number of potential targets for therapeutic intervention exist, including inhibition of *BCL2* expression or protein activity; upregulation of neutralizing proteins such as mdm-2 or BAX that inhibit *p53* or *BCL2*, respectively; suppression of mutant *p53* or increased normal *p53* expression, or both; and suppression of other oncogenes such as c-*myc*. Specific therapeutic approaches, some of which are under active investigation, include development of antiidiotype therapy and immunotherapy with cytotoxic T cells that can induce *BCL2*-independent PCD, and biologic therapy with agents such as TGF-β and TNF that may induce PCD.[64, 65] Ultimately, novel approaches such as these, when used in combination with conventional chemotherapy, may lead to a significant increase in the cure rate of non-Hodgkin's lymphomas.

NEW DIRECTIONS FOR ANTILYMPHOMA THERAPY

Table 12–2 contains a summary of the primary pharmacologic properties of the commonly used agents. However, it is not the purpose of this chapter to describe in depth the pharmacologic properties of the important anticancer drugs, as has been done in the major textbooks of pharmacology and cancer medicine.[66, 67] Rather, the important future directions for chemotherapy research related to lymphomas are indicated.

The most promising new compounds for treatment of lymphoid malignancies belong to the general class of antipurines.[68] 2'-Deoxycoformycin, an inhibitor of adenosine deaminase, has particular effectiveness in hairy cell leukemia but little activity in other lymphoid cancer.[69] Two newer compounds, fludarabine phosphate (FDA) and 2-chloro-2'-deoxyadenosine (CdA), have a broader activity range that includes the low-grade lymphomas and CLLs.[70–76] Both the latter compounds are resistant to deamination and share a common mechanism of activation (deoxycytidine kinase converts them to a monophosphate).[77] As triphosphates, CdA and fludarabine inhibit ribonucleotide reduction, inhibit DNA repair and DNA elongation during DNA synthesis, and become incorporated into DNA.[76] However, the ultimate cause of cell death of these two drugs remains obscure. From studies of their effect in CLL, these two analogues appear to be clinically cross resistant in some but not all cases.[76, 78, 79] In addition to its cytotoxic properties, fludarabine also potentiates radiation damage by inhibiting repair of strand breaks, the greatest effect occurring when the drug was administered to tumor-bearing mice 24 hours prior to radiation therapy.[80] The synergy observed between radiation therapy and fludarabine may also result from blockade of cells at the G_1/S boundary by fludarabine, with release of a synchronized population and enhanced sensitivity of S-phase cells to subsequent inactivation. Neither CdA nor fludarabine has yet been used in combination with other drugs or with irradiation for treatment of lymphoma; however, because of their level of activity as single agents and lack of cross resistance with other agents, they certainly deserve careful evaluation in primary regimens. The only exception to their lack of cross resistance with standard agents may be potential cross resistance with cytosine arabinoside, which is also activated by deoxycytidine kinase.

Among other promising agents, only the camptothecins and paclitaxel (Taxol) have shown evidence of activity in lymphoma. Early phase II trials of CPT-11, a camptothecin analogue and prodrug for an active metabolite (SN-38), disclosed a 38% response rate in a pretreated group of lymphoma patients with both indolent and aggressive histology.[81] The camptothecins attack a unique target (topoisomerase I) and, with the exception of topotecan, are not subject to classic MDR.[82] Interest in these drugs as antilymphoma agents is likely to grow as clinical experience in their use for treating other solid tumors such as colon cancer, non–small cell lung cancer, and leukemia accumulates.

A second group of interesting new agents, the taxanes, have at least minimal activity in lymphomas. One recent phase II trial describes a 17% response rate to paclitaxel in patients with relapsed low- and intermediate-grade lymphoma, but the experience is too limited to draw any final conclusions.[83] Experimental studies of cross resistance indicate that paclitaxel, which stabilizes microtubules and prevents the continuous dynamic remodeling of this key structural protein, remains active against cells that develop resistance to the vinca alkaloids on the basis of tubulin mutations.[84] However, the taxanes and vinca alkaloids do share cross resistance in cells expressing MDR-type resistance.[85] Despite extensive evidence of activity of paclitaxel and docetaxel (Taxotere) as single agents in ovarian cancer, breast cancer, and other solid tumors, little is known about the use of these drugs in combination therapy. Experimental evidence suggests that their interaction with cisplatin, anthracyclines, and alkylating agents may be highly schedule dependent and often antagonistic, particularly when paclitaxel is given simultaneously with or following cisplatin or anthracyclines.[86]

PROSPECTS FOR NEW AGENTS

Although the pace for identification of new agents for treating lymphomas has been slow, strategies for drug discovery are changing. At the National Cancer Institute (NCI), human cell line screens have replaced traditional murine leukemias as the primary discovery tool, and although lymphomas are not part of the primary panel, active new drugs identified in the primary 60-cell line panel are then screened against a set of acquired immunodeficiency syndrome–related lymphoma cell lines to expedite the recognition of agents active in this set of neoplasms.[87] The emphasis of NCI screening has shifted from synthetic chemicals to natural products, and a series of novel structures with unique sites of action have shown sufficient preclinical activity to warrant preclinical evaluation. The NCI screening approach has been supplemented by the development of computer-based programs that allow recognition of patterns of cell line response that reflect drug interactions with specific molecular targets, identify specific mechanisms of drug action, and provide clues to mechanisms of drug resistance.[88] In this way, the initial screening information, derived from responses of the primary 60 cell lines, provides important leads that determine NCI's interest in further compound evaluation and development.

Complementary to the NCI discovery effort, biotechnology companies have targeted specific molecular processes as

Table 12–2. Dose, Toxicity, and Mechanism of Resistance of Major Antineoplastic Agents for Lymphomas

Class	Dose[a] (mg/m²)	Dose Frequency	Acute Toxicity — Leukocyte	Platelet	Nausea and Vomiting	Other Toxicity	Mechanism of Drug Resistance
Tubulin Binding Agents							
Paclitaxel	130–250 IV	q 3 wk	Marked	Moderate	Mild	Anaphylactoid response, sensory neuropathy, alopecia	Transport, tubulin mutants
Vincristine	1–1.4 IV	q wk	Mild	Mild	Mild	Distal neuropathy, inappropriate ADH	Transport, tubulin mutants
Vinblastine	6 IV	q wk	Marked	Moderate–marked	Mild	Mucositis	Transport, tubulin mutants
Topoisomerase II Inhibitors							
Etoposide	100–200 IV	q 3–4 wk	Moderate	Mild	Mild	Mucositis	Transport, target modulation
Mitoxantrone	12–14 IV	q 3–4 wk	Marked	Moderate	Mild	Cholestasis, cardiac	Transport, target modulation
Doxorubicin	25–75 IV	q 3–4 wk	Marked	Marked	Moderate	Alopecia, cardiomyopathy	Transport, target modulation
Idarubicin	10–15 IV	q 3–4 wk	Marked	Marked	Moderate	Alopecia, mucositis, cardiomyopathy	Transport, target modulation
Antimetabolites							
Methotrexate	100–400 IV	q 3–4 wk	Moderate–marked	Moderate	Mild	Stomatitis	↓Polyglutamation, transport, ↑DHFR
Cytarabine (cytosine arabinoside)	300–4000 IV	q 3–4 wk	Marked	Marked	Moderate	Cholestasis, mucositis, neurotoxicity	↓Activation, ?transport
Deoxycoformycin	4 IV	q 1–2 wk	Mild	Mild	Mild	Neurotoxicity (at high doses), conjunctivitis	Not known, ?↑adenosine deaminase
2-Chloro-2′-deoxyadenosine	4 IV	qd × 7	Mild	Moderate	Mild	Immune suppression	Not known
Fludarabine	20–25 IV	qd × 5	Moderate–marked	Mild	Mild	Neurotoxicity, stomatitis, hepatitis	↓Activation
Alkylating Agents							
Cyclophosphamide	350–1500 IV	q 3–4 wk	Marked	Mild	Moderate	Cystitis, pulmonary fibrosis, water retention	↑Metabolic detoxification, repair of DNA
Ifosfamide	1000 IV	qd × 5 with mesna	Moderate–marked	Moderate	Mild	Nephrotoxicity, cystitis, neurotoxicity	↑Metabolic detoxification, repair of DNA
Mechlorethamine	6 IV	q 2–4 wk	Marked	Moderate	Moderate	Leukemia	Detoxification, repair of DNA
Chlorambucil	1–3 PO	qd	Moderate	Moderate	Mild	Leukemia	Detoxification, repair of DNA
Dacarbazine	150 IV	qd × 5	Mild	Mild	Marked	Flulike syndrome, venoocclusive	⎫
Procarbazine	100 PO	qd × 7–14 d	Moderate	Moderate	Mild	Sensitivity to amines, sterility, leukemia	⎬ Detoxification, repair of DNA by guanine alkyl transferase
CCNU	100–150 PO	q 4 wk	Marked	Marked	Moderate	Leukemia, pulmonary fibrosis, renal failure	⎭
Miscellaneous							
Bleomycin	5–10 IV	q 2–4 wk	Rare	Rare	Mild	Skin, pulmonary fibrosis, fever, hypersensitivity reactions	Metabolism repair
Cisplatin	50–100 IV	q 3–4 wk	Mild	Moderate	Severe	Renal failure, Mg²⁺ wasting, peripheral neuropathy, anemia	Transport, detoxification, repair of DNA

[a]Doses per cycle are typical of those used in combination regimens, but appropriate modification must be made depending on other drugs used, organ dysfunction, and other considerations.
ADH, antidiuretic hormone; DHFR, dihydrofolate reductase.

Table 12–3. Drug-Biologic Interactions

Biologic	Combined With	Effect of Biologic	Reference No.
IL-1	Chemotherapy	Enhanced cytotoxicity	94
Anti-her2/neu	Cisplatin	Enhanced cytotoxicity	95
Anti-EGF	Cisplatin	Enhanced cytotoxicity	96
GM-CSF, IL-3	Cytarabine	Enhanced cytotoxicity for AML	9
TGF-β	Chemotherapy	Protects bone marrow	97
IFN	5-Fluorouracil	Decreases compensatory rise in target enzyme (TS)	93

IL-1, interleukin-1; anti-EGF, anti-epidermal growth factor; AML, acute myelocytic leukemia; TS, thymidylate synthase; GM-CSF, granulocyte-macrophage colony-stimulating factor; TGF-β, transforming growth factor-β; IFN, interferon.

the foundation for their drug discovery strategy. These targets include tyrosine kinases that transduce growth signals and regulate cell cycle progression, and proteins that control apoptosis and other important pathways in growth, differentiation, and cell death.[89] To simplify the process of finding lead compounds that interact with these targets, companies have developed automated processes for detecting interactions of a target protein, peptide or nucleic acid sequence with large libraries of randomly generated peptides, oligonucleotides, or synthetic chemicals.[90, 91] The lead ligand thus identified then becomes the object of rational chemical design to enhance its binding to the target and to incorporate desirable pharmacologic features such as stability, solubility, and a favorable toxicologic profile. The success of approaches directed at a specific molecular target obviously depends on the wisdom of the initial choice of a suitable target, a choice that may be based on compelling logic but may prove elusive or unimportant in practice. In addition to the complexity of finding new molecules that interact with these targets, these efforts must successfully refine lead compounds so that they have requisite pharmacologic properties and are able to pass the cell membrane and persist as active agents in the living host.

PROTOCOL DESIGN

Historically, combination chemotherapy empirically evolved out of a need for more effective treatments than were produced by single agents. The development of combination chemotherapy regimens has been and continues to be largely empiric, particularly for the non-Hodgkin's lymphomas. More recently, however, strategies based on pharmacologic considerations such as drug intensification and reversal of drug resistance, and biologic and immunologic approaches are increasingly incorporated into the design of new regimens.

When developing a new chemotherapy regimen, several basic principles should be followed. First and foremost, drugs with the best single-agent activity should be chosen, and attention must be paid to both potential synergism and antagonism.[11] Experimentally, for example, combinations of ifosfamide and etoposide, and cytarabine and etoposide are synergistic, whereas paclitaxel and doxorubicin, and camptothecin and etoposide are antagonistic. Selection of drugs with nonoverlapping toxicities will allow the administration of higher doses with less toxicity. The choice of dose, rate, and route of drug administration (e.g., oral, or intravenous bolus or infusion) should be based on the pharmacokinetics of the drugs in question and on existing information regarding the maximal tolerated doses for any given schedule. Experimental modeling of administration schedules (e.g., bolus or continuous infusion), timing of administration, and drug interactions can be useful. For example, cisplatin significantly affects the clearance of paclitaxel when administered first, thereby increasing the toxicity of the combination.[92]

A promising area of research in clinical treatment involves the modulation of drug resistance. Theoretically, following the entry of a cytotoxic agent into a tumor cell, any of the multiple events that lead to cell death are potential targets for modulation (see Fig. 12–1). For example, clinical strategies to block the efflux of natural products by the P-170 pump, or to inhibit the detoxification of alkylating agents by glutathione transferase may potentially increase the sensitivity of tumor cells to chemotherapy, and are under active investigation. Furthermore, agents that modulate the levels of the intracellular drug targets for specific cytotoxic drugs are being investigated in vitro, and candidate drugs such as interferon-γ, a modulator of thymidylate synthase, are being clinically tested.[93] As previously discussed, modulation of cell cycle checkpoints can also significantly affect drug sensitivity, and regulation of these checkpoints is another important strategy for future therapies. Finally, biologically oriented therapies (such as immunotherapy with lymphokine-activated cells, natural killer cells and cytotoxic T cells, free antibodies, immunotoxins, vaccines, cytokines, and other proteins such as TNF and TGF-β) are in early stages of clinical evaluation. Some of these (e.g., IL-1, anti-epidermal growth factor, and anti-her 2/neu antibodies) sensitize experimental tumor to cytotoxic agents and may have value in combination with drugs.[94–96] Others (e.g., marrow stimulating and suppressing factors) may enhance recovery of normal tissues or protect them from drug or radiation damage (Table 12–3). Ultimately, however, treatment regimens are judged by results, and since so many variables impact on the outcome of chemotherapy, it must be recognized that there still remains a large element of empiricism in protocol design.

REFERENCES

1. El Rouby S, Thomas A, Costin D, et al: p53 gene mutation in B-cell chronic lymphocytic leukemia is associated with drug resistance and is independent of MDR1/MDR3 gene expression. Blood 1993; 82:3452.

2. O'Connor PM, Jackman J, Jondle D, et al: Role of the p53 tumor suppressor gene in cell cycle arrest and radiosensitivity of Burkitt's lymphoma cell lines. Cancer Res 1993; 53:4776.

3. Lowe SW, Schmitt EM, Smith SW, et al: p53 is required for radiation-induced apoptosis in mouse thymocytes. Nature 1993; 362:847.

4. Skipper HE, Schabel F, Wilcox WS: Experimental evaluation of potential anticancer agents: XIII. On the criteria and kinetics associated with "curability" of experimental leukemia. Cancer Chemother Rep 1964; 35:1.

5. Longo DL, Wilson WH: Follicular lymphomas. In Magrath IT (ed): The Non-Hodgkin's Lymphomas. Baltimore, Williams & Wilkins, 1990, pp 293–308.

6. Schabel FM Jr, Simpson-Herren L: Cell kinetics and pharmacodynamics of anticancer drugs. Fundam Cancer Chemother Antibiot Chemother 1978; 23:113.

7. Magrath IT, Lwanga S, Carswell W, Harrison N: Surgical reduction of tumour bulk in management of abdominal Burkitt's lymphoma. Br Med J 1974; 2:308.

8. Frei E III, Teicher BA, Holden SA, et al: Effect of alkylating agent dose: Preclinical studies and possible clinical correlation. Cancer Res 1988; 48:6417.

9. Aglietta M, DeFelice L, Stacchini A, at al: In vivo effect of granulocyte-macrophage colony-stimulating factor on the kinetics of human acute myeloid leukemia cells. Leukemia 1991; 5:979.

10. Fisher RI, Gaynor ER, Dahlberg S, et al: Comparison of a standard regimen (CHOP) with three intensive chemotherapy regimens for advanced non-Hodgkin's lymphoma. N Engl J Med 1993; 328:1002.

11. DeVita VT Jr: Principles of chemotherapy. In DeVita VT Jr, Hellman S, Rosenberg SA (eds): Cancer: Principles and Practice of Oncology. Philadelphia, JB Lippincott, 1988, pp 257–285.

12. DeVita VT Jr, Hubbard SM, Longo DL: The chemotherapy of lymphomas: Looking back, moving forward. Cancer Res 1987; 47:5810.

13. Kwak LW, Halpern J, Olshen RA, Horning SJ: Prognostic significance of actual dose intensity in diffuse large cell lymphoma: Results of a tree-structured survival analysis. J Clin Oncol 1990; 8:963.

14. Meyer RM, Quirt IC, Skillings JR, et al: Escalated as compared with standard doses of doxorubicin in BACOP therapy for patients with non-Hodgkin's lymphoma. N Engl J Med 1993; 329:1770.

15. Cooper IA, Wolf MM, Robertson TI, et al: Randomized comparison of MACOP-B with CHOP in patients with intermediate-grade non-Hodgkin's lymphoma. J Clin Oncol 1994; 12:769.

16. Dana BW, Dahlberg S, Miller TP, et al: m-BACOD treatment for intermediate- and high-grade malignant lymphomas: A Southwest Oncology Group phase II trial. J Clin Oncol 1990; 8:1155.

17. Longo DL, DeVita VT Jr, Duffey PL, et al: Superiority of ProMACE over ProMACE-MOPP in the treatment of advanced diffuse aggressive lymphoma: Results of a prospective randomized trial. J Clin Oncol 1991; 9:25.

18. Hagenbeek A, Verdonck L, Sonneveld P, et al: CHOP chemotherapy versus autologous bone marrow transplantation in slowly responding patients with intermediate- and high-grade malignant non-Hodgkin's lymphoma: Results from a prospective randomized phase III clinical trial in 294 patients [Abstract]. Proc Am Soc Hematol (Blood) 1994; 82:332a.

19. Haioun C, Lepage E, Gisselbrecht C, et al: Autologous bone marrow transplantation (ABMT) versus sequential chemotherapy in first complete remission of aggressive non-Hodgkin's lymphoma (NHL): First interim analysis on 370 patients (LNH87 protocol) [Abstract]. Proc Am Soc Clin Oncol 1992; 11:316.

20. Wilson WH, Bryant G, Bates S, et al: EPOCH chemotherapy: Toxicity and efficacy in relapsed and refractory non-Hodgkin's lymphoma. J Clin Oncol 1993; 11:1573.

21. Lai G-M, Chen Y-N, Mickley LA, et al: P-glycoprotein expression and schedule dependence of Adriamycin cytotoxicity in human colon carcinoma cell lines. Int J Cancer 1991; 49:696.

22. Ema H, Suda T, Sakamoto S, et al: Effects of the in vivo administration of recombinant human granulocyte colony-stimulating factor following cytotoxic chemotherapy on granulocytic precursors in patients with malignant lymphoma. Jpn J Cancer Res 1989; 80:577.

23. Gerhartz HH, Engelhard M, Meusers P, et al: Randomized, double-blind, placebo-controlled, phase III study of recombinant human granulocyte-macrophage colony-stimulating factor as adjunct to induction treatment of high-grade malignant non-Hodgkin's lymphomas. Blood 1993; 82:2329.

24. Goldie JH, Coldman AJ: A mathematic model for relating the drug sensitivity of tumors to their spontaneous mutation rate. Cancer Treat Rep 1979; 63:1717.

25. Luria SE, Delbruck M: Mutations of bacteria from virus sensitivity to virus resistance. Genetics 28:491, 1943.

26. Harris CC, Hollstein M: Clinical implications of the p53 tumor-suppressor gene. N Engl J Med 1993; 329:1318.

27. Moscow JA, Cowan KH: Multidrug resistance. J Natl Cancer Inst 1988; 80:14.

28. Gros P, Ben Neriah YB, Croop JM, Housman DE: Isolation and expression of a complementary DNA that confers multidrug resistance. Nature 1986; 323:728.

29. Ling V, Thompson LH: Reduced permeability in CHO cells as a mechanism of resistance to colchicine. J Cell Physiol 1974; 83:103.

30. Bech-Hansen NT, Till JE, Ling V: Pleiotropic phenotype of colchicine-resistant CHO cells: Cross resistance and collateral sensitivity. J Cell Physiol 1976; 88:23.

31. Gros P, Croop J, Housman D: Mammalian multidrug resistance gene: Complete cDNA sequence indicates strong homology to bacterial transport proteins. Cell 1986; 47:371.

32. Fojo AT, Ueda K, Slamon DJ, et al: Expression of a multidrug-resistance gene in human tumors and tissues. Proc Natl Acad Sci U S A 1987; 84:265.

33. Goldstein LJ, Galski H, Fojo A, et al: Expression of a multidrug resistance gene in human cancers. J Natl Cancer Inst 1989; 81:116.

34. Nichans GA, Jaszcz W, Brunetto V, et al: Immunohistochemical identification of P-glycoprotein in previously untreated, diffuse large cell, and immunoblastic lymphomas. Cancer Res 1992; 52:3768.

35. Miller TP, Grogan TM, Dalton WS, et al: P-glycoprotein expression in malignant lymphoma and reversal of clinical drug resistance with chemotherapy plus high-dose verapamil. J Clin Oncol 1991; 1:17.

36. Bates SE, Denicoff AM, Cowan K, et al: A study of MDR-1 expression and pharmacologic reversal in human breast cancer [Abstract]. Proc Am Soc Clin Oncol 1991; 10:68.

37. Fojo T, McAtee N, Allegra C, et al: Use of quinidine and amiodarone to modulate multidrug resistance mediated by the mdr-1 gene [Abstract]. Proc Am Soc Clin Oncol 1989; 8:68.

38. Eliason JF, Ramuz H, Kaufmann F: Human multidrug-resistant cancer cells exhibit a high degree of selectivity for stereoisomers of verapamil and quinidine. Int J Cancer 1990; 46:113.

39. Dalton WS, Grogan TM, Meltzer PS, et al: Drug-resistance in multiple myeloma and non-Hodgkin's lymphoma: Detection of P-glycoprotein and potential circumvention by addition of verapamil to chemotherapy. J Clin Oncol 1989; 7:415.

40. List AF, Spier C, Greer J, et al: Phase I/II trial of cyclosporine as a chemotherapy-resistance modifier in acute leukemia. J Clin Oncol 1993; 11:1652.

41. Wilson WH, Bates S, Fojo A, et al: A controlled trial of dexverapamil, a modulator of multidrug resistance, in lymphomas refractory to EPOCH chemotherapy. J Clin Oncol 1995; 13:1995.

42. Sachs L, Lotem J: Control of programmed cell death in normal and leukemic cells: New implications for therapy. Blood 1993; 82:15.

43. Walton MI, Whysong D, O'Connor PM, et al: Constitutive expression of human Bcl-2 modulates nitrogen mustard and camptothecin-induced apoptosis. Cancer Res 1993; 53:1853.

44. Solary E, Bertrand R, Kohn K, Pommier Y: Differential induction of apoptosis in undifferentiated and differentiated HL-60 cells by DNA topoisomerase I and II inhibitors. Blood 1993; 81:1359.

45. Hockenberry D, Nunez G, Milliman C, et al: Bcl-2 is an inner mitochondrial membrane protein that blocks programmed cell death. Nature 1990; 348:334.

46. Clarke AR, Purdie CA, Harrison DJ, et al: Thymocyte apoptosis induced by p53-dependent and -independent pathways. Nature 1993; 362:849.

47. Dancescu M, Rubio-Trujillo M, Biron G, et al: Interleukin 4 protects chronic lymphocytic leukemic B cells from death by apoptosis and upregulates Bcl-2 expression. J Exp Med 1992; 176:1319.

48. Gaidano G, Ballerini P, Gong JZ, et al: p53 mutations in human lymphoid malignancies: Association with Burkitt lymphoma and chronic lymphocytic leukemia. Proc Natl Acad Sci U S A 1991; 88:5413.

49. Zutter M, Hockenberry D, Silverman GA, Korsmeyer SJ: Immunolocalization of the Bcl-2 protein within hematopoietic neoplasms. Blood 1991; 78:1062.

50. Arends MJ, Wyllie AH: Apoptosis: Mechanisms and roles in pathology. Int Rev Exp Pathol 1991; 32:223.

51. Tsujimoto Y, Gorham G, Cossman J, et al: The t(14;18) chromosome translocations involved in B-cell neoplasms result from mistakes in VDJ joining. Science 1985; 229:1390.

52. Yunis JJ, Frizzera G, Oken MM, et al: Multiple recurrent genomic defects in follicular lymphoma: A possible model for cancer. N Engl J Med 1987; 316:79.

53. Kondo E, Nakamura S, Onoue H, et al: Detection of bcl-2 messenger RNA in normal and neoplastic lymphoid tissues by immunohistochemistry and in situ hybridization. Blood 1992; 80:2044.

54. Pezzella F, Tse AGD, Cordell JL, et al: Expression of the bcl-2 oncogene protein is not specific for the 14;18 chromosomal translocation. Am J Pathol 1990; 137:225.

55. Oltvai ZN, Milliman CL, Korsmeyer SJ: Bcl-2 heterodimerizes in vivo with a conserved homolog, Bax, that accelerates programmed cell death. Cell 1993; 74:609.

56. Lotem J, Sachs L: Regulation by bcl-2, c-myc, and p53 of susceptibility to induction of apoptosis by heat shock and cancer chemotherapy compounds in differentiation of competent and defective myeloid leukemic cells. Cell Growth Differ 1993; 4:41.

57. Farrugia MM, Duan L-J, Reis MD, et al: Alterations of the p53 tumor suppressor gene in diffuse large-cell lymphomas with translocations of the c-MYC and BCL-2 proto-oncogenes. Blood 1994; 83:191.

58. Fujiwara T, Grimm EA, Mukhopadhyay T, et al: Induction of chemosensitivity in human lung cancer cells in vivo by adenovirus-mediated transfer of the wild-type p53 gene. Cancer Res 1994; 54:2287.

59. Fanidi A, Harrington EA, Evan GI: Cooperative interaction between c-myc and bcl-2 proto-oncogenes. Nature 1992; 359:554.

60. Shivdasani RA, Hess JL, Skarin AT, Pinkus GS: Intermediate lymphocytic lymphoma: Clinical and pathologic features of a recently characterized subtype of non-Hodgkin's lymphoma. J Clin Oncol 1993; 11:802.

61. O'Connor PM, Ferris DK, Pagano M, et al: G_2 delay induced by nitrogen mustard in human cells affects cyclin A/cdk2 and cyclin B1/cdc2-kinase complexes differently. J Biol Chem 1993; 268:8298.

62. Acker B, Hoppe RT, Colby TV, et al: Histologic conversion in the non-Hodgkin's lymphomas. J Clin Oncol 1983; 1:11.

63. Wilson WH, Teruya-Feldstein J, Harris C, et al: P53, but not bcl-2, overexpression is independently associated with drug resistance in relapsed non-Hodgkin's lymphomas treated with EPOCH chemotherapy [Abstract]. Proc Am Soc Clin Oncol 1995; 14:1225.

64. Vaux DL, Aguila HL, Weissman IL: Bcl-2 prevents death of factor-deprived cells but fails to prevent apoptosis in targets of cell-mediated killing. Int Immunol 1992; 4:821.

65. Vuist WMJ, Levy R, Maloney DG: Lymphoma regression induced by monoclonal anti-idiotypic antibodies correlates with their ability to induce Ig signal transduction and is not prevented by tumor expression of high levels of bcl-2 protein. Blood 1994; 83:899.

66. Chabner BA, Collins JM (eds): Cancer Chemotherapy: Principles and Practice. Philadelphia, JB Lippincott, 1990.

67. Chabner BA, Grever MR, Morrow CS, et al: Anticancer drugs. In DeVita VT Jr, Hellman S, Rosenberg SA (eds): Cancer: Principles and Practice of Oncology. Philadelphia, JB Lippincott, 1993, pp 325–417.

68. Cheson BD: The purine analogs–a therapeutic beauty contest [Editorial]. J Clin Oncol 1992; 10:371.

69. Grever MR, Kopecky K, Head D, et al: A randomized comparison of deoxycoformycin versus alpha-2a interferon in previously untreated patients with hairy cell leukemia: An NCI-sponsored intergroup study. N Engl J Med. Submitted for publication.

70. Leiby JM, Snider KM, Kraut EH, et al: Phase II trial of 9-β-D-arabinosyl-2-fluoroadenine 5′-monophosphate in non-Hodgkin's lymphoma: Prospective comparison of response with deoxycytidine kinase activity. Cancer Res 1987; 47:2719.

71. Keating MJ, Kantarjian H, Talpaz M, et al: Fludarabine: A new agent with major activity against chronic lymphocytic leukemia. Blood 1989; 74:19.

72. Whelan JS, Davis CL, Rule S, et al: Fludarabine phosphate for the treatment of low-grade lymphoid malignancy. Br J Cancer 1991; 64:120.

73. Redman JR, Cabanillas F, Velasquez WS, et al: Phase II trial of fludarabine phosphate in lymphoma: An effective new agent in low-grade lymphoma. J Clin Oncol 1992; 10:790.

74. Zinzani PL, Lauria F, Rondelli D, et al: Fludarabine—an active agent in the treatment of previously treated and untreated low-grade non-Hodgkin's lymphoma. Ann Oncol 1993; 4:575.

75. Hidderman W, Unterhalt M, Pott C, et al: Fludarabine single-agent therapy for relapsed low-grade non-Hodgkin's lymphomas—a phase II study of the German low-grade non-Hodgkin's Lymphoma Study Group. Semin Oncol 1993; 20(Suppl 7):28.

76. Saven A, Piro LD: 2-Chlorodeoxyadenosine: A newer purine analog active in the treatment of indolent lymphoid malignancies. Ann Intern Med 1994; 120:784.

77. Kawasaki H, Carrera CJ, Piro LD, et al: Relationship of deoxycytidine kinase and cytoplasmic 5′-nucleotidase to the chemotherapeutic efficacy of 2-chlorodeoxyadenosine. Blood 1993; 81:597.

78. O'Brian S, Kantarjian H, Estey E, et al: Lack of effect of 2-chlorodeoxyadenosine therapy in patients with chronic lymphocytic leukemia refractory to fludarabine therapy. N Engl J Med 1994; 330:319.

79. Juliusson G, Einhorn-Rosenberg A, Liliemark J: Response to 2-chlorodeoxyadenosine in patients with B-cell chronic lymphocytic leukemia resistant to fludarabine. N Engl J Med 1992; 327:1056.

80. Gregoire V, Hunter N, Milas L, et al: Potentiation of radiation-induced regrowth delay in murine tumors by fludarabine. Cancer Res 1994; 54:468.

81. Ohno R, Okada K, Masaoka T, et al: An early phase II study of CPT-11: A new derivative of camptothecin, for the treatment of leukemia and lymphoma. J Clin Oncol 1990; 8:1907.

82. Hendricks CB, Rowinsky EK, Grochow LB, et al: Effect of p-glycoprotein expression on the accumulation and cytotoxicity of topotecan (SK&F 104864), a new camptothecin analogue. Cancer Res 1992; 52:2268.

83. Wilson WH, Chabner BA, Bryant G, et al: A phase II study of paclitaxel (Taxol) in relapsed non-Hodgkin's lymphomas. J Clin Oncol 1995; 13:381.

84. Minotti AM, Barlow SB, Cabral F: Resistance to antimitotic drugs in Chinese hamster ovary cells correlates with changes in the level of polymerized tubulin. J Biol Chem 1991; 266:3987.

85. Greenberger LM, Williams SS, Horwitz SB: Biosynthesis of heterogeneous forms of multidrug resistance–associated glycoproteins. J Biol Chem 1987; 262:1.

86. Citardi M, Rowinsky EK, Schaefer KL, et al: Sequence-dependent cytotoxicity between cisplatin and the antimicrotubule agents taxol and vincristine [Abstract]. Proc Am Assoc Cancer Res 1990; 31:2431.

87. Boyd MR: Status of the NCI preclinical antitumor drug discovery screen. PPO Updates 1989; 3:1.

88. Paull KD, Hodes L, Plowman J, et al: Reproducibility and response patterns of the IC50 values and relative cell line sensitivities from the NCI human tumor cell line drug screening project [Abstract]. Proc Am Assoc Cancer Res 1988; 29:488.

89. Powis G, Kozikowski A: Growth factor and oncogene signalling pathways as targets for rational anticancer drug development. Clin Biochem 1991; 24:385.

90. Ohlmeyer MHJ, Swanson RN, Dillard LW, et al: Complex synthetic chemical libraries indexed with molecular tags. Proc Natl Acad Sci U S A 1993; 90:10922.

91. DeWitt SH, Kiely JS, Stankovic CJ, et al: "Diversomers": an approach to nonpeptide, nonoligomeric chemical diversity. Proc Natl Acad Sci U S A 1993; 90:6909.

92. Huizing MT, Keung ACF, Rosing H, et al: Pharmacokinetics of paclitaxel and metabolites in a randomized comparative study in platinum-pretreated ovarian cancer patients. J Clin Oncol 1993; 11:2127.

93. Chu E, Zinn S, Boarman D, Allegra J: Interaction of gamma-interferon and 5-fluorouracil in the H630 human colon carcinoma cell line. Cancer Res 1990; 50:5834.

94. Nakamura S, Kashimoto S, Kajikawa F, Nakata K: Combination effect of recombinant human interleukin-1 alpha with antitumor drugs on syngeneic tumors in mice. Cancer Res 1991; 51:215.

95. Hancock MC, Langton BC, Chan T, et al: Monoclonal antibody against the c-erb B-2 protein enhances the cytotoxicity of cis-diammine-dichloro-platinum against human breast and ovarian tumor cell lines. Cancer Res 1991; 51:4575.

96. Fan Z, Masui H, Baselgna J, Mendelsohn J: Antitumor effect of anti-EGF receptor monoclonal antibody is enhanced by combination treatment with cis-platinum [Abstract]. Proc Ann Meet Am Assoc Cancer Res 1993: 34:2037a.

97. Ruscetti F, Dubois C, Folk LA, et al: In vivo and in vitro effects of TGF-beta 1 on normal and neoplastic hemopoiesis. Ciba Found Symp 1991; 157:212.

Thirteen

═══ Bone Marrow Transplantation ═══ for Malignant Lymphoma

Julie M. Vose
James O. Armitage

Many effective chemotherapeutic agents used for cancer therapy are destructive to normal hematopoietic cells. With bone marrow toxicity being the dose-limiting factor to the administration of many agents, bone marrow transplantation from an autologous source or from a donor offers the possibility of avoiding the lethal consequences of marrow damage and makes it possible to give "supralethal" chemotherapy and radiation therapy in an effort to kill a greater fraction of malignant cells. This is predicated on the "dose-response effect" exhibited by many malignancies.[1] Additionally, the healthy new cells transplanted may allow the replacement of an intact immune system to provide an antitumor effect.

The modern era of bone marrow transplantation was initiated with the identification of various histocompatibility antigens (human leukocyte antigens [HLAs]) and the ability to cryopreserve autologous hematopoietic cells. Allogeneic bone marrow transplantation was first successfully used as treatment for malignant disease by E. Donnall Thomas and colleagues in the late 1960s.[2] Throughout the 1970s this technology was defined and evaluated further for the treatment of various malignancies. For those few patients with HLA-identical twin siblings, syngeneic bone marrow transplantation was also developed during this period.[3] The first reports of autologous bone marrow transplantation (ABMT) being successfully employed to treat patients with lymphoma appeared in the late 1970s.[4] The use of this treatment modality has become widespread over the past 2 decades.

In the mid-1980s the use of peripheral blood progenitors as an alternative source for hematopoietic reconstitution was reported.[5, 6] Although transplantation using peripheral blood progenitors was originally used for patients who could otherwise not receive an ABMT owing to bone marrow tumor contamination or hypocellularity, the technology has now been applied to many patients undergoing autologous transplantation.

A proportion of patients with newly diagnosed aggressive non-Hodgkin's lymphoma (NHL) achieve complete remission (CR) with combination chemotherapy. However, 30% to 60% of the patients either do not attain an initial CR or they relapse later despite being treated with multi-

agent chemotherapy such as CHOP (cyclophosphamide, hydroxydaunomycin, Oncovin, prednisone), M-BACOD (methotrexate, bleomycin, Adriamycin, cyclophosphamide, Oncovin, dexamethasone), MACOP-B (methotrexate, Adriamycin, cyclophosphamide, Oncovin, prednisone, bleomycin), or ProMACE-CytaBOM (prednisone, methotrexate [with leucovorin rescue], Adriamycin, cyclophosphamide, etoposide; cytarabine, bleomycin, Oncovin).[7–10] Additionally, most patients with advanced low-grade NHL eventually relapse after any conventional therapy with no evidence of a disease-free survival plateau in most trials.[11, 12]

Although many conventional salvage chemotherapy programs have been developed, such as the IMVP-16 (ifosfamide, methotrexate, etoposide), MIME (methyl-GAG, ifosfamide, mitoxantrone, etoposide), and DHAP (dexamethasone, high-dose ara-C, Platinol) regimens, only a small percentage of patients have been reported to be disease free at 2 years posttherapy.[13–15] The clinical use of high-dose chemotherapy and bone marrow transplantation for the treatment of NHL was initially performed in the setting of recurrent or refractory disease that was not believed to be otherwise curable by standard methods. Therapy with bone marrow transplantation for each histologic subtype is discussed in the following sections.

BONE MARROW TRANSPLANTATION FOR LOW-GRADE NHL

It has traditionally been thought that virtually no patients with advanced-stage low-grade lymphoma were curable with conventional therapy. Although a high percentage of patients with stage III or IV follicular lymphoma can obtain a clinical CR with conventional therapy, this is usually of limited duration, a median of 1.5 to 3.0 years being the normal range.[16, 17] Most studies have disease-free survival rates of 25% or less at 5 years following diagnosis and treatment of advanced follicular lymphoma.[18] The use of aggressive conventional chemotherapy such as ProMACE/CytaBOM has increased the CR rate in this group of patients; however,

Table 13–1. Trials Evaluating High-Dose Chemotherapy and Autologous Transplantation for Follicular Non-Hodgkin's Lymphoma

Reference No.	No. of Patients	Regimen°	Complete Remission No. (%)	Disease Free Survival (%)
23	69	Cy/TBI	—	53
24	33	Cy/TBI (28)		
		BEAC (5)	22 (67)	42
25	35	Cy/VP/TBI (24)	23 (66)	N/A
		Cy/VP/BCNU (11)		
26	64	Cy/TBI	—	40

°See text for abbreviations. Numbers in parentheses are the number of patients receiving each regimen.
N/A, not applicable.

no increase in the overall survival has been seen with 7 years of followup.[19] With each therapy, the duration of CR in patients with follicular lymphoma typically decreases by approximately half.[20] In addition, a high percentage of patients eventually transform to a more aggressive intermediate- or high-grade histology that becomes difficult to treat.[21, 22]

The use of high-dose chemotherapy and allogeneic or autologous transplantation has only recently been investigated for the treatment of patients with low-grade NHL. Physicians have been hesitant to use bone marrow transplantation in this patient population because it is known that some patients with low-grade NHL can survive for a number of years with good performance status despite having lymphoma that is not curable with standard measures. Because low-grade NHL is inevitably fatal, high-dose therapy and bone marrow transplantation have now been attempted for patients with relapsed NHL and recently as part of their initial management.

Several single-arm trials have now been published evaluating the use of high-dose chemotherapy, radiation therapy, and autologous transplant in patients with follicular low-grade NHL at the time of first or subsequent relapse or second remission. The CR rates in these trials range from 40% to 75%; however, because of the relatively short followup period, it is unknown how many of these will be durable. The published studies report disease-free survival rates of 40% to 55% and overall survival rates of 50% to 75% at 3 to 4 years posttherapy (Table 13–1).[23–26] Rohatiner and associates[26] demonstrated an improved failure-free survival in transplanted patients compared with historical control groups (Fig. 13–1). The use of transplantation for patients with transformed follicular NHL has been found to have poor results in some, but not all, series.[23, 27]

Recently, a few trials using high-dose chemotherapy and ABMT in patients with extensive follicular NHL as part of their initial therapy following standard induction therapy have been reported.[28, 29] Horning[28] reported 25 of 29 patients transplanted in first remission to be alive and of disease-free status at a median of 13 months (range 3 to 48 months) posttransplant. In another study at the Dana-Farber Cancer Institute, patients with extensive follicular lymphoma received CHOP chemotherapy for six to eight cycles until CR, then were given cyclophosphamide/total body irradiation (TBI) and purged ABMT in first CR. Freedman and colleagues[29] reported, with a median followup of 22 months, that 48 of 73 patients were alive and disease free. The overall survival at the time of evaluation was 95%. Prolonged followup of these patients will be necessary to compare these results with conventional treatment.

Fewer reports of the use of high-dose chemotherapy and

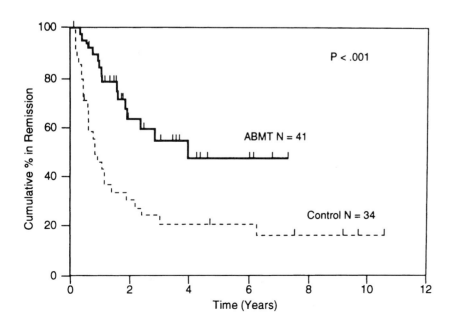

Figure 13–1. Freedom from recurrence for patients with follicular lymphoma receiving Cy/TBI/ABMT in second remission compared with results for a historical control group. See text for abbreviations. (From Rohatiner AZS, Johnson PWM, Price CGA, et al: Myeloablative therapy with autologous bone marrow transplantation as consolidation therapy for recurrent follicular lymphoma. J Clin Oncol 1994; 12:1177.)

bone marrow transplant for unusual subtypes in the low-grade category such as mantle cell lymphoma and small cell lymphocytic NHL/chronic lymphocytic leukemia (CLL) are available for review. A review of the literature and International Bone Marrow Transplant Registry (IBMTR) data by Bandini and coworkers[30] in 1991 showed that 26 patients have received either allogeneic or syngeneic bone marrow transplantation for CLL. At the time of the evaluation, 11 of 26 patients were alive and disease free, with followup of between 5 and 48 months. A subsequent report by Rabinowe and associates[31] evaluated 20 patients with poor-prognosis CLL who received purged ABMT (N = 12) or allogeneic bone marrow transplantation (N = 8). Seventeen of the patients were in clinical CR following bone marrow transplantation, and at 12 months posttransplant, the predicted disease-free survival was 82%.[31] Transplantation for another rare low-grade NHL, mantle cell lymphoma, has only rarely been reported in the literature. At the University of Nebraska Medical Center, seven patients with relapsed mantle cell lymphoma have undergone high-dose chemotherapy and autologous bone marrow or peripheral blood progenitor transplantation.[32] The 2-year failure-free survival of seven patients transplanted for mantle cell lymphoma was 44%, compared with an 11% failure-free survival rate in a group of patients with mantle cell NHL receiving conventional chemotherapy. Larger studies and longer followup will be necessary to validate these initial results.

BONE MARROW TRANSPLANTATION FOR INTERMEDIATE-GRADE NHL

Most patients with lymphoma who have received high-dose chemotherapy and ABMT have been transplanted for relapsed diffuse large cell or immunoblastic NHL (Table 13–2).[33–37] A few series have also reported on the use of high-dose chemotherapy and ABMT for other intermediate-grade histologies such as diffuse small cleaved or diffuse mixed small and large cell NHL.[38, 39]

One of the most important prognostic factors that has been identified by these studies is the chemotherapy sensitivity status of the patient's lymphoma at the time of transplantation. This important characteristic was identified by Philip and colleagues[40] in an evaluation of 100 patients receiving high-dose chemotherapy and ABMT in a multiinstitution trial. In this trial, patients who had not achieved a CR prior to the transplant had no chance of long-term disease-free survival following the transplant. Of the patients who had achieved an initial CR and later relapsed but were resistant to salvage chemotherapy, 14% had long-term disease-free survival. However, the patients who had relapsed from an initial CR but had chemotherapy-sensitive disease at the time of relapse had a 36% 4-year disease-free survival.[40] The importance of this prognostic factor has now been identified in multiple trials evaluating high-dose chemotherapy and ABMT in relapsed or progressive NHL. The European Bone Marrow Transplant Group (EBMTG) registry has evaluated the effect of chemotherapy sensitivity in a large number of patients who were transplanted beyond first remission and found that patients with chemotherapy-

Table 13–2. Studies Evaluating High-Dose Chemotherapy and Bone Marrow Transplantation for Relapsed Aggressive Non-Hodgkin's Lymphoma

Reference No.	Status at Transplantation	Regimen*	Survival %
33	Induction failure	Cy/TBI	10
	Refractory relapse		28
	Sensitive relapse		50
34	Induction failure	Variable	0
	Refractory relapse		10
	Sensitive relapse		45
35	Resistant relapse	Variable	10
	Sensitive relapse		50
36	Complete remission	VP/Cy/TBI	80
	Sensitive relapse		60
	Progressive disease		11
37	All patients	Variable	40

*See text for abbreviations.

sensitive disease had a projected 42% survival at 6 years posttransplant compared with a projected 20% survival at the same period in patients with chemotherapy-resistant disease (Fig. 13–2).[41]

Many transplant centers accept only patients who have been demonstrated to have a chemotherapy-sensitive relapse for consideration of high-dose chemotherapy and ABMT. However, other programs are continuing to evaluate the use of alternative preparative regimens or other adjuvant therapies in the resistant-relapse population or those that have never been in CR. Since most series are published by large transplant referral centers, the patients in the series are often highly selected—only the patients believed to have good chances with the transplant procedure are sent on a referral basis.

Other important prognostic factors identified in transplant series include the number of prior chemotherapy regimens a patient has received, a large tumor mass or bulk present at the time of transplant, and an elevated lactate dehydrogenase (LDH) level present at the time of transplant.[42] Many of these prognostic factors are identical to those predictive of a poor outcome in patients being treated at the initial diagnosis of NHL.[43–46] A multivariate analysis of 158 patients being transplanted for relapsed or primary refractory intermediate or immunoblastic NHL at the University of Nebraska Medical Center identified a good- and poor-prognosis group of patients based on these characteristics.[42] The poor-prognosis group had either a mass 10 cm or larger in diameter present at the time of transplant or two or three of these three characteristics: three or more prior chemotherapy regimens, an elevated LDH level, or chemotherapy-resistant disease. The patients in the poor-prognosis group had only a 10% chance of failure-free survival at 3 years post-ABMT (Fig. 13–3). The good-prognosis group had no mass 10 cm or larger in diameter and no more than one of the characteristics noted earlier. The good-prognosis group had a 40% chance of failure-free survival at 4 years post-ABMT.

Probably the most important area of current research is in the selection of patients for high-dose chemotherapy and ABMT in first partial or CR who are classified at the time of diagnosis as high risk for relapse. Many different prognostic factors have been identified as important in predicting the

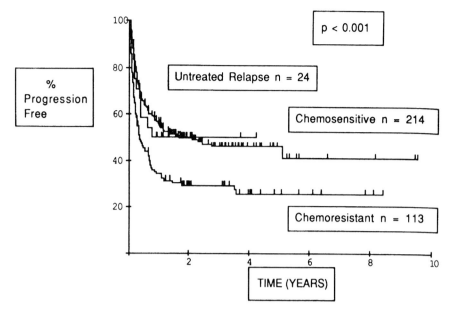

Figure 13–2. Effect of chemotherapy sensitivity in patients transplanted for non-Hodgkin's lymphoma beyond first remission (data from the European Bone Marrow Transplant Group Registry). (From Armitage JO, Antman K [eds]: High-Dose Cancer Therapy: Pharmacology, Hematopoietins, Stem Cells. Baltimore, Williams & Wilkins, 1992, pp 662–676.)

outcome of high-risk patients. These include bulk disease, number of extranodal sites, high LDH level, stage at diagnosis, and rapidity of achieving a CR.[43–49] The International Prognostic Index, recently developed by Shipp and other members of the International NHL Prognostic Factors Project, has identified a group of patients younger than 60 years of age who are at high risk for relapse with doxorubicin-based therapy.[50] In this analysis, patients who have two or three of the following characteristics at the time of diagnosis had a 25% to 30% chance of 5-year disease-free survival: stage III or IV, Karnofsky performance status of 70 or less, or a higher-than-normal LDH level.[50] Many centers are now using these prognostic factors to choose patients at the time of diagnosis who are believed to be at a very high risk for relapse and entering them into clinical trials with the use of high-dose chemotherapy and autologous transplant in first partial or CR. Several pilot trials have now been initiated in this patient group, with many studies reporting between 60% and 80% of the patients to be long-term disease-free survivors (Table 13–3).[51–53]

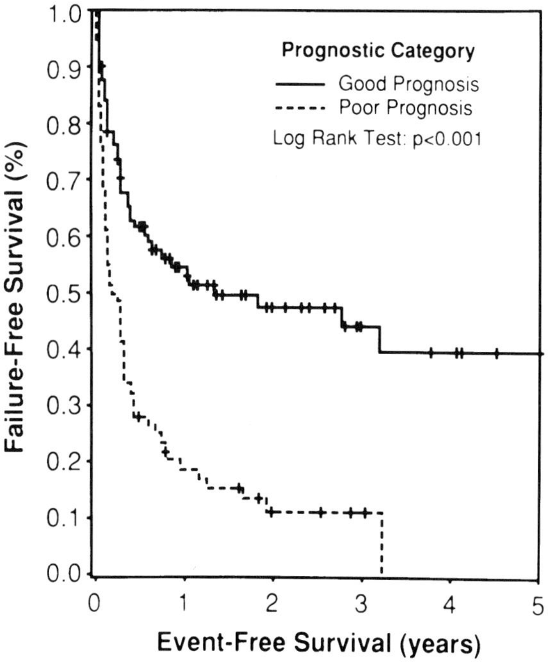

BONE MARROW TRANSPLANTATION FOR HIGH-GRADE NHL

Lymphoblastic NHL and small noncleaved cell lymphoma often present with an aggressive clinical history. Conventional chemotherapy regimens specifically designed

Figure 13–3. Failure-free survival in patients within the poor-prognosis group or the good-prognosis group receiving high-dose chemotherapy and autologous transplantation for intermediate-grade non-Hodgkin's disease. (From Vose JM, Anderson JR, Kessinger A, et al: High-dose chemotherapy and autologous hematopoietic stem cell transplantation for aggressive non-Hodgkin's lymphoma. J Clin Oncol 1993; 11:1846.)

Table 13–3. Results of High-Dose Chemotherapy and Bone Marrow Transplantation in First CR for High-Risk Non-Hodgkin's Lymphoma

Reference No.	No. of Patients	Disease Status	Outcome
51	20	First CR	17 CCR (35–73 mo) 84% actuarial DFS
52	17	First PR	13 CCR (8–75 mo) 75% actuarial survival
53	12	First CR	8 CCR (8–52 mo) 66% actuarial DFS

CR, complete remission; PR, partial remission; DFS, disease-free survival; CCR, continuous complete remission.

for lymphoblastic NHL that encompass central nervous system (CNS) prophylaxis and protocols similar to those designed for acute lymphoblastic leukemia have improved the overall survival of patients diagnosed with this subtype of NHL.[54, 55] However, certain prognostic features such as stage IV disease with bone marrow or CNS disease, or a significantly elevated LDH level have been associated with a long-term disease-free survival of less than 20%.[56] This group of patients has been targeted by many studies as the patient population eligible for the use of high-dose chemotherapy and transplantation as part of their overall treatment strategy.

The small noncleaved lymphomas are most often treated with induction regimens containing dose-intensive cyclophosphamide and methotrexate. In addition, many protocols for small noncleaved NHL also specify the use of CNS prophylaxis in the management.[57, 58] The data would suggest that patients with small noncleaved NHL who have CNS disease do have a poor prognosis with standard therapy.[59] Patients that have bone marrow involvement or a high LDH level are also believed to have a poorer prognosis with conventional treatment.[60] Children with high-grade NHL demonstrate improved results when compared with adult patients in most conventional chemotherapy trials.

The use of high-dose chemotherapy and autologous or allogeneic transplantation for patients with relapsed high-grade NHL has been disappointing with only a small number of patients disease-free following transplant.[61, 62] A major concern in using autologous bone marrow for hematopoietic reconstitution in patients being transplanted for high-grade NHL is the possibility of infusing occult tumor cells that contribute to relapse. Reports of early disseminated relapse following autologous transplantation suggest that this may be a possibility.[63] However, early disseminated relapse in some patients receiving an allogeneic source of bone marrow can also occur.

Most recent studies of transplantation for patients with high-grade NHL have focused on the selection of high-risk patients at the time of diagnosis with the use of high-dose chemotherapy and transplant as consolidative therapy. Several pilot studies have indicated that in the case of patients with high-risk lymphoblastic NHL, the use of high-dose chemotherapy and transplantation may increase the survival to approximately 60% to 75% in many studies.[64, 65] High-risk patients with a high LDH level and bone marrow or CNS involvement are now considered for transplantation in first complete or partial remission at many centers. Although there are no randomized studies in this patient population, this survival appears to be improved over historical studies of conventional therapy in these risk groups. Some studies have indicated that younger patients may benefit more from the use of allogeneic bone marrow over autologous bone marrow as the hematopoietic rescue product.[66] There is little information available evaluating the use of high-dose chemotherapy and bone marrow transplantation in patients with small noncleaved NHL in first remission and at high-risk for relapse. However, many transplant centers would consider such patients for transplantation if they had an elevated LDH level and stage IV disease at the time of diagnosis.

ISSUES IN BONE MARROW TRANSPLANTATION

SOURCE OF STEM CELLS

The best source of hematopoietic stem cells for use in transplantation following high-dose chemotherapy is an unanswered question. The number of reports using syngeneic bone marrow are few[67, 68]; however, the use of allogeneic marrow from HLA-identical siblings has been reported with more frequency.[68–70] Because of the relatively small size of the family in Western countries, only approximately 25% to 30% of patients can expect to find an HLA-identical match within their family. As an alternative, partially matched family donors or HLA-matched unrelated donors have been used in a small number of patients being transplanted for lymphoma. The relatively aggressive behavior of some lymphomas and the extremely large number of possible HLA phenotypes makes searching for an unrelated donor difficult. Results from transplantation of partially mismated related donors is directly related to the degree of matching.[71] The use of a hematopoietic stem cell source other than an autologous source can be associated with the additional risks of graft-versus-host disease (GVHD) or graft rejection. Both of these complications are immune mediated (see the section on transplant complications).

Because of the lack of allogeneic sources of bone marrow in all patients and the increased complications associated with allogeneic transplantation, autologous sources of hematopoietic stem cells for transplantation have gained popularity over the past decade. Autologous transplantation has the relative advantage of being able to be performed in a larger number of patients and in older persons compared with allogeneic transplantation. Autologous transplantation for lymphoma has now been reported in patients about 65 to 70 years of age with comparative safety and a low early mortality rate.[72] For patients with bone marrow tumor involvement or hypocellular bone marrow, peripheral blood progenitors have been used as an alternative source of hematopoietic stem cells.[73–75] Because of the ease of obtaining peripheral blood progenitor cells and reports of rapid engraftment, this form of transplantation has rapidly expanded to most transplant centers.

A primary concern with autologous sources of hematopoietic stem cells is to ensure that the graft contains no viable tumor cells. Cells consistent with lymphoma can be cultured from histologically negative bone marrows and, to a lesser extent, peripheral blood progenitors, and such patients do have a higher relapse rate posttransplant.[76] However, relapses occur at sites of previous disease in most patients, raising the question of whether resistance to treatment rather than the reinfusion of clonogenic tumor cells is the cause of the relapse. Controlled clinical trials have not yet definitively answered this question. There has been some evidence to suggest that using peripheral blood progenitors may be associated with an enhanced natural killer cell activity present following transplantation.[77] In one nonrandomized trial the patients undergoing high-dose chemotherapy who received peripheral blood progenitors had an improved long-term disease-free survival compared with those patients receiving autologous bone marrow transplants within the same prognostic groups.[42] This association is currently being tested in a prospective, randomized trial to confirm the potential differences in relapse rates associated with the different types of autologous transplants.

The successful use of cord blood as a hematopoietic rescue product has been reported.[78] Although this technique can be particularly useful in pediatric patients, an inadequate number of cells can currently be collected to ensure engraftment in adult patients. Ex vivo expansion of a small amount of bone marrow, peripheral blood, or cord blood with an optimal cytokine mixture may soon offer an alternative. This approach may allow the ex vivo expansion of an otherwise inadequate cell collection. In addition, the expansion of postprogenitor myeloid cells infused may allow a decrease in the time of absolute neutropenia from 9 to 12 days as it currently stands with mobilized peripheral blood progenitors. An expansion of 21-fold to 66-fold in colony-forming units has been achieved using this technique; however, whether this will allow for any improvement in engraftment time over currently available techniques is unknown.[79]

The relative roles of autologous and allogeneic bone marrow transplantation after the administration of high-dose therapy have not been clearly defined. There have been a few reports comparing allogeneic and autologous transplants for lymphoma.[67, 68] However, no randomized trials are available for comparison. Chopra and associates[66] reported a case-controlled study comparing 101 NHL patients allografted with 101 matched patients in the EBMTG registry, taking into account prognostic factors important by multivariate analysis for outcome after transplantation. Patients were matched for status at transplant, stage at transplant, histology, conditioning therapy, age, sex, and length of time between diagnosis and transplantation. The results of this analysis show that using these closely matched patients, there was no difference in the progression-free survival between autologous and allogeneic bone marrow transplantation for all histologic types of NHL. In the subgroup of patients undergoing transplant for lymphoblastic NHL, the relapse and progression rates were greater for the autologous transplant patients (48% autologous versus 24% allogeneic; $P = 0.0035$). However, the progression-free survival was not different owing to an increased mortality in the allogeneic transplant group, which offset the advantage for the allogeneic group.[66] This implies either that infused tumor cells in the autologous graft contribute to the relapse of the patient or that a graft-versus-lymphoma effect is apparent. Improvements in GVHD prophylaxis and other supportive care measures could potentially change this outcome.

HODGKIN'S DISEASE

Although a high percentage of patients with advanced Hodgkin's disease can experience long-term disease-free survival with combination chemotherapy, some either fail to go into an initial CR or relapse quickly following the initial therapy. Conventional salvage regimens for patients with induction failure may put a small number of patients into remission; however, few experience long-term disease-free survival.[80, 81] For patients who relapsed following an initial CR lasting more than 12 months, a high CR rate with salvage therapy of 85% was obtainable, compared with a 24% CR rate for those patients with remissions of less than 12 months.[80] Despite this, the overall survival of patients with long initial remissions was projected to be 24%, and only 11% of patients with short initial remissions survived longer than 10 years.

The use of high-dose therapy and autologous hematopoietic stem cell transplantation for patients with advanced refractory Hodgkin's disease has been shown to produce long-term disease-free survival in selected patients.[82–85] Issues that are still controversial with respect to transplantation for Hodgkin's disease include the optimal timing of transplantation, best transplant regimen, optimal source of hematopoietic stem cells, and the potential use of localized radiotherapy or immunologic methods to decrease post-transplant relapse.

Because of the long natural history of Hodgkin's disease, transplantation studies need to have long followup to ensure that the results demonstrate the full picture of this patient population. The study with the longest followup is a combined study of 128 patients transplanted at the University of Nebraska Medical Center and M. D. Anderson Cancer Center.[86] All patients in this study received the "standard-dose" CBV regimen consisting of cyclophosphamide, 1.5 g/M^2 × 4 days (day −6 to −3); carmustine, 300 mg/M^2 × 1 day (day −6); and etoposide, 125 mg/M^2 × 4 days (day −6 to −3); this was followed on day 0 by either autologous bone marrow or peripheral blood progenitor transplantation. At the time of the last published report, this cohort had a median followup of 77 months with a minimum followup of 48 months for all patients.

In this study of 128 patients with long-term followup, the overall and failure-free survival were projected to be 45% and 25%, respectively, at 48 months. Multivariate analysis revealed performance status and the number of failed chemotherapy regimens to be most predictive for failure-free survival. The failure-free survival at 48 months was projected to be 53% for good performance status patients (European Cooperative Oncology Group stage 0–1) who had failed only one chemotherapy regimen prior to transplant.[86]

Another large series published by Nademanee and colleagues[87] evaluated 85 patients with relapsed or refractory Hodgkin's disease who underwent either VP-CY-TBI (etoposide, 60 g/kg; cyclophosphamide, 100 mg/kg; and TBI, 1200 cGy) or high-dose CBV (cyclophosphamide, 100 mg/kg; etoposide, 60 mg/kg; and carmustine, 450 mg/M^2) followed by autologous bone marrow or peripheral blood progenitor transplantation. At the time of analysis, 44 (52%) of the patients were alive in continuous CR with a median followup for the surviving patients of 28 months (range 7 to 66 months). Thirty (35%) of the patients relapsed at a median of 9 months (range 1 to 43 months). Eleven patients died of transplant-related complications, including venoocclusive disease of the liver in five, acute and late interstitial pneumonitis in three, graft failure in one, cerebral hemorrhage in one, and myelodysplasia syndrome (MDS)/acute leukemia in one patient. At a median followup of 25 months (range 1 to 66 months), the cumulative probability of 2-year overall and disease-free survival of all 85 patients was 75% and 58%, respectively. The only significant prognostic factor identified by multivariate analysis was the number of prior chemotherapy regimens received. There was no significant difference in the outcome of patients with respect to the transplant regimen received.

The optimal timing of transplantation for patients with Hodgkin's disease remains controversial. The use of transplantation for patients who fail to obtain an initial CR with induction therapy can improve their long-term disease-free survival.[83, 88] Additionally, patients with an initial CR duration of less than 12 months can demonstrate an improved long-term disease-free survival with transplantation.[88, 89]

The role of transplantation in patients with an initial CR of longer than 12 months is debated. Seventeen patients in the study by Nademanee and colleagues[87] whose initial CR was 12 months or longer received transplants in the first relapse or second CR. The 2-year disease-free survival in that group of patients was 76%, which is comparable to those results reported by other studies.[86, 90] However, with longer followup, these initially promising results may demonstrate a decline in the long-term disease-free survival.

The early identification of high-risk patients at the time of diagnosis for the use of high-dose chemotherapy and transplantation as part of their initial treatment strategy has also been evaluated. Carella[91] has evaluated 21 patients with high-risk Hodgkin's disease who received high-dose chemotherapy and autologous transplantation as part of their initial treatment. At the time of analysis, a progression-free survival of 70% was seen in these patients, with a median followup of 27 months. Compared with similar high-risk patients used as historical control groups, the progression-free survival was improved. Selection biases must always be kept in mind when historical control groups are used.

GENERAL PRINCIPLES OF BONE MARROW TRANSPLANTATION FOR LYMPHOMA

TRANSPLANT PREPARATIVE REGIMEN

The chemotherapeutic agents that can be used for dose escalation and autologous transplantation for patients with lymphomas are limited. The ideal regimen would have only myelotoxicity with no associated nonhematopoietic toxicity. Unfortunately, most high-dose regimens do have associated extramedullary toxicities that are dose limiting. Furthermore, the anthracyclines, which are one of the most active group of agents available for lymphoma therapy, cannot be dose escalated to a great extent. Most high-dose preparative regimens used in patients with lymphoma include one or more alkylating agents, etoposide, and occasionally other agents such as cytarabine, carmustine, or platinum compounds. TBI has been used in preparative regimens for patients undergoing transplant for lymphoma as well.

There have been no prospective studies comparing transplant regimens for NHL. The optimal dosing of agents is also unknown. For example, the CBV regimen is widely used for patients undergoing transplantation for Hodgkin's disease or NHL. However, the doses of the drugs in the CBV regimen vary widely. Regimens that contain the highest doses may be associated with an increased CR rate; however, an increase in the mortality rate is also apparent.[83] Comparative trials are necessary to resolve these issues.

The role of radiation therapy in transplantation for lymphoma is equally unclear. TBI is widely used for transplantation in patients with low-grade and lymphoblastic lymphoma. However, most patients undergoing transplantation for intermediate-grade and small noncleaved NHL do not receive TBI. Unfortunately, there are no prospective, randomized trials to evaluate the need for TBI in preparative regimens. Most nonrandomized comparisons have not found a clear-cut benefit for those patients receiving TBI, although irradiation does appear to be associated with an increased toxicity, primarily related to pulmonary complications.[40, 93] In addition, one transplant center has recently reported an increased incidence of secondary MDSs and acute myelogenous leukemia (AML) following transplantation using TBI-based regimens.[93]

Involved-field irradiation either pretransplant or posttransplant as "consolidative treatment" to areas of bulky tumor involvement is also frequently used. Although no comparative studies are available for the use of this technique either, it is widely believed that this decreases the chance of local recurrence in the radiation field. Whether this changes the overall outcome of patients transplanted for lymphoma is unclear. An extension of this concept is the use of radiolabeled antibody therapy along with high-dose chemotherapy transplant regimens.[94] This concept is attractive owing to the potential additive therapeutic value of the radiolabeled antibody without additive toxicity other than the hematopoietic toxicity. Further evaluation of this technique is ongoing at some centers.

MARROW PURGING

The use of purging for ABMT for NHL is a controversial issue. A wide variety of methods have been developed to accomplish this goal, including the use of chemotherapeutic agents, immunologic agents such as monoclonal antibodies, and mechanical separation devices. Both chemotherapy and monoclonal antibody purging techniques appear to decrease tumor cell contamination between two and five logs.[95] However, it is not clear which marrow needs to be purged to increase the clinical benefit from transplant. Occult lymphoma can be detected in histologically negative bone marrow specimens; however, whether the cells contribute directly to lymphoma relapse following transplantation has not been proved.[76] Most relapses following transplantation for lymphoma occur at sites of previous disease rather than at new locations. This suggests that relapse following transplantation results from inadequacies of the preparative regimen rather than from reinfusion of contaminated marrow. There have been several nonrandomized studies that have failed to demonstrate a benefit from purging.[36, 92, 96, 97]

The antibody most commonly used for purging of follicular B-cell lymphomas has been the anti-B$_1$. Additional antibodies are sometimes added in a cocktail such as anti-B$_5$, J$_5$, and J$_2$, along with complement. In a report by Gribben and associates,[98] patients with follicular lymphoma and evidence of t(14;18) in their marrow at the time of harvest were purged using a cocktail of monoclonal antibodies. Following purging, patient samples were studied to determine whether lymphoma cells were still detectable in the marrow. The results of transplantation were significantly better in those patients without lymphoma cells following purging, compared with those believed to have residual lymphoma cells in their marrow. In a more recent publication by Johnson and colleagues,[99] 29 patients with follicular lymphoma who were undergoing high-dose chemotherapy and ABMT had their harvested bone marrow tested by polymerase chain reaction (PCR) to test the efficacy of purging. In 25 of the 29 cases, the same t(14;18) was detected after the antibody purge. Three of the four patients treated with PCR-negative marrow subsequently developed recurrent lymphoma, compared with 11 of 25 in the PCR-positive group. Even with these data, the role of purging for follicular lymphoma remains unclear.

Another alternative to direct chemical or antibody purging is the use of peripheral blood progenitor or CD34 "positive" selection of autologous bone marrow or peripheral blood. By some methods, fewer lymphoma cells are detected in the blood compared with the bone marrow.[100] However, for follicular lymphomas, it is unclear that blood has less tumor contamination compared with bone marrow. For tumors such as the NHLs that have no CD34 antigen on their surface, the use of "positive selection" with the CD34 column is an alternative form of purging. Pilot series of patients transplanted with CD34-selected cells have now demonstrated the feasibility of this technique.[101] Further evaluation of the use of this technique is warranted in lymphoma transplantation.

TIMING OF TRANSPLANTATION

Perhaps one of the most important issues for physicians caring for lymphoma patients is that of the proper timing for the use of high-dose chemotherapy and transplantation. Patients with a high probability of cure using conventional treatments should not be subjected to the possibility of morbidity and mortality associated with high-dose chemotherapy and transplant. Similarly, the transplant should not be withheld until the lymphoma is chemotherapy resistant and dose escalation could no longer cure patients and/or they would have an increased risk of mortality because of their poor performance status.

Early studies such as the one by Philip and coworkers[40] demonstrated that for those patients undergoing transplantation for intermediate-grade NHL who had never been in a CR had virtually no chance of long-term disease-free survival. Outside of research protocols, most primary chemotherapy-refractory patients are no longer recommended for transplant. Patients who have had an initial CR to induction therapy and relapsed later but are chemotherapy resistant can still have a small chance of long-term disease-free survival with transplant.[33, 40, 42] However, many transplant centers are only accepting patients who have a "chemotherapy-sensitive" relapse for transplantation. It has now clearly been demonstrated in multiple trials that these patients can have a 30% to 50% chance of long-term disease-free survival with transplant.[33, 35, 40, 42] Other factors such as the tumor bulk, LDH level, and number of prior chemotherapies administered have also been found to have prognostic importance in patients undergoing high-dose chemotherapy and transplant.[42]

Many transplant centers are now attempting to direct high-risk lymphoma patients identified at the time of their initial diagnosis into programs using high-dose chemo-

therapy and transplantation as an integrated part of their initial therapy. Several prognostic factor analyses have now identified patient groups that have a poor outcome with doxorubicin-containing induction regimens.[44, 46, 50] Pilot trials using high-dose chemotherapy and transplantation when these high-risk patients are in first CR or partial response have demonstrated an improved disease-free survival to between 60% to 80% in most series.[51–53] Recent randomized trials from Europe compared the use of high-dose chemotherapy and transplant in first CR for patients who completed an initial induction therapy and then were randomized to receive an intensive consolidation regimen or CBV and ABMT.[102] Although there was no difference between the two groups overall, the patients in the high-risk group according to the international prognostic index did show an improvement in disease-free survival in the transplant group. An additional study evaluating a conventional salvage regimen versus ABMT for residual lymphoma after induction therapy has demonstrated an improved result for patients in the ABMT arm.[103] Further study of the use of early high-dose chemotherapy and transplantation early in the disease course of high-risk patients is ongoing in the United States.

Another area of controversy regarding the timing of transplant centers around the use of high-dose chemotherapy and ABMT for treatment of follicular lymphomas. Only within the past few years has this form of therapy been offered to patients with follicular lymphoma. Because of the relatively long life span (median 5 to 8 years) of patients diagnosed with follicular lymphomas, physicians have been hesitant to offer this therapy to these patients. However, reports in the literature of follicular lymphoma patients being transplanted in first or subsequent relapse have recently been published. Although the CR rates in many series are impressive (60% to 80%), it is unknown at this time if it is possible to change the natural history of the disease by this approach.[24, 25] Several trials have now been published with disease-free survivals of 40% to 55% and overall survivals of 50% to 75% at 3 to 4 years posttransplant.[23–26] The use of high-dose chemotherapy and ABMT for patients with transformed follicular NHL have been evaluated and found to have poor results in some but not all series.[26, 27]

In addition, some centers are also using high-dose chemotherapy and transplantation in patients with extensive follicular NHL as part of their initial management following induction of CR with a standard regimen.[28, 29] These studies have only recently been initiated, and much longer followup is necessary to evaluate the efficacy of this approach. These studies are not randomized but need to be compared with historical control groups to evaluate the possibility of change in the natural history of newly diagnosed follicular lymphoma patients.

ACUTE TRANSPLANT COMPLICATIONS

High-dose chemotherapy and bone marrow transplantation can be associated with several unusual complications.

GVHD. Patients undergoing allogeneic transplantation can develop variable symptoms associated with GVHD. This is usually manifested primarily by skin rash, oral mucosal lesions, gastrointestinal symptoms such as diarrhea, or elevated liver enzyme and bilirubin levels. The severity of the condition is graded according to the involvement of these organs (Table 13–4). The immunosuppression associated with GVHD and its therapy is the most life-threatening acute complication associated with transplantation. Even with adequate prophylaxis, most adult patients still develop some degree of GVHD following allogeneic transplant.[104–106] Treatment for established GVHD such as high-dose corticosteroids, antithymocyte globulin, and various monoclonal antibodies are available but not always totally successful.[107–109]

Graft Rejection. Rejection of an allogeneic bone marrow graft typically results from immunologically mediated host cells directed against transplanted cells. This phenomenon most often is associated with patients receiving a higher degree of mismatch or aplastic anemia patients who have had a large number of prior transfusions, using less immunosuppressive transplant regimens, or T-cell–depleted grafts.[110, 111]

Pancytopenia. Because of the high doses of chemotherapy and/or radiation therapy administered in patient preparative regimens, prolonged pancytopenia is present following transplant. Prior to the era of hematopoietic growth factors, morbidity and mortality associated with prolonged myelosuppression and infectious complications were frequent following transplant. With currently available cytokines such as granulocyte colony-stimulating factor (G-CSF) and granulocyte-macrophage CSF (GM-CSF), the period of myelosuppression can be decreased by 1 week in many circumstances.[112, 113] Further testing has confirmed this in multiple studies and demonstrated decreased infection rates in cytokine-treated patients.[114, 115] The need for platelet and packed red blood cell transfusions has not been altered by the currently available cytokines. However, some of the earlier acting cytokines such as interleukin-6, interleukin-3 with G-CSF or GM-CSF, or the fusion molecule PIXY321 may be able to decrease the transfusion requirements.[116–118]

Pulmonary Complications. Pulmonary complications associated with high-dose chemotherapy and transplantation include infectious complications such as bacterial pneumonia, fungal agents (including *Aspergillus*), cytomegalovirus (CMV) infection, diffuse alveolar hemorrhage, or nonspecific interstitial pneumonia. The risk of bacterial infection has been diminished greatly by the use of hematopoietic growth factors. The rate of fungal infections varies greatly depending on the transplant environment and the patient population. The risk of symptomatic CMV pneumonia is much higher in patients undergoing allogeneic transplant, particularly those with severe GVHD.[119] The use of CMV-negative blood products in patients who lack CMV antibodies at the time of transplant and the administration of immune globulin,[120, 121] prophylactic acyclovir,[122] or ganciclovir[123] to patients at high risk both have potential for reducing this complication. Diffuse alveolar hemorrhage or interstitial pneumonia of unknown cause occasionally occurs in both allogeneic and autologous transplant patients. High-dose corticosteroids may reduce the mortality associated with this condition.[124]

Venoocclusive Disease. The three primary symptoms associated with venoocclusive disease include jaundice, tender hepatomegaly, and ascites with unexplained weight gain. As many as 40% to 50% of patients undergoing transplant may have one or all of these symptoms to a variable extent. Severe venoocclusive disease with progressive hepatic failure is fatal in a high percentage of patients. Predisposing factors include prior hepatic injury, the use of very high-dose regimens, or the use of unrelated donors.[125] There are a few reports of thrombolytic therapy with tissue plasminogen activator followed by heparin therapy that showed some benefit for treatment.[126]

Hemorrhagic Cystitis. This toxicity is associated with the oxazaphosphorine class of chemotherapeutic agents such as high-dose cyclophosphamide and ifosfamide. Various methods of prevention have been used, including intravenous hydration, continuous bladder irrigation, or intravenous mesna. Bladder irrigation or the use of mesna has been found to be equally efficacious as far as the prevention of severe hemorrhagic cystitis; however, bladder irrigation was found to be associated with an increased incidence of urinary tract infections.[127]

CHRONIC TRANSPLANT COMPLICATIONS

Chronic GVHD. GVHD occurring after the first 100 days posttransplant is referred to as "chronic GVHD" and often presents with distinct clinical findings such as sicca syndrome, chronic sinusitis, skin thickening, scarring, and contractures similar to scleroderma.[128] Adverse prognostic factors include the presence of thrombocytopenia, a progressive presentation, and an elevated bilirubin level.[129] Treatment options include alternate-day cyclosporine and prednisone or thalidomide.[130, 131] However, total control of chronic GVHD with immunosuppressive agents can be difficult without creating excessive opportunistic infections.

Cataract Formation. Patients receiving a TBI-containing regimen have a high associated risk of developing cataracts. In one study, at 3.5 years posttransplant, 100% of the living patients who received single-dose TBI had

Table 13–4. Clinical Grading of Acute Graft-Versus-Host Disease

Organ	Extent of Involvement		Stage	I	II$_{SLI}$	II$_S$	II$_{LI}$	III	IV
Skin	Rash (% of body surface)	<25	+						
		25–50	++						
		>50	+++						
	Bullae, desquamation		++++						
Liver	Bilirubin (mg/dL)	2–3	+						
		3.1–6	++						
		6.1–15	+++						
		>15	++++						
Intestine	Diarrhea (mL/day)	>500	+						
		>1000	++						
		>1500	+++						
	Pain/ileus		++++						
—	Impairment of performance		+						
			++						
			+++						

The clinical grade subscripts indicate the following: S = skin only; SLI = skin, liver, and intestine; and LI = liver and intestine.

developed cataracts.[132] Twenty percent of the patients who received fractionated TBI developed cataracts, and only 3% of the patients who received a chemotherapy-only regimen developed cataracts posttransplant.[132]

Pulmonary Fibrosis. Chronic restrictive pulmonary changes have been reported in a small number of patients who survive for extended periods following transplantation.[133] There is an increased risk of this complication in patients who have received high doses of carmustine, a TBI-containing transplant regimen, or have received mantle irradiation prior to transplant. Although some component of this may be reversible, progressive fibrotic changes can occur.

Cardiac Insufficiency. In a small number of patients diminished cardiac function manifested by symptomatic congestive heart failure can occur posttransplant. This finding has been associated with high doses of anthracyclines administered prior to transplant and/or high-dose cyclophosphamide–containing transplant regimens.[134] Medical management is usually capable of controlling the symptoms associated with this toxicity.

Secondary Malignancy. Several studies have now identified an increased risk of secondary solid tumors, MDS, and AML in long-term survivors of bone marrow transplantation.[26, 93] As with secondary malignancies following conventional chemotherapy, the risk of MDS/AML peaks at 4 to 7 years posttreatment, with the full extent of the risks of secondary solid tumors probably not yet fully identified owing to inadequate long-term followup of survivors. Most cases of MDS/AML have been associated with chromosomal abnormalities seen with alkylating agent–associated leukemias such as chromosome 5 or 7 abnormalities.[93] Treatment of the secondary MDS/AML cases has not been successful in most cases.[26, 93] An association with the use of TBI-containing regimens and an age of 40 years or older at the time of transplant has been identified in one study.[93]

Psychosocial Changes. Although most long-term survivors posttransplant return to a normal lifestyle, an increased risk for psychosocial changes posttransplant has been identified.[135, 136] Fear of disease relapse or long-term complications associated with cancer therapy can lead to a difficult adjustment posttransplant. Sexual dysfunction has also been reported by a moderate number of patients posttransplant.[135, 137]

CHANGING OUTCOME OF TRANSPLANTATION FOR LYMPHOMA

Although high-dose chemotherapy and transplantation has been demonstrated to be successful in subsets of patients with NHL, improvements in long-term disease-free survival are certainly needed. Various options are currently being explored in an attempt to decrease the relapse rate associated with high-dose chemotherapy and transplantation. One possible additional treatment is the use of "consolidative" radiation therapy to sites of bulk tumor either prior to or following transplantation. Although this technique has not been studied in a prospective, randomized fashion, studies have demonstrated a decreased relapse rate

in sites of prior involved-field radiation therapy.[138] Along similar treatment patterns, the addition of radiolabeled antibodies to the high-dose chemotherapy preparative regimen has preliminarily been explored in an attempt to add antitumor effect without additive nonhematopoietic toxicity.[94] Several radiolabeled antibodies have now shown promise in phase I trials in treating NHL.[139, 140] An eventual application of these agents with high-dose chemotherapy and transplantation may decrease the relapse rate by treating the tumor with the addition of another treatment modality.

The treatment of minimal residual disease with posttransplant immunomodulation has also been initially explored with agents such as interleukin-2, interferon, or bestatin.[141–143] It is hoped that with the addition of an immunomodulating agent, a small amount of minimal residual disease could be eliminated if residual tumor is still present in the patient. Immunomodulation of the graft itself by interleukin-2 is also being evaluated in an attempt to decrease the possible tumor contamination.[144]

CONCLUSIONS

High-dose chemotherapy and hematopoietic stem cell transplantation has now become the standard of care for eligible patients with recurrent aggressive NHL or Hodgkin's disease. The most appropriate clinical context in which transplantation should be performed for patients with follicular lymphomas or high-risk aggressive lymphomas has not yet been well established. As supportive care measures for transplantation continue to develop, the use of this treatment modality may be expanded to alternative patient groups.

REFERENCES

1. Frei E III, Canellos G: Dose: A critical factor in cancer chemotherapy. Am J Med 1980; 69:584.
2. Thomas ED, Storb R, Clift RA, et al: Bone marrow transplantation. N Engl J Med 1975; 292:832.
3. Appelbaum FR, Sullivan KM, Buckner CD, et al: Treatment of malignant lymphoma in 100 patients with chemotherapy, total-body irradiation, and marrow transplantation. J Clin Oncol 1987; 5:1340.
4. Appelbaum FR, Herzig GP, Ziegler JL, et al: Successful engraftment of cryopreserved autologous bone marrow in patients with malignant lymphoma. Blood 1978; 52:85.
5. Kessinger A, Armitage JO, Landmark JD, et al: Autologous peripheral hematopoietic stem cell transplantation restores hematopoietic function following marrow ablative therapy. Blood 1988; 71:723.
6. Korbling M, Martin H: Autologous blood stem cell transplantation: A new treatment concept for patients with malignant lymphohematopoietic disorders. *In* Dicke KA, Spitzer G (eds): Autologous Bone Marrow Transplantation: Proceedings of the Third International BMT Symposium, 1987, pp 615–617.
7. DeVita VT Jr, Canellos GP, Chabner B, et al: Advanced diffuse histiocytic lymphoma, a potentially curable disease. Lancet 1975; 1:248.
8. Shipp MA, Harrington DP, Klatt MM, et al: Identification of major prognostic subgroups of patients with large-cell lymphoma treated with m-BACOD or M-BACOD. Ann Intern Med 1986; 104:757.
9. Klimo P, Connors JM: MACOP-B chemotherapy for the treatment of diffuse large-cell lymphoma. Ann Intern Med 1985; 102:596.
10. Fisher RI, DeVita VT Jr, Hubbard SM, et al: Randomized trial of ProMACE-MOPP vs. ProMACE-CytaBOM in previously untreated, advanced stage, diffuse aggressive lymphomas. Proc Am Soc Clin Oncol 1984; 3:242a.

11. Dana BW, Dahlberg S, Nathwani BN, et al: Long-term follow-up of patients with low-grade malignant lymphomas treated with doxorubicin-based chemotherapy or chemoimmunotherapy. J Clin Oncol 1993; 11:644.

12. Anderson JR, Vose JM, Bierman PJ, et al: Clinical features and prognosis of follicular large-cell lymphoma: A report from the Nebraska Lymphoma Study Group. J Clin Oncol 1993; 11:218.

13. Cabanillas F, Hagemeister FB, Bodey GP, Freireich EJ: IMVP-16: An effective regimen for patients with lymphoma who have relapsed after initial combination chemotherapy. Blood 1982; 60:693.

14. Cabanillas F, Hagemeister FB, McLaughlin P, et al: Results of MIME salvage regimen for recurrent or refractory lymphoma. J Clin Oncol 1987; 5:407.

15. Velasquez WS, Cabanillas F, Salvador P, et al: Effective salvage therapy for lymphoma with cisplatin in combination with high-dose Ara C and dexamethasone (DHAP). Blood 1988; 71:117.

16. Gallagher CJ, Gregory WM, Jones AE, et al: Follicular lymphoma: Prognostic factors for response and survival. J Clin Oncol 1986; 4:1470.

17. Morrison VA, Peterson BA: Combination chemotherapy in the treatment of follicular low-grade lymphoma. Leuk Lymphoma 1993; 10:29.

18. Spinolo JA, Cabanillas F, Dixon DO, et al: Therapy of relapsed or refractory low-grade follicular lymphomas: Factors associated with complete remission, survival, and time to treatment failure. Ann Oncol 1992; 3:227.

19. Young RC, Longo DL, Glatstein E, et al: The treatment of indolent lymphomas: Watchful waiting vs. aggressive combined modality treatment. Semin Hematol 1988; 25:11.

20. Portlock CS: Management of the low-grade non-Hodgkin's lymphomas. Semin Oncol 1990; 17:51.

21. Armitage JO, Dick FR, Corder MP: Diffuse histiocytic lymphoma after histologic conversion: A poor prognostic variant. Cancer Treat Rep 1981; 65:413.

22. Cullen MH, Lister TA, Brearley RL, et al: Histologic transformation of non-Hodgkin's lymphoma: A prospective study. Cancer 1979; 44:645.

23. Freedman AS, Ritz J, Neuberg D, et al: Autologous bone marrow transplantation in 69 patients with a history of low-grade B-cell non-Hodgkin's lymphoma. Blood 1991; 77:2524.

24. Bierman P, Vose J, Armitage JO: High-dose therapy followed by autologous hematopoietic rescue for follicular low-grade non-Hodgkin's lymphoma (NHL). Proc ASCO 1992; 11:1074a.

25. Molina A, Nademanee A, Schmidt GM, et al: High-dose therapy (HDT) followed by autologous hematopoietic stem cell transplantation (AGSCT) for follicular low-grade and transformed lymphoma. In Proceedings of the Fifth International Conference on Lymphoma, 1993, 130a.

26. Rohatiner AZS, Johnson PWM, Price CGA, et al: Myeloablative therapy with autologous bone marrow transplantation as consolidation therapy for recurrent follicular lymphoma. J Clin Oncol 1994; 12:1177.

27. Shouten HC, Bierman PJ, Vaughan WP, et al: Autologous bone marrow transplantation in follicular non-Hodgkin's lymphoma before and after histologic transformation. Blood 1989; 74:2579.

28. Horning SJ: Low-Grade Lymphoma, 1993: State of the Art. In Proceedings of the Fifth International Conference on Lymphoma, 1993, 24a.

29. Freedman A, Gribben J, Rabinowe S, et al: Autologous bone marrow transplantation in advanced low-grade B-cell non-Hodgkin's lymphoma in first remission. Blood 1993; 82:1313a.

30. Bandini G, Michallet M, Rosti G, et al: Bone marrow transplantation for chronic lymphocytic leukemia. Bone Marrow Transplant 1991; 7:251.

31. Rabinowe SN, Soiffer RJ, Gribben JG, et al: Autologous and allogeneic bone marrow transplantation for poor prognosis patients with B-cell chronic lymphocytic leukemia. Blood 1993; 82:1366.

32. Vose JM, Weisenburger DD, Anderson JR, et al: Mantle cell lymphoma (MCL) has a poorer prognosis than follicular non-Hodgkin's lymphoma (F-NHL); however, high-dose therapy (HDC) and autologous stem cell transplantation (ASCT) may overcome treatment resistance in MCL. Blood 1993; 82:527a.

33. Phillips GL, Fay JW, Herzig RH, et al: The treatment of progressive non-Hodgkin's lymphoma with intensive chemoradiotherapy and autologous marrow transplantation. Blood 1990; 75:831.

34. Vose JM, Armitage JO, Bierman PJ, et al: Salvage therapy for relapsed or refractory non-Hodgkin's lymphoma utilizing autologous bone marrow transplantation. Am J Med 1989; 87:285.

35. Gribben JG, Goldstone AH, Linch DC, et al: Effectiveness of high-dose combination chemotherapy and autologous bone marrow transplantation for patients with non-Hodgkin's lymphomas who are still responsive to conventional-dose therapy. J Clin Oncol 1989; 7:1621.

36. Gulati S, Yahalom J, Acaba L, et al: Treatment of patients with relapsed and resistant non-Hodgkin's lymphoma using total-body irradiation, etoposide, and cyclophosphamide and autologous bone marrow transplantation. J Clin Oncol 1992; 10:936.

37. Bosly A, Coiffier B, Gisselbrecht C, et al: Bone marrow transplantation prolongs survival after relapse in aggressive lymphoma patients treated with the LNH-84 regimen. J Clin Oncol 1992; 10:1615.

38. Freedman AS, Takvorian T, Neuberg D, et al: Autologous bone marrow transplantation in poor-prognosis intermediate-grade and high-grade B-cell non-Hodgkin's lymphoma in first remission: A pilot study. J Clin Oncol 1993; 11:931.

39. Gordon B, Warkentin PI, Weisenburger DD, et al: Bone marrow transplantation for peripheral T-cell lymphoma in children and adolescents. Blood 1992; 80:2938.

40. Philip T, Armitage JO, Spitzer G, et al: High-dose therapy and autologous bone marrow transplantation after failure of conventional chemotherapy in adults with intermediate-grade or high-grade non-Hodgkin's lymphoma. N Engl J Med 1987; 316:1493.

41. Goldstone AH, McMillan AK, Chopra R: High-dose therapy for the treatment of non-Hodgkin's lymphoma. In Armitage J, Antman K (eds): High-Dose Cancer Therapy: Pharmacology, Hematopoietins, Stem Cells. Baltimore, Williams & Wilkins, 1992, pp 662–676.

42. Vose JM, Anderson JR, Kessinger A, et al: High-dose chemotherapy and autologous hematopoietic stem cell transplantation for aggressive non-Hodgkin's lymphoma. J Clin Oncol 1993; 11:1846.

43. Jagannath S, Velasquez WS, Tucker SL, et al: Tumor burden assessment and its implications for a prognostic model in advanced diffuse large-cell lymphoma. J Clin Oncol 1986; 4:859.

44. Coiffier B, Gisselbrecht C, Vose JM, et al: Prognostic factors in aggressive malignant lymphomas: Description and validation of a prognostic index that could identify patients requiring a more intensive therapy [The Groupe d'Etudes des Lymphomes Agressifs]. J Clin Oncol 1991; 9:211.

45. Kwak LW, Halpern J, Olshen RA, et al: Prognostic significance of actual dose intensity in diffuse large cell lymphoma: Results of a tree-structured survival analysis. J Clin Oncol 1990; 8:963.

46. Hoskins PJ, Ng V, Spinelli JJ, et al: Prognostic variables in patients with diffuse large cell lymphoma treated with MACOP-B. J Clin Oncol 1991; 9:220.

47. Armitage JO, Weisenburger DD, Hutchins M, et al: Chemotherapy for diffuse large cell lymphoma: Rapidly responding patients have more durable remissions. J Clin Oncol 1986; 4:160.

48. Shipp MA, Harrington DP, Klatt MM, et al: Identification of major prognostic subgroups of patients with large cell lymphoma treated with m-BACOD or M-BACOD. Ann Intern Med 1986; 104:757.

49. Coiffier B, Shipp MA, Cabanillas F, et al: Report of the first workshop in prognostic factors in large cell lymphomas. Ann Oncol 1991; 2:213.

50. International Non-Hodgkin's Lymphoma Prognostic Factors Project: A predictive model for aggressive non-Hodgkin's lymphoma. N Engl J Med 1993; 329:987.

51. Nademanee A, Schmidt GM, O'Donnell MR, et al: High-dose chemoradiotherapy followed by autologous bone marrow transplantation as consolidation therapy during first complete remission in adult patients with poor-risk aggressive lymphoma: A pilot study. Blood 1992; 80:1130.

52. Philip T, Hartmann O, Biron P, et al: High-dose therapy and autologous bone marrow transplantation in partial remission after first-line induction therapy for diffuse non-Hodgkin's lymphoma. J Clin Oncol 1988; 6:1118.

53. Baro J, Richard C, Calavia J, et al: Autologous bone marrow transplantation as consolidation therapy for non-Hodgkin's lymphoma patients with poor prognostic features. Bone Marrow Transplant 1991; 8:283.

54. Anderson JR, Derek R, Jenkin T, et al: Long-term follow-up of patients treated with COMP or LSA₂L₂ therapy for childhood non-Hodgkin's lymphoma: A report of CCG-551 from the Children's Cancer Group. J Clin Oncol 1986; 11:1024.

55. Slater DE, Mertelsmann R, Koziner B, et al: Lymphoblastic lymphoma in adults. J Clin Oncol 1986; 4:57.

56. Coleman CN, Picozzi VJ, Cox RS, et al: Treatment of lymphoblastic lymphoma in adults. J Clin Oncol 1986; 4:1628.

57. Bernstein JI, Coleman CN, Strickler JG, et al: Combined modality therapy for adults with small noncleaved cell lymphoma (Burkitt's and non-Burkitt's) types. J Clin Oncol 1986; 4:847.

58. Sullivan MP, Ramirez I: Curability of Burkitt's lymphoma with high-dose cyclophosphamide, high-dose methotrexate therapy and intrathecal chemoprophylaxis. J Clin Oncol 1985; 3:627.

59. MaGrath IT, Shiramizu B: Biology and treatment of small noncleaved cell lymphoma. Oncology 1989; 3:41.

60. Lopez TM, Hagemeister FB, McLaughlin P, et al: Small noncleaved cell lymphoma in adults: Superior results for stages I-III disease. J Clin Oncol 1990; 8:615.

61. Appelbaum FR, Deisseroth AB, Graw RG, et al: Prolonged complete remission following high-dose chemotherapy of Burkitt's lymphoma in relapse. Cancer 1978; 41:1059.

62. O'Leary M, Ramsay NK, Nesbit ME, et al: Bone marrow transplantation for non-Hodgkin's lymphoma in children and young adults. Am J Med 1983; 74:497.

63. Vaughan WP, Weisenburger DD, Sanger W, et al: Early leukemic recurrence of non-Hodgkin's lymphoma after high-dose antineoplastic therapy. Bone Marrow Transplant 1987; 1:373.

64. Troussard X, Leglond V, Kuentz M, et al: Allogeneic bone marrow transplantation in adults with Burkitt's lymphoma or acute lymphoblastic leukemia in first complete remission. J Clin Oncol 1990; 8:809.

65. Santini G, Coser P, Chisesi T, et al: Autologous bone marrow transplantation for advanced-stage adult lymphoblastic lymphoma in first complete remission: A pilot study of the Non-Hodgkin's Lymphoma Cooperative Study Group (NHLCSG). Bone Marrow Transplant 1989; 4:399.

66. Chopra R, Goldstone AH, Pearce R, et al: Autologous versus allogeneic bone marrow transplantation for non-Hodgkin's lymphoma: A case-controlled analysis of the European Bone Marrow Transplant Group registry data. J Clin Oncol 1992; 10:1690.

67. Santos GW, Saral R, Burns WH, et al: Allogeneic, syngeneic, and autologous marrow transplantation in the acute leukemias and lymphomas—Baltimore experiences. Acta Haematol 1987; 78:175.

68. Appelbaum FR, Sullivan KM, Buckner CD, et al: Treatment of malignant lymphoma in 100 patients with chemotherapy, total-body irradiation, and marrow transplantation. J Clin Oncol 1987; 5:1340.

69. Phillips GL, Herzig RH, Lazarus HM, et al: High-dose chemotherapy, fractionated total-body irradiation, and allogeneic marrow transplantation for malignant lymphoma. J Clin Oncol 1986; 4:480.

70. Shepherd JD, Barnett MJ, Connors JM, et al: Allogeneic bone marrow transplantation for poor-prognosis non-Hodgkin's lymphoma. Bone Marrow Transplant 1993; 12:591.

71. Beatty PG, Clift RA, Mickelson EM, et al: Marrow transplantation from related donors other than HLA-identical siblings. N Engl J Med 1985; 313:765.

72. Stewart D, Bierman P, Anderson J, et al: High dose chemotherapy (HDC) with autologous hematopoietic rescue in patients (Pts) age 60 and over. Proc ASCO 1994; 13:1260a.

73. Brice P, Marolleau JP, Dombret H, et al: Autologous peripheral blood stem cell transplantation after high-dose therapy in patients with advanced lymphomas. Bone Marrow Transplant 1992; 9:337.

74. Dreyfus F, Leblond V, Velanger C, et al: Peripheral blood stem cell collection and autografting in high-risk lymphomas. Bone Marrow Transplant 1992; 10:409.

75. Kessinger A, Vose JM, Bierman PJ, et al: High-dose therapy and autologous peripheral stem cell transplantation for patients with bone marrow metastases and relapsed lymphoma: An alternative to bone marrow purging. Exp Hematol 1991; 19:1013.

76. Sharp JG, Joshi SS, Armitage JO, et al: Significance of detection of occult non-Hodgkin's lymphoma in histologically uninvolved bone marrow by a culture technique. Blood 1992; 79:1074.

77. Kiesel S, Pezzutto A, Korbling M, et al: Autologous peripheral blood stem cell transplantation: Analysis of autografted cells and lymphocyte recovery. Transplant Proc 1989; 21:3084.

78. Wagner JE, Broxmeyer JE, Byrd RL, et al: Transplantation of umbilical cord blood after myeloablative therapy: Analysis of engraftment. Blood 1992; 79:1874.

79. Koller MR, Emerson SG, Palsson BO: Large-scale expansion of human stem and progenitor cells from bone marrow mononuclear cells in continuous perfusion cultures. Blood 1993; 82:378.

80. Longo DL, Duffey PL, Young RC, et al: Conventional-dose salvage combination chemotherapy in patients relapsing with Hodgkin's disease after combination chemotherapy: The low probability for cure. J Clin Oncol 1992; 10:210

81. Santaro A, Bonfante V, Bonadonna G: Salvage chemotherapy with ABVD in MOPP-resistant Hodgkin's disease. Ann Intern Med 1982; 96:139.

82. Jagannath S, Dicke KA, Armitage JO, et al: High-dose cyclophosphamide, carmustine, and etoposide and autologous bone marrow transplantation for relapsed Hodgkin's disease. Ann Intern Med 1986; 104:163.

83. Reece DE, Barnett MJ, Connors JM, et al: Intensive chemotherapy with cyclophosphamide, carmustine, and etoposide followed by autologous bone marrow transplantation for relapsed Hodgkin's disease. J Clin Oncol 1991; 9:1871.

84. Carella AM, Congiu AM, Gaozza E, et al: High-dose chemotherapy with autologous bone marrow transplantation in 50 advanced resistant Hodgkin's disease patients: An Italian study group report. J Clin Oncol 1988; 6:1411.

85. Armitage JO, Bierman PJ, Vose JM, et al: Autologous bone marrow transplantation for patients with relapsed Hodgkin's disease. Am J Med 1991; 91:605.

86. Bierman PJ, Bagin RG, Jagannath S, et al: High-dose chemotherapy followed by autologous hematopoietic rescue in Hodgkin's disease: Long-term follow-up in 128 patients. Ann Oncol 1993; 4:767.

87. Nademanee A, O'Donnell MR, Snyder DS, et al: High-dose chemotherapy with or without total-body irradiation followed by autologous bone marrow and/or peripheral blood stem cell transplantation for patients with relapsed and refractory Hodgkin's disease: Results in 85 patients with analysis of prognostic factors. Blood 1995; 85:1381.

88. Gianni AM, Siena S, Bregni M, et al: Prolonged disease-free survival after high-dose sequential chemoradiotherapy and hemopoietic autologous transplantation in poor-prognosis Hodgkin's disease. Ann Oncol 1991; 2:645.

89. Yahalom J, Gulati SC, Toia M, et al: Accelerated hyperfractionated total-lymphoid irradiation, high-dose chemotherapy, and autologous bone marrow transplantation for refractory and relapsing patients with Hodgkin's disease. J Clin Oncol 1993; 11:1062.

90. Reece DE, Connors JM, Spinelli JJ, et al: Intensive therapy with cyclophosphamide, carmustine, etoposide ± cisplatin, and autologous bone marrow transplantation for Hodgkin's disease in first relapse after combination chemotherapy. Blood 1994; 83:1193.

91. Carella AM: The place of high-dose therapy with autologous stem cell transplantation in primary treatment of Hodgkin's disease. Ann Oncol 1993; 4:s15.

92. Petersen FB, Appelbaum FR, Hill R, et al: Autologous marrow transplantation for malignant lymphoma: A report of 101 cases from Seattle. J Clin Oncol 1990; 8:638.

93. Vose JM, Darrington D, Bierman P, et al: Myelodysplastic syndrome (MDS)/acute myelogenous leukemia (AML) following high-dose chemotherapy and autologous stem cell transplantation for lymphoid malignancy: Characterization and relative risk. *In* Proceedings of the Fifth International Conference on Malignant Lymphoma, 1993, 42a.

94. Bierman PJ, Vose JM, Leichner PK, et al: Yttrium 90-labeled antiferritin followed by high-dose chemotherapy and autologous bone marrow transplantation for poor-prognosis Hodgkin's disease. J Clin Oncol 1993; 11:698.

95. Treleaven JG, Kemshead JT: Removal of tumour cells from bone marrow: An evaluation of the available techniques. Hematol Oncol 1985; 3:65.

96. Colombat P, Gorin NC, Lemonnier MP, et al: The role of autologous bone marrow transplantation in 46 adult patients with non-Hodgkin's lymphomas. J Clin Oncol 1990; 8:630.

97. Weisdorf DJ, Haake R, Miller WJ, et al: Autologous bone marrow transplantation for progressive non-Hodgkin's lymphoma: Clinical impact of immunophenotype and in vitro purging. Bone Marrow Transplant 1991; 8:135.

98. Gribben JG, Freedman AS, Neuberg D, et al: Immunologic purging of marrow assessed by PCR before autologous bone marrow transplantation for B-cell lymphoma. N Engl J Med 1991; 325:1525.

99. Johnson PWM, Price CGA, Smith T, et al: Detection of cells bearing the t(14;18) translocation following myeloablative treatment and autologous bone marrow transplantation for follicular lymphoma. J Clin Oncol 1994; 12:798.

100. Sharp JG, Crouse DA: Marrow contamination: Detection and significance. *In* Armitage J, Antman K (eds): High-Dose Cancer Therapy: Pharmacology, Hematopoietins, Stem Cells. Baltimore, Williams & Wilkins, 1992, pp 226–248.

101. Berenson RJ, Shpall EJ, Franklin W, et al: Transplantation of CD34 positive (+) marrow and/or peripheral blood progenitor cells (PBPC) into breast cancer patients following high-dose chemotherapy (HDC). Blood 1993; 82:678a.

102. Haioun C, Lepage E, Gisselbrecht C, et al: Comparison of autologous bone marrow transplantation (ABMT) with sequential chemotherapy for aggressive non-Hodgkin's lymphoma (NHL) in first complete remission: A study of 464 patients (LNH87 protocol). Blood 1993; 82:334a.

103. Zinzani PL, Tura S, Mazza P, et al: ABMT versus DHAP in residual disease following third-generation regimens for aggressive non-Hodgkin's lymphomas. *In* Proceedings of the Fifth International Conference on Malignant Lymphoma, 1993, 41a.

104. Storb R, Deeg HJ, Whitehead J, et al: Methotrexate and cyclosporine compared with cyclosporine alone for prophylaxis of graft-versus-host disease in patients given HLA-identical marrow grafts for leukemia: Long-term follow-up of a controlled trial. Blood 1989; 73:1729.

105. Ramsay NKC, Kersey JH, Robison LL, et al: A randomized study of the prevention of acute graft-versus-host disease. N Engl J Med 1982; 306:392.

106. Mitsuyasu RT, Champlin RE, Gale RP, et al: Treatment of donor bone marrow with monoclonal anti-T-cell antibody and complement for the prevention of graft-versus-host disease: A prospective, randomized, double-blind trial. Ann Intern Med 1986; 105:20.

107. Martin PJ, Schoch G, Fisher L, et al: A retrospective analysis of therapy for acute graft-versus-host disease: Initial treatment. Blood 1990; 76:1464.

108. Kennedy MS, Deeg HJ, Storb R, et al: Treatment of acute graft-versus-host disease after allogeneic marrow transplantation: Randomized study comparing corticosteroids and cyclosporine. Am J Med 1985; 78:978.

109. Herve P, Wijdenes J, Bergerat JP, et al: Treatment of corticosteroid-resistant acute graft-versus-host disease by in vivo administration of anti-interleukin-2 receptor monoclonal antibody (B-B10). Blood 1990; 75:1017.

110. Champlin RE, Horowitz MM, van Bekkum DW, et al: Graft failure following bone marrow transplantation for severe aplastic anemia: Risk factors and treatment results. Blood 1989; 73:606.

111. Anasetti C, Doney KC, Storb R, et al: Marrow transplantation for severe aplastic anemia: Long-term outcome in fifty "untransfused" patients. Ann Intern Med 1986; 104:461.

112. Nemunaitis J, Rabinowe SN, Singer JW, et al: Recombinant granulocyte-macrophage colony-stimulating factor after autologous bone marrow transplantation for lymphoid cancer. N Engl J Med 1991; 324:1773.

113. Taylor KM, Jagannath S, Spitzer G, et al: Recombinant human granulocyte colony-stimulating factor hastens granulocyte recovery after high-dose chemotherapy and autologous bone marrow transplantation in Hodgkin's disease. J Clin Oncol 1989; 7:1791.

114. Link H, Boogaerts MA, Carella AM, et al: A controlled trial of recombinant human granulocyte-macrophage colony-stimulating factor after total-body irradiation, high-dose chemotherapy, and autologous bone marrow transplantation for acute lymphoblastic leukemia or malignant lymphoma. Blood 1992; 80:2188.

115. Gorin NC, Coiffier B, Hayat M, et al: Recombinant human granulocyte-macrophage colony-stimulating factor after high-dose chemotherapy and autologous bone marrow transplantation with unpurged and purged marrow in non-Hodgkin's lymphoma: A double-blind, placebo-controlled trial. Blood 1992; 80:1149.

116. Lazarus HM, Winton EF, Williams SF, et al: Phase I study of recombinant human interleukin-6 (IL-6) after autologous bone marrow transplant (ABMT) in patients with poor-prognosis breast cancer. Blood 1993; 82:677a.

117. Fay J, Bernstein S, Herzig R, et al: A phase I study of sequential rhil-3 and rhgm-CSF following autologous bone marrow transplantation therapy for lymphoma. Blood 1993; 82:334a.

118. Vose JM, Anderson J, Bierman PJ, et al: Initial trial of PIXY321 (GM-CSF/IL-3) fusion protein following high-dose chemotherapy and autologous bone marrow transplantation (ABMT) for lymphoid malignancy. Proc ASCO 1993; 12:37a.

119. Miller W, Flynn P, McCullough H, et al: Cytomegalovirus infection after bone marrow transplantation: An association with acute graft-versus-host disease. Blood 1986; 67:1162.

120. Bowden RA, Sayers M, Flournoy N, et al: Cytomegalovirus immune globulin and seronegative blood products to prevent primary cytomegalovirus infection after marrow transplantation. N Engl J Med 1986; 314:1006.

121. Winston DJ, Ho WG, Lin CH, et al: Intravenous immune globulin for prevention of cytomegalovirus infection and interstitial pneumonia after bone marrow transplantation. Ann Intern Med 1987; 106:12.

122. Meyers JD, Feed EC, Shepp DH, et al: Acyclovir for prevention of cytomegalovirus infection and disease after allogeneic marrow transplantation. N Engl J Med 1988; 318:70.

123. Goodrich JM, Mori M, Gleaves CA, et al: Early treatment with ganciclovir to prevent cytomegalovirus disease after allogeneic bone marrow transplantation. N Engl J Med 1991; 325:1601.

124. Chao NJ, Duncan SR, Long GD, et al: Corticosteroid therapy for diffuse alveolar hemorrhage in autologous bone marrow transplant recipients. Ann Intern Med 1991; 114:145.

125. Shulman HM, Hinterberger W: Hepatic veno-occlusive disease–liver toxicity syndrome after bone marrow transplantation. Bone Marrow Transplant 1992; 10:197.

126. Bearman SI, Shuhart MC, Hinds MS, et al: Recombinant human tissue plasminogen activator for the treatment of established severe venoocclusive disease of the liver after bone marrow transplantation. Blood 1992; 80:2458.

127. Vose JM, Reed EC, Pipert G, et al: A randomized trial of mesna versus continuous bladder irrigation for prevention of hemorrhagic cystitis associated with high-dose therapy and autologous bone marrow transplantation. J Clin Oncol 1993; 11:1306.

128. Shulman HM, Sullivan KM, Weiden PL, et al: Chronic graft-versus-host syndrome in man: A long-term clinicopathologic study of 20 Seattle patients. Am J Med 1980; 69:204.

129. Wingard JR, Piantadosi S, Vogelsang GB, et al: Predictors of death from chronic graft-versus-host disease after bone marrow transplantation. Blood 1989; 74:1428.

130. Sullivan KM, Witherspoon RP, Storb R, et al: Alternating-day cyclosporine and prednisone for treatment of high-risk chronic graft-versus-host disease. Blood 1988; 72:555.

131. Vogelsang GB, Farmer ER, Hess AD, et al: Thalidomide for the treatment of chronic graft-versus-host disease. N Engl J Med 1992; 326:1055.

132. Tichelli A, Gratwohl A, Egger T, et al: Cataract formation after bone marrow transplantation. Ann Intern Med 1993; 119:1175.

133. Badier M, Guillot C, Delpierre S, et al: Pulmonary function changes 100 days and one year after bone marrow transplantation. Bone Marrow Transplant 1993; 12:457.

134. Braverman AC, Antin JH, Plappert MT, et al: Cyclophosphamide cardiotoxicity in bone marrow transplantation: A prospective evaluation of new dosing regimens. J Clin Oncol 1991; 9:1215.

135. Vose JM, Kennedy BC, Bierman PJ, et al: Long-term sequelae of autologous bone marrow transplantation or peripheral stem cell transplantation for lymphoid malignancies. Cancer 1992; 69:784.

136. Chao NJ, Tierney DK, Bloom JR, et al: Dynamic assessment of quality of life after autologous bone marrow transplantation. Blood 1992; 80:825.

137. Wingard JR, Curbow B, Baker F, et al: Sexual satisfaction in survivors of bone marrow transplantation. Bone Marrow Transplant 1992; 9:185.

138. Pezner RD, Nademanee A, Niland J, et al: Involved-field radiation therapy in the management of Hodgkin's disease patients undergoing autologous bone marrow transplantation regimens. Proc ASCO 1994; 13:1313a.

139. Kaminski MS, Zasadny KR, Francis IR, et al: Radioimmunotherapy of B-cell lymphoma with [131I] Anti-B1 (Anti-CD20) antibody. N Engl J Med 1993; 329:459.

140. Press OW, Eary JR, Appelbaum FR, et al: Radiolabeled-antibody therapy of B-cell lymphoma with autologous bone marrow support. N Engl J Med 1993; 329:1219.

141. Lauria F, Raspadori D, Zinzani PL, et al: Clinical and immunologic effects of IL-2 in non-Hodgkin's lymphoma patients after autologous bone marrow transplantation. Blood 1993; 82:566a.
142. Smalley RV, Andersen JW, Hawkins MJ, et al: Interferon alfa combined with cytotoxic chemotherapy for patients with non-Hodgkin's lymphoma. N Engl J Med 1992; 327:1336.
143. Urabe A, Mutoh Y, Mizoguchi H, et al: Ubenimex in the treatment of acute nonlymphocytic leukemia in adults. Ann Hematol 1993; 67:63.
144. Mazumder A, Verma U, Areman E, et al: Peripheral blood stem cell (PBSC) transplantation in breast cancer patients with interleukin-2 (IL-2)–activated PBSC leads to visceral graft-versus-host disease (GVHD). Proc ASCO 1994; 13:91a.

━━ Biologic Therapy for Lymphomas ━━

Derek Crowther

Biologic therapy for lymphoma has involved the use of natural products designed to augment the host's own defense mechanisms. Approaches used for treating patients with lymphoma have included natural proteins such as the interferons, antibodies and cytokines, or growth factors and have been attended by some success. Methods of inducing and enhancing immune defenses against the tumor using techniques of tumor vaccination and transfusion of immune cells have also been employed, although the therapeutic effects have been relatively modest. In the last few years a more scientifically directed approach to biotherapy has been possible with improvements in the understanding of the mechanisms involved and the development of molecular genetic procedures that have allowed the production of specific therapeutic agents.

THE INTERFERONS

In 1957, two scientists at the National Institute of Medical Research in London discovered that virus-infected cells became resistant to secondary infection. Drs. Alick Isaacs and Jean Lindenmann found that influenza virus–infected chick embryo cells released a substance that conferred on cells on the same species resistance to a wide range of viruses. This substance was named "interferon," which is now known to be secreted in small amounts by most vertebrate cells when they are appropriately stimulated.

The interferons have significant antiviral activity, and it is likely that they have a role in controlling infection by many types of virus. They also have a role in immune function and act as negative regulators of cell growth. Interferon-α has been found to have a role in the treatment of certain forms of lymphoid malignancy.

CLASSIFICATION

The interferons belong to a family of extracellular signaling proteins with some degree of overlapping activities. The type I interferons (α and β) have predominant antiviral effects and negative effects on cell growth, whereas type II interferon (γ)—produced by T cells when they are stimulated by antigens or mitogens—has a role in immune modulation. Interferons α and β are induced following viral infection, with the α interferons predominating in leukocytes and epithelial cells and interferon-β in fibroblasts.

At least 24 different interferon-α genes have been located on chromosome 9 that encode 15 functional proteins. A high degree of homology exists between these molecules (about 92%), and they are functionally indistinguishable. The interferon-α2 proteins differ from the interferon-α_1 in having six or seven more amino acids and being glycosylated. Interferon-β is encoded by a single gene on chromosome 9 close to the interferon-α gene cluster and is structurally related to interferon-α (about 45% homology). The α and β interferons share a receptor, but interferon-γ has little homology with other interferons, is located as a single gene on chromosome 12, and has a distinct receptor (Table 14–1).

Initial preparations of interferon for use in humans were prepared from blood leukocytes or lymphoblastoid cell lines. The classification of recombinant interferons is given in Table 14–2.

PHYSIOLOGIC ROLE

The physiologic role of the several types of interferon is largely unknown, although a considerable amount is known about their properties. They act as a family of extracellular signaling proteins influencing the expression of many genes. The cellular responses evoked vary with the type of interferon and the cells involved. Undoubtedly, the inhibition of viral reproduction and packaging early during infection plays an important role in recovery from viral infection, and the interferon immunomodulatory properties are likely to play a part in other forms of infections. Immune modulation with enhancement of major histocompatibility complex (MHC) class I proteins by interferon α, β, and γ and increased cell surface expression of MHC class II molecules by interferon-γ may well play an important part in assisting the presentation of cell-associated antigens to cells of the immune system. These and other effects on immune function are listed in Table 14–3.

ANTITUMOR PROPERTIES

During the 1960s interferon was recognized to have antitumor effects in experimental systems, but only in the 1970s were interferons derived from human leukocytes and lymphoblastoid cell lines made available for clinical trials.

Table 14–1. Chromosome Location of Interferons (IFNs) and Their Receptors

	IFN-α	IFN-β	IFN-γ
Number of genes	24+	1	1
Chromosome location	9	9	12
Receptor type	α/β	α/β	γ
Chromosome location of IFN receptors	21	21	6

New molecular technology allowed the manufacture of recombinant human interferon-α in 1982, and subsequently human recombinant interferon β and γ became available for therapy. The introduction of these pure recombinant proteins permitted a more specific and quantitative approach to laboratory and human studies. More than 15 years have passed since recombinant interferons were first used as antitumor therapy in humans, but we remain unsure of the mechanisms regulating the most desirable attributes of the interferons and uncertain as to the best ways of exploiting them clinically.

The interferons have been shown to have direct antitumor effects on human tumor xenografts in athymic (nude) mice. The human interferons do not bind to murine interferon receptors, and the tumor regressions seen in these models cannot be attributed to host interactions.[1] Murine interferons, however, can have antitumor effects against human xenografts in nude mice.

INTERFERON THERAPY

The antiproliferative effects of the interferons demonstrated on tumor cell lines in vitro and their antitumor properties in animal models led the way to clinical studies in humans. In animal studies interferons used as single agents are capable of causing tumor regression and prolonged survival, but they seldom achieve cure. The species specificity of the interferons was an added difficulty in preclinical evaluation, and as is the case for other anticancer agents, animal model systems have not been good predictors of clinical outcome. Early studies were hampered by the use of impure preparations available only in small quantities. Despite this, anticancer effects were soon demonstrated in humans.

Interferon preparations studied clinically include mixed interferon-α subtypes purified from virus-stimulated lymphoblastoid cell lines (e.g., "Wellferon") and from virus-stimulated buffy coat cells, in addition to the single α

Table 14–2. Recommended Nomenclature of the Recombinant Human Interferons (IFNs)

Nomenclature		Peptide Sequences	
New	**Old**	**Position 23**	**Position 24**
IFN-α2a	IFN-αA	Lys	His
IFN-α2b	IFN-α2	Arg	His
IFN-α2c	IFN-α2arg	Arg	Arg
IFN-β	Fibroblastoid IFN		
IFN-γ	Immune IFN		

Table 14–3. Immunomodulating Effects of the Interferons

	Interferon-α/β	Interferon-γ
Class I MHC protein expression	+	++
Class II MHC protein expression	0	++
Macrophage activation	+	++
Granulocyte activation	0	++
Natural killer cell activation	+	++
Increased antibody-dependent cellular cytotoxicity	+	++
Cytotoxic T-cell activation	0	++
Immunoglobulin class switch	0	++
B-cell activation	+	+
IgG Fc receptor expression	+	+
β2-microglobulin induction	+	+
Cytokine expression	±	+

subtypes produced by recombinant DNA technology (e.g., interferon-α2a "Roferon" and interferon-α2b "Intron-A"). Natural human interferon-β is unstable in vitro, so the recombinant preparation in clinical use has serine substituted for cysteine at amino acid position 17 (interferon-βser). This compound is stable for prolonged periods.

The interferons have been found to be active as single agents in inducing remissions in patients with follicular lymphoma, low-grade T-cell lymphoma, and hairy leukemia/lymphoma. They are generally ineffective as single agents in intermediate-grade or high-grade lymphoma, although transient responses may be observed.

The first licensed application for interferon-α was for the therapy of hairy cell leukemia/lymphoma. Since 1984, numerous clinical studies have confirmed its usefulness in this rare disease. Although highly active in hairy cell leukemia, interferons do not cure the disease, and prolonged therapy is necessary for most patients. In a large multicenter study, 195 patients received interferon-α2b 2 megaunits (MU) m² three times weekly by subcutaneous injection for 12 or 18 months.[2] The overall response rate (complete responses plus pathologic partial responses plus hematologic partial responses) was 87%, with significant improvement in anemia, neutropenia, and thrombocytopenia. Among 91 patients evaluable for the maintenance phase of treatment, relapse was more common in those assigned to observation only, but a further partial response to interferon was seen in about half of those retreated at relapse. Another study showed that after remission induction with interferon-α2a, approximately half the patients relapsed at a median interval of 10 months, and these relapses could be predicted by a persistently low platelet count on completion of primary treatment.[3] The CD25 molecule that corresponds to the p55 α chain of the interleukin-2 (IL-2) receptor is highly expressed by neoplastic cells in hairy cell leukemia and is released in large amounts in the soluble form, which is detectable in the serum. The amount of CD25 in the circulation correlates with tumor burden and can be used as a disease marker.[4] Treatment is well tolerated if paracetamol is given prophylactically, and most patients with hairy cell leukemia are symptomatically improved. Disease can be controlled for long periods using repeated courses of therapy, although there have been few complete remissions. In a followup report of 69 patients receiving their primary treatment from 1983 to 1986, only 11 patients had died before 1991, with 16 of 57 patients who completed the initial course of interferon continuing in remission without further therapy.[5]

Interferon-α has been used as first-line therapy in patients with hairy cell leukemia/lymphoma for several years, but the recently introduced agent 2-chlorodeoxyadenosine is associated with a higher remission rate. The comparative role of these two approaches needs further assessment.[6]

Initial studies of the antilymphoma effects of interferon involved the use of polyclonal interferon derived either from the leukocytes of the peripheral blood buffy coat or from lymphoblastoid cell lines. In the first report, three heavily treated patients with diffuse large cell lymphoma received interferon but showed no response. Three other patients with follicular lymphoma, however, were partial responders, with two responses lasting 6 and 9 months.[7] Subsequently, other series of patients with follicular lymphoma were reported, and of a total of 55 patients treated, 17 (31%) showed a complete or partial response (Table 14–4). The interferon used in these trials was not highly purified (it consisted of a variable mixture of different types of interferon), and the specific activity varied depending on the production batch.

The advent of recombinant technology resulted in the commercial production of pure, monoclonal proteins with defined specific activity for clinical use, allowing evaluation on a more systematic basis. These studies of recombinant interferon-α confirmed the efficacy in low-grade lymphoma (Table 14–5). In one of the earliest studies, responses were seen in 13 of 24 patients with follicular lymphoma (four complete and nine partial), but responses were only seen in two of six patients with intermediate-grade lymphoma and one of seven patients with a high-grade lymphoma.[13] In general, responses in patients with intermediate- and high-grade lymphoma have been few in number and transient, whereas the overall response rate for follicular lymphoma has been consistently higher and more durable, with a response rate of 50% in a collected series of 115 patients (see Table 14–5).

Interferon-α has also been shown to be effective in patients with cutaneous T-cell lymphoma, and response rates ranging from 30% to 85% have been reported.[19] Both newly diagnosed patients with early disease and those with advanced disease refractory to chemotherapy have been treated, resulting in a response rate of 65% in 86 patients pooled from six reported series. Responses lasted from 3 months to more than 2 years. Interferon-γ has also been shown to be effective in this condition, with response rates of 30% to 60% being reported.[20, 21]

Table 14–4. Studies of Therapy Using Polyclonal Leukocyte Interferon in Follicular Lymphoma

Reference	No. of Patients	Complete + Partial Response
Merigan et al, 1978[7]	3	3
Gutterman et al, 1980[8]	6	3
Louie et al, 1981[9]	8	4
Gamms et al, 1984[10]	20	4
Horning et al, 1985[11]	18	3
Total	**55**	**17 (31%)**

Table 14–5. Recombinant Human Interferon-α in Follicular Non-Hodgkin's Lymphoma

Reference	No. of Patients	Complete + Partial Response	Interferon
Quesada et al, 1984[12]	17	6	rh IFN-α2a
Foon et al, 1984[13]	24	13	rh IFN-α2a
Wagstaff et al, 1986°, [14]	30	15	rh IFN-α2b
O'Connell et al, 1986°, [15]	9	4	rh IFN-α2a
Leavitt et al, 1983[16]	15	10	rh IFN-α2b
Mantovani et al, 1989°, [17]	8	5	rh IFN-α2a
Billard et al, 1991[18]	12	5	rh IFN-α2a
Total	**115**	**58 (50%)**	

°Previously untreated patients.
IFN, interferon.

Dose and Schedule

The relationship between dose and response remains unclear, and an optimum schedule has not been defined. One study attempted to address this issue using a randomized trial, but only 40 patients were included with a variety of low-grade lymphomas and different amounts of previous chemotherapy.[22] Of the 19 patients randomized to low-dose therapy (3 MU subcutaneously daily), five achieved a partial response. Of 20 patients treated with the high-dose schedule (50 MU intramuscularly twice weekly), seven responded and two achieved a complete response. The discrepancy in response rates was not significant between the two schedules, and no patient who was crossed to high-dose from the low-dose therapy had a further response. All eventually progressed on the high-dose regimen.

In general, the induction of remission in patients with low-grade lymphoma is less rapid than with conventional chemotherapy. Responses often take more than 1 month to develop, with a median time to maximal response of about 3 months and a median time to disease progression of approximately 6 months. Since the toxic side effects are dose related, and no significant differences in response rates have been seen between doses ranging from 2 MU/m² up to 50 MU/m² given three times weekly, the current recommendation for treatment is at the lower dose of 2 to 5 MU/m² given three times weekly by subcutaneous injection.

Some authors have suggested that downregulation of interferon-α receptors and the induction of 2'-5' oligoadenylate synthetase in tumor B cells may be correlated with an increase in response rates, but the evidence is weak.[18, 23] Further work on the mechanism of action in lymphoma is required.

Side Effects

The most commonly described side effect of interferon treatment is a flulike syndrome of fever, headache, myalgia, and fatigue. These symptoms begin within hours of interferon administration and typically resolve within 12 hours. For this reason many patients prefer to be treated in the evening. Nausea and vomiting occur occasionally and may lead to weight loss. These side effects frequently reduce in severity with time in patients receiving continuous treatment. Transient elevation of liver enzyme levels may sometimes occur. Hypotension has also been reported, particularly when high doses are used, and may be related to increased vascular permeability.

Bone marrow depression with neutropenia and thrombocytopenia is more serious and can limit administration (particularly when the interferons are used in association with cytotoxic chemotherapy), and anemia can occur with chronic administration. Central nervous system toxicity, including lassitude, depression, and temporary memory loss, is fairly common. Neurotoxicity may accompany high-dose therapy and can include encephalopathy, ataxia, and cortical blindness,[24, 25] but severe neurotoxicity is unusual at conventional doses. Because the interferons do not readily cross the blood-brain barrier, these side effects are believed to be indirect and may be related to the cascade of other cytokines released following interferon therapy. Cardiac changes have been reported in patients receiving interferon, but it is not clear whether these are direct or indirect effects.[26] A history of epilepsy and angina is a relative contraindication to its use. In view of the effects of the interferons on MHC antigen expression, patients have been closely monitored for the development of autoantibodies. A high incidence of thyroid autoantibodies has been reported, with some patients developing overt hypothyroidism[27]

Some patients develop antibodies to recombinant interferon during therapy, and this seems to be more common for interferon-α2a than for interferon-α2b.[28] In this study, of 33 patients treated with interferon-α2b, only 2 developed antibodies, and these were at low titer. Of 50 patients treated with interferon-α2a, however, 14 (28%) developed antibodies and 10 were at high titer.

Interferon with Chemotherapy

Most of the responses to interferon in patients with lymphoma have been only partial, slow to develop, and of relatively short duration. In addition, the patients benefiting most have been those with follicular lymphoma—a group known to have relatively high complete and partial response rates with single alkylating agent therapy. Experiments in murine models of leukemia and lymphoma[29, 30] and studies of human breast cancer xenografts in nude mice[31] have

suggested that alkylating agents and interferon-α may act synergistically. These observations have led to several studies in which interferon has been used in conjunction with chemotherapy.

In previously untreated follicular lymphoma, two randomized trials have compared interferon-α in combination with chemotherapy with chemotherapy only (Table 14–6). In the United States, the Eastern Cooperative Oncology Group compared 8 to 10 cycles of COPA (cyclophosphamide, Oncovin, prednisolone, Adriamycin) with COPA plus interferon-α2a at 6 MU/m[2] given for the last 5 days of each 28 day cycle. Of the 291 patients randomized, 42 were ineligible, 83 had diffuse, well-differentiated lymphocytic lymphoma or diffuse, poorly differentiated lymphocytic lymphoma, and 166 had follicular lymphoma (28 of these were nodular histiocytic). The response rates were similar in the two groups, but patients in the interferon group had significant prolongation of time to treatment failure and overall survival at 3 years.[33] However, a later 5-year followup showed no significant survival difference.[34] The second study was conducted by the Group d'Etudes des Lymphomes des l'Adulte (a French/Belgian group).[32] This randomized trial involved 242 previously untreated patients with follicular lymphoma and adverse prognostic features. All patients were treated with a regimen of CHVP (cyclophosphamide, hydroxydaunomycin, VM-26, and prednisone) given monthly for six cycles and then every 2 months for 1 year. One hundred nineteen patients were randomized to the chemotherapy-alone arm, and 123 patients received CHVP plus interferon-α2b at a dose of 5 MU three times weekly for 18 months. The patients treated with interferon had a significantly higher response rate, event-free survival, and overall survival at 3 years (see Table 14–6). This is the only report demonstrating a benefit in terms of overall survival for interferon-treated patients.

A British trial has addressed the role of interferon-α in combination with single-agent chemotherapy for remission induction and as maintenance following chemotherapy using double randomization.[35] This study has not yet been fully reported. Patients with follicular lymphoma requiring treatment were randomized at trial entry to receive chlorambucil alone or chlorambucil plus interferon-α2b (2 MU/m[2] three times weekly), and those who responded were further

Table 14–6. Two Large, Randomized Trials Comparing Chemotherapy with or without Interferon-α in Previously Untreated Patients with Follicular Lymphoma

Group (Reference)	Diagnosis	No. Enrolled	Randomization	No. Evaluable	Response	EFS	3-yr Survival
GELA (Solal-Celigny et al, 1993[32])	Follicular lymphoma	242	CHVP alone (18 mth)	119	69%	19 mth	69%
			P value		0.006	<0.001	0.02
			CHVP + IFN-α (5 MU three times weekly)	123	85%	35 mth	86%
ECOG (Smalley et al, 1992[33])	Mostly follicular	291	COPA alone (8–10 cycles)	127	86%	19 mth	68%
			P value		NS	<0.001	0.014
			COPA + IFN-α (6 MU/m[2] last 5 d of each cycle)	122	86%	30 mth	76%

NS, no significance; EFS, event-free survival. See text for other abbreviations.

randomized to maintenance interferon for up to 12 months or no further treatment. There was no significant difference in the response rate or overall survival, but patients receiving interferon throughout had a significantly longer duration of response. Another randomized study investigating the role of maintenance interferon following eight cycles of CVP (cyclophosphamide, vincristine, prednisolone) in patients with follicular lymphoma has been reported in preliminary form.[36] Of the 331 patients in the study, 231 were randomized for maintenance therapy or control. Although there was no difference in overall survival, the progression-free survival was 135 weeks for the interferon-treated patients and 86 weeks for the control group ($p = 0.02$).

Despite these randomized trials the case for treating low-grade lymphoma with interferon, either in combination with chemotherapy or as maintenance following remission induction, remains unproven. Only one such study has shown an improvement in survival for patients with follicular lymphoma treated with interferon in combination with chemotherapy, and the followup in this study was relatively brief (3 years). Already, one trial initially showing an improvement in survival at 3 years has shown no significant advantage after a median followup of 5 years.[34] Four studies have shown an improvement in event-free survival associated with the use of interferon, but the agent is toxic and commonly causes fatigue and malaise. In addition there is increased myelodepression when interferon is used with cytotoxic chemotherapy, and patients find the prolonged course of injections unpleasant. Identification of the mechanisms involved in inducing a response or prolonging remission would be of advantage in deciding on an appropriate dose or schedule of administration and might help in tailoring improved treatment for a particular group of patients with lymphoma.

Interferon with Retinoic Acid

Both interferons and retinoids have been shown to have antilymphoma effects, and although these agents are known to have antiproliferative, immunomodulating, and differentiating activity, they probably exert their antitumor effects through different molecular mechanisms. Experimental data support the concept that the simultaneous use of both retinoids and interferons may be synergistic in inducing differentiation and antiproliferative effects in a variety of target cells, including lymphoma cell lines.[37] The synergistic mechanisms are largely unknown, although all-*trans* retinoic acid (ATRA) is known to enhance the induction of 2′-5′-oligoadenylate synthetase by interferon-γ in various cell lines, including the lymphoma cell line U937.[38] Although these in vitro studies used doses of these agents higher than those usually achieved during therapy in humans, they have stimulated their clinical use.

IMMUNOTHERAPY

BIOLOGY OF THE IMMUNE SYSTEM

Immunotherapy involves an attempt to augment the host's immune defense against the tumor. This approach depends on the tumor cells being sufficiently "foreign" to enable an immune response to be mounted. Tumor-specific antigens

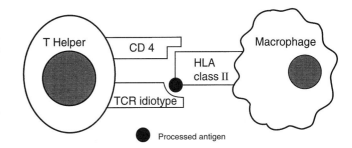

Figure 14–1. Helper T-cell activation by macrophage.

have been difficult to demonstrate in humans, but human tumors have been shown to be sufficiently different from their normal cellular counterparts to allow immunologic approaches to be of value in diagnosis and therapy. Tumor-associated transplantation antigens have been demonstrated in many chemically or virally induced tumors in experimental mice by studying their rejection when transplanted into genetically similar animals. Although tumor-specific antigens have not been demonstrated in humans, tumor-associated antigens that are preferentially expressed by tumor cells have been described. Such antigens may be encoded by genetic alterations that form an integral part of malignant transformation and are expressed by the malignant clone. Some of these antigens are expressed in the cell surface and are potentially immunogenic.

The immune reaction to an antigen has two components—antibody mediated (humoral immunity) and cell mediated—but the mechanisms involved are closely integrated. In addition, soluble proteins or glycoproteins (cytokines) produced by cells of the immune system have important regulatory effects on immune reactivity. An understanding of these mechanisms is leading to the development of new immunotherapeutic approaches for patients with lymphoma.

Humoral Immunity

Humoral immunity involves the formation of antibody by cells of B lineage that originate from hematopoietic stem cells in the bone marrow and differentiate into plasma cells under the influence of antigens and T-cell factors. The response to most antigens involves a macrophage presenting a processed antigen to a T-helper cell, which in turn interacts with specific B lymphocytes, resulting in the production of antibody (Fig. 14–1). Although cytotoxic antibodies capable of binding complement may cause direct lysis of a target tumor cell, antibody-dependent cell-mediated cytotoxicity (ADCC) may be more important in vivo. The latter process involves the binding of tumor antigen with the antigen-combining site of the immunoglobulin molecule and activating ADCC by binding macrophages, neutrophils, or activated natural killer (NK) cells using the Fc end of the molecule. Cell-mediated tumor cell killing can involve a number of effector cells, including macrophages, granulocytes, and lymphocytes.

Antibodies are large molecules formed by the covalent linkage of two heavy and two light chains. The amino terminal end of the Ig molecule comprises variable (V) regions of the heavy and light chains. The variable regions

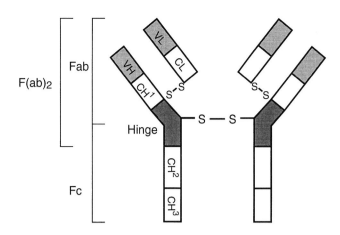

Figure 14–2. Structure of the immunoglobulin molecule.

and the first constant domains together form the Fab region where the Ig molecule binds to antigen. The other end of the Ig molecule is composed of the constant domains that make up the Fc portion, which is crucial in determining biologic effector functions such as complement activation and ADCC (Fig. 14–2).

Cell-Mediated Immunity

Macrophages, lymphocytes, and cells of the granulocytic series all are derived from hematopoietic stem cells in the bone marrow and play an important part in cell-mediated immunity. Macrophages originating in the bone marrow circulate as monocytes in the blood and differentiate into tissue macrophages, which have an important role in antigen processing. These cells bear Fc and C3 receptors capable of binding antibody and complement on the surface of a tumor cell and inducing cell death. T cells originate in the bone marrow before migrating to the thymus, where they proliferate and differentiate into mature T cells, which are then distributed throughout the immune system. Of the three major subsets of T cells, cytotoxic T lymphocytes are capable of direct tumor cell lysis, helper T cells stimulate the immune response by interacting with processed antigen or macrophages, and suppressor T cells are important in regulating the immune response.

Some macrophages process antigens, presenting them at the cell surface in association with human leukocyte antigen (HLA) class II molecules, where they are recognized by helper (CD4+) T cells (see Fig. 14–1). Antigen recognition occurs through the T-cell receptor (the CD3 molecule complexed with the T-idiotype molecule). Antigen presentation leads to T-cell activation, cytokine release (e.g., IL-2, IL-4, and IL-6), and clonal proliferation of T-cell subsets. Macrophages also secrete cytokines tumor necrosis factor ([TNF-α] and IL-1) during this process. Cytotoxic T cells (CD8+) recognize antigenic determinants in association with HLA class I molecules; the T cell receptor attaching to the tumour antigen and the CD8 molecule attaching to the class I molecule (Fig. 14–3). Tumor lysis is induced by cytokines such as tumor necrosis (TNF-α and -β) secreted by the T cell. Other types of T cells exist that are less restricted by self-MHC molecules, and these are capable of killing a range of tumor cell types. NK cells, for example, are capable of

killing tumor cells directly without prior sensitization, and their activity may be greatly augmented using IL-2.

A number of other molecules that bind to T cells may act as costimulatory factors following antigen binding. These include the membrane protein B7, a member of the immunoglobulin gene superfamily that is present on activated B cells, antigen-presenting cells, repeatedly activated T cells, and stimulated monocytes. B7 is the natural ligand for CD28, a membrane receptor on T cells, and the interaction enhances T-cell activation with expression of cytokine genes. Other costimulatory molecules include the adhesion molecules ICAM-1, which binds to LFA-1 on T cells, and LFA-3, which binds the T-cell ligand CD2.

Helper T cells are an important source of cytokines and augment the immune response by interacting with B cells to induce antibody production and with other T cells in cell-mediated responses. The cytotoxic and suppressor T lymphocytes also produce cytokines, such as interferon-γ, that are capable of attracting macrophages to the tumor site and nonspecifically activating them.

The induction and potentiation of these immune processes, both humoral and cell mediated, might be expected to augment host defense against lymphoma, and a great deal of effort is currently being directed toward this objective. The main approaches are listed in Table 14–7.

ANTIBODY THERAPY

The use of antibody as anticancer therapy was first described almost 100 years ago, but the antibody preparations were poorly defined and experiments in humans were difficult to repeat. The development of a technique for producing monoclonal antibodies in pure form with well-defined characteristics by Kohler and Milstein[38a] in 1975 enabled a more rigorous assessment of their clinical role in anticancer therapy. In addition, new molecular engineering techniques have allowed the development of specific antibody molecules with more desirable characteristics for therapy in humans. These antibodies have been found to have a role in therapy, purging bone marrow of malignant cells, and in other aspects of supportive care.[39] Tumors of B-cell origin have frequently been used to evaluate antibody-based therapies since they often express well-characterized antigens at the cell surface and are susceptible to damage by immune mechanisms and a wide range of cytotoxic agents. Furthermore, patients with B-cell malignancies develop antimouse Ig antibodies less frequently than patients with T-cell malignancies or with solid tumors.[40]

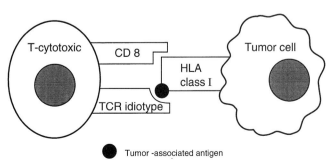

Figure 14–3. Cytotoxic T-cell interaction with tumor cell.

Antibody Alone

The use of antibody directed against a tumor-associated surface antigen may result in tumor cell lysis involving complement-mediated cytotoxicity or ADCC in which the patient's own immune system attacks and removes the malignant cells. Mouse monoclonal antibodies directed against the immunoglobulin idiotype expressed on the surface of human B-cell lymphoma cells have been used as antilymphoma therapy with these mechanisms in mind. Levy and colleagues at the Stanford Medical Center treated 16 patients with relapsed, chemotherapy refractory lymphoma using individually prepared antiidiotypic antibody.[41] One patient achieved a complete response lasting up to 6 years, and partial responses were seen in an additional 7 patients. The dose of antibody administered to the patient who achieved a complete remission for 6 years was considered too low to have caused direct destruction of the tumor mass; therefore, an explanation involving indirect mechanisms must be involved. Subsequently, these workers have used a panel of antiidiotypic antibodies to define a reactive population of lymphoma patients with shared idiotypes, and partial remissions in patients with low-grade lymphoma have also been observed using this approach that circumvents the necessity of preparing a specific antiidiotypic antibody for each individual patient.

A number of problems were recognized to be associated with this type of antibody therapy. In some patients lymphoma regrew with the tumor cells expressing idiotypic variants not recognized by the antiidiotypic antibodies.[42] Shedding of surface immunoglobulin also led to binding of the injected antibody, preventing its interaction with the lymphoma cell target. In addition, murine antibodies were recognized to be less effective than human antibodies in recruiting human effector functions and are inactivated by human antimouse antibody.

Monoclonal antibodies directed against normal differentiation antigens expressed on the surface of the lymphoma cells have also been used to treat patients with lymphoma. One example of this approach is the use of a mouse monoclonal antibody directed against CD19, which is one of the earliest B-cell antigens appearing during differentiation. The CD19 antigen has other advantages in that it does not appear to be shed or secreted by normal or malignant B cells and is known to be internalized.[43] In this study, six patients with progressive B cell lymphoma were treated, and one patient achieved a partial remission on two occasions, with

an interval of 8 months between treatments. The second remission lasted 9 months.

Monoclonal antibodies prepared against normal T-cell differentiation antigens have also been used to treat patients with T-cell lymphoma involving the skin. In one study eight patients with cutaneous T-cell lymphoma were treated with anti-Leu-1 resulting in one complete and one partial remission.[44] Another study using anti-Leu-1 resulted in two minor regressions in four patients.[45] Chimeric anti-CD4 was used to treat seven patients with mycosis fungoides, and of these, two achieved a partial response.[46]

Monoclonal antibodies directed against the CAMPATH-1H antigen (a differentiation antigen designated CDw52 expressed on most benign and malignant lymphoid cells) developed by Herman Waldmann and colleagues at Cambridge University in the United Kingdom have also been used to treat patients with lymphoma. The initial rodent monoclonal antibody studied was of IgM type (CAMPATH-1M). This antibody was capable of binding T and B lymphocytes but not hematopoietic colony-forming cells and showed high titer in a complement-mediated cytotoxicity assay. CAMPATH-1M resulted in only transient reduction in circulating tumor cell counts in two patients; one with lymphoma and the other with chronic lymphocytic leukemia. A class switch variant secreting an IgG2b antibody (CAMPATH-1G) was subsequently developed for clinical evaluation.[47] In a series of 29 patients with a variety of CDw52 antigen-positive lymphoid malignancies, the treatment cleared both normal and malignant lymphoid cells from the circulation, marrow infiltration was significantly reduced in 10 of 19 cases, and splenomegaly was significantly reduced (7 of 7 cases). However, palpable lymph nodes showed little or no regression. A chimeric humanized antibody (CAMPATH-1H) has been engineered more recently in which the six hypervariable complementarity-determining regions (CDRs) of the heavy and light chain variable domains of the rodent IgG2a monoclonal antibody were grafted into a human IgG1 κ variable framework.[48] This humanized antibody, produced for clinical evaluation by Wellcome Research, is equivalent in potency to CAMPATH-1G in terms of complement-mediated lysis and two to four times more potent in ADCC assays with normal and malignant human lymphocytes. CAMPATH-1H has been used to treat two patients with relapsed low-grade lymphoma, and both patients achieved a durable complete response without developing a human antirat antibody response.[49] The evaluation of CAMPATH-1H is continuing in a large international phase II trial.

Antibody fragments may penetrate tumor tissue better than the entire Ig molecule, but they tend to be more rapidly cleared from the circulation. Fragments include enzymatic digestion products (F(ab'$)_2$ and Fab) and Fv—a single chain molecule containing the variable heavy (^{V}H) and light (^{V}L) chains joined by a bridging peptide (see Fig. 14–2). Small recombinant parts of the immunoglobulin molecule hold promise for diagnosis and therapy, but their clinical value for patients with lymphoma remains to be evaluated.

A key feature of malignant transformation is the production of a tumor cell capable of survival and self-renewal. Environmental damage may induce necrosis, but an alternative form of cell death, an energy-driven process of programmed cell death termed "apoptosis," is operative during fetal development and in the control of cell turnover in organs such as the immune system, bone marrow, skin, and gastrointestinal tract. During the development of the nematode *Caeorhabitidis elegans*, 131 of 1090 somatic cells die from apoptosis.[50] The functions of two genes, *CED*3 and *CED*4, have been shown to be necessary for programmed cell death in these cells but a third gene (*CED*9) protects cells from this type of cell death.[51] The BCL2 oncogene associated with follicular B-cell lymphoma appears to have similarities to the *CED*9 gene, and expression of the BCL2 protein has been shown to enhance survival by blocking apoptosis and can extend the lifetime of memory B cells.[52] BCL-2 expression in transgenic mice blocks apoptosis in the B-cell population, allowing transformation following secondary genetic abnormalities and, after a long latent period, leads to the development of malignant lymphoma.[53] Apoptosis seems to be controlled by factors also responsible for cell transformation, differentiation, and cell cycle progression and represents a legitimate target in the search for a new approach to cancer therapy.

Alternative cell surface targets are currently being exploited in the search for more effective antilymphoma monoclonal antibodies. These include antibodies directed against cell surface receptors regulating growth, such as the receptors for IL-2, IL-6, and epidermal growth factor. Such antibodies would be expected to block cytokine-induced signal transduction, but some monoclonal antibodies have also been found to bind to lymphoid surface antigens, inducing apoptosis. One antibody in the latter category was raised against a human B-cell lymphoblastic cell line surface antigen and named APO-1. Nanogram qualities of anti-APO-1 completely block proliferation and induce apoptotic cell death with intravenous administration in nude mice bearing a xenograft of a human B-cell tumor, causing regression.[54] Another antibody capable of inducing apoptosis is the monoclonal antibody raised against the Fas antigen, which belongs to the protein family of TNF receptors and is present on chronically activated lymphocytes.[55]

The MDR1 gene product, a p glycoprotein mediating multidrug resistance, is another possible target for antibody therapy, but any clinical role for these antibodies remains to be determined. Overall, the results of using naked antibody in advanced disease have been relatively disappointing, with low numbers of tumor responses that are usually incomplete and short lived. Studies in an adjuvant setting with patients bearing fewer residual tumor cells after initial chemotherapy may prove more fruitful.

Conjugated Antibody

Monoclonal antibodies that may not have the capacity to kill tumor cells when used alone can, nevertheless, be used to target tumor cells and carry a cytocidal agent to the tumor site using an immunoconjugate. Using this method, cytotoxic drugs, irradiation, and toxins may be preferentially located at the tumor site, improving anticancer specificity.[56] Conjugates with cytokines have also been used in an attempt to augment immune reactivity to the tumor. In addition, antibody heteroconjugates (bispecific antibodies) able to react with both the tumor cell and host effector cells have been developed in the hope that cytokine release and antitumor reactivity will be enhanced. Antitumor antibodies

Table 14–8. Antibody Conjugates

Radionuclide conjugates
Immunotoxins
Cytotoxic drug conjugates
Enzyme conjugates
Cytokine conjugates

conjugated with enzymes capable of converting a prodrug into a cytotoxic derivative are also being developed. Some of the different forms of antibody conjugated for use as immunotherapy are listed in Table 14–8.

Radionuclide-Antibody Conjugates. Antibodies conjugated to radionuclides may be used to locate tumor deposits or as therapy. This type of targeted radiation therapy is attractive in lymphoma treatment in view of the tumors' radiosensitivity. Radionuclides used for therapy include both α and β emitters, whereas γ emitters are used in diagnosis. α particles have a short range (50 to 80 μm) that limits the cytotoxic effect to the immediate vicinity of the bound tumor cell. Examples of α-emitting radionuclides include ^{211}A and ^{212}B. β emitters have a wider range (1 to 10 mm) and allow the irradiation of tumor cells in the neighborhood that may not have bound the immunoconjugate. Examples of β-emitting radionuclides include ^{90}Yt and ^{31}P. A number of conjugates used for lymphoma therapy have involved immunoconjugates with ^{131}I, which has the disadvantage of a long half-life and high-energy γ emission in addition to its β emission.

^{131}I conjugated to the antibody OKB7, which reacts with CD21, the Epstein-Barr virus receptor, has been used to treat 18 patients with recurrent malignant lymphoma expressing the antigen.[57] Tumor uptake visualized using whole-body γ camera imaging was observed in 8 of 18 patients. Lymphoma regression was observed in 13 patients, but most of these were mixed responses of short duration, and only 1 patient achieved a defined partial response. Most patients in this series had low-grade B-cell lymphoma. It was noted in this study that more responses were associated with the higher total doses of immunoconjugate.

High-dose radioimmunotherapy using ^{131}I-labeled anti-CD20 and anti-CD37 antibodies followed by autologous bone marrow support has been used to treat 19 patients with B-cell lymphoma selected if they expressed the CD20 or CD37 antigen and had a favorable antibody biodistribution.[58] In this study therapeutic infusions of 234 to 777 mCi ^{131}I-labeled antibodies (58 to 1168 mg) resulted in 16 of the 19 patients achieving a complete remission, with a partial remission in an additional 2 patients. Nine patients remained in continuous complete remission for 3 to 53 months.

Kaminski and colleagues have used a more modest dose of irradiation, delivered using an ^{131}I immunoconjugate directed against the B-cell–associated membrane antigen CD20. Six of nine treated patients responded with four complete remissions lasting more than 8 months.[59] Others have shown responses in patients with B-cell lymphoma using ^{131}I-labeled Lym-1 antibody, an immune conjugate with a Burkitt's cell antigen,[60] and a chimeric anti-CD20 monoclonal antibody.[61]

Iodinated antibody is a substrate for deiodinases, and this leads to the accumulation of free iodine in the thyroid and gastrointestinal tract, reducing the specificity of imaging and therapy. This problem is being circumvented by the development of new methods of linking iodine with antibody and the use of alternative β-emitting radionuclides such as ^{90}Yt. Clinical studies using ^{90}Yt attached to antibody have been started, and responses have been observed in patients treated with lymphoma using ^{90}Yt-labeled humanized antibody. The potential of alternative radionuclides of ^{212}Bi and ^{211}A is also being explored.

Toxin Antibody Conjugates. A number of highly potent toxins from a wide variety of sources have been used as immunoconjugates for therapy in lymphoma. Diphtheria toxin and *Pseudomonas* exotoxin A represent a class of toxins that kill cells by catalyzing the adenosine diphosphate–ribosylation and inactivation of elongation factor 2 (an essential cofactor in protein synthesis). Another class of toxins includes ricin, abrin, gelonin, and saporin, which act by modifying the ribosome such that it can no longer interact with elongation factor 2. Ricin, a lectin derived from the seeds of the castor bean, has been one of the most popular toxins used in anticancer therapy. This toxin consists of a B chain with a capacity for binding galactose-containing carbohydrate receptors at the cell surface and an A chain that is the toxic moiety, inactivating protein synthesis by ribosomal binding on cell entry. To prevent unwanted toxicity due to nonspecific cellular binding by the B chain, either immunoconjugates have been prepared with blocked galactose-binding sites, or only the A-chain has been used.

New molecular techniques have been used to design molecules linking a toxin to targeting vehicles such as antibodies, growth factors, and cytokines. In this way unwanted domains in the toxin gene may be deleted or inactivated, and rapid clearance of the immunotoxin may be reduced by fusion with nonimmunogenic human serum albumin or chimeric antibody.

During the past decade these first-generation ricin A-chain–containing immunoconjugates have been used with modest success in treating patients with malignant lymphoma. However, these molecules were often unstable and short-lived in vivo, generally had low potency, were immunogenic, and damaged normal tissues. Patients with cutaneous T-cell lymphoma have been treated with an anti-CD5 ricin A-chain immunoconjugate, and partial responses lasting 3 to 8 months were seen in 11 of 14 patients treated.[62] Responses were seen in 6 of 24 patients given the IgG conjugate and 6 of 14 patients given a Fab fragment linked with deglycosylated ricin A chain.[63, 64] Researchers at the Dana-Farber Cancer Institute have linked blocked ricin to an antibody directed against CD19 as a therapeutic immunotoxin for patients with B-cell lymphoma.[65, 66] In these studies some patients responded (mainly those with low tumor burdens), but complete remissions were infrequent. Studies are being conducted in patients with minimal residual disease following myeloablative chemotherapy, but the evaluation of clinical efficacy in this setting requires an appropriate randomized study.[66]

Second-generation immunotoxins with improved stability, potency, and specificity have been produced and are being evaluated clinically. Constructs involving an anti-CD22 antibody attached to deglycosylated ricin A chain have been shown to be more toxic than ricin itself and many logs more specific. Clinical trials using Fab′–A chain and IgG–A chain constructs have resulted in a modest number of transient partial response. Responses were seen in 6 of 24 patients with B-cell lymphoma given the IgG conjugate and 6 of 14 patients given the Fab fragment linked with deglycosylated ricin A chain.[63, 64] Bispecific F(ab′)2 antibody linking the delivery of saporin (a ribosome-inactivating protein from the seeds of *Saponaria*) to the CD22 antigen has also been shown to induce a response in a patient with lymphoma.[67]

The potential of bacterial toxins such as *Pseudomonas* exotoxin and diphtheria toxin attached to antibody is also being explored. Molecular engineering techniques have allowed the production of these toxins with deleted binding domains that are noncytocidal unless conjugated with antibody directed against the tumor cell target. Fusion of an anti-Tac monoclonal antibody against the IL-2 receptor to a modified portion of the *Pseudomonas* toxin PE40 has resulted in a construct that was cytotoxic in vitro to IL-2 receptor–positive cells but not for IL-2 receptor–negative cells.[68] The PE40 construct lacks the toxin cell-binding site and is not toxic unless linked to a delivery molecule such as a monoclonal antibody and another ligand. A similar strategy has been used to construct a fusion protein linking PE40 to IL-6.[69] This protein is being evaluated as a cytotoxic agent for tumor cells expressing the IL-6 receptor.

Cytotoxic Drug–Antibody Conjugates. Conjugating cytotoxic drugs with antibody has proved to be more difficult than linking radionuclides or toxic proteins. The cytotoxic drugs effective against lymphoma are usually hydrophobic and result in precipitation if too many molecules are linked with the antibody. In addition, these molecules are less potent than plant and bacterial toxins, in which the entry of one molecule into the cell can result in lysis. The drug-antibody complex may be fivefold to 100-fold more toxic for the antigen-bearing cell lines, but the toxicity is often less than free drug owing to poor internalization and inefficient release of active drug within lysosomes.

An approach using antibody-dependent enzyme-prodrug therapy (ADEPT) has been developed to overcome these difficulties.

Antibody Heteroconjugates. The cytolytic effects of antibody used alone are believed to be mediated by host ADCC and complement-mediated cell killing. Heteroconjugates have been designed to react with both the tumor cell surface and a host effector cell to enhance tumor cell lysis by invoking cytokine release and host effector cell killing without requiring specific receptor–tumor cell attachment. Examples of these bispecific antibodies include antibodies binding to the T-cell receptor for antigen or to the Fc γ receptor in addition to the tumor antigen.[70–73] Another interesting heteroconjugate consists of an antitumor antibody and a superantigen. Superantigens are proteins of mostly microbial origin with a unique ability to activate a substantial proportion of T lymphocytes, regardless of their antigen specificity. Whether these approaches will have a role in the development of new antilymphoma therapy in humans is unknown.

Antibody-Directed Enzyme Prodrug Therapy (ADEPT). An interesting new approach involving the use of an enzyme conjugated with an antibody directed against the tumor has been developed by Bagshawe and colleagues.[74, 75] In this concept an enzyme is directed to the tumor with the capacity to activate a prodrug producing a cytotoxic agent at the tumor site, sparing normal tissues elsewhere. The enzyme linked with antibody is administered intravenously, and after the conjugate is cleared from the blood but is still retained in the tumor, a prodrug, which is a substrate for the enzyme, is given. The active cytotoxic component is then generated from the prodrug at the tumor site. This technique overcomes the problem of poor tumor penetration by antibody since the generated low-molecular-weight cytotoxic product is able to diffuse through the tumor mass, producing a considerable bystander effect. Moreover, since the enzyme can catalyze the activation of many substrate molecules, a high concentration of cytotoxic drug can be produced in the tumor vicinity.

Studies in mice xenografted with human cancers have shown that ADEPT is more effective than conventional cytotoxic chemotherapy in experimental models and has the capacity to eradicate established xenografted tumors.[76] A pilot study in eight patients with colorectal cancer has resulted in four partial or mixed tumor responses using this approach.[77] The availability of antibodies directed against lymphoma cells means that the technique could also be used in patients with lymphoma.

Antibody in Combination with Cytokines

Interferon and TNF can augment expression of MHC classes I and II antigens and some tumor-associated antigens.[78, 79] The use of interferon in conjunction with antiidiotype monoclonal antibody has been shown to be synergistic in murine lymphoma.[80] Two complete responses and 7 partial responses have been observed in 11 patients with B-cell lymphoma treated with monoclonal antiidiotypic antibody and interferon-α, but this study was too small to indicate whether the two agents acted synergistically.[41]

Activated NK cells have been implicated in tumor responses observed with IL-2 therapy, and these cells can also mediate ADCC. Interferon-α can also activate NK cells, and activation of neutrophils, monocytes, and macrophages by granulocyte colony-stimulating factor (G-CSF), granulocyte-macrophage (GM) CSF, and macrophage (M-CSF) also augments ADCC. Clinical trials are required to evaluate these agents in combination with monoclonal antibody. Another form of targeted therapy involves the use of a cytokine-toxin fusion protein to direct a toxin to a tumor cell with appropriate receptors on the cell surface. Several fusion proteins have been produced using conjugates between various interleukins or growth factors and diphtheria or *Pseudomonas* toxins.[81] An example of this approach is the IL-2–diphtheria toxin fusion protein DAB_{486} IL-2.[82–84] Several forms of leukemia and lymphoma express high-affinity IL-2 receptors and are potentially susceptible to this form of therapy. The genetic construct was made by deleting the receptor-binding domain from the gene encoding native diphtheria toxin and replacing it with a synthetic gene for human IL-2. The fusion protein undergoes rapid endocytosis on binding to IL-2 receptors, and subsequent acidification within the endosome allows the delivery of the cytotoxic A fragment into the cytosol, causing an inhibition of protein synthesis. Preliminary clinical studies have shown responses in patients with lymphoma, including three of five patients with cutaneous

T-cell lymphoma, one of whom had a complete remission sustained for more than 33 months.

Side Effects and Difficulties Associated with Antibody Therapy

The clinical efficacy of immunoconjugates is hindered by a number of problems, including low antigen density at the tumor cell surface, poor tumor access, and production of human antirodent antibodies (HARA). Lack of specificity of the antibody results in damage to normal tissues, and damage to tumor cells may be limited by heterogeneity of antigen expression within the tumor or antigenic modulation by capping, antigen shedding, or endocytosis. A considerable amount of effort has been devoted to solving these problems by selecting appropriate antibodies for an individual tumor, and some of these (e.g., antiCD20) are not associated with antigenic modulation.[85]

Monoclonal antibodies produced by rodent cells are immunogenic in humans, and side effects associated with HARA may become prominent, particularly after repeated administration, resulting in allergic reactions including anaphylaxis, fever, rigors, rashes, and hypotension. The production of HARA is also associated with increased antibody clearance and metabolism and a reduction in antitumor effect. Some of these problems are being circumvented by using chimeric or humanized antibodies prepared using recombinant technology, but these antibodies may remain weakly immunogenic. One approach has been to use CDRs involved in specific antigen-antibody interaction grafted onto the human antibody framework, resulting in antibodies that are about 95% human. Humanization of the Fc domain would be expected to confer optimal Fc receptor binding and activation of host effector cells. In addition, these humanized molecules have a better pharmacokinetic profile, with reduced metabolism and excretion and a more prolonged half-life in the circulation.

Tumor penetration by whole antibody or immunoconjugates may be poor, and the smaller-molecular-weight F(ab) fragments have been used to improve access, but these molecules are not only cleaved rapidly but lack the important Fc fraction responsible for complement activation and ADCC. Monovalent monoclonal antibodies may also be more penetrating, and in vitro work with monovalent CD3 has indicated that complement-mediated lysis may also be enhanced.[86] Vasoactive agents have also been employed to increase tumor uptake.[87]

The rapid clearance of immunotoxins as foreign proteins is also a problem, and the fusion of nonimmunogenic human serum albumin sequences has been used in an attempt to solve this difficulty.

Side effects associated with the use of antibody may occur acutely following the first dose and commonly involve fever, rigors, nausea, and headache; however, some tolerance may develop on repeated administration. More severe reactions may also occur. These include dyspnea, diarrhea, edema, myalgia, cardiopulmonary dysfunction, and abnormalities of liver function with elevated liver enzyme levels, jaundice, and hypoalbuminemia. Such features are usually short-lived and disappear after treatment is discontinued, but immunodeficiency can be more prolonged with an increased incidence of infection.

Myelosuppression may be a major feature associated with therapy using radionuclide conjugates, and bone marrow support may be required at high-dose levels. This complication may be controlled by individualizing the dose and titrating the dose delivered to normal tissues such as the bone marrow using trace doses to assess biodistribution. Latent hypothyroidism may occur in patients treated with ^{131}I immunoconjugates, and this may rise to 42% when high doses are used.[58] In this study patients treated with doses that delivered 23 to 75 Gy or less to normal organs had few nonhematologic toxic effects, whereas 11 patients who received higher doses had marked asthenia, nausea, diarrhea, and anorexia, with further dose escalation limited by life-threatening cardiopulmonary and gastrointestinal toxicity.

There is some evidence that tumor response is related to the dose delivered, and fewer responses have also been observed in patients with a high tumor burden. For these reasons better results might be expected in patients who have already achieved a complete remission using conventional therapy and have few remaining tumor cells. However, there are no reported randomized trials of antibody therapy in an adjuvant setting, and clinical efficacy in this context remains unassessed. Improved manufacturing techniques for antibody production, including the introduction of phage expression libraries, and the production of large quantities of monoclonal antibodies in other systems, including plants and transgenic animals, are likely to make an important impact on the availability of these new treatments.

TUMOR VACCINATION

Lymphoma cells have been shown to express tumor-specific antigens at the cell surface, but the fact that these tumors develop in their presence means that host immune mechanisms have not been effective in rejecting the tumor. The variable regions of the immunoglobulin molecules expressed on malignant B cell (idiotypes) are tumor specific but are weak immunogens, and there are additional constraints inhibiting the development of an appropriate immune response to self-protein. To induce an immune response the immunogeneic protein mixed with an adjuvant must be injected. The resulting response can protect animals from subsequent tumor challenge and cure animals with established tumors in combination with chemotherapy.

Some of the problems associated with passive antibody administration might be overcome by actively immunizing the patient with idiotypic immunoglobulin. This would have the advantage of inducing a polyclonal antiidiotypic antibody response against multiple idiotypic determinants on the lymphoma surface and would be expected to reduce the likelihood of regrowth of tumor cells with mutated unreactive idiotype.[88] In addition, the production of natural antibody should be more effective in recruiting human effector functions (complement and ADCC). The immunization, hopefully, would also stimulate appropriate cytotoxic and helper T-cell responses.

Kwak and colleagues have reported a trial of idiotype vaccination in nine patients with follicular lymphoma in whom a remission had previously been induced using conventional chemotherapy.[89] The idiotypic immunoglobulin prepared in heterohybridomas was purified and conjugated to an immunogenic carrier protein before administra-

tion. Idiotype-specific humoral or cell-mediated immune responses were seen in seven of the nine vaccinated patients, and a complete tumour regression was seen in the two patients who had measurable disease.

Idiotype vaccination is also possible using gene transfer technology.[90] This group has developed a method of identifying the idiotypic immunoglobulin based on DNA sequencing, which can be used to isolate the idiotypic antibody V genes from a lymphoma biopsy specimen within a few days. This technique avoids the need for production screening and characterization of multiple patient-specific hybridomas. The plasmid containing the required DNA sequences for the individual patient can be inoculated directly into muscle. The encoded idiotype is expressed by muscle cells near the injection site.[90, 91] This form of genetic immunization in animal models is as effective as vaccination with purified protein plus adjuvant and is currently under evaluation in patients with follicular lymphoma. Monoclonal antibodies that bind to idiotypic determinants are also being evaluated as tumor vaccines. This strategy is based on the observation that some antiidiotype antibodies can mimic the structure of the target antigen.[92]

The recognition that local cytokine activity is of importance in augmenting the immune response to a tumor vaccine has led to the development of engineered fusion proteins in which the tumor-associated antigen is linked to an appropriate cytokine. The local production of cytokines by genetically engineered tumor cells can decrease tumorigenicity and induce a protective immune response against the parental tumor.[93, 94] GM-CSF augments antigen presentation in a variety of cells, and a fusion protein linking GM-CSF with a murine lymphoma–derived idiotype has been constructed that is capable of eliciting a strong antibody response, protecting animals from a subsequent challenge with tumor cells.[95] Coadministration of the antigen and cytokine or a fusion protein containing species-specific human GM-CSF are both ineffective. This approach avoids the requirement for more toxic immunologic adjuvants, but evaluation in humans is required. Studies of various cytokines are necessary to optimize tumor antigen presentation, and it is of note that a study of irradiated murine tumor cells that had been transduced with retroviruses encoding 10 different cytokines or immunomodulators showed that cells expressing murine GM-CSF were the most effective at stimulating long-lasting and specific immunity.[96] In addition, constructs including HLA and costimulatory factors could be incorporated to augment immune reactivity, but these new approaches remain to be evaluated in the future.

NONSPECIFIC IMMUNOPOTENTIATION USING BACTERIAL PRODUCTS

In the mid nineteenth century, regression of malignant skin tumors was observed in the wake of bacterial infection involving the tumor in an inflammatory response, and since then there have been many studies where bacterial products have been used to induce regressions in various forms of human cancer.[97] The local induction of an inflammatory response following the injection of bacterial products directly into the tumor or the induction of a delayed hypersensitivity reaction using chemical agents such as dinitrochlorobenzene were shown capable of inducing a regression in a variety of tumors, including lymphoma of the skin.[98] Although local regression was frequently seen following direct injection of these agents, effects on distant tumor deposits proved to be more difficult to demonstrate. Mathe and associates[99] reported a favorable effect of bacille Calmette-Guérin (BCG) in children with acute lymphoblastic leukemia in remission, and subsequent studies of this agent suggested that there may be a modest antitumor effect in patients with malignant lymphoma.[100–103] Other trials of BCG in lymphoma have reported no significant advantage.[104, 105]

The largest randomized studies have been reported by the Southwest Oncology Group. In their first trial involving 652 patients using BCG administered by a scarification technique between cycles of induction chemotherapy, a beneficial effect was seen in two groups of patients.[101] Patients with large cell lymphoma more often achieved a complete response and had a better survival if treated with CHOP-BCG compared with CHOP-bleomycin or COP-bleomycin. Survival of patients with follicular lymphoma was also better in patients treated with CHOP-BCG, but there was no apparent effect of BCG on remission rate or duration. The effects of BCG in this trial were relatively modest and the chemotherapy used was different in the BCG-treated patients, making interpretation difficult. In their second trial, involving 696 evaluable patients, a comparison was made between chemotherapy alone (CHOP) and chemotherapy given with levamisole or levamisole plus BCG during remission induction.[104] A further randomization following induction of remission compared levamisole therapy as maintenance with a group receiving no further therapy. Chemoimmunotherapy with levamisole-BCG offered no advantage in terms of survival or remission rate and duration compared with CHOP chemotherapy alone.

Other studies suggesting an advantage for BCG used as maintenance therapy for patients with minimal residual disease have been flawed by the inadequate number of patients treated.[102] BCG therapy cannot be recommended at this time.

Any nonspecific effects of BCG are likely to be mediated by cytokine production, and the introduction of pure recombinant protein into clinical practice has made further studies of this approach less attractive.

INTERLEUKIN-2

Interleukin-2 is a naturally occurring cytokine first identified in 1976 as a growth promoter of activated T lymphocytes.[106] Following purification of the native glycoprotein, it became apparent that the agent has pleotropic activity with an important role regulating the complex network of immune function. These properties suggested a possible role in cancer therapy.

Properties

The IL-2 gene, located in humans on chromosome 4q, mediates the production of a glycoprotein with a molecular weight of 14 to 17 kilodaltons, depending on differences in glycosylation. Glycosylation is not required for biologic activity, and the *Escherichia coli*–derived recombinant

protein is as active as the native glycosylated product. IL-2 is an α-helical protein that binds to a specific receptor composed of at least three protein chains with variable affinity.[107]

Biologic Effects

IL-2 is mainly produced by activated T-helper cells and has a mitogenic effect on T, NK, and B cells. Differentiation and functional activation of lymphocytes and monocytes lead to the induction of T-helper function and the augmentation in cytotoxicity of NK cells, monocytes, and previously generated cytotoxic T-lymphocytes. Following incubation with IL-2, subpopulations of lymphocytes can generate *lymphocyte-activated killer* (LAK) cells, effectors capable of lysing tumor cells, including those which are NK resistant.[108] The LAK cytotoxicity is MHC independent and more effective against tumor cells than normal cells. Direct cytocidal effects of IL-2 have not been reported, and any antitumor effects of IL-2 are believed to be indirect and mediated through the immune system.

Following leukapheresis LAK activity may be generated in culture using IL-2, and the amplified LAK effectors may be used as adoptive immunotherapy. Expanded populations of tumor-infiltrating lymphocytes (TILs) may also be produced in culture from lymphocytes derived from the tumor mass, and these cells have increased specific cytolytic activity against their autologous tumors and require less IL-2 to support their activity than LAK cells. TIL and LAK effectors recognize their targets by different mechanisms, LAK activity being without MHC restriction, whereas TILs may show specific MHC-restricted killing and are generally more effective than LAK cells.[109]

A further important property of IL-2 is the induction of cytokine release. Stimulation of T cells in vitro results in increased production of interferon-γ, TNF-α, IL-2, IL-3, IL-4, IL-5, and GM-CSF. Thus, T cells can be activated to release tumor-cytotoxic cytokines both by tumor antigens recognized by the T-cell receptor complex or by IL-2 resulting in the augmentation of specific and nonspecific tumoricidal effects.[110] IL-2 also has a chemotactic function, recruiting lymphocytes to the site of IL-2 production. The increased expression of adhesion molecules on endothelial cells induced by the cytokine cascade also contributes to the accumulation of inflammatory cells.

Antitumor Effects in Experimental Animals

The administration of IL-2 with or without LAK or TIL effectors has been shown to be accompanied by antitumor effects in several animal models, including lymphoma and leukemia.[111] In one study using intraperitoneal administration in mice transplanted with lymphoma, high doses of IL-2 exerted an antitumor effect via LAK cells, whereas a low-dose effect, not observed in nude mice, was attributed to an antitumor effect of host T cells.[112] More effective responses have been recorded by combining IL-2 with TIL rather than LAK cells in some tumor models.[113]

IL-2 also promotes a graft-versus-lymphoma (GVL) effect in experimental allograft models and exerts a protective effect against relapse from the EL4 leukemia in situations where the transplant has been rendered tolerant to the host.[114, 115] Sykes and colleagues have shown that GVL can be dissociated from graft-versus-host disease (GVHD) using the EL4 leukemia/lymphoma model in mice.[116] They have demonstrated in this system that IL-2 treatment inhibits the activity of CD4 + T cells and markedly reduces GVHD without compromising the GVL effect. This protective effect of IL-2 occurred independently of NK cells or LAK activity. The recognition that LAK cells generated following autologous bone marrow transplantation in humans are able to recognize and lyse autologous lymphoma cells suggests that this method might be used to improve relapse-free survival in patients with minimal residual disease following myeloablative chemotherapy and hematopoietic rescue.[117, 118]

The potential use of IL-2 in situations where minimal residual disease is left following chemotherapy in humans has been investigated in an elegant series of experiments by Slavin and colleagues using a spontaneous nonimmunogenic murine B-cell leukemia/lymphoma model.[119] In this model a short course of IL-2 shortly after inoculating 10^2 to 10^4 leukemia cells prevented the development of leukemia. The same IL-2 therapy was not effective in mice inoculated with 10^6 cells. However, spleens from apparently healthy mice 2 to 3 months after IL-2 therapy were shown to harbor dormant leukemia cells capable of causing leukemia when injected into susceptible animals. This implies that a natural defense mechanism is operable during the state of tumor dormancy. When tested again 9 months after IL-2 therapy, clonogenic leukemia cells could no longer be demonstrated, suggesting that the dormant tumor cells eventually die without additional treatment in this model. Mice inoculated with a higher dose of leukemia cells may be cured following cyclophosphamide/total-body irradiation and allogeneic marrow transplantation. Again, some of these apparently cured chimeras were shown to bear dormant tumor cells but did not experience GVHD, and the GVL effect appears to be separable. In stable chimeras the GVL effect may be reduced by the administration of cyclosporin A, resulting in the development of leukemia. Similar experiments using syngeneic marrow following chemotherapy plus radiation therapy showed that IL-2 was also effective in treating animals with minimal residual leukemia under these conditions and that this effect could be enhanced by coadministration of interferon-α. The GVL effects may also be induced by the administration of allogeneic lymphocytes following initial transplantation with T-lymphocyte–depleted allografts, an effect also potentiated by low-dose IL-2 in vivo.

IL-2 Therapy in Humans

IL-2 has been used alone and combined with other cytokines in combination with cells of the immune system in the treatment of patients with non-Hodgkin's lymphoma. Therapeutic benefit has been slight for patients with lymphoma, although more favorable results have been consistently documented in patients with renal cell carcinoma or malignant melanoma.

The rationale for using IL-2 as a therapeutic agent in lymphoma is based on its immune-stimulating properties; however, autocrine or paracrine effects of IL-2 are postulated to have a role in tumor growth in some forms of T-cell lymphoma, and this could be a disadvantage. The persis-

tence of certain viruses in the cell clones they infect may lead to a predisposition to malignant transformation. In the case of human T-cell leukemia/lymphoma type I (HTLV-I) and HTLV-II, the *tax* gene transactivates several T-cell activation genes, including the genes for IL-2 and its receptor, creating an autocrine loop.[120] Furthermore, it is possible that IL-2 can promote tumor growth indirectly by releasing other growth-promoting cytokines such as IL-1 and IL-6.

Native glycosylated IL-2 derived from the Jurkatt cell line was first evaluated clinically in 1980, but subsequently recombinant IL-2 was cloned, allowing the manufacture of sufficient quantities of nonglycosylated recombinant protein for clinical trial. A considerable amount of work evaluating the clinical effects of IL-2 has been carried out by Rosenberg and colleagues.[121]

A number of different IL-2 dosages and schedules have been investigated since the recombinant protein became available for large-scale use in 1984. Cetus was the first company to produce recombinant IL-2 (Proleukin), but Hoffmann-La Roche also has a recombinant product (Teceleukin) for clinical use. The two products have different specific activity: 1 Cetus unit is equivalent to 6 IU, and 1 Roche unit is 2.6 IU. Continuous infusion appears to result in greater biologic effects than the equivalent total dose given by bolus infusion.[122] However, despite large numbers of different doses, schedules, and routes of administration being tested clinically, the optimal approach is unknown. The single-agent response rate in patients with lymphoma has been too low and inconsistent to provide useful information regarding the appropriate dose or schedule of administration for patients with lymphoma, and current modes of administration are based on information from patients treated for renal cell cancer and malignant melanoma. In Europe, an approved dosage regimen for patients with renal cell cancer is a 24-hour infusion of 18×10^6 IU/m^2 for 5 days followed by 2 to 6 days without drug, then 5 days of the same infusion regimen followed by a 3-week rest period. In the United States higher doses have been recommended with 6×10^5 IU/kg given intravenously using a 15-minute bolus every 8 hours for up to a total of 14 doses, followed by a further cycle after a variable interval. Subcutaneous and regional methods of administration have also been used, but appropriate doses and schedules have not yet been defined, although surgical reports demonstrate that low-dose subcutaneous IL-2 given by continuous infusion is tolerated well as an outpatient treatment and may be associated with tumor responses.

Most reported clinical trials have involved patients with renal cell cancer and malignant melanoma with the most favorable results in renal cell cancer.[109] Approximately 20% of patients with metastatic renal cancer and 13% of patients with melanoma achieve objective responses using IL-2 alone. In renal cell cancer about 5% of patients achieved a complete remission, and some of these are durable, persisting in many instances for more than 12 months and in some patients for more than 5 years. Complete response rates for patients with malignant melanoma are low (approximately 2.5%) but show a similar durability.

IL-2 Therapy in Patients with Lymphoma. A number of studies have been reported in which patients with lymphoma have been treated with IL-2 alone, in combination with other cytokines, or with immune effector cells. In four early studies using low-dose IL-2 intravenously given alone, 12 evaluable patients with advanced lymphoma were treated and 7 responded, although there were no complete responses. Both low- and high-grade lymphoma patients were represented in the responding groups.[121, 123–125] In most series, however, responses in patients with lymphoma have been only occasional when IL-2 is used alone, and some reports showed no evidence of response. There is a suggestion that patients with low-grade disease may respond more frequently to IL-2 alone than patients with intermediate- or high-grade lymphoma, but reports are conflicting. Levy and colleagues[126] reported one complete and four partial responses in 10 patients with follicular lymphoma, whereas 7 patients with diffuse large cell lymphoma progressed on therapy. In contrast, others have reported no responses in patients with low- or intermediate-grade lymphoma treated with IL-2 alone.[127]

IL-2 used in conjunction with LAK cells has also been used to treat both the low grade and the higher grades of lymphoma, but few patients have responded. In one series in which 11 patients with lymphoma were treated with IL-2 alone, there were no responses, but one complete response and three partial responses were seen in 8 patients treated with IL-2 plus LAK cells.[127] A study from France in which cycles of IL-2 were given by intravenous infusion with or without LAK cells resulted in only one complete remission in 22 patients with low-grade lymphoma, but three complete and two partial remissions in 22 patients with high-grade lymphoma.[128] Two complete and two partial remissions were seen in 4 patients with mycosis fungoides treated in the same study, and in one of these patients, the remission lasted more than 12 months. The low response rate observed in most series and the increased incidence of side effects associated with the use of LAK cells in addition to IL-2 mean that this form of therapy cannot be recommended for use in lymphoma outside the confines of a research study. The expense involved in the production of LAK cells in vitro and the lack of a defined advantage over IL-2 alone in any form of cancer have also resulted in less research effort in this direction.

The use of IL-2 alone or with other cytokines in some experimental systems has provided evidence for a nonlinear dose-response curve.[129] This allows for optimal biologic and therapeutic effects of IL-2 at doses far below the maximum tolerated dose. Improved therapeutic effects have been observed in patients with renal cell cancer and malignant melanoma when reducing IL-2 by more than 90% of the maximum tolerated dose and combining IL-2 with other cytokines such as interferon-α. The combined use of IL-2 with interferon is based on the concept of augmenting cytolytic effectors and antiproliferative activity. However, there is no evidence that IL-2 given in conjunction with any of the interferons is associated with improvement in response rate, although relatively few patients with lymphoma have been treated in this way. In a randomized trial comparing IL-2 alone (5 IU × 10^6/m^2 intravenous bolus 3 times weekly) with interferon-β (5 × 10^6 IU/m^2 intravenous bolus 3 times weekly) followed by IL-2 using the same schedule, an overall response rate of 17%, lasting 83 to 402 days, in 41 evaluable patients with lymphoma was reported by the Cancer and Leukaemia Group B.[130] There was no significant difference between the randomized arms (Table 14–9), and severe life-threatening toxicity was experienced in 17 patients with three treatment-related deaths. Responses in patients with lymphoma have also been reported using IL-2 with interferon-γ, but it is not known whether there is any advantage in combining these two agents.[131]

Adverse Effects. The side effects of IL-2 administration are dose and schedule dependent, and the addition of LAK cells increases the toxicity significantly.[132] The mechanisms involved are largely unknown, although the release of secondary cytokines may play a part. The incidence and severity of adverse effects have been used to define appropriate methods of administration. Adverse effects may be severe and affect most organ symptoms but tend to be rapidly reversible when treatment is stopped (Table 14–10).

High-dose schedules ($\geq 50 \times 10^6$ IU/m^2 given daily as bolus infusions or $\geq 15 \times 10^6$IU/m^2 daily as continuous infusion for several days) are likely to be attended by severe toxicity, and the patients may require intensive support for vascular leak syndrome and features resembling septic shock, which can be lethal. Mortality rates have been 1% to 6% in reported trials. Low-dose schedules ($\leq 7 \times 10^6$ IU/m^2 daily as a continuous intravenous infusion for 2 to 5 days or by subcutaneous injection) can often be given on an outpatient basis, but constitutional symptoms are common and dose limiting for ambulatory patients.[133] A lower dose of IL-2 (5.2 IU/m^2 daily) administered by continuous intravenous infusion over 90 days was not accompanied by serious side effects in patients following allogeneic bone marrow transplantation.[134]

Table 14–9. Randomized Phase II Trial Comparing IL-2 Alone with IL-2 + IFN-β in Patients with Relapsed or Refractory Non-Hodgkin's Lymphoma

| Randomization | No. of Patients Working Formulation Grade | | | | No. Responding | Intravenous Schedule |
	Low	Intermediate	High	Unclassified		
IL-2 alone	6	11	1	1	1CR, 1PR	5 × 10^6 IU/m^2 IV bolus
IL-2 + IFN-β	9	10	1	1	1CR, 2PR	Il-2 5 × 10^6 IU/m^2 bolus IFN-β 5 × 10^6 IU/m^2 bolus 3 times per week

IL-2, interleukin-2; IFN, interferon; CR, complete response; PR, partial response.
Data from Duggan DB, Santarelli MT, Zamkoff K, et al: A phase II study of recombinant interleukin-2 with or without recombinant interferon beta in non-Hodgkin's lymphoma: A study of the cancer of leukaemia group. Br J Immunother 1992; 12:115.

Table 14–10. Adverse Events Following IL-2 Administration

Category	Signs and Symptoms
General	Malaise, fatigue, fever, myalgia
Gastrointestinal Cardiopulmonary	Anorexia, nausea, vomiting, mucositis and diarrhea that may be severe; tachycardia, hypotension with renal failure, capillary leak syndrome with fluid retention, pulmonary edema, pleural effusions, and ascites. These may be life threatening
Hepatic dysfunction	Elevated bilirubin and liver enzyme levels
Neurologic	Mental disturbance, agitation, somnolence, seizures, and coma; these features may progress during the first few days after treatment is discontinued
Skin	Mostly erythema or a macular rash with pruritus that may desquamate
Hematologic	Anemia, eosinophilia, thrombocytopenia and coagulation disorders; lymphopenia may occur during therapy but usually rebounds when treatment is discontinued
Infection	Increased susceptibility to infection, which may be severe, can occur on both low- and high-dose schedules
Autoimmune phenomena	Thyroid dysfunction and exacerbation of preexisting autoimmune disease

IL-2, interleukin-2.

IL-2 Therapy for Patients with Minimal Residual Disease. Although lymphoma cells are sensitive to IL-2–generated effector mechanisms in vitro, most efforts to treat advanced lymphoma patients using IL-2 have been associated with little effect on tumor masses. There is some suggestion that in patients with certain forms of cancer such as malignant melanoma, improved therapeutic effects are seen using a combination of IL-2 with cytotoxic chemotherapy compared with either modality used alone.[133] IL-2 is more likely to be effective when given to patients at a time of minimal residual disease following chemotherapy. Animal models predict that it is at this time that biologic approaches are most likely to be effective.

High-dose myeloablative chemotherapy followed by bone marrow or peripheral blood progenitor cell rescue can be associated with sustained remissions or even cure in some patients with high-grade lymphoma. However, a significant proportion of patients with high-risk features relapse following high-dose therapy. Studies with leukemia patients have shown that recipients of allogeneic transplants have a lower incidence of relapse than recipients of syngeneic grafts and that the development of GVHD is associated with a reduced frequency of recurrent disease.[135–137] There is some evidence that this GVL effect may be separated from the overt effects of GVHD, although the target antigens and mechanisms involved are unknown. Comparison of relapse rates among patients with acute myelogenous leukemia (AML) receiving identical twin transplants with those receiving HLA-compatible bone marrow grafts who did not develop GVHD shows that reactivity to the minor histocompatibility antigens expressed on the leukemia cells can be associated with a GVL effect.[136] In addition, patients with chronic granulocytic leukemia treated using bone marrow grafts depleted of T cells have a lower incidence of GVHD but a higher relapse rate than patients treated with unmodified bone marrow grafts.[138] Intensification of immunosuppressive regimens to prevent GVHD has also been associated with a higher risk of relapse following allogeneic bone marrow transplantation,[139] and remissions have been reported in patients relapsing following allogeneic bone marrow transplantation using an infusion of donor lymphocytes.[140, 141]

In humans, LAK cells generated following autologous transplantation are able to recognize and lyse autologous lymphoma cells in vitro, and a marked expansion in the number of NK and LAK effector cells occurs during low-dose IL-2 infusion after both autologous and T-cell–depleted allogeneic transplantation.[118, 134] The low-dose IL-2 infusion (5.2×10^5 IU/m^2 daily) over 90 days in the study from the Dana-Farber Cancer Institute was accompanied by minimal toxicity, and no patient developed GVHD. The absence of T-cell stimulation at these low doses probably accounts for the low incidence of GVHD in this study. These and other studies have shown that in patients treated with myeloablative therapy followed by hematopoietic progenitor cell rescue, IL-2 infusion is associated with an amplification of lymphocytes expressing a cytotoxic phenotype, substantial augmentation of NK and LAK activity, and the release of various cytokines, including TNF and interferon-γ. These effects might be expected to augment any GVL effect that could result in the elimination of minimal residual disease.[142]

The clinical application of this approach in patients with lymphoma has been limited, and no randomized trials have been carried out to determine whether IL-2 has a role in improving relapse-free survival or in reducing infectious complications following transplantation. However, one group has suggested that IL-2 with or without LAK cells is associated with a lower relapse rate in patients undergoing autologous bone marrow transplantation for AML.[143] Research continues in an attempt to maximize any antilymphoma effects in this setting by examining the dose, route of administration, schedule, and duration of therapy and the effects of additional immunomodulating agents.

A mild form of GVHD has been reported to occur spontaneously in 8% of patients receiving autologous or syngeneic bone marrow transplants. The use of cyclosporin A following myeloablative therapy and autologous bone marrow transplantation in patients with non-Hodgkin's lymphoma or Hodgkin's disease resulted in the induction of grade 2 GVHD in all five patients treated in this study.[144] This effect seems to be mediated by autoreactive lymphocytes directed against HLA class II histocompatibility antigens and raises the possibility of using interferon-γ to increase the effect. The approach deserves further exploration as a possible therapeutic measure for patients left with a small amount of residual disease after intensive chemotherapy and autologous hematopoietic progenitor cell rescue.

TARGETED THERAPY USING AUTOLOGOUS LYMPHOCYTES AS VECTORS

The migratory properties of the lymphocyte render it an ideal vector for the selective deposition of therapeutic agents at sites of disease along the lymphocyte migration pathway. Within an hour of intravenous injection, lymphocytes leave the vascular compartment and localize in lymphoid tissue at concentrations approximately 10,000 times that of nonlymphatic tissue.[145] Although the pathways for lymphocyte migration and recirculation were established using small experimental animals, lymphocyte radionuclide-labeling studies in humans have confirmed these patterns of migration and allowed quantitative kinetic evaluation of lymphocyte traffic.[146, 147]

Lymphoma deposits in patients are usually composed of one clone of malignant cells, and different sites of disease in the same patient result from tumor cell migration. The pattern of spread in patients with lymphoma is extremely varied and does not correlate well with predictions based on anatomic considerations of blood or lymph circulation. There appears to be a degree of organ specificity characteristic for certain types of lymphoma, and the microenvironment in which lymphoma cells lodge seems to be an important factor determining their accumulation and proliferation. The surface phenotype may determine the metastatic pattern.[148]

Ford and colleagues developed lymphocyte-targeting systems fulfilling three important criteria: (1) the cytotoxic agent should be incorporated into the lymphoid cells in vitro; (2) the labeled lymphocytes remain capable of normal migratory behavior for at least 1 hour after intravenous injection to allow penetration of lymphatic tissue; and (3) having reached the target site, the material must be released in a form causing damage to neighboring cells with minimal systemic effect.[146, 149]

In view of the marked radiosensitivity of lymphoma cells a radionuclide has been incorporated into this lymphocyte delivery system. Based on previous experience using indium 111 oxine for lymphocyte migration studies, the β-emitting radionuclide indium 114m was substituted for therapy. The carrier lymphoid cells die approximately 12 hours after injection, and the indium 114m is transferred to neighboring nonmigratory, relatively radioresistant macrophages where the source of radiation remains "fixed" in the lymphocyte traffic areas. A pharmacokinetic study in seven patients with lymphoid malignancy showed a consistent in vivo distribution of activity, permitting dose estimations for critical organs.[150] Patients with chronic lymphocytic leukemia and low-grade lymphoma have been treated using this approach, and responses have been seen in chemotherapy refractory cases. Autologous lymphocytes were labeled using indium 114m, and following intravenous infusion these cells actively migrated to lymphoid tissues, creating a localized field of irradiation within the lymphocyte migration pathways for several weeks. Responses were seen in five of the seven patients with chronic lymphocytic leukemia (one complete response and four partial responses) of 2 to 24 months' duration. The therapy was associated with myelosupression but no subjective toxicity.[151]

Targeting lymphoma using lymphocyte-ricin complexes has also been suggested, but no studies have been carried out in humans.[152] The use of a lymphocyte delivery system to target cytotoxic agents to the site of lymphoma is an attractive concept, but present methodology is too crude, and therapeutic efficacy needs further evaluation before lymphocyte vectors can be recommended for general use.

VITAMINS

Vitamin deficiencies may occur in patients with many forms of cancer, including lymphoma, and dietary correction is beneficial. Therapeutic administration of certain vitamins in doses above normal physiologic requirements has been attended by tumor regression in patients with some forms of leukemia, lymphoma, and solid tumors.

VITAMIN D THERAPY

$1,25(OH)_2D_3$ (calcitriol) is the biologically active metabolite of vitamin D_3 that combines with the vitamin D receptor in the cytoplasm. Following this, the complex passes to the nucleus where it interacts with DNA. The gene encoding the vitamin D receptor has homology with other steroid receptors, indicating that it is a member of the same supergene family. $1,25(OH)_2D_3$ is a steroid-type hormone with important developmental and immunoregulatory functions.[153] The recognition that $1,25(OH)_2D_3$ has the capacity to promote differentiation and arrest proliferation in a variety of cell lines (including those derived from the immunohematopoietic system) provided a rationale for its use in the therapy of lymphoma, although its mechanism of action is unknown.[154, 155]

α-Calcidiol (alfacalcidol), which is metabolized to $1,25(OH)_2D_3$ in the liver, has been used to treat patients with low-grade lymphoma.[156] Four of 28 patients with follicular small, cleaved cell lymphoma achieved complete remission with response durations of 36, 14, 12, and 10 months. The response to therapy in these patients was attained between 6 and 8 weeks after starting treatment with alfacalcidol 1 µg daily orally for a minimum of 8 weeks. The overall response rate for 36 patients with follicular lymphoma and malignant lymphocytic lymphoma was 24% with disease stabilization in a further 29%. Most of the patients were previously untreated.

The dose-limiting toxicity of alfacalcidol is hypercalcemia. However, vitamin D_3 analogues are available that have the antiproliferative properties of $1,25(OH)_2D_3$ but do not have an effect on calcium metabolism.[157, 158] Such analogues could prove to be beneficial.

VITAMIN A THERAPY

The retinoids are vitamin A (retinol) and related derivatives that have a critical role in growth, reproduction, epithelial cell differentiation, immune function, and vision.[159] Vitamin A and ATRA are derived from carotenoids in the diet; unlike ATRA, vitamin A accumulates in the liver, where it may cause chronic hepatic damage when used in large amounts. Cytoplasmic proteins bind vitamin A and ATRA before transfer to the α, β, and γ nuclear retinoic acid receptors (members of the steroid superfamily of nuclear receptors). Multiple isoforms of these receptors exist that have tissue-specific and developmental stage–specific expression, suggesting distinctive functional roles.

The α nuclear receptor gene maps to the q21 band of chromosome 17, which is located at the breakpoint associated with acute promyelocytic leukemia. ATRA is a powerful inducer of differentiation and apoptosis in the promyelocytic cell line HL-60, and oral therapy is associated with a high complete remission rate in patients with acute promyelocytic leukemia. Other preclinical and clinical studies have suggested a wider therapeutic action with at least some antitumor activity in squamous cell carcinoma of the head, neck, cervix, and skin.

Patients with mycosis fungoides have been treated with a range of retinoids, and some useful clinical responses have been observed. In one series of 25 patients treated with 13-*cis*-retinoic acid, 11 patients responded and 3 achieved complete remission.[160] The Scandinavian Mycosis Fungoides Group reported complete remissions in 21% of patients, with responses occurring within 2 to 4 weeks of starting treatment.[161] Unfortunately, subsequent studies have shown that remissions are not sustained, but studies in combination with other agents such as interferon-α are being carried out in an attempt to improve results. There are also cooperative interactions between members of the steroid superfamily of nuclear receptors (e.g., vitamins A and D_3) that could be exploited.

Toxicity of retinoic acid therapy includes features of hypervitaminosis A syndrome with cheilitis, dry skin and mucous membranes with erythema and desquamation, pruritus, lethargy, nausea, and anorexia. Headache, dry eyes with visual disturbance, and psychological changes may also be seen.

Initial doses of 1 to 2 mg/kg/day of 13-*cis* retinoic acid have been used to treat patients with mycosis fungoides, and peak plasma levels of 1 μmol/L occur 1.5 to 3 hours following an oral dose, although there is considerable individual variation. There is a biphasic elimination profile with a terminal-phase half-life of about 17 hours. As with other oral agents, bioavailability is affected by drug formulation and the relationship of dosing to food intake. The pharmacokinetics of ATRA are somewhat different with more rapid elimination (terminal half-life of about 45 minutes), and chronic administration is associated with lower peak concentrations and total systemic exposure.[162] In a recent phase I study using oral doses ranging from 45 to 200 mg/m^2 over 4 weeks, dose-limiting toxicity was seen at 175 mg/m^2 daily and doses of 150 mg/m^2 were recommended.[163] Lower doses are advised using a more prolonged schedule of administration. Account needs to be taken of these pharmacokinetic issues in future studies.

THERAPEUTIC APPROACHES USING GENE TRANSFER

A better understanding of the molecular changes responsible for the development of a lymphoma and host resistance mechanisms against the tumor has raised the possibility of using genetic techniques for treatment. Applications of gene transfer technology relating to therapy are listed in Table 14–11.

Advances in the technology of gene transfer have led to the development of clinical protocols designed to evaluate the technical feasibility and efficacy of this form of therapy. The aim of most approaches has been to enhance host defenses against malignant cells. However, such studies are only beginning, and the role of these procedures in the therapy of any form of cancer is unassessed. Suggested approaches include the genetic modification of tumor cells or host cells in vitro resulting in the expression of cytokines and tumor-associated antigens in an attempt to generate and augment an immune response to the tumor following injection in vivo.

Experimental studies have established the feasibility of transferring genes coding for a variety of cytokines, including IL-2,[164, 165] IL-4,[185] IL-6,[167] IL-7,[94, 168] interferon-γ,[169] TNF-α,[170, 171] G-CSF,[166] and GM-CSF.[96] In some model systems tumor cells transfected with these genes constitutively express and release the encoded protein over a prolonged period following injection, leading to the generation and amplification of an antitumor immune response and the development of antitumor memory.

Several experiments have involved the transfer of the IL-2 gene into tumor cells in an attempt to circumvent the limitations associated with the use of relatively high doses of IL-2 in vivo; namely, the disturbing side effects of treatment and the lack of a particularly effective antitumor response. Evidence that tumor growth is inhibited by the injection of tumor cells transfected with the IL-2 gene and that specific T-cell–mediated cytotoxicity and durable antitumor memory may develop has been provided by examining a number of murine model systems.[164, 165] The studies by Fearson and colleagues involved the use of IL-2–transduced CT26 murine colon cancer cells to immunize BALB/c mice.[164] The inhibition of tumor growth was associated with the produc-

Table 14–11. Somatic Cell Gene Transfer: Applications Designed to Improve Patient Management

Category	Actions
Immunotherapeutic	Increase the immunogenicity of tumor cells by improving the presentation of tumor-associated antigens or by augmenting immune-effector systems using immune cells, antibody, or cytokines
Correction of genetic abnormality	Replace missing genes such as tumor suppressor genes or inhibit the overexpression of oncogenes
Gene-directed enzyme prodrug therapy	Transfer of genes to the tumor-encoding enzymes capable of activating a prodrug
Gene transfer of drug resistance	Transfer of genes encoding enzymes responsible for drug resistance (e.g., multidrug resistance, DNA repair) to hematopoietic stem cells, allowing a more dose-intensive therapy
Gene marking	Genetic marking of host normal cells (hematopoietic progenitors or immune cells, tumor cells, and their progeny to follow their migration and survival to evaluate therapy

tion of an MHC class I–restricted cytotoxic lymphocyte response against the tumor mediated by CD8+ cells and did not require the presence of CD4 + T-helper cells. Immunized animals were resistant to a further challenge by parental tumor cells. A murine B lymphoblastic lymphoma was used by Gansbacher and colleagues[165] demonstrating that lymphoma regression was possible using gene transfer–mediated, localized IL-2 secretion. It is hoped that a similar approach in humans might lead to the expression and release of IL-2 in amounts likely to generate specific cytotoxicity against the tumor cells, increase NK and LAK effectors, and stimulate the local release of TNF-α and interferon-γ.

Other gene products expressed in tumor cells are also being used to induce levels of antitumor immunity that cannot be achieved with tumor cells alone, and the use of transfected cells that express more than one cytokine could be available for future study. The rodent tumor models used in preclinical studies often involved weakly immunogenic tumors, and it should be remembered that such models may not mimic spontaneous tumors in humans. Nevertheless, these studies do provide a rationale for testing the concept in patients with lymphoma.

Successful gene transfer has been accomplished in human tumor cells in culture, and production of encoded protein has been maintained following irradiation to inhibit proliferation. Clinical vaccination is being attempted in patients with solid tumors using genetically engineered malignant cells. It remains to be seen whether this approach is feasible in patients with lymphoma.

PROBLEMS ASSOCIATED WITH GENE TRANSFER

The development of gene transfer as a therapeutic tool in patients with lymphoma depends on the feasibility of the technique, the safety of the procedure, and an assessment of the efficacy of therapy. Potential products for gene transfer therapy include nucleic acid containing the cloned gene ligated into appropriate plasmids or cassettes, nucleic acid complexed with polymers or encapsulated in liposomes, replication-deficient viral vectors, and genetically modified cells containing the cloned genes that can be introduced into the patients. Problems associated with technical feasibility have been reviewed.[172] Gene transfer is frequently carried out using retroviral vectors, and some of these have the ability to produce stable transduction in almost 100% of certain target cells with the appropriate viral receptor. However, human target cells may lack these receptors, and any tumor cell population may be heterogeneous in this respect. Successful transduction by a retroviral vector also depends on the ability to induce proliferation in the target cell, and both these factors may be significant in the difficulties encountered in transducing hematopoietic stem cells. In addition, these vectors are labile, and this accounts for an important difficulty in using viral-mediated gene transfer directly in vivo.

A further problem is the possibility of reconstructing replication-competent virus either in vitro or in vivo. High titers of replication-defective recombinant virus can be produced in "packaging cells," which are free of genetic information for virus production, and these cells would not be expected to form wild-type virus; however, this has

occurred using some cell lines, and lymphomas have occurred in primates following the transplantation of hematopoietic stem cell transduced by a retroviral vector contaminated with replication-competent virus.[173]

Adenovirus vectors have been introduced because of their potential for in vivo gene delivery since, unlike retroviral vectors, they can infect nondividing cells, express large amounts of encoded product, and are relatively stable. However, integration into the DNA of the target cell is not a characteristic feature of infection, and it is possible that existing adenovirus vectors may be partially replication competent. This could explain the persistence of gene expression in vivo. If replication is found in vivo, this would be of concern in terms of safety.

Studies of other possible viral vectors such as adenoassociated viruses, herpesvirus, vaccinia virus, and several RNA viruses are continuing to circumvent some of these difficulties.

Ideally, gene transfer in vivo should be appropriately targeted. This has not as yet proved possible using viral vectors alone, but complexes between plasmid DNA and specific polypeptide ligands can be constructed with an affinity for defined receptors on the cell surface. The use of these complexes for receptor-mediated gene transfer appears promising, but a great deal of further work is required to solve problems of stability and escape of DNA following endocytosis. Methods of targeting the integration of DNA to specific regions of the chromosome DNA also need to be developed for the risks of random insertion to be minimized.

Adequate expression and release of the encoded product following gene transfer is of obvious importance. However, gene expression tends to be transient, and although transduced material may be delivered repeatedly, improved methods for stable transduction are required.

Safety issues are of particular importance in situations where the patients to be treated are potentially long-term survivors as is the case when treating patients with intermediate- or high-grade lymphoma with minimal residual disease. In spite of these difficulties, therapy for lymphoma based on genetic techniques remains an attractive possibility, and a great deal of work is being carried out in an attempt to evaluate novel therapeutic approaches using these techniques.

GENETIC TARGETS IN THE TUMOR CELL

Molecular genetic techniques have provided information concerning characteristic genetic abnormalities present in lymphoma cells and their functional consequences. In the future it may be possible to use this information to develop specific therapeutic strategies for patients with lymphoma.[174, 175] Defined genetic events must take place for malignant cell transformation and clonal evolution of a malignant cell population to occur. Characteristic functional changes are a consequence of a cascade of molecular genetic events leading to increased survival, the capacity to self-renew, proliferation, and often a differentiation block in the transformed malignant cells. It is probably that a preneoplastic phase occurs in which there is an increased life span of a cell associated with increased proliferation resulting in a further risk of genomic damage leading to neoplastic transformation. Inherited predisposition and environmental factors influence these events to a variable extent.

The discovery that certain genes important in the pathogenesis of cancer are involved in the regulation of programmed cell death is leading to approaches designed to trigger apoptosis in the malignant cell population. *BCL2* is a protooncogene with an important role in the development of follicular lymphoma. The t (14;18) translocation is present in most but not all follicular lymphomas and a proportion of other forms of lymphoma. The *BCL2* gene was identified by its translocation site on chromosome 18q21 and is inappropriately expressed because of its juxtaposition to the immunoglobulin heavy chain sequence on chromosome 14q32. The *BCL2* gene has been identified as one of the genes regulating apoptosis and has the capacity to extend the survival of cells in which it is expressed. Mice, transgenic for *BCL2*, develop a polyclonal expansion of mature follicle B cells that have extended survival, and a proportion of these mice develop malignant lymphoma.[53, 175] In the lymphoid system, programmed cell death is an efficient mechanism for elim-inating cells that develop unwanted antigen specificity (e.g., against "self") or fail to synthesize an appropriateantigen receptor at certain points in the differentiation process. Any therapy designed to block the production of the *BCL2*-encoded protein in an attempt to trigger apoptosis in lymphoma must therefore take account of these physiologic effects on the immune system and other organs. Nevertheless, the *BCL2* gene does provide a potential target for biologic therapy in those patients with lymphoma in which the *BCL2*-encoded functional product is expressed.

The presence of a chromosome translocation involving lineage-specific genes, such as an immunoglobulin or T-cell antigen receptor locus on one chromosome and a transcription factor on the partner chromosome, is a frequent occurrence in several forms of lymphoma. The resulting deregulation of transcription factors such as c-*myc*, *pbx*, the rhombotin genes, and *scl* may provide an important step in the development of a malignant lymphoma. These transcription factors also provide the possibility for targeted therapy specific for the chimeric molecules.

Chromosome translocations involving the immunoglobulin heavy chain gene on chromosome 14q32 provide a critical lesion for the development of various B-cell neoplasms, including mantle zone lymphoma and other lymphomas of small and large cell types. The highly malignant B-cell neoplasms characterized by translocation of chromosome 8 at the site of the c-*myc* protooncogene are further examples of this principle. In these translocations the c-*myc* becomes located next to the site of the heavy chain immunoglobulin gene on chromosome 14 or, less commonly, adjacent to the light chain genes on chromosome 2 or 22. In this situation c-*myc* transcription becomes abnormally regulated by the immunoglobulin gene–enhancing sequences. In T-cell neoplasms a number of translocations have been described where a transcription factor is brought into juxtaposition with a chromosome 14 breakpoint in band q11, the location of the α and δ T-cell receptor gene loci or with 7q35, the site of the β T-cell receptor gene. These translocations provide specific targets for lymphoma therapy that could involve techniques designed to kill those cells containing the translocation or inhibit function of the fused sequences.

Antisense Oligonucleotides

Antisense molecules are stretches of DNA or RNA capable of binding specifically to DNA or a selected messenger RNA preventing its translation.[176, 177] The mechanisms involved have not been completely elucidated, but degradation by ribonuclease H in the case of DNA:RNA hybrids and ribonuclease L in the case of RNA:RNA hybrids may be involved. Ribozymes are also candidates for use as antisense molecules in the therapy of lymphoma since these molecules are designed to cleave substrate RNA molecules in a sequence-specific manner. Single-stranded oligonucleotides can also recognize specific sequences in double-stranded DNA and inhibit the expression of a particular gene by forming a stable triplex molecule.[178, 179] However, these studies have been carried out only in vitro, and this potential therapeutic approach is in its infancy.

Some antisense nucleotide sequences have been synthesized that are capable of binding specifically to selected messenger RNA, blocking the production of encoded protein, and ablating gene function. The use of antisense sequences has been suggested as a therapeutic approach in patients with lymphoma when a genetic abnormality has been identified that is considered to be critical in the pathogenesis of the disease. The *BCL2* gene provides an example for this strategy since it is commonly rearranged and overexpressed in follicular lymphoma and appears to be functionally related to cell survival.

The consequence of inappropriate *BCL2* expression has been investigated using the gene transfer approach. A *BCL 2* transgene is capable of preventing apoptotic cell death in an IL-3–dependent lymphoid cell line when deprived of IL-3.[180] Antisense oligodeoxynucleotides complementary to strategic sites in *BCL2* messenger RNAs have been shown to suppress the growth and survival of lymphoma cells in culture in a sequence-specific manner.[181]

Antisense oligonucleotides could also be used against unique stretches of nucleotides generated by chromosome translocations involving the c-*myc* protooncogene. In a high proportion of Burkitt's lymphomas, transcription of the c-*myc* gene is initiated from a cryptic promoter in the first intron, creating abnormal messenger RNA molecules in which intron sequences, normally spliced out, persist. An antisense oligodeoxynucleotide directed against these sequences has been shown to inhibit the proliferation of Burkitt's lymphoma cell lines containing the abnormal transcripts but not that of cell lines containing normal c-*myc* transcripts.[182] A marked reduction in intracellular c-*myc* encoded protein was observed in cells with the aberrant transcripts but not in control cells.

Unfortunately, there are many problems in the path of a useful therapy involving antisense molecules in vivo. These include lack of specificity, failure to target and access the tumor population, and the rapid degradation of oligonucleotides by nucleases present in the serum. These issues are currently being addressed, and strategies are available for overcoming at least some of the problems. These include the use of chemical modification of the backbone structure of the nucleotide sequence coupling with other molecules, liposomal packaging, or viral transfer. These approaches may prevent degradation and enhance tumor uptake, but lack of specificity remains a problem. In the future it may be possible to deliver nucleotide sequences directed against structurally unique genes or inhibitory sequences under the control of regulatory molecules operating in a particular type of tumor cell. Lymphoid lineage–specific enhancers could be useful in this respect. Receptor-mediated oligonucleotide transfer is a further possibility, but again the specificity of this approach remains questionable, and the possibility of transfecting more than a small proportion of the targeted tumor cells is remote.

Although characteristic genetic changes have been observed in several forms of lymphoma that could provide a therapeutic target, and problems of delivery of appropriate molecules might be overcome, it remains to be seen whether blocking one step in the evolution of a malignant tumour will result in a useful tumor response. Several steps in such a cascade could be made redundant during clonal evolution, rendering the tumor cell resistant to such a specific genetic approach. In spite of these problems, this type of genetic approach to the treatment of cancer remains attractive and deserves continued emphasis.

Gene-Directed Enzyme Prodrug Therapy

A new therapeutic strategy for treating cancer involves the possible transfer of genes encoding enzymes capable of converting a nontoxic prodrug into a cytotoxic drug within the tumor. The administration of the prodrug could then be associated with enzymatic activation within the tumor cell resulting in cytotoxicity that may also damage tumor cells in the neighborhood. Examples include the herpes thymidine kinase that is capable of converting gancyclovir to its active triphosphate and a bacterial cytosine deaminase that converts the inactive 5-fluoro-cytosine to its cytotoxic metabolite, 5-fluorouracil. However, these approaches require effective methods for targeting the tumor, perhaps by inducing transferred gene expression using tumor-related promotor sequences. Such techniques remain only a possibility for lymphoma therapy.

Gene Transfer of Drug Resistance

There is evidence in lymphoma that increasing the dose intensity of cytotoxic therapy is associated with an increased relapse-free survival. Dose-intensive cytotoxic drug therapy is limited mainly by hematopoietic toxicity. Gene transfer technology raises the possibility of transplanting hematopoietic stem cells that have been transfected in vitro with genes conferring resistance to certain types of cytotoxic drugs. This method would be expected to increase the therapeutic index of the cytotoxic agent and allow a more efficacious dose-intensive approach to therapy. However, technical difficulties in transfecting hematopoietic stem cells are delaying the introduction of clinical protocols.

CONCLUSION

The application of new molecular techniques in the design of biologic therapeutic approaches in the management of lymphoma is in its infancy. The scientific advances made in understanding the molecular genetic changes occurring during the development and clonal evolution of lymphoma and host defense mechanisms have already led to new biologic approaches undergoing clinical trial. Some of these biologic treatments have been shown to be effective in shrinking measurable tumor masses, and there is every hope that such methods will be of greater advantage in the management of patients with minimal residual disease. Therapeutic strategies in the context of minimal residual disease require controlled, randomized study.

REFERENCES

1. Balkwill FR: Interferons. *In* Cytokines in Cancer Therapy. Oxford, Oxford University Press, 1984, pp 8–53.
2. Golomb H, Fefer A, Golde D, et al: Update of a multi-institutional study of 195 patients (pts) with hairy cell leukaemia (HCL) treated with interferon-alfa2b (IFN). Proc Am Soc Clin Oncol 1990; 9:215.
3. Berman E, Heller G, Kempin S, Gee T, et al: Incidence of response and long-term follow-up in patients with hairy cell leukemia treated with recombinant interferon alfa-2a. Blood 1990; 75:839.
4. Ambrosetti A, Nadali G, Vinante F, et al: Soluble interleukin-2 receptor in hairy cell leukaemia: A reliable marker of disease. Int J Clin Lab Res 1993; 23(1):34.
5. Golomb HM, Ratain MJ, Mick R, et al: Interferon treatment for hairy cell leukaemia: An update on a cohort of 69 patients treated from 1983–1986. Leukaemia 1992 (6):1177.
6. Golomb HM, Ratain MJ, Mick R, et al: The treatment of hairy cell leukaemia: An update. Leukaemia 1992; 6(Suppl 2):24.
7. Merigan TC, Sikora K, Breeden JH, et al: Preliminary observations on the effect of human leukocyte interferon in non-Hodgkin's lymphoma. N Engl J Med 1978; 299:1449.
8. Gutterman JU, Blumenschein GR, Alexanian R: Leukocyte interferon-induced tumor regression in human metastatic breast cancer, multiple myeloma and malignant lymphoma. Ann Intern Med 1980; 93:399.
9. Louie AC, Gallagher JC, Sikora K, et al: Follow-up observations on the effect of human leukocyte interferon in non-Hodgkin's lymphoma. Blood 1981; 58:71.
10. Gams R, Gordon B, Guaspari A, Tuttle R: Phase II trial of human polyclonal lymphoblastoid interferon (Welferon) in the management of malignant lymphomas. ASCO Abstracts 1984; C-253.
11. Horning SJ, Merigan TC, Krown SE: Human interferon alpha in malignant lymphoma and Hodgkin's disease. Cancer 1985; 56:1305.
12. Queseda GR, Hawkins M, Horning SJ, et al: Collaborative phase I-II study of recombinant DNA–produced leukocyte interferon (clone A) in metastatic breast cancer, malignant lymphoma, and multiple myeloma. Am J Med 1984; 77:427.
13. Foon KA, Sherwin SA, Abrams PG, et al: Treatment of advanced non-Hodgkin's lymphoma with recombinant leukocyte A interferon. N Engl J Med 1984; 311:1148.
14. Wagstaff J, Loynds P, Crowther D: A phase II study of human recombinant DNA-a2 interferon in patients with low-grade non-Hodgkin's lymphoma. Cancer Chemother Pharmacol 1986; 18:54.
15. O'Connell MJ, Colgan JP, Oken MM, et al: Clinical trial of recombinant leukocyte A interferon as initial therapy for favorable histology non Hodgkin's lymphomas and chronic lymphocytic leukemia. J Clin Oncol 1986; 4:128.
16. Leavitt RD, Ratanatharathorn V, Ozez H, et al: A phase II study of recombinant alpha 2 interferon in patients with malignant lymphoma with unfavorable histology. Proc Am Soc Clin Oncol 1983; 2:54.
17. Mantovani L, Gugliemi C, Martelli M, et al: Recombinant alpha-interferon in the treatment of low-grade non-Hodgkin's lymphoma: Results of a cooperative phase II trial in 31 patients. Haematologica 1989; 74:571.
18. Billard C, Ferbus D, Diez RA, et al: Correlation between the biological and therapeutic effects of interferon-alpha in low-grade nodular non-Hodgkin's lymphoma: Lack of in vivo down-regulation and reduced affinity of IFN-alpha receptors in unresponsive patients. Leuk Res 1991; 15:121.
19. Rohatiner AZS: Interferon alpha in lymphoma. Br J Haematol 1991; 79:26.

20. Kaplan EH, Rosen ST, Norris DB, et al: Phase II study of recombinant human interferon gamma for treatment of cutaneous T cell lymphoma. J Natl Cancer Inst 1990; 82:208.

21. Kobayashi Y, Urabem A: Gamma interferon therapy of cancer patients. Gan To Kagaku Ryoho 1988; 15:804.

22. VanderMolen LA, Steis RG, Duffey PL, et al: Low- versus high-dose interferon alfa-2a in relapsed indolent non-Hodgkin's lymphoma. J Natl Cancer Inst 1990; 82(3):235.

23. Ferbus D, Khosravi S, Dumont J, Billard C: In vivo and in vitro induction of 2'-5' oligoadenylate synthetase by interferon alpha in nodular non-Hodgkin's lymphoma and correlations with the clinical response. J Biol Regul Homeost Agents 1990; 4(4):127.

24. Adams F, Quesada JR, Gutterman JU: Neuropsychiatric manifestations of human leucocyte interferon therapy in patients with cancer. JAMA 1984; 252:938.

25. Merimsky O, Reider-Groswasser I, Inbar M, et al: Interferon-related mental deterioration and behavioural changes in patients with renal cell carcinoma. Eur Cancer 1990; 26:596.

26. Cohen MC, Huberman MS, Nesto RW: Recombinant alpha-2 interferon–related cardiomyopathy. Am J Med 1988; 85:549.

27. Fentiman IS, Balkwill FR, Thomas BS, et al: An autoimmune aetiology for hypothyroidism following interferon therapy for breast cancer. Eur J Cancer Clin Oncol 1988; 24:1299.

28. Von Wussow P, Hehlmann R, Hochhaus T, et al: Roferon (rIfN-alpha 2a) is more immunogenic than intron A (rIFN-alpha 2b) in patients with chronic myelogenous leukemia. J Interferon Res 1994; 14:217.

29. Chirgios MA, Pearson JW: Cure of murine leukaemia with drugs and interferon treatments. J Natl Cancer Inst 1973; 14:97.

30. Gresser I, Maury C, Tovey M: Efficacy of combined interferon-cyclophosphamide therapy after diagnosis of lymphoma in KR mice. Eur J Cancer 1978; 14:97.

31. Balkwill RF, Moodie EM: Positive interactions between human interferon and cyclophosphamide or Adriamycin in a human tumour model system. Cancer Res 1984; 44:904.

32. Solal-Celigny P, Lepage E, Brousse N, et al: Recombinant interferon alpha-2b combined with a regimen containing doxorubicin in patients with advanced follicular lymphoma. N Engl J Med 1993; 329:1608.

33. Smalley RV, Anderson JW, Hawkins MJ, et al: Interferon alfa combined with cytotoxic chemotherapy for patients with non-Hodgkin's lymphoma. N Engl J Med 1992; 327:1336.

34. Anderson JW, Smalley RV: Interferon alfa plus chemotherapy for non-Hodgkin's lymphoma: Five-year follow-up. N Engl J Med 1993; 329:1821.

35. Price CGA, Rohatiner AZS, Steward W, et al: Interferon alpha-2b in addition to chlorambucil in the treatment of follicular lymphoma: Preliminary results of a randomised trial in progress. Eur J Cancer 1991; 27:S34.

36. Hagenbeek A, Carde P, Somers R, et al: Maintenance of remission with human recombinant alpha-2 interferon (roferon-A) in patients within stages III and IV low-grade malignant non-Hodgkin's lymphoma: Results from a prospective randomised phase III clinical trial in 331 patients [Abstract]. Blood 1992; 79(suppl 1):288A.

37. Lippman SM, Glisson BS, Kavanagh JA, et al: Retinoic acid and interferon combination studies in human cancer. Eur J Cancer 1993; 29A(Suppl 5):S9.

38. Ho CK, Want SY, Ou BR, et al: Enhancement of interferon-induced 2-5 oligoadenylate synthetase activity by retinoic acid in human histiocytic lymphoma U937 cells and WISH cells. Differentiation 1989; 40:70.

38a. Kohler G, Milstein C: Continuous cultures of fused cells secreting antibody of predefined specificity. Nature 1975; 256:475.

39. Lim SH, Marcus RE: Monoclonal antibody (MoAb) therapy in non-Hodgkin's lymphomas. Blood Rev 1992; 6:157.

40. Dillman RO: Human antimouse and antiglobulin responses to monoclonal antibodies. Antibody Immunoconjugates Radiopharmaceut 1992; 3:1.

41. Brown S, Miller R, Horning SJ, et al: Treatment of B-cell lymphomas with anti-idiotypic antibodies alone and in combination with alpha-interferon. Blood 1989; 73:651.

42. Bahler DW, Levy R: Clonal evolution of a follicular lymphoma: Evidence for antigen selection. Proc Natl Acad Sci U S A 1993; 89:6770.

43. Hekman A, Honselaar A, Vuist WM, et al: Initial experience with treatment of human B-cell lymphoma with anti-CD19 monoclonal antibody. Cancer Immunol Immunother 1991; 32:364.

44. Bertram JH, Gill PS, Levin AM, et al: Monoclonal antibody T101 in T-cell malignancies: A clinical, pharmacokinetic, and immunological correlation. Blood 1986; 68:752.

45. Dillman RO, Shawlier DL, Dillman JB, et al: Therapy of chronic lymphocytic leukaemia and cutaneous T cell lymphoma with T101 monoclonal antibody. J Clin Oncol 1984; 2:881.

46. Knox SJ, Levy R, Hodgkinson S, et al: Observations on the effects of chimeric anti-CD4 monoclonal antibody in patients with mycosis fungoides. Blood 1991; 77:20.

47. Dyer MJS, Hale H, Marcus R, et al: Remission induction in patients with lymphoid malignancies using unconjugated CAMPATH-1 monoclonal antibodies. Leuk Lymphoma 1992; 2:179.

48. Riechmann L, Clark MR, Waldman H, et al: Reshaping human antibodies for therapy. Nature 1988; 332:323.

49. Hale G, Clark MR, Marcus R, et al: Remission induction in non-Hodgkin's lymphoma with reshaped human monoclonal antibody CAMPATH-1H. Lancet 1988; 1:1394.

50. Ellis RE, Yaun J, Horovitz H: Mechanisms and functions of cell death. Annu Rev Cell Biol 1991; 7:663.

51. Hengarter MO, Ellis RE, Horovitz HR: *Caeorhabitidis elegans* gene *ced 9* protects cells from programmed cell death. Nature 1992; 352:494.

52. Nunez G, London L, Hockenbury D, et al: Deregulated *Bcl-2* gene expression selectively prolongs survival of growth factor–deprived haemopoietic cell lines. J Immunol 1990; 144:3602.

53. McDonnell TJ, Deane N, Platt FM, et al: *bcl-2* immunoglobulin transgenic mice demonstrate extended B cell survival and follicular lymphoproliferation. Cell 1989; 57:79.

54. Trauth BC, Klas C, Peters AMJ, et al: Monoclonal antibody–mediated tumour regression by induction of apoptosis. Science 1989; 245:301.

55. Owen-Shaub LB, Yonehara S, Crump WL, et al: DNA fragmentation and cell death is selectively triggered in activated human lymphocytes by Fas antigen engagement. Cell Immunol 1992; 140:197.

56. Pietersz GA, McKenzie IFC: Antibody conjugates for the treatment of cancer. Immunol Rev 1992; 129:57.

57. Czuczman MS, Straus DJ, Divgi CR, et al: Phase I dose escalation trial of iodine 131-labelled monoclonal antibody OKB7 in patients with non-Hodgkin's lymphoma. J Clin Oncol 1993; 10:2021.

58. Press OW, Eary JF, Appelbaum FR, et al: Radiolabeled-antibody therapy of B-cell lymphoma with autologous marrow support. N Engl J Med 1993; 329:1219.

59. Kaminski MS, Zasadny KR, Francis IR, et al: Radioimmunotherapy of B-cell lymphoma with [131I]anti-B1 (anti CD20) antibody. N Engl J Med 1993; 329:459.

60. Gobuty A, De Nardo G, De Nardo SJ: Lym-1 radioimmunotherapy: A case history of how we do it. Antibody Immunoconjugates Radiopharmaceut 1992; 5:13.

61. Maloney DG, Liles TM, Czerwinski DK, et al: Phase I clinical trial using escalating single-dose infusion of chimeric anti-CD20 monoclonal antibody (IDEC-C2B8) in patients with recurrent B cell lymphoma [Abstract]. Blood 1993; 82(Suppl 1):176.

62. Le Maistre CF, Rosen S, Frankel A, et al: Phase I trial of H65-RTA immunoconjugates in patients with T-cell lymphoma. Blood 1991; 78:1173.

63. Vitella ES, Stone M, Amlot P, et al: Phase I immunotoxin trial in patients with B-cell lymphoma. Cancer Res 1991; 51(15):4052.

64. Amlot PL, Stone MJ, Cunningham D, et al: A phase I study of an anti-CD22–deglycosylated ricin-A chain immunotoxin in the treatment of B-cell lymphoma resistant to conventional therapy. Blood 1993; 82:2624.

65. Grossbard ML, Freedman AS, Ritz J, et al: Serotherapy of B-cell neoplasms with anti-B4–blocked ricin: A phase I trial of daily bolus infusion. Blood 1992; 79:576.

66. Grossbard ML, Gribben JG, Freedman AS, et al: Adjuvant immunotoxin therapy with anti-B-4–blocked ricin after autologous bone marrow transplantation for patients with B-cell non-Hodgkin's lymphoma. Blood 1993; 81(9):2263.

67. Bonardi M, Bell A, French RR, et al: Initial experience in treating human lymphoma with a combination of bispecific antibody and saporin. Int J Cancer 1992; 7:73.

68. Chaudhary VK, Queen C, Junghans RP: A recombinant immunotoxin consisting of two antibody variable domains fused to pseudomonas exotoxin. Nature 1989; 339:394.

69. Siegall CB, Chaudhary FK, Fitzgerald DJ: Cytotoxic activity of an interleukin 6 *Pseudomonas* exotoxin fusion protein on human myeloma cells. Proc Natl Acad Sci U S A 1988; 85:9738.

70. Kapovsky B, Titus JA, Stephany DA, et al: Production of target-specific effector cells using hetero-cross-linked aggregates containing anti-target cell and ant-Fc receptor antibodies. J Exp Med 1984; 160:1686.

71. Perez P, Titus JA, Lotze MT, et al: Specific lysis of human tumour cells by T cells coated with anti-T3 cross-linked to anti-tumour antibody. J Immunol 1986; 137:2069.

72. Weiner GJ, Hillstrom J: Bispecific anti-idiotype anti CD3 antibody therapy of murine B cell lymphoma. J Immunol 1991; 147:4035.

73. Brissinck J, Demanet C, Moser M, et al: Treatment of mice-bearing *bcl 1* lymphoma with bispecific antibodies. J Immunol 1991; 147:4019.

74. Bagshawe KD: Antibody-directed enzymes revive anti-cancer pro-drugs concept. Br J Cancer 1987; 56:531.

75. Bagshawe KD, Springer CJ, Searle F, et al: A cytotoxic agent can be generated selectively at cancer sites. Br J Cancer 1988; 58:700.

76. Springer CJ, Bagshawe KD, Sharma SK, et al: Ablation of human choriocarcinoma xenografts in nude mice by antibody-directed enzyme prodrug therapy (ADEPT) with three novel compounds. Eur J Cancer 1991; 27:1361.

77. Bagshawe KD, Sharma SK, Springer CJ, et al: Antibody-directed enzyme prodrug therapy (ADEPT): A pilot scale clinical trial. Ann Oncol 1994; 5:879.

78. Houghton AN, Thomson TM, Gross D, et al: Surface antigens of melanoma and melanocytes: Specificity of induction of Ia antigens by human gamma-interferon. J Exp Med 1984; 160:255.

79. Pfizenmaier K, Scheurich P, Schluter C, et al: Tumour necrosis factor enhances HLA-A, B, C and HLA-DR gene expression in human tumor cells. J Immunol 1987; 138:975.

80. Basham TY, Kaminski MS, Kitamura K, et al: Synergistic antitumour effect of interferon and anti-idiotypic monoclonal antibody in murine lymphoma. J Immunol 1986; 137:3019.

81. Pastan I, Fitzgerald D: Recombinant toxins for cancer treatment. Science 1991; 254:1173.

82. Le Maistre CF, Meneghetti C, Rosenblum M, et al: Phase I trial of an interleukin-2 (IL-2) fusion toxin (DAB$_{486}$ IL-2) in haematologic malignancies expressing the IL-2 receptor. Blood 1992; 79:2547.

83. Hesketh P, Caguioa P, Koh H, et al: Clinical activity of a cytotoxic fusion protein in the treatment of cutaneous T-cell lymphoma. J Clin Oncol 1993; 11:1682.

84. Williams DP, Parker K, Bacha P, et al: Diphtheria toxin receptor–binding domain substitution with interleukin-2: Genetic construction and properties of a diphtheria toxin–related interleukin-2 fusion protein. Protein Eng 1987; 1:493.

85. Press PW, Farr AG, Borroz KI, et al: Endocytosis and degradation of monoclonal antibodies targeting human B cell malignancies. Cancer Res 1989; 49:4906.

86. Routledge E, Lloyd I, Gorman SD, et al: A humanised monovalent CD3 antibody which can activate homologous complement. Eur J Immunol 1991; 21:2717.

87. Smyth MJ, Pietersz GA, McKenzie IFC: The use of vasoactive agents to increase tumour perfusion and the antitumour efficacy of drug monoclonal antibody conjugates. J Natl Cancer Inst 1987; 79:1367.

88. George AJ, Stevenson FK: Prospects for the treatment of B cell tumours using idiotypic vaccination. Int Rev Immunol 1989; 4:271.

89. Kwak LW, Campbell MJ, Czerwinski DK, et al: Induction of immune responses in patients with B-cell lymphoma against the surface immunoglobulin idiotype expressed by their tumour. N Engl J Med 1992; 327:1209.

90. Hawkins RE, Ovecka M, Russell SJ, et al: Idiotypic vaccination against B-cell lymphoma: A genetic approach. Br J Cancer 1993; 67(Suppl 20):13.

91. Jiao S, Williams P, Berg RK, et al: Direct gene transfer into nonhuman primate myofibers in vivo. Hum Gene Ther 1992; 3:21.

92. Herlyn D, Sears H, Illiopolous D, et al: Anti-idiotypic antibodies to monoclonal antibody CO17-1A. Hybridoma 1986; S51.

93. Tepper RI, Pattengale RK, Leder P: Murine interleukin-4 displays potent and antitumour activity in vivo. Cell 1989; 57:503.

94. Hock H, Dorsch M, Diamanstein T, et al: Interleukin 7 induces CD4+ T cell–dependent tumour rejection. J Exp Med 1991; 174:1291.

95. Tao MH, Levy R: Idiotype/granulocyte-macrophage colony-stimulating factor fusion protein as vaccine for B-cell lymphoma. Nature 1993; 362:755.

96. Dranoff G, Jaffee E, Lazenby A, et al: Vaccination with irradiated tumour cells engineered to secrete murine granulocyte-macrophage colony-stimulating factor stimulates potent specific and long-lasting anti-tumour immunity. Proc Natl Acad Sci U S A 1993; 90:3539.

97. Currie JA: Eighty years of immunotherapy. Br J Cancer 1972; 26:141.

98. Klein E: Tumors of the skin: X. Immunotherapy of cutaneous and mucosal neoplasms. N Y State J Med 1968; 68:900.

99. Mathe G, Amiel JL, Schwarzenberg L, et al: Active immunotherapy for acute lymphoblastic leukaemia. Lancet 1969; 1:697.

100. Sokal JE, Aungst CN, Synderman M: Delay in progression of malignant lymphoma after BCG vaccination. N Engl J Med 1974; 291:1226.

101. Jones SE, Grozea PN, Metz EN, et al: Improved complete remission rates and survival for patients with large cell lymphoma treated with chemoimmunotherapy: A Southwest Oncology Group study. Cancer 1983; 51:1083.

102. Ravaud A, Ebhbali E, Trojani M, et al: Adjuvant bacillus Calmette-Guérin therapy in non-Hodgkin's malignant lymphomas: Long-term results of a randomized trial in a single institution. J Clin Oncol 1990; 8:608.

103. Hoerni B, Eghbali H, Durand M, et al: Adjuvant BCG therapy of non-Hodgkin's malignant lymphomas stages I and II. *In* Salmon SE, Jones SE (eds): Adjuvant Therapy of Cancer, 4th ed. Philadelphia, Grune & Stratton, 1984, pp 653–660.

104. Jones SE, Grozea PN, Miller TP, et al: Chemotherapy with cyclophosphamide, doxorubicin, vincristine, and prednisolone alone or with levamisole or with levamisole plus BCG for malignant lymphoma: A Southwest Oncology Group study. J Clin Oncol 1985; 3:1318.

105. Thomas JW, Plenderleith IH, Landi S, et al: Bacille Calmette-Guérin as maintenance for non-Hodgkin's lymphoma. Can Med Assoc J 1983; 129:539.

106. Morgan DA, Ruscetti FW, Gallo R: Selective in vitro growth of T lymphocytes from normal bone marrows. Science 1976; 193:1007.

107. Minami Y, Kono T, Yamada K, et al: The interleukin-2 receptors: Insights into a complex signalling mechanism. Biochem Biophys Acta 1992; 1114:163.

108. Grimm EA, Mazumder A, Zhang HZ, et al: Lymphokine-activated killer cell phenomenon: Lysis of natural killer–resistant fresh solid tumour cells by interleukin-2–activated autologous human peripheral blood lymphocyte. J Exp Med 1982; 155:1823.

109. Whittington R, Faulds D: Interleukin-2: A review of its pharmacological properties and therapeutic use in patients with cancer. Drugs 1993; 46(3):446.

110. Parmiani G, Gambacorti-Passerini C: Interleukin-2 biology and immunology. *In* Wagstaff J (ed): The Role of Interleukin-2 in the Treatment of Cancer Patients. The Netherlands, Kluwer, 1993, pp 71–80.

111. Barrett AJ, Gordon MY: Bone Marrow Disorders: The Biological Basis of Treatment. Oxford, Blackwell Scientific, 1983.

112. Talamadge JE, Phillips H, Schindler J: Systematic preclinical study on the therapeutic properties of recombinant human interleukin-2 for the treatment of metastatic disease. Cancer Res 1987; 47:5725.

113. Rosenberg SA. Immunotherapy and gene therapy of cancer. Cancer Res 1991; 51(Suppl 1):5074s.

114. Slavin SA, Ackerstein E, Naparstek R, et al: Hypothesis: The graft-versus-leukaemia (GVL) phenomenon: Is GVL separable from GVHD? Bone Marrow Transplant 1990; 6:155.

115. Sachs DH, Sharibi Y, Sykes M: Chimerism and the induction of transplant tolerance. *In* Gale R, Champlin RK (eds): New Strategies in Bone Marrow Transplantation. New York, Wiley-Liss, 1991, p 21.

116. Sykes M, Abraham VS, Harty MW, et al: IL-2 reduces graft-versus-host disease and preserves a graft-versus-leukaemia effect by selectively inhibiting CD4+ T cell activity. J Immunol 1993; 150(1):197.

117. Oshimi K, Oshimi Y, Akutsu M, et al: Cytotoxicity of interleukin-2–activated lymphocytes for leukaemia and lymphoma cells. Blood 1986; 68:938.

118. Schlegel PG, Schmidt-Wolf G, Schmidt-Wolf IGH, et al: Lymphokine-activated killer cell activity against autologous lymphoma cells following bone marrow transplantation. Cancer Res Ther Control 1993; 3:145.

119. Slavin S, Ackerstein A, Vourka-Karussis U, Nagler A, et al: Control of relapse due to minimal residual disease (MRD) by cell-mediated cytokine-activated immunotherapy in conjunction with bone marrow transplantation. Baillieres Clin Haematol 1991; 4(3):715.

120. Siekevitz M, Feinberg MB, Holbrook N, et al: Activation of interleukin-2 and interleukin-2 receptor (Tac) promoter expression by the transactivator (tat) gene product of human T cell leukaemia virus type I. Proc Natl Acad Sci U S A 1987; 84:5389.

121. Rosenberg SA, Lotze MT, Yang JC, et al: Experience with the use of

high-dose interleukin-2 in the treatment of 652 cancer patients. Ann Surg 1990; 210:474.

122. Thompson JA, Lee DJ, Lindgren CG, et al: Influence of dose and duration of infusion of interleukin-2 on toxicity and immunomodulation. J Clin Oncol 1988; 6:669.

123. West WH, Tauer KW, Yannelli JR, et al: Constant-infusion recombinant interleukin-2 in adoptive immunotherapy of advanced cancer. N Engl J Med 1987; 316(15)898.

124. Allison MAK, Jones SE, McGuffey P: Phase II trial of outpatient interleukin-2 in malignant lymphoma, chronic lymphocytic leukaemia, and selected solid tumours. J Clin Oncol 1989; 7(1):75.

125. Luria F, Zinzani PL, Rondelli D, et al: Continuous infusion of interleukin-2 in two relapsed high-grade non-Hodgkin's lymphoma patients: Effectiveness and tolerability. Eur J Cancer 1991; 27(4):5241.

126. Levy R, Tourani JM, Andrieu JM: Interleukin-2 therapy with or without lymphokine-activated killer cell infusions for low-grade non-Hodgkin's lymphomas? [Letter]. J Clin Oncol 1992; 10:1366.

127. Weber JS, Yang JC, Topalian SL, et al: The use of interleukin-2 and lymphokine-activated killer cells for the treatment of patients with non-Hodgkin's lymphoma. J Clin Oncol 1992; 10(1):33.

128. Gisselbrecht C, Maraninchi D, Puico JL, et al: Interleukin 2 (IL2) in lymphoma: A phase II multicentre study. Proc Am Soc Cancer Res 1992; 33:227.

129. Atzpodien J, Schomburg A, Kirchner H, et al: Interleukin-2 and other cytokines. *In* Wagstaff J (ed): The Role of Interleukin-2 in the Treatment of Cancer Patients. The Netherlands, Kluwer, 1993, pp 141–167.

130. Duggan DB, Santarelli MT, Zamkoff K, et al: A phase II study of recombinant interleukin-2 with or without recombinant interferon beta in non-Hodgkin's lymphoma: A study of the cancer and leukaemia group. Br J Immunother 1992; 12:115.

131. Redman BG, Flaherty L, Chou TH, et al: A phase I trial of recombinant interleukin-2 combined with recombinant interferon gamma in patients with cancer. J Clin Oncol 1990; 8(7):1269.

132. Palmer PA, Vinke J, Evers P, et al: Continuous infusion of recombinant interleukin-2 with or without autologous lymphokine-activated killer cells for the treatment of advanced renal cell carcinoma. Eur J Cancer 1992; 28A:1038.

133. von Rohr A, Thatcher N: Clinical applications of interleukin-2. Prog Growth Factor Res 1992; 4:229.

134. Soiffier RJ, Murray C, Cochran K, et al: Clinical and immunologic effects of prolonged infusion of low-dose recombinant interleukin-2 after autologous and T-cell–depleted allogeneic bone marrow transplantation. Blood 1992; 79(2):517.

135. Weiden PL, Fluornoy N, Thomas ED, et al: Antileukemia effect of graft-versus-host disease in human recipients of allogeneic marrow granfts. N Engl J Med 1979; 300:1068.

136. Horowitz MM, Gale RP, Sondel PM, et al: Graft-versus-leukemia reactions following bone marrow transplantation. Blood 1990; 75:555.

137. Sullivan KM, Weiden PL, Storb R, et al: Influence of acute and chronic graft-versus-host disease on relapse and survival after bone marrow transplantation from HLA-identical siblings as treatment of acute and chronic leukaemia. Blood 1989; 73:1720.

138. Goldman JM, Gale RP, Horowitz MM, et al: Bone marrow transplantation for chronic myelogenous leukemia in chronic phase: Increased risk for relapse associated with T-cell depletion. Ann Intern Med 1988; 108:806.

139. Bacigalupo A, Van Lint MT, Occhini D, et al: Increased risk of leukemia relapse with high-dose cyclosporine A after allogeneic marrow transplantation for acute leukemia. Blood 1991; 77:1423.

140. Szer J, Grigg AP, Phillips GL, Sheridan WP: Donor leukocyte infusions after chemotherapy for patients relapsing with acute leukemia following allogeneic BMT. Bone Marrow Transplant 1993; 11:109.

141. Drobyski WR, Keever CA, Roth MS, et al: Salvage immunotherapy using donor leukocyte infusions as treatment for relapsed chronic myelogenous leukemia after allogeneic bone marrow transplantation: Efficacy and toxicity of a defined T-cell dose. Blood 1993; 82:2310.

142. Foa R: Does interleukin-2 have a role in the management of acute leukaemia? J Clin Oncol 1993; 11:1817.

143. Benyunes MC, Massumoto C, York A, et al: Interleukin 2 with or without lymphokine-activated killer cells as consolidative immunotherapy after autologous bone marrow transplantation for acute myelogenous leukaemia. Bone Marrow Transplant 1993; 12:159.

144. Hood AF, Vogelsang GB, Black LP, et al: Acute graft-versus-host disease: Development following autologous and syngeneic bone marrow transplantation. Arch Dermatol 1987; 123:745.

145. Smith ME, Ford WL: The recirculating lymphocyte pool of the rat: A systematic description of the migratory behavior of recirculating lymphocytes. Immunology 1983; 49:83.

146. Wagstaff J, Gibson C, Thatcher N, et al: A method for following human lymphocyte traffic using indium-111 oxine labelling. Clin Exp Immunol 1981; 43:435.

147. Wagstaff J, Gibson C, Thatcher N, et al: Human lymphocyte traffic assessed by indium-111 oxine labelling: Clinical observations. Clin Exp Immunol 1981; 43:443.

148. Crowther D, Wagstaff J: Lymphocyte migration in malignant disease. Clin Exp Immunol 1983; 51:413.

149. Birch M, Sharma HL, Bell EB, Ford WL: The carriage and delivery of substances to lymphatic tissue by recirculating lymphocytes: II. Long-term selective irradiation of the spleen and lymph nodes by deposition on In-114m. Immunology 1986; 58:359.

150. Hamilton D, Cowan RA, Sharma HL, et al: The behaviour of autologous indium-114m–labelled lymphocytes in patients with lymphoid cell malignancy. J Nucl Med 1988; 29:485.

151. Cowan RA, Drayson M, Sharma H, et al: Autologous lymphocytes as vectors to target therapeutic radiation in patients with chronic lymphocytic leukaemia. Submitted.

152. Ramsden CS, Drayson M, Bell EB: Lymphocyte-targeted ricin as a potential therapy for lymphoid malignancy. In: Targeting efficiency. Br J Cancer 1991.

153. Studizinski GP, McLane JA, Uskovic MR: Signalling pathways for vitamin D–induced differentiation: Implications for therapy of proliferative and neoplastic diseases. Crit Rev Eukaryot Gene Expr 1993; 3(4):229.

154. Abe E, Miyaura C, Sakagumi H, et al: Differentiation of mouse myeloid leukaemia cells induced by 1α25-dihydroxyvitamin D. Proc Natl Acad Sci U S A 1981; 78:4990.

155. Hicklish T, Cunningham D, Colston K, et al: The effect of 1,25-dihydroxyvitamin D_3 on lymphoma cell lines and expression of vitamin D receptor in lymphoma. Br J Cancer 1993; 68:668.

156. Raina V, Cunningham D, Gilchrist N, et al: Alfacalcidol is a nontoxic effective treatment of follicular small-cleaved cell lymphoma. Br J Cancer 1991; 63:463.

157. Binderup L, Bram E: Effects of a novel vitamin D analogue MC903 on cell proliferation and differentiation in vitro and on calcium metabolism in vivo. Biochem Pharmacol 1988; 37:880.

158. Colston KW, Chander SK, Mackey AG, Coombes RC: Effects of synthetic vitamin D analogues on breast cancer cell proliferation in vivo and in vitro. Biochem Pharmacol 1992; 44:693.

159. Smith MA, Parkinson DR, Cheson BD, et al: Retinoids in cancer therapy. J Clin Oncol 1992; 10:839.

160. Kessler J, Jones S, Levine N, et al: Isotretinoin and cutaneous helper T-cell lymphoma (mycosis fungoides). Arch Dermatol 1987; 123:201.

161. Molin L, Thomsen K, Volden G, Lange-Wantzin G: Retinoid dermatitis mimicking progression in mycosis fundgoides: A report from the Scandinavian Mycosis Fungoides Group. Acta Derm Venereol 1985; 65:69.

162. Muindi J, Frankel S, Miller W, et al: Continuous treatment with all-*trans* retinoic acid causes a progressive reduction in plasma drug concentrations: Implications for relapse and retinoid resistance in patients with acute promyelocytic leukaemia. Blood 1992; 79:299.

163. Lee JS, Newman RA, Lippman SM, et al: Phase I evaluation of all-*trans* retinoic acid in adults with solid tumours. J Clin Oncol 1993; 11:959.

164. Fearson E, Pardoll D, Itaya T, et al: Interleukin-2 produced by tumour cells bypasses T-helper function in the generation of an antitumour response. Cell 1990; 60:397.

165. Gansbacher B, Zier K, Daniels B, et al: Interleukin-2 gene transfer into tumour cells abrogates tumorigenicity and induces protective immunity. J Exp Med 1990; 172:1217.

166. Golomb M, Ferrari G, Stoppancciaro A, et al: Granulocyte colony-stimulating factor gene transfer suppresses tumourogenicity of a murine adenocarcinoma in vivo. J Exp Med 1991; 173:889.

167. Porgador A, Gansbacher B, Bannerji R, et al: Antimetastatic vaccination of tumour-bearing mice with IL-2 gene inserted tumour cells. Int J Cancer 1993; 53:471.

168. McBride W, Thacker J, Comora S, et al: Genetic modification of a murine fibrosarcoma to produce interleukin-7 stimulates host cell infiltration and tumour immunity. Cancer Res 1992; 52:3931.

169. Esumi N, Hung B, Itaya T, et al: Reduced tumourogenicity of murine

tumour cells secreting gamma interferon is due to nonspecific host responses and is unrelated to class I major histocompatibility complex expression. Cancer Res 1991; 51:1185.

170. Asher A, Mule J, Kasid A, et al: Murine tumour cells transduced with the gene for tumour necrosis factor-α. J Immunol 1991; 146:3227.

171. Blankenstein T, Qin Z, Überla K, et al: Tumour suppression after tumour cell targeted tumour necrosis factor α gene transfer. J Exp Med 1991; 173:1047.

172. Mulligan RC: The basic science of gene therapy. Science 1993; 260:926.

173. Donahue RE, Kessler SW, Bodine D, et al: Helper virus–induced T-cell lymphoma in nonhuman primates after retroviral-mediated gene transfer. J Exp Med 1992; 176:1125.

174. Magrath I: Molecular basis of lymphomagenesis. Cancer Res 1992; 52(Suppl 1):5529.

175. McDonnell TJ, Korsmeyer SJ: Progression from lymphoid hyperplasia to high-grade malignant lymphoma in mice transgenic for the t(14;18). Nature 1991; 349:254.

176. Neckers L, Whitesell L, Rosolen A, et al: TI antisense inhibition of oncogene expression. Crit Rev Oncog 1992; 3:175.

177. Castanotto D, Rossi JJ, Deshler JO: Biological and functional aspects of catalytic RNAs. Crit Rev Eukaryot Gene Expr 1992; 2:331.

178. Toulme JJ, Helen C: Antimessenger oligodeoxyribonucleotides: An alternative to antisense RNA for artificial regulation of gene expression—a review. Gene 1988; 82:51.

179. Sun, 1989

180. Hockenberry D, Nunez G, Milliman C, et al: *Bcl-2* is an inner mitochondrial membrane protein that blocks programmed cell death. Nature 1990; 348:334.

181. Reed JC, Stein C, Subasingh C, et al: Antisense-mediated inhibition of *bcl2* protooncogene expression and leukaemia cell growth and survival: Comparisons of phosphodiester and phosphorothioate oligodeoxynucleotides. Cancer Res 1990; 50:6565.

182. McManaway ME, Neckers LM, Loke SL, et al: Tumour-specific inhibition of lymphoma growth by an antisense oligodeoxynucleotide. Lancet 1990; 335:808.

HODGKIN'S DISEASE

Chapter Fifteen

Biology of Hodgkin's Disease

Harald Stein
Michael Hummel
Horst Dürkop
Hans-Dieter Foss
Hermann Herbst

Hodgkin's disease (HD) is one of the few lymphoprolif-erative disorders that, despite intensive research, evades clarification of even the most basic questions. These include the cell lineage relation, the clonality, and the isolated distribution of the dysplastic cells in HD, that is, the Hodgkin and Reed-Sternberg (HRS) cells. There are also differing opinions as to whether the Reed-Sternberg (RS) cells become multinucleated by cell fusion or endomitosis. Additionally, it is unclear why nondysplastic cells of various types in HD predominate in number and not the dysplastic cells, as in the case with other lymphoproliferative disorders, like non-Hodgkin's lymphomas (NHLs). It remains to be clarified whether the different histotypes of HD represent different disease entities or variants of one disease. There is no understanding why attempts to establish cell lines from HD tissue are usually successful only in terminal phases of the disease and why the results of antigen receptor gene rearrangement studies are so variable and do not correlate with the concentration of HRS cells present in the tissue samples investigated. Furthermore, the question remains as to why study results are unsettled, such as those on the metaphase and interphase karyotypes, DNA content, and mutation patterns in the p53 locus, and why terminal repeats of EBV genomes were so heterogeneous in HRS cells.

This review does not reiterate all the data previously discussed in detail in several excellent reviews,[1–8] but it does address most of the questions mentioned and focuses on findings that appear relevant to answer these unresolved questions.

CELL LINES

Research on HD has been hampered because it was practically impossible to isolate HRS cells from tissue biopsies. This is due to the fragility of HRS cells and the abundance of contaminating normal bystander cells present in the tissue affected by HD. Consequently, in vitro cultivation techniques have been applied in attempts to enrich and purify HRS cells in temporary or permanent cultures.[9–14] Few of these attempts have been successful since the 1970s, resulting in approximately 10 HD-derived cell lines that are available today (Table 15–1).[5, 15–26] These HD cell lines have enabled the generation of new antibodies, leading to the detection of HRS cell–associated antigens, such as CD30,[27] CD70,[28] and Ki-27.[28–30] The availability of the HD cell lines has also allowed in vitro immunopheno-typic and genotypic studies. The results summarized in Table 15–1 show that all but one of the available cell lines have the same antigen profile as in situ HRS cells. The exception is the HD-MyZ cell line, which lacks all antigenic character-istics of HRS cells, such as CD30, CD70, and CD15, but instead expresses the monocyte/macrophage CD68 epi-tope.[31] Since the immunophenotypic analysis (performed in our laboratory) of the HRS cells in the biopsy from which the HD-MyZ cell line has been established revealed the expected expression of CD30 and CD15 but not of CD68, it appears highly likely that the cell line mentioned is not derived from HRS cells but from other cells, such as macrophages or their precursors. All other cell lines ex-hibit immunophenotypic and/or genotypic features of either B cells or T cells, suggesting that HRS cells are lymphocytic in origin and that HRS cells are related to either B cells or T cells. However, this conclusion is not generally accepted because it has been impossible to demonstrate that the HD cell lines were really derived from HRS cells and not from other cells present in the tissue or effusion samples. On the other hand, it has been proved that a recently established cell line with B-cell features does derive from HRS cells because the same immunoglobulin (Ig) gene rearrangement was demonstrated in both the in situ HRS cells and in the cell line cells.[32]

In spite of the growing body of evidence that favors a derivation of most HD cell line from HRS cells, it is repeatedly questioned whether these cell lines are repre-sentative for HD. This reservation appears to be justified in view of the fact that the HRS cells in 50% of HD cases are Epstein-Barr virus (EBV) infected, whereas only 1 of the available 11 HD-derived cell lines harbors the EBV genome. A major reason for the rarity of EBV-infected HD-derived cell lines might be that before the discovery of EBV in HRS cells, all EBV-infected cell lines were regarded as

This work was completed with financial support from the Consultation and Reference Center for Lymph Node Pathology and Haematopathology sponsored by the Deutsche Krebshilfe at the Institute of Pathology, Klinikum Benjamin Franklin, Free University Berlin, Hindenburgdamm 30, 12200 Berlin, Germany.

Table 15–1. Immunophenotype and Genotype of Classic Hodgkin's Disease Cell Lines

Cell Lines	CD30	CD70	CD15	CD68	B-AG	T-AG	Rearranged AGR Gene	AGR Chain	References
L428°	+	+	+	–	–CD19?	–	IgH, (L)	–	15, 16
L591°	+	+	+/–	–	CD19, 20	CD2	IgH, L	IgA λ	14
KM-H2°	+	+	+	–	–	–	IgH, L	–	26
L540°	+	+	(+)	–	–	–	TCR-α, β, δ	–	14, 17
CO°	+	–	+	–	–	cyCD3, 7	TCR-β, δ	–	18, 21
HO°	+	+	–	–	–	CD3, 5, 7	TCR-β, δ	TCR-β ?	21
HDLM2°	+		+	–	–	CD2	TCR-α, β, δ	–	20, 22
DEV†	+		+		CD20, 22	–	IgH, L	cyIgA	19, 24
HD-70†	+		+		–	–	IgH, L	cyIgA κ	25
ZO†	+		+		–	–	IgH, L	–	24
SUP-HD1†	–		+	–	–	–	IgH, L, TCR-β	κ	23
HD-MyZ‡	–		–	+	–	–		–	31

°Permanently growing and available.
†It is not known whether these lines are still alive or whether the diagnosis of the primary material was correct; most of these cell lines have not been made available.
‡This line has been established from a patient with nodular sclerosis Hodgkin's disease. However, it is highly unlikely that the cell line is derived from the Hodgkin and Reed-Sternberg (HRS) cells because the HRS cells in the tissue biopsy proved to be CD30+, CD15+, and CD68–, whereas the cell line cells are CD30–, CD15–, and CD68+.
B-AG, B-cell antigen; T-AG, T-cell antigen; AGR, antigen receptor; Ig, immunoglobulin; cy, cytoplasmic; TCR, T-cell receptor.
+ = constantly positive; (+) = faintly positive; +/– = variably positive; – = constantly negative; ? = uncertain expression.

being derived from EBV-carrying bystander B cells and not from HRS cells. The consequence is that many EBV-positive cell lines established from HD-affected tissue samples were not submitted for publication or were rejected in the reviewing process as possible candidates for being direct HRS cell derivatives (Stein H, unpublished observations).

MORPHOLOGY, IMMUNOPHENOTYPING, AND IN SITU HYBRIDIZATION

Immunohistologic studies of HD biopsies have proved to be of relevance in two areas: one area concerns the subtyping of HD and the other the elucidation of the nature of HRS

cells. However, in a third area, namely, whether the proliferation of the HRS is clonal, immunohistologic studies have produced more confusion than clarification.

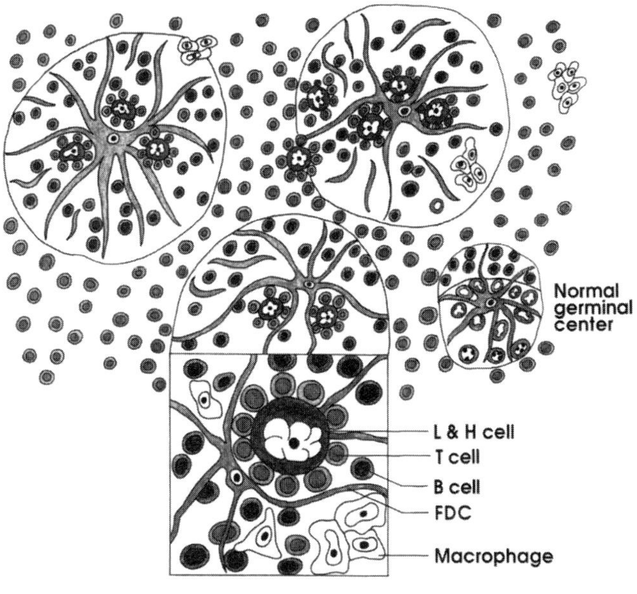

HISTOTYPES

Figures 15–1 to 15–4 show the histotypes of HD that have been generally distinguished since the Rye Conference in 1966, and Figure 15–5 shows the areas in which the histologic criteria of the histotypes overlap with each other or with other lymphoid neoplasms (reviewed by Lukes and Butler[33] and Harris and colleagues[34]). Immunohistologic studies using antibodies discovered in the 1980s[27, 28, 30, 35–37] (Table 15–2) have shown that HRS cells present in nodular sclerosis (NS), mixed cellularity (MC), and lymphocyte depletion (LD) of HD resemble each other in terms of antigen profile but differ from the lymphocyte and histiocyte (L&H) type of HRS cells (which are also called "popcorn cells") present in lymphocyte-predominant Hodgkin's disease (LPHD).[34, 37–39] This adds to the clinical and morphologic differences between LPHD and the other histotypes of HD. The distinction between LPHD and the non-LPHD

Figure 15–1. Nodular lymphocyte-predominant Hodgkin's disease. See text for abbreviations.

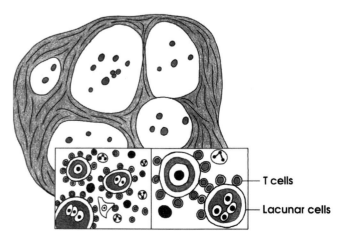

Figure 15–2. Nodular sclerosing Hodgkin's disease.

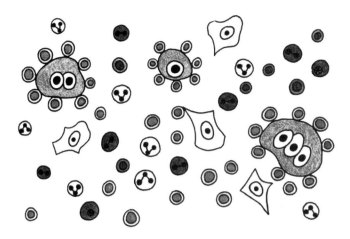

Figure 15–3. Mixed cellular Hodgkin's disease.

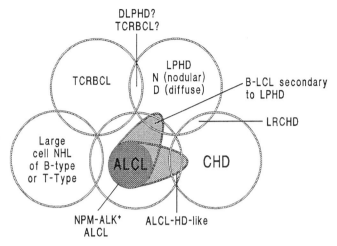

Figure 15–5. Morphologic overlaps of Hodgkin's disease with anaplastic large cell lymphoma (ALCL) and other lymphomas. See text for additional abbreviations.

forms is important because LPHD is indolent and in most instances shows little or no progression with or without therapy, in contrast with the other HD forms, which are fatal without treatment.[1, 8, 34, 40, 41] To emphasize the close relation between NS, MC, and LD forms of HD and their differences from LPHD, the International Lymphoma Study Group (ILSG) proposed the combination of NS, MC, and LD under the generic term "classic HD" (cHD).[34]

LYMPHOCYTE-RICH HISTOTYPES

Although the features of LPHD appear distinct, data available in literature on the frequency and clinical features of LPHD vary greatly.[2, 38, 41] This stems from a relatively frequent confusion of LPHD with other lymphoid disorders (see Fig. 15–5), especially lymphocyte-rich variants of cHD (see later) and T-cell-rich B-cell lymphoma (TCR-BCL).[34, 41–43] Most of the differential diagnostic problems could be avoided with the knowledge that there are two subtypes of LPHD, that is, nodular (nLPHD) and diffuse (dLPHD), and that the nodular form is well-defined, whereas the diffuse form is not. A characteristic feature of nLPHD is the presence of large, usually circular meshworks

of follicular dendritic cells (FDCs)[35, 44] that contain, in addition to the popcorn-type HRS cells, mainly B cells and scattered T cells.[45] A relatively large proportion of the latter contain a great number of CD57-positive T cells that are distributed in a nodular arrangement, in most instances.[45] In dLPHD, nodules with FDCs and B cells are missing, and their cellular background is dominated by diffusely distributed T cells. Immunophenotypic studies have confirmed that there are also cHD cases that resemble dLPHD in their lymphocyte (T-cell) richness but are more similar to cHD in terms of antigen profile of the HRS cells and of clinical behavior (reviewed by Harris and associates[34]). Thus, correctly grouping these cases together with cHD has not only theoretical relevance but also clinical importance. The ILSG proposed calling the cHD cases with a lymphocyte-rich background "classic lymphocyte-rich HD" (cLRHD)[34] with the intent that it might help further proper typing. Whether cLRHD represents a distinct subtype of cHD or merely a variant is not answered, nor is it intended to be

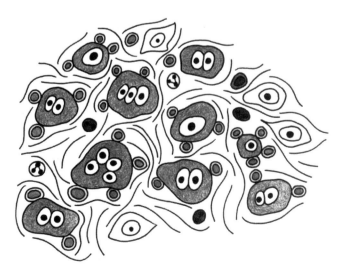

Figure 15–4. Lymphocyte-depleted Hodgkin's disease.

Table 15–2. Immunophenotype of Classic Hodgkin's Disease Histotypes, TCR-BCL, and ALCL

Marker	TCR-BCL	LPHD	NS, MC, LD	cLRHD	ALCL
CD30	−(+)	−	+	+	+
CD70	−(+)	−(+)	+	+	−+
CD15	−	−	+(−)	+(−)	−+
EMA	+−	+−	−(+)	−	+−
CD20(L26)	+	+	−+	−+	−
CD79a(JCB117)	+	+	−+	−+	−
J chain	+	+	−	−	−
CD3	−	−	−+	−+	+−
TCR-β	−	−	−+	−+	+−

HD, Hodgkin's disease; TCR-BCL, T-cell-rich B-cell lymphoma; LPHD, lymphocyte-predominant HD; NS, nodular sclerosing; MC, mixed cellular; LD, lymphocyte-depleted; cLRHD, classic lymphocyte-rich HD; ALCL, anaplastic large cell lymphoma; EMA, epithelial membrane antigen; TCR-β, β chain of the T-cell receptor.

− = all cases negative; −(+) = most cases negative; −+ = majority of cases negative; +− = majority of cases positive; +(−) = most cases positive; + = all cases positive.

answered by this proposal. The solution of this problem requires further research.

DISTINCTION BETWEEN dLPHD AND TCR-BCL

The distinction of dLPHD from TCR-BCL seems to be of even more importance clinically than the issue discussed earlier because TCR-BCL is usually associated with bone marrow involvement at presentation, is extremely aggressive, and requires immediate treatment, whereas dLPHD does not.[34, 43] In spite of great efforts, neither morphologic nor immunophenotypic criteria have been found that allow a distinction between dLPHD and TCR-BCL. This was confirmed by a workshop organized by the European Association of Hematopathology (EAHP) in Toledo, Spain, in October 1994. In consequence, some authors doubt the existence of dLPHD as a distinct disease entity and thus believe that in most instances dLPHD in reality represents TCR-BCL.[43] In a recent article there is speculation that TCR-BCL might represent a variant of dLPHD rather than a separate entity related to large B-cell NHL.[46] On the other hand, there is evidence that TCR-BCLs are heterogeneous, because forms exist that are related to dLPHD and forms that are related to diffuse large B-cell lymphoma.

DISTINCTION BETWEEN HD AND ANAPLASTIC LARGE CELL LYMPHOMA

Another area where an overlap occurs is between cHD and anaplastic large cell lymphoma (ALCL)[47] (see Fig. 15–5). The cases considered to be in this overlapping area possess features of both cHD and ALCL.[48–51] It is not known whether these borderline cases represent ALCL that mimic cHD or vice versa. Since the ILSG believed that the first possibility is more likely, it proposed calling these borderline cases "ALCL-HD-like," at least for the time being. There is accumulating evidence that ALCL-HD-like is more aggressive than cHD and responds better to treatment modalities used for the management of high-grade NHL than to cHD treatment.[34, 48] In the earlier mentioned Toledo EAHP workshop, a lot of time was devoted to the question of whether immunophenotypic criteria are available that can reliably distinguish cHD from ALCL; however, no convincing conclusions were reached. Consequently, the observation of a characteristic translocation involving chromosomes 2 and 5 in ALCL attracted interest,[52–55] which increased when Orscheschek and associates reported the presence of the ALCL characteristic t(2;5) in 11 of 13 cHD cases.[56] However, other studies using both identical and different methods failed to demonstrate the t(2;5) in all of the 250 cHD cases studied,[57–63] suggesting that (1) Orscheschek and associates' results represent a technical artifact and (2) ALCL carrying the t(2;5) and HD are not related.

THE NATURE OF HRS CELLS

LPHD is generally regarded as a distinct type of B-cell lymphoma because of the highly constant expression of a range of B-cell-specific antigens (J chain, CD20, CD79a, and others) on the popcorn variant of HRS cells of LPHD.[2, 7, 8, 30, 34, 37, 38, 47, 64–68] In contrast, the derivation of HRS cells of cHD is, because of the heterogeneity of published research data, still an enigma. As Tables 15–2 through 15–4 show, immunohistologic results are uniform in cHD because all or most HRS cells express CD30,[30, 34, 35, 47, 65, 69–71] CD70,[28, 30] and CD15[36, 72–74] and lack markers specific or characteristic for macrophages[47, 49, 75–78] and interdigitating cells (IDCs),[30, 35, 48, 79] making a close relationship between HRS cells and these cells highly unlikely. This conclusion is, however, not generally accepted, since there are conflicting reports and interpretations in the literature on the specificity of the HRS cell–associated antigens CD30 and CD15 and the significance of lymphocyte markers on HRS cells (reviewed in Drexler[2]). For example, the so-called IDC marker IRAC is claimed to be selectively expressed on HRS cells and IDC.[80] However, Hsu and Hsu[80] ignored the fact that this molecule is much more widely expressed. In addition to IDC, it has been detected on many macrophages and lymphoid cells in immunolabeling experiments performed in our laboratory[49] and in others. This makes IRAC irrelevant as a cell lineage marker. The confusion is all the greater because the expression of B-cell and T-cell antigens in cHD proved to be very heterogeneous[49] (reviewed in Pileri and coworkers[1]) (Table 15–5). Because of this heterogeneity, the presence of the markers mentioned earlier on HRS cells is frequently regarded as an aberrant gene expression rather than an indication that HRS cells originate from B cells or T cells. Considering the conflicting reports on the cellular expression of the markers mentioned and the differing opinions on their value as cell lineage indicators, the most relevant markers of HRS cells are briefly discussed in the following sections.

Table 15–3. Range of Expression of the CD30 Molecule: Updated Results

Cell Types	CD30 Positivity
Classic HRS cells	100% +
Popcorn variant HRS cells	– or weakly +
Interfollicular/perifollicular blasts	+
Activated B cells	subset +
Activated T cells	subset +
Activated T_{HO}	(+)
Activated T_{H1}	–+
Activated T_{H2}	+–
Activated CD8 T cells producing T_{H2} type cytokines	+–
Resting B and T cells	–
Precursor B and T cells	–
Myeloid precursor cells	–
Monocytes and macrophages	–
Cultivated monocytes	–°
Accessory cells (FDC, IDC)	–
Fat cells	–†
Decidua cells	–†
Soft tissue tumors	–†
Embryonal carcinoma cells	+

°Repeat experiments showed that the CD30 expression as evidenced by binding of the Ki-1 antibody to activated monocytes (Andreesen et al[83, 84]) represents an artifact mediated by the IgG3 Fc fragment since anti-CD30 antibodies of another isotype, e.g., IgG1, did not bind to the cultivated monocytes.

†The reported immunostaining of fat cells, decidua, and soft tissue tumors proved to be an artifact with rare exceptions in the field of poorly differentiated soft tissue neoplasms.

HRS, Hodgkin and Reed-Sternberg; FDC, follicular dendritic cell; IDC, interdigitating cell.

Table 15–4. Immunophenotype of HRS Cells of cHD in Comparison with that of Macrophages, FDCs, and IDCs as Revealed by the Study of More Than 300 Cases of Hodgkin's Disease

Marker	Classic HRS Cells	Macrophages	FDC	IDC
CD30	+	–	–	–
CD70	+	–(+)	–	–
Ki-27	+	–+	–	–
CD15	+	–+	–	–
CD25[199]	+–	+	–	–
CD68	–	+	–	– or weakly +
Lysozyme	–	+	–	– or weakly +
Desmosomes	–	–	+	–
CD21	–+	–	+	–
R4/23	–	–	+	–
S100	–	–	–	+
CD1a	–	–	–	+
IRAC	–+	–+	–	+
CD20	–+	–	– or weakly +	–
CD79a	–+°	–	–	–
CD40	+	–+	–	+
CD3	–+°	–	–	–
TCR-β	–+°	–	–	–

°Few to many positive HRS cells are detectable in approximately 20% of the cHD cases.

For an explanation of the symbols, refer to Table 15–2.

cHD, classic Hodgkin's disease; FDC, follicular dendritic cell; IDC, interdigitating cell; HRS, Hodgkin and Reed-Sternberg.

CD30

Molecular cloning identified the CD30 molecule as a member of the tumor necrosis factor receptor/nerve growth factor receptor (TNFR/NGFR) superfamily.[81] Detailed information about the structural and functional characteristics of the CD30 molecule were provided in a recent review.[82] Therefore, only those features are discussed here that appear to be relevant to the elucidation of the nature of HRS cells (see Table 15–4). There is agreement that CD30 expression can be induced on B cells, T cells, and natural killer (NK) cells following mitogen activation or viral transformation.[47, 83] However, the restriction of the CD30 molecule to the three lineages of activated lymphoid cells has been repeatedly thrown into doubt. Some authors have reported the presence of CD30 on activated monocytes,[84] macrophages,[84] fat cells,[85] myoepithelial cells,[86] various soft tissue tumors,[87] decidua,[88] and embryonal carcinoma cells,[89] among others.[69] This has resulted in much doubt about the

Table 15–5. B-Cell and T-Cell Markers on HRS Cells of Hodgkin's Disease

Histotype	Averaged Percentage of Cases	CD20 and/or CD79a	TCR-β and/or CD3
nLPHD	100	+	–
cHD	20	+	–
	20	–	+
	3	+	+
	57	–	–

HRS, Hodgkin and Reed-Sternberg; nLPHD, nodular lymphocyte-predominant Hodgkin's disease; cHD, classic Hodgkin's disease.

specificity of CD30 as a lymphoid activation marker and thus the justification for regarding the CD30 expression on HRS cells as evidence for their lymphoid origin. However, repeat experiments performed in our laboratories using CD30-type antibodies of high affinity and a different isotype (e.g., the IgG1 isotype antibody Ber-H2 instead of the IgG3 isotype antibody Ki-1) (see Table 15–3), revealed that, with the exception of embryonal carcinoma type of testicular germ cell tumors, the earlier mentioned demonstration of the CD30 expression outside the lymphoid system represented an artifact, owing to either interactions of the murine γ3 chain of the Ki-1 antibody with human Fc receptors or unspecific stickiness of this antibody.[82]

Great confusion was generated also by the finding that the original Ki-1 antibody reacted not only to the membrane bound CD30 antigen but also to a nuclear molecular structure.[90] It was even more confusing that the nuclear antigen was demonstrable in cells without the membrane staining.[91] Molecular studies were able to clarify the puzzle. The nuclear molecule recognized by the Ki-1 antibody proved to be different in molecular weight (57 kilodaltons [kD])[91] and amino acid sequence from that of CD30 (120 kD),[81] indicating that both structures represent different, unrelated molecules. The nonrelationship between these two molecules was confirmed by the fact that CD30 antibodies recognizing epitopes different from the ones seen by the Ki-1 antibody do not bind to the 57-kD nuclear protein.[69] Considering this cross-reactivity and the earlier mentioned stickiness, the Ki-1 antibody should no longer be used for the identification of the CD30 molecule.

Considerable doubt about the usefulness of the CD30 molecule as a lymphoid activation marker and/or HRS cell marker also came from immunostainings of paraffin sections. A reproducible immunostaining of paraffin sections was seen only after proteolytic treatment, even when high-affinity CD30 antibodies such as Ber-H2 were applied. The confusing observation was that the Ber-H2 antibody, as well as other CD30-type antibodies, did label not only the same cells as in frozen sections (i.e., HRS cells, ALCL cells, and interfollicular-perifollicular blasts in normal lymphoid tissue) but also plasma cells and, in some instances, endothelial cells, macrophages, and even epithelial cells.[69] This additional immunostaining seen especially in overdigested paraffin sections also represents an artifact because it could be removed by the introduction of the new antigen retrieval procedure (Stein H and coauthors, unpublished data) in which the paraffin sections are boiled in citrate buffer,[92] and also because of the fact that in frozen sections, high-affinity CD30 antibodies such as Ber-H2 do not bind to plasma cells, macrophages, endothelial cells, or epithelial cells.[69, 82]

It can be concluded that the CD30 molecule is only rarely expressed outside of the lymphoid cell population and thus represents the most specific lymphoid activation marker presently available. Hence, it follows that the constant CD30 positivity of classic HRS cells is a strong indication of their lymphoid origin.

CD40

The CD40 molecule has been identified as a 50-kD member of the TNFR family[93] that is constantly expressed on B cells.[94, 95] It plays a key role in the regulation of the B cell's survival in the germinal center reaction (reviewed by McLennan and associates[96]). CD40 is also expressed on IDCs, macrophages, many carcinomas, and thymic epithelium.[95] HRS cells have been demonstrated to be constantly positive for CD40.[97, 98] The significance of this finding for the origin of the HRS cells is unclear, considering the broad cellular expression of the CD40 molecule. In conjunction with the absence of specific or characteristic markers for IDCs (CD1a, S100), macrophages (e.g., CD68, lysozyme, Ber-MAC3), and epithelial cells (e.g., cytokeratins) on HRS cells, the presence of CD40 on HRS cells is at least not in disharmony with the derivation of HRS cells from lymphoid cells (see Table 15–4). The ligand for CD40 is not detectable on HRS cells but on some intermingled T cells[97] (Stein H and colleagues, unpublished findings). Experiments with cultured HRS cells[97] showed that the CD40 ligand has pleomorphic activities on HRS cells; for example, it enhances the expression of costimulatory molecules, such as the intracellular adhesion molecule 1 (ICAM-1) and B7-1, and it reduces the expression of CD30. Thus, the CD40-CD40 ligand interaction might be involved in the deregulated cytokine network (for details see the section on cytokines) and the activation status of the HRS cells characteristic for cHD.

MYELOID MARKERS

CD15 antibodies (e.g., TÜ9,[36] 3C4,[72] C3D1,[64] Leu-M1[73, 74]) recognize the trisaccharide antigen lacto-N-fucopentaose III, also termed "X-hapten."[64, 99] The analysis of CD15 in cHD has achieved diagnostic significance because it is detectable on HRS cells of most cHD cases but usually not on L&H cells of LPHD (see Table 15–4).[1, 2, 34, 37, 100] CD15, however, has no value as a lineage marker because it is expressed not only on late cells of the granulopoiesis but also by various epithelial cells,[72, 99] some macrophages (e.g., a subpopulation of epithelioid cells), and, more important, by a subpopulation of B cells and T cells following mitogen activation and/or transformation by EBV (Stein H and colleagues, unpublished observations) and on activated neoplastic T cells.[101] It can also be found on some of the RS-like cells occurring in infectious mononucleosis (Stein H and colleagues, unpublished observations) and in some NHLs.[74, 100–103] Thus, the expression of CD15 by classic HRS cells is not in conflict with the lymphoid origin of these cells but rather indicates, in conjunction with other markers, a special lymphoid activation/transformation stage of the classic HRS cells.

LYMPHOID MARKERS

As mentioned earlier, there is a common consensus that the L&H (popcorn) cells express the B-cell antigens CD20 and J chain in most cases.[2, 4, 7, 34, 64] Use of the recently generated monoclonal anti-CD79 antibody JCB117 has demonstrated that the L&H cells of most LPHD cases also carries the CD79a molecule on the surface.[104] This molecule has a similar function in B cells to CD3 in T cells. It is involved in the signal transduction induced by the binding of antigen to surface Ig.[105] CD79a appears to be the most B-cell–specific antigen known.[106] The detection of CD79a further confirms the B-cell nature of the L&H cells present in nLPHD and dLPHD.

In contrast with LPHD, reports on the expression of lymphoid markers on HRS cells of cHD are less homogeneous.[47, 49, 65] One reason is that the staining for these antigens is usually weak and variable within the same cases. Thus, the detection of the lymphoid antigen on HRS cells requires an optimal, intense immunostaining with no background. Another reason is that the evaluation of the immunostaining is frequently quite difficult. This applies especially to T-cell antigen immunostainings because HRS cells are usually ringed by T cells, making it impossible in frozen sections and often even in paraffin sections to determine whether a T-cell antigen staining stems from surrounding (ringing) T cells or from the surface of the HRS cells themselves. Because of these problems, the expression of B-cell and T-cell markers has been investigated using differently processed tissue sections (frozen, paraffin, plastic), cases with clusters of HRS cells lacking ringing T cells between the HRS cells and on cytospins.[37, 78, 100, 104, 107–111] The carefully performed studies agree in that there are four patterns of B-cell and T-cell marker expressions on HRS cells of cHD (see Table 15–5): (1) cases with B-antigen positive, T-antigen negative HRS cells; (2) cases with T-antigen positive, B-antigen negative HRS cells; (3) cases with B-antigen and T-antigen double-positive HRS cells; and (4) cases with B- and T-antigen double-negative HRS cells. However, there is disagreement about the frequency of these patterns (reviewed by Pileri and associates[1]). For example, Schmid and colleagues[67] reported B-cell antigens to be present on HRS cells in up to 80% of cHD cases. In paraffin sections CD20 and/or CD79a are detectable in at least 20% of cases and T-cell receptor β (TCR-β) and/or CD3 on a further 20%.[110]

Altogether, the immunophenotypic studies strongly suggest that the HRS cells in cHD are lymphocytic in origin in at least 40% of cases and that cHD is, in comparison with LPHD, heterogeneous in that B-cell and T-cell types exist analogous to NHLs. The existence of cHD cases with B-cell-related HRS cells is further supported by the detection of a lymphoid-associated molecule, designated "BLA.36," that is expressed only by HRS cells, neoplastic cells of certain B cells, NHLs, and a subset of B cells.[112] The existence of B-cell-derived HRS cells could be recently confirmed by the demonstration of rearranged Ig genes in single HRS cells (see the section on single cell analysis for details). There is also further evidence for the existence of cHD cases with T-cell-related HRS cells. Two research groups[113, 114] detected in cases with T-cell antigen positive HRS and in some cases with double-negative HRS cells cytotoxic molecules (perforin and/or granzyme B). The occurrence of the mentioned cytotoxic molecules is restricted in normal lymphoid tissue to cytotoxic T cells and NK cells. A close relation of the HRS cells carrying cytotoxic molecules to NK cells is, however, not likely because the NK cell characteristic molecule CD56 is not expressed.[114] The lineage assignment of the HRS cells in most cHD cases with double-negative HRS cells is also beginning to become clearer. Many of these might be B-cell–related because HRS cells with rearranged Ig genes were demonstrable (see the section on single cell analysis for details), and some of these cases might be cytotoxic T-cell related because of the expression of the earlier mentioned cytotoxic molecules.

CLONALITY

Immunolabeling for Ig heavy and light chains failed to clarify whether HRS cells are derived from many cells (polyclonal) or from only one cell (monoclonal). In frozen sections, HRS cells are immunoglobulin negative, apart from rare exceptions.[35] In paraffin sections, HRS cells frequently stain positively for both Ig κ light chains and Ig λ light chains.[115–119] This is an odd staining pattern because reactive B cells and reactive plasma cells may react either with anti-κ or anti-λ antibodies, but not with both. The paradoxical immunostaining of HRS cells for both Ig κ and Ig λ light chains, therefore, appears to be due to uptake of Ig from the serum during the formol fixation process.[115, 116, 119, 120] Supporting this interpretation is the nondetectability of Ig light-chain–specific transcripts in classic HRS cells.[121, 122] In LPHD, a double-positive staining for both Ig light chains also occurs[35] but is less pronounced. Poppema and colleagues reported the presence of Ig κ+λ– and Ig λ+κ– popcorn-type HRS cells within the same cases, which they interpreted as an indication of polyclonality.[123] In contrast, Schmid and colleagues reported expression of only Ig κ light chains by the dysplastic cells in 19 of 20 LPHD cases and on the basis of these findings deduced a clonal proliferation of the dysplastic popcorn cells in LPHD.[67] The latter finding was in part supported by two in situ hybridization studies in which monotypic Ig κ mRNA was detected in the popcorn cells in 50% to 80% of the nLPHD cases.[124, 125]

GENOTYPING

ANTIGEN RECEPTOR GENE REARRANGEMENTS

As a result of the immunophenotypic evidence for the B-cell or T-cell origin of HRS cells, most genotypic studies on cHD have focused on the detection of clonally rearranged antigen receptor genes. However, these studies, which were carried out on whole-tissue DNA from cHD biopsies, were inconclusive because in most instances a clonal rearrangement was not demonstrable.[2, 126–128] It was not clear whether this nondetectability was due to the scarcity of clonally rearranged HRS cells or to a real absence of clonal rearrangements. The latter could mean that HRS cells

represent nonlymphoid cells or NK cells, or polyclonal lymphoid cells or lymphoid progenitor cells being arrested in a maturation stage before antigen receptor gene rearrangement takes place. Since polyclonally proliferating malignancies are exceptions (at least according to current research), usually occurring only in immunocompromised conditions; since all cell lines established from patients with HD were apparently monoclonal from the beginning; and since cHD is associated with the development of large tumor masses and progression, we favored the view that the HRS cells harbor identically rearranged antigen receptor gene rearrangements but that these cells are in most instances too rare to be detected by Southern blot techniques in whole-tissue DNA.[127] Therefore, a larger number of cHD cases were reinvestigated by applying a polymerase chain reaction (PCR) assay with increased sensitivity for the detection of clonal IgH rearrangements. With this method, clonal IgH rearrangements could be demonstrated in whole-tissue DNA for approximately 70% of the LPHD cases and in 28% of the cHD cases (Table 15–6).[128] Evaluating the presence of B-cell and T-cell markers on HRS cells revealed a strikingly positive correlation between the expression of CD20 by the HRS cells and the detectability of clonally rearranged IgH genes, suggesting that the HRS cells of at least 60% of the cHD cases of B-cell immunophenotype represented clonally proliferating B-cell derivatives.

SINGLE CELL ANALYSIS

Since whole-tissue DNA investigations could not determine whether the detected clonal rearrangements were really derived from HRS cells and not from other cells present in the biopsy samples and could not explain why a clonal IgH rearrangement is frequently not demonstrable in cHD of B-cell immunophenotype,[1, 126–129] methods were developed that allow analysis of single HRS cells isolated from tissue blocks or tissue sections. In the first study of this kind, cells were picked with a micropipette from suspended cHD biopsied tissue and subsequently assayed by PCR for the presence of cell type–specific transcripts.[130] The results of this study were inconclusive because of the great heterogeneity of the findings.[130] The weak point of the study was that the identification of the putative HRS cells was based on cell size only. To avoid this disadvantage, Roth and

Table 15–6. Frequency of IgH Rearrangements in Hodgkin's Disease in Relation to the Immunophenotype of HRS Cells and in Comparison to NHL[128]

Histologic Type	B−AG+ No.	B−AG+ Percentage	T−AG+ (No.)	B−/T− No.	B−/T− Percentage	Total No.	Total Percentage
LPHD	11/16	69	0	3/5	60	14/21	67
cHD	5/8	64	0/3	8/35	23	13/46	28
B-CLL	7/7	100					
MCL	6/6	100					
FCL (CB-CC)	8/12	67					
B-LCL	6/10	60					

HRS, Hodgkin and Reed-Sternberg; NHL, non-Hodgkin's lymphoma; LPHD, lymphocyte-predominant Hodgkin's disease; cHD, classic Hodgkin's disease; B-CLL, B-type chronic lymphocytic leukemia; MCL, mantle cell lymphoma; FCL, follicle center lymphoma (CB-CC, centroblastic); B-LCL, B-cell large cell lymphoma.

colleagues[131] modified the method in that the suspended cells were cytospun, immunostained for CD30, and then scratched from the slides. The second technique developed by Delabie with Chan and coworkers[132, 133] is the isolation of L&H or HRS cells from paraffin section–derived cell suspensions stained for epithelial membrane antigen (EMA) or CD30 cells that were picked with a manually operated pipette.[132, 133] The third technique, introduced by Küppers and associates,[134] is a much more straightforward technique for the isolation of single cells. In this method, single cells are picked from immunostained frozen sections using a hydraulic micromanipulator. This method allows the identification of cells that are to be isolated on the basis of morphology, antigen profile, and tissue localization because the architecture of the tissue is not destroyed. It also avoids any loss of certain cell types that regularly occurs when tissue is suspended. By picking B cells from germinal centers and follicle mantles, the authors were able to convincingly demonstrate the reliability and high efficiency of this direct single cell isolation method, that is, they proved that cutting does not significantly contaminate the tissue sections with released DNA. They also showed that (1) few B-cell clones are multiplied in the germinal center; (2) somatic IgV region gene mutations are introduced in the germinal center; and (3) the follicle mantle is a reservoir for naive (unmutated) unrelated B cells. Küppers and associates[135] also applied this method with success to three cases of cHD using CD30 immunostained frozen sections affected by cHD. Encouraged by these results, we (Hummel and colleagues[136, 137]) investigated 12 cases of cHD with HRS cells of a B-cell immunophenotype for IgH rearrangement using the same method (Fig. 15–6). The results generated by the different approaches mentioned earlier are summarized in Table 15–7. The group of Trümper (Roth and associates[131] and Daus and coworkers[138]) was unable to detect Ig and T-cell receptor rearrangements in the material that was believed to be derived from HRS cells in any of the 13 cases investigated. In contrast, the results of the three other studies agreed in that they found rearranged Ig genes in HRS-cell–derived DNA but differed in terms of clonality of the rearranged genes.[132, 133, 135, 136] The Ig rearrangements detected by Delabie and colleagues in all four LPHD cases[132] and in three of six cHD cases[133] were different from each other within the same cases, indicating polyclonality of popcorn/HRS cells. Contrary to these results, Küppers and associates[135] found only identical Ig rearrangements in the HRS-cell–derived DNA, a finding that is consistent with a monoclonal origin of HRS cells. We observed in our first cHD series both types of Ig rearrangements: in six cases all or most of the Ig rearrangements of the HRS cells were identical (clonal), and in the other six cases they were different from each other (polyclonal).[136] These varying results were intensively discussed at the Third International Symposium on Hodgkin's Lymphoma in Cologne, Germany, in September 1995. Klaus Rajewsky argued that the monoclonal tumor cell population escaped detection in the reported polyclonal cHD cases because the HRS cells carry highly mutated V region genes, which makes the primers being homologous to unmutated Ig gene sequences unable to bind to their target sequences. To test this possibility, we reinvestigated the single HRS cells of our 12 cHD cases with additional primer sets.[137, 139] The results are shown in Table

15–8. The existence of HRS cells with clonal rearrangements were confirmed for all six cases. From the six polyclonal cases, only four could be reinvestigated since in two cases the DNA was deteriorated. In two of the four cases left, the application of family-specific primers led to the detection of a clonal population of HRS cells, one carrying a clonal VH5 rearrangement and one a clonal Vκ3 rearrangement.[137, 139] The latter case had also been investigated by Klaus Rajewsky's group (Küppers and associates[140, 141]), and the same Vκ3 rearrangement was found in the single HRS cells. The sequence analysis of the clonal HRS cell rearrangements of Küppers and associates' and our series indeed revealed a high load of somatic mutations in the V region genes, indicating that Klaus Rajewsky was correct in his assumption that clonal populations can be missed if one applies only one set of primers. In the meantime, Küppers and associates studied nine additional cHD cases and found clonally rearranged HRS cells in eight of these cases (see Table 15–7). Altogether, the data presented indicate that (1) the HRS cells in most cHD cases represent a clonal proliferation of B-cell–derived tumor cells; (2) the existence of polyclonal populations of HRS cells needs to be confirmed by further investigations; and (3) the inability of Roth and

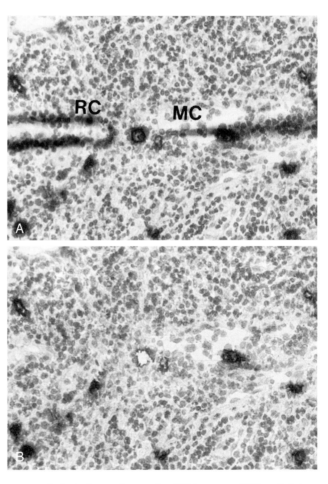

Figure 15–6. Picking of a single CD30-positive HRS cell from a Hodgkin's disease tissue section (×600) before *(A)* and after *(B)* extraction. Note that the cell extraction with the manipulation capillary (MC) did not damage the surrounding cells and tissue. The picked immunostained HRS cell was subsequently transferred to a reception capillary (RC).

Table 15–7. Summary of Analyses of Single L&H and HRS Cells of Hodgkin's Disease for Rearranged Ig and TCR-γ Genes

			Cases with:				
References	Histotype	Total No. of Cases	All Ig-R	Clonal Ig-R	Polyclonal Ig-R	Mixed Polyclonal and Clonal Ig-R	TCR-γ-R
Roth et al, 1994[131]	LPHD	1	0†				0†
Daus et al, 1995[138]	cHD°	12	0†				0†
Küppers et al, 1994[135]	LPHD	1	1	1	0	0	NA‡
	cHD	2	2	2			NA
Delabie et al, 1994[132]	LPHD	4	4	0	4	0	NA
Chan et al, 1996[133]	cHD†	6	3	0	3		NA
Hummel et al, 1995[136]	CD20 + cHD°	12	12	3	6	3	NA
Küppers et al, 1996[140]	cHD°	9	8	8	0		NA
Hummel et al, 1996[137]	CD20 + cHD	10	10	8	2		NA

°Classic types of Hodgkin's disease comprising nodular sclerosis, mixed cellularity, and lymphocyte depletion.
†Includes only nodular sclerosing types of cHD.
‡NA = not analyzed.
LPHD, lymphocyte-predominant Hodgkin's disease; cHD, classic Hodgkin's disease; TCR, T-cell receptor; HRS, Hodgkin and Reed-Sternberg; Ig, immunoglobulin; Ig-R, Ig gene rearrangement; TCR-γ-R, TCR-γ gene rearrangement.

colleagues to demonstrate rearranged Ig genes in isolated HRS cells represents an artifact, probably owing to technical reasons. In addition, the data obtained by the single cell assays make it highly unlikely that the multinuclear RS cells are generated by fusion of different B cells because most of the clonal Ig rearrangements were found to be monoallelic.

RELATION OF HRS CELLS TO NORMAL B-CELL DIFFERENTIATION: IMPLICATIONS FOR HD PATHOGENESIS

In the past, many researchers have convincingly demonstrated that HRS cells in most cases of cHD do not express Ig chains or Ig-specific transcripts. In light of the single cell assay finding that the HRS cells from most cHD cases are B-cell related, two questions arise. First, why is Ig usually not expressed by HRS cells, although these cells have rearranged their Ig genes? And second, does the nonexpression of Ig by HRS cells have an impact on the pathogenesis of cHD?

To answer the first question, the sequences of all available clonal Ig rearrangements demonstrated in HRS cells were analyzed.[135–137, 139–141a] The results of this analysis revealed that in up to 40% of the cases the IgH genes and in 50% the IgL genes contained stop codons, deletions, or frame shifts, rendering the Ig genes nonfunctional in most instances. These genomic alterations in the Ig gene locus appear to be

a highly characteristic feature of the tumor cells in cHD because such alterations were not at all or seldom demonstrable in the clonally rearranged Ig genes of low- and high-grade B-NHL. The second question as to whether the nonexpression of Ig by HRS cells contributes to the pathogenesis of cHD grows in light of the finding that HRS cells of cHD are B-cell derived in most instances. Different experiments have shown that normal B cells are unable to survive if their capacity to express Ig is lost.[142] The pattern of the DNA alterations that could be detected as the reason for the nonexpression of Ig in cHD suggests that these mentioned alterations developed as a result of the mutation process taking place during the germinal center reaction. Therefore, it might well be that the germinal center reaction plays a crucial role in the pathogenesis of cHD as outlined in the schematic representation in Figure 15–7. After entering a germinal center, an antigen-reactive B cell transforms into rapidly proliferating centroblasts. Simultaneously with proliferation and differentiation of the centroblasts toward centrocytes, somatic mutations are introduced into the V region of the Ig gene. Since this mutational process is to a certain extent random, the centrocytes are checked as to whether their mutations have changed the V region gene in a favorable or unfavorable way. Favorable mutations are when they have increased the affinity of the Ig chains toward the antigen that has evoked the germinal center reaction. In the case of favorable mutations, the

Table 15–8. Reinvestigation of Single CD30+ HRS Cells of the Hummel et al Series of cHD with Additional Primer Sets°

Type of Ig Rearrangements in HRS Cells Found in the First Analysis	No. of Cases	Type of Ig Rearrangements in HRS Cells Found in the Reinvestigation	No. of Cases
Clonal†	6	Clonal	6
Polyclonal	6	DNA deterioration	2
		Polyclonal	2
		Clonal (1 × V_{H5}; 1 × V_{κ3}‡)	2

°CDR3 consensus and FW1 family-specific primers.
†Includes the cases with mixed polyclonal and clonal Ig rearrangements in the HRS cells.
‡The same clonal V_{κ3} rearrangement was found in the HRS cells of this cHD case, which was sent to Küppers et al for a parallel analysis.
CDR3, complementarity determining region 3; FW1, framework 1; HRS, Hodgkin and Reed-Sternberg; cHD, classic Hodgkin's disease.

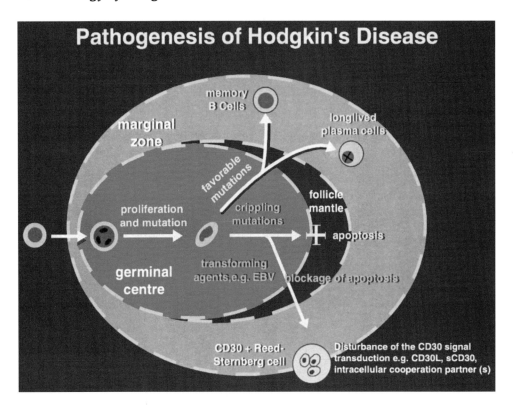

Figure 15–7. Pathogenetic model for Hodgkin's disease.

acentrocytes are selected by their antigen-binding capacity to survive and to differentiate into memory B cells or long-lived plasma cells. If the mutations are unfavorable by causing reduction or loss of the antigen binding affinity or by blocking the expression of Ig chains, the centrocytes are eliminated by apoptosis.[142] As mentioned earlier, the analysis of the rearranged Ig genes in HRS cells revealed high loads of somatic mutations in the V region genes that have often crippled the coding capacity. Thus, HRS cells appear to be derivatives of germinal center cells with unfavorable mutations, meaning that HRS cells should die of apoptosis. Since this is not the case, the apoptotic pathway must be blocked in HRS cells. This prompts the conclusion that factors exist that are responsible for the blockage of the apoptic pathway. The postulated factors include viruses such as EBV, dysfunction of genes that monitor cells for unfavorable genetic alterations and/or mediate apoptosis like the *p53* gene, and others. The CD30 cytokine receptor might also be involved because there are now more and more lines of evidence showing that the CD30 cytokine receptor is able to induce apoptosis.[143–145] It is tempting to speculate that the HRS cells overexpress CD30 because the signal transduction of the CD30 receptor is also blocked. Whatever is correct, the data collected indicate that in most instances cHD represents a clonal proliferation of late, that is, germinal center–derived, B cells that have lost their capacity to express Ig.

CHROMOSOME ABERRATIONS AND HRS CELLS

Conventional cytogenetic studies on cHD have proved to be disappointing. Chromosome aberrant clones were detected in only 100 of the 250 cHD cases studied. The comparison of the aberrant clones of the different cHD cases revealed that some chromosome regions are recurrently affected by structural alterations.[146–148] These include chromosomes 3, 6, 7, 8, 11, 12, 13, and 15. Most of these findings could be confirmed in a recent study by Deerberg-Wittram and associates, and the recurrent breakpoints could be located in 1p13, 7q32/34, 2p16/21, 19p13, 4q25/28, 6q15/21, 12q22/23, and 14q11/32.[149, 149a] The location of the breakpoints in chromosome 14 is of interest because they are the sites of the TCR-α and -δ genes and the Ig heavy genes. In addition, the pericentric regions of the chromosomes 1, 4, 7, 9, 16, 17, 21, and 22 were recurrently affected.

The results mentioned earlier cannot ignore that the most frequent finding in conventional chromosome analysis of cHD is metaphases with a regular karyotype. Conventional cytogenetic techniques, however, do not allow the assignment of the chromosome features to a certain cell type. This causes a problem in cHD because in this disorder normal bystander cells by far exceed HRS cells in number. Therefore, it is not clear as to whether the metaphases with a normal karyotype found in cHD are derived from the normal bystander cells or from the HRS cells themselves. The first successful attempt to overcome this dilemma was made by Teerenhovi and coworkers.[150] These authors combined classic chromosome banding with immunophenotyping of metaphase cells. With this technically taxing and time-consuming method, few cases of cHD could be analyzed. Chromosome aberrations were found only in CD30-positive cells, that is, HRS cells, suggesting that HRS cells represent clonally proliferating and cytogenetically aberrant cells.

Recently, further significant improvements could be introduced for cytogenetic investigations. This was achieved by combining fluorescence immunophenotyping plus fluorescence interphase hybridization called "FICTION."[151]

Using this new FICTION method, numerically aberrant tumor cells can be identified in nonmitotic (interphase) cells. The application of this technique to 30 cHD cases using the CD30 antigen as a label for HRS cells and different centromeric DNA probes specific for the chromosomes 1, 8, 12, 15, 17, X, and Y revealed that (1) all CD30-positive HRS cells in each of the 30 cases contained numerical chromosome aberrations and (2) at least some of the detected aberrations were identical throughout all HRS cells in the same single case.[152] These findings strongly suggest that HRS cells in cHD are derived from one single precursor cell. In one of the 30 cHD cases, 1500 HRS cells could be analyzed, revealing that some chromosome aberrations were constant throughout the total tumor cell population, whereas other chromosomes showed highly variable copy numbers; for example, the copies of chromosome 1 varied between 2 and 8. Similar findings were obtained by conventional cytogenetic analysis, indicating that karyotype type variability is a real phenomenon of cHD. Another important finding of the quoted FICTION study was that the cells that were CD30 negative and thus appeared normal were devoid of chromosome aberrations.

EPSTEIN-BARR VIRUS

In 1987 Weiss and colleagues demonstrated EBV DNA in 4 of 19 cHD cases and provided evidence that the EBV DNA detected was monoclonal in 3 of the 4 EBV-positive cases.[153] When sensitive methods allowing the demonstration of an EBV infection at the single cell level became available, it could be demonstrated that approximately 50% rather than 20% of cHD cases are EBV infected and that the virus is indeed present in the HRS cells themselves.[154, 155] The many analyses performed agree that the frequency of EBV infection of HRS cells is dependent on the histotype with LPHD being negative, or only rarely positive, and with MCHD being positive most frequently.[154, 156–162] (The results of one representative study are shown in Table 15–9.) Although the EBV infection of HRS cells was always found to be accompanied by the expression of LMP1,[154, 158, 159, 161] a protein with transforming and antiapoptotic potential,[163] the virus cannot be the transforming factor in all cHD cases, because it is absent in half of all cases published. Most studies of EBV genomes in cHD, such as the one by Weiss and coworkers[153, 155] and Anagnostopoulos and associates,[164] have

Table 15–9. Frequency of EBV-Infected HRS Cells and EBV Gene Expression in cHD*

Histotype	EBER (%)	LMP1 (%)	EBNA2 (%)
LPHD	14	14	0
NSHD	41	41	0
MCHD	68	68	0

*Data from Hummel et al[154]: The results of other studies showed in part differing frequencies, but all agreed in that EBV infection of HRS cells is most frequently seen in MCHD and least frequently in LPHD.

EBV, Epstein-Barr virus; EBER, EBV-encoded nuclear RNA; LMP1, EBV-encoded latent membrane protein; EBNA2, EBV-encoded nuclear antigen 2; HRS, Hodgkin and Reed-Sternberg; cHD, classic Hodgkin's disease; LPHD, lymphocyte-predominant HD, NSHD, nodular sclerosis HD; MCHD, mixed cellularity HD.

Table 15–10. Presence of EBV in Human Cells as Revealed by EBER In Situ Hybridization

Cell Type	EBV	References
Epithelial Cells		
Hairy leukoplakia	+	Young et al[200]
Nasopharyngeal cancer	+	Zur Hausen et al[201]
10% of gastric cancer	+	Shibata et al[202]
Undifferentiated salivary gland carcinoma°	+	Hamilton-Dutoit et al[203]
Myocytes		
Immunodeficiency related leiomyomas	+	McClain et al[204]
Immunodeficiency related leiomyosarcoma	+	Lee et al[205]
Lymphoid Cells		
Extrafollicular B and T cells	Rarely +†	Niedobitek et al[206]
B-cell lymphoma	Some +‡	Hummel et al[207]
T-cell lymphoma	Some +	Korbjuhn et al[208]
Germinal center B cells	Rarely +‡	Niedobitek et al[206]
Myeloid Cells	–	Stein et al§
Macrophages	–	Anagnostopoulos et al[167]
Interdigitating Cells	–	Anagnostopoulos et al[167]
Follicular Dendritic Cells	–	Anagnostopoulos et al[167]

°Occurring in Greenland.
†Frequent in infectious mononucleosis.
‡Frequent in human immunodeficiency virus infection.
§Unpublished observations.
EBV, Epstein-Barr virus; EBER, EBV-encoded nuclear RNA.

found evidence of monoclonal EBV episomes, using a molecular probe of the virus terminal repeat region.[153, 155, 162, 164–166] This finding is in harmony with the studies of single HRS cells by Küppers and colleagues[135, 140, 141] and Hummel and coworkers,[137, 139] indicating that most cases of cHD represent a clonal B-cell proliferation.

The detection of EBV in HRS cells is important not only because of the possible pathogenic role of this virus in cHD but also in terms of the nature of the HRS cells. Careful investigations, such as that of Anagnostopoulos and associates,[167] of a large range of normal tissues and malignancies for EBV-specific DNA and EBV-encoded gene products (e.g., EBER, LMP1, EBNA2, BHLF1, and ZEBRA) revealed that infection by EBV is restricted to neoplastic epithelial cells, neoplastic muscle cells, and B cells and T cells (Table 15–10). An EBV infection of myeloid cells, macrophages, interdigitating cells, and follicular dendritic cells has not yet been observed.[164] In several investigations by our group (reference 167 and unpublished observations), HRS cells were found to be constantly devoid of epithelial and myogenic markers, such as cytokeratins, desmosomes, epithelial cell–specific molecule HEA125/Ber-EP4, and desmin. The EBV infection of HRS cells strongly favors a derivation of HRS cells from lymphoid cells of either B-cell or T-cell type rather than from other cells present in lymph nodes.

CYTOKINES

HD differs from other malignancies in that in its tumor masses, nonneoplastic and nondysplastic cells of various types exceed the putative tumor cells by a factor of 10 to 1000. In addition, there is often a marked collagen fibrosis that is ringlike in the NSHD type. Clinically, fever and night sweats in patients are frequently present. For a long time it has been assumed that these features and symptoms are caused by an increased and unbalanced secretion of cytokines. There have been numerous attempts to prove this hypothesis, but the studies were hampered by the fact that most cytokines cannot be reliably demonstrated by immunohistologic means. Reasons for this difficulty appear to include lack of specific antibodies suitable for immunohistology and fast diffusion of the usually small cytokine molecules. Most of our knowledge on cytokine production in cHD is based on (1) the demonstration of cytokine transcripts at the single cell level; (2) studies on cHD-derived cell lines,[168] which are not necessarily representative of cHD; and (3) analysis of serum levels.[169] Table 15–11 summarizes the available data on the expression of cytokines by HRS cells and neoplastic cells in monomorphic NHL in tissues. This comparison shows that cHD is indeed associated with an increased expression of cytokines, whereas monomorphic NHLs are not. This supports the view that

cytokines released by HRS cells may indeed be involved in the accumulation of reactive cells in the vicinity of HRS cells. The most interesting cytokine in this respect appears to be interleukin-7 (IL-7),[170] since injection of various cell lines that had been transfected with the IL-7 gene into mice resulted in a prominent admixture of various non-malignant cell types around and in between the neoplastic cell line cells and reduced tumorigenesis. Similar, but apparently less dramatic, effects have also been observed in transfection studies with other cytokines,[171, 172] for example, interferon-γ,[173, 174] tumor necrosis factor,[175, 176] IL-2,[177, 178] and IL-4.[179] Therefore, the expression of IL-7 by HRS cells in synergism with other released cytokines might be involved in the generation of the reactive infiltrate and the low aggressiveness of cHD.[170]

With some limitation, expression of cytokines by HRS cells may also permit a conclusion as to the nature of these cells. In vitro, production of cytokines is in most instances achieved only following exposure to mitogens. Therefore, expression of cytokines by HRS cells in vivo supports the concept that these cells represent transformed, activated cells. The expression of lymphotoxin, IL-9, and interferon-γ

Table 15–11. Cytokine Expression by Neoplastic Cells in Hodgkin's Disease and Monomorphic NHL°

Cytokine	In Situ Hybridization		Immunohistology		References
	Hodgkin's Disease	Monomorphic NHL	Hodgkin's Disease	Monomorphic NHL	
IL-1			20/20	0/86	Hsu & Zhao[209]
IL-1α	0/25 10/19	0/10			Herbst & Foss† Xerri et al[210]
IL-1β	0/20	0/10			Herbst & Foss†
IL-4	0/50	0/5	0/33		Herbst et al[211] Hsu et al[212]
IL-5	16/17				Samoszuk & Nansen[213]
IL-6	81/125	0/20	27/34		Foss et al[214]; Herbst et al‡ Hsu et al[212]
IL-7	24/31	0/14			Foss et al[214]
IL-8	3/33	0/8			Foss et al[215]
IL-9	8/64 6/13	1/10 (ALCL) 2/6 (ALCL) 0/29 (others)			Herbst et al† Merz et al[216] Merz et al[216]
IL-10	15/52	11/17 (ARL)			Herbst et al[211]
LT	26/26	0/8			Foss et al[214]
TNF-α	26/26 10/19 6/8	0/8	3/10 10/10		Foss et al[214] Xerri et al[210] Kretschmer et al[217] Hsu & Hsu[218]
IFN-γ	17/45		14/30		Foss et al† Gerdes et al[219]
CSF-1			13/13		Moreau et al[220]
TGF-β	20/20				Herbst et al†

°Values refer to cytokine expression in tumor cells.
†Unpublished observations.
‡Submitted for publication.
ARL, AIDS-related lymphoma; LT, lymphotoxin; TNF-α, tumor necrosis factor-α; CSF-1, colony-stimulating factor-1; IFN-γ, interferon-γ; TGF-β, transforming growth factor-β; IL, interleukin; NHL, non-Hodgkin's lymphoma; ALCL, anaplastic large cell lymphoma.

in HRS cells fits best to a lymphoid nature of HRS cells because the production of these cytokines appears to be largely confined to activated lymphoid cells.[180]

It is clear that morphologic demonstration of cytokine transcripts is only the first step toward an elucidation of the role of the cytokine network in cHD and that future studies have to address the expression of these molecules at the level of translation, the release of these molecules, and their interaction with receptor molecules. There are controversial data concerning the expression of some cytokines, such as transforming growth factor β and IL-5, the discussion of which is beyond the scope of this chapter.

ONCOGENES AND SUPPRESSOR GENES

PCR studies on the occurrence of rearranged *BCL2* genes in cHD have generated heterogeneous results.[181–186] The *BCL2* rearrangement detected in whole-tissue DNA by some authors might reflect technical artifacts or the presence of bystander cells (found in reactive lymphoid tissue such as tonsils) carrying the *BCL2* rearrangement. Because of the new availability of an efficient single cell assay, the elucidation of the cellular source and the frequency of the *BCL2* rearrangement in cHD is in sight. The mutation and/or expression of other oncogenes, including c-*myc*, c-*jun*, c-*raf*, and N-*ras*, have also been investigated.[2, 7, 187–190] However, so far no characteristic expression or mutation pattern has emerged.

The possible involvement of the *p53* tumor suppressor gene in the pathogenesis of cHD is suggested by the finding of a frequent abnormal accumulation of *p53* in the nuclei of HRS cells in most cases.[183, 191–193] The accumulation of *p53* protein in the HRS cells might be a consequence of *p53* gene mutations and/or other mechanisms including inactivating interactions between the *p53* protein and *p53* binding proteins such as certain viral products or the mouse double-minute 2 oncogene *(MDM2)* gene product. It can generate multiple transcripts giving rise to *MDM2* proteins capable of binding to *p53* molecules and acting as a specific antagonist of *p53* gene activity by concealing its activation domain.[194–196] Data on *p53* gene mutations in cHD are scarce and inconclusive.[130, 193, 197] Furthermore, point mutations of *p53* have been demonstrated in only one of six cHD cell lines.[193] However, there is evidence for an involvement of the *MDM2* gene because its product is overexpressed in the HRS cells in most cases, whereby a coexpression of both *MDM2* and *p53* proved to be common in the same cells.[198] Since the cells of normal lymphoid tissue do not contain immunohistologically detectable amounts of *p53* and/or *MDM2* (with rare exceptions), the overexpression and asymmetric distribution of *p53* and *MDM2* in HRS cells point toward a severely disordered cell cycle in these cells. This conclusion fits in well with the model of cHD pathogenesis described earlier and that is outlined in Figure 15–7. Studies on the single cell level using a reliable cell isolation technique are needed to clarify the presence and frequency of mutations in the *p53* and *MDM2* gene and other suppressor genes, as well as genes regulating and managing DNA repair.

CONCLUSION

The fog surrounding unsettled questions about HD is beginning to dissipate. It is now clear that HD, in spite of common features that include the presence of characteristic dysplastic cells and an abundant reactive cellular infiltrate, is not a single disease with variants, but rather a group of at least two diseases, namely nLPHD and cHD. nLPHD is a uniform lymphoproliferative disorder of B cells showing slow or no progression. What is not yet clear is whether patients with nLPHD benefit from polychemotherapy. It is also not clear as to whether the B-cell-derived dysplastic cells in nLPHD, that is, the L&H or popcorn cells, are monoclonal or polyclonal. Evidence has been provided for both possibilities. In contrast, the classic types of HD are more heterogeneous. This concerns the histology, the clinical course, and the origin of the neoplastic HRS cells. Within cHD, four histotypes can be distinguished: NSHD, MCHD, LDHD, and cLRHD. The distinction of the latter histotype is relevant because it might be confused with nLPHD. The different histotypes vary in their clinical presentation and disease course. All classic types of HD require treatment because otherwise they are fatal. Immunohistologic and molecular biologic studies of cHD at the single cell level strongly suggest that the HRS cells in most cHD cases are monoclonal derivatives of late germinal center B cells, and in a few cases are derivatives of cytotoxic T cells and, although less likely, of NK cells. At least the B-cell-derived HRS cells should die of apoptosis because they are unable to express Ig. As this does not happen, it is likely that a major event in the pathogenesis of B-cell-related cHD is the blockage of the apoptotic pathway. EBV, as well as genes monitoring the human genome for damaged DNA, such as *p53*, might be involved in the postulated hindrance of the apoptotic pathway, leading to the genesis of classic HRS cells. This is a hypothesis that is in harmony with the morphologic and molecular biologic evidence for a disturbance of the mitotic process in classic HRS cells.

Acknowledgment

We thank Joannah Caborn for her editorial contributions during the preparation of this chapter.

REFERENCES

1. Pileri S, Sabattini E, Tazzari PL, et al: Hodgkin's disease: Update of findings. Haematologica 1991; 76:175.
2. Drexler HG: Recent results on the biology of Hodgkin and Reed-Sternberg cells: I. Biopsy material. Leuk Lymphoma 1992; 8:283.
3. Said JS: The immunohistchemistry of Hodgkin's disease. Semin Diagn Pathol 1992; 9:265.
4. Poppema S, Kaleta J, Hepperle B, Visser L: Biology of Hodgkin's disease. Ann Oncol 1992; 3(Suppl 4):5.
5. Drexler HG: Recent results on the biology of Hodgkin and Reed-Sternberg cells: II. Continuous cell lines. Leuk Lymphoma 1993; 9:1.
6. Hsu SM, Waldron JW, Hsu PL, Hough AJ: Cytokines in malignant lymphomas: Review and prospective evaluation. Hum Pathol 1993; 24:1040.
7. Haluska FG, Brufsky AM, Canellos GP: The cellular biology of the Reed-Sternberg cell. Blood 1994; 84:1005.

8. Wolf J, Diehl V: Is Hodgkin's disease an infectious disease? Ann Oncol 1994; 5(Suppl 1):105.

9. Sykes JA, Dmochowski B, Shullenberger CC, Howe CD: Tissue culture studies on human leukemia and malignant lymphoma. Cancer Res 1962; 22:21.

10. Trujillo JM, Drewinko B, Ahearn MJ: The ability of tumor cells of the lymphoreticular system to grow in vitro. Cancer Res 1972; 32:1057.

11. Pretlow TG, Luberoff DE, Hamilton LJ, et al: Pathogenesis of Hodgkin's disease: Separation and culture of different kinds of cells from Hodgkin's disease in a sterile isokinetic gradient of Ficoll in tissue culture medium. Cancer 1973; 31:1120.

12. Boecker WR, Hossfeld DK, Gallmeier WM, Schmidt CG: Clonal growth of Hodgkin's cells. Nature 1975; 258:235.

13. Kaplan HS, Gartner S: Sternberg-Reed giant cells of Hodgkin's disease cultivation in vitro, heterotransplantations, and characterization as neoplastic macrophages. Int J Cancer 1977; 19:511.

14. Diehl V, Kirchner HH, Burrichter H, et al: Characteristics of Hodgkin's disease–derived cell lines. Cancer Treat Rep 1982; 66:615.

15. Schaadt M, Fonatsch C, Kirchner H, Diehl V: Establishment of a malignant Epstein-Barr virus (EBV)-negative cell line from the pleural effusion of a patient with Hodgkin's disease. Blut 1979; 38:185.

16. Schaadt M, Diehl V, Stein H, et al: Two neoplastic cell lines with unique features derived from Hodgkin's disease. Int J Cancer 1980; 26:723.

17. Diehl V, Kirchner HH, Schaadt M, et al: Hodgkin's disease: Establishment and characterization of four in vitro cell lines. J Cancer Res Clin Oncol 1981; 101:111.

18. Jones DB, Scott CS, Wright DH, et al: Phenotypic analysis of an established cell line derived from a patient with Hodgkin's disease (HD). Hematol Oncol 1985; 3:133.

19. Poppema S, De Jong B, Atmosoerodjo J, et al: Morphologic, immunologic, enzymehistochemical, and chromosomal analysis of a cell line derived from Hodgkin's disease. Evidence for a B-cell origin of Reed-Sternberg cells. Cancer 1985; 55:683.

20. Drexler HG, Gaedicke G, Lok MS, et al: Hodgkin's disease–derived cell lines HDLM-2 and L428: Comparison of morphology, immunological, and isoenzyme profiles. Leuk Res 1986; 10:487.

21. Jones DB, Furley AJW, Gerdes J, et al: Phenotypic and genotypic analysis of two cell lines derived from Hodgkin's disease tissue biopsies. In Diehl V, Pfreundschuh M, Loeffler M (eds): New Aspects in the Diagnosis and Treatment of Hodgkin's Disease. Berlin, Springer, 1989, pp 62–66.

22. Drexler HG, Gignac SM, Hoffbrand AV, et al: Characterisation of Hodgkin's disease–derived cell line HDLM-2. In Diehl V, Pfreundschuh M, Loeffler M (eds): New Aspects in the Diagnosis and Treatment of Hodgkin's Disease. Berlin, Springer, 1989, pp 75–82.

23. Naumovski L, Lutz PJ, Bergstrom SK, et al: SUP-HD1: A new Hodgkin's disease–derived cell line with lymphoid features produces interferon-γ. Blood 1989; 74:2733.

24. Poppema S, Visser L, De Jong B, et al: The typical Reed-Sternberg phenotype and Ig gene rearrangement of Hodgkin's disease–derived cell line ZO indicating a B-cell origin. In Diehl V, Pfreundschuh M, Loeffler M (eds): New Aspects in the Diagnosis and Treatment of Hodgkin's Disease. Berlin, Springer, 1989, pp 67–74.

25. Kanzaki T, Kubonishi I, Eguchi T, et al: Establishment of a new Hodgkin's cell line (HD-70) of B-cell origin. Cancer 1992; 69:1034.

26. Kamesaki H, Fukuhara S, Tatsumi E, et al: Cytochemical, immunologic, chromosomal, and molecular genetic analysis of a novel cell line derived from Hodgkin's disease. Blood 1986; 68:285.

27. Schwab U, Stein H, Gerdes J, et al: Production of a monoclonal antibody specific for Hodgkin and Reed-Sternberg cells of Hodgkin's disease and a subset of normal lymphoid cells. Nature 1982; 299:65.

28. Stein H, Gerdes J, Schwab U, et al: Evidence for the detection of the normal counterpart of Hodgkin's and Sternberg-Reed cells. Haematol Oncol 1983; 1:21.

29. Stein H, Gerdes J, Schwarting R, et al: Three new lymphoid activation antigens (A2.12). In McMichael AJ (ed): Leucocyte Typing III: White Cell Differentiation Antigens. Oxford, Oxford University Press, 1987, p 574.

30. Stein H, Gerdes J, Lemke H, et al: Immunohistological classification of Hodgkin's disease and malignant histiocytosis. In Ford RJ, Fuller LM, Hagermeister FB, et al (eds): MD Anderson Clinical Conference on Cancer: New Perspectives in Human Leukemia, Vol 27. New York, Raven Press, 1984, pp 35–47.

31. Bargou RC, Mapara MY, Zugck C, et al: Characterization of a novel Hodgkin cell line, HD-MyZ, with myelomonocytic features mimicking Hodgkin's disease in severe combined immunodeficient mice. J Exp Med 1993; 177:1257.

32. Kanzler H, Hansmann ML, Kapp U, et al: Molecular single cell analysis demonstrates the derivation of a peripheral blood–derived cell line (L1236) from the Hodgkin/Reed-Sternberg cells of a Hodgkin's lymphoma patient. Blood 1996; 87:3429.

33. Lukes RJ, Butler JJ: The pathology and nomenclature of Hodgkin's disease. Cancer Res 1966; 26:1063.

34. Harris NL, Jaffe E, Stein H, et al: A revised European-American classification of lymphoid neoplasms: A proposal from the International Lymphoma Study Group. Blood 1994; 84:1361.

35. Stein H, Gerdes J, Schwab U, et al: Identification of Hodgkin and Sternberg-Reed cells as a unique cell type derived from a newly detected small cell population. Int J Cancer 1982; 30:445.

36. Stein H, Uchanska-Ziegler B, Gerdes J, et al: Hodgkin and Sternberg-Reed cells contain antigens specific to late cells of granulopoiesis. Int J Cancer 1982; 29:283.

37. Pinkus GS, Said JW: Hodgkin's disease, lymphocyte predominance type, nodular: Further evidence for a B-cell derivation. Am J Pathol 1988; 133:211.

38. Mason DY, Banks PM, Chan J, et al: Nodular lymphocyte predominance Hodgkin's disease: A distinct clinico-pathological entity [Editorial]. Am J Surg Pathol 1994; 18:526.

39. Stein H, Hansmann MI, Lennert K, et al: Reed-Sternberg and Hodgkin cells in lymphocyte-predominant Hodgkin's disease of nodular subtype contain J chain. Am J Clin Pathol 1986; 86:292.

40. Regula D, Hoppe R, Weiss L: Nodular and diffuse types of lymphocyte predominance Hodgkin's disease. N Engl J Med 1988; 318:214.

41. Poppema S: Lymphocyte-predominance Hodgkin's disease. Semin Diagn Pathol 1992; 9:257.

42. Ramsay AD, Smith WJ, Isaacson PG: T-cell–rich B-cell lymphoma. Am J Surg Pathol 1988; 12:433.

43. Chittal SM, Brousset P, Voigt JJ, Delsol G: Large B-cell lymphoma rich in T cells and simulating Hodgkin's disease. Histopathology 1991; 19:211.

44. Abdulaziz Z, Mason DY, Stein H, et al: An immunohistological study of the cellular constituents of Hodgkin's disease using a monoclonal antibody panel. Histopathology 1984; 8:1.

45. Poppema S: The nature of the lymphocytes surrounding Reed-Sternberg cells in nodular lymphocyte predominance and in other types of Hodgkin's disease. Am J Pathol 1989; 135:351.

46. Schmidt U, Metz KA, Leder LD: T-cell-rich B-cell lymphoma and lymphocyte-predominant Hodgkin's disease: Two closely related entities? Br J Haematol 1995; 90:398.

47. Stein H, Mason DY, Gerdes J, et al: The expression of the Hodgkin's disease–associated antigen Ki-1 in reactive and neoplastic lymphoid tissue: Evidence that Reed-Sternberg cells and histiocytic malignancies are derived from activated lymphoid cells. Blood 1985; 66:848.

48. Pileri S, Bocchia M, Baroni CD, et al: Anaplastic large cell lymphoma (CD30+/Ki–1+): Results of the prospective clinicopathologic study of 69 cases. Br J Haematol 1994; 86:513.

49. Stein H, Herbst H, Anagnostopoulos I, et al: The nature of Hodgkin and Reed-Sternberg cells, their association with EBV, and their relationship to anaplastic large-cell lymphoma. Ann Oncol 1991; 2(Suppl 2):33.

50. Stein H, Dallenbach F: Diffuse large cell lymphomas of B and T cell type. In Knowles D (ed): Neoplastic Hematopathology. Baltimore, Williams & Wilkins, 1992, pp 675–714.

51. Leoncini L, Del Vecchio MT, Kraft R, et al: Hodgkin's disease and CD30-positive anaplastic large cell lymphomas—a continuous spectrum of malignant disorders: A quantitative morphometric and immunohistologic study. Am J Pathol 1990; 137:1047.

52. Mason DY, Bastard C, Rimokh R, et al: CD30-positive large cell lymphoma ("Ki-1 lymphoma") are associated with a chromosomal translocation involving 5q35. Br J Haematol 1990; 74:161.

53. Bitter MA, Franklin WA, Larson RA, et al: Morphology in Ki-1 (CD30)-positive non-Hodgkin's lymphoma is correlated with clinical features and the presence of a unique chromosomal abnormality t(2;5)(p23;q35) Am J Surg Pathol 1990; 14:305.

54. Rimokh R, Magaud JP, Berger F, et al: A translocation involving a specific breakpoint (q35) on chromosome 5 is characteristic of anaplastic large cell lymphoma ("Ki-1 lymphoma"). Br J Haematol 1989; 71:31.

55. LeBeau MM, Bitter MA, Franklin RA, et al: The t(2;5)(p23;q35): A

recurring chromosomal abnormality in sinsoidal Ki-1+ non-Hodgkin's lymphoma. Blood 1988; 72(Suppl):247.

56. Orscheschek K, Merz H, Hell J, et al: Large cell anaplastic lymphoma-specific translocation (t[2;5][p23;q35]) in Hodgkin's disease: Indication of a common pathogenesis? Lancet 1995; 345:87.

57. Ladyani M, Cavalchire G, Morris SW, et al: Reverse transcriptase polymerase chain reaction for the Ki-1 anaplastic large cell lymphoma–associated t(2;5) translocation in Hodgkin's disease. Am J Pathol 1994; 145:1296.

58. Shioto M, Fujimoto J, Takenaga M, et al: Diagnosis of t(2;5)(p23; q35)-associated Ki-1 lymphoma with immunohistochemistry. Blood 1994; 84:3648.

59. Lucey DR, Shoarer GM: Large cell anaplastic lymphoma-specific translocation in Hodgkin's disease [Letter to the Editor]. Lancet 1995; 345:919.

60. Herbst H, Anagnostopoulos I, Heinze B, et al: ALK gene products in anaplastic large cell lymphomas and Hodgkin's disease. Blood 1995; 86:1694.

61. Delsol G: NPM/ALK-positive B-cell lymphomas and Hodgkin's disease. Session on Anaplastic Large Cell Lymphoma: Controversial Aspects at the Fifth International Lymphoma Study Group Meeting, Hong Kong, April 1995.

62. Jaffe E: NPM/ALK data on anaplastic large cell lymphoma, T-cell lymphoma, and HD. Session on Anaplastic Large Cell Lymphoma: Controversial Aspects at the Fifth International Lymphoma Study Group Meeting, Hong Kong, April 1995.

63. Weiss LM, Lopategui JR, Sun LH, et al: Absence of the t(2;5) in Hodgkin's disease. Blood 1995; 85:2845.

64. Stein H, Hansmann ML, Lennert K, et al: Reed-Sternberg and Hodgkin cells in lymphocyte-predominant Hodgkin's disease of nodular subtype contain J chain. Am J Clin Pathol 1986; 86:292.

65. Chittal SM, Cavariviere P, Schwarting R, et al: Monoclonal antibodies in the diagnosis of Hodgkin's disease. Am J Surg Pathol 1988; 12:9.

66. Nicholas DS, Harris S, Wright DH: Lymphocyte predominance Hodgkin's disease—an immunohistochemical study. Histopathology 1990; 16:157.

67. Schmid C, Sargent C, Isaacson PG: L and H cells of nodular lymphocyte-predominant Hodgkin's disease show immunoglobulin light chain restriction. Am J Pathol 1991; 139:1281.

68. Tesch H, Gorschlüter M, Hasenclever D, et al: Correlations of cytokine levels with clinical parameters in patients with Hodgkin's disease. Ann Haematol 1993; 67S:A124.

69. Schwarting R, Gerdes J, Dürkop H, et al: A new anti-Ki-1 (CD30) monoclonal antibody directed at a formol-resistant epitope. Blood 1989; 74:1678.

70. Kadin ME: Hodgkin's disease: Immunobiology and pathogenesis. *In* Knowles DM (ed): Neoplastic Hematopathology. Baltimore, Williams & Wilkins, 1992, pp 535–554.

71. Ree HJ, Neiman RS, Martin AW, et al: Paraffin-section markers for Reed-Sternberg cells: A comparative study of PNA, Leu-M1, LN-2, and Ber-H2. Cancer 1989; 63:2030.

72. Schienle HW, Stein H, Müller-Ruchholtz W: Neutrophil granulocytic cell antigen defined by a monoclonal antibody: Its distribution within normal hematological and non-hematological tissue. J Clin Pathol 1982; 35:959.

73. Hsu SM, Jaffe ES: Leu-M1 and peanut agglutinin stain the neoplastic cells of Hodgkin's disease. Am J Clin Pathol 1984; 82:29.

74. Pinkus GS, Thomas P, Said JW: Leu-M1—a marker for Reed-Sternberg cells in Hodgkin's disease: An immunoperoxidase study of paraffin-embedded tissues. Am J Pathol 1985; 119:244.

75. Falini B, Flenghi L, Pileri S, et al: PG-M1: A new monoclonal antibody directed against a fixative-restricted epitope on the macrophage-restricted form of the CD68 molecule. Am J Pathol 1993; 142:1359.

76. Backe E, Schwarting R, Gerdes J, et al: Ber-MAC3: New monoclonal antibody that defines human monocyte/macrophage differentiation antigen. J Clin Pathol 1991; 44:936.

77. Strauchen JA, Dimitriu-Bona A: Immunopathology of Hodgkin's disease: Characterization of Reed-Sternberg cells with monoclonal antibodies. Am J Pathol 1986; 123:293.

78. Casey TT, Olson SJ, Cousar JB, Collins RD: Immunophenotypes of Reed-Sternberg cells: A study of 19 cases of Hodgkin's disease in plastic-embedded sections. Blood 1989; 74:2624.

79. Stein H, Gerdes J, Falini B: Phenotypic and genotypic markers in malignant lymphomas: Cellular origin of Hodgkin and Sternberg-Reed cells and implications for the classification of T-cell and B-cell lymphomas. *In* Seifert G, Hübner K, Gustav F (eds): Pathology

80. Hsu PL, Hsu SM: Identification of an M_r 70,000 antigen associated with Reed-Sternberg cells and interdigitating reticulum cells. Cancer Res 1990; 50:350.

81. Dürkop H, Latza U, Hummel M, et al: Molecular cloning and expression of a new member of the nerve growth factor receptor family that is characteristic for Hodgkin's disease. Cell 1992; 68:421.

82. Falini B, Pileri S, Pizzolo G, et al: CD30 (Ki-1) molecule: A new cytokine receptor of the tumor necrosis factor receptor superfamily as a tool for diagnosis and immunotherapy. Blood 1995; 85:1.

83. Andreesen R, Osterholz J, Löhr GW, Bross KJ: A Hodgkin's cell specific antigen is expressed on a subset of auto- and alloactivated T (helper) lymphoblasts. Blood 1984; 63:1299.

84. Andreesen R, Brugger W, Löhr GW, Bross KJ: Human macrophages can express the Hodgkin's cell–associated antigen Ki-1 (CD30). Am J Pathol 1989; 134:187.

85. Sohail D, Simpson RH: Ber-H2 staining of lipoblasts [Letter]. Histopathology 1990; 18:409.

86. Mechtesheimer G, Kruger KH, Born IA, Moller P: Antigenic profile of mammary fibroadenoma and cystosarcoma phyllodes: A study using antibodies to estrogen and progesterone receptors and to a panel of cell surface molecules. Pathol Res Pract 1990; 186:427.

87. Mechtersheimer G, Möller O: Expression of Ki-1 antigen (CD30) in mesenchymal tumors. Cancer 1990; 66:1732.

88. Ito K, Watanabe T, Horie R, et al: High expression of the CD30 molecule in human decidual cells. Am J Pathol 1994; 145:276.

89. Pallesen G, Hamilton-Dutoit SJ: Ki-1 (CD30) antigen is regularly expressed by tumor cells of embryonal carcinoma. Am J Pathol 1988; 133:446.

90. Hansen H, Lemke H, Berdfeldt G, et al: The Hodgkin-associated Ki-1 antigen exists in an intracellular and a membrane-bound form. Biol Chem Hoppe Seyler 1989; 370:409.

91. Rohde D, Hansen H, Hafner M, et al: Cellular localizations and processing of the two molecular forms of the Hodgkin-associated Ki-1 (CD30) antigen: The protein kinase Ki-1/57 occurs in the nucleus. Am J Pathol 1992; 140:473.

92. Catroretti G, Pileri S, Parravicini C, et al: Antigen unmasking on formalin-fixed, paraffin-embedded tissue sections. J Pathol 1993; 171:83.

93. Stamenkovic I, Clark EA, Seed B: A B-lymphocyte activation molecule related to the nerve growth factor receptor and induced by cytokines in carcinomas. EMBO J 1989; 8:1403.

94. Clark EA, Ledbetter JA: Activation of human B cells mediated through two distinct cell surface differentiation antigens, Bp35 and Bp50. Proc Natl Acad Sci U S A 1986; 83:4494.

95. Ledbetter JA, Clark EA, Norris NA, et al: Expression of a functional B-cell receptor CDw40(Bp50) on carcinomas. *In* McMichael AJ (ed): Leukocyte Typing III: White Cell Differentiation Antigens. Oxford, Oxford University Press, 1987, pp 432–435.

96. McLennan ICM, Liu YJ, Oldfield S, et al: The evolution of B cell clones. Curr Top Microbiol Immunol 1990; 159:37.

97. Gruss HJ, Hirschstein D, Wright B, et al: Expression and function of CD40 on Hodgkin and Reed-Sternberg cells and the possible relevance for Hodgkin's disease. Blood 1994; 84:2315.

98. O'Grady, Stewart S, Lowrey J, et al: CD40 expression in Hodgkin's disease. Am J Pathol 1994; 144:21.

99. Knapp W, Dörken B, Gilks WR, et al: (Organizing Committee of the Fourth International Workshop on Human Leucocyte Differentiation Antigens): CD guide. *In* Knapp W, Dörken B, Gilks WR, et al (eds): Leucocyte Typing IV. Oxford, Oxford University Press, 1989, pp 1074–1093.

100. Agnarsson BA, Kadin ME: The immunophenotype of Reed-Sternberg cells: A study of 50 cases of Hodgkin's disease using fixed frozen tissues. Cancer 1989; 63:2083.

101. Chadburn A, Inghirami G, Knowles DM: T-cell activation antigen expression by neoplastic T cells [Abstract 89]. Lab Invest 1990; p 17a.

102. Wieczorek R, Burke JS, Knowles DM: Leu-M1 antigen expression in T-cell neoplasia. Am J Pathol 1985; 121:374.

103. Sheibani K, Battifora H, Burke JS, Rappaport H. Leu-M1 antigen in human neoplasms: An immunohistological study of 400 cases. Am J Surg Pathol 1986; 10:227.

104. Korkolopoulou P, Cordell JL, Jones M, et al: The expression of the B-cell marker mb-1 (CD79a) in Hodgkin's disease. Histopathology 1994; 24:511.

105. Cambier JC, Campbell KS: Membrane immunoglobulin and its accomplices: New lessons from an old receptor. FASEB J 1992; 6:3207.

106. Mason DY, Cordell JL, Tse AGD, et al: The IgM-associated protein mb-1 as a marker of normal and neoplastic B cells. J Immunol 1991; 147:1474.

107. Stein H, Gerdes J, Lemke H, Mason DY: Hodgkin's disease: A neoplasm of activated lymphoid cells of either T-cell or B-cell type. *In* Grignani F, Martelli MF, Mason DY (eds): Monoclonal Antibodies in Haematopathology: Serono Symposia, Vol 26. New York, Raven Press, 1985, pp 265–269.

108. Angel CA, Warford A, Campbell AC, et al: The immunohistology of Hodgkin's disease—Reed-Sternberg cells and their variants. J Pathol 1987; 153:21.

109. Dallenbach FE, Stein H: Expression of T-cell receptor β chain in Reed-Sternberg cells. Lancet 1989; 2:828.

110. Falini B, Stein H, Pileri S, et al: Expression of lymphoid-associated antigens in Hodgkin's disease: An immunohistochemical study on lymph node cytospins using monoclonal antibodies. Histopathology 1987; 11:1229.

111. Cibull ML, Stein H, Gatter KC, Mason DY: The expression of the CD3 antigen in Hodgkin's disease. Histopathology 1989; 15:599.

112. Della Croce DR, Imam A, Brynes RK, et al: Anti-BLA.36 monoclonal antibody shows reactivity with Hodgkin's cells and B lymphocytes in frozen and paraffin-embedded tissues. Hematol Oncol 1991; 9:103.

113. Oudejans JJ, Kummer JA, Jiwa M, et al: Granzyme B expression in Reed-Sternberg cells of Hodgkin's disease. Am J Pathol 1996; 148:233–240.

114. Foss HD, Anagnostopoulos I, Araujo I, et al: Anaplastic large cell lymphoma of T-cell and null-cell phenotype express cytotoxic molecules. Blood 1996; 88:4005.

115. Stein H, Staudinger M, Tolksdorf G, Lennert K: Immunological markers in the differential diagnosis of non-Hodgkin's lymphomas. J Cancer Res Clin Oncol 1981; 101:29.

116. Stein H, Gerdes J, Kirchner H, et al: Immunohistological analysis of Hodgkin and Sternberg-Reed cells: Detection of a new antigen and evidence for selective IgG uptake in absence of B-cell, T-cell, and histiocytic markers. J Cancer Res Clin Oncol 1981; 101:125.

117. Taylor CR: Immunohistological study of lymphoma. Eur J Cancer 1976; 12:61.

118. Kadin M, Stites DP, Levy R, Warnke R: Exogenous immunoglobulin and the macrophage origin of Reed-Sternberg cells in Hodgkin's disease. N Engl J Med 1978; 299:1208.

119. Papadimitriou CS, Stein H, Lennert K: The complexity of immuno-histochemical staining pattern of Hodgkin and Reed-Sternberg cells: Demonstration of immunoglobulin, albumin, anti-alpha₁-chymo-trypsin, and lysozyme. J Cancer 1978; 21:531.

120. Mason DY, Stein H, Naiem M, Abdulaziz Z: Immunohistological analysis of human lymphoid tissue by double immunoenzymatic labelling. J Cancer Res Clin Oncol 1981; 101:13.

121. Lauritzen AP, Pluzek KJ, Kristensen IE, Nielsen HW: Detection of immunoglobulin light-chain mRNA in nodular sclerosing Hodgkin's disease by in situ hybridization with biotinylated oligonucleotide probes compared with immunohistochemical staining with poly- and monoclonal antibodies. Histopathology 1992; 21:353.

122. Ruprai AK, Pringle JH, Angel CA, et al: Localization of immunoglob-ulin light-chain mRNA expression in Hodgkin's disease by in situ bybridization. J Pathol 1991; 164:37.

123. Poppema S, Kaiserlin E, Lennert K: Nodular paragranuloma and progressively transformed germinal centers. Virchows Arch B Cell Pathol 1979; 31:211.

124. Hell K, Pringle JH, Hansmann ML, et al: Demonstration of light chain mRNA in Hodgkin's disease. J Pathol 1993; 171:137.

125. Stoler MH, Nichols GE, Symbula Weiss LM: Lymphocyte-predominance Hodgkin's disease—evidence for a kappa light chain–restricted monotypic B-cell neoplasm. Am J Pathol 1995; 146:812.

126. Weiss LM, Strickler JG, Hu E, et al: Immunoglobulin gene rearrangements in Hodgkin's disease. Hum Pathol 1986; 17:1009.

127. Herbst H, Tippelmann G, Anagnostopoulos I, et al: Immunoglobulin and T-cell receptor gene rearrangements in Hodgkin's disease and Ki-1 positive anaplastic large cell lymphoma: Dissociation between phenotype and genotype. Leuk Res 1989; 13:103.

128. Tamaru J, Hummel M, Zemlin M, et al: Hodgkin's disease with a B-cell phenotype often shows a VDJ rearrangement and somatic mutations in the V_H genes. Blood 1994; 84:708.

129. Knowles DM, Neri A, Pelicci PG, et al: Immunoglobulin and T-cell receptor beta-chain gene rearrangement analysis of Hodgkin's disease: Implications for lineage determination and differential diagnosis. Proc Natl Acad Sci U S A 1986; 83:7942.

130. Trümper LH, Brady G, Bagg A, et al: Single-cell analysis of Hodgkin and Reed-Sternberg cells: Molecular heterogeneity of gene expression and p53 mutation. Blood 1993; 81:3097.

131. Roth J, Daus H, Trümper L, et al: Detection of immunoglobulin heavy-chain gene rearrangement at the single-cell level in malignant lymphomas: No rearrangement is found in Hodgkin and Reed-Sternberg cells. Int J Cancer 1994; 57:1.

132. Delabie J, Tierens A, Wu G, et al: Lymphocyte-predominance Hodgkin's disease: Lineage and clonality determination using single-cell assay. Blood 1994; 84:3291.

133. Chan WC, Delabie J: Single-cell analysis of H/RS cells. Ann Oncol 1996; 7(Suppl 4):41.

134. Küppers R, Zhao M, Hansmann ML, Rajewski K: Tracing B-cell development in human germinal centres by molecular analysis of single cells picked from histological sections. EMBO J 1993; 12:4955.

135. Küppers R, Rajewsky K, Zhao M, et al: Hodgkin's disease: Hodgkin and Reed-Sternberg cells picked from histological sections show clonal immunoglobulin gene rearrangements and appear to be derived from B cells at various stages of development. Proc Natl Acad Sci U S A 1994; 91:10962.

136. Hummel M, Ziemann K, Lammert H, et al: Hodgkin's disease with monoclonal and polyclonal populations of Reed-Sternberg cells. N Engl J Med 1995; 333:901.

137. Hummel M, Marafioti T, Ziemann K, Stein H: Ig rearrangements in isolated Reed-Sternberg cells: Conclusions from four different studies. Ann Oncol 1996; 7(Suppl 4):31.

138. Daus H, Trümper L, Roth J, et al: Hodgkin and Reed-Sternberg cells do not carry T-cell receptor γ gene rearrangements: Evidence from single-cell polymerase chain reaction examination. Blood 1995; 85:1590.

139. Hummel M, Marafioti T, Stein H: Response to the Letter to the Editor. N Engl J Med 1996; 334:405.

140. Küppers R, Kanzler H, Hansmann M-L, Rajewsky K: Single-cell analysis of Hodgkin/Reed-Sternberg cells. Ann Oncol 1996; 7(Suppl 4):27.

141. Küppers R, Kanzler H, Hansmann M-L, Rajewsky K: Letter to the Editor. N Engl J Med 1996; 334:404.

141a. Kanzler H, Küppers R, Hansmann M-L, et al: Hodgkin and Reed-Sternberg cells in Hodgkin's disease represent the outgrowth of a dominant tumor clone derived from (crippled) germinal center B cells. J Exp Med 1996; 184:1.

142. Rajewsky K: Clonal selection and learning in the antibody system. Nature 1996; 381:751.

143. Gruss HJ, Boiani N, Williams DE, et al: Pleiotropic effects of the CD30 ligand on CD30-expressing cells and lymphoma cell lines. Blood 1994; 83:2045.

144. Smith CA, Gruss HJ, Davis T, Anderson D, et al: CD30 antigen, a marker for Hodgkin's lymphoma, is a receptor whose ligand defines an emerging family of cytokines with homology to TNF. Cell 1993; 73:1349.

145. Amakawa R, Hakem A, Kundig TM, et al: Impaired negative selection of T cells in Hodgkin's disease antigen CD30-deficient mice. Cell 1996; 84:551.

146. Fonatsch C, Diehl V, Schaadt M, et al: Cytogenetic investigations in Hodgkin's disease: I. Involvement of specific chromosomes in marker formation. Cancer Genet Cytogenet 1986; 20:39.

147. Döhner H, Bloomfield CD, Frizzera G, Arthur DC: Recurring chromosome abnormalities in Hodgkin's disease. Blood 1989; 74:82a.

148. Tilly H, Bastard C, Delastre T, et al: Cytogenetic studies in untreated Hodgkin's disease. Blood 1991; 77:1298.

149. Schlegelberger B, Weber-Matthiesen K, Himmler A, et al: Cytogenetic findings and results of combined immunophenotyping and karyotyping in Hodgkin's disease. Leukemia 1994; 8:72.

149a. Deerberg-Wittram J, Weber-Matthiesen K, Schlegelberger B: Cytogenetics and molecular cytogenetics in Hodgkin's disease. Ann Oncol 1996; 7(Suppl 4):49.

150. Teerenhovi L, Lindholm C, Pakkala A, et al: Unique display of a pathologic karyotype in Hodgkin's disease by Reed-Sternberg cells. Cancer Genet Cytogenet 1988; 34:305.

151. Weber-Matthiesen K, Winkemann M, Muller-Hermelink A, et al: Simultaneous fluorescence immunophenotyping and interphase cytogenetics: A contribution to the characterization of tumor cells. J Histochem Cytochem 1992; 40:171.

152. Weber-Matthiesen K, Deerberg J, Poetsch M, et al: Numerical chromosome aberrations are present within the CD30-positive Hodgkin and Reed-Sternberg cells in 100% of analyzed cases of Hodgkin's disease. Blood 1995; 86:1464.

153. Weiss LM, Strickler JG, Warnke RA, et al: Epstein-Barr viral DNA in tissues of Hodgkin's disease. Am J Pathol 1987; 129:86.

154. Hummel M, Anagnostopoulos I, Dallenbach F, et al: EBV infection patterns in Hodgkin's disease and normal lymphoid tissue: Expression and cellular localization of EBV gene products. Br J Haematol 1992; 82:689.

155. Weiss LM, Movahed AM, Warnke RA, Sklar J: Detection of Epstein-Barr viral genomes in Reed-Sternberg cells of Hodgkin's disease. N Engl J Med 1989; 320:502.

156. Herbst H, Niedobitek G, Kneba M, et al: High incidence of Epstein-Barr virus genomes in Hodgkin's disease. Am J Pathol 1990; 137:13.

157. Brousset P, Chittal S, Schlaifer D, et al: Detection of Epstein-Barr virus messenger RNA in Reed-Sternberg cells of Hodgkin's disease by in situ hybridization with biotinylated probes on specially processed modified acetone methyl benzoate xylene (ModAMeX) sections. Blood 1991; 77:1871.

158. Herbst H, Dallenbach F, Hummel M, et al: Epstein-Barr virus latent membrane protein expression in Hodgkin- and Reed-Sternberg cells. Proc Natl Acad Sci U S A 1991; 88:4766.

159. Pallesen G, Hamilton-Dutoit SJ, Rowe M, Young LS: Expression of Epstein-Barr virus latent gene products in tumor cells of Hodgkin's disease. Lancet 1991; 337:320.

160. Weiss LM, Chen YY, Lui XF, Shibata D: Epstein-Barr virus and Hodgkin's disease: A correlative in situ hybridization and polymerase chain reaction study. Am J Pathol 1991; 139:1259.

161. Delsol G, Brousset P, Chittal S, Rigal-Huguet F: Correlation of the expression of Epstein-Barr virus latent membrane protein and in situ hybridization with biotinylated BamHI-W probes in Hodgkin's disease. Am J Pathol 1992; 140:247.

162. Gulley ML, Eagan OA, Quintanilla-Martinez L, et al: Epstein-Barr virus is abundant and monoclonal in the Reed-Sternberg cells of Hodgkin's disease: Association with mixed cellularity subtype and Hispanic American ethnicity. Blood 1994; 83:1595.

163. Henderson S, Rowe M, Croom-Carter D, et al: Induction of bcl-2 expression by Epstein-Barr virus latent membrane protein 1 protects infected B cells from programmed cell death. Cell 1991; 65:1107.

164. Anagnostopoulos I, Herbst H, Niedobitek G, Stein H: Demonstration of monoclonal EBV genomes in Hodgkin's disease and Ki-1-positive anaplastic large cell lymphoma by combined Southern and in situ hybridization. Blood 1989; 74:810.

165. Uccini S, Monardo F, Stoppacciaro A, et al: High frequency of Epstein-Barr virus genome detection in Hodgkin's disease of HIV-positive patients. Int J Cancer 1990; 46:581.

166. Boiocchi M, Dolcetti R, De Re V, et al: Demonstration of a unique Epstein-Barr virus–positive cellular clone in metachronous multiple localizations of Hodgkin's disease. Am J Pathol 1993; 142:33.

167. Anagnostopoulos I, Hummel M, Kreschel C, Stein H: Morphology, immunophenotype, and distribution of latently and/or productively Epstein-Barr virus–infected cells in acute infectious mononucleosis: Implications for the interindividual infection route of Epstein-Barr virus. Blood 1995; 85:744.

168. Gruss H-J, Brach MA, Bonifer R, Mertelsmann RH: Expression of cytokine genes, cytokine receptor genes, and transcription factors in cultured Hodgkin and Reed-Sternberg cells. Cancer Res 1992; 52:3353.

169. Trümper L, Jung W, Dahl G, et al: Interleukin-7, interleukin-8, soluble TNF receptor, and p53 protein levels are elevated in the serum of patients with Hodgkin's disease. Ann Oncol 1994; 5(Suppl 1):93.

170. Foss HD, Hummel M, Gottstein S, et al: Frequent expression of IL-7 gene transcripts in tumor cells of classical Hodgkin's disease. Am J Pathol 1995; 146:33.

171. Aoki T, Tashiro K, Miyatake S, et al: Expression of murine interleukin 7 in a murine glioma cell line results in reduced tumorgenicity in vivo. Proc Natl Acad Sci U S A 1992; 89:3850.

172. Hock H, Dorsch M, Diamantstein T, Blankenstein T: Interleukin 7 induces CD4+ T cell–dependent tumor rejection. J Exp Med 1991; 174:1291.

173. Watanabe Y, Kuribayashi K, Miyatake S, et al: Exogenous expression of mouse IFN gamma cDNA in mouse neuroblastoma C1300 cells results in reduced tumorigenicity by augmented anti-tumor immunity. Proc Natl Acad Sci U S A 1989; 86:9456.

174. Gansbacher B, Bannerji R, Daniels B, et al: Retroviral vector-mediated gene transfer into tumor cells generates potent and long lasting anti-tumor immunity. J Exp Cancer Res Med 1990; 50:7820.

175. Asher AL, Mule JJ, Kasid A, et al: Evidence for a paracrine immune effect of tumor necrosis factor against tumors. Immunology 1991; 146:3227.

176. Blankenstein T, Qin Z, Uberla K, et al: Tumor suppression after tumor cell–targeted tumor necrosis factor a gene transfer. J Exp Med 1991; 173:1047.

177. Gansbacher B, Zier K, Daniels B, et al: Interleukin 2 gene transfer into tumor cells abrogates tumorigenicity and induces protective immunity. J Exp Med 1990; 172:1217.

178. Levitsky JW, Simons H, Vogelstein B, Frost P: Interleukin 2 production by tumor cell bypasses T helper function in the generation of an antitumor response. Cell 1990; 60:397.

179. Tepper RI, Pattengale PK, Leder P: Murine interleukin 4 displays potent anti-tumor activity in vivo. Cell 1989; 57:503.

180. Paul NL, Ruddle NH: Lymphotoxin. Am Rev Immunol 1988; 6:407.

181. Stetler-Stevenson M, Crush-Stanton S, Cossman J: Involvement of the bcl-2 gene in Hodgkin's disease. J Natl Cancer Inst 1990; 82:855.

182. Reid AH, Cunningham RE, Frizzera G, O'Leary TJ: Bcl-2 rearrangement in Hodgkin's disease: Results of polymerase chain reaction, flow cytometry, and sequencing on formalin-fixed, paraffin-embedded tissue. Am J Pathol 1993; 142:395.

183. Gupta RK, Whelan JS, Lister TA, et al: Direct-sequence analysis of the t(14;18) chromosomal translocation in Hodgkin's disease. Blood 1992; 79:2084.

184. Louie CD, Kant JA, Brooks JJ, Reed JC: Absence of t(14;18) major and minor breakpoints and of bcl-2 protein over-production in Reed-Sternberg cells of Hodgkin's disease. Am J Pathol 1991; 139:1231.

185. Athan E, Chadburn A, Knowles DM: The bcl-2 gene translocation is undetectable in Hodgkin's disease by Southern blot hybridization and polymerase chain reaction. Am J Pathol 1992; 141:193.

186. Said JW, Sassoon AF, Shintaku IP, et al: Absence of bcl-2 major breakpoint region and JH gene rearrangement in lymphocyte-predominance Hodgkin's disease: Results of Southern blot analysis and polymerase chain reaction. Am J Pathol 1991; 138:261.

187. Sklar M, Kitchingham G: Isolation of activated *ras* transforming genes from two patients with Hodgkin's disease. Int J Radiat Oncol Biol Phys 1985; 11:49.

188. Mitani S, Sugawara I, Shiku H, Mori S: Expression of c-*myc* oncogene product and *ras* family oncogene products in various human malignant lymphomas defined by immunohistochemical techniques. Cancer 1988; 62:2085.

189. Steenvoorden AC, Janssen JW, Drexler HD, et al: *Ras* mutations in Hodgkin's disease. Leukemia 1988; 2:325.

190. Jucker M, Schaadt M, Diehl V, et al: Heterogeneous expression of proto-oncogenes in Hodgkin's disease–derived cell lines. Hematol Oncol 1990; 8:191.

191. Doglioni C, Pelosio P, Mombello A, et al: Immunohistochemical evidence of abnormal expression of the antioncogene-encoded p53 phosphoprotein in Hodgkin's disease and CD30+ anaplastic lymphomas. Hematol Pathol 1991; 5:67.

192. Doussis IA, Pezzella F, Lane DP, et al: An immunocytochemical study of p53 and bcl-2 protein expression in Hodgkin's disease. Am J Clin Pathol 1993; 99:663.

193. Gupta RK, Patel K, Bodmer WF, Bodmer JG: Mutation of p53 in primary biopsy material and cell lines from Hodgkin's disease. Proc Natl Acad Sci U S A 1993; 90:2817.

194. Oliner JD: Discerning the function of p53 by examining its molecular interactions. Bioessays 1993; 15:703.

195. Zauberman A, Barak Y, Ragimov N, et al: Sequence-specific DNA binding by p53: Identification of target sites and lack of binding to p53-MDM2 complexes. EMBO J 1993; 12:2799.

196. Haines DS, Landers JE, Engle LJ, George DL: Physical and functional interaction between wild-type p53 and mdm2 proteins. Mol Cell Biol 1994; 14:1171.

197. Inghirami G, Macri L, Rosati S, et al: The Reed-Sternberg cells of Hodgkin's disease are clonal. Proc Natl Acad Sci U S A 1994; 91: 9842.

198. Chilosi M, Doglioni C, Menestrina F, et al: Abnormal expression of the p53-binding protein MDM2 in Hodgkin's disease. Blood 1994; 84:4295.

199. Pizzolo G, Chilosi M, Semenzato G, et al: Immunohistological analysis of Tac antigen expression in tissues involved in Hodgkin's disease. Br J Cancer 1984; 50:415.

200. Young IS, Lau R, Rowe M, et al: Differentiation-associated expression of the Epstein-Barr virus BZLF1 transactivator protein in oral hairy leukoplakia. J Virol 1991; 65:2868.
201. Zur Hausen H, Schulte-Holthausen H, Klein G, et al: EBV DNA in biopsies of Burkitt tumours and anaplastic carcinomas of the nasopharynx. Nature 1970; 228:1056.
202. Shibata D, Weiss LM: Epstein-Barr virus–associated gastric adenocarcinoma. Am J Pathol 1992; 140:769.
203. Hamilton-Dutoit SJ, Hamilton-Therkildsen M, Nielsen NH, et al: Undifferentiated carcinoma of the salivary gland in Greenland Eskimos: A demonstration of Epstein-Barr virus DNA by in situ nucleic acid hybridization. Hum Pathol 1991; 22:811.
204. McClain KL, Leach CT, Jenson HB, et al: Association of Epstein-Barr virus with leiomyosarcomas in children with AIDS. N Engl J Med 1995; 332:12.
205. Lee ES, Locker J, Nalesnik M, et al: The association of Epstein-Barr virus with smooth muscle tumors occurring after organ transplantation. N Engl J Med 1995; 332:19.
206. Niedobitek G, Herbst H, Young LS, et al: Pattern of Epstein-Barr virus infection in non-neoplastic lymphoid tissue. Blood 1992; 79:2520.
207. Hummel M, Anagnostopoulos I, Korbjuhn P, Stein H: Epstein-Barr virus in B-cell non-Hodgkin's lymphomas: Unexpected infection patterns and different infection incidence in low- and high-grade types. J Pathol 1995; 175:263.
208. Korbjuhn P, Anagnostopoulous I, Hummel M, et al: Frequent latent Epstein-Barr virus infection of neoplastic T cells and bystander B cells in HIV-negative European peripheral pleomorphic T-cell lymphomas. Blood 1993; 82:217.
209. Hsu S-M, Zhao X: Expression of interleukin 1 in Reed-Sternberg cells and neoplastic cells from true histiocytic malignancies. Am J Pathol 1986; 125:221.
210. Xerri L, Birg F, Guigou V, et al: In situ expression of the IL-1-α and TNF-α genes by Reed-Sternberg cells in Hodgkin's disease. Int J Cancer 1992; 50:689.
211. Herbst H, Foss HD, Samol J, et al: Frequent expression of interleukin 10 by Epstein-Barr virus–harboring tumor cells of Hodgkin's disease. Blood 1996; 87:2918.
212. Hsu SM, Xie SS, Hsu PL, Waldron JA: Interleukin 6 but not interleukin 4 is expressed by Reed-Sternberg cells in Hodgkin's disease with or without histologic features of Castleman's disease. Am J Pathol 1992; 141:129.
213. Samoszuk M, Nansen L: Detection of interleukin 4 messenger RNA in Reed-Sternberg cells of Hodgkin's disease with eosinophilia. Blood 1990; 75:13.
214. Foss HD, Herbst H, Oelman E, et al: Lymphotoxin, tumour necrosis factor, and interleukin-6 gene transcripts are present in Hodgkin and Reed-Sternberg cells of most Hodgkin's disease cases. Br J Haematol 1993; 84:627.
215. Foss HD, Herbst H, Gottstein S, et al: Interleukin 8 in Hodgkin's disease: Preferential expression by reactive cells and association with neutrophil density. Blood 1996; 148:1229.
216. Merz H, Housiau FA, Orscheschek K, et al: Interleukin-9 expression in human malignant lymphomas: Unique association with Hodgkin's disease and large cell anaplastic lymphoma. Blood 1991; 78:1311.
217. Kretschmer C, Jones DB, Morrison K, et al: Tumor necrosis factor-α and lymphotoxin production in Hodgkin's disease. Am J Pathol 1990; 137:341.
218. Hsu PL, Hsu SM: Production of tumor necrosis factor-α and lymphotoxin by cells of Hodgkin's neoplastic cell lines HDLM-1 and KM-H2. Am J Pathol 1989; 135:735.
219. Gerdes J, Kretschmer C, Zahn G, et al: Immunoenzymatic assessment of interferon-γ in Hodgkin and Sternberg-Reed cells. Cytokine 1990; 2:307.
220. Moreau A, Praloran V, Berrada L, et al: Immunohistochemical detection of cells positive for colony-stimulating factor 1 in lymph nodes from reactive lymphadenitis and Hodgkin's disease. Leukemia 1992; 6:126.

Sixteen

Hodgkin's Disease

Saul A. Rosenberg
George P. Canellos

Clinical Aspects

Hodgkin's disease (HD) has been a fascinating challenge for physicians and investigators since its recognition during the nineteenth century. As the disease became recognized, histologically and clinically, characteristics of an infection or inflammation and also of a neoplasm have long been known. Although it is now widely accepted that HD belongs in the general disease category of "malignant lymphomas," it is considered unique among the neoplasms derived from lymphoid tissues.

Some of the most fascinating, often controversial, characteristics of HD are described in other chapters of this book. These include the epidemiology, genetics, histopathology, immunology, biology, and theories of etiology and pathogenesis of the disease. These important subjects are not covered in this chapter. Other chapters present in detail the diagnostic methods used to identify the extent of the disease and the principles of radiation therapy and chemotherapy in treating HD.

This chapter describes the major clinical characteristics of HD, including the usual and the occasional manifestations of the disease. However, the spectrum of the clinical picture of HD is great, and a textbook chapter cannot include all possible clinical manifestations found in the literature.[1]

In addition, the modern therapy of HD has greatly influenced its clinical course and prognosis. The natural history of HD is almost never seen in modern medical practice. This disease, almost always fatal if untreated and before the time of currently available therapies, is now curable in most patients throughout the world.[2]

CLINICAL SIGNS AND SYMPTOMS

HD is diagnosed in approximately 7500 new patients per year in the United States. Population-based registries indicate an age distribution somewhat different from the experience at large referral centers or groups. At Stanford University Medical Center, the age and sex distribution of more than 2000 patients treated at the institution over a 30-year period are shown in Figure 16–1. The median age is 27.0 years, and the male to female sex ratio is 1.4:1.

HD presents as an illness in two general forms: one that might be called overt and the other, much more uncommon, occult. Even in patients who present with overt HD, the presenting signs and symptoms may be relatively nonspecific, often suggesting an infection rather than a neoplasm. Only after their persistence and progression for weeks to months are these symptoms recognized as consistent with HD.

The most characteristic clinical presentation of HD is a young adult discovering an asymptomatic lymph gland swelling. The enlarged gland, which is usually nontender, occurs most frequently in the neck, often in the supraclavicular fossa, but it may also be discovered in the mid or high neck or in the axilla. Less often, the lymphadenopathy is initially noticed in the ilioinguinal-femoral region. These abnormal glandular enlargements may not be noticed by the patient or their significance appreciated and may be discovered on a routine physical examination.

Another common presentation of the illness is the discovery of an anterior mediastinal mass on a routine chest radiographic examination. The mediastinal mass may be quite large without producing local symptoms. Less commonly, an intrathoracic presentation of HD may be discovered after the symptoms of substernal chest pain, cough, or shortness of breath. Rarely, the intrathoracic HD may be so large and invasive that it results in effusions of the pericardium or the pleura. Occasionally, a parasternal mass may be evident to the patient or physician from involvement of an internal mammary lymph node and invasion of the chest wall. The syndrome of superior vena caval syndrome can be seen in patients with intrathoracic HD but is more common in patients with one of the non-Hodgkin's lymphomas or in carcinoma of the lung.

A significant proportion of patients with undiscovered HD develop systemic symptoms before or along with the discovery of lymphadenopathy. The characteristic symptoms of HD are fever, night sweats, pruritus, fatigue, and weight loss. None of these are specific for HD, but when they are persistent, severe, and otherwise unexplained, they should always suggest the diagnosis of HD that might be overt or occult.

The fever of HD, much like that of an infection, appears or is more noticeable in the evening and is usually continuous, becoming more severe with time. Night sweats are usually associated with the fever or may be present without a recorded temperature elevation. Sometimes the

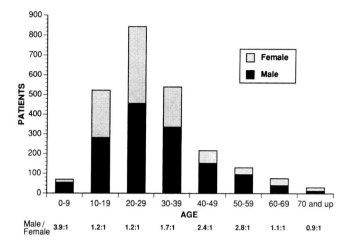

Figure 16–1. Age and sex distribution of 2424 patients with Hodgkin's disease at Stanford University Medical Center, 1960 to 1993. The male/female sex ratio is shown for each age group.

night sweats are brought about by the patient's using antipyretics for fever or malaise. In their mildest form, night sweats may be hardly noticed, with a slight increase in perspiration of the head and/or neck. When they are severe, patients may become soaked with perspiration, requiring a change of bedclothes and linens.

Much has been written about the intermittent or cyclic fever of HD as characteristic of the disease. This type of fever, which is not common, recurs at variable intervals of several days to many weeks and may build to a peak over several days, last 1 to 2 weeks, and then wane. This is the so-called Pel-Ebstein fever, which may have been described by other authors as well.

The pruritus of HD, although not specific for the disease, can be a severe symptom of the disease, often antedating the disease recognition for months to 1 or more years. Although the itching may start in a local area, if caused by HD, it becomes generalized and may result in severe excoriations, hyperpigmentation, and other secondary changes in the skin if the HD is not recognized and successfully treated.

Patients with undiscovered HD may also complain of fatigue and anorexia as symptoms of the disease. These are usually mild at the onset and do not often progress to significant disability or weight loss unless other systemic and local symptoms are also present. In patients with the occult form of the disease, systemic symptoms may predominate, without explanation, even after detailed medical investigation.

An uncommon presenting symptom of HD is pain. A few patients have lymphadenopathy that is painful and tender, especially with their initial enlargement. As a general rule, painful and tender lymphadenopathy is more suggestive of an infectious disease process than HD. Enlarged lymph glands due to HD may compress sensitive structures within the chest, in the neck, and especially in the paravertebral regions. Nerve roots may be impinged on, producing severe pain and radicular symptoms and signs. When HD involves osseous sites, pain is common. Although this a rare presenting manifestation, the vertebrae, pelvis, and sternum are most frequently involved.

A rare but fascinating and unexplained cause of pain in HD, and occasionally a presenting symptom, is pain induced

by alcohol ingestion. This pain is characteristic in that it is severe, occurring within a few minutes of the ingestion of even a small amount of alcohol, and it localizes to a site of HD involvement. This occurs more often at a site of osseous involvement but also may occur at a site of lymphadenopathy. Sometimes this alcohol-induced pain calls attention to a site of disease not detected by ordinary diagnostic studies. Patients may suffer so severely from this alcohol-induced pain that they fall to the floor from the dinner table after drinking a sip of wine.

Pain resulting from retroperitoneal lymphadenopathy is quite characteristic. The discomfort, often felt in the paravertebral or flank regions, is greatest when the patient is supine with the legs extended. In contrast to musculoskeletal causes for back pain, patients with retroperitoneal adenopathy prefer to be sitting or standing rather than lying in bed.

There are many uncommon presentations of HD. Some of these clinical problems occur more frequently as this disease progresses, or with recurrence after unsuccessful initial therapy; these presentations are described in more detail subsequently. These include signs and symptoms secondary to anemia or thrombocytopenia or infections secondary to neutropenia and immunosuppression. Patients may present with abdominal swelling secondary to hepatic or splenic enlargement or, rarely, ascites. Even more rare is a presentation with jaundice, usually obstructive in character.

Patients may present with neurologic deficits due to nerve root compression and occasionally as a result of epidural spinal cord compression. Intracranial presentations are extremely rare, although paraneoplastic neurologic syndromes are well known and sometimes are a presenting problem. Other paraneoplastic presentations, such as the nephrotic syndrome and idiopathic thrombocytopenia purpura (ITP), are detailed in other chapters.

Virtually all patients with HD have occult disease beyond that which is initially discovered, even with the most sensitive investigations. Rare patients, however, have an occult form of HD that is difficult to diagnose even if the patients are exhaustively studied. These patients tend to be older and have the poorer prognostic histologic subtypes (mixed cellularity or lymphocyte depletion). These patients may experience prolonged systemic symptoms, weight loss, and liver and/or bone marrow dysfunction and have minimal or no significant lymphadenopathy. If a lymphogram is obtained, occult retroperitoneal HD may be recognized or suspected. Liver or bone marrow involvement may produce these problems but be difficult to document with the usual needle biopsy procedures. Diagnostic laparotomy and splenectomy may be necessary to reveal the cause of the clinical problems, and occasionally only an autopsy reveals the occult HD.

PATTERNS OF DISEASE AT PRESENTATION

The nature of HD, whether a systemic disease at presentation, such as the leukemias, or unifocal in its clinical onset, such as in solid tumors, has been a subject of debate. Radiation therapists, such as Rene Gilbert, Vera Peters, and Henry Kaplan, believed the disease started in a single site, usually a lymph node, and clinically progressed to adjacent lymphoid tissues before it became disseminated to distant, nonadjacent sites and tissues. Others believed the disease was usually disseminated and unpredictable in its distribution from the onset.

As patients were evaluated more completely, with improved diagnostic methods, such as lower extremity lymphography and exploratory laparotomy with splenectomy, data supported the view that HD was usually unicentric in its origin and progressed in an orderly, predictable manner.[3] This appeared to be the case in most patients in the younger age groups and with the favorable histologic subtypes.

There are also patterns of HD at presentation that are relatively common and have important therapeutic implications, especially when radiation therapy is to be the treatment of choice.[1] It is rare, for example, for HD to be evident in the neck and also in the lower abdomen or groin regions without disease in the upper abdomen. It is unusual to have HD in bilateral axillary regions without having the disease evident in the low neck regions as well. It is extremely unusual to have HD involvement of the liver or bone marrow without having disease in the spleen, although the splenic involvement might require its removal to be demonstrated. It is unusual to have HD involve the lung at presentation without having the disease demonstrable in the intrathoracic lymph nodes, usually on the ipsilateral side.

There are patients who present with a clinical pattern of disease combining HD in the low supraclavicular lymph nodes, perhaps more often on the left than on the right side, with demonstrable disease in the upper abdomen, the lymph nodes, and/or the spleen without evident intrathoracic HD. If one accepts the theory that HD spreads or has patterns of initial involvement explained by contiguity along lymphatic channels, then one has to accept that the disease can spread via the thoracic duct, possibly in either direction, without clinical involvement of the mediastinum. The opposite, or "reciprocal," is also true. Patients may present with modest or extensive HD in the chest, usually in the anterior mediastinum, with no evident disease in the neck or axillae, and a low risk of clinical or occult disease in the abdomen.

After primary management, sites and patterns of disease at recurrence are also relatively predictable. This is especially true after initial treatment with radiation therapy and if the time after initial treatment is relatively brief. Recurrences, which might best be described as or called "extensions of new disease," are usually in unirradiated sites adjacent to the initial treatment fields. This may be in lymphoid tissues or extranodal sites, such as the lung or bone, which are connected by lymphatic channels. Recurrences after initial chemotherapy management, however, are more often true recurrences within sites of initial involvement, often those that were initially bulky or most significant in their size.

Figure 16–2 illustrates the most common patterns of disease documented in 100 consecutive patients at Stanford, at a time when lymphography, laparotomy with splenectomy, and bone marrow biopsy were done in all patients. If one considers the upper abdominal lymph nodes "contiguous" to the low neck via the thoracic duct, patterns of HD presentation were contiguous in more than 90% of the patients.[3]

GENERAL CLINICAL FEATURES

All the presenting signs or symptoms of HD described previously may occur in patients during the course of their disease. As the disease progresses in patients who have had several courses of therapy, the orderly progression and predictable sites of involvement are much less. Virtually any organ or tissues have been described as being involved by HD at some time in the course of the disease.

Lymph glands remain the most common site of the disease, even in patients with one or more recurrences. The lymphadenopathy is usually nontender, rubbery, or firm. As the nodes enlarge they may coalesce, forming large fixed tumor masses. When this occurs on one or both sides of the neck, a so-called bull-neck appearance of HD is characteristic of untreated or uncontrolled HD (Fig. 16–3). This kind of tumor mass may cause tracheal deviation and partial obstruction, dysphagia, or peripheral neuropathy. In extreme cases large underlying tumor masses may involve and irritate the skin, resulting in redness, skin nodules, and ulceration.

The lymphadenopathy of HD is found in locations somewhat different from those of other lymphoid neoplasms. The most common sites of the disease are in the neck, the axillae, and the paraaortic and ilioinguinal regions. Intrathoracic nodal involvement, described later, is also common. In the neck, supraclavicular locations are characteristic, but the disease may occur in the deep cervical, midcervical, and posterior cervical nodes as well. Less common is involvement of the high submandibular, occipital, and periauricular regions. Infraclavicular nodal involvement occurs and is best appreciated by palpating patients who are in the supine position. Axillary nodal involvement is common but must be distinguished from nonpathologic axillary lymph nodes that are often palpated and may reach

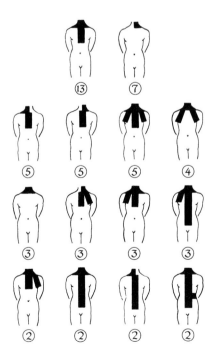

Figure 16–2. Most common anatomic patterns of Hodgkin's disease in 100 consecutive patients who underwent staging laparotomy. The circled numbers are the numbers of patients. (From Rosenberg SA, Kaplan HS: Evidence of an orderly progression in the spread of Hodgkin's disease. Cancer Res 1966; 26:1255.)

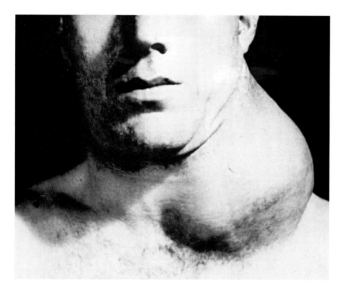

Figure 16–3. Massive cervical lymphadenopathy in a patient with Hodgkin's disease.

2 to 3 cm in diameter, especially in more obese patients. Epitrochlear nodal involvement occurs, but less commonly than in the low-grade non-Hodgkin's lymphomas, and if small, that is, smaller than 1 cm, may not be due to HD. In the axilla, the disease is usually in the apex of the region, palpated best with the patient in the sitting position. Recurrences, or extensions of the disease after radiation therapy, may be found lower in the axilla, along the chest wall, in the tail of the breast or subpectoral region.

Within the abdomen, computed tomographic (CT) studies and laparotomy data indicate that the nodal disease is predominately in the celiac, paraaortic, splenic hilar, and ilioinguinal regions. Involvement of porta hepatis and mesenteric nodes occurs, but only rarely. Femoral nodal involvement is found less often than in the non-Hodgkin's lymphomas. HD involvement of the inguinal lymph nodes is often difficult to determine, unless the nodes are extremely large, because of the frequent inflammatory lymphadenopathy found at that site.

The disease within the chest is usually in the anterior mediastinum, often at the site of the thymus gland. When minimal in size, the mediastinal disease may be difficult to recognize on the routine posteroanterior (PA) chest radiograph, but more evident on chest CT scans and on the gallium scan. The intrathoracic disease may also be obvious and in patients with the nodular sclerosis subtype may be massive. When extensive, the disease may involve all the lymphoid sites within the chest, including the hilar, subcarinal, and cardiophrenic lymph nodes. The disease may extend to the pericardium, the pleura, the lung, and the chest wall. Often these extensions are only demonstrated on CT scans or magnetic resonance imaging (MRI) studies. The pleural and pericardial effusions associated with intrathoracic HD may be difficult to document as "malignant" when examined cytologically. They usually have a high protein content and a nonspecific cytologic appearance. In some instances these may be due to lymphatic or venous obstruction by the central tumor masses, but they always

must be suspect as being secondary to direct tumor involvement, although possibly localized. There are examples of modest pleural effusions, cytologically negative, that permanently regress after irradiation of mediastinal HD, suggesting that, at least in some patients, the tumor involvement is central and the pleural involvement localized or obstructive in its pathogenesis.

The lung is one of the most common nonlymphoid tissues involved by HD. Patients may present with pulmonary involvement, or it may develop in the course of the disease. There are rare cases of so-called primary HD of the lung without documented disease in lymph nodes or any other site. As a rule, however, pulmonary HD is associated with intrathoracic nodal HD at presentation.

There are several forms of pulmonary HD. Direct extension to the lung is the most common, with linear infiltrations sometimes difficult to distinguish from atelectasis, pneumonitis, or lymphatic obstruction. Other patients have discrete fibronodular infiltrates, separate from the intrathoracic nodal disease. These are usually multiple but not often numerous. Occasionally these cavitate and suggest a granulomatous infection. Sometimes this cavitation is only seen after therapy as the disease resolves.

Despite the large masses that may result from intrathoracic HD, with involvement of extranodal structures such as the lung and pericardium, it is not common to see superior vena caval syndrome, recurrent laryngeal nerve paralyses, or pericardial tamponade. Airway obstruction can occur, however, although even this problem occurs less often than might be expected from the size and location of the tumor. The relative infrequency of these complications suggests that HD in its typical form is less invasive, locally, than other neoplasms such as lung carcinoma and some of the non-Hodgkin's lymphomas.

The spleen is one of the most frequent sites of HD involvement and was described as characteristic of the disease in Thomas Hodgkin's original report.[4] Involvement of the spleen may be obvious with significant splenomegaly but much more often is occult and difficult to demonstrate clinically. At laparotomy and splenectomy, involvement of the spleen can be demonstrated by the pathologist in approximately 30% of the patients who undergo the procedure.[5] Unless quite large, the size of the spleen is not a reliable predictor of splenic involvement. Unfortunately, no imaging technique is reliable in identifying minimal splenic HD.

The bone marrow may be involved with HD, rarely at the presentation of the disease, more commonly later in its course. Bone marrow involvement is usually focal, demonstrable reliably only with adequate biopsy techniques. Bone marrow aspirates, even with sectioning of bone marrow clots, do not often demonstrate the disease. Rarely, patients present with bone marrow dysfunction and cytopenias secondary to HD involvement. In the natural history of the unsuccessfully treated patient, this becomes a much more common problem.

Involvement of the liver by HD is also difficult to demonstrate clinically. When the liver is extensively involved, abnormal liver function, often with an obstructive biliary picture, is found. Elevation of the serum alkaline phosphatase level is the most sensitive indicator of HD of the liver, but unfortunately elevation up to twice the normal level may be found nonspecifically in patients with the disease. Macroscopic hepatic nodules may be evident on CT scan or abdominal ultrasonography, but the diffuse periportal infiltrates characteristic of HD are usually not evident on these studies.

STAGING OF HODGKIN'S DISEASE

The staging system generally accepted as useful for patients with HD is the four-stage system agreed on after a conference in Ann Arbor in 1974.[6] This proposal was a modification of several three- or four-stage definitions in use at that time that acknowledged the value of the lymphogram and laparotomy with splenectomy. It also defined the so-called E lesion, accepting that limited extranodal extension of the disease from lymph node sites was not an unfavorable prognostic factor. The Ann Arbor system and definitions are shown in Table 16–1.

The Ann Arbor system was validated with survival data available from several centers and series employing the best available treatment programs of the 1960s. The prognoses of patients with HD have changed dramatically since then, such that the prognostic value of the Ann Arbor system has largely been lost. However, the system, with several modifications described later, is still of value in planning treatment programs for individual patients and in comparing series that have been managed by different or new methods. The Ann Arbor system and recommendations attempt to clarify the differences between "clinical" stage and "pathologic" stage, with letter designations of CS and PS, respectively. The clinical stage refers to the extent of disease determined by all the diagnostic methods employed after a single diagnostic biopsy. The pathologic stage, developed primarily to acknowledge the greater accuracy of disease extent determination after staging laparotomy, is employed if a second biopsy, of any kind, has been obtained. A bone marrow biopsy, or even a second lymph node biopsy, requires that the stage designation be shown as pathologic

stage according to the Ann Arbor recommendations. A complex system is used to show which secondary biopsies have been obtained, whether positive (+) or negative (−), and the resulting change, if any, from clinical stage to pathologic stage. Practically, however, most clinicians use the designation PS to indicate the stage determined after exploratory laparotomy with splenectomy. The laparotomy procedure is being performed more rarely, and most patients and reported series can be considered clinically staged, even if a bone marrow biopsy or second lymph node biopsy has been obtained.

Several proposed modifications of the Ann Arbor staging system have found variable acceptance by clinicians and clinical investigators. Data are available that demonstrate the heterogeneity of patients with stage IIIA HD. Patients with limited upper abdominal disease, treated with irradiation only, have a better prognosis in some series than patients who have more extensive abdominal disease throughout the retroperitoneal region and into the pelvis. The former patients have been designated stage III_1, and the latter III_2. The extent of involvement of the spleen has also been shown to predict the success of radiation therapy for the same group of stage IIIA patients and is discussed in more detail subsequently.

There have also been proposals to substage patients according to the acknowledged prognostic significance of the bulk of disease. This has been best documented and used for patients with mediastinal HD. There have been different definitions of "bulk" in the mediastinum. The definition that has found the greatest acceptance states that a mediastinal mass whose transverse diameter on a standing PA chest radiograph exceeds one third of the greatest intrathoracic diameter of the chest wall is unfavorable, when irradiation is the sole modality of therapy. This substage was proposed to be designated with a subscript "x."[7]

All staging systems of HD acknowledge the prognostic importance of certain systemic symptoms. The Ann Arbor system recognizes only three systemic symptoms as prognostically important: unexplained persistent fever, unexplained persistent night sweats, and unexplained significant weight loss. These are defined in more detail in Table 16–1. When one or more of these symptoms have been present, the patient's stage is designated as "B" and if absent as "A." There are other characteristic systemic symptoms of HD, such as generalized pruritus or fatigue, but there is not a consensus to accept them as prognostically important. It is also likely that there is a spectrum of severity of systemic symptoms varying from hardly noticeable night sweats to all three symptoms of a severe degree and a spectrum of prognostic significance that is correlated.

Figure 16–4 shows the stage distribution of 2421 patients in the Stanford series. There is an increasing proportion of patients with B symptoms with advancing disease (8% of stage I, 23% of stage II, 37% of stage III, and 68% of stage IV).

HEMATOLOGIC FINDINGS

Most patients present with normal blood counts at the onset of their HD. During the course of the disease, and

Table 16–1. Ann Arbor Staging System

Stage	Criteria
I	Involvement of single lymph node region (I) or of single extralymphatic organ or site (I_E)
II	Involvement of ≥2 lymph node regions on same side of the diaphragm alone (II) or with involvement of limited, contiguous extralymphatic organ or tissue (II_E)
III	Involvement of lymph node regions on both sides of diaphragm (III), which may include spleen (III_S), or limited, contiguous extralymphatic organ or site (III_E), or both (III_{ES})
IV	Multiple or disseminated foci of involvement of ≥1 extralymphatic organs or tissues, with or without lymphatic involvement

All cases are subclassified to indicate the absence (A) or presence (B) of the systemic symptoms of significant fever, night sweats, or unexplained weight loss exceeding 10% of normal body weight. The clinical stage (CS) denotes the stage as determined by all diagnostic examinations and a single diagnostic biopsy only. If a second biopsy of any kind has been obtained, whether negative or positive, the term "pathologic stage" (PS) is used.

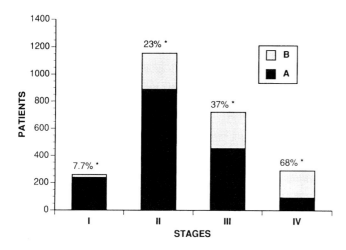

Figure 16–4. Ann Arbor stage distribution of 2424 patients with Hodgkin's disease at Stanford University Medical Center, 1960 to 1993. The percentage of systemic symptoms (B) for each stage is shown.

especially as a result of therapy, there may be profound abnormalities. Some patients have a leukocytosis and elevated platelet count at the time of their presentation. A mild anemia may be present and is usually normochromic and normocytic in type. Severe anemia, if it occurs at presentation, may be multifactorial and secondary to bone marrow infiltration, hemolysis, and/or hypersplenism.

The leukocytosis, which may be noted at presentation or during other episodes of disease activity until influenced by therapy, is usually modest in the 10,000 to 25,000 per mL range with a predominance of neutrophils. A mild eosinophilia is not unusual and rarely is marked. A relative lymphopenia has been noted in some patients with HD and when unassociated with therapy is believed to be a poor prognostic sign. Rare patients have marked leukocytosis with a leukemoid blood picture that may present a difficult differential diagnostic problem.

An elevation in the erythrocyte sedimentation rate (ESR) is quite characteristic of HD. It may be the only hematologic abnormality and the only sign of disease activity or recurrence in a previously treated patient. The level of the ESR elevation is often correlated with the extent of disease and, as such, has been used as a prognostic factor. The test has found more favor in Europe than in the United States.

Thrombocytopenia may occur for a variety of reasons in patients with HD. By far the most common cause is as a result of therapy. In some patients extensive bone marrow involvement causes or contributes to the platelet count depression, and some patients with splenomegaly have characteristic hypersplenism. The ITP syndrome is also associated with HD. The ITP may precede, coexist with, or follow the HD activity by years. In patients who are in remission after treatment, ITP does not usually indicate or herald a recurrence of the disease.

Severe autoimmune hemolytic anemia is unusual in patients with HD. The Coombs' test is usually negative, and only rarely is the reticulocyte response significant or indirect bilirubinemia noted. On the other hand, when studied carefully, patients with active HD can be shown to have a relatively shortened red cell survival of a modest degree.

As mentioned earlier, bone marrow involvement by HD is not common at disease presentation and rarely causes peripheral blood abnormalities. Occasional patients, however, have extensive bone marrow involvement, diffusely involving the marrow and often associated with extensive fibrosis. These patients may present with cytopenias and a myelophthisic picture, as may be seen in carcinomatosis or tuberculosis.

OTHER LABORATORY ABNORMALITIES

Numerous laboratory abnormalities have been described in patients with HD. Most of them are nonspecific, although some can be shown to be of some prognostic value. Table 16–2 lists many of the prognostic variables that have been reported.

When elevated, the serum alkaline phosphatase level is probably the most valuable blood chemistry abnormality in patients with the disease. Modest elevations (less than twice the upper limit of normal in postpubertal patients) may be nonspecific and merely reflect the general activity of HD. Elevations above that level, however, are usually meaningful and should direct the physician to the bones, bone marrow, and/or liver as sites of involvement by the disease.

The serum copper level has been used, much as the ESR, as an indicator of HD activity. In some centers, the normal and abnormal levels are more clearly separable than the ESR levels and thus more useful. Elevations of the serum copper level, however, also occur during pregnancy and when exogenous hormones are administered and in these situations lose their value.

Patients may develop chemical or clinical jaundice, as a result of HD, by a variety of mechanisms. Diffuse involvement of the liver may result in obstructive jaundice. This must be distinguished from extrahepatic biliary obstruction resulting from lymph node compression at the porta hepatis, although the two may coexist. Jaundice rarely is caused by severe hemolysis, with its characteristic laboratory findings. Jaundice in a patient with HD may also result from hepatitis, viral or drug induced. A rare syndrome of intrahepatic cholestasis has been described in patients with HD as a paraneoplastic or indirect manifestation of the disease. Thus, the causes of jaundice in a patient with HD may have widely different prognostic and therapeutic implications and should be ascertained as accurately as possible.

Table 16–2. Proposed Prognostic Variables in Hodgkin's Disease

- Nodular L&H subtype
- Nodular sclerosis subtypes
- Erythrocyte sedimentation rate
- Hemoglobin level
- Serum albumin level
- Serum lactate dehydrogenase level
- Serum β_2-microglobulin level
- Generalized pruritus
- Absolute lymphocyte count
- Number of sites
- Tumor burden

L&H, lymphocytic and histiocytic.

IMMUNE ABNORMALITIES

Some aspects of the immune abnormalities associated with HD are reviewed in other chapters. The immune deficit found in patients with this disease has been known for many years and represents one of its unique features.[1]

It has long been known that patients with HD do not have normal cellular immunity. This was first noted when patients with the disease were found to be anergic to antigens that normally produce cutaneous delayed hypersensitivity, that is, the tuberculin test. This was a general phenomenon to all antigens and found to be a basic defect in cellular immunity, similar to that seen in patients with sarcoidosis.

Studies of this immune defect have become more sophisticated and quantitative in recent years. It has become realized that the therapy for HD, especially wide-field irradiation, can contribute to the cellular immunity defect, and the effects of the therapy had to be separated from those of the disease. Sensitive tests, such as quantitative in vitro phytohemagglutinin stimulation, have shown that virtually all patients with HD, even those with minimal and early-stage disease, have T-cell dysfunction. This abnormality is not totally corrected by therapy, in some cases is aggravated by it, and persists for many years despite the continuous disease-free status of the individual.

There have been studies that suggest that a humoral factor or factors may play a role in the T-cell dysfunction and may transfer the defect to T cells from normal persons in vitro. The identification and purification of cytokines have provided further characterization of immune and histologic abnormalities of patients with HD. This is a field of intensive research and promise for the better understanding of many clinical and biologic aspects of HD.

Patients with HD, especially when the disease is advanced and/or recurrent, are susceptible to certain infections. These infections are those associated with defects in cellular immunity: tuberculosis and fungal and viral diseases. These infectious complications of the disease are subsequently discussed in more detail.

Patients with HD often have granulomatous histologic reactions associated with their tumor, and also in tissues not involved with the disease. HD itself has been called a granuloma, and clinicopathologic entities such as "granulomatous thymoma" and "lymphogranulomatosis" are, in fact, synonyms for HD. Tissues uninvolved with HD, however, may show noncaseating granulomas similar to those of sarcoidosis. Their pathogenesis or significance is largely unknown but may well be related to the immune defect found in these clinical conditions.[8]

SELECTED CLINICAL PROBLEMS

Within the myriad of clinical problems that patients with HD may present with or develop, several are worthy of special emphasis and description:

- Pulmonary infiltrates
- Epidural cord compression
- Herpes zoster
- Postsplenectomy sepsis
- Coexistent non-Hodgkin's lymphoma
- Infectious mononucleosis

PULMONARY INFILTRATES IN HODGKIN'S DISEASE

The pulmonary infiltrate can present a difficult diagnostic problem for physicians managing patients with HD. This is especially true for infiltrates that appear during or after the initiation of therapy.

As previously discussed, HD may involve the lung as a presenting site or, more commonly, as a site of extension of the disease later in its course. The radiologic appearance of pulmonary HD is not usually so characteristic as to be diagnostic. An infiltrate extending from bulky mediastinal or hilar lymphadenopathy is typical of HD but may have to be distinguished from areas of atelectasis or lymphatic obstruction. Nodular infiltrates separate from the nodal masses are also typical of HD, especially when multiple, with ipsilateral hilar adenopathy. They must be distinguished from old, or occasionally active, granulomatous infectious disease. Finally, coexistent malignant disease must be considered, especially when the total clinical circumstances raise that suspicion. In certain clinical settings a lung biopsy by the least morbid technique may be necessary to distinguish these possibilities and especially when their documentation would change the therapeutic plan significantly.

During the course of the disease, the problem becomes more complicated. In addition to the likely causes and appearances of pulmonary infiltrates listed earlier, the effects and complications of therapy and pulmonary infections become more common.

Radiation therapy in the doses employed for treating HD virtually always results in radiation pneumonitis. This is usually evident on routine chest radiographs and readily seen on chest CT scans. The infiltrates generally are confined fairly closely within the irradiation ports and appear several weeks after the radiation has been completed. Their initial appearance is as soft infiltrates that over the course of several months "harden," that is, they become more dense with clearer margins and eventually appear to partially regress as fibrosis takes place. Patients almost always have symptoms from radiation pneumonitis, varying from very mild to severe. These include cough, fever, and dyspnea. In some patients, infection of the lung appears to complicate the problem, producing increased fever, productive sputum, and frank pneumonia. The experienced physician will recognize the time course and radiologic appearance and not confuse radiation pneumonitis for HD or more serious infections. Chronic changes of radiation fibrosis may be quite extensive. Measurable pulmonary dysfunction with restrictive and diffusion abnormalities is characteristic of acute and chronic radiation pneumonitis.

Treated HD in the chest results in calcification within sites of previous disease. This usually is within mediastinal lymph node sites and usually is not seen before approximately 5 years after therapy. It is of no prognostic significance.

Patients treated for HD are susceptible to a wide range of pulmonary infections. Bacterial pneumonia is common, especially in the neutropenic patient. Viral, *Pneumocystis,* cytomegalovirus, *Legionella,* and atypical pneumonias can present difficult, and occasionally serious, diagnostic and clinical problems. Tuberculosis was a common infection found in patients with HD. This is much less common today but does occur in patients from settings where tuberculosis is found. Fungal infections of all kinds are common in HD patients, especially late in their course when patients are maximally immunosuppressed from their disease and therapy.

Cavitary lung disease may occur in HD of the lung without infection but must always raise the possibility of acid-fast, fungal, or suppurative bacterial infection. The clinical setting and appropriate culture efforts usually clarify and identify the cause of the lesion.

EPIDURAL CORD COMPRESSION

The problem of spinal cord compression by an epidural mass occurs in patients with HD, occasionally as a presenting problem with the disease; rarely, is it the sole manifestation of HD, requiring biopsy of the epidural tumor to identify the cause. The symptom complex, however, is more common in patients with non-Hodgkin's lymphomas, multiple myeloma, and metastatic carcinomas.

The epidural tumor usually arises from paravertebral lymphoid masses of HD and less often from vertebral osseous tumor. The dura is usually an effective barrier to the spread of the disease so that meningeal HD is rare, in contrast with the non-Hodgkin's lymphomas.

The clinical features of epidural cord compression are well known and easily recognized when the process has produced major neurologic deficits. The challenge to the physician is to recognize the problem early in its course so that appropriate therapy, usually irradiation, can prevent serious and permanent neurologic dysfunction.

Back pain of several types may be the first indication of cord compression. The pain may be radicular because of compression of sensory nerve roots; it may be retroperitoneal in its nature, aggravated by lying supine; or it may be vertebral, increased on standing or with movement.

More uncommon is a presentation with motor weakness of the extremities, sensory deficits, or bowel and bladder dysfunction. It is not unusual for the patient to have radicular and lower motor neuron signs and symptoms at the level of the epidural tumor and cord signs below this level.

Modern imaging techniques have greatly facilitated the demonstration and recognition of spinal cord compression. MRI is the diagnostic method of greatest value, but the CT scan may also be diagnostic. Myelography is almost never required currently and has associated morbidity that does not justify its use in the usual case. If the spinal fluid is examined, the protein level is characteristically elevated without an abnormal cytologic appearance.

Spinal cord compression is an oncologic emergency. The diagnosis must be considered and made promptly. Only rarely is surgery required either to make the diagnosis or to relieve the problem. Needle biopsy material may be adequate to recognize HD if there is no accessible tumor elsewhere in a patient not known to have the disease. Appropriate irradiation almost always reverses the neurologic progression and controls epidural HD permanently.

HERPES ZOSTER

Herpes zoster, or varicella-zoster, is a complication of the immunocompromised state. Although this characteristic infection may occur sporadically, without evident illness, especially with advancing age, it occurs frequently in patients with HD and other lymphomas.

The typical dermatome presentation of vesicular lesions on an erythematous base is usually not difficult to recognize by experienced clinicians. Occasionally shingles present with radicular pain before the cutaneous lesions appear or are recognized. Older descriptions of lymphoma suggest that herpes zoster may antedate the clinical diagnosis of HD or other lymphomas and always should suggest its presence. This is, in fact, a rare occurrence and has not been statistically established.

On the other hand, after the onset of the lymphoma, perhaps influenced by the therapies employed, herpes zoster occurs in up to one third of patients. It should be recognized promptly because in the immunocompromised patient, especially in older age, the local infection may be severe with prolonged postherpetic neuralgia, or dangerous dissemination may occur if not treated promptly. When varicella-zoster becomes disseminated, involving nondermatomal skin regions, the patient may develop serious, even fatal involvement of the lungs, central nervous system, and other viscera. It has been suggested that herpes zoster involves dermatomes that are involved with the malignant lymphomas, but this is unproved.

Fortunately, antiviral chemotherapy with acyclovir, if given in proper dosage and early in the course of the disease, reduces local morbidity, probably reduces postherpetic neuralgia, and reduces the incidence and severity of dissemination.

POSTSPLENECTOMY SEPSIS

The serious syndrome of overwhelming postsplenectomy bacterial sepsis is seen in a small percentage of HD patients. Almost all these patients have undergone diagnostic laparotomy and splenectomy as part of their initial staging procedures for the disease. There are rare patients who may develop this problem because of functional hyposplenism as a result of splenic irradiation.

The bacterial sepsis after splenectomy has been well described in the literature and is usually seen in children after splenectomy or in persons who are functionally hyposplenic. The infection is due to encapsulated bacteria, *Streptococcus pneumoniae* (pneumococcus), *Meningococcus,* or *Haemophilus influenzae.* The pneumococcal organisms are the most common agent, especially in adults. It is possible that this syndrome, which is usually seen in children, occurs in adults with HD because of the additional defects in immunity associated with HD and is aggravated by therapy. In this author's experience, the syndrome is recognized less often in adults with the non-Hodgkin's lymphoma who have undergone splenectomy.

The clinical picture is that of overwhelming bacterial sepsis, with bacteremia, easily demonstrable, and usually pneumonia, often with meningitis. The onset is rapid, with high fever, shaking chills, headache, extreme malaise, and hypotension. The blood usually shows a granulocytosis or a shift to the left in the granulocyte series, with normal or low total white blood cell counts. Sometimes encapsulated bacteria are evident on routine blood smears. The complications of disseminated intravascular coagulation (DIC) and/or adult respiratory distress syndrome (ARDS) may develop and add to the very poor prognosis of the infection.

Successful therapy depends on its prompt recognition, administration of appropriate antibiotics intravenously, and excellent fluid and intensive care support. Patients and their families must be educated about the signs and symptoms of this rare complication of splenectomy and seek medical attention very promptly if it is suspected.

The proper use of polyvalent pneumococcal vaccine as early as possible before splenectomy and before therapy for HD may well reduce the incidence of this overwhelming infectious complication. The vaccine does not protect against all pneumococcal strains, and because other bacteria may cause the infection, the patient remains at risk. There is controversy whether patients should receive pneumococcal vaccine after splenectomy and/or therapy since their immune response is unpredictable and vaccination may actually reduce antibody levels in rare instances.[9]

This catastrophic complication of the management of HD may be seen much less often as the use of diagnostic laparotomy with splenectomy is performed more infrequently. Management programs that do not require the more precise identification of occult disease in the abdomen, possible only with the surgical procedure, are evolving for treating HD. However, as long as some patients have in the past or will undergo splenectomy or splenic irradiation in their management, the syndrome must be prevented, if possible, and treated promptly, if recognized.

COEXISTENT NON-HODGKIN'S LYMPHOMA

Patients may present with two different histologic types of lymphomas: composite lymphoma or discordant lymphoma (if the two types are within the same site or from separate sites and biopsy specimens). Of the various combinations that have been observed, HD combined with low-grade follicular lymphoma or with intermediate-grade diffuse large cell lymphoma has been the most common.

The presence of two different types of lymphomas complicates the diagnostic and staging studies and their interpretation. It also complicates the therapeutic recommendations. As a generalization, the treatment is directed to the disease with the poorest prognosis, and if precise staging or extent of disease cannot be ascertained, chemotherapy, rather than irradiation therapy only, is preferred.

Non-Hodgkin's lymphoma may also develop in patients with HD long after the onset and treatment of the HD and often in patients apparently cured of HD.[10] The non-Hodgkin's lymphoma is usually of an intermediate- or high-grade type, often involving the viscera of the abdomen. The probability of this type of non-Hodgkin's lymphoma being diagnosed in patients treated for HD increases with time and reached a level of approximately 5% at 20 years in a series at Stanford.[11]

This type of non-Hodgkin's lymphoma may develop in a patient with HD. Unusual sites for HD, long disease-free intervals, and rapid growth of disease should alert the physician and be indications for biopsy to differentiate recurrent HD from a de novo non-Hodgkin's lymphoma.

The cause of non-Hodgkin's lymphomas appearing late in the course of patients with HD has been likened to non-Hodgkin's lymphomas occurring after organ transplantation, acquired immunodeficiency syndrome (AIDS), or other immunodeficient states. Although there are some similarities in these various clinical settings, there also are clinical, biologic, and viral differences.

INFECTIOUS MONONUCLEOSIS

Pathologists have pointed out that there are some histologic similarities between infectious mononucleosis and HD. Very reactive immunoblasts in reactive lymph nodes from infectious mononucleosis may appear, superficially, like HD. In general, however, pathologists can make the appropriate distinction.

Clinically, perhaps epidemiologically, recent biologic studies suggest a relationship between infectious mononucleosis, or at least Epstein-Barr virus (EBV) infection, and HD. Occasionally young patients have a well-documented case of infectious mononucleosis that merges, almost without interruption, with the signs and symptoms and diagnosis of HD. Much more common is the finding of a well-documented case of infectious mononucleosis in the recent or more distant past medical history of a patient who subsequently develops HD. In some instances, the diagnosis of infectious mononucleosis is presumed and not documented, and, in fact, the signs and symptoms all were the result of HD. Since infectious mononucleosis is a common disease, especially in an age group in which HD is also common, the etiologic relationship is difficult to establish. Epidemiologic studies relating the two diseases are inconclusive and are reviewed in Chapter 3.

Perhaps more provocative have been the biologic and viral studies that demonstrate the EBV genome and viral particles in Reed-Sternberg cells of a significant number of HD patients.

In general, lymph node biopsy is not recommended for patients with infectious mononucleosis. However, the clinician must remain alert to the possibility that what appears to be infectious mononucleosis may, in fact, be HD or become HD after a variable period.

CLINICAL PROBLEMS AFTER THERAPY

A more detailed description of various complications of therapy is found later in this chapter. Some of these complications are quite specific for the treatment modality or individual chemotherapeutic agent used. Others are a result of the total therapy given or are more poorly understood. Several of the problems have already been discussed. Some general considerations are worthy of emphasis.

Gradually, with increased time after therapy, the clinical problems of the patient and the attention of the physician change from recurrence of the HD to late effects of the therapy.

Radiation effects progress from acute inflammatory reactions to chronic effects, usually manifested by fibrosis, scarring, and vascular damage. Many of the late vascular effects of irradiation are difficult to separate from those commonly seen with aging. Coronary artery disease is one of these, but vascular endothelial damage from irradiation can also produce cardiac valvular damage as well as major arterial problems in the chest, neck, kidney, liver, bone, pericardium, and other sites. The clinical signs, symptoms, and laboratory and radiologic abnormalities of these late effects should be recognized. Often they are minor in their significance and reassurance is all that is required. In other situations, the problem can be serious—even fatal—as the process progresses.

Secondary malignancies are serious problems of which patients with treated and cured HD and their physician must be aware.[11] These include radiation-induced carcinomas and sarcomas within treated fields, chemotherapy-induced acute leukemia, and non-Hodgkin's lymphoma (previously described).

Sterility is not a life-threatening complication of the therapy of HD, but it is a "problem of success." Relatively young patients are cured of their HD and have a relatively normal life span and aspirations after treatment. Irradiation and several of the chemotherapeutic agents employed for the treatment of the disease produce sterility in most patients, depending on the doses administered. Until alternative treatments are developed and tested, patients must be aware of the sterility risks of the therapy. Men should be given the opportunity to store semen before initiating therapy or undergoing extensive diagnostic tests. Advances in the field of fertility make it possible for women to anticipate in vitro fertilization in specialized centers.

As a general philosophy, the author advises patients, especially women, to avoid pregnancy and parenting for at least 2 years after completion of the initial HD therapy. This is to allow the close diagnostic radiologic followup desirable to recognize early recurrence and to allow secondary or salvage treatments to be administered without concern for the fetus. This time of freedom from recurrence usually takes the patients through a significant portion (perhaps 75%) of their risk period.

Chemical and clinical hypothyroidism is a common problem of patients who have received neck irradiation for HD. Since this occurs more commonly in HD patients than in others who have received this kind of therapy, other factors, such as lymphangiography, may play a role; perhaps it is because more of the HD patients live longer after treatment and clinicians are aware of the potential problem. The usual finding is a significant and persistent elevation of the thyroid-stimulating hormone (TSH) level in a clinically euthyroid patient. Less commonly, patients have the clinical signs of hypothyroidism; even more rarely, they present with exophthalmos while euthyroid or hypothyroid. In all instances, the patient should receive thyroid replacement therapy. If necessary, this should be supervised by an endocrinologist. The need for replacement therapy is not only to reverse or prevent the appearance of clinical hypothyroid symptoms but to protect the irradiated thyroid from prolonged TSH stimulation and the development of thyroid nodules, both benign and malignant.

Psychosocial problems are always present for patients with a malignant disease and their families. This is especially true for young patients in the HD age group. The patients may still be in school or college, recently married and starting a family, or near the prime of their occupational career, all of which are seriously interrupted by the diagnosis and required management of their HD.

Appearance and physical capacity are significantly changed, as much or more from the treatment required than from the disease itself. After therapy, questions of fertility, sexuality, insurability, and prognosis become important issues for HD patients and their families. Unfortunately, too often, the physician does not have the awareness, time, or skills to appreciate and properly help solve these difficulties. Other support personnel and systems are often needed to provide for the complete needs of HD patients and their families, so they can enjoy the benefits of modern curative therapy.

Management

The treatment of patients with HD has been one of the most significant successes in twentieth century clinical medicine. This once uniformly fatal disease is now curable in approximately 75% of patients at many major medical centers, worldwide. The management of these patients, however, is often difficult and requires meticulous attention to details of the staging and treatment program. This is necessary to achieve the excellent results that are possible while keeping to a minimum the potential serious toxicities and morbidities of the therapy.

Some of the serious effects of the therapy of HD are not evident for at least 5 years and often not for 10 to 20 years or more after treatment is completed. These might be described as problems of success since they require many years of survival, free of HD recurrence, to be recognized. As they have become evident, treatment programs have been modified in an effort to reduce their incidence and severity to a minimum. Thus, the management of patients with HD continues to evolve. Treatment recommendations may differ, somewhat, even among physicians and investigators experienced in the management of HD patients. This chapter draws heavily from the experience and treatment results of the authors and whenever appropriate calls attention to major controversies that may exist.

The therapeutic program for a patient with HD should not be initiated without a definitive diagnosis by an experienced hematopathologist. Appropriate diagnostic studies and stage determination should be made before one embarks on therapy. Almost all patients benefit from consultation with both an experienced medical oncologist or hematologist and a radiation oncologist to jointly plan the treatment program, although not all patients require both modalities—chemotherapy and radiation therapy—in their initial management. Appropriate consultation between the subspecialties, however, ensures that the best possible result will be achieved in the most efficient and least toxic manner available.

PRIMARY AND SECONDARY (SALVAGE) THERAPY

Unlike patients with other cancers, patients with HD have a significant probability of being cured of their disease after a recurrence or relapse following their initial treatment. This is dependent on the type of primary therapy used and the response and duration of that response before the recurrence. For example, if a patient is treated with radiation therapy only and a recurrence occurs after an interval that allows recovery of good bone marrow function, combination chemotherapy may be successful in achieving permanent control of the disease.[12, 13] In selected cases, the opposite may apply. Chemotherapy may have been used for relatively favorable stages of the disease, and recurrence after a significant interval, usually more than 1 year, is documented within limited lymph node sites only. Such a patient may be managed, with curative intent, with secondary or so-called salvage irradiation.[14, 15] Thus, there are situations in which the physician may choose to accept a higher relapse rate with single-modality therapy (usually radiation therapy) than would be possible with combined-modality therapy, preferring to reserve the other modality (usually chemotherapy) for those who have a recurrence. In general, this is not a recommended approach if the recurrence after single-modality therapy can be predicted to be 50% or greater.

Patients with HD may also achieve prolonged control of their disease after two or more recurrences by means of intensive therapy supported by autologous bone marrow infusions or peripheral stem cell regimens. These methods and results are discussed in more detail subsequently.

When patients are not cured of their HD and have exhausted all standard treatment programs that might permanently control their disease, they should be managed with palliation as the goal or be considered for experimental therapies. Some patients with persistent HD, despite multiple courses of treatment, tolerate their disease relatively well for prolonged periods. Experience with the disease is required to apply appropriate palliative treatment, or no treatment at all, for periods that may extend for years after curative treatment methods have failed. This subject is discussed in more detail later in this chapter.

SELECTION OF TREATMENT BY STAGE

In general, the standard and recommended treatment for patients with HD depends on the stage of the disease. There are special clinical situations and settings in which the standard approach must be modified, and these are reviewed in detail. As noted previously, new management programs are being developed that are likely to require modifications of the standard methods currently accepted. However, it is useful to describe the general approach to patients as of 1994. The details of radiation therapy technique, fields, and dosage and of chemotherapy regimens and administration are found in Chapters 11 and 12 and later in this chapter.

STAGES IA AND IIA
Supradiaphragmatic

Adult patients who are found to have the most limited disease settings, without unfavorable systemic symptoms and without unusual bulky disease, are managed with full-dose, extended-field irradiation without chemotherapy. The radiation fields are usually the mantle and upper abdominal fields for supradiaphragmatic disease. As a rule, these patients should have undergone staging laparotomy and splenectomy to be more certain the disease is limited in extent. Lower extremity lymphography is strongly recommended to stage these patients properly, although some centers rely on abdominopelvic CT scanning and gallium scanning for this purpose (see Chapter 9).

Bulky

Patients with otherwise favorable disease settings but who have large tumor masses, usually in the mediastinum, are best managed with combined-modality therapy. Although irradiation alone may control about half of these patients, it is generally accepted that the initial cure rate can be improved to the 75% to 85% range by preceding the irradiation with combination chemotherapy.[16, 17]

The definition of "bulk" is somewhat confusing in the literature and is usually quantified only in the mediastinum. The data that identified this subgroup of patients are derived from a relatively simple method of measuring the greatest transverse diameter of the mediastinal mass on a standard PA chest radiograph and dividing by the maximal diameter of the chest wall at its pleural surfaces. A ratio of the mass to chest wall greater than 1:3 is considered "bulky" and unfavorable and can be designated with a subscript x by the Cotswold agreement.[7] There are more sophisticated methods of determining the bulk of tumors, by calculating their true volume, that could improve the selection of these patients, especially in borderline situations. But these methods have not been widely reported or used. Similarly, it is likely that large tumor masses in other sites, such as the neck, axilla, abdomen, or pelvis, are also unfavorable for irradiation management alone. There is no agreement, however, on how these sites of bulky disease should be defined.

Infradiaphragmatic

Patients occasionally present with otherwise favorable disease limited to the pelvis and/or abdomen. A typical presentation is lymphadenopathy in the femoral–inguinal–external iliac region. After full staging, preferably with lymphography and staging laparotomy and splenectomy, these patients can achieve excellent control of their disease with radiation therapy alone. Some patients are found to have involvement of their spleen with HD at laparotomy. These patients often have paraaortic involvement evident on the lymphogram. Patients with upper abdominal HD should have irradiation to supradiaphragmatic sites in their initial management. Those rare stage IIA patients who have extensive involvement of their spleen, or documented involvement of porta hepatis or mesenteric lymph nodes, should receive combined-modality therapy.

STAGES I AND IIB

There is more controversy in the recommendation of standard therapy for patients who have otherwise favorable extent of disease, with documented systemic symptoms. If complete staging is performed with the use of lymphography and laparotomy with splenectomy, subtotal nodal irradiation for supradiaphragmatic disease and total nodal irradiation for infradiaphragmatic disease can provide good results, in the 60% to 80% range.[18] A significant proportion of patients with clinical stage I or IIB disease have occult disease in the abdomen and/or extensive involvement of the spleen. This probability is increased if all the B symptoms are present and severe. Those patients with infradiaphragmatic presentation of clinical stage IIB disease often are found to have splenic involvement at staging laparotomy. Therefore, it is justified in certain subgroups of clinically staged patients to avoid staging laparotomy and use combination chemotherapy, either alone or in a combined-modality program.

It is quite rare for patients to present with stage IB disease. Occasional patients with bulky disease limited to the mediastinum have documented systemic symptoms. More often, as detailed diagnostic studies are obtained, the disease is found to be more widespread, or the systemic symptoms are found to be undocumented or caused by some other process.

As a rule, no patient should be presumed to have stage I or IIB disease and be treated with irradiation alone without documentation of the limited extent of disease with lymphography and staging laparotomy.

STAGE IIIA

The management of patients with clinical or pathologic stage IIIA disease is also controversial. Patients with nonbulky disease and limited upper abdominal disease, usually identified at staging laparotomy, can achieve 60% to 80% cure rates with total nodal irradiation alone. Equally good results can be achieved with appropriate combination chemotherapy. In some centers, combined-modality programs are used with excellent results. The choice among these management plans depends on the kind and duration of toxicity, acute and long term, that is acceptable to the patient and physician.

Patients with clinical or pathologic stage IIIA disease who have extensive involvement of the spleen (five or more nodules)[19] or widespread lymph node involvement in the paraaortic and pelvic regions have relatively poor cure rates when treated with irradiation alone.[20, 21] These patients, if their extent of disease is well documented, are best treated with combination chemotherapy or a combined-modality program.

STAGE IIIB

There is general agreement that chemotherapy should be the primary treatment for patients with stage IIIB disease. In some patients the extent of disease is clearly evident and documentation by staging laparotomy is not necessary. In others, the abdominal imaging studies are equivocal and the value of the lymphogram and/or staging laparotomy is greater. Even patients with only upper abdominal disease and/or minimal splenic involvement (fewer than five nodules) should be managed with primary combination chemotherapy. However, in such patients with an otherwise favorable extent of disease, the documentation and acceptance of the B symptoms becomes more important.

It is more controversial to use irradiation to limited or extended fields for patients with stage IIIB disease, combined with their chemotherapy. In general, this is probably indicated to sites of initial bulky disease, and/or sites of incomplete regression. The indications, timing, dose, and clinical settings for combined-modality therapy are discussed in more detail subsequently.

STAGE IV

Patients with stage IV disease, defined and documented according to the Ann Arbor system, require combination chemotherapy as their primary modality of treatment. As with stage IIIB patients, there may be selected situations in which irradiation should be used as well.

EXTRANODAL INVOLVEMENT: THE E LESION

Patients with stages I, II, or III disease may have limited extranodal extension of their disease, as defined by the Ann Arbor system. The definition of the E lesion is somewhat ambiguous and interpreted differently by various experts and centers. These sites of involvement are usually found in patients with moderate or bulky mediastinal disease. The most common extranodal sites that are E lesions are the lungs, pericardium, pleura, chest wall, and bone. In general, extranodal disease that is limited in extent, adjacent to or near known nodal involvement, and can be encompassed within radiation fields without undue morbidity does not change the prognosis or the recommended management.

HISTOLOGIC SUBTYPE

There is no doubt that the various histologic subtypes (see Chapter 5) identify patients with different clinical characteristics and natural histories. In general, however, patients are managed the same whether they have the nodular sclerosis or mixed cellularity subtypes. This is the case even for the subdivisions of the nodular sclerosis group that have been proposed by some authors. These two major subtypes, nodular sclerosis and mixed cellularity, account for most (≥90%) patients with HD.

Patients with the subtype of lymphocyte predominance are different in several important features from other patients with HD. As described in Chapters 6 and 7, their tumors differ immunologically, genetically, and probably clinically from those of other patients. Most cases of the lymphocyte-predominance subtype according to the Rye classification are more properly characterized as the nodular, lymphocytic, and histiocytic subtype (nodular L&H) as first described by Lukes and Butler. These subtypes are found more often in boys and men than other subtypes, and these patients have relatively favorable stages of disease and have a good prognosis. They may have a risk of recurrence for a more prolonged period than other patients with HD, a plateau in the relapse-free survival curve being later and lower than is typical for the major subtypes of the disease.[22]

Therefore, it is difficult to recommend standard treatment programs, by stage, for this uncommon type of HD. Since these patients usually have relatively favorable stages of the disease, radiation therapy is recommended, but with more restricted fields than might be indicated for other patients. These patients should not be managed without consultation at a center with major experience with HD to confirm the histologic subtype and recommend the therapy.

RADIATION THERAPY

A detailed review and description of the history, role, techniques, and complications of radiation therapy for HD are found in Chapter 11. Radiation therapy was the first effective treatment discovered for patients with HD and remains an important modality of therapy for many patients.

Radiation therapy as a single modality can result in the cure of patients with relatively favorable stages of the disease. Radiation therapy can improve the cure probabilities for selected patients treated with combination chemotherapy. Radiation therapy can be highly effective in managing clinical emergencies and can be an effective means of palliation for patients who are no longer curable. Total-body irradiation is often a component of high-dose therapy (HDT) for patients undergoing bone marrow transplantation and/or peripheral stem cell support.

As effective combination chemotherapy has been discovered and become available for patients with HD, the role of radiation therapy has become more limited and, in some situations, controversial and difficult to prove. In some settings the two modalities are equivalent in value when used singly and, as such, are "competitive." It would be preferable to consider each modality as an alternative, rather than competitive, since the choice between them should depend on the different acute and long-term toxicities and morbidities of each modality rather than differences in their effectiveness. As described earlier in this chapter, it may be sufficient to accept a lower initial cure rate, induced by a shorter, well-tolerated irradiation approach, knowing that the fraction of patients not cured can be effectively controlled with subsequent combination chemotherapy. This is an acceptable course only when the eventual long-term survival rate is not reduced by accepting a higher relapse rate and if the combination chemotherapy program is more toxic and dangerous. This is the case for most of the original combination drug regimens used for HD, such as six or more cycles of MOPP (mechlorethamine, Oncovin [vincristine], procarbazine, prednisone) and/or ABVD (Adriamycin [doxorubicin], bleomycin, vinblastine, dacarbazine), but it may not be the case in the future if different effective regimens become available.

Radiation therapy should always be considered in managing patients with emergency situations resulting from the disease. These include

- Airway obstruction
- Superior vena caval obstruction
- Pericardial tamponade
- Epidural spinal cord compression
- Ureteral obstruction
- Extrahepatic biliary obstruction
- Cranial and peripheral neuropathies

Some of these clinical problems are relatively rare in patients with HD, but all may occur. Occasionally, they are among the presenting symptoms of the disease. It is almost never necessary, or indicated, to initiate emergency radiation therapy for these conditions without an accurate histologic diagnosis. Combination chemotherapy may also be beneficial in some of these situations but may interfere with the accurate staging of patients who present with disease in this way. Radiation therapy in full dose is also more likely to

effect permanent control of disease in these critical sites than is chemotherapy.

The role of radiation therapy as an adjuvant to chemotherapy is finding increasing use. Its role for patients with large mediastinal masses is generally accepted, although it is difficult to prove its value in randomized trials. It may also be of value as an adjuvant for patients with limited bone lesions, for those with significant residual masses other than in the mediastinum, and for those with disease in certain extranodal sites such as the breast, skin, thyroid, and, rarely, brain.

COMBINED-MODALITY THERAPY

The use of both radiation therapy and chemotherapy, or combined-modality therapy, is referred to earlier in this chapter. Until recently, the use of both modalities in the primary management of patients with HD was restricted to the few following clinical settings:

- Clinical emergency situations
- Disease in children, usually younger than 16 years of age
- Bulky disease, usually in the mediastinum

Physicians were appropriately cautious in using both modalities because morbidities, both acute and long term, were increased, secondary or "salvage" therapy was more difficult, and randomized clinical studies had failed to show a survival advantage for the combined-modality approach. These considerations remain valid if full doses and courses of each modality are used.

The situation in children, detailed subsequently, is different. Less than full-dose irradiation is prescribed for children who have not obtained their full skeletal and muscular development. Chemotherapy is required to supplement the radiation effect, and excellent therapeutic results can be achieved.

In the case of bulky mediastinal disease, it is generally agreed that when used alone, each modality does not provide greater than 50% cure rates, and combined-modality therapy can significantly improve the results. Even in that setting, no study has yet demonstrated a survival advantage of the combined modality.

Recent studies, again generally nonrandomized, have demonstrated high initial control and projected cure rates when less than maximal or full-course single-modality regimens are combined. For example, two to four cycles of standard chemotherapy have been combined with limited-field irradiation with excellent results in patients with favorable clinical settings of HD.[23, 24] These approaches should reduce the long-term complications of each of the modalities, because cumulative drug and radiation dosages are significantly smaller than those previously employed. Major organ dysfunction and late complications such as sterility, cardiotoxicity, and acute leukemia can be reduced or eliminated as problems by combining low-dose irradiation (or limited fields) with relatively brief courses of chemotherapy. Longer followup and greater experience will be necessary to establish more firmly the value of these novel combined-modality treatment programs, especially for patients with early-stage, favorable disease.

Patients with advanced, relatively unfavorable settings of HD may also benefit from combined-modality therapy. Those with bulky mediastinal disease have already been mentioned. Stanford studies have demonstrated the value and tolerance of alternating chemotherapy and irradiation in controlling at least 75% of patients with the most unfavorable settings of the disease. These are difficult treatment programs to carry out for both the patient and the medical team and should not be undertaken by groups unfamiliar with the approach and techniques.

The availability of hematopoietic growth factors has allowed the safer use of greater dose intensity of chemotherapy and combined-modality treatment programs. Preliminary studies have shown that intensive, relatively brief combined-modality therapy can be safely administered to patients with advanced disease with excellent results, assisted by the use of growth factors. This could well be the future approach for most patients with other than the most favorable presentations of HD.

PROGNOSIS

Estimates and general comments about the prognosis for patients with HD are described in other sections of this and other chapters. Available data for describing the prognosis of HD must be qualified, depending on their source, because of several important factors.

The prognosis for patients with HD has been changing over the last several decades owing to changes and modifications in treatment programs. The most reliable data derived from adequate patient numbers (e.g., those followed for at least 10 years) represent the outcome of therapies administered 10 to 15 years ago. Advances have been made in the treatment of HD patients since that time, but the data available to demonstrate and quantify these advances are not yet statistically reliable.

There are differences in statistics derived from single institutions, cooperative groups, and geographic or population-based registries. As a rule, single-institution studies are most reliable in terms of accuracy of diagnosis, uniformity of therapy programs, and availability of multiple prognostic variable information. However, single-institution data suffer from patient selection, small patient numbers, and difficulty of translation from the setting of heavily experienced management teams to more average community settings. Geographic or population-based statistics contain diagnostic and staging inaccuracies, limited prognostic variable data, and nonuniform, or even unknown, therapy information. Cooperative group or metaanalysis data provide some of the needs of patient numbers, accuracy of diagnoses, and applicability to more typical and relevant management settings. They suffer, however, from relative nonuniformity in patient management skills and experience, variable degrees of patient selection, and use of treatment methods somewhat outdated when compared with those of the leading single institutions.

The most recent Surveillance, Epidemiology, and End Results (SEER) data from The Surveillance Program of the National Cancer Institute provide an excellent population-based picture of the prognosis of HD from 1973 to 1990. The

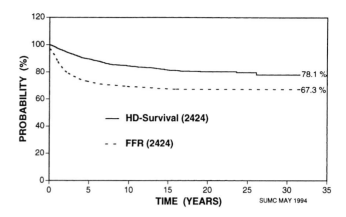

Figure 16–5. Actuarial freedom from recurrence (FFR) and survival in 2424 patients with Hodgkin's disease (HD) treated at Stanford University Medical Center (SUMC), 1960 to 1993.

median age of patients in the SEER data base is 32 years, with peak risks in the age groups of 20 to 24 and 80 to 84 years. The 5-year relative survival rate is 78.1% for all cases diagnosed from 1983 to 1989. The prognosis is somewhat better for whites than for blacks (78.6% versus 74.1%) and for women than for men (81.3% versus 75.7%). The 5-year survival has risen from 61% for patients diagnosed in 1973 to 80.5% for those diagnosed in 1985. The 10-year survival has risen from 52.5% in 1973 to 68.1% in 1980. The age at diagnosis is a highly significant prognostic variable, with 5-year relative survival rates of 82.4% for patients younger than 65 years of age and 40.3% for those aged 65 years and older diagnosed between 1983 and 1989.

Single-institution data from 2424 patients treated at Stanford from 1960 to 1993 provide valuable prognostic information. Figure 16–5 shows the actuarial disease-specific survival and freedom from recurrence after initial therapy for the entire group of patients. At 30 years, 67.3% of all patients remain in their first remission and 78.1% have survived their HD. The median age of the total group of patients is 27 years, with a range of 1 to 83 years.

Figures 16–6 and 16–7 show the improvement in freedom from recurrence and HD survival during three periods: 1960

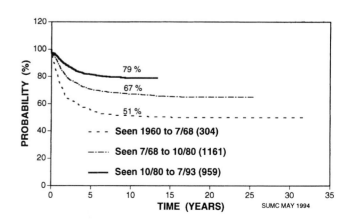

Figure 16–6. Actuarial freedom from recurrence of Hodgkin's disease after initial treatment during three periods—1960 to 1968 (304 patients), 1968 to 1980 (1161 patients), and 1980 to 1993 (959 patients)—at Stanford University Medical Center (SUMC).

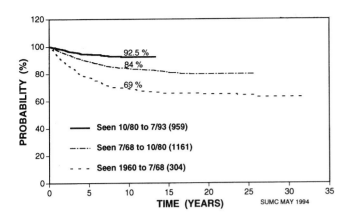

Figure 16–7. Actuarial disease-specific survival of patients with Hodgkin's disease during three periods—1960 to 1968 (304 patients), 1968 to 1980 (1161 patients), and 1980 to 1993 (959 patients)—at Stanford University Medical Center (SUMC).

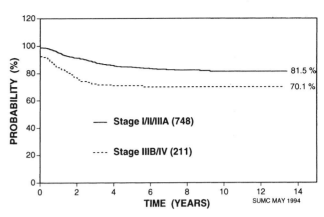

Figure 16–9. Actuarial freedom from recurrence of Hodgkin's disease after initial treatment of 959 patients at Stanford University Medical Center (SUMC) between 1980 and 1993 according to stage of disease.

to 1968, 1968 to 1980, and 1980 to 1993. The 10-year freedom from recurrence has risen from 51% in the earliest era to 79% in the most recent. Survival from HD has risen at 10 years from 69% to 92.5%. The overall 10-year survival, which includes deaths from all causes, disease specific, disease related, and disease apparently unrelated, is shown in Figure 16–8; it has risen from 59% to 75% to 85% during these three periods. The median age of patients during these three eras was 28.5, 26.0, and 27.0 years with comparable ranges.

The freedom from recurrence and HD survival actuarial probabilities according to initial stages of the disease for patients treated from 1980 to 1993 are shown in Figures 16–9 and 16–10. Stages I, II, and IIIA are grouped, as are stages IIIB and IV, since there are no significant differences among the stages grouped together. It can be seen that at 10 years 81.5% of the more favorable stages of the disease and 70.1% of the unfavorable stages remain in their first remission. The 10-year survival of HD is 95.6% and 81.2% for these groups, respectively.

Figure 16–11 shows the actuarial freedom from recurrence and overall survival of a similar group of 1770 patients treated at Stanford between 1974 and 1993, according to

histologic subtype. There are no major prognostic differences between the two major subtypes, nodular sclerosis and mixed cellularity, and a somewhat better recurrence-free survival, but not survival, for the 5% of patients who have the lymphocyte-predominance subtype. Figure 16–12 demonstrates the important differences in prognoses for these 1770 patients according to their age at diagnosis.

SPECIAL CLINICAL PROBLEMS

Several clinical settings require different therapeutic approaches than those used in patients with uncomplicated HD. These are HD in

- Children
- Pregnant patients
- Clinical emergencies
- Patients with AIDS

IN CHILDREN

HD is relatively uncommon in children younger than 16 years of age. Therefore, it is preferable that children with

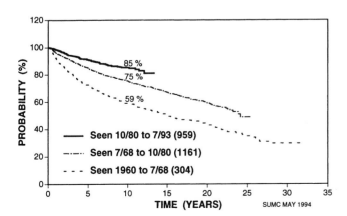

Figure 16–8. Actuarial overall survival of patients with Hodgkin's disease during three periods—1960 to 1968 (304 patients), 1968 to 1980 (1161 patients), and 1980 to 1993 (959 patients)—at Stanford University Medical Center (SUMC).

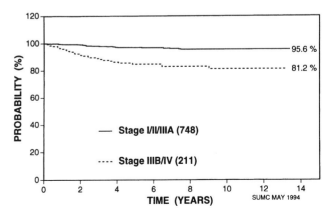

Figure 16–10. Actuarial disease-specific survival of patients with Hodgkin's disease after initial treatment of 959 patients at Stanford University Medical Center (SUMC) between 1980 and 1993 according to stage of disease.

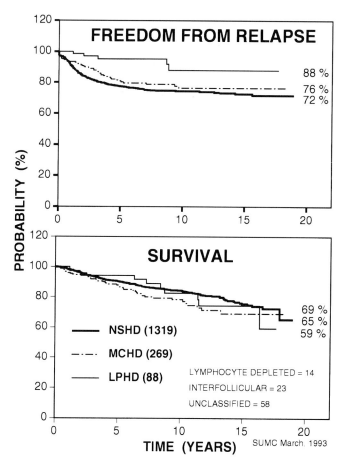

Figure 16–11. Actuarial freedom from relapse (*upper*) and overall survival (*lower*) of 1771 consecutive patients treated at Stanford University Medical Center (SUMC) from 1974 to 1993 according to histologic subtype of Hodgkin's disease. NSHD, nodular-sclerosing Hodgkin's disease; MCHD, mixed cellularity Hodgkin's disease; LPHD, lymphocyte-predominant Hodgkin's disease. (From Rosenberg SA: The treatment of Hodgkin's disease. Ann Oncol 1994; 5[Suppl 2]:S17.)

HD be managed at centers experienced in pediatric oncology.

The main problem in managing children is the growth inhibitory effect of irradiation on bone and muscle. If full-dose irradiation in the range of 30 Gy or higher is used, skeletal and muscle development is seriously impaired, leading to unacceptable long-term morbidity. Therefore, combination chemotherapy is indicated as the primary form of therapy, even for children with favorable early stages of the disease. These children do not require staging laparotomy and splenectomy to detect otherwise occult disease. Adjuvant radiation therapy in a dose range of 15 to 25 Gy is often used, without interfering with bone and muscle development.

The combined-modality treatment, as described previously, results in excellent control of HD, with cure rates reported in the 90% to 95% range from various centers. The precise role and contribution of irradiation to the excellent control of the disease in children have not been demonstrated in controlled clinical trials.

Because children have an excellent prognosis, it is desirable to minimize other serious late treatment effects. Sterility and acute leukemia can be reduced by avoiding full

courses of the MOPP or MOPP-like regimens. The anthracycline cumulative dosage should be kept to a minimum because of significant cardiotoxicity effects reported for children cured of acute leukemia. The Stanford group has used three cycles each of MOPP and ABVD, in an alternating sequence, followed by 15 to 25 Gy adjuvant radiation therapy, with excellent disease control and minimal morbidity.[25]

IN PREGNANCY

Women who develop HD during pregnancy pose special therapeutic problems.[26, 27] The potential damage to the developing fetus from radiologic diagnostic studies, therapeutic irradiation, and chemotherapy is an important consideration. Patients and families have philosophic and religious differences in approaching these problems that must be considered.

Generally, women who develop HD in the first trimester of pregnancy are advised to undergo therapeutic abortion. During the first trimester, the embryo and fetus would be seriously damaged by the effects of the diagnostic studies and therapy required for the optimal control of the woman's HD. It is rare that a woman should be allowed to delay the

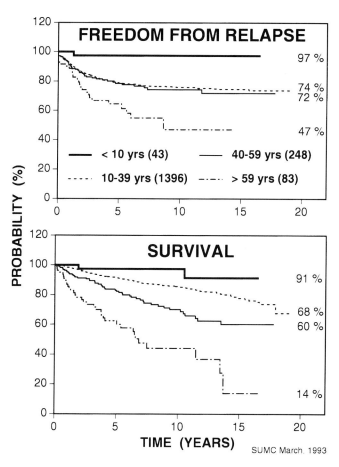

Figure 16–12. Actuarial freedom from relapse (*upper*) and overall survival (*lower*) of 1770 consecutive patients treated at Stanford University Medical Center (SUMC) from 1974 to 1993 according to age at onset. (From Rosenberg SA: The treatment of Hodgkin's disease. Ann Oncol 1994; 5[Suppl 2]:S17.)

6 or more months for the pregnancy to be completed without an effort to stage and treat the HD. In exceptional cases, this can be done, but it is not generally recommended.

Women in the third trimester of pregnancy are generally able to carry the fetus to near full term without difficulty. Patients with clinically favorable disease can undergo a minimum of diagnostic studies (i.e., PA chest radiograph, abdominal ultrasonography, or abdominal MRI) without serious risk to the fetus. Often HD treatment can be delayed until vaginal delivery can be safely induced. Women who have bulky or symptomatic supradiaphragmatic disease can receive partial-dose, or even full-dose, radiation therapy to the neck, axillae, and/or upper mediastinum without serious risk to the developing fetus. Chemotherapy, either a single agent, such as vinblastine, or full-combination chemotherapy, can also be given during the third trimester without damage to the fetus. This is recommended only when the clinical situation demands therapy and cannot be managed temporarily with limited-field irradiation.

The most difficult management decisions arise for women in the second term of their pregnancy. It is difficult to generalize about the range of clinical and emotional issues that are relevant for individual patients. Some women early in the second trimester with advanced or serious disease may accept the recommendation to undergo a therapeutic abortion. Others, because of more favorable disease presentations or patient decisions, can be observed closely, delaying intervention or full diagnostic studies as long as possible. These women are best managed with the advice of a medical team experienced in dealing with these special HD problems.

IN CLINICAL EMERGENCIES

The major clinical emergencies of airway, superior vena caval, ureteral, and biliary obstruction as well as epidural spinal cord and peripheral nerve compression are discussed in previous sections dealing with radiation therapy.

In selected patients and situations, combination chemotherapy or combined-modality therapy more rapidly and completely resolves these emergencies than single-modality approaches. If chemotherapy is used in emergency situations, full diagnostic staging studies may be less reliable. The chemotherapy may also result in relatively serious blood count depressions, predisposing to infectious or bleeding complications that may be dangerous when other serious clinical problems are present.

The physician is cautioned against attempting to reverse the clinical emergency too rapidly or completely if maximal treatment programs are required. Gradual control of these clinical situations usually suffices and allows the full benefit of standard diagnostic and therapeutic programs.

Patients who present with large mediastinal and/or hilar masses pose special problems when they undergo general anesthesia. Even without symptomatic airway obstruction, intubation and especially extubation may be extremely difficult, even catastrophic. Patients may not be easily extubated after general anesthesia or may develop major lung collapse in the presence of large mediastinal HD. It is preferable to obtain the necessary diagnostic biopsy in such patients from sites other than the mediastinum, if possible, or with the patient under local anesthesia, if necessary.

IN ACQUIRED IMMUNE DEFICIENCY SYNDROME

It is not accepted, or established, that patients who are human immunodeficiency virus (HIV) positive have a higher incidence of developing HD. There is a general experience, however, that when HD does occur in these patients, it is more advanced clinically and more difficult to manage.[28]

Occasional patients have only positive HIV serologic tests, have not had opportunistic infections, and have no demonstrable immunodeficiency. Such patients can be managed with the same protocols as HIV-negative patients, but with caution. If unusual or unexpected blood count depressions or opportunistic infections occur, the treatment program should be modified.

In patients with opportunistic infections or significant T4-lymphocyte depression, it is generally preferable to use limited treatment programs primarily oriented to provide palliation. The AIDS patient's prognosis in these settings is usually sufficiently poor to be more grave than the HD. These clinical situations can be quite diverse and challenging and require considerable experience and judgment.

TREATMENT COMPLICATIONS

The acute and long-term complications of the treatment of HD have been discussed in other chapters. These may be secondary to the diagnostic studies used (i.e., postsplenectomy sepsis), irradiation (see Chapter 11), and chemotherapy (see Chapter 12).

Although all the complications are important to recognize and minimize, if possible, the most serious are those that are life threatening. Of those, the secondary malignancies are the most important.[11, 29–32] They include acute nonlymphocytic leukemia, radiation-induced carcinomas and sarcomas, and non-Hodgkin's lymphoma.

Ionizing irradiation is a well-established cause of acute nonlymphocytic leukemia. However, the most important cause of this secondary malignancy after the treatment of HD is chemotherapy. The chemotherapeutic agents responsible are the alkylating agents, including procarbazine. Studies have indicated that the leukemia risk is increased with increasing doses of alkylating agents and with the age of the patient (greater in older age). The data are conflicting as to the role of irradiation in adding to the leukemia risk but generally show little or no contribution to the chemotherapy risk.[33] Studies with adequate numbers and followup indicate that the risk period to develop acute leukemia after treatment of HD is approximately 10 years, with few cases diagnosed after that time. The secondary acute leukemia after treatment of HD often presents after a variable period of myelodysplasia. Patients may have an unexplained anemia and/or thrombocytopenia, and erythroid dysplasia seen on bone marrow examination. The picture is often clarified if cytogenetic studies are done. Characteristic abnormalities of chromosomes 5 and 7 are frequent in the drug-induced secondary leukemia and myelodysplasia. Rarely, the acute leukemia does not evolve completely, and the patient experiences prolonged, often severe, hypoplasia.

The management of HD patients who develop secondary acute leukemia is difficult and usually unsuccessful. If the patient is in remission from HD, the usual treatment of acute nonlymphocytic leukemia is recommended. If bone marrow transplantation is to be considered, it must be with an allogeneic matched donor.

Occurrence of radiation-induced carcinomas and sarcomas after treatment for HD remains one of the most serious problems in managing these patients. Now evolving and being tested are new clinical protocols that are designed to reduce the dose and volume of irradiation while not reducing the excellent HD cure rates that are possible. Solid tumors of a wide variety can be caused by irradiation, and most have been described in patients with HD. One of the most important is secondary carcinoma of the breast. The relative risk of developing breast cancer is not seen until approximately 15 years after treatment. The risk is greatly increased in girls and young women who have received mantle irradiation. Girls younger than 15 years of age when treated have been estimated to have a greater than 100-fold increased risk, those aged 15 to 25 years an approximately 20-fold increased risk, those 25 to 29 years a sevenfold increased risk, and those 30 years of age and over no increased risk.[34] Therefore, these women should have more intensive breast cancer screening performed at an earlier age than for the general population.

Carcinoma of the lung has been the most common secondary cancer documented in various series. In the Stanford series, the risk of this complication was increased in patients who smoked cigarettes. Other major sites of irradiation-induced secondary cancers have been the stomach, thyroid, soft tissues, bones, and skin.

Non-Hodgkin's lymphomas seen in patients treated for HD have been discussed previously. The incidence of this secondary malignancy increases with time after treatment and has reached an actuarial risk of approximately 5% at 25 years, without an apparent plateau, or reduced risk with time. The cause of the non-Hodgkin's lymphoma is unknown, but it is likely to be multifactorial and largely the result of immunosuppression of the disease and therapy.

CHEMOTHERAPY

The history of combination chemotherapy for HD began with the MOPP regimen, and this program has been slowly replaced by attempts to improve results and/or decrease its toxicity. The evolution of this effort has gone from replacing MOPP with an entirely different regimen; alternating MOPP or its variants with other regimens; hybridizing with a half-cycle of MOPP and half of another active regimen; and alternating schedules of weekly administration of chemotherapeutic agents for a total period shorter than the usual 6 to 8 months to escalated doses of active agents requiring stem cell growth factor support. This panoply of chemotherapeutic efforts has resulted in some new information, and for the most part the goal of superiority over MOPP therapy and/or less toxicity has been achieved. There are many unanswered questions, some of which are under investigation; others require prospective clinical trials to solve. Furthermore, there is a continuing need for identification of new agents as well as clarification of the biologic factors in the genesis and maintenance of HD to develop newer biotherapeutic strategies.

CURRENT STATUS OF THE CHEMOTHERAPY OF HODGKIN'S DISEASE IN ADVANCED STAGES

The wide variety of cytotoxic drugs with activity against HD has led to a maze of different regimens for primary and salvage therapy. The biochemical and kinetic bases for the action of these agents are described in Chapter 12. The range is from corticosteroids, alkylating agents, vinca alkaloids, DNA intercalating agents (doxorubicin and mitoxantrone), etoposide, bleomycin, antimetabolites, dacarbazine, and procarbazine. The following review attempts to summarize the current status of the chemotherapy of HD in advanced stages and to define the unanswered questions.

PRIMARY SYSTEMIC THERAPY WITH COMBINATION CHEMOTHERAPY

The clinician has a selection of therapeutic regimens, any of which are appropriate for the systemic treatment of advanced disease or high-risk localized disease. In the latter circumstance, issues of chronic toxicity and interaction with radiation therapy may influence the choice of approach.

The options include single combination chemotherapy given over 6 to 8 months; alternating cycles of two or three regimens; hybrid regimens such as MOPP/ABV; or intensive weekly regimens of short duration. In the setting of localized but high-risk disease, the options could be brief courses of established regimens or regimens altered to avoid the toxicity of alkylating agents and doxorubicin.

Until a few years ago, MOPP or its variants were the standard regimens that demonstrated a cure rate of approximately 50% for previously untreated patients with stage IIIB/IV disease.[12] As with all regimens, the outcome was influenced by clinical prognostic factors; stage, symptoms, performance status, and bulk of tumor; age; and number of extranodal sites in stage IV patients. The major problem with MOPP was its acute toxicity, which was significantly improved by substituting chlorambucil for mechlorethamine (Mustargen), resulting in ChlVPP (chlorambucil, vinblastine, procarbazine, prednisone), or LOPP (Table 16–3).[35] The latter regimens are equivalent to MOPP but without the hair loss, nausea, and vomiting, and with ChlVPP the peripheral neuropathy of vincristine is avoided. The long-term toxicity of sterility and secondary myelodysplasia/leukemia was not corrected and thus prompted a need for an alternative program.

Nonalkylating regimens used as primary or salvage therapy are shown in Table 16–4. The ABVD regimen was developed in Milan and compared with MOPP in various stages with or without radiation therapy.[13, 36–38] In both instances, it was shown to be superior in response and progression-free survival. The ABVD regimen that was the standard second-line regimen became the major front-line regimen on the basis of this data and the fact that permanent sterilization and secondary myelodysplasia were not seen.[28] The major unique toxicities of ABVD were nausea and vomiting induced by dacarbazine and the threat of cardiopulmonary toxicity due to doxorubicin and bleomycin, especially when used with mantle irradiation. The toxicity of the latter circumstance has been quite minimal, and, as such, ABVD is used with irradiation quite generally for lower-stage HD.[39–41]

Table 16–3. Alkylating Agent–Containing Regimens Active in the Treatment of Hodgkin's Disease

Protocol	Dose (mg/m^2)	Days	Reference
MOPP			Longo et al[12]
Mechlorethamine	6	1, 8	
Vincristine	1.4	1, 8	
Procarbazine	100	1–14	
Prednisone	40	1–14	
ChlVPP			International
Chlorambucil	6 (total) PO	1–14	ChlVPP Treatment
Vinblastine	6 (max. 10)	1, 8	Group[35]
Procarbazine	100	1–14	
Prednisone	40	1–14	
LOPP			Hancock et al[44]
Chlorambucil	10 (total)	1–10	
Vincristine	1.4	1, 8	
Procarbazine	100 PO	1–10	
Prednisone	25 PO	1–14	
MOPP/ABV hybrid			Klimo and
Mechlorethamine	6	1	Connors[107]
Vincristine	1.4	1	
Procarbazine	100 PO	1–7	
Prednisone	40 PO	1–14	
Doxorubicin	35	8	
Bleomycin	10	8	
Vinblastine	6	8	
LOPP/EVA hybrid			Hancock et al[47]
Vinblastine	10 (total)	1	
Chlorambucil	10 (total)	1–7	
Procarbazine	50	1–7	
Prednisolone	50	1–7	
Vincristine	2	8	
Doxorubicin	50	8	
Etoposide	200	8	

ALTERNATING AND HYBRID COMBINATION CHEMOTHERAPY

The alternation of MOPP with ABVD for 12 monthly cycles by the Milan group was shown to be superior to MOPP in progression-free survival.[42] This was confirmed in trials by Cancer and Leukemia Group B (CALGB) and the European Organization for the Research and Treatment of Cancer (EORTC), in which progression-free survival was also superior for the alternating regimen.[38, 43] In both trials, there was no difference in overall survival, indicating the chronicity of HD and the ability of salvage therapy to prolong survival. A British National Lymphoma Investigation (BNLI) trial compared LOPP with LOPP alternating with EVAP (etoposide, vinblastine, doxorubicin, prednisone) and found the latter to be superior in relapse-free and overall survival.[44] The alternation of combination chemotherapy regimens entailed a somewhat greater spectrum of toxicity, but they were otherwise well tolerated. All the trials, except the National Cancer Institute (NCI) MOPP/CABS (CCNU, Adriamycin, bleomycin, streptozocin) versus MOPP, showed a superiority for alternating programs over MOPP (Table 16–5). The CALGB trial comparing ABVD alone with MOPP alone or with MOPP alternating with ABVD failed to show a superiority of the alternating program to ABVD alone, although both were superior to MOPP alone in progression-free survival.[38]

The hybrid approach originated with the Vancouver group.[36] Their MOPP/ABV regimen (see Table 16–3) was given for six cycles and generated early excitement. The alternating MOPP/ABVD regimen was promptly compared with the hybrid, and in three published trials no difference was noted (Table 16–6).[37, 45, 46] The BNLI terminated a trial comparing LOPP/EVAP alternating with hybrid LOPP/EVA because of no differences after 160 patients were randomized.[47] The North American Intergroup Trial is currently comparing the MOPP/ABV hybrid with ABVD alone. The large number of patients accrued to that trial suggests no significant early differences. The added risk of mechlorethamine toxicity would require a superiority for the hybrid regimen.

Recently a regimen (Stanford V) has been developed that intensifies the frequency of chemotherapy with weekly administration of drugs over a relatively short period.[48, 49] This program is relatively early in its evaluation and has not achieved wide acceptance, but reduction in the duration of therapy may have a great deal of appeal. A similar approach in the salvage setting is the VAPEC-B regimen (vincristine, doxorubicin, prednisolone, etoposide, cyclophosphamide, bleomycin, prophylactic co-trimoxazole and ketoconazole) (Christie Hospital, Manchester) (Table 16–7). The dose intensity is increased by shortening the interval between drug administrations. Another option would be to increase dose intensity by increasing the doses but retain a traditional schedule. The ultimate dose intensification is high-dose myeloablative therapy with bone marrow or stem cell support (see later).

For patients with compromise of pulmonary function by previous radiation therapy or a premorbid condition such as emphysema and pulmonary fibrosis, the bleomycin compo-

Table 16–4. Nonalkylating Combination Chemotherapy Regimens

Protocol	Dose (mg/m^2)	Days	Reference
ABVD			Bonfante et al[13]
Doxorubicin	25 IV	1, 15	
Bleomycin	10 units	1, 15	
Vinblastine	6	1, 15	
Dacarbazine	375	1, 15	
EVA			Canellos et al[50]
Etoposide	100	1, 2, 3	
Vinblastine	6	1	
Doxorubicin	50	1 q 28 days	
EVAP			Hancock et al[44]
Etoposide	150 PO (200 mg max)	1–3	
Vinblastine	6 (10 mg max)	1, 8	
Doxorubicin	25	1, 8	
Prednisone	25	1, 8	
VEEP			Hill et al[51]
Vincristine	1.4 (2.0 max)	1, 8	
Epirubicin	50	1 q 21 days	
Etoposide	100	1–4	
Prednisolone	100 PO	1–8	
NOVP			Hill et al[51]
Mitoxantrone	10	1	
Vincristine	1.4	8 q 21 days	
Vinblastine	6	1	
Prednisone	100 PO	1–5	

Table 16–5. Randomized Trials Comparing Alternating Combination Chemotherapy Regimens to MOPP or a Variant

Trial	CR Rate	RFS	PFS	Survival	Reference
Milan					Bonadonna[37]
MOPP	74%	46%	37%	58%	
MOPP/ABVD	89%	68%	61%	69%	
P value	NS	.002	.005	NS at 10 yr	
CALGB					Canellos et al[38]
MOPP	67%	48%	50%	64%	
ABVD	82%	64%	62%	72%	
MOPP/ABVD	83%	64%	65%	75%	
P value	.006	—	.02	NS	
ECOG					Glick et al[45]
BCVPP	73%	56%	49%	68%	
MOPP/ABVD	80%	61%	61%	75%	
P value	NS	NS	NS	NS	
EORTC					Somers et al[43]
MOPP	57%	61%	43%	57%	
MOPP/ABVD	59%	69%	60%	65%	
P value	NS	NA	.013	NS	
UK/BNLI					Hancock et al[44]
LOPP	57%	52%	32%	66%	
LOPP/EVAP	64%	72%	47%	75%	
P value	NS	<.001	—	<.05	
NCI/Bethesda					Longo et al[108]
MOPP	91%	65%	68%	80%	
MOPP/CABS	92%	72%	54%	72%	
P value	NS	NS	NS	NS	
Manchester/Bart's					Radford et al[109]
MVPP	55%	—	66%	71%	
ChlVPP/EVA	68%	—	80%	80%	
P value	—	—	NS	NS	

CR, complete response; RFS, relapse-free survival; PFS, progression-free survival; NS, not significant; NA, not applicable; MOPP, ChlVPP, LOPP, see Table 16–3; ABVD, EVAP, EVA, see Table 16–4; BCVPP = BCNU, cyclophosphamide, vinblastine, procarbazine, prednisone; CABS = lomustine, doxorubicin, bleomycin, streptozocin; MVPP = mechlorethamine, vinblastine, procarbazine, prednisone; CALGB, Cancer and Leukemia Group B; ECOG, Eastern Cooperative Oncology Group; EORTC, European Organization for the Research and Treatment of Cancer; UK/BNLI, United Kingdom/British National Lymphoma Investigation; NCI, National Cancer Institute.

nent of ABVD represents a potential threat of pulmonary toxicity, especially when used with mantle irradiation. There are a number of anti-HD regimens without bleomycin that can be given with radiation therapy (see Table 16–4). These include EVA,[50] EVAP,[44] VEEP (vincristine, epirubicin, etoposide, prednisolone),[51] and NOVP (mitoxantrone, vincristine, vinblastine, prednisone).[51] These regimens have had limited investigation but could substitute in the setting in which there is serious concern for pulmonary toxicity due to bleomycin.

The optimal duration of therapy is uncertain even in patients with advanced disease. The duration of chemotherapy plus radiation therapy for patients with poor-prognosis stage I/II disease has varied in numerous series from one cycle of MOPP/ABVD, two cycles of MOPP to more recently demonstrated three cycles of ABVD plus ra-

Table 16–6. Trials in Which Hybrid Regimens of MOPP/ABVD Are Randomized Against Alternating or Sequential Therapy

Trial	CR	RFS	PFS	OS	Reference
Milan					Bonadonna[37]
MOPP/ABVD hybrid	89%	78%	71%	75% (8 yr)	
MOPP/ABVD alternating	91%	76%	69%	74%	
P value	NS	NS	NS	NS	
ECOG					Glick et al[45]
MOPP/ABV	81%	70%	80%	90% (30 mo)	
Sequential MOPP × 6–8, ABVD × 3	76%	56%	67%	85%	
P value	NS	.04	.007	.04	
NCI/Canada					Connors et al[46]
MOPP/ABV	85%	—	75%	84% (5 yr)	
MOPP/ABVD alternating	82%	—	70%	84%	
P value	—	—	NS	NS	

MOPP, see Table 16–3; ABV, ABVD, see Table 16–4; CR, complete remission; RFS, relapse-free survival; PFS, progression-free survival; OS, overall survival; ECOG, Eastern Cooperative Oncology Group; NCI, National Cancer Institute.

Table 16–7. Experimental Dose-Intense Regimens of Short Duration*

Protocol	Dose Regimens	Reference
VAPEC-B—*relapsed patients only*		Radford and
(Manchester University, Christie Hospital)		Crowther[48]
Vincristine	1.4 mg/m² weeks 2, 4, 6, 8, 10	
Doxorubicin	35 mg/m² weeks 1, 3, 5, 7, 9, 11	
Prednisolone	50 mg/day PO weeks 1–6, 25 mg/day weeks 7–11	
Etoposide	100 mg/m² PO days 1–5, weeks 3, 7, 11	
Cyclophosphamide	350 mg/m² IV weeks 1, 5, 9	
Bleomycin	10 mg/m² IV weeks 2, 6, 10	
Prophylactic co-trimoxazole, ketoconazole		
Stanford V (per cycle)—*primary treatment only*		Bartlett et al[49]
Doxorubicin	25 mg/m² days 1, 15	
Vinblastine	6 mg/m² days 1, 15	
Nitrogen mustard	6 mg/m² day 1	
Etoposide	60 mg/m² IV days 15, 16	
Vincristine	1.4 mg/m² (max. 2.0 mg) days 8, 22	
Bleomycin	5 U/m² days 8, 22	
Prednisone	40 mg/m² every other day	
Prophylactic co-trimoxazole, ketoconazole, acyclovir		

*For a total of three cycles over 12 weeks.

diation.[52] The question has not been addressed in prospective trials with the exception of a Canadian trial in which three cycles of MOPP were compared with six cycles of MOPP with extensive radiation therapy in stage III patients. There was an advantage to six cycles of MOPP.[53] The CALGB trial of ABVD or MOPP for six cycles compared with 12 cycles of alternating therapy again showed no advantage for the alternating (12 months) therapy over ABVD (6 months) in patients with stages III₂A/IVB.[38] The newer, more intensified 12-week regimen such as Stanford V appears to be as active as 6 months of ABVD or MOPP/ABV, although it has not been compared in a prospective trial.

The issue of substituting chemotherapy for radiation therapy in stage I/II disease was addressed in several randomized trials comparing MOPP alone with primary radiation therapy. The results of two different randomized trials are conflicting, with MOPP superior in the NCI trial but decidedly inferior in an Italian trial.[54, 55] The use of MOPP alone for localized disease has not been accepted, but the need remains for an effective and nontoxic regimen that can be used alone or with minimal radiation therapy for localized disease. The current use of ABVD for three cycles plus radiation therapy is becoming more widely used for patients with stage I/II disease but with unfavorable prognostic features—without a staging laparotomy.[40]

In almost all series, prognostic factors in advanced-stage disease usually predict the benefits of systemic therapy. Negative prognostic effects were attributable to age older than 40 or 50 years; male sex; a lymphocyte count less than 0.75 × 10⁹/L; stage III or IV; B symptoms; multiple extranodal sites; reduced hemoglobin levels; low serum albumin levels; an increased sedimentation rate; size of mediastinal mass; high serum lactic dehydrogenase levels; and inguinal node involvement. All these have been identified as negative factors by multivariate analyses in various studies.[56–59]

A better definition of the risk for relapse would assist in the planning for innovative or intensive therapies in well-defined patients with poor prognostic features, since the latter in many series have a long-term cure rate of less than 30%.

The results of chemotherapy regimens used in the past suffer from the fact that current imaging technology has improved its sensitivity so that "unconfirmed CR" refers to patients who achieve a prompt regression of tumor masses but with a residual mass on CT or MRI scan. Radionuclide scans with gallium citrate Ga 67 have been useful in assessing residual masses.[60–62] Residual gallium uptake predicts a higher likelihood of relapse at that site in the absence of complementary radiation therapy. However, patients with positive gallium uptake in multiple sites after a full course of chemotherapy have a high chance of relapse. Patients with mediastinal masses (bulky stage II) who achieve a status whereby the gallium uptake is negative despite a residual mass are likely to have a longer disease-free period, especially after complementary radiation therapy.

The role of complementary radiation therapy after a full course (six to eight cycles) of chemotherapy for stage IIIB/IV is still a matter of some debate. The randomized trials are few and conflicting, but it would appear that low doses of irradiation to involved sites in stages IIIB/IV have not been shown to enhance survival. A trial from Argentina showed a significant advantage to adding 3000 cGy to a modification of MOPP as part of initial therapy of stage III/IV compared with chemotherapy alone, but no overall survival advantage was noted at 7 years.[63] The Southwest Oncology Group (SWOG) randomized trial of adjuvant low-dose radiation therapy (2000 cGy) to nodal sites and 1000 to 1500 cGy to other sites after achieving complete remission (CR) with chemotherapy in stage III/IV failed to prolong remission duration or survival. In fact, the results of salvage therapy in the radiation group that relapsed were clearly inferior to the results in the chemotherapy-alone group. The remission duration advantage without a survival effect resided in those patients with nodular sclerosis histologic types or bulky (>6 cm) disease.[64] There are many studies in advanced disease in which combined-modality therapy is used with "good" results, but the long-term toxicity of radiation added to chemotherapy is worthy of concern. Definitions of "bulk" vary from 5 to 10 cm throughout the literature. There may be a clearer role for involved-field radiation therapy to sites of prior bulky disease, especially mediastinal masses more than one third of the thoracic diameter or any mass larger than 10 cm in diameter.[65] Most workers agree that relapse in irradiated sites is unusual, and subsequent relapse tends to occur in unirradiated sites after combination chemotherapy.[66] Despite that, it is difficult to discern a survival advantage from the routine irradiation of all known sites of disease, regardless of extent.

TOXICITY ISSUES IN CHEMOTHERAPY

Acute toxicity of most chemotherapy used in the treatment of HD entails myelosuppression, nausea, vomiting, mucositis, and neurologic sequelae of the vinca alkaloids. In almost all circumstances, the acute toxicity is reversible in time.

Pronounced cumulative myelosuppression resulting in dose modification is more likely in alkylating agent–

containing regimens such as MOPP when compared with a nonalkylating agent–containing regimen such as ABVD.[38] Although hematopoietic growth factors enhance the recovery of neutrophils between cycles, there has been no trial comparing a given regimen with or without a growth factor in the chemotherapy of HD. Trials in other diseases, including large cell lymphoma, have not shown a survival advantage to using growth factors with combination chemotherapy.

UNIQUE CHRONIC TOXICITIES OF ALKYLATING AGENT–CONTAINING REGIMENS

The two major chronic toxicities of the MOPP era were sterilization and secondary myelodysplasia/leukemia. The extent to which procarbazine contributed to these side effects as well has never been clarified, but nitrogen mustard has been considered the major offender.

Azoospermia should be expected in all instances with increased serum follicle-stimulating hormone (FSH) levels, confirming the effect on germinal epithelium. Serum testosterone levels are usually normal, suggesting intact Leydig's cell function.[67] Impaired spermatogenesis appears to be irreversible in most cases after six cycles of chemotherapy, and pretreatment sperm banking is recommended. About three fourths of menstruating women become amenorrheic after treatment with MOPP. Menstrual and reproductive function can return in women in their teens and twenties, but amenorrhea usually persists in women older than 25 years of age. Treated women who retain or return to menstrual function might sustain a premature ovarian failure. At least half of all treated women might require hormone replacement because of estrogen deficiency.[68, 69] Those women who do conceive after systemic therapy appear to have no increased risk of adverse outcomes in the pregnancy.[70]

The alkylating agent–related or historically the MOPP-related myelodysplasia or leukemia syndrome represents the first of the treatment-induced bone marrow disorders. It is usually characterized by a myelodysplastic syndrome with cytogenetic abnormalities in chromosome 5 and/or 7. It usually occurs 3 to 8 years after treatment, and the incidence decreases beyond that time. The risk is determined by the cumulative dose of alkylating agent and an age above 40 years.[29] When the overall risk is considered, other factors, such as the extent of radiation therapy in some series and the absence of splenic function, also contributed to the risk.[30] The cumulative probability of developing leukemia over 20 years is approximately 2%, whereas the overall second solid cancer increases to 18% by 20 years. The late-appearing solid tumors, especially lung and breast cancer, are strongly related to radiation therapy independent of chemotherapy.[31, 32] The risk for non-Hodgkin's lymphoma is also increased.

TOXICITY OF REGIMENS OTHER THAN MOPP

The absence of permanent sterility and secondary myelodysplasia after ABVD regimens and the demonstration of effectiveness equivalent to that of MOPP regimens have led to the widespread use of ABVD and similar regimens without alkylating agents.

Regimens that include doxorubicin and/or bleomycin such as ABVD and BCAVe (bleomycin, CCNU, Adriamycin, Velban) are widely employed, often with radiation therapy, especially in high-risk low-stage disease. Overall, the incidence of clinically significant pulmonary toxicity is low, although most patients who receive radiation and bleomycin have a decrease in carbon monoxide diffusion capacity to less than 70% and abnormalities in total vital capacity. These variables tend to improve in time. The most sensitive test of pulmonary damage is the carbon monoxide diffusion capacity. A recent study of 1145 patients from Stanford, however, showed that despite the absence of clinically severe pulmonary toxicity, mantle irradiation was the major factor associated with persistent mild reduction of forced vital capacity and diffusion capacity. Nonetheless, fatal pulmonary toxicity continues to be seen rarely and unexpectedly in patients treated with radiation and ABVD.[71] The total dose of bleomycin also influences the likelihood of pulmonary toxicity that would be manifest by radiologic changes, minor restrictive defects (~40%), decreases in the diffusion of carbon monoxide (~25%), and some dyspnea on exertion. In the absence of radiation therapy, bleomycin-induced changes are mild and reverse in time. The cardiac toxicity of doxorubicin alone without mediastinal irradiation is minimal, but some abnormalities, such as pericarditis and some decrease in left ventricular ejection, are enhanced in combined-modality treatment. Studies in 49 patients with pulsed Doppler echocardiography 2 to 10 years after chemotherapy with doxorubicin noted pericardial (38%) and valvular thickening (43%) but no cardiomyopathy and no impact on cardiac function.[72]

Cardiac toxicity unique to doxorubicin and separate from radiation therapy is rare. In one study of 40 patients treated with three cycles of ABVD and mantle irradiation, only two had a low ventricular ejection fraction (~50%) with no cardiac symptoms.[73] The cumulative dose of doxorubicin in six cycles of ABVD is 300 mg/m^2, well below the cardiotoxic level when the drug is given independently of radiation. Myocardial infarctions are not increased with ABVD alone, although mediastinal irradiation increases the risk.[74]

The vinca alkaloid–associated peripheral neuropathy is usually reversible. The constipation may require stool softeners and/or other cathartics. Rarely, the steroid-containing regimens may be complicated by avascular necrosis of the femoral head.[75]

High cumulative dosage of etoposide has been associated with a new (epipodophyllin) leukemic syndrome that occurs early (<3 years), without myelodysplasia, monocytoid morphology, and chromosomal abnormality at 11q23 with rearrangement of the acute lymphoblastic leukemia (ALL) gene. This has not been reported in HD series, since etoposide is not widely used except in salvage regimens.

GENERAL PRINCIPLES OF SALVAGE THERAPY

Most patients who relapse after primary radiation therapy for early-stage HD are considered candidates for systemic chemotherapy. This relapse occurs in about 30% of early-stage patients, usually within 3 years after treatment. The

Stanford series, however, showed 13% of patients relapsing late, from 3 to 20 years.[76] The EORTC series showed 37 of 1082 (3.5%) relapsing after 5 years.[77] The ability to successfully treat patients in relapse who originally had localized disease (I/II) treated only with radiation therapy is high. These patients usually relapse in previously unirradiated sites. The overall CR rate is high, and in three series the long-term (10-year) overall event-free survival was 53% to 56% when all patients were considered.[78–80] Special precautions may be necessary for pulmonary toxicity when bleomycin is given to patients who have had extensive thoracic radiation. Prior pelvic radiation may compromise bone marrow reserve. Otherwise, in most series, the ability of cytotoxic therapy to salvage such patients is similar to or better than that in patients presenting in advanced stages previously untreated.

Generally, patients who relapse after systemic therapy have a poorer outcome with conventional-dose second-line chemotherapy. Most second-line chemotherapy trials in patients whose first remission lasts less than 12 months achieve an approximately 20% 5-year failure-free survival, and this is the best that one can expect for conventional-dose therapy.[81–83] The variable results with second-line chemotherapy reflect the varied prognostic factors that may predict outcome after salvage therapy. These factors have been reviewed for several series and include the duration of first CR; whether a second-line CR is achieved; age; B symptoms; bulk; and number of extranodal sites.

In the NCI/Bethesda series, the group that achieved a second CR (49% of the whole group) had a 34% disease-free survival (45% in those whose first remission lasted more than a year).[81] This is still a small fraction of overall salvage, 16% at 20 years.

The Vancouver group analyzed a series of 71 patients receiving second-line therapy and found that stage IV at initial diagnosis, first remission at less than 1 year, and B symptoms at relapse predicted a 5-year failure-free survival of 17%, whereas the absence of these features had an associated 82% second-line failure-free survival.[82] Unfavorable prognostic factors predict a relatively poor second-line outcome regardless of primary therapy (four drugs, or seven or eight drugs). Poor prognostic features might direct patients to high-dose chemotherapy programs with supportive stem cell therapy. However, it remains to be seen whether this more intensive therapy can overcome poor risk factors.

The choice of second-line therapy is probably less important than the prognostic features, since even a repeat of the same induction regimen, such as MOPP and alternating with ABVD or a hybrid, can achieve a second CR in favorable (long first CR) patients.[81–84] Most patients who relapse after chemotherapy for advanced disease have effectively received MOPP (or variants) and ABVD (or variants) in sequence, alternating, or as a hybrid. Consideration of third-line therapy is for either treatment or preparation for HDT. Many varieties of third-line regimens have been employed containing etoposide and nitrosoureas (Table 16–8). The CR rate varies between 20% and 40%, with most third-line responses lasting a median of 12 to 18 months with rare long-term survivors.[85–91] It is impossible to ascertain the superiority of one therapy over the other. In the era when MOPP or its variants were the sole primary chemotherapy, ABVD was the main second-line regimen. The changing face of primary chemotherapy to using ABVD alone as primary therapy would presuppose the use of MOPP-like regimens as second-line salvage. In the CALGB prospective, randomized trial comparing MOPP with ABVD, there was a crossover for early failure showing that MOPP after ABVD is somewhat superior to ABVD after MOPP for achieving second-line failure-free survival (33% versus 17% 5-year failure-free survival).[38]

Rarely, late isolated failure in limited lymph node sites in asymptomatic (selected) patients may be salvaged by radiation therapy alone, resulting in 30% to 50% 5-year relapse-free survival.[14, 92, 93]

HIGH-DOSE THERAPY WITH AUTOLOGOUS BONE MARROW AND/OR PERIPHERAL STEM CELL TRANSPLANTATION

HDT is discussed in greater detail in Chapter 13. The principle of residual drug sensitivity in some patients with relapsing HD is the basis for HDT. The presumed dose-responses for certain escalatable drugs such as alkylating agents (cyclophosphamide, melphalan, bis-chloroethyl-nitrosourea [BCNU], and etoposide) have been the basis for their incorporation into myeloablative regimens.

Since a large fraction of patients will have received prior mediastinal or extensive nodal radiation therapy, "drug only" regimens have been the mainstay of high-dose ablative regimens (Table 16–9).

Table 16–8. Third-Line Etoposide-Containing Salvage Regimens for Patients Who Failed MOPP/ABVD

Protocol	No. Evaluable	CR (%)	CR + PR (%)	Reference
Lomustine/etoposide/prednimustine	58	40	54	Santoro et al[86]
Lomustine/etoposide/methotrexate	32	13	47	Tseng et al[87]
Methyl-GAG/ifosfamide/methotrexate/etoposide (MIME)	43	23	60	Hagemeister et al[88]
Etoposide/vincristine/doxorubicin (EVA)	19	32	58	Richards et al[89]
Vincristine/prednisolone/etoposide/chlorambucil (OPEC)	15	7	27	Barnett et al[90]
Lomustine/etoposide/vindesine/dexamethasone (CEVD)	32	44	56	Pfreundschuh et al[91]
CCNU/melphalan/etoposide (CAV)	58	29	48	Brusamolino et al[92]
Etoposide/doxorubicin/cyclophosphamide/vincristine/bleomycin/prednisolone (VAPEC-B)	20	30	50	Radford and Crowther[48]

CR, complete response; PR, partial response; MOPP, see Table 16–3; ABVD, see Table 16–4; methyl-GAG = methylglyoxal-bis-guanylhydrazone.

Table 16–9. Myeloablative Regimens with Peripheral or Bone Marrow Stem Cell Support Used in the Salvage Therapy of Hodgkin's Disease

Protocol	Dose Regimen	Reference
CBV		Bierman et al[95]
Cyclophosphamide	1.5 g/m²/days × 4 days (day −6 to −3)	
BCNU (carmustine)	300 mg/m²/day × 1, day −6	
VP-16 (etoposide)	125–150 mg/m² b.i.d. × 3, days −6 to −4	
Augmented CBV (Vancouver)		
C	1.8 g/m²	
B	600 mg/m²	
V	400 mg/m²	
CBVP (Vancouver)		Reece et al[96]
Cyclophosphamide	1.8 g/m²/day, days −6 to −3	
Cisplatin	50 mg/m²/day, days −7 to −5	
BCNU	500 mg/m²/day × 1, day −2	
preceded by		
Etoposide	2400 mg/m² infused over 34 hr, day −7	
BEAM		Chopra et al[97]
BCNU	300 mg/m² × 1, day −6	
Etoposide	200 mg/m² b.i.d. days −5 to −2	
Cytarabine (Ara-C)	200 mg/m² b.i.d., days −5 to −2	
Melphalan	140 mg/m² × 1, day −1	
BEAC		Rapoport et al[98]
BCNU	300 mg/m² × 1, day −7	
Etoposide	100 mg/m² b.i.d., days −6 to −3	
Ara-C	100 mg/m² b.i.d., days −6 to −3	
Cyclophosphamide	35 mg/kg/day × 4, days −6 to −3	
Other Regimens		
Etoposide	60 mg/kg × 1 infused over 5 hr, day −4	Crump et al[99]
Melphalan	160 mg/m² × 1, day −3	
Total body irradiation	1200 cGy: 120 cGy × 10 or 200 cGy × 6, days −8 to −5	Nademanee et al[100]
Followed by		
Etoposide	60 mg/kg × 1, day −4	
Cyclophosphamide	100 mg/kg × 1, day −2	

The impact of high-dose myeloablative therapy was assessed in six publications from 1993 to 1995 with a total of 546 patients (Table 16–10).[94–99] The continuous progression-free survival varied from 64% at 4 years (Vancouver) with a median followup of 28 months when autologous bone marrow transplantation (ABMT) was performed at first relapse to 25% at 4 years (Nebraska) with a median followup time of 77 months. It is impossible to say which myeloablative regimen is optimal. The ABMT-associated lethal toxicity rate was 11%. The survival curves have not achieved a clear plateau because of late relapses and unexpected deaths. All these issues as well as the clinical status of the patients enter into the decision to offer HDT. Clinical prognostic factors and patient selection influence the outcome of all salvage therapies, including ABMT. These are outlined for conventional-dose chemotherapy as well as ABMT in Table 16–11. The definition of bulk varied from 2 to 10 cm, depending on the series. The major prognostic factors that are determined by multivariate analysis and are relatively consistent among series include the remission status; a relapse in prior radiated sites; the number of prior chemotherapy regimens; the performance status; the bulk of disease; B symptoms; extranodal relapse; and a first remission at less than 12 months.

Patients with bulky disease, refractory to multiple regimens and producing compromising constitutional symptoms, do extremely poorly with ABMT. In light of the favorable effects of second-line conventional chemotherapy in some patients whose first relapse occurs at more than 12 months in nodal sites and without symptoms, the advantage of HDT in such patients is uncertain, and HDT may be best reserved for the second relapse.[101]

The poor results of unconventional-dose salvage in most other settings would suggest that HDT might be considered after preparative conventional-dose chemotherapy to assess the responsiveness of the disease. Whether there is a place for HDT as part of the initial therapy of advanced HD will be determined by prospective trials in patients who are universally accepted to have poor prognostic features at presentation.

The adjunctive use of HDT has already been investigated within a pilot trial in a small number of patients.[102] The encouraging results should be a stimulus to develop a prognostic scheme for poor outcomes with conventional-dose therapy to avoid HDT in patients already cured of their disease.

Table 16–10. Overall Results of ABMT in Hodgkin's Disease (1993 to 1995)

Series	Date	Total No. of Patients	Progression-Free Survival (%)	Time (Yr)	Median Followup (Mo)	Toxic Deaths (No.)	Reference
City of Hope	1995	85	52	3	28	11	Nademanee et al[100]
Vancouver	1994	58	64	4	27	3	Reece et al[96]
Toronto	1993	73	38.6	4	30	7	Crump et al[99]
Nebraska	1993	128	25	4	77	11	Bierman et al[95]
Rochester	1993	47	49	3	24	8	Rapoport et al[98]
UCH/London	1993	155	50	5	36	20	Chopra et al[97]
Total		546				60	

UCH, University College Hospital; ABMT, autologous bone marrow transplantation.

Table 16–11. Poor Prognostic Risk Factors in Salvage Therapy After Relapse from Primary Systemic Therapy

Conventional-dose therapy
Duration of first complete response <12 mo
B symptoms at relapse
Performance status at relapse
New extranodal sites at relapse

High-dose therapy with autologous marrow or peripheral cell support (multivariate analysis of two series)
Number of prior chemotherapy regimens
B symptoms at relapse
Bulk disease
Length of complete response <1 yr
Extranodal disease at relapse
Performance status

GENERAL RECOMMENDATION OF SALVAGE THERAPY

As a general approach, early failure or late failure with poor prognostic features might be considered for HDT and ABMT. Patients who present with asymptomatic late relapses can be treated with conventional-dose chemotherapy to achieve a CR. If CR or maximal partial remission is *not* obtained, then ABMT should be considered. The choice of salvage regimen should be determined by prior chemotherapy.

If ABVD, VEEP, EVAP, or EVA fails, then an alkylating agent–containing regimen would be appropriate. Patients in whom early alternating MOPP-ABVD or hybrid regimens fail might benefit from a third-line regimen containing etoposide. Varied chemotherapeutic approaches have been applied to preparing patients for HDT. They include lower doses of the ablative regimen known as BEAM(-miniBEAM) (BCNU, 60 mg/m^2/day on day 1; etoposide, 75 mg/m^2/day on days 2 to 5; cytarabine [ara-C], 100 mg/m^2 twice a day on days 2 to 5; melphalan, 30 mg/m^2/day on day 6) with a high response rate of 84%[103]; the DHAP (dexamethasone, high-dose ara-C, cisplatin) regimen used for non-Hodgkin's lymphoma[104]; high-dose ara-C, 3 g/m^2 every 12 hours on days 1 and 2 and mitoxantrone, 10 mg/m^2 on days 3 to 5[105]; and the VAPEC-B regimen (see Table 16–7).

Few trials have investigated biologic agents. Interferon has been generally discarded as a salvage agent. Immunotoxins entailing a fusion of a cytotoxin to antibodies have had limited experience. DAB$_{486}$ IL-2 is a fusion between interleukin-2 (IL-2) and diphtheria toxin targeted to cells containing an IL-2 receptor. One of four patients responded with a prolonged remission.[106]

REFERENCES

Clinical Aspects

1. Kaplan HS: Hodgkin's disease, 2d ed. Cambridge, Harvard University Press, 1980.
2. Rosenberg SA: Hodgkin's disease: No stage beyond cure. Hosp Pract 1986; 21:91.
3. Rosenberg SA, Kaplan HS: Evidence for an orderly progression in the spread of Hodgkin's disease. Cancer Res 1966; 26:1255.
4. Hodgkin T: On some morbid appearances of the absorbed glands and spleen. Med Chir Trans 1832; 17:68.
5. Kaplan HS, Dorfman RF, Nelsen T, et al: Staging laparotomy and splenectomy in Hodgkin's disease: Analysis of indications and patterns of involvement in 285 consecutive, unselected patients. Natl Cancer Inst Monogr 1973; 36:291.
6. Carbone PP, Kaplan HS, Musshoff K, et al: Report of the committee on Hodgkin's disease staging classification. Cancer Res 1971; 31:1860.
7. Lister TA, Crowther D, Sutcliffe SB, et al: Report of a committee convened to discuss the evaluation and staging of patients with Hodgkin's disease: Cotswolds Meeting. J Clin Oncol 1989; 7:1630.
8. Kadin ME, Donaldson SS, Dorfman RF: Isolated granulomas in Hodgkin's disease. N Engl J Med 1970; 283:895.
9. Siber GR, Weitzman SA, Aisenberg AC, et al: Impaired antibody response to pneumococcal vaccine after treatment for Hodgkin's disease. N Engl J Med 1978; 299:442.
10. Krikorian JG, Burke JS, Rosenberg SA, et al: Occurrence of non-Hodgkin's lymphoma after therapy for Hodgkin's disease. N Engl J Med 1979; 300:452.
11. Tucker MA, Coleman CN, Cox RS, et al: Risk of second cancers after treatment for Hodgkin's disease. N Engl J Med 1988; 318:76.

Management

12. Longo DL, Young RC, Wesley M, et al: Twenty years of MOPP therapy for Hodgkin's disease. J Clin Oncol 1986; 4:1295.
13. Bonfante V, Santoro A, Viviani S, et al: ABVD in the treatment of Hodgkin's disease. Semin Oncol 1992; 19(Suppl 5):38.
14. Roach M III, Kapp DS, Rosenberg SA, Hoppe RT: Radiotherapy with curative intent: An option in selected patients relapsing after chemotherapy for advanced Hodgkin's disease. J Clin Oncol 1987; 5:550.
15. Brada M, Eeles R, Ashley S, et al: Salvage radiotherapy in recurrent Hodgkin's disease. Ann Oncol 1992; 3:131.
16. Hoppe RT: The management of bulky mediastinal Hodgkin's disease. Hematol Oncol Clin North Am 1989; 3:265.
17. Bonadonna G, Valagussa P, Santoro A: Prognosis of bulky Hodgkin's disease treated with chemotherapy alone or combined with radiotherapy. Cancer Surv 1985; 4:439.
18. Crnkovich MJ, Leopold K, Hoppe RT, Mauch PM: Stage I to IIB Hodgkin's disease: The combined experience at Stanford University and the Joint Center for Radiation Therapy. J Clin Oncol 1987; 5:1041.
19. Hoppe RT, Rosenberg SA, Kaplan HS, Cox RS: Prognostic factors in pathological stage IIIA Hodgkin's disease. Cancer 1980; 46:1240.
20. Stein RS, Hilborn RM, Flexner JM, et al: Anatomical substages of stage III Hodgkin's disease: Implications for staging, therapy, and experimental design. Cancer 1978; 42:429.
21. Stein RS, Golomb HM, Diggs CH, et al: Anatomic substages of stage IIIA Hodgkin's disease: A collaborative study. Ann Intern Med 1980; 92:159.
22. Regula DP Jr, Hoppe RT, Weiss LM: Nodular and diffuse types of lymphocyte predominance Hodgkin's disease. N Engl J Med 1988; 318:214.
23. Bonfante V, Santoro A, Viviani S, et al: ABVD plus radiotherapy (subtotal nodal versus involved field) in early-stage Hodgkin's disease [Abstract]. Proc ASCO 1994; 13:373.
24. Klasa RJ, Connors J, Hoskins P, et al: Early-stage Hodgkin's disease: Impact of brief chemotherapy together with radiotherapy without staging laparotomy [Abstract]. Proc ASCO 1994; 13:372.
25. Donaldson SS: Hodgkin's disease in children. Semin Oncol 1990; 17:36.
26. Ward FT, Weiss RB: Lymphoma and pregnancy. Semin Oncol 1989; 16:397.
27. Jacobs CD, Donaldson SS, Rosenberg SA, Kaplan HS: Management of the pregnant patient with Hodgkin's disease. Ann Intern Med 1981; 95:669.
28. Prior E, Goldberg AF, Conjaka MS, et al: Hodgkin's disease in homosexual men: An AIDS-related phenomenon? Am J Med 1986; 81:1085.
29. Van Leeuwen FE, Chorus AMJ, van den Belt-Dusebout AW, et al: Leukemia risk following Hodgkin's disease: Relation to cumulative dose of alkylating agents, treatment with teniposide combinations, number of episodes of chemotherapy, and bone marrow damage. J Clin Oncol 1994; 12:1063.

30. Dietrich P-Y, Henry-Amar M, Cosset J-M, et al: Second primary cancers in patients continuously disease-free from Hodgkin's disease: A protective role for the spleen? Blood 1994; 84:1209.

31. Van Leeuwen FE, Klokman WJ, Hagenbeek A, et al: Second cancer risk following Hodgkin's disease: A 20-year follow-up study. J Clin Oncol 1994; 12:312.

32. Henry-Amar M: Second cancer after the treatment for Hodgkin's disease: A report from the International Database on Hodgkin's Disease. Ann Oncol 1992; 3(4):S117.

33. Kaldor JM, Day NE, Clarke EA, et al: Leukemia following Hodgkin's disease. N Engl J Med 1990; 322:7.

34. Hancock SL, Tucker MA, Hoppe RT: Breast cancer after treatment of Hodgkin's disease. J Natl Cancer Inst 1993; 85:25.

35. The International ChlVPP Treatment Group: ChlVPP therapy for Hodgkin's disease: Experience of 960 patients. Ann Oncol 1995; 6:167.

36. Santoro A, Bonadonna G, Valagussa P, et al: Long-term results of combined chemotherapy-radiotherapy approach in Hodgkin's disease: Superiority of ABVD plus radiotherapy versus MOPP plus radiotherapy. J Clin Oncol 1987; 5:27.

37. Bonadonna G: Modern treatment of malignant lymphomas: A multidisciplinary approach? Ann Oncol 1994; 5:25.

38. Canellos GP, Anderson JR, Propert KJ, et al: Chemotherapy of advanced Hodgkin's disease with MOPP, ABVD, or MOPP alternating with ABVD. N Engl J Med 1992; 327:1478.

39. Eghbali H, Bonichon F, David B, et al: Combination of ABVD and radiotherapy in early stages of Hodgkin's disease: Analysis of a series of 94 patients. Radiother Oncol 1990; 18:127.

40. Carde P, Hagenbeek A, Hayat M, et al: Clinical staging versus laparotomy and combined modality with MOPP versus ABVD in early-stage Hodgkin's disease: The H6 twin randomized trials from the European Organization for Research and Treatment of Cancer Lymphoma Cooperative Group. J Clin Oncol 1993; 11:2258.

41. Brusamolino E, Lazzarino M, Orlandi E, et al: Early-stage Hodgkin's disease: Long-term results with radiotherapy alone or combined radiotherapy and chemotherapy. Ann Oncol 1994; 5:2101.

42. Bonadonna G, Valagussa P, Santoro A: Alternating noncross-resistant combination chemotherapy or MOPP in stage IV Hodgkin's disease. Ann Intern Med 1986; 104:739.

43. Somers R, Carde P, Henry-Amar M, et al: A randomized study in stage IIIB and IV Hodgkin's disease comparing eight courses of MOPP versus an alternation of MOPP with ABVD: A European Organization for Research and Treatment of Cancer Lymphoma Cooperative Group and Groupe Pierre-et-Marie-Curie controlled clinical trial. J Clin Oncol 1994; 12:279.

44. Hancock BW, Vaughan Hudson G, Vaughan Hudson B, et al: LOPP alternating with EVAP is superior to LOPP alone in the initial treatment of advanced Hodgkin's disease: Results of a British National Lymphoma Investigation trial. J Clin Oncol 1992; 10:1252.

45. Glick J, Tsiatis A, Schilsky R, et al: A randomized phase III trial of MOPP/ABV hybrid versus sequential MOPP-ABVD in advanced Hodgkin's disease: Preliminary results of the Intergroup trial [Abstract 941]. Proc ASCO 1991; 10:271.

46. Connors JM, Klimo P, Adams G, et al: MOPP/ABV hybrid versus alternating MOPP/ABVD for advanced Hodgkin's disease [Abstract 1073]. Proc ASCO 1992; 11:317.

47. Hancock BW, Vaughan Hudson G, Vaughan Hudson B, et al: Hybrid LOPP/EVA is not better than LOPP alternating with EVAP: A prematurely terminated British National Lymphoma Investigation randomized trial. Ann Oncol 1994; 5(2):S117.

48. Radford JA, Crowther D: Treatment of relapsed Hodgkin's disease using a weekly chemotherapy of short duration: Results of a pilot study in 20 patients. Ann Oncol 1991; 2:505.

49. Bartlett NL, Rosenberg SA, Hoppe RT, et al: Brief chemotherapy, Stanford V, and adjuvant radiotherapy for bulky or advanced stage Hodgkin's disease: A preliminary report. J Clin Oncol 1995; 13:1080.

50. Canellos GP, Petroni GR, Barcos M, et al: Etoposide, vinblastine, and doxorubicin: An active regimen for the treatment of Hodgkin's disease in relapse following MOPP. J Clin Oncol 1995; 13:2005.

51. Hill M, Milan S, Cunningham D, et al: Evaluation of the efficacy of the VEEP regimen in adult Hodgkin's disease with assessment of gonadal and cardiac toxicity. J Clin Oncol 1995; 13:387.

52. Hagemeister FB, Purugganan R, Fuller L, et al: Treatment of early stages of Hodgkin's disease with Novantrone, vincristine, vinblastine, prednisone, and radiotherapy. Semin Hematol 1994; 31:36.

53. Preti A, Hagemeister FB, McLaughlin P, et al: Hodgkin's disease with a mediastinal mass greater than 10 cm: Results of four different treatment approaches. Ann Oncol 1994; 5(2):S97.

54. Yelle L, Bergsagel D, Basco V, et al: Combined modality therapy of Hodgkin's disease: Ten-year results of National Cancer Institute of Canada clinical trials group multicenter clinical trial. J Clin Oncol 1991; 9:1983.

55. Longo DL, Glatstein E, Duffey PL, et al: Radiation therapy versus combination chemotherapy in the treatment of early-stage Hodgkin's disease: Seven-year results of a prospective, randomized trial. J Clin Oncol 1991; 9:906.

56. Biti GP, Cimino G, Cartoni C, et al: Extended-field radiotherapy is superior to MOPP chemotherapy for the treatment of pathologic stage I-IIA Hodgkin's disease: Eight-year update of an Italian prospective randomized study. J Clin Oncol 1992; 10:378.

57. Straus DJ, Gaynor JJ, Myers J, et al: Prognostic factors among 185 adults with newly diagnosed advanced Hodgkin's disease treated with alternating potentially noncross-resistant chemotherapy and intermediate-dose radiation therapy. J Clin Oncol 1990; 8:1173.

58. Proctor SJ, Taylor P, Dopnnan P, et al: A numerical prognostic index for clinical use in identification of poor-risk patients with Hodgkin's disease at diagnosis. Eur J Cancer 1991; 27:624.

59. Wagstaff J, Gregory WM, Swindell R, et al: Prognostic factors for survival in stage IIIB and IV Hodgkin's disease: A multivariate analysis comparing two specialist treatment centres. Br J Cancer 1988; 58:487.

60. Oza AM, Ganesan TS, Leahy M, et al: Patterns of survival in patients with Hodgkin's disease: Long follow-up in a single centre. Ann Oncol 1993; 4:385.

61. Cooper DL, Caride VJ, Zloty M, et al: Gallium scans in patients with mediastinal Hodgkin's disease treated with chemotherapy. J Clin Oncol 1993; 11:1092.

62. Hagemeister FB, Purugganan R, Podoloff DA, et al: The gallium scan predicts relapse in patients with Hodgkin's disease treated with combined modality therapy. Ann Oncol 1994; 5(2):S59.

63. Front D, Israel O: The role of GA-67 scintigraphy in evaluating the results of therapy of lymphoma patients. Semin Nucl Med 1995; 25:60.

64. Pavlovsky S, Santarelli MT, Sackmann Muriel F, et al: Randomized trial of chemotherapy versus chemotherapy plus radiotherapy for stage III-IV A and B Hodgkin's disease. Ann Oncol 1992; 3:533.

65. Fabian CJ, Mansfield CM, Dahlberg S, et al: Low-dose involved-field radiation after chemotherapy in advanced Hodgkin's disease. Ann Intern Med 1994; 120:90.

66. Longo DL, Russo A, Duffey PL, et al: Treatment of advanced-stage massive mediastinal Hodgkin's disease: The case for combined modality treatment. J Clin Oncol 1991; 9:227.

67. Yahalom J, Ryu J, Straus DJ, et al: Impact of adjuvant radiation on the patterns and rate of relapse in advanced-stage Hodgkin's disease treated with alternating chemotherapy combinations. J Clin Oncol 1991; 9:2193.

68. Clark ST, Radford JA, Crowther D, et al: Gonadal function following chemotherapy for Hodgkin's disease: A comparative study of MVPP and a seven-drug hybrid regimen. J Clin Oncol 1995; 13:134.

69. Andrieu JM, Ochoa-Molina ME: Menstrual cycle, pregnancies and offspring before and after MOPP therapy for Hodgkin's disease. Cancer 1983; 52:435.

70. Whitehead E, Shalet SM, Blackledge G, et al: The effect of combination chemotherapy on ovarian function in women treated for Hodgkin's disease. Cancer 1983; 52:988.

71. Janov AJ, Anderson J, Cella DF, et al: Pregnancy outcome in survivors of advanced Hodgkin disease. Cancer 1992; 70:688.

72. Horning SJ, Adhikari A, Rizk N, et al: Effect of treatment for Hodgkin's disease on pulmonary function: Results of a prospective study. J Clin Oncol 1994; 12:297.

73. Kreuser E-D, Vller H, Behles C, et al: Evaluation of late cardiotoxicity with pulsed Doppler echocardiography in patients treated for Hodgkin's disease. Br J Haematol 1993; 84:615.

74. Brice P, Tredanie LJ, Monsuez JJ, et al: Cardiopulmonary toxicity after three courses of ABVD and mediastinal irradiation in favorable Hodgkin's disease. Ann Oncol 1991; 2:273.

75. Cosset JM, Henry-Amar M, Meerwaldt JH for the EORTC Lymphoma Cooperative Group: Long-term toxicity of early stages of Hodgkin's disease therapy: The EORTC experience. Ann Oncol 1991; 2:277.

76. Thorne JC, Evans WK, Alison RE, Fournasier V: Avascular necrosis

of bone complicating treatment of malignant lymphoma. Am J Med 1981; 71:751.

77. Herman TS, Hoppe RT, Donaldson SS, et al: Late relapse among patients treated for Hodgkin's disease. Ann Intern Med 1985; 102:292.

78. Bodis S, Henry-Amar M, Bosq J, et al: Late relapse in early-stage Hodgkin's disease patients enrolled on European Organization for Research and Treatment of Cancer protocols. J Clin Oncol 1993; 11:225.

79. Healey EA, Tarbell NJ, Kalish LA, et al: Prognostic factors for patients with Hodgkin's disease in first relapse. Cancer 1993; 71:2613.

80. Olver IN, Wolf MM, Cruickshank D, et al: Nitrogen mustard, vincristine, procarbazine, and prednisolone for relapse after radiation in Hodgkin's disease. Cancer 1988; 62:233.

81. Roach M III, Brophy N, Cox R, et al: Prognostic factors for patients relapsing after radiotherapy for early-stage Hodgkin's disease. J Clin Oncol 1990; 8:623.

82. Longo DL, Duffey PL, Young RC, et al: Conventional-dose salvage combination chemotherapy in patients relapsing with Hodgkin's disease after combination chemotherapy: The low probability for cure. J Clin Oncol 1992; 10:210.

83. Lohri A, Barnett M, Fairey RN, et al: Outcome of treatment of first relapse of Hodgkin's disease after primary chemotherapy: Identification of risk factors from the British Columbia experience, 1970 to 1988. Blood 1991; 77:2292.

84. Harker GW, Kushlan P, Rosenberg SA: Combination chemotherapy for advanced Hodgkin's disease after failure of MOPP: ABVD and B-CAVe. Ann Intern Med 1984; 101:440.

85. Viviani S, Santoro A, Negretti E, et al: Salvage chemotherapy in Hodgkin's disease. Ann Oncol 1990; 1:123.

86. Santoro A, Viviani S, Valagussa P, et al: CCNU, etoposide, and prednimustine (CEP) in refractory Hodgkin's disease. Semin Oncol 1986; 13:23.

87. Tseng A Jr, Jacobs C, Coleman CN, et al: Third-line chemotherapy for resistant Hodgkin's disease with lomustine, etoposide, and methotrexate. Cancer Treat Rep 1987; 71:475.

88. Hagemeister FB, Tannir N, McLaughlin P, et al: MIME chemotherapy (methyl-GAG ifosfamide, methotrexate, etoposide) as treatment for recurrent Hodgkin's disease. J Clin Oncol 1987; 5:556.

89. Richards MA, Waxman JH, Man T, et al: EVA treatment for recurrent or unresponsive Hodgkin's disease. Cancer Chemother Pharmacol 1986; 18:51.

90. Barnett MJ, Man AM, Richards MA, et al: OPEC chemotherapy (vincristine, prednisolone, etoposide and chlorambucil) for refractory and recurrent Hodgkin's disease. Hematol Oncol 1987; 5:79.

91. Pfreundschuh MG, Schoppe WD, Fuchs R, et al: Lomustine, etoposide, vindesine, and dexamethasone (CEVD) in Hodgkin's lymphoma refractory to cyclophosphamide, vincristine, procarbazine, and prednisone (COPP) and doxorubicin, bleomycin, vinblastine, and dacarbazine (ABVD): A multicenter trial of the German Hodgkin Study Group. Cancer Treat Rep 1987; 71:1203.

92. Brusamolino E, Orlandi E, Canevari A, et al: Results of CAV regimen (CCNU, melphalan, and VP-16) as third-line salvage therapy for Hodgkin's disease. Ann Oncol 1994; 5:427.

93. Brada M, Eeles R, Ashley S, et al: Salvage radiotherapy in recurrent Hodgkin's disease. Ann Oncol 1992; 3:131.

94. Uematsu M, Tarbell NJ, Silver B, et al: Wide-field radiation therapy with or without chemotherapy for patients with Hodgkin disease in relapse after initial combination chemotherapy. Cancer 1993; 207.

95. Bierman PJ, Bagin RG, Jagannath S, et al: High-dose chemotherapy followed by autologous hematopoietic rescue in Hodgkin's disease: Long-term follow-up in 128 patients. Ann Oncol 1993; 4:767.

96. Reece DE, Connors JM, Spinelli JJ, et al: Intensive therapy with cyclophosphamide, carmustine, etoposide ± cisplatin, and autologous bone marrow transplantation for Hodgkin's disease in first relapse after combination chemotherapy. Blood 1994; 83:1193.

97. Chopra R, McMillan AK, Linch DC, et al: The place of high-dose BEAM therapy and autologous bone marrow transplantation in poor-risk Hodgkin's disease: A single-center eight-year study of 155 patients. Blood 1993; 81:1137.

98. Rapoport AP, Rowe JM, Kouides PA, et al: One hundred autotransplants for relapsed or refractory Hodgkin's disease and lymphoma: Value of pretransplant disease status for predicting outcome. J Clin Oncol 1993; 11:2351.

99. Crump M, Smith AM, Brandwein J, et al: High-dose etoposide and melphalan, and autologous bone marrow transplantation for patients with advanced Hodgkin's disease: Importance of disease status at transplant. J Clin Oncol 1993; 11:704.

100. Nademanee A, O'Donnell MR, Snyder DS, et al: High-dose chemotherapy with or without total-body irradiation followed by autologous bone marrow and/or peripheral blood stem cell transplantation for patients with relapsed and refractory Hodgkin's disease: Results in 85 patients with analysis of prognostic factors. Blood 1995; 85:1381.

101. Desch CE, Lasala MR, Smith TJ, Hillner BE: The optimal timing of autologous bone marrow transplantation in Hodgkin's disease patients after a chemotherapy relapse. J Clin Oncol 1992; 10:200.

102. Carella AM, Carlier P, Congiu A, et al: Autologous bone marrow transplantation as adjuvant treatment for high-risk Hodgkin's disease in first complete remission after MOPP/ABVD protocol. Bone Marrow Transplant 1991; 8:99.

103. Colwill R, Crump M, Couture F, et al: Mini-BEAM as salvage therapy for relapsed or refractory Hodgkin's disease before intensive therapy and autologous bone marrow transplantation. J Clin Oncol 1995; 13:396.

104. Brandwein JM, Callum J, Sutcliffe SB, et al: Evaluation of cytoreductive treatment prior to high-dose treatment with autologous bone marrow transplantation in relapsed and refractory Hodgkin's disease. Bone Marrow Transplant 1990; 5:99.

105. Hiddemann W, Schmitz N, Pfreundschuh M, et al: Treatment of refractory Hodgkin's disease with high-dose cytosine arabinoside and mitoxantrone in combination. Cancer 1990; 66:838.

106. Tepler I, Schwartz G, Parker K, et al: Phase I trial of an interleukin-2 fusion toxin (DAB$_{486}$ IL-2) in hematologic malignancies: Complete response in a patient with Hodgkin's disease refractory to chemotherapy. Cancer 1994; 73:1276.

107. Klimo P, Connors JM: An update on the Vancouver experience in the management of advanced Hodgkin's disease treated with the MOPP/ABV hybrid program. Semin Hematol 1988; 25:34.

108. Longo DL, Duffey PL, DeVita VT Jr, et al: Treatment of advanced-stage Hodgkin's disease: Alternating noncross-resistant MOPP/CABS is not superior to MOPP. J Clin Oncol 1991; 9:1409.

109. Radford JA, Crowther D, Rohatiner AZS, et al: Results of a randomized trial comparing MVPP chemotherapy with a hybrid regimen, ChlVPP/EVA, in the initial treatment of Hodgkin's disease. J Clin Oncol 1995; 13:2379.

NON-HODGKIN'S LYMPHOMAS

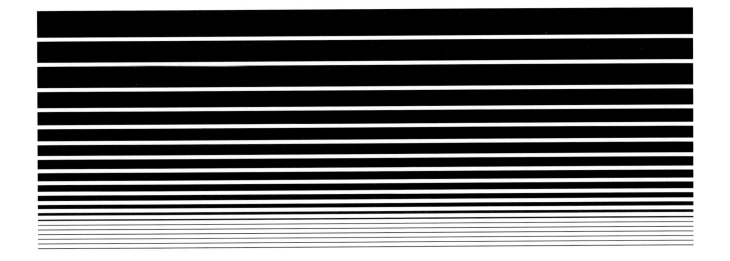

Part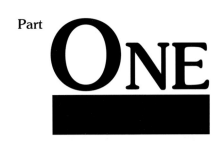

BIOLOGIC ASPECTS

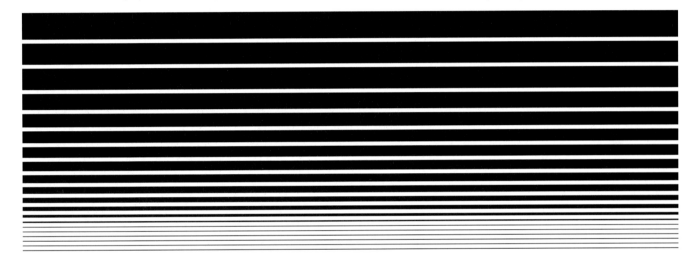

Seventeen

The Biology of Low-Grade — Malignant Lymphoma

Mary M. Zutter
Stanley J. Korsmeyer

Over the past 20 years, the field of hematologic oncology has blossomed with an increase in the understanding of malignant lymphoma and leukemia. During this period, the once disparate and confusing classification system for malignant lymphoma has been refined for simple clinical usage as well as broadened with the recognition of distinctive subtypes of malignant lymphoma.[1, 2] Malignant hematologic neoplasms were originally subdivided based on morphologic parameters and were later subclassified based on immunologic markers.[3, 4] We now recognize that these subclasses define subsets of malignant neoplasms with distinct molecular genetic alterations and biologic potential. To review the biology of low-grade lymphomas, we begin with an overview of the classification scheme for malignant lymphoma and then focus on the subtypes of "low-grade" malignant lymphoma.

CLASSIFICATION SCHEMES FOR MALIGNANT LYMPHOMA

HISTORICAL PERSPECTIVE

The non-Hodgkin's lymphomas (NHLs) constitute a heterogeneous group of malignant neoplasms that are diverse in their cellular origin, morphology, cytogenetic abnormalities, response to treatment, and prognosis. Since the early 1970s, when Rappaport devised his first classification scheme for malignant lymphoma based on morphologic criteria, numerous other schemes and revisions of the schemes based on a rapidly increasing data base have been published. These different classifications include the original Rappaport, Lukes and Collins, Kiel, British National Lymphoma Investigation, Dorfman, World Health Organization (WHO) classification scheme, and Working Formulation for Clinical Usage.[1, 3–7] Rappaport's original and most important contribution to the understanding of malignant lymphoma was identifying the importance of overall architecture. In the Rappaport scheme, lymphomas are subclassed as either follicular or diffuse. Other characteristics important in classification of malignant lymphomas include cell size, cell shape, nuclear and nucleolar appearance, chromatin distri-

bution, and cytoplasmic characteristics.[1] Later, a classification system of Lukes and Collins included features of cellular differentiation and cell origin (B cell versus T cell) and began to synthesize morphology with immunology.[4, 8, 9]

As knowledge of the immune system advanced, the Rappaport classification scheme has undergone numerous modifications by Berard, Dorfman, and Rappaport himself.[10, 11] A considerable amount of descriptive terminology has been retained, even though more biologically important subsets have been defined. The modified Rappaport system divides NHLs into 12 morphologic subtypes (Table 17–1). The nodular and/or diffuse subtypes include (1) nodular, poorly differentiated lymphocytic, (2) mixed, (3) histiocytic, (4) Burkitt's, and (5) undifferentiated non-Burkitt's. The modified Rappaport system has seven morphologic subtypes of NHLs characterized by diffuse involvement of the lymph node, including (1) well-differentiated lymphocytic, (2) intermediate lymphocytic, (3) lymphoblastic, (4) immunoblastic, (5) NHL with a diffuse epithelioid histiocytic reaction (Lennert's type), (6) mycosis fungoides, and (7) unclassified. The diffuse lymphomas appear to be more heterogeneous in respect to their cellular origin and clinical characteristics than the nodular lymphomas.

The existence of multiple classification schemes and the inability to clearly translate one type of classification to another has generated confusion over the years. The confusion generated frustration in the analysis of clinical trials and treatment response in NHLs. Therefore, in 1975, the National Cancer Institute sponsored a multiinstitutional clinicopathologic study to assess the usefulness of the different classification systems. The unified system generated is entitled "The Working Formulation of Non-Hodgkin's Lymphoma for Clinical Usage" (Table 17–2). The major advantage of the Working Formulation is stratification of malignant lymphoma into low-grade, intermediate-grade, and high-grade categories. Since the original publication of the Working Formulation in 1982, significant additions and modifications have evolved to include developments in molecular immunology and oncology.[12, 13] For most clinical trials, subclassification of lymphomas into low-grade, intermediate-grade, and high-grade categories is important to treatment decisions and prognosis. In the original

Table 17–1. The Rappaport Classification of Non-Hodgkin's Lymphomas

Type and Subtype	Cell of Origin	Growth Pattern and Morphology
Nodular and/or diffuse		
Poorly differentiated lymphocytic (NPDL)	Follicular center (B cell)	Small cleaved lymphoid cells
Mixed		Small and large lymphoid cells in nodular or nodular and diffuse growth pattern
Histiocytic		Large cleaved or noncleaved cells, frequent mitoses
		Rarely purely nodular pattern
Burkitt's	Early B cell	Undifferentiated
		Rarely nodular
		Small noncleaved cells, prominent nucleoli
		Starry-sky appearance
Undifferentiated, non-Burkitt's		Pleomorphic, noncleaved nuclei
		Starry-sky appearance
		Diffuse growth pattern
Diffuse		
Well-differentiated lymphocytic (DWDL)1	Small B-cell medullary cords of lymph nodes	Small round lymphoid cells, "pseudofollicular growth centers"
Intermediate lymphocytic	B cells of primary follicles and mantle zones of lymph nodes	Intermediate differentiation between DWDL and PDL
		Small cleaved and noncleaved cells
Lymphoblastic	T cell/thymocyte, rarely pre-B cell	Lymphoblastic
		Convoluted and nonconvoluted nuclei with fine chromatin
		No nucleoli
		Starry-sky appearance
Immunoblastic	B cell	Plasmacytoid
	Peripheral T cell of T-dependent areas of lymph nodes and spleen	Polymorphous or clear cell or epithelioid
Non-Hodgkin's lymphoma with diffuse epithelioid histiocytic reaction (Lennert's type)	Peripheral T cell	Mixed cells and transitional forms
Mycosis fungoides	Mature peripheral T helper cell	Cerebriform nuclei
		Aggregates in the epidermis (Pautrier's) microabscesses
Unclassifiable		

cell (intermediate lymphocytic lymphoma) and the marginal zone (either nodal or extranodal of mucosal-associated lymphoid tissue [MALT]) B-cell lymphoma.[12, 13]

Advances in cellular immunology have provided insight into the normal pathways of lymphocyte development and the cellular origin of lymphoid neoplasms. With the development of monoclonal antibodies directed against cell-surface antigens that distinguish B and T lymphocytes at defined differentiation stages, it became apparent that most low-grade malignant lymphomas considered in the Working Formulation were of mature B-cell origin.[8, 9, 14–19] Only in 1988, with the updated Kiel classification, were a small percentage (15% to 20%) of T-cell NHLs added to this group.[20] The Kiel classification for low-grade T-cell malignancies included lymphocytic (chronic lymphocytic and prolymphocytic leukemia), small cerebriform cell (mycosis fungoides), Sézary syndrome, lymphoepithelioid (Lennert's lymphoma), immunoblastic (angioimmunoblastic lymphadenopathy) T-zone, and pleomorphic small cell (human T-cell lymphotropic virus, type I, positive [HTLV-I+] or HTLV-I–). The widespread usage of monoclonal antibodies directed at differentiation stages of T-cell maturation demonstrated that the low-grade T-cell lymphomas also originated from mature lymphoid cells. These mature lymphoid cells have a low

Table 17–2. Working Formulation of Non-Hodgkin's Lymphomas for Clinical Usage

Low grade
  A. Small lymphocytic
      Consistent with chronic lymphocytic leukemia
      Plasmacytoid
  B. Follicular small cleaved cell
      Diffuse areas
      Sclerosis
  C. Follicular mixed small cleaved and large cell
      Diffuse areas
      Sclerosis
Intermediate grade
  D. Follicular predominantly large cell
      Diffuse areas
      Sclerosis
  E. Diffuse small cleaved cell
      Sclerosis
  F. Diffuse mixed, small and large cell
      Sclerosis
      Epithelial cell component
  G. Diffuse large cell
      Cleaved cell
      Noncleaved cell
      Sclerosis
High grade
  H. Large cell, immunoblastic
      Plasmacytoid
      Clear cell
      Polymorphous
      Epithelial cell component
  I. Lymphoblastic
      Convoluted cell
      Nonconvoluted cell
  J. Small noncleaved cell
      Burkitt's
      Follicular areas
Miscellaneous
  Composite
  Mycosis fungoides
  Histiocytic
  Extramedullary plasmacytoma
  Unclassifiable

Working Formulation in 1982, low-grade malignant lymphomas comprised small lymphocytic lymphoma; plasmacytoid lymphocytic lymphoma (immunocytoma); and either follicular lymphoma, small cleaved, or mixed cell type. Revisions of the low-grade category allow the inclusion of the mantle

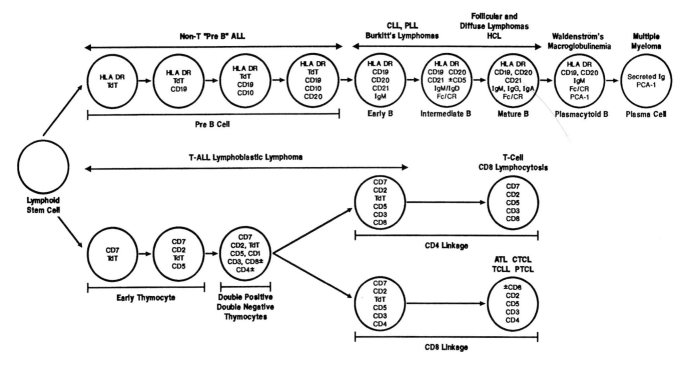

Figure 17–1. Schematic diagram of human lymphocyte differentiation and accompanying antigen expression as depicted by the CD nomenclature. The approximate location of lymphoid neoplasms within this scheme is denoted above the cells. ALL, acute lymphoblastic leukemia; CLL, chronic lymphocytic leukemia; PLL, prolymphocytic leukemia; HCL, hairy cell leukemia; HLA DR, human leukocyte antigen DR; TdT, terminal deoxynucleotidyl transferase; Ig, immunoglobulin; PCA-1, plasma cell antigen-1; CR, complement receptor; ATL, acute T-cell leukemia/lymphoma; CTCL, cutaneous T-cell lymphoma; TCLL, T-cell chronic lymphocyte leukemia; PTCL, Peripheral T-cell lymphoma; T-All, T-cell acute lymphoblastic leukemia.

proliferative potential that correlates with their low-grade malignant potential. The maturation stage of low-grade B- and T-cell lymphoid malignancies contrasts with the immature stage of T- or B-cell maturation that defined the high-grade acute lymphoblastic leukemia, high-grade lymphoblastic lymphoma, and high-grade small, noncleaved cell (Burkitt's type) lymphoma.

MALIGNANT LYMPHOMAS ORIGINATE FROM DEFINED ANATOMIC COMPARTMENTS

Malignant lymphomas originate from defined anatomic compartments of the lymph node or extranodal site. The architecture and cytologic features of malignant lymphoma correlate with the anatomic compartment from which the particular malignant lymphoma originated. For example, follicular small cleaved- and mixed cell lymphoma are probably derived from the follicular center cell; mantle cell (intermediate lymphocytic) lymphoma derived from the follicular mantle zone; and marginal zone B-cell lymphoma derived from the marginal zone, recirculating memory B cell. The architecture of each distinct malignant lymphoma mimics the architectural organization displayed by its normal lymphoid counterpart.

CELL SURFACE ANTIGENS DEFINE STAGES OF B-CELL MATURATION

Advances in cellular immunology have provided insight into the normal pathways of lymphocyte development. Monoclonal antibodies against cell surface antigens define stages of lymphocyte differentiation from the hematopoietic

progenitor cell (Fig. 17–1). B-cell commitment is recognized by the expression of leukocyte common antigen (CD45) and CD19.[21, 22] CD19 is expressed at all stages of B-cell maturation, is the earliest detectable B-cell antigen, and is expressed until the plasma cell stage.[23] The immunoglobulin (Ig) molecule is unique to B cells, and its expression and location is useful in defining the stage of B-cell maturation.[24–26] Pluripotent lymphoid progenitor cells maintain the Ig gene in germline configuration. When progenitor cells commit to B-lymphoid differentiation, they enter the stage of Ig gene rearrangement. Immature B cells (pre-pre-B and pre-B), which are in the process of rearranging the Ig heavy- and light-chain genes, cannot yet express Ig protein but express terminal deoxynucleotidyl transferase (Tdt).[27] Expression of Tdt defines a stage of immature B- or T-lymphoid development. Tdt functions as a DNA polymerase to catalyze the addition of a random number of deoxynucleotides at the junction during normal Ig or T-cell receptor (TCR) gene rearrangement; this allows additional diversity in the Ig or TCR genes.[27–29] At this same stage of B-cell maturation, the "common acute lymphoblastic leukemia antigen" (CALLA) (CD10), a cell surface endopeptidase, is expressed; CD10 is expressed on the majority of immature B cells as well as on a subset of follicular center cells and malignancies derived from follicular center cells.[30, 31] Other mature B cells, plasma cells, and B-cell lymphomas fail to express the CD10 antigen. A small subset of pre-B cells immediately before the mature B-cell stage coexpress Tdt and cytoplasmic Ig; this defines not only a stage of normal B-cell maturation but a subtype of acute lymphoblastic leukemia.[30, 31] Mature B cells are defined as those that express surface Ig and CD20.[32–34] The

IgM is expressed first on early mature B cells. Later, both IgM and IgD are expressed on the cell surface.[33] After genomic switching, a mature Ig (either IgM, IgD, IgA, or IgG) is expressed. Some cells progress and become antibody-forming cells; others become memory B cells.[35]

In addition, B cells express a wide number of additional cell surface antigens. In order to organize the rapidly expanding repertoire of monoclonal antibodies to cell surface antigens on lymphoid cells as well as other cells of the hematopoietic system, immunologists organized the International Workshop on Human Leukocyte Differentiation Antigens.[36] Through this workshop, monoclonal antibodies are clustered into cluster differentiation (CD) groups based on biochemical and immunoprecipitation data, functional analyses, flow cytometric studies, and immunohistochemistry. In 1994, the Fifth International Workshop proposed 136 CD groups, of which 55 are expressed by B lymphocytes.[37]

T-cell maturation occurs in a manner similar to that of B-cell maturation. T cells also express antigens that again define distinct stages of T-cell maturation. The earliest recognized T-cell-specific antigen is CD7.[38] As T cells mature, they progressively express CD2, the CD3 TCR complex, and CD4 and/or CD8.[39-41] Mature T cells express all these antigens but restrict expression to either the CD4 or the CD8 molecule.

IMMUNOGLOBULIN GENE SUBSEGMENTS REARRANGE TO GENERATE ANTIBODY DIVERSITY

The molecular dissection of the immune response has revealed the mechanisms that enable humans to generate a seemingly unlimited number (10^6 to 10^9) of different antibody specificities.[42, 43] The final antibody molecule comprises two identical heavy (H) chains disulfide-linked to two identical light (L) chains. The N-terminal variable (V) portion of each chain possesses the antigen recognition site, while the C-terminal constant (C) portion is invariant in sequence and performs effector functions. In 1965, Dreyer and Bennett examined very limited peptide map information and correctly surmised that this unusual Ig molecule would be encoded by at least two separate gene segments.[44] Studies by Tonegawa and Leder and their colleagues using recombinant DNA technology discovered that in their embryonic or germline form Ig genes are organized as discontinuous DNA segments that are assembled during B-cell development.[42, 43]

The variable portion of the human H-chain gene is generated from families of variable (V_H) regions, a set of internal diversity (D_H) regions, and a strip of six alternative joining (J_H) gene segments located on chromosomal segment 14q32 (Fig. 17–2). The first step of Ig gene assemblage is usually to rearrange a D_H region together with a J_H region to produce a D_H/J_H intermediate rearrangement.[45] Subsequently, a V_H region fuses with that D_H/J_H combination to create the functional $V_H/D_H/J_H$ responsible for the cell's H-chain protein. Inserted extranucleotides are frequently found at the site of each juncture and have been referred to as "N" segments.[27] These bases contribute to antibody diversity in that they are located at a site within the antibody molecule that has contact with an antigen. In addition, a somatic hypermutation mechanism is activated at a later stage of B-cell development that alters the V/D/J sequence and can improve the antigen-binding affinity.[46, 47] Most human B cells need to rearrange both their Ig H-chain alleles in order to create a workable $V_H/D_H/J_H$ recombination. The other allele often possesses an intermediate D_H/J_H or invalid rearrangement. The earliest recognizable B cells display only surface IgM and thus utilize the most proximal constant (C_H) region, C_μ (Fig. 17–2). Subsequently, they exploit an alternative splicing mechanism to place either C_μ or C_δ with the same V/D/J specificity and display simultaneous surface IgM and IgD.[48, 49] Finally, an H-chain class

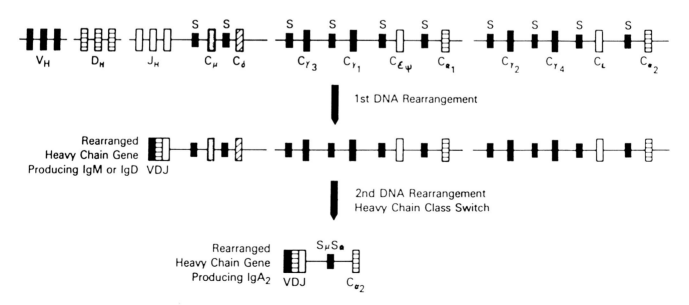

Figure 17–2. Schematic representation of human embryonic or germline heavy chain gene locus on chromosome segment 14q32. The first DNA rearrangement assembles the variable (V), diversity (D), and joining (J) segments to complete the variable portion of the molecule. Later in development, a second DNA rearrangement may occur between the homologous switch (S) sites flanking each construct (C) region. The heavy chain class switch moves a distal C region next to the assembled V/D/J.

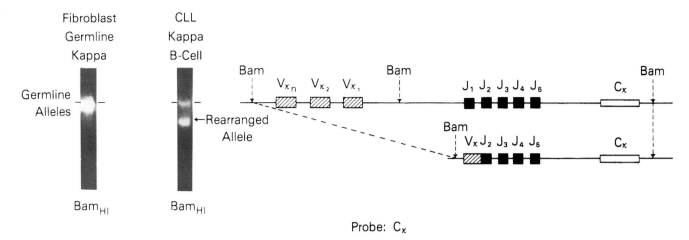

Figure 17–3. Southern blot detection of a rearranged human κ gene. The upper schematic denotes a germline configuration of the κ gene in which a C_κ probe recognizes a 12-kilobase-sized *Bam*HI fragment. Activation of a κ allele juxtaposes one of many V_κ regions with one of five alternative J_κ segments. This V_κ/J_κ rearrangement introduces a new 5′*Bam*HI restriction site. Consequently, a rearranged κ allele is altered in size compared with a germline allele. CLL, chronic lymphocytic leukemia.

switch may occur that moves a more distal constant region of C_γ, C_ϵ, or C_α next to that same V/D/J (see Fig. 17–2).[50–52] The H-chain class switch enables the same antigen specificity to be linked with a new constant region, providing the different physiologic function of an IgG, IgE, or IgA molecule.

Mature B cells produce only one of the two available L-chain classes, κ or λ, referred to as "isotypic exclusion." Moreover, of that selected L-chain class, the cell expresses only the maternal or paternal allele, referred to as "allelic exclusion." Human B cells display κ 60% of the time and λ 40% of the time. If a B cell is to ultimately produce κ L chain, it rearranges its κ-gene locus after H-chain rearrangement. The human κ-gene locus is located on the short arm of chromosome 2 at band 2p11 (Fig. 17–3).[53] Multiple different V_κ segments exist in humans, but each is foreshortened, contributing only the N-terminal 95 amino acids of the 108 that constituted the variable portion of the protein. The remaining 13 amino acids are contributed by one of five alternative joining (J_κ) gene segments. There is but one constant (C_κ) gene region on each allele. Once again, a process of V/J rearrangement completes the coding sequence for the variable portion and activates this gene. The alternative λ L-chain gene is located on chromosome segment 22q11.[54] Similarly, it assembles V_λ/J_λ segments to activate this gene. However, it is slightly more complex in that it is constituted of multiple J_λ/C_λ clusters (6 to 9 in humans) that have a common pool of V_λ regions.

DEVELOPMENTAL SEQUENCE OF T-CELL RECEPTOR GENE ACTIVATION

The T cells also demonstrate antigen-specific recognition through a cell surface T_3-Ti (idiotype) complex.[41] The Ti portion of the antigen receptor is constituted of either α plus β TCR chains or alternative γ plus δ heterodimeric TCR chains. The genes for α-, β-, γ-, and δ-TCR chains have been cloned and characterized. These genes are evolutionarily related but distinct from Ig genes yet also rearrange to assemble gene subsegments. The β TCR, located on

chromosome segment 7q35, is diagrammed in Figure 17–4.[41, 55] It has two available constant regions, $C_\beta 1$ and $C_\beta 2$, and sets of diversity (D_β) and joining (J_β) segments as well. The γ-TCR complex is located on chromosome segment 7p15 and is rearranged and expressed early in T-cell development.[56–58] The α- and δ-TCR loci have the most novel organization. The δ TCR is a gene within a gene located within the heart of the α-TCR complex on chromosome segment 14q11.[59, 60] An important advantage must exist for embracing this complexity. The rationale is not immediately obvious in that the δ and the α locus most often use unique rather than shared sets of V's, D's, and J's. One enticing possibility is that the δ within α TCR design is intentional to ensure that an early T cell can make only α or δ. A number of lines of evidence are emerging that suggest that the γδ and αβ TCR pathways are distinct rather than sequential lineages.[61] Since the δ-TCR locus is located between the V_α and the J_α region, any V_α/J_α rearrangement would loop out and delete the δ-TCR locus. Moreover, specialized sequences known as δ-deleting elements flank the δ-TCR locus and rearrange in thymus to eliminate the possibility of making δ but not α. One intriguing possibility is that an early decision to effectively rearrange versus eliminate the δ-TCR locus may provide a pivotal event in choosing between the γδ versus αβ lineages.

IMMUNOGLOBULIN GENE REARRANGEMENTS REVEAL THE CLONALITY, LINEAGE, AND TRANSLOCATIONS OF LYMPHOID NEOPLASMS

The molecular event that moves and combines a V and J segment results in the relocation of restriction endonuclease sites at the DNA level. Consequently, the DNA restriction fragment that bears an Ig gene in its rearranged form is of altered size compared with the germline form of the gene (see Fig. 17–2). Classic B-cell malignancies represent clonal expansions of a single progenitor cell. Each tumor possesses multiple copies of an identical V/J rearrangement. This expanded copy number makes it possible to detect such

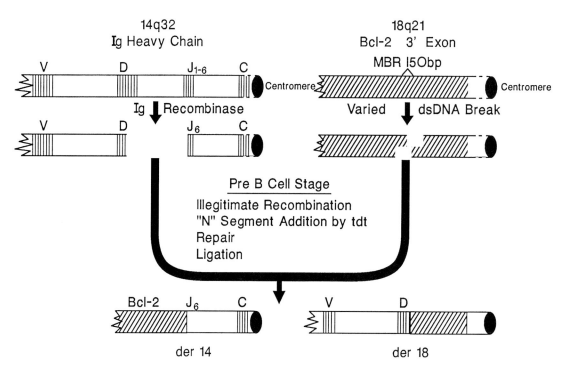

Figure 17–4. Mechanism of the t(14;18) recombination. Der(14) chromosomes demonstrate breakpoints at J segments, while der(18) breakpoints are at D segments. This suggests the translocation occurs at a pre-B-cell stage when Ig recombinase has cleaved at a D and J segment and these ends recombine with a break at 18q21 within the major breakpoint region (MBR) of *bcl*-2 exon III. tdt, terminal deoxynucleotidyl transferase.

rearrangements by routine Southern blots. Since each B cell uses but one V and one J of the many possibilities, the pattern of its gene rearrangement proves unique to that cell. Thus, these rearrangements serve as tumor-associated molecular markers useful in determining clonality and lineage commitment.[62–64]

The TCR genes provided the first uniformly applicable clonal markers for T cells and proved that most T-cell neoplasms are of clonal origin.[62, 65–72] The TCR genes enable issues of lineage commitment, clonality, stage of development, and site of translocation to be addressed in T-cell neoplasms parallel to the use of Ig genes in B cells. The assessment of TCR genes has been useful in addressing whether T-cell lymphoproliferations are polyclonal expansions of regulatory T cells or monoclonal proliferations. TCR genes were instructive in the CD8 (T_γ) lymphocytosis often associated with hematocytopenias, especially granulocytopenia. The regulatory capacities of these large granular lymphocytes and the often indolent course raised questions as to whether this was a chronic leukemia or reactive process. The majority of such patients (approximately 80%) have revealed clonal β- and/or γ-TCR rearrangements indicating a clonal neoplasia.[67, 70, 72]

The detection of an Ig or a TCR gene rearrangement is a moderately sensitive as well as specific marker, capable of identifying minor populations (1% to 5%) of clonal cells in tissues of mixed cellularity. However, clonality is not necessarily tantamount to a verdict of malignancy. Lymphoproliferation, particularly in the setting of immunodeficiency, can result in the emergence of transient clones that need not result in malignancy.[63, 73] Importantly, the molecular rearrangement markers are unique to these cells and provide the capacity to follow the natural history of such clones.

Since DNA rearrangement markers do not require the production of the final protein, they are applicable to the entire spectrum of neoplasia including pre-B- and pre-T-cell neoplasms. Gene rearrangements have proved instructive when the cellular origin of lymphoid neoplasms lacking lineage-restricted surface antigens is examined. Moreover, a developmental hierarchy for both the Ig and TCR gene rearrangements is manifest during early B- and T-cell maturation, providing a means to categorize the developmental stage of each neoplasm. Finally, a number of the unexpected rearrangements of Ig and TCR genes noted in lymphoid tumors have proved to be the sites of interchromosomal translocation.

"LOW-GRADE" MALIGNANT LYMPHOMA BASED ON THE WORKING FORMULATION

We have reviewed the historical development and classification schemes of malignant lymphoma, detailed the cell surface antigens that define distinct stages of lymphocyte maturation, and discussed the molecular biology of lymphoid differentiation. We now focus on the different subtypes of low-grade malignant lymphoma, based on the revised classification scheme of the Working Formulation for Clinical Usage.[12, 13]

SMALL LYMPHOCYTIC LYMPHOMA

Small lymphocytic lymphoma (SLL) is a low-grade malignant lymphoma that occurs predominantly in middle- and older-aged individuals.[1, 74, 75] The nomenclature "small lymphocytic lymphoma" describes the cytologic features of the malignant cell, which is the "small mature lymphocyte."[76] SLL, also termed "well-differentiated lymphocyte lymphoma" in Rappaport's classification, is closely related to chronic lymphocytic leukemia and Waldenström's macroglobulinemia.[75, 76] Although SLL is a low-grade malignancy, 61% to 90% of patients present with stage IV disease, and 69% to 82% of these patients have bone marrow involvement at diagnosis.[77–79]

Pathology

Lymph node biopsies in patients with SLL show diffuse effacement of the nodal architecture by small, mature-appearing lymphocytes.[74, 78] The disease is always diffuse, with the caveat that pseudofollicles can mimic follicular architecture. In the majority of cases, the cells are uniform in size and shape, are small (6 to 12 μm in diameter), and are mature in appearance. The earlier terminology "well-differentiated" arose from the round and regular shape of each cell, the clumped chromatin with a small amount of cytoplasm, and only slightly irregular nuclei. At low power, clusters of pale zones representing proliferation centers produce the pseudofollicles. Within these pseudofollicles, the cells have a higher proliferative rate and the appearance of transformed cells, including larger nuclei, prominent nucleoli, and a greater amount of pale cytoplasm.[76–79] In addition to transformed lymphocytes, proliferation centers can be composed of prolymphocytes, immunoblasts, and occasional small cleaved cells.

Immunologic Studies

Immunologically, SLL is almost identical to the other lymphoproliferative disorders, chronic lymphocytic leukemia (CLL) and Waldenström's macroglobulinemia. Many patients with SLL present with an absolute lymphocytosis and bone marrow involvement indistinguishable from CLL. CLL also represents a low-grade malignancy, and the clinical courses of SLL and CLL are similar. In most cases, manifestations of the two diseases overlap, and the diagnosis is based on the site of the primary involvement (i.e., if the primary feature is "lymph node involvement," the case is considered an "SLL"; if the primary involvement is "peripheral blood and bone marrow," the disease is considered "CLL"). Not only do these diseases share biologic and morphologic similarities, but the mature B cell in SLL and CLL represents a clonal expansion of a similar novel B-cell subset.

The majority of cells in CLL and SLL (>95% or 80%, respectively) are monoclonal B cells that express CD5 (Leu-1, OKT-1), a 67-kilodalton (kD) surface protein.[12, 13, 76, 80–83] A CD5-positive subset of B cells accounts for only about 15% of B cells in normal individuals. CD5-positive B cells are associated with the production of autoantibodies such as rheumatoid factor (RF) and anti-DNA antibodies, frequently of the spontaneously secreted IgM type. The $_\kappa$-producing CLL cells have been shown to express a single V_κIIIb variable region in approximately 25% of cases.[84] Curiously, this Hum κ 325 subgroup encodes the idiotype found in most monoclonal RFs. Recently, other cross-reactive idiotypes found on human IgM RF paraproteins have also been found to be overrepresented in CLL.[85]

Moreover, CLLs do not appear to possess hypermutational activity for Ig genes and retain the germline sequence for these Ig's. These findings indicate that CLL arises from a distinct subpopulation of B cells possessing a restricted Ig gene repertoire.

As discussed earlier, B cells during maturation express a number of B-cell-restricted or nonrestricted antigens; these antigens are useful in distinguishing distinct subtypes of B-cell lymphomas. SLL expresses the pan-B-cell antigens CD19 and CD22, low-density CD20, and surface Ig. Comparison of SLL to mantle zone lymphoma to follicular small cleaved cell lymphoma shows a gradient of surface Ig expression, with SLL expressing the least surface Ig and follicular small cleaved cell lymphoma expressing the most. The gradient of surface Ig parallels the normal development of mature B-cell maturation and suggests that these lymphomas reflect sequential stages of B-cell differentiation. SLLs are restricted in expression of surface IgM and IgD.[86, 87] In addition to the pan-B-cell antigens, it has recently been demonstrated that SLLs and CLL express CD23 (Blast-2a, a 50-kD membrane glycoprotein), which serves as the low-affinity receptor for IgE (Fc$_\epsilon$RII) and CD43 (L60), a 95-kD highly-sialated integral membrane protein known as "leukosialin." Coexpression of CD5, CD23, and CD43 and lack of expression of CD10 typify SLL and CLL.[13, 87]

Molecular Biology

The B cells in SLL and CLL represent a clonal expansion of a single B cell and therefore exhibit rearrangement of both the Ig H- and L-chain genes. The molecular changes described in SLL and CLL are heterogeneous. Rearrangements involving a number of different chromosomal sites and oncogenes, including *bcl*-1, *bcl*-2, and *bcl*-3, in addition to deletions, additions, and translocations of chromosomes 14, 11, 12, 13, and 16,[88–94] have all been described in CLL and SLL.

The molecular hallmark of CLL is not an interchromosomal translocation, but trisomy 12. Trisomy 12 is seen in SLL but not limited to this subtype.[95] Trisomy 3 and trisomy 16 are also observed in greater than 10% of cases. Although a number of cytogenetic and molecular changes have been reported in cases of CLL and SLL, no single cytogenetic or molecular change is pathognomonic of this lymphoproliferation.

One of the first interchromosomal breakpoints to be cloned was the t(11;14)(q13;q32), *bcl*-1, identified originally in B-cell CLL. Although originally noted in B-cell CLL, *bcl*-1 rearrangements have been found in only a minority of patients with CLL or SLL but are found in many cases (50%) of mantle cell lymphomas, as discussed later. Rearrangements of the *bcl*-2 protooncogene are characteristic of follicular lymphomas, seen rarely in B-cell CLL, and almost never identified in SLL.

A case of CLL with a t(14;19)(q32;q13) translocation allowed the identification of a novel protooncogene *bcl*-3 on chromosome 19 adjacent to the breakpoint.[96] Sequence analysis of the *bcl*-3 gene identified a CDC 10 motif, suggesting a role for *bcl*-3 in cell cycle control.[97, 98] The *bcl*-3 gene is expressed at high levels in normal blood cells after mitogenic stimulation and in leukemic cells with the translocation.

Recently identified cytogenetic abnormalities define discrete subsets of SLL with histomorphologic differences.[99–103] Del(6q) is generally associated with progression in follicular lymphomas but has been identified in some diffuse SLLs as well. In one recent series, deletion of 6(q21;q23) was the most common cytogenetic abnormality in SLL.[99, 100] The del(6) abnormality was associated with the subset of SLLs with circulating prolymphocytes. In this setting, no difference in clinical behavior was appreciated between lymphomas with or without the karyotypic abnormality. The t(9;14)(p13;q32), an infrequent abnormality, is highly correlated with the subset of SLL with plasmacytoid differentiation.[101] Among a series of 426 karyotypically abnormal NHLs, the t(9;14)(p13;q32) was identified in eight cases. Seventy-five percent of these cases had the identical histologic appearance and immunophenotype of SLL with plasmacytoid differentiation.[102] In addition, other less common karyotypic abnormalities have been identified in isolated cases of CLL.

FOLLICULAR LYMPHOMA

Follicular lymphoma, composed of small cleaved cells or a mixture of small cleaved and large cells, constitutes approximately 40% to 45% of NHLs in adults.[103, 104] The term "follicular small cleaved cell lymphoma" is descriptive of the pathologic findings and replaces Rappaport's classification of "nodular, poorly differentiated lymphocytic lymphoma."[1, 3] Although the initial clinical course is often indolent, the neoplastic cells are usually widely distributed, including bone marrow and blood. Follicular lymphoma presents with disseminated disease (stage III or IV) in the majority of patients.[103] Only 10% to 20% of patients at the time of diagnosis have stage I or II disease. Indeed, 10% of patients with follicular lymphoma have an elevated lymphocyte count with circulating malignant cells. The circulating cells are slightly larger than mature lymphocytes and have nuclear clefts distinguishing them from the round, uniform cells of CLL. In fact, with more sensitive studies using the polymerase chain reaction, 75% of patients with follicular small cleaved cell lymphoma had malignant cells detectable in their peripheral blood or bone marrow at the time of diagnosis and after therapy.[105]

Pathology

Follicular lymphomas are monoclonal expansions of B cells derived from the normal germinal center. Follicular lymphomas primarily involve the lymph nodes at the time of presentation.[106, 107] Lymph node biopsies reveal crowded, round-to-oval follicles that efface the normal nodal architecture and replace the nonmalignant nodal compartments. The malignant follicles can be surrounded by residual small T cells, or malignant cells can extrude from the follicles to produce a diffuse pattern. Malignant follicles, in contrast to normal germinal centers, are monotonous and are composed strictly of follicular center cells. The normal T cells and reactive histiocytes present in a reactive follicle are absent. In all follicular center cell lymphomas, there is a mixture of small cleaved cells, large cleaved cells, and large noncleaved cells. Follicular lymphomas composed either predominantly of small cleaved cells or a mixture of small cleaved and large cells, representing 25% to 50% of the cells, are both included in the low-grade category in the Working Formulation.[1]

Immunologic Studies

The immunophenotype of malignant lymphocytes in follicular lymphoma suggests that they are derived from normal germinal center cells. The cells express either surface IgM, often with low levels of IgD, or occasionally IgG, and monoclonal Ig L chain. In addition to the other B-cell lineage markers, CD19, CD20, CD22, they frequently express CD10 and fail to express CD5.

Follicular Lymphoma as a Hypermutational B-Cell Stage

During a normal primary immune response within the germinal center, a population of memory B cells is generated that is relatively long-lived and enables a higher-affinity secondary response upon reexposure to antigen. Part of this maturation of the Ig response is related to the presence of extensive somatic mutation within variable regions. Importantly, follicular lymphomas have been shown to display clonal variation with respect to their Ig idiotype (a measurement of the uniqueness of an antibody molecule). This has been shown to result in a high rate of variable region somatic mutation that is ongoing within the tumors.[108] Unfortunately, this often enables these tumors to escape from anti-idiotype antibody therapy.[109] In contrast, the rate of somatic mutation in other B-cell tumors including CLL, pre-B acute lymphoblastic leukemia, and Burkitt's lymphoma/leukemia have been shown to be quite low.[110–112] This suggests that follicular B-cell lymphoma represents a neoplasm of a developmental stage characterized by selective hypermutation of Ig genes.

Translocation (14;18) of Follicular Lymphoma Reveals the bcl-2 Protooncogene

The t(14;18)(q32;q21) is the most common translocation in hematologic malignancies. Approximately 85% of follicular and 20% of diffuse B-cell lymphomas possess this translocation.[113, 114] The location of the Ig H-chain locus at 14q32 and the B-cell phenotype provided the rationale for cloning this chromosomal breakpoint. Molecular cloning of the t(14;18) breakpoint revealed a putative protooncogene, bcl-2, at 18q21.[115–117] Despite the mature B-cell phenotype of t(14;18)-bearing lymphomas, the translocation appears to occur earlier in development at a pre-B-cell stage. Immunoglobulin recombinase initiates the first attempt at rearrangement in pre-B development by cleaving at a D and J Ig segment (see Fig. 17–4). Instead of completing that recombination, however, progenitor cells of follicular lymphoma introduce a broken bcl-2 gene from 18q21 into these sites.[115, 118, 119]

Approximately 70% of the breakpoints on chromosome 18 are clustered within a major breakpoint region (MBR) in the 3' untranslated region of the bcl-2 gene (Fig. 17–5). Curiously, neither the MBR nor the more distant minor cluster region (mcr)[120] of bcl-2 possesses the typical heptamer-spacer-nonamer motif recognized by Ig recombinase. Of interest, 8–base pair (bp) chi-like consensus

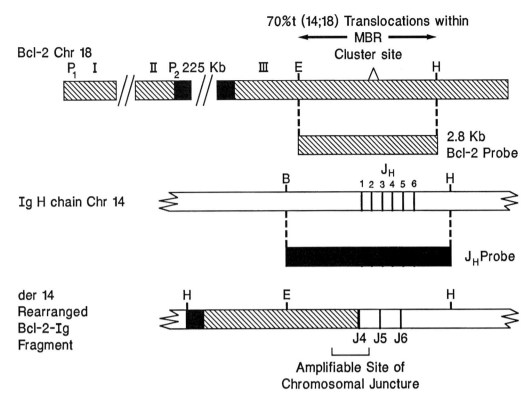

Figure 17–5. Schematic representation of a molecular marker for the t(14;18) interchromosomal breakpoint. The der(14) chromosome possesses an altered size *Hind*III (H) DNA fragment that will hybridize to both a chromosome 18 *bcl-2* probe or a chromosome 14 J$_H$ probe. The focusing of the breakpoints on chromosomes 14 and 18 results in an amplifiable site of chromosomal juncture. MBR, major breakpoint region.

sequences have been noted adjacent to *bcl-2* breakpoints, raising the possibility that such variable tandem repeats may participate.[121] However, the precise mechanisms responsible for the localized DNA breaks in *bcl-2* and its recombination with the Ig locus remain uncertain.

The cloning of this second-generation breakpoint provided a new gene, *bcl-2*. The gene *bcl-2* demonstrates the novel function of blocking programmed cell death rather than promoting proliferation.[122–124] Overexpressed *bcl-2* prevents apoptosis in selected hematopoietic cell lines after deprivation of growth factors.[124] In retrospect, the indolent clinical course of follicular lymphoma provided many clues concerning the ultimate function of *bcl-2*.

The contribution of the t(14;18) to neoplasia was directly assessed by generating transgenic mice bearing a *bcl-2*-Ig minigene that recapitulated the molecular consequences of the human translocation.[125, 126] These mice uniformly developed a polyclonal follicular lymphoproliferation that selectively expanded small resting B cells. These recirculating B cells accumulate due to extended survival rather than increased proliferation. Like patients with follicular lymphoma, these mice progress from indolent follicular hyperplasia to diffuse large cell lymphoma.[127] This satisfies a molecular Koch's postulate for the t(14;18) in B-cell lymphoma. Moreover, this also indicates that prolonged cell survival is oncogenic. Thus, *bcl-2* represents the first member of a new category of oncogenes, regulators of programmed cell death. Extended cell survival may prove to be a key event in carcinogenesis that enables the acquisition of further genetic changes.

The spatial distribution of *bcl-2* within organized tissues was examined to obtain clues concerning its normal physiologic roles. The *bcl-2* protein displayed a remarkably restricted topographic distribution with immature tissues that are characterized by apoptotic cell death.[128] One of the most dramatic examples was provided by secondary germinal centers (Fig. 17–6). Immunohistochemical assessment revealed that the follicular mantle composed of

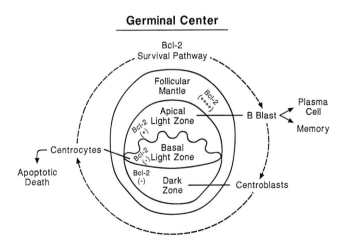

Figure 17–6. Distribution of *bcl-2* protein with secondary germinal centers as determined by immunoperoxidase staining using an anti-*bcl-2* MoAb, monoclonal antibody. Proposed *bcl-2* survival pathway operative within the light zone enables secondary immune responses.

long-lived recirculating IgM-IgD B cells possessed abundant *bcl*-2.[128, 129] Of note, *bcl*-2 was essentially absent from the dark zone of proliferating centroblasts and from the basal portion of the light zone where centrocytes die by apoptosis. Yet, *bcl*-2 expression returns in B cells in the more apical portion of the light zone, where it has been proposed that a subset of B cells is selected for survival by their affinity for residual antigen present on follicular dendritic cells. In contrast to the absent or focal expression of *bcl*-2 by normal germinal centers, the malignant follicles in malignant lymphoma strongly express the *bcl*-2 protein.[130] The use of monoclonal antibodies to the *bcl*-2 protein are helpful in distinguishing atypical follicular hyperplasia from malignant follicular lymphoma.

The progression of low-grade follicular lymphoma to a high-grade process is usually associated with histologic transformation to either a diffuse large cell immunoblastic lymphoma or a small, noncleaved cell lymphoma; both subtypes represent transformation of follicular center cells. These transformations are usually associated with additional cytogenetic and molecular alterations.[93, 131] Additional cytogenetic changes associated with progression to diffuse mixed or large cell lymphoma include del(6q), dup(7p), der(18), breakpoints at 1p36, 6q13, 1q21, 2q21, or gains of X, 7, 12, 20, 21, and 22. Transformation to a small, noncleaved cell lymphoma is often associated with the typical t(8;14)(q24; q32) of Burkitt's lymphoma. Defects in the tumor suppressor genes *p53*, retinoblastoma, and/or the protooncogene *rel* are also typical of advanced stages of follicular lymphoma.[126]

MANTLE CELL LYMPHOMA

Revisions to the original Working Formulation Classification include the addition of two subtypes of low-grade malignant lymphoma.[12, 13] The first to be discussed is the mantle cell lymphoma, also known as "diffuse or nodular intermediate lymphocytic lymphoma," "lymphocytic lymphoma of intermediate differentiation," or "centrocytic lymphoma." Mantle cell lymphoma is named for the morphologic and immunophenotypic similarities to lymphocytes found in the mantle zone of secondary germinal centers and to the small resting B lymphocytes of primary germinal centers.[132–135]

As with other subtypes of low-grade lymphoma, this is a disease of older individuals, with a median age of approximately 60 years.[135–139] Patients usually present with advanced-stage disease (stage III/IV), generalized lymphadenopathy, and involvement of the peripheral blood, bone marrow, and liver. Median survival ranges from 30 to 56 months, but patients with the nodular variant of mantle cell lymphoma had a significantly longer median survival than those with diffuse mantle cell lymphoma.[135–139]

Pathology

In early stages of mantle cell lymphoma, the neoplastic proliferation maintains the normal nodal architecture with a distinctly nodular pattern. The neoplastic mantle zone cells surround, expand, and gradually obliterate the central reactive germinal center.[135–139] As the disease progresses, the nodularity is lost and the process becomes diffuse. Mantle cell lymphoma is composed of a predominant population of small- to medium-sized lymphoid cells with irregular and slightly indented nuclei, moderately coarse chromatin, inconspicuous nucleoli, and scant cytoplasm.[139]

Immunology

The malignant lymphocytes of mantle cell lymphoma have a mature B-cell phenotype and express monoclonal Ig L chain with surface IgM often coexpression of surface IgD, and express the B-cell antigens CD19, CD20, CD22, CD24, and HLA-DR.[135–139] In addition, the cells immunophenotypically resemble cells of SLL/CLL in the expression of CD5 and the absence of CD10.[135, 140–142] Mantle cell lymphoma and SLL are immunophenotypically similar except for the lack of expression of CD23 by mantle cell lymphoma.[140–143]

Molecular Biology

One of the first interchromosomal breakpoints to be cloned was the t(11;14)(q13;q32).[144, 145] Once again the Ig H-chain locus at 14q32 recombined with a region on chromosome segment 11q13 entitled the *bcl*-1 locus. Despite intensive searches surrounding the breakpoint and substantial chromosomal walks, no deregulated transcriptional unit was identified. The *bcl*-1 rearrangements were noted in a few percent of myelomas, diffuse large cell lymphomas, and CLLs.[146–148] However, mantle cell lymphomas have a much higher incidence (30% to 50%) of *bcl*-1 rearrangement.[149] This suggests that *bcl*-1 rearrangement is involved in the pathogenesis of this subset of low- to intermediate-grade lymphoma.

A back door approach identified a candidate protooncogene for *bcl*-1. A number of parathyroid adenomas had been noted to bear clonal rearrangements of their phenotypic landmark gene, parathyroid hormone *(PTH)*.[150] This proved to be an interchromosomal translocation with 11q13 that overexpressed a newly identified gene located there, *PRAD-1* (parathyroid adenomatosis-1).[151] *PRAD-1* encodes a novel cyclin that has been shown to complex with $p34^{cdc2}$ and to induce its kinase activity. It is tantalizing that the same gene has been identified in two other systems. A $p36^{cyl}$ has been observed in mouse macrophages and is induced by CSF-1 in the G1 phase of the cell cycle.[152] The $p36^{cyl}$ is the murine equivalent of *PRAD-1* and also associates with a cdc2-related polypeptide. Moreover, a powerful selection scheme in which genes from a human glioblastoma were introduced into budding yeast lacking classic CLN1 and CLN2 cyclins revealed a new subclass, cyclin D1.[153] Cyclin D1 is abundant in human glioblastoma and is identical to PRAD-1. This gene provides an avenue to determine how a cyclin that appears to act at the G1/S boundary influences cell growth and neoplasia.

Equipped with this new information concerning *PRAD-1*, $p36^{cyl}$, and cyclin D1, the *bcl*-1 locus identified in t(11; 14)(q13;q32)-bearing B-cell tumors was revisited. Pulsed field gel electrophoresis suggested that *bcl*-1 breakpoints and *PRAD-1* are both located within 130 kilobase (kb). In addition, *PRAD-1* mRNA was abundant in CLLs bearing *bcl*-1 rearrangements and in seven of seven mantle cell lymphomas but was not detected in related tumor types lacking *bcl*-1 rearrangement.[154] Thus, *PRAD-1*, or conceivably a gene flanking it, represents an attractive candidate for the oncogene at 11q13 that participates in some tumors.

MARGINAL ZONE B-CELL LYMPHOMA

The most recent addition to the Working Formulation is the marginal zone lymphoma, of either extranodal or nodal origin.[12, 13] This entity encompasses the monocytoid B-cell lymphoma (MBCL) and lymphomas of mucosal-associated lymphoid tissue (MALT).[155] These two entities, derived from the marginal zone B-cell compartment, outside the lymphoid follicle, share features of cellular composition and immunophenotype.

MBCL is a low-grade lymphoma found predominantly in the elderly.[156–160] In many respects, MBCL demonstrates morphologic features of SLL or mantle cell lymphoma; however, the biology, immunophenotype, and clinical course differ. The majority of patients present with stage I and stage II disease with primary nodal involvement or localized involvement of extranodal sites.[158–160]

In contrast to MBCL, MALT lymphomas present at extranodal sites and are usually localized. Recent clinico-pathologic studies suggest a relationship between marginal zone B-cell lymphoma and autoimmune diseases, such as Sjögren's syndrome.[160, 161] Patients with Sjögren's syndrome present with MBCL involving the salivary glands and adjacent cervical lymph nodes. In addition to Sjögren's syndrome, MBCL has been frequently associated with acquired immunodeficiency syndrome–related lymphadenopathy and other autoimmune diseases, such as Hashimoto's thyroiditis. On the other hand, the majority of MALT lymphomas are associated with chronic gastritis secondary to *Helicobacter pylori* infection.[162] The normal gastric mucosa is devoid of MALT. Infection with *H. pylori* induces ulceration and chronic gastritis. Chronic infection with *H. pylori* begins early in life in developing countries, with 80% of the population infected by their 20th birthday. In contrast, the infection occurs at a slower pace in developed countries, where only 50% of the population is infected by the age of 50 years.[163] Of the two major types of *H. pylori* isolated, type I and type II, only type I causes gastric abnormalities.[164] MALT lymphomas and indeed gastric adenocarcinomas arise in the setting of ulceration and reactive lymphoid hyperplasia.[165–168] Gastric MALT lymphomas may be dependent on antigen stimulation by *H. pylori* since malignant lymphoid cells respond specifically to *H. pylori* antigens. The lymphoma has been shown to regress with eradication of the infection.[169, 170] In a recently described mouse model of *H. pylori* infection, oral immunization with *H. pylori* antigens prevented bacterial infection.[171]

Malignant monocytoid B cells of nodal origin commonly involve the lymph node sinuses and extend into the interfollicular region surrounding residual normal follicular centers.[157, 159] By surrounding the normal germinal center, the malignant cells produce a pseudomantle zonelike pattern. Neoplastic monocytoid B cells have moderate pale, clear cytoplasm and bland nuclei. Extranodal sites of involvement include predominantly the salivary glands, spleen, stomach, liver, and breast. The monocytoid B cell of extranodal lymphoma is similar to the nodal subtype except for the primary site of involvement.[156]

MALT lymphomas most commonly arise in the stomach, and less often in the salivary glands or thyroid.[169] The MALT lymphomas often arise in inflamed areas with associated ulceration. The malignant B cells, probably arising in the marginal zone region, expand around reactive germinal centers and spread into the surrounding glands and invade the epithelium to form lymphoepithelial lesions. The cells are small with pale cytoplasm and small, slightly indented nuclei.

Immunology

The B cells of marginal zone lymphoma, either nodal or extranodal monocytoid, express the B-cell-restricted antigens including surface Ig with monoclonal L-chain, CD19, and CD20, and fail to express CD5, CD10, or CD23.[155, 169] In addition to these pan-B-cell antigens, marginal zone B-cell lymphoma differs from the other SLLs by the expression of CD11c (a member of the β_2-integrin family) and PCA-1 (a plasma cell–associated antigen). The similarities in antigen expression, anatomic location, and morphology suggest that marginal zone B-cell lymphomas arise from the normal follicular marginal zone B cell. The cell has the capacity to differentiate into both monocytoid B cells and plasma cells and to recirculate to extranodal lymphoid sites.[156, 158]

Sjögren's Syndrome as a Preneoplastic Model

Sjögren's syndrome, long regarded as an autoimmune disorder, is a disease that is also characterized by lymphoid infiltrations and lymphoproliferations. The salivary and lacrimal glands are the initial sites of an infiltrate of B and T cells that results in a glandular destruction entitled the "benign lymphoepithelial lesion." Some patients develop extraglandular lymphoid aggregates termed "pseudolymphoma" that usually follow a benign course. However, over time, Sjögren's syndrome patients also demonstrate an increased incidence of NHLs. Application of molecular technology has indicated that Ig gene rearrangements, and thus clonal B cells, are already present at the stage of the benign lymphoepithelial lesion.[172] Provocatively, the L-chain rearrangements are disproportionately κ and not λ in type. Moreover, the lymphomas from Sjögren's patients usually display κ rather than λ L chain.[161] Curiously, evidence is emerging that Sjögren's patients' sera often possess a V_κ-encoded RF and their B-cell lymphomas often utilized the same RF-encoding V_κIIIb region associated with CLL.[173] Thus, molecular genetic data suggest that Sjögren's syndrome may provide a model of multistep malignancy. The early benign lymphoepithelial lesion already possesses a clonal outgrowth of a distinct B-cell subset. These clones may be subject to continued proliferation providing the opportunity for genetic alterations that account for the high incidence of lymphoma in Sjögren's syndrome. Similar clonal evolution is likely to be demonstrated for lymphomas of MALT.

REFERENCES

1. The non-Hodgkin's lymphoma pathologic classification: National Cancer Institute sponsored study of classification of non-Hodgkin's lymphomas—Summary and description of a working formulation for clinical usage. Cancer 1982; 49:2112.

2. Lukes RJ, Collins RD: Tumors of the hematopoietic system. *In* Hartmann WH, Sobin LH (eds): Atlas of Tumor Pathology, 2nd Series, Fasc 28. Washington DC, Armed Forces Institute of Pathology, 1988, pp 1–38.

3. Warnke RA, Weiss LM, Chan JKC: *In* Rosai J, Sobin LH (eds): Atlas of Tumor Pathology, Sec III, Fasc 14. Washington DC, Armed Forces Institute of Pathology, 1966, pp 43–51.

4. Lukes RJ, Collins RD: Immunologic characterization of human malignant lymphomas. Cancer 1974; 34:1488.

5. Lennert K, Stein H, Kaiserling E: Cytological and functional criteria for the classification of malignant lymphomata. Br J Cancer 1975; 31(II):29.

6. Dorfman RF: Classification of non-Hodgkin's lymphomas. Lancet 1974; 1:1295.

7. Mathe G, Rappaport H, O'Conor GT, Torloni H: Histological and cytological typing of neoplastic diseases of hematopoietic and lymphoid tissues. *In* WHO International Histological Classification of Tumors, No. 14. Geneva, World Health Organization, 1976.

8. Foon KA, Todd RF: Immunologic classification of leukemia and lymphoma. Blood 1986; 68:1.

9. Aisenberg AC: Cell surface markers in lymphoproliferative disease. N Engl J Med 1978; 304:331.

10. Rappaport H, Braypan RC: Changing concepts in the classification of malignant neoplasms of the hematopoietic system. *In* Rebuck J, Berard CW, Abell MR (eds): The Reticuloendothelial System. Baltimore, Williams & Wilkins, 1975, pp 1–19.

11. Mann RB, Jaffe ES, Berard CW: Malignant lymphomas—A conceptual understanding of morphologic diversity: A review. Am J Pathol 1979; 94:105.

12. Harris NL, Jaffe ES, Stein H, et al: A revised European-American classification of lymphoid neoplasms: A proposal from the International Lymphoma Study Group. Blood 1994; 84:1361.

13. Chan JKC, Banks PM, Cleary ML, et al: A proposal for classification of lymphoid neoplasms (by the International Lymphoma Study Group). Histopathology 1994; 25:517.

14. Spier CM, Grogan TM, Fielder K, et al: Immunophenotypes in "well-differentiated" lymphoproliferative disorders, with emphasis on small lymphocytic lymphoma. Hum Pathol 1986; 17:1126.

15. Harris NL, Bhan AK: B-cell neoplasms of the lymphocytic lymphoplasmacytoid, and plasma cell types: Immunohistologic analysis and clinical correlation. Hum Pathol 1985; 16:829.

16. Medeiros LJ, Strickler JG, Picker LJ, et al: "Well-differentiated" lymphocytic neoplasms: Immunologic findings correlated with clinical presentation and morphologic features. Am J Pathol 1987; 129:523.

17. Stein H, Gerdes J, Mason DY: The normal and malignant germinal centre. Clin Haematol 1982; 11:531.

18. Stein H, Lennert K, Feller A, et al: Immunological analysis of tissue sections in diagnosis of lymphoma. *In* Hoffbrand AV (ed): Recent Advances in Haematology. New York, Churchill Livingstone, 1985, p 127.

19. Bhan AK, Nadler LM, Stashenko P, et al: Stages of B cell differentiation in human lymphoid tissues. J Exp Med 1981; 154:737.

20. Lennert K, Feller AC: Histopathology of Non-Hodgkin's Lymphomas (Based on the Updated Kiel Classification), 2nd ed. Berlin, Springer-Verlag, 1992.

21. Nadler LM, Korsmeyer SJ, Anderson KC, et al: The B cell origin of non-T acute lymphoblastic leukemia: A model for discrete stages of neoplastic and normal pre-B cell differentiation. J Clin Invest 1984; 74:332.

22. LeBien TW, McCormack RT: The common acute lymphoblastic leukemia antigen (CD10)—Emancipation from a functional enigma. Blood 1989; 73:625.

23. Nadler LM, Anderson KC, Marti LG, et al: B4, a human B lymphocyte–associated antigen expressed on normal mitogen activated, and malignant B lymphocytes. J Immunol 1983; 131:244.

24. Campana D, Janossy G, Bofill M, et al: Human B cell development: I. Phenotypic differences of B lymphocytes in the bone marrow and peripheral lymphoid tissue. J Immunol 1985; 134:1524.

25. Moldenhauer G, Dorken B, Schwartz R, et al: Characterization of a human B lymphocyte specific antigen defined by monoclonal antibodies HD6 and HD39. *In* Reinherz EL, Haynes BF, Nadler LM, Bernstein ID (eds): Leucocyte Typing II: Human B lymphocytes. Berlin, Springer-Verlag, 1986, p 97.

26. Mason DY, Stein H, Gerdes J, et al: Value of monoclonal anti-CD22 (p135) antibodies for the detection of normal neoplastic B lymphoid cells. Blood 1987; 69:836.

27. Desiderio S, Yancopoulos GD, Paskind M, et al: Insertion of N regions into heavy-chain genes is correlated with expression of terminal deoxytransferase in B cells. Nature 1984; 311:752.

28. McCaffrey R, Smoler DF, Baltimore D: Terminal deoxynucleotidyl transferase in a case of childhood acute lymphoblastic leukemia. Proc Natl Acad Sci USA 1973; 70:521.

29. Bollum FJ: Terminal deoxynucleotidyl transferase as a hematopoietic cell marker. Blood 1979; 54:1203.

30. Greaves MF, Brown G, Rapson NT, et al: Antisera to ALL cells. Clin Immunol Immunopathol 1975; 4:67.

31. Vogler LB, Crist WB, Bockman DE, et al: Pre-B cell leukemia: A new phenotype of childhood lymphoblastic leukemia. N Engl J Med 1978; 298:872.

32. Pernis B: Lymphocyte membrane immunoglobulins: An overview. *In* Littman GW, Good RA (eds): Immunoglobulins. New York, Plenum Press, 1978, p 359.

33. Abney ER, Cooper MD, Kearney JF, et al: Sequential expression of immunoglobulin on developing mouse B lymphocytes: A systematic survey that suggests a model for the generation of immunoglobulin isotype diversity. J Immunol 1978; 120:2041.

34. Fu SM, Winchester RJ, Kunkel HG: Occurrence of IgM, IgD, and free light chains on human lymphocytes. J Exp Med 1974; 139:451.

35. Black SJ, Van der Loo W, Loken MR, et al: Expression of IgD by murine lymphocytes. Loss of surface IgD indicates maturation of memory B cells. J Exp Med 1978; 147:984.

36. Dorken B, Moller P, Pezzutto R, et al: B-cell antigens. *In* Knapp W, Dorken B, Rieber EP, et al (eds): Leucocyte Typing IV, White Cell Differentiation Antigens. Oxford, Oxford University Press, 1989, p 15.

37. Shaw S, Luce GG, Gilks WR, et al: Leucocyte differentiation antigen database. *In* Schlossman SF, Boumsall L, Gilles W, et al (eds): Leucocyte Typing V. Oxford, Oxford University Press, 1995, pp 483–783.

38. Kurtzberg J, Waldmann TA, Davey MP, et al: CD7+, CD4–, CD8– acute leukemia: A syndrome of malignant, pluripotent lymphohematopoietic cells. Blood 1989; 73:381.

39. Reinherz EL, Kung PC, Goldstein G, et al: Discrete stages of human intrathymic differentiation. Analysis of normal thymocytes and leukemic lymphoblasts of T-cell lineage. Proc Natl Acad Sci USA 1980; 77:1588.

40. Royston I, Majda JA, Baird SM, et al: Human T cell antigens defined by monoclonal antibodies: The 65,000-dalton antigen of T cells (T65) is also found on chronic lymphocytic leukemia cells bearing surface immunoglobulin. J Immunol 1980; 125:725.

41. Yanagi Y, Yoshikai Y, Leggett K, et al: A human T-cell specific cDNA clone encodes a protein having extensive homology to immunoglobulin chains. Nature 1984; 308:145.

42. Leder P: The genetics of antibody diversity. Sci Am 1982; 246:102.

43. Tonegawa S: Somatic generation of antibody diversity. Nature 1983; 302:575.

44. Dreyer WJ, Bennett JC: The molecular basis of antibody formation: A paradox. Proc Natl Acad Sci USA 1965; 54:864.

45. Ravetch JV, Siebenlist U, Korsmeyer SJ, et al: The structure of the human immunoglobulin μ locus: Characterization of embryonic and rearranged J and D genes. Cell 1981; 27:583.

46. Cook WD, Scharff MD: Antigen-binding mutants of mouse myeloma cells. Proc Natl Acad Sci USA 1977; 74:5687.

47. Kim S, David M, Sinn E, et al: Antibody diversity: Somatic hypermutation of rearranged VH genes. Cell 1981; 27:573.

48. Knap MR, Liu C-P, Newell N, et al: Simultaneous expression of immunoglobulin μ and heavy chains by a cloned B cell lymphoma: A single copy of the VH gene is shared by two adjacent CH genes. Proc Natl Acad Sci USA 1982; 79:2996.

49. Moore KW, Rogers J, Hunkapiller T, et al: Expression of IgD may use both DNA rearrangement and RNA splicing mechanisms. Proc Natl Acad Sci USA 1981; 78:1800.

50. David MM, Kim SK, Hood LE: DNA sequences mediating class switching in α-immunoglobulins. Science 1980; 209:1360.

51. Kataoka T, Miyata T, Honjo T: Repetitive sequences in class switch recombination regions of immunoglobulin heavy chain genes. Cell 1981; 23:357.

52. Ravetch JV, Kirsch IR, Leder P: Evolutionary approach to the question of immunoglobulin heavy chain switching: Evidence from cloned human and mouse genes. Proc Natl Acad Sci USA 1980; 77:6734.

53. Malcolm S, Barton P, Murphy C, et al: Localization of human immunoglobulin K light chain variable region genes to the short arm of chromosome 2 by in situ hybridization. Proc Natl Acad Sci USA 1982; 79:4957.

54. Hieter PA, Hollis GF, Korsmeyer SJ, et al: Clustered arrangement of immunoglobulin λ constant region genes in man. Nature 1981; 294:536.

55. Hedrick SM, Cohen DI, Nielson EA, et al: Isolation of cDNA clones encoding T-cell specific membrane-associated proteins. Nature 1984; 308:149.

56. Hayday AC, Saito H, Gillies SD, et al: Structure, organization, and somatic rearrangement of T-cell γ genes. Cell 1985; 40:259.

57. Lefranc MP, Rabbitts TH: Two tandemly organized human genes encoding the T-cell γ constant region sequences show multiple rearrangement in different T-cell lines. Nature 1985; 316:464.

58. Quertermous T, Murre C, Dialynas D, et al: Human T-cell chain gamma genes: Organization, diversity and rearrangement. Science 1986; 231:252.

59. Chien Y, Iwashima M, Kaplan KB, et al: A new T-cell receptor gene located within the alpha locus and expressed early in T-cell differentiation. Nature 1987; 327:677.

60. Hockett RD, deVillartay JP, Pollock K, et al: Human T-cell antigen receptor (TCR) delta-chain locus and elements responsible for its deletion are within the TCR alpha-chain locus. Proc Natl Acad Sci USA 1988; 85:9694.

61. Brenner MB, McLean J, Dialynas DP, et al: Identification of a putative second T-cell receptor. Nature 1986; 322:145.

62. Korsmeyer SJ, Hieter PA, Ravetch JV, et al: Developmental hierarchy of immunoglobulin gene rearrangements in human leukemic pre-B cells. Proc Natl Acad Sci USA 1981; 78:7096.

63. Arnold A, Cossman J, Bakhshi A, et al: Immunoglobulin gene rearrangement as unique clonal markers in human lymphoid neoplasms. N Engl J Med 1983; 309:1593.

64. Cleary ML, Chao J, Warnke R, et al: Immunoglobulin gene rearrangement as a diagnostic criterion of B cell lymphoma. Proc Natl Acad Sci USA 1984; 81:593.

65. Griesser H, Tkachuk D, Reis MD, et al: Gene rearrangements and translocations in lymphoproliferative diseases. Blood 1989; 73:1402.

66. Waldmann TA: The arrangement of immunoglobulin and T cell receptor genes in human lymphoproliferative disorders. Adv Immunol 1987; 40:247.

67. Waldmann TA, Davis MM, Bongiovanni KF, et al: Rearrangements of genes for the antigen receptor on T cells as markers of lineage and clonality in human lymphoid neoplasms. N Engl J Med 1985; 313:776.

68. Minden MD, Toyonaga B, Ha K, et al: Somatic rearrangement of T-cell antigen receptor gene in human T-cell malignancies. Proc Natl Acad Sci USA 1985; 82:1224.

69. Rabbitts TH, Stinson A, Forster A, et al: Heterogeneity of T-cell β chain rearrangements in human leukemias and lymphomas. EMBO J 1985; 4:2217.

70. Aisenberg AC, Krontiris TG, Mak T, et al: Rearrangement of the gene for the beta chain of the T-cell receptor in T-cell chronic lymphocytic leukemia and related disorders. N Engl J Med 1985; 313:529.

71. Bertness V, Kirsch I, Hollis G, et al: T-cell receptor gene rearrangements as clinical markers of human T-cell lymphomas. N Engl J Med 1985; 313:534.

72. Flug F, Pelicci P-G, Bonetti F, et al: T-cell receptor gene rearrangements as markers of lineage and clonality in T-cell neoplasms. Proc Natl Acad Sci USA 1985; 82:3460.

73. Cleary ML, Warnke R, Sklar J: Monoclonality of lymphoproliferative lesions in cardiac-transplant recipients on immunoglobulin gene rearrangements. N Engl J Med 1984; 310:477.

74. Pangalis GA, Nathwani BN, Rappaport H: Malignant lymphoma, well differentiated type: Its relationship with chronic lymphocytic leukemia and macroglobulinemia of Waldenström. Cancer 1977; 39:999.

75. Evans HL, Butler JJ, Youness EL: Malignant lymphoma, small lymphocytic type: A clinicopathologic study of 84 cases with suggested criteria for intermediate lymphocytic lymphoma. Cancer 1978; 41:1440.

76. Spier CM, Grogan TM, Fielder K, et al: Immunophenotypes in "well-differentiated" lymphoproliferative disorders, with emphasis on small lymphocytic lymphoma. Hum Pathol 1986; 17:1126.

77. Ben-Ezra J, Burke JS, Swartz WG, et al: Small lymphocytic lymphoma: A clinicopathologic analysis of 268 cases. Blood 1989; 73:579.

78. Icli F, Ezdinli EZ, Costello W, et al: Diffuse well-differentiated lymphocytic lymphoma (DLWD): Response and survival. Cancer 1978; 42:1936.

79. Morrison WH, Hoppe RT, Weiss LM, et al: Small lymphocytic lymphoma. J Clin Oncol 1989; 7:598.

80. Harris NL, Bhan AK: B-cell neoplasms of the lymphocytic, lympho-plasmacytoid, and plasma cell types: Immunohistologic analysis and clinical correlation. Hum Pathol 1985; 16:829.

81. Medeiros LJ, Strickler JG, Picker LJ, et al: "Well-differentiated" lymphocytic neoplasms: Immunologic findings correlated with clinical presentation and morphologic features. Am J Pathol 1987; 129:523.

82. Thaler J, Denz H, Gattringer C, et al: Diagnostic and prognostic value of immunohistological bone marrow examination. Results in 212 patients with lymphoproliferative disorders. Blut 1987; 54:213.

83. Sundeen JT, Longo DL, Jaffe ES: CD5 expression in small lymphocytic malignancies: Correlations with clinical presentation and sites of disease. Am J Surg Pathol 1992; 16:130.

84. Kipps TJ, Fong S, Tomhove E, et al: High frequency expression of a conserved K light chain variable-region gene in chronic lymphocytic leukemia. Proc Natl Acad Sci USA 1987; 84:2916.

85. Kipps TJ, Robbins BA, Kuster P, et al: Auto-antibody associated cross-reactive idiotypes expressed at high frequency in chronic lymphocyte leukemia relative to B cell lymphomas of follicular center cell origin. Blood 1988; 72:422.

86. Zukerberg LR, Medeiros JL, Ferry JA, et al: Diffuse low-grade B-cell lymphomas: Four clinically distinct subtypes defined by a combination of morphologic and immunophenotypic features. Am J Clin Pathol 1993; 100:373.

87. Balata A, Shen B: Immunophenotyping of subtypes of B-chronic (mature) lymphoid leukemia. Cancer 1992; 70:2436.

88. Levine EG, Arthur DC, Frizzera G, et al: There are differences in cytogenetic abnormalities among the histologic subtypes of the non-Hodgkin's lymphomas. Blood 1985; 66:1414.

89. Koduru PRK, Filippa DA, Richardson ME, et al: Cytogenetic and histologic correlations in malignant lymphomas. Blood 1987; 69:97.

90. Fifth International Workshop on Chromosomes in Leukemia-Lymphoma: Correlation of chromosome abnormalities with histologic and immunologic characteristics in non-Hodgkin's lymphoma and adult T cell leukemia-lymphoma. Blood 1987; 70:1554.

91. Whang-Peng J, Knutsen T, Jaffe ES, et al: Sequential analysis of 43 patients with non-Hodgkin's lymphoma: Clinical correlations with cytogenetic histologic immunophenotyping, and molecular studies. Blood 1995; 85:203.

92. Offit K, Chaganti RSK: Chromosomal aberrations in non-Hodgkin's lymphoma: Biological and clinical correlations. Hematol Oncol Clin North Am 1991; 5:853.

93. Offit K, Parsa NZ, Filippa D, et al: t(9;14)(p13;q32) denotes a subset of low-grade non-Hodgkin's lymphoma with plasmacytoid differentiation. Blood 1992; 80:2594.

94. Schouten HC, Sanger WG, Weisenberger DD, et al: Chromosomal abnormalities in untreated patients with non-Hodgkin's lymphoma: Association with histology, clinical characteristics, and treatment outcome. Blood 1990; 75:1841.

95. Crossen PE: Cytogenetic and molecular changes in chronic B-cell leukemia. Cancer Genet Cytogenet 1989; 43:143.

96. Ueshima Y, Bird ML, Vardiman J, et al: A 14;19 translocation in B-cell chronic lymphocytic leukemia: A new recurring chromosome aberration. Int J Cancer 1985; 36:287.

97. Ohno H, Takimoto G, McKeithan TW: The candidate proto-oncogene *bcl-3* is related to genes implicated in cell lineage determination and cell cycle control. Cell 1990; 60:991.

98. Cleary ML: Transcription factors in human leukaemias. Cancer Surv 1992; 15:89.

99. Offit K, Louis DC, Parsa NZ, et al: Clinical and morphologic features of B-cell small lymphocytic lymphoma with del(6)(q21q23). Blood 1994; 83:2611.

100. Datta T, Baughinger M, Emmerich B, et al: Chromosome analyses in chronic lymphocytic leukemia and related B-cell neoplasms. Cancer Genet Cytogenet 1991; 55:49.

101. Offit K, Parsa NZ, Filippa DA, et al: t(9;14)(p13;q32) denotes a subset of low-grade non-Hodgkin's lymphoma with plasmacytoid differentiation. Blood 1992; 80:2594.

102. Offit K, Jhanwar SC, Ladanyi M, et al: Cytogenetic analysis of 434 consecutively ascertained specimens of non-Hodgkin's lymphoma: Correlations between recurrent aberrations, histology, and exposure to cytotoxic treatment. Genes Chromosom Cancer 1991; 3:189.

103. Jones SE, Fuks Z, Bull M, et al: Non-Hodgkin's lymphomas IV: Clinicopathologic correlation in 405 cases. Cancer 1973; 31:806.

104. Newell JR, Cabanillas FG, Hagemeister FJ, et al: Incidence of lymphoma in the US classified by the Working Formulation. Cancer 1987; 59:857.

105. Lambrechts AC, Hupkes PE, Dorssers LCJ: Translocation (14;18)-

positive cells are present in the circulation of the majority of patients with localized (stage I and II) follicular non-Hodgkin's lymphoma. Blood 1993; 82:2510.

106. Mann RB, Jaffe ES, Berard CW: Malignant lymphomas: A conceptual understanding of morphologic diversity. Am J Pathol 1979; 94:105.

107. Jaffe ES: Follicular lymphomas: Possibility that they are benign tumors of the lymphoid system. J Natl Cancer Inst 1983; 70:401.

108. Cleary ML, Meeker TC, Levy S, et al: Clustering of extensive somatic mutations in the variable region of an immunoglobulin heavy chain gene from a human B cell lymphoma. Cell 1986; 44:97.

109. Meeker T, Lowder J, Cleary ML, et al: Emergence of idiotype variants during treatment of B cell lymphoma with anti-idiotype antibodies. N Engl J Med 1985; 312:1658.

110. Meeker TC, Grimaldi JC, O'Rourke R, et al: Lack of detectable somatic hypermutation in the V region of the IgH chain gene of a human chronic B lymphocytic leukemia. J Immunol 1988; 141:3994.

111. Bird J, Galili N, Link M, et al: Continuing rearrangement but absence of somatic hypermutation in immunoglobulin genes of human B cell precursor leukemia. J Exp Med 1989; 168:229.

112. Carroll WL, Yu M, Link MP, et al: Absence of Ig V region gene somatic hypermutation in advanced Burkitt's lymphoma. J Immunol 1989; 143:692.

113. Fukuhara S, Rowley JD, Varrakojis D, et al: Chromosome abnormalities in poorly differentiated lymphocytic lymphoma. Cancer Res 1979; 39:3119.

114. Yunis JJ, Frizzera G, Oken MM, et al: Multiple recurrent genomic defects in follicular lymphoma. N Engl J Med 1987; 316:79.

115. Tsujimoto Y, Gorham J, Cossman J, et al: The t(14;18) chromosome translocations involved in B-cell neoplasms result from mistakes in VDJ joining. Science 1975; 229:1390.

116. Bakhshi A, Jensen JP, Goldman P, et al: Cloning the chromosomal breakpoint of t(14;18) human lymphomas: Clustering around J$_H$ on chromosome 14 and near a transcriptional unit on 18. Cell 1985; 41:889.

117. Cleary ML, Sklar J: Nucleotide sequence of a t(14;18) chromosomal breakpoint in follicular lymphoma and demonstration of a breakpoint cluster region near a transcriptionally active locus on chromosome 18. Proc Natl Acad Sci USA 1985; 82:7439.

118. Bakhshi A, Wright JJ, Graninger W, et al: Mechanism of the t(14;18) chromosomal translocation: Structural analysis of both derivative 14 and 18 reciprocal partners. Proc Natl Acad Sci USA 84:2396.

119. Tsujimoto Y, Louis E, Bashir MM, et al: The reciprocal partners of both the t(14;18) and the t(11;14) translocations involved in B-cell neoplasms are rearranged by the same mechanism. Oncogene 1988; 2:345.

120. Ngan B-Y, Nourse J, Cleary ML: Detection of chromosomal translocation t(14;18) within the minor cluster region of *Bcl-2* by polymerase chain reaction and direct genomic sequencing of the enzymatically amplified DNA in follicular lymphomas. Blood 1989; 73:1759.

121. Krowczynska AM, Rudders RA, Krontiris TG: The human minisatellite consensus at breakpoints of oncogene translocations. Nucleic Acids Res 1989; 18:1121.

122. Vaux DL, Cory S, Adams JM: *Bcl-2* gene promotes haemopoietic cell survival and cooperates with c-*myc* to immortalize pre-B cells. Nature 1988; 335:440.

123. Hockenbery D, Nunez G, Milliman C, et al: *Bcl-2* is an inner mitochondrial membrane protein that blocks programmed cell death. Nature 1990; 348:334.

124. Nunez G, London L, Hockenbery D, et al: Deregulated *Bcl-2* gene expression selectively prolongs survival of growth factor–deprived hemopoietic cell lines. J Immunol 1990; 144:3602.

125. McDonnell TJ, Deane N, Platt FM, et al: *Bcl-2* immunoglobulin transgenic mice demonstrate extended B-cell survival and follicular lymphoproliferation. Cell 1989; 57:79.

126. McDonnell TJ, Nunez G, Platt FM, et al: Deregulated *Bcl-2*-immunoglobulin transgene expands a resting but responsive immunoglobulin M- and D-expression B cell population. Mol Cell Biol 1990; 10:1901.

127. McDonnell TJ, Korsmeyer SJ: Progression from lymphoid hyperplasia to high-grade malignant lymphoma in mice transgenic for the t(14;18). Nature 1991; 349:254.

128. Hockenbery D, Zutter M, Hickey W, et al: *Bcl-2* protein is topographically restricted in issues characterized by apoptotic cell death. Proc Natl Acad Sci USA 1991; 88:6961.

129. Pezzella F, Tse AG, Cordell JL, et al: Expression of the *Bcl-2* oncogene protein is not specific for the 14;18 chromosome translocation. Am J Pathol 1990; 137:225.

130. Zutter M, Hockenbery D, Silverman GA, et al: Immunolocalization of the *bcl-2* protein within hematopoietic neoplasms. Blood 1991; 78:1062.

131. Yunis JJ, Tanzer J: Molecular mechanisms of hematologic malignancies. Crit Rev Oncogen 1993; 4:161.

132. Weisenburger DD, Kim H, Rappaport H: Mantle-zone lymphoma. A follicular variant of intermediate lymphocytic lymphoma. Cancer 1982; 49:1429.

133. Weisenburger DD: Mantle-zone lymphoma. An immunohistologic study. Cancer 1984; 53:1073.

134. Palutke M, Eisenberg L, Mirchandani I, et al: Malignant lymphoma of small cleaved lymphocytes of the follicular mantle zone. Blood 1982; 59:317.

135. Weisenburger DD, Nathwani BN, Diamond LW, et al: Malignant lymphoma, intermediate lymphocytic type. A clinicopathologic study of 42 cases. Cancer 1981; 48:1415.

136. Lardelli P, Bookman MA, Sundeen J, et al: Lymphocytic lymphoma of intermediate differentiation. Morphologic and immunophenotypic spectrum and clinical correlations. Am J Surg Pathol 1990; 14:752.

137. Bookman MA, Lardelli P, Jaffe ES, et al: Lymphocytic lymphoma of intermediate differentiation. Morphologic, immunophenotypic, and prognostic factors. J Natl Cancer Inst 1990; 82:742.

138. Brittinger G, Bartels H, Common H, et al: Clinical and prognostic relevance of the Kiel classification of non-Hodgkin's lymphomas. Results of a prospective multicenter study by the Kiel Lymphoma Study Group. Hematol Oncol 1984; 2:269.

138a. Lo Coco F, Gaidano G, Louis DC, et al: *p53* mutations are associated with histologic transformation of follicular lymphoma. Blood 1993; 82:2289.

139. Swerdlow SH, Habeshaw JA, Murray LJ, et al: Centrocytic lymphoma. A distinct clinicopathologic immunologic entity. A multiparameter study of 18 cases at diagnosis and relapse. Am J Pathol 1983; 113:181.

140. Hollema H, Poppema S: Immunophenotypes of malignant lymphoma centroblastic-centrocytic and malignant lymphoma centrocytic: An immunohistologic study indicating a derivation from different stages of B cell differentiation. Hum Pathol 1988; 19:1053.

141. Harris NL, Bhan AK: Mantle-zone lymphoma. A pattern produced by lymphomas of more than one cell type. Am J Surg Pathol 1985; 9:872.

142. Salter DM, Krajewski AS, Cunningham S: Activation and differentiation antigen expression in B-cell non-Hodgkin's lymphoma. J Pathol 1988; 154:209.

143. Stein H, Mason DY: Immunological analysis of tissue sections in diagnosis of lymphoma. *In* Hoffbrand AV (ed): Recent Advances in Haematology. Edinburgh, Churchill Livingstone, 1985, p 127.

144. Tsujimoto Y, Yunis J, Onorato-Showe L, et al: Molecular cloning of the chromosomal breakpoint of B-cell lymphomas and leukemias with the t(11;14) chromosome translocation. Science 1984; 224:1403.

145. Tsujimoto Y, Jaffe D, Cossman J, et al: Clustering of breakpoints on chromosome 11 in human B-cell neoplasms with the t(11;14) chromosome translocation. Nature 1985; 315:340.

146. Ince C, Blick M, Lee M, et al: *Bcl-1* gene rearrangements in B cell lymphoma. Leukemia 1988; 2:343.

147. Rabbitts PH, Douglas J, Fischer P, et al: Chromosome abnormalities at 11q13 in B cell tumours. Oncogene 1988; 3:99.

148. Medeiros LJ, Van Krieken JH, Jaffe ES, et al: Association of *bcl-1* rearrangements with lymphocytic lymphoma of intermediate differentiation. Blood 1990; 76:2086.

149. Williams ME, Swerdlow SH, Rosenberg CL, et al: Chromosome 11 translocation breakpoints at the *PRAD1/Cyclin D1* gene locus in centrocytic lymphoma. Leukemia 1993; 7:241.

150. Arnold A, Kim HG, Gaz RD, et al: Molecular cloning and chromosomal mapping of DNA rearranged with the parathyroid hormone gene in a parathyroid adenoma. J Clin Invest 1989; 83:2034.

151. Motokura T, Bloom T, Kim HG, et al: A novel cyclin encoded by a *bcl-1* linked candidate oncogene. Nature 1991; 350:512.

152. Matsushima H, Roussell MF, Ashmun RA, et al: Colony-stimulating factor 1 regulates novel cyclins during the G1 phase of the cell cycle. Cell 1991; 65:701.

153. Xiong Y, Connolly LT, Futcher B, et al: Human D-type cyclin. Cell 1991; 65:691.

154. Rosenberg CL, Wong E, Petty EM, et al: *PRAD-1*, a candidate *Bcl-1*

oncogene: Mapping and expression in centrocytic lymphoma. Proc Natl Acad Sci USA 1991; 88:9638.

155. Harris NL: Low-grade B-cell lymphoma of mucosa-associated lymphoid tissue and monocytoid B-cell lymphoma. Related entities that are distinct from other low grade B-cell lymphoma. Arch Pathol Lab Med 1993; 117:771.

156. Ngan B-Y, Warnke RA, Wilson M, et al: Monocytoid B-cell lymphoma: A study of 36 cases. Hum Pathol 1991; 22:409.

157. Piris M, Rivas C, Morente M, et al: Monocytoid B-cell lymphoma, a tumour related to the marginal zone. Histopathology 1988; 12:383.

158. Nathwani B, Mohrmann R, Byrnes R, et al: Monocytoid B-cell lymphomas: An assessment of diagnostic criteria and a perspective on histogenesis. Hum Pathol 1992; 23:1061.

159. Sheibani K, Burke JS, Swartz WG, et al: Monocytoid B-cell lymphoma. Clinicopathologic study of 21 cases of unique type of low-grade lymphoma. Cancer 1988; 62:1531.

160. Shin SS, Sheibani K, Fishleder A, et al: Monocytoid B-cell lymphoma in patients with Sjögren's syndrome: A clinicopathologic study of 13 patients. Hum Pathol 1991; 22:422.

161. Zulman J, Jaffe R, Talal N, et al: Evidence that the malignant lymphoma of Sjögren's syndrome is a monoclonal B cell neoplasm. N Engl J Med 1978; 299:1215.

162. Isaacson PG: Pathology of malignant lymphomas. Curr Opin Oncol 1992; 4:811.

163. Megraud F: Epidemiology of *Helicobacter pylori* infections. Gastroenterol Clin North Am 1993; 22:73.

164. Xiang A, Censini S, Bayeli PF, et al: Analysis of expression of CagA and VacA virulence factors in 43 strains of *Helicobacter pylori* reveals that clinical isolates can be divided into two major types and that CagA is not necessary for the expression of the vacuolating cytotoxin. Infect Immun 1995; 63:94.

165. NIH Consensus Development Panel on *Helicobacter pylori* in peptic ulcer disease. JAMA 1994; 272:65.

166. Parsonnet J, Hansen S, Rodriguez L, et al: *Helicobacter pylori* infection and gastric lymphoma. N Engl J Med 1994; 330:1267.

167. Isaacson PG, Spencer J: Malignant lymphoma of mucosa-associated lymphoid tissue. Histopathology 1987; 11:445.

168. Isaacson PG: Lymphomas of mucosa-associated lymphoid tissue (MALT). Histopathology 1990; 16:617.

169. Isaacson PG: Gastrointestinal lymphoma. Human Pathol 1994; 25:1020.

170. Wotherspoon AC, Doglioni C, Diss TC, et al: Regression of primary low-grade B-cell gastric lymphoma of mucosa-associated lymphoid tissue after eradication of *Helicobacter pylori*. Lancet 1993; 342:575.

171. Marchetti M, Ariso B, Burroni D, et al: Development of a mouse model of *Helicobacter pylori* infection that mimics human disease. Science 1995; 267:1655.

172. Fishleder A, Tubbs R, Hesse B: Uniform detection of immunoglobulin gene rearrangement in benign lymphoepithelial lesions. N Engl J Med 1987; 316:118.

173. Fong S, Chen PP, Gilbertson TA, et al: Expression of three crossreactive idiotypes on rheumatoid factor autoantibodies from patients with autoimmune diseases and sero-positive adults. J Immunol 1986; 137:122.

Eighteen

The Biology of High-Grade Non-Hodgkin's Lymphoma

Gianluca Gaidano
Riccardo Dalla-Favera

GENERAL CONCEPTS

Non-Hodgkin's lymphomas (NHLs) conventionally classified as high-grade lymphomas include diffuse large cell lymphoma (DLCL), Burkitt's lymphoma (BL), anaplastic large cell lymphoma (ALCL), and lymphoblastic lymphoma (LBL).[1] Acquired immunodeficiency syndrome (AIDS)-related NHLs (AIDS-NHLs) also consistently display a high-grade of malignancy and thus belong to this category of lymphomas.[2] Recently, the clinicopathologic spectrum of high-grade NHL recognized by the Revised European-American Lymphoma (REAL) classification has been expanded to include a rare NHL type provisionally termed "body-cavity–based lymphoma" (BCBL).[3, 4]

This chapter summarizes knowledge on the pathogenesis of those high-grade NHL categories for which some information exists, including DLCL, BL, and AIDS-NHL among B-cell NHLs, and, among mature T-cell NHLs, ALCL. Although formally a high-grade NHL, LBL, particularly cases of T-cell origin, closely reflects the pathogenesis of acute lymphoblastic leukemias (ALLs) of similar phenotype. Thus, the reader is referred to one of the many existing reviews on this subject.

The pathogenesis of high-grade NHL is most likely a highly complex process involving lesions at the DNA level, deregulation of cytokine loops, and stimulation of B-cell receptors by antigens. At present, most established knowledge concerns the involvement of genetic lesions, which are the focus of this chapter. Analogous to human cancers, the genetic lesions involved in high-grade NHL are represented by the activation of protooncogenes, disruption of tumor suppressor genes, and infection of the tumor clone by oncogenic viruses. In contrast with many types of epithelial cancers, the genome of lymphoma cells tends to be relatively stable and is not subject to the generalized random instability that characterizes many types of epithelial cancers.[5] In addition, lymphomas generally lack microsatellite instability, which denotes the presence of molecular defects in DNA mismatch repair genes observed in some hereditary cancer predisposition syndromes as well as in a large fraction of sporadic solid cancers.[6, 7]

ACTIVATION OF PROTOONCOGENES

Analogous to low-grade NHL, the main mechanism of protooncogene activation in high-grade NHL is represented by chromosome translocations. Analogous to most types of lymphoid neoplasms, chromosome translocations of high-grade NHL are constituted by reciprocal and balanced recombination events between two specific chromosome sites. These translocations are recurrently associated with a specific NHL subtype and are clonally represented in each tumor case (Table 18–1). All chromosome translocations of NHL share a common denominator, that is, the presence of a protooncogene mapping to the proximity of the chromosome recombination sites. In most instances, translocations associated with NHL do not lead to coding fusions between two genes, as is commonly the case for ALL.[8] Rather, the translocations alter the expression pattern of the target protooncogene by juxtapositioning it to heterologous regulatory sequences derived from the partner chromosome, a mechanism called "protooncogene deregulation." The heterologous regulatory regions responsible for protooncogene deregulation in high-grade NHL frequently derive from antigen receptor loci and are consistently characterized by high levels of expression in the normal cellular population from which lymphoma is believed to arise. The only exception to the deregulation model is represented by t(2;5)(p23;q35) of T-cell ALCL, in which the translocation fuses two genes, giving rise to a chimeric transcript.

The mechanism by which chromosome translocations occur is still unclear. With respect to chromosome translocations involving antigen receptor loci, indirect evidence suggests that translocations may constitute errors of the machinery involved in antigen receptor gene rearrangement in normal lymphoid cells.[9] Further support to this hypothesis may be derived from the observation that, in B-cell NHL, chromosome breakpoints within the immunoglobulin (Ig) loci are frequently located within joining (J) or switch (S) sequences, which are the DNA regions normally implicated in Ig gene rearrangements during B-cell development. Thus, it is possible that chromosome translocations may result from mistakes in the enzymatic apparatus that, in physiologic conditions, mediates the recombination of antigen receptor genes and, in pathologic conditions, would join sequences

Table 18–1. Chromosome Breaks of B-Cell Non-Hodgkin's Lymphomas

Lymphoma	Translocation	Protooncogene	Function
Lymphoplasmacytoid	9p13	PAX-5	Transcription factor
Mantle cell	11q13	BCL-1	Cyclin D1
Follicular	18q22	BCL-2	Prevents apoptosis
Diffuse large cell	3q27	BCL-6	Transcription factor
Burkitt's	8q24	c-MYC	Transcription factor

from different chromosomes instead of sequences within the same antigen receptor locus.

The pathogenetic role of chromosome translocations is demonstrated by in vitro transformation studies and by tumorigenicity assays in experimental animal models. However, chromosome translocations commonly occur at a certain rate also in normal lymphoid cells when investigated with high-sensitivity techniques, suggesting that these abnormalities lead to tumor development only when associated with other genetic lesions and/or when developing in a permissive microenvironment.[10–13]

In addition to chromosome translocation, other mechanisms of protooncogene activation can also occur in high-grade NHL. Protooncogene amplification is substantially less common than in epithelial cancers,[5] yet it occurs in some cases of high-grade NHL, as exemplified by the instance REL amplifications of B-DLCL.[14] Point mutations may alter the coding sequence of the protooncogene, as in the case of c-MYC and BCL-2,[15–20] or may affect the protooncogene regulatory sequences, as in the case of c-MYC and BCL-6.[21, 22] Although mutations of c-MYC and BCL-2 are virtually restricted to translocated alleles of the protooncogenes, mutations of BCL-6 may occur both in translocated and germline copies of the gene.[22] In contrast with many other types of human neoplasia, mutations of the RAS genes are virtually always absent among NHLs.[23]

INACTIVATION OF TUMOR SUPPRESSOR LOCI

Disruption of tumor suppressor loci in high-grade NHL occurs through mechanisms similar to those associated with other human cancers, that is, deletion of one allele and inactivation of the other allele by mutation. At present, the only tumor suppressor gene known to be consistently implicated in the pathogenesis of high-grade lymphomas is p53.[24, 25] In addition, high-grade NHLs frequently carry specific chromosome deletions, which conceivably are the site of tumor suppressor genes that have not been identified.[5] The most frequent of these deletions involves the long arm of chromosome 6 (6q).[26] The putative pathogenetic role of 6q deletions in high-grade NHL is suggested by the observation that 6q deletions may occur as the sole cytogenetic abnormality in some cases.[5] In addition, 6q deletions may harbor prognostic value as a marker of poor outcome in B-cell NHL.[27]

VIRAL INFECTION

An additional molecular mechanism implicated in high-grade NHL development is represented by infection of the tumor clone by oncogenic viruses. Oncogenic viruses of high-grade NHL are mainly represented by two herpesviruses: Epstein-Barr virus (EBV)[28] and human herpesvirus, type 8 (HHV-8).[29] Both of these viruses display their transforming activity by introducing potential oncogenes genes into the host cells.

EBV represents the prototype of an oncogenic virus implicated in lymphomagenesis.[28] Historically, EBV was initially identified in cases of endemic BL (eBL) of African children, although the spectrum of EBV-infected NHLs includes also sporadic BL (sBL) and AIDS-NHL, in addition to eBL.[28, 30–33] On infection of a B cell, the EBV genome is transported into the nucleus, where it is predominantly present as an extrachromosome circular molecule (episome).[28] The cohesive terminal repeats of EBV, constituted by a variable number of tandem repeats (VNTR) sequence, mediate the formation of the circular episomes.[34] Because of the heterogeneity of the EBV termini, the precise number of VNTR sequences enclosed in the newly formed episomes displays a marked degree of variation, thus providing a constant clonal marker of the episome and, consequently, of a single infected cell.[34]

The pathogenetic relevance of EBV in lymphomagenesis is substantiated by at least two sets of data. First, EBV is able to significantly alter the growth of B cells in vitro and in vivo.[28] Second, EBV-infected NHLs generally harbor one single form of fused EBV termini, consistent with the hypothesis that infection has preceded and may thus have been contributing to clonal expansion.[30, 32] Finally, a fraction of EBV-infected NHLs expresses the EBV-encoded proteins LMP-1 and EBNA-2, which are well-known transforming agents for B cells.[31] Despite this body of evidence, two observations make the pathogenetic role of EBV in lymphomagenesis difficult to understand. First, most healthy people are infected by EBV, whereas the risk of NHL in the general population is low.[35] Second, EBV-infected cases of BL generally fail to express the EBV-encoded transforming proteins LMP-1 and EBNA-2.[31]

HHV-8 is a novel γ-herpesvirus initially identified in tissues of AIDS-related Kaposi's sarcoma and subsequently found to infect virtually 100% of cases of Kaposi's sarcoma, a substantial fraction of multicentric Castleman's diseases, and all cases of BCBL.[3, 4, 29, 36–38] Phylogenetic analysis has shown that the closest relative of HHV-8 is herpes virus saimiri (HVS), a γ2-herpesvirus of primates associated with T-cell lymphoproliferative disorders.[39] Like the other γ-herpesviruses,[40, 41] HHV-8 is also lymphotropic, since it can be found in lymphocytes both in vitro and in vivo.[3, 4, 36, 38 42, 43] Lymphoma cells naturally infected by HHV-8 harbor the HHV-8 genome in its episomal configuration and display a marked restriction of viral gene expression, suggesting a pattern of latent infection.[39, 44] On the application of appropriate stimuli, infected cells may switch from latent to productive, or lytic, replication of the virus.[44] HHV-8 carries several genes that may putatively behave as oncogenes, including a gene homologous to the cellular D-type cyclins, a G-protein–coupled receptor displaying constitutive activation, and several genes encoding for molecules displaying high homology with cellular cytokines (interleukin-6 [IL-6]) and chemokines (MIP-1α, MIP-2).[45–48] The precise pathogenetic role of these HHV-8 genes in human tumors is not yet fully clarified.

B-CELL DIFFUSE LARGE CELL LYMPHOMA

B-cell diffuse large cell lymphoma (B-DLCL) is the most common type of NHL in the Western world, accounting for approximately 40% of all B-cell NHLs occurring in the general population.[49] According to the REAL classification, the term "B-DLCL" is likely to include more than one disease entity, as suggested by the striking heterogeneity of morphology, clinical presentation, and response to treatment.[1] Part of this heterogeneity may reflect the heterogeneous natural history of the disease, which may arise de novo or, alternatively, may develop from the histologic transformation of a progressed follicular lymphoma (FL).[1, 50–56] Despite this heterogeneity, all B-DLCLs represent clonal expansions of mature B cells, with many phenotypic features of germinal center (GC) centroblasts.[1] Because of the extreme complexity of the biologic interactions regulating the physiologic proliferation and differentiation of mature B cells residing in the GC,[57] it is conceivable that a multitude of complex and poorly understood epigenetic alterations may be implicated in the pathogenesis of B-DLCL. However, analogous to most other types of NHL, it is now clearly established that development of B-DLCL associates with specific molecular lesions involving protooncogenes and tumor suppressor genes.

Until a few years ago, no genetic alteration was known to associate specifically and at high frequency with B-DLCL. In fact, alterations of *BCL-2* and *p53*, which do occur in B-DLCL, are not specific for this category of lymphomas and are detected at higher frequencies in other types of B-NHL. Recently, however, our understanding of the molecular pathogenesis of B-DLCL has made a substantial progress with the cloning of 3q27 chromosome breakpoints and with the identification of the *BCL-6* gene. In contrast with the genetic lesions previously detected in B-DLCL, alterations of *BCL-6* display a close association with B-DLCL and may therefore be viewed as a specific pathogenetic element in the development of these disorders.

ROLE OF *BCL-6* IN B-DLCL PATHOGENESIS

Cytogenetic studies of NHL have demonstrated that chromosome alterations affecting band 3q27 are a frequent recurrent abnormality in B-DLCL.[5, 58, 59] These alterations are predominantly represented by reciprocal translocations between the 3q27 region and several alternative partner chromosomes, including, although not restricted to, the sites of the Ig genes at 14q32 (IgH), 2p11 (Igκ), and 22q11

(Igλ).[5, 58, 59] The variability of the partner chromosomes juxtaposed to 3q27 in B-DLCL translocations suggests that these abnormalities belong to the group of "promiscuous" translocations, which involve a fixed chromosome breakpoint on one side and, on the other side, different chromosome partners in different cases.[8]

The recurrency of 3q27 breaks in B-DLCL, as well as the relative specificity of this cytogenetic abnormality for this lymphoma category, suggested that a gene mapping to 3q27 might be pathogenetically implicated in B-DLCL development.[5, 58, 59] The cloning of the chromosome breakpoints of several cases of translocations between 3q27 and Ig loci led to the identification of a genomic region involved in the overwhelming majority of B-DLCL cases harboring 3q27 breaks, irrespective of the partner chromosome participating in the translocation.[60–64] Detailed analysis of such region led to the discovery of a gene, termed "BCL-6," which was expressed in B-DLCL and which was structurally altered by the chromosome breakpoints.[60–64]

Function of the BCL-6 Protein

The *BCL-6* gene codes for a novel protein containing six zinc-finger motifs that are present in a number of related transcription factors and are able to mediate the protein binding to specific DNA sites (Fig. 18–1).[65–68] The amino-terminal region of the *BCL-6* protein contains a domain, termed "POZ," which is homologous to domains found also in several other zinc-finger transcription factors, including several *Drosophila* developmental regulators, the human KUP protein, and the human PLZF protein, which is occasionally involved in chromosome translocations of human promyelocytic leukemia.[69, 70] Apparently, the POZ domain acts as a protein-protein interface implicated in homodimerization-heterodimerization processes.[69] These structural features of the *BCL-6* protein are consistent with functional studies indicating that *BCL-6* can indeed function as a transcription factor that binds a specific DNA sequence and represses transcription from linked promoters.[71] Thus, in physiologic conditions, the *BCL-6* protein

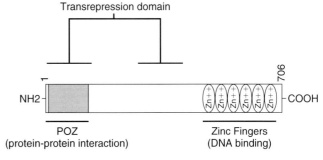

Figure 18–1. Structure of the BCL-6 protein. BCL-6 is a transcription factor composed of 706 amino-acidic residues (residues 1 and 706 are indicated by numbers).[63] The main functional domains of the BCL-6 protein are schematically represented in the figure, including the six zinc-finger motifs at the carboxy-terminus of the protein and the POZ domain at the amino-terminus of the protein. The zinc-finger domain of BCL-6 mediates DNA binding, whereas the POZ domain mediates protein-protein interactions. The portion of the BCL-6 protein responsible for the transrepressor function of BCL-6 is also indicated (transrepression domain).

acts as a transcriptional repressor that inhibits the expression of genes carrying its specific DNA-binding motif.

Insights into the physiologic function of *BCL-6* may be gained from its expression pattern in normal tissues.[72] Indeed, the pattern of *BCL-6* expression in human tissues is highly specific. Although minimal amounts of *BCL-6* RNA and protein can be found in numerous tissues, high levels of expression are specifically restricted to the B-cell lineage.[72] Notably, expression of *BCL-6* within the B-cell compartment is specifically regulated during differentiation, since *BCL-6* is expressed in mature B cells but not in immature bone marrow precursors or terminally differentiated cells such as plasma cells.[72] Furthermore, *BCL-6* expression is highly compartmentalized among mature B cells, since its expression is topographically restricted to the GC, where *BCL-6* is expressed by virtually all proliferating cells (the centroblasts) as well as nonproliferating elements (the centrocytes).[72] This expression pattern, that is, expression within the GC, but not before entrance into (mantle zone) or after exit from (memory B cells, plasma cells) the GC, suggests that *BCL-6* may be needed for GC development and sustainment, whereas its downregulation may be necessary for differentiation of B cells into plasma cells or, alternatively, memory B cells (Fig. 18–2).

The role of *BCL-6* in physiologic immune processes has been further clarified by animal models in which the *BCL-6* gene has been biallelically disrupted.[73] Mice carrying the *BCL-6–/–* phenotype display normal B- and T-cell counts, yet they consistently fail to form GC after injection of T-cell–dependent antigens, an immunologic defect typically associated with the inability of B cells to proliferate and acquire the GC phenotype. Consistent with lack of GC formation, *BCL-6–/–* mice also display an impaired antigen-specific IgG response. The defect in GC formation in *BCL-6*–deficient mice is the result of an intrinsic defect in the lymphoid compartment rather than of an abnormality of accessory cells. Lack of GC formation induced by *BCL-6* disruption is associated with a high incidence of infectious diseases and inflammatory processes, which cause premature death in *BCL-6*–deficient mice. Overall, these animal models unequivocally demonstrate that *BCL-6* is a key regulator of GC formation and B-cell immune response.

Mechanism of *BCL-6* Deregulation in B-DLCL: Promoter Substitution

Chromosome translocations involving band 3q27 truncate the *BCL-6* gene within its 5′ flanking region, within the first exon, or within the first intron (Fig. 18–3), making these alterations readily detectable as rearrangements by Southern blot hybridization analysis of tumor DNA.[60–64, 74] The coding domain of the *BCL-6* gene is left intact in all cases displaying *BCL-6* rearrangements, whereas the 5′ regulatory sequences, which contain the *BCL-6* promoter, are either truncated or, alternatively, completely removed, as in the case of truncation within the *BCL-6* first exon or first intron.[60–64, 74] In all *BCL-6* rearrangements, the entire coding sequence of *BCL-6* is juxtaposed downstream to heterologous sequences that, based on cytogenetic data, may originate from different chromosome sites in different patients.[60–64, 74]

The rearranged *BCL-6* genes and related transcription products have been analyzed in high detail in a few cases of B-DLCL.[75, 76] These studies have revealed that the common functional consequence of these alterations is the juxtaposition of heterologous promoters to the *BCL-6* coding domain, a mechanism called "promoter substitution" (Fig. 18–4). These recombinatory events generate chimeric transcripts that initiate from promoters derived from one of the various chromosome loci recombining with 3q27 and juxtaposed to normal *BCL-6* coding sequences. The resulting chimeric transcript encodes a normal *BCL-6* protein.

In a small fraction of B-DLCLs carrying *BCL-6* rearrangements, the breakpoint location maps to the immediate vicinity of the 5′ promoter region and, consequently, only the

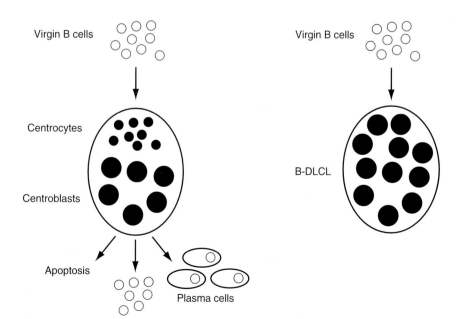

Figure 18–2. Model of BCL-6 involvement in normal mature B-cell subsets *(A)* and in B-DLCL *(B)*. *A,* In mature B cells that have not yet entered the germinal center (GC)—the virgin B cells—expression of BCL-6 is consistently absent.[72] On entering the GC, B cells express high levels of BCL-6, which is detectable in both proliferating (i.e., the centroblasts) and nonproliferating (i.e., the centrocytes) cells.[72] On exit from the GC, B cells switch off BCL-6 expression independent of their fate (memory B cells, plasma cells, apoptosis). *B,* In the case of B-DLCL carrying rearrangements of BCL-6, the expression of BCL-6 is constitutively activated by heterologous promoters juxtaposed to the BCL-6 coding sequence as a result of chromosome translocation.[72, 76] The constitutive activation of BCL-6 in B-DLCL prevents its physiologic downregulation and, consequently, prevents further maturation of B-DLCL cells, which are thus "frozen" at the stage of GC B cells.

A

B

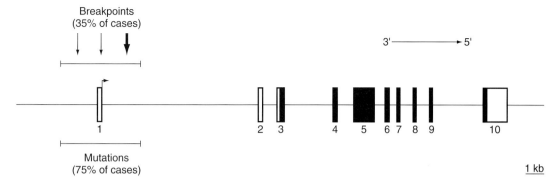

Figure 18–3. Schematic representation of genetic lesions affecting the *BCL-6* gene in high-grade NHL. In its germline configuration, the *BCL-6* gene is composed of 10 exons.[63] The coding region of *BCL-6* is indicated by black boxes, and the noncoding exons (or portions of exons) are indicated by white boxes. The physiologic *BCL-6* promoters are indicated by an arrow. Rearrangements of *BCL-6* occur in approximately 35% of B-DLCL cases and the breakpoint sites (indicated by *arrows*) span the *BCL-6* first exon and its adjacent sequences on both sides.[60–64, 74, 78, 79] The majority of breakpoints map to 3′ sequences in the immediate vicinity of the *BCL-6* first exon (indicated by *thick arrow*). In addition to rearrangements, *BCL-6* may also be affected by small mutations clustering in the proximity of the *BCL-6* first exon/first intron border.[22]

putative 5′ regulatory sequences are removed.[60–64, 74] Conceivably, the consequence of the translocation in such cases may be the substitution of these regulatory sequences with enhancers or with other distantly acting regulatory elements derived from other chromosomes.

In functional terms, the substitution of the *BCL-6* promoter by heterologous regulatory sequences implies that *BCL-6* expression is deregulated in B-DLCL carrying *BCL-6* rearrangements. One feature shared by the heterologous promoters linked to rearranged *BCL-6* alleles is that they are physiologically active in normal B cells and are not downregulated during the late stages of B-cell differentia-

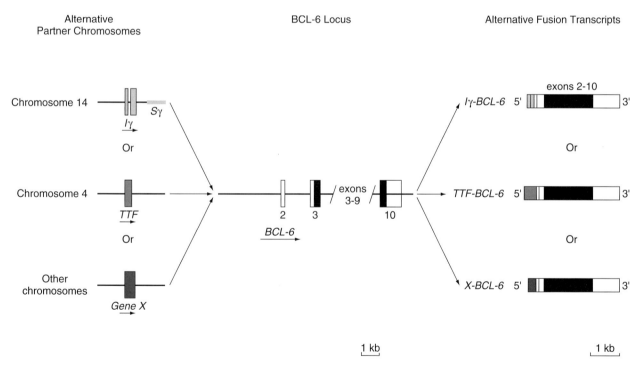

Figure 18–4. Schematic representation of promoter substitution caused by chromosome translocations involving the *BCL-6* gene. The figure shows the example of t(3;14), juxtaposing *BCL-6* to Ig_{H},[76] and t(3;4), juxtaposing *BCL-6* to *TTF*.[75] Various other chromosome sites (designated as "other chromosomes") may be involved. The putative genes implicated by these other translocations are designated as "genes X." Regardless of the partner chromosome involved, most *BCL-6* translocated alleles are deprived of their exon 1 and their endogenous promoters. The novel sequences derived from chromosome 14, chromosome 4, or other chromosomes are thus juxtaposed 5′ to the *BCL-6* first intron. These novel sequences provide a heterologous promoter to *BCL-6*, such as the Ig_{H} germline transcript promoter Iγ (or alternatively Iμ) in the case of t(3;14) and the *TTF* promoter in the case of t(3;4).[75, 76] Other chromosome sites can follow the pattern of t(3;14) and t(3;4), thus contributing a heterologous promoter (gene X in the figure) to the juxtaposed *BCL-6* gene. The translocations leave intact the genomic configuration of the *BCL-6* gene downstream to the breakpoint site. The far right of the figure represents the transcripts resulting from t(3;14), t(3;4), and translocations of 3q27 with other chromosome sites. In all cases, the translocation gives rise to a fusion transcript, represented by Ig/*BCL-6* in the case of t(3;14), *TTF/BCL-6* in the case of t(3;4), and X/*BCL-6* in the case of *BCL-6* translocations with other chromosome sites.[75, 76] These chimeric transcripts initiate from heterologous promoters provided by the chromosome site juxtaposed to *BCL-6* and retain the entire normal *BCL-6* coding domain, which translates into a normally sized *BCL-6* protein.

tion.[75, 76] Thus, one common consequence of *BCL-6* rearrangements may be that of preventing downregulation of *BCL-6* and, in turn, blocking the differentiation of GC B cells toward the stage of plasma cells (see Fig. 18–2). According to this model, B-DLCL cells carrying *BCL-6* rearrangements would thus be "frozen" at the stage of GC cells. This model needs to be substantiated by studies aimed at defining the behavior of B cells transfected with activated *BCL-6* alleles both in vitro and in vivo.

Distribution of BCL-6 Rearrangements Throughout the Spectrum of NHLs

By conventional molecular assays, *BCL-6* rearrangements are detectable in 35% of cases of B-DLCL and in a small fraction of FLs.[60–64, 74, 78, 79] Conversely, *BCL-6* rearrangements are consistently absent in all other types of NHL or in other lymphoid neoplasms, including ALL, chronic lymphocytic leukemia, multiple myeloma, and T-cell malignancies.[60–64, 74, 78, 79]

Among B-DLCLs, the frequency of *BCL-6* rearrangements detected by molecular investigations far exceeds the frequency of 3q27 cytogenetic abnormalities, suggesting that *BCL-6* rearrangements may occur as a consequence of submicroscopic chromosome aberrations.[63] On the other hand, however, not all B-DLCL cases carrying a 3q27 cytogenetic abnormality display a rearrangement of *BCL-6* when assessed with current available molecular assays.[63] Most likely, this is due to the presence of more than one breakpoint cluster in the proximity of the *BCL-6* gene.

Hypermutation of the 5' Noncoding Regions of BCL-6

In addition to rearrangements, the *BCL-6* gene may be altered by other mechanisms in B-DLCL as well as in other types of B-cell NHL. In approximately 70% of B-DLCLs and 50% of FLs, the *BCL-6* gene is affected by multiple, often biallelic, mutations that selectively cluster within the 5' noncoding regions of the gene (see Fig. 18–3).[22] The mutations detected in *BCL-6* 5' noncoding sequences differ from the mutations affecting the c-*MYC* and *BCL-2* protooncogenes when translocated to Ig loci in NHL, since *BCL-6* mutations frequently occur independently of translocation to Ig loci or in the absence of any recognizable chromosome abnormality affecting band 3q27 or rearrangement of the *BCL-6* locus.[15–22] The DNA sequences most frequently affected by mutations lie in closer proximity to the *BCL-6* promoter region and overlap with the major cluster of chromosome breaks at 3q27, suggesting that mutations and rearrangements may be selected for their ability to alter the same region that conceivably regulates the normal expression of *BCL-6*.[22] The cumulative frequency of mutations and rearrangements approaches 100% of B-DLCL cases, indicating that structural alterations of the 5' noncoding regions of *BCL-6* might be a *sine qua non* for the development of these lymphomas.[22] Studies involving in vitro cell transformation systems and in vivo expression in transgenic mice are needed to determine the exact role played by mutated *BCL-6* alleles in lymphomagenesis.

OTHER GENETIC LESIONS OF B-DLCL

Several other genetic lesions have been detected in B-DLCL. In contrast with *BCL-6* rearrangements, however, these additional lesions either are not specific for B-DLCL, being detected also in other NHL types, or occur at low frequencies in B-DLCL cases.

A variable fraction of B-DLCL cases display chromosome rearrangements of *BCL-2*.[78, 80–82] These translocations are entirely similar to the ones associated with FL and lead to the deregulated expression of *BCL-2*, thus preventing apoptosis.[83–86] These alterations appear to be mutually exclusive with *BCL-6* rearrangements and tend to associate with B-DLCL cases deriving from the histologic transformation of FL (see later).[78, 80]

Several initial reports had described a certain rate of c-*MYC* rearrangements among B-DLCLs.[87, 88] These rearrangements appeared to be structurally similar to those of sBL (see later). However, subsequent studies have unequivocally defined that c-*MYC* activation among B-DLCLs is extremely rare[78] and preferentially associates with small numbers of extranodal B-DLCL or B-DLCL transformed from a previous FL phase.[89, 90]

Two members of the *NF-kB/REL* family of transcription factors appear to be involved in the pathogenesis of a fraction of B-DLCLs, including *NF-kB2* and *REL*.[14, 91] The *NF-kB2* gene maps to 10q24 and occasionally has been found to undergo rearrangements in B-DLCL.[91] These rearrangements are structurally similar to those more frequently found in T-cell NHL and cause the production of altered proteins that are unable to repress transcription and behave as constitutional transactivators.[92, 93] Genetic alterations of *REL* appear to be a more frequent event, since they occur in 20% of B-DLCLs, preferentially in cases with extranodal involvement.[14]

Among tumor suppressor genes, inactivation of *p53* is virtually absent in B-DLCL arising de novo, whereas it frequently associates with cases resulting from the histologic transformation of FL.[77, 78, 94] In these cases, mutations of *p53* are presumably acquired during transformation from FL to B-DLCL. Given the role of *p53* in controlling cell proliferation and genomic stability,[25] it is likely that disruption of normal *p53* functions may contribute to tumor progression directly, by providing FL cells with a high proliferative rate, or indirectly, by allowing the accumulation of additional genetic lesions. Finally, deletions of the long arm of chromosome 6 are also frequently detected in B-DLCL, although the gene (or genes) involved is not known.[26]

MOLECULAR HETEROGENEITY OF B-CELL DLCL

The REAL classification has established that with current knowledge and methods it is impractical to histologically subclassify B-DLCL into the morphologic variants recognized by previous classifications, that is, diffuse centroblastic lymphoma (Working Formulation category G), diffuse immunoblastic lymphoma (Working Formulation category H), and diffuse mixed, small and large cell lymphoma (Working Formulation category F).[1, 95] However, clinicians and pathologists converge in stating that B-DLCL does represent a highly heterogeneous disease. Conceivably, B-DLCL

Transformation Pathway

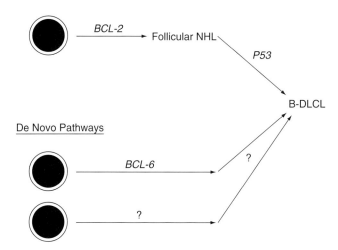

De Novo Pathways

Figure 18–5. Model of molecular pathways in B-DLCL development. Three main pathogenetic pathways may be recognized in B-DLCL.[77, 78, 80, 94] The first pathway, designated as the "transformation pathway," implicates the transformation of a preexisting follicular NHL to a B-DLCL histology. Cases of B-DLCL belonging to this pathway harbor rearrangements of *BCL-2* and mutations of *p53*. Whereas the *BCL-2* rearrangement is already present in the follicular NHL phase, *p53* mutations are gained during histologic transformation. The other two molecular pathways are designated as "de novo pathways," since in these instances B-DLCL develops without a preexistent follicular lymphoma. The first de novo pathway implicates the *BCL-6* gene and, possibly, additional genetic lesions presently unknown (indicated by the question mark). The second de novo pathway involves presently unknown genetic lesions (indicated by the question marks), although some cases may harbor alterations of *REL* or *NF*-kB2.[14, 91]

heterogeneity may reflect pathogenetic heterogeneity, including the association with distinct genetic alterations.

The identification of several distinct molecular types of B-DLCL corroborates the hypothesis that the heterogeneity of the disease relies on its pathogenetic heterogeneity. At least three distinct molecular pathways have been identified in association with B-DLCL.[77, 78, 80, 94, 96] The first molecular type of B-DLCL, accounting for approximately 40% of the cases, displays rearrangements of *BCL-6*, whereas all other known genetic alterations of NHL are absent. Cases of B-DLCL harboring *BCL-6* rearrangements are de novo lymphomas, presenting without a previous history of FL (Fig. 18–5). The second B-DLCL type involves activation of *BCL-2*, either alone or in association with *p53* mutations. Cases of B-DLCL carrying both *BCL-2* and *p53* rearrangements derive from the histologic transformation of a previous FL phase (see Fig. 18–5), whereas the natural history of *BCL-2+/p53−* B-DLCL is still debated. The third molecular type of B-DLCL displays germline *BCL-2* and *BCL-6* alleles. No genetic lesion has been found to consistently associate with this B-DLCL type, although rearrangements of *REL* or *NF*-kB2 may occur in selected cases.

The distinction of B-DLCL categories based on the tumor genotype may prove to be practically relevant, since one study has shown that cases with *BCL-6* rearrangements display the most favorable prognosis, whereas cases carrying *BCL-2* translocations have the poorest outcome.[80] The third group—cases without any known genetic alteration—appear to have an intermediate prognosis.[80]

BURKITT'S LYMPHOMA

BL is classified into two main epidemiologic variants: sBL and eBL.[1] Cases of sBL occur in North America and Europe, where sBL accounts for approximately one third of pediatric lymphomas. Cases of eBL occur primarily in Equatorial Africa and Papua-New Guinea, where BL accounts for approximately 50% of childhood cancer. Although sBL and eBL display many morphologic similarities, the two BL variants differ in their natural history and clinical behavior, particularly with respect to the involvement of body sites.[1] Further clinical heterogeneity of BL is due to the fact that some cases present with massive involvement of the bone marrow and peripheral blood. Such cases had been traditionally termed ALL, L_3 type according to the French-American-British (FAB) classification of ALL. During the last few years, however, several investigators believed that such leukemic cases should be classified as BL because of their biologic features and their response to therapy. In 1994, the REAL classification of B-cell neoplasia has formally acknowledged that L_3-ALL and classic BL represent different manifestations of the same disease.[1]

Despite the epidemiologic and clinical heterogeneity of BL, all BL variants, including sBL, eBL, and L_3-ALL, consistently share a common genetic background represented by chromosome translocations between c-*MYC* and one of the Ig loci. Other genetic lesions associate at variable frequencies with cases of BL and include infection of the tumor clone by EBV and mutations of *p53*.

BREAKS AT 8q24 AND c-*MYC*

Chromosome breaks at 8q24 are found in 100% of sBLs, eBLs, and L_3-ALLs.[1] Historically, translocations of 8q24 have provided the first example of the involvement of protooncogenes in tumor-associated chromosome abnormalities and have thus constituted the model for the study of other chromosome translocations involving antigen receptor loci.[97] The study of 8q24 translocations in human tumors has been paralleled by that of analogous translocations in tumors of several animal species, thus corroborating the pathogenetic relevance of these genetic lesions.[98–100] In human BL, all 8q24 breaks lead to a common final consequence: deregulation of the expression of the c-*MYC* protooncogene.[97] Depending on the Ig locus concerned, the c-*MYC* gene may be involved in three distinct translocations (Fig. 18–6).[97, 101–105] In 80% of cases the translocation involves IgH, leading to t(8;14)(q24;q32). In the remaining 20% of cases, c-*MYC* juxtaposes either to Igκ, leading to t(2;8)(p11;q24) (15% of cases), or to Igλ, leading to t(8;22)(q24;q11) (5% of cases). Throughout the spectrum of B-cell neoplasms recognized by the REAL classification, breaks at 8q24 selectively cluster with all BL variants, whereas they are virtually absent in all other NHL categories.[1]

Structure and Function of the c-MYC Protein

The product of the c-*MYC* protooncogene is a ubiquitously expressed nuclear phosphoprotein that functions as a transcriptional regulator controlling cell proliferation, differentiation, as well as apoptosis.[97] Expression of c-*MYC* is higher in proliferating cells and is rapidly induced in

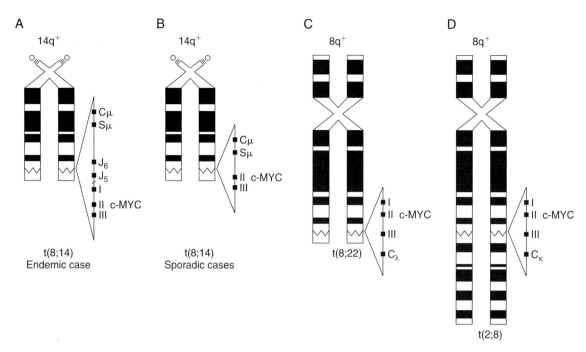

Figure 18–6. Schematic representation of chromosome translocations involving c-*MYC*. The t(8;14) of eBL and sBL is shown in *A* and *B*, respectively. The variant translocations t(8;22) and t(2;8) are shown in *C* and *D*, respectively. Black boxes indicate functional regions of the Ig$_H$ (Cμ, Sμ, J), Igκ, (Cκ), and Ig$_L$ (Cλ) genes as well as exons of the c-*MYC* gene.

quiescent cells on mitogenic induction, suggesting that c-*MYC* plays a role in mediating the transition from quiescence to proliferation.[106] In addition to mediating cell proliferation, c-*MYC* is also implicated in blocking the cellular programs of differentiation, as demonstrated by the observation that cells constitutively harboring sustained levels of c-*MYC* protein are unable to achieve a terminally differentiated status.[106] In the absence of a supportive microenvironment providing adequate concentrations of growth stimuli, however, proliferation and block of differ-

entiation, or both, are replaced by cellular apoptosis.[107–110] Given that c-*MYC* expression is necessary for proliferation and that downregulation of c-*MYC* is necessary for growth arrest and differentiation, the c-*MYC* protooncogene appears to be an important central regulator determining the alternative fates of a cell: proliferation, differentiation, and death.

The biochemical mechanisms through which c-*MYC* achieves its various functions have been clarified to a certain extent. In physiologic in vivo settings, c-*MYC* is mainly en-

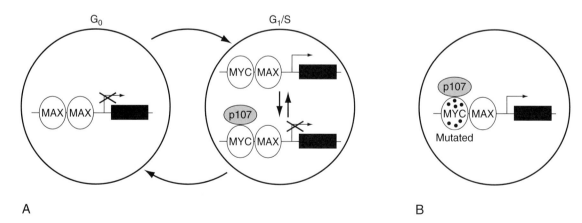

Figure 18–7. Interactions between c-*MYC*, *MAX*, and p107 in normal cells *(A)* and in BL *(B)*. c-*MYC*, *MAX*, and p107 are represented by open circles (c-*MYC* and *MAX*) or gray circles (p107). Downstream genes regulated by c-*MYC* are schematically represented by a black rectangle. The arrow indicates the site of transcriptional initiation of c-*MYC* downstream genes. In normal cells, expression of *MAX* is stable throughout the cell cycle, whereas, in G$_0$, c-*MYC* expression is absent or extremely low.[106, 111–116] In this context, *MAX* homodimers predominate, whereas no *MYC/MAX* heterodimers are formed, resulting in inhibited transcription of genes regulated by c-*MYC*. On entering the cell cycle (G$_1$/S phase), c-*MYC* levels rise and *MYC/MAX* heterodimers are formed, thus promoting transcription of c-*MYC* downstream genes.[106, 111–116] Active *MYC/MAX* complexes are in equilibrium with complexes in which c-*MYC* binds to p107, a pRb-related protein that represses the transcriptional activity of c-*MYC*.[130, 131] In BL, activation of c-*MYC* occurs through two distinct mechanisms. First, transcription of the c-*MYC* gene is deregulated, leading to constitutive levels of c-*MYC* mRNA and protein.[97, 121–123] Second, c-*MYC* translocated alleles frequently carry mutations in the c-*MYC* transactivation domain (indicated by black dots within the c-*MYC* circle).[15, 16] As a consequence of these mutations, p107 is no longer able to suppress c-*MYC* transcriptional activity, leading to constitutive transcription of c-*MYC* downstream genes.[130–132]

gaged in heterodimeric complexes with the related protein *MAX* (Fig. 18–7).[111–116] The interaction between c-*MYC* and *MAX* is mediated by basic helix-loop-helix (bHLH) and leucine-zipper (LZIP) domains present in both proteins. Heterodimers composed of c-*MYC* and *MAX* stimulate transcription and cell proliferation through DNA binding to the core hexanucleotide CACGTG.[111–116] In addition to c-*MYC*, *MAX* can also form homodimers as well as heterodimers with *MAD* and *MXI*1, two bHLH-LZIP proteins that act as negative regulators of transcription.[117, 118] Since the levels of *MAX* tend to be stable throughout the cell cycle, the ratio of c-*MYC*/*MAX* heterodimers is controlled by the relative abundance of c-*MYC*, *MAD*, and *MXI*1.[111–118] As the ratio of c-*MYC* to *MAD* or *MXI*1 varies, the promoter activity of target genes is expected to be modulated in either a positive

(when c-*MYC* levels are high) or negative (when *MAD* or *MXI*1 levels are high) fashion. Therefore, in lymphoid tumors associated with c-*MYC* deregulation (see later), it is conceivable that constitutive expression of c-*MYC* leads to the prevalence of *MYC*/*MAX* heterodimers, thus inducing positive growth regulation.[115]

Deregulation of c-MYC by Chromosome Rearrangement

Although fairly homogeneous at the microscopic level, c-*MYC* translocations display a high degree of heterogeneity when dissected at the molecular level (Fig. 18–8). The t(8;14) breakpoints are located 5′ and centromeric to c-*MYC*, whereas they map 3′ to c-*MYC* in t(2;8) and t(8;22).[97, 101–105]

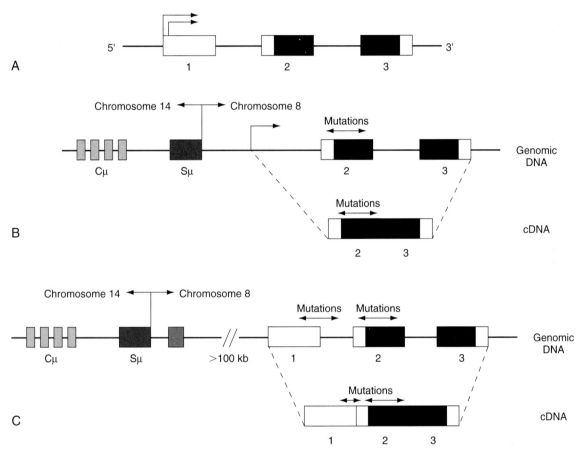

Figure 18–8. Schematic representation of chromosome translocations involving the c-*MYC* gene. In its germline configuration *(A)*, c-*MYC* is composed of three exons. The coding region of c-*MYC* is indicated by black boxes, and noncoding exons (or portions of exons) are indicated by white boxes. The c-*MYC* promoters are indicated by arrows. The molecular consequences of the most frequent c-*MYC* translocation, that is, t(8;14), are depicted in *B* and *C*. Two molecular subtypes of t(8;14) are recognized, which tend to associate with sBL *(B)* and eBL *(C)*, respectively. For each molecular subtype of t(8;14), both the genomic configuration and the resulting cDNA of a representative translocated c-*MYC* allele are shown. In the case of t(8;14) of sBL *(B)*, the chromosome 8 breakpoint involves sequences within c-*MYC*, which is deprived of its exon 1. Since the physiologic promoters are removed by the translocation, transcription is driven by an otherwise silent promoter located within c-*MYC* intron 1 (indicated by an *arrow* in the figure). On chromosome 14, the breakpoint maps in the proximity of the switch μ (S$_\mu$) region. Notably, the translocation leaves intact the gross configuration of the coding sequence of c-*MYC*. However, at the nucleotide level, c-*MYC* translocated alleles frequently harbor point mutations within the exon 2 coding sequence, leading to amino acid substitutions in the c-*MYC* protein. The cDNA encoded by translocated c-*MYC* alleles includes the exons 2 and 3 of the gene, as well as an abnormally transcribed sequence of intron 1, starting from the novel transcriptional initiation site within c-*MYC* intron 1. Since the c-*MYC* coding region is intact, a normally sized c-*MYC* protein is translated by t(8;14) of sBL. In the case of t(8;14) of eBL *(C)*, the c-*MYC* breakpoint involves sequences on chromosome 8 at an undefined distance (>100 kb) 5′ to c-*MYC* and sequences on chromosome 14 within or in proximity to the Ig J$_H$ region. The internal genomic configuration of the translocated c-*MYC* allele is thus apparently preserved. However, c-*MYC* alleles involved by t(8;14) of eBL consistently harbor small mutations mapping to the exon 1–intron 1 border, where c-*MYC* regulatory regions are located. In addition, point mutations within exon 2 coding sequence are also present. The cDNA transcribed by translocated c-*MYC* alleles of eBL includes c-*MYC* exons 1 through 3 and gives rise to a normally sized c-*MYC* protein.

In the instance of t(8;14), the exact location of the breakpoint sites of chromosomes 8 and 14 contributes further heterogeneity. In eBL, the breakpoint sites on chromosome 8 preferentially involve sequences at an undefined distance (>1000 kilobases [kb]) 5' to c-*MYC*, whereas, on chromosome 14, the breakpoints fall within or in proximity of the Ig J_H region.[119, 120] In sBL, the t(8;14) breakpoints fall within or immediately 5' (<3 kb) to c-*MYC* on chromosome 8 and within the Ig S regions on chromosome 14.[119, 120]

The common functional effect of t(8;14), t(2;8), and t(8;22) is that c-*MYC* translocated alleles undergo constitutive expression in tumor cells, whereas in physiologic conditions c-*MYC* levels are tightly regulated during B-cell proliferation and differentiation.[121–123] Chromosome translocations cause c-*MYC* deregulation by at least two distinct mechanisms. First, translocated c-*MYC* alleles are juxtaposed to heterologous regulatory elements derived from Ig loci.[97, 101–105] For example, in the case of t(8;14), the enhancer region Eμ and 3'αE have been proposed as the relevant sequences responsible for c-*MYC* deregulation.[124, 125] Second, the 5' regulatory regions of c-*MYC* are consistently affected by structural alterations that are supposed to modify their responsiveness to cellular factors regulating c-*MYC* expression. In the case of sBL and L_3-ALL, the t(8;14) chromosome translocation decapitates the c-*MYC* gene of its first exon.[120] Conversely, in cases carrying breakpoints located either 5' or 3' to the c-*MYC* gene, that is, eBL harboring t(8;14) and all cases carrying t(2;8) or t(8;22), a 400-base pair region spanning the first exon–first intron junction is selectively and consistently mutated in translocated c-*MYC* alleles.[21] This region contains potentially relevant regulatory domains, including (1) the sequences involved in the block of transcriptional elongation, a mechanism modulating c-*MYC* expression during proliferation and differentiation[126, 127]; and (2) the domain involved in the differentiation-regulated binding of *MYC* intron factor (MIF), a protein believed to regulate c-*MYC* expression.[128]

In addition to transcriptional deregulation, oncogenic conversion of c-*MYC* is also believed to stem from amino acid substitutions in c-*MYC* exon 2 affecting the *N*-terminal transcriptional activation domain of the gene.[15, 16] These mutations, which are found in comparable positions in retroviral v-*MYC*, occur in more than 50% of BL and cluster in hot spots involving Glu-39, Thr-58, Ser-62, and Phe-138.[15, 16, 129] The high prevalence of these mutations suggests a biologic role for these alterations in lymphomagenesis. Although in normal conditions the activity of the c-*MYC* transactivation domain is suppressed by protein-protein interactions with the pRB-related protein p107, c-*MYC* proteins carrying exon 2 mutations are able to escape the p107-mediated modulation (see Fig. 18–7).[130, 131] The mechanism of resistance of mutant c-*MYC* proteins to p107-mediated suppression is not known, although it is not caused by the disruption of the physical interactions between c-*MYC* and p107. Rather, c-*MYC* exon 2 mutations may confer resistance to p107-mediated phosphorylation, which is essential for the p107 suppression effect (see Fig. 18–7).[132]

Several lines of experimental evidence document that the deregulated expression of c-*MYC* can influence the growth of B cells in vitro and in vivo. In vitro, the expression of c-*MYC* oncogenes transfected into EBV-immortalized human B cells, a potential natural target for c-*MYC* activation in EBV-positive BL, leads to their malignant transformation.[133] In addition, antisense oligonucleotides directed against translocated c-*MYC* alleles are able to revert the tumorigenicity of BL.[134–136] In vivo, the targeted expression of c-*MYC* oncogenes in the B-cell lineage of transgenic mice leads to the development of B-cell malignancies at a high rate.[137]

OTHER GENETIC LESIONS OF BURKITT'S LYMPHOMA

In addition to c-*MYC* translocations, the molecular pathogenesis of BL also involves infection of the tumor clone by EBV, inactivation of the *p53* tumor suppressor gene, and deletions of 6q.

Infection by EBV occurs in virtually all cases of eBL and in approximately 30% of cases of sBL.[28, 31] The consistent monoclonality of EBV infection in BL, as assessed by molecular analysis of EBV terminal repeats, suggests that infection precedes clonal expansion of the tumor, consistent with a pathogenetic role of the virus.[32] Notably, however, BL cells fail to express the EBV-encoded antigens LMP-1 and EBNA-2, which are transforming for B cells.[28, 31]

Inactivation of *p53* is detected in approximately 30% to 40% of BL cases, independent of their geographic origin or of the presence of EBV infection.[24] As in other human cancers,[25] *p53* inactivation in BL occurs most commonly through deletion of one allele and mutation of the other.

As in many other NHL types, BL is also associated with deletions of 6q.[26] The genes involved in this cytogenetic abnormality have not yet been identified.

AIDS-RELATED LYMPHOMAS

AIDS-NHLs invariably derive from B cells and are primarily classified into two broad groups: systemic AIDS-NHL and AIDS-related primary central nervous system lymphoma (AIDS-PCNSL).[2] Systemic AIDS-NHLs are histologically heterogeneous and may be morphologically distinguished into two major categories: AIDS-related DLCL (AIDS-DLCL) and AIDS-related BL (AIDS-BL). Conversely, AIDS-PCNSLs display a uniform morphology consistent with a diffuse architecture of large cells. In addition to AIDS-DLCL, AIDS-BL, and AIDS-PCNSL, the spectrum of AIDS-NHL has been recently expanded by the inclusion of AIDS-related BCBL (AIDS-BCBL), which, however, accounts for a small fraction (<1%) of cases.[3, 4, 37]

The different categories of AIDS-NHL associate with distinctive molecular pathways.[2] Cases of AIDS-BL consistently display activation of c-*MYC* by chromosome translocations that show structural similarities to those found in patients with sBL.[2, 30, 138] Rearrangements of *BCL-6* are consistently absent in this AIDS-NHL type.[139] AIDS-BL also frequently harbors mutations of *p53* (60%) and, in 30% of cases, infection of the tumor clone by EBV.[30] The EBV-encoded antigens LMP-1 and EBNA-2 are consistently downregulated in AIDS-BL.[31, 140] Overall, these genetic features of AIDS-BL suggest that it is closely related to sBL rather than eBL. One puzzling feature of AIDS-BL is that AIDS is the only immunodeficiency condition associated with this type of lymphoma.[2] In fact, patients affected by other types of immunodeficiency syndromes, such as congenital and iatrogenically induced immunodeficiencies, do have a high relative risk of NHL development, but these NHLs are consistently DLCL or PCNSL and not BL.

AIDS-DLCLs display several genotypic differences compared with DLCLs of the immunocompetent host.[2, 78] First, the most frequent genetic alteration detected in AIDS-DLCL is infection by EBV, which occurs in approximately 70% of the cases, whereas it is virtually always negative in B-DLCL of the immunocompetent host.[30, 78] The status of EBV infection of AIDS-DLCL differs from that of AIDS-BL (see earlier) and AIDS-PCNSL (see later), since AIDS-DLCLs frequently express LMP-1 but only in rare instances express EBNA-2.[31, 140] A second major feature distinguishing AIDS-DLCL from B-DLCL of the immunocompetent host is represented by the consistent absence of *BCL-2* translocations in the AIDS setting.[2] This finding suggests that AIDS-DLCL originates de novo and does not represent the transformation phase of a preexistent low-grade NHL. Finally, AIDS-DLCL shares with B-DLCL of the immunocompetent host the involvement of *BCL-6* rearrangements, although at a lower frequency (20%).[139] Recently, it has been demonstrated that AIDS-DLCL can be segregated into two distinct categories based on biologic features, in particular the expression pattern of the BCL-6 protein and the EBV-encoded antigen LMP-1.[140] Apparently, *BCL-6* and LMP-1 are expressed in a mutually exclusive fashion by AIDS-DLCL cases. AIDS-DLCLs associated with the *BCL-6+/LMP-1–* phenotype tend to display a centroblastic-like morphology with few or no signs of immunoblastic differentiation.[140] Conversely, *BCL-6–/LMP-1+* AIDS-DLCLs display a clearly immunoblastic morphology with plasmacytoid differentiation.[140] The clinical implications of this biologic heterogeneity of AIDS-DLCL is still unclear.

AIDS-PCNSL has not been widely investigated at the molecular level. Despite these limitations, it is well established that all AIDS-PCNSL cases harbor EBV infection that generally associates with expression of both LMP-1 and EBNA-2.[2] Although some reports have suggested that HHV-8 may be related to PCNSL pathogenesis in immunocompromised patients, extensive analysis of AIDS-PCNSL has unequivocally ruled out this hypothesis.[141, 142]

Finally, BCBL is an additional rare type of AIDS-NHL. The term "BCBL" designates a lymphoma entity characterized by HHV-8 infection and clinically presenting as effusions in the serosal cavities of the body (pleura, pericardium, peritoneum) in the absence of solid tumor masses.[3, 4, 37] The term "primary effusion lymphoma" has also been proposed as an equivalent of BCBL.[143] Immunogenotypic analysis has shown that BCBL consistently derives from B cells, although it usually fails to express the most common B-cell–associated antigens on the cell surface.[3, 4, 37, 143] The epidemiologic distribution of BCBL is peculiar, since it occurs preferentially, although not exclusively, in the AIDS setting. Among immunocompetent hosts, BCBL is extremely rare, since it has been estimated that it accounts for less than 1% of the cases of high-grade NHL.[3] BCBL is characterized by peculiar genetic features. Infection of the tumor clone by HHV-8 occurs in 100% of cases and is a *sine qua non* for the diagnosis of BCBL.[3, 4, 36–38, 143] Tumor cells carry a high number of

HHV-8 copies (40 to 60 copies per cell), suggesting a pathogenetic role of the virus in lymphomagenesis.[3, 4] The virus carries several potential oncogenes that may be implicated in BCBL development, including a gene homologous to the cellular D-type cyclins, a G-protein–coupled receptor displaying constitutive activation, and a gene encoding for a cytokine with high homology to the cellular IL-6 and termed "viral IL-6."[45–48] Preliminary studies of small panels of BCBL suggest that these genes are expressed by the lymphoma cells, thus corroborating their potential relevance to BCBL development. In addition to HHV-8, cases of BCBL frequently carry coinfection of the tumor clone by EBV.[3, 4, 36–38, 143] Finally, it is notable that BCBLs are consistently devoid of all genetic lesions associated with other types of B-cell NHL, including rearrangements of *BCL-1*, *BCL-2*, *BCL-6*, c-*MYC*, and mutations of *p53*.[3, 4, 36, 37, 143]

ANAPLASTIC LARGE CELL LYMPHOMA

ALCL is a distinct clinicopathologic category of NHL composed of large pleomorphic cells that usually express the CD30 antigen and is characterized by frequent cutaneous and extranodal involvement.[1] Classic cytogenetic analysis of ALCL cases has shown a unique translocation involving bands 2p23 and 5q35 in a substantial fraction of ALCL cases, namely cases expressing T-cell or null phenotypes.[5] The cloning of the t(2;5)(p23;q35) translocation has demonstrated that it involves the fusion of the nuclephosmin/B23 (*NPM*) gene on 5q35 to a novel anaplastic lymphoma kinase (*ALK*) on 2p23.[144] As a consequence of this translocation, the *NPM* and *ALK* genes are fused to form a chimeric transcript that encodes a hybrid protein (p80) in which the amino-terminus of *NPM* is linked to the catalytic domain of *ALK*.[144] The oncogenic effect of t(2;5) is supposed to be twofold. First, *ALK*, which is not normally expressed in T lymphocytes, undergoes ectopic expression in lymphoma cells, most likely due to its juxtaposition to the promoter sequences of *NPM*, which are physiologically expressed in T cells.[144, 145] Second, based on the activation model of other tyrosine kinase oncogenes, one would predict that the truncated *ALK* constitutively phosphorylates intracellular targets to trigger malignant transformation.[144–146]

The pathogenetic role of *NPM/ALK* is substantiated by functional evidence both in vitro and in vivo. In vitro, overexpression of p80 induces neoplastic transformation of target cells, corroborating the notion that the p80 kinase is aberrantly activated.[147] In vivo, retroviral-mediated gene transfer of *NPM/ALK* causes lymphoid malignancies in mice that are similar to human disease, since they consistently express a T-cell phenotype.[148] In such animal models, *NPM/ALK* selectively transforms lymphoid cells of T-cell lineage, whereas other hematopoietic cells concomitantly transduced with the *NPM/ALK* chimeric genes do not undergo neoplastic transformation.[148]

The distribution of *NPM/ALK* rearrangements throughout the spectrum of NHL is highly selective, being virtually restricted to ALCL expressing T-cell or null phenotypes.[149–152] Within this category, *NPM/ALK* rearrangements seem to preferentially associate with cases of childhood (88% positivity), although they are also detected in a large fraction of cases of adulthood (60%).[149–152]

REFERENCES

1. Harris NL, Jaffe ES, Stein H, et al: A Revised European-American classification of lymphoid neoplasms: A proposal from the International Lymphoma Study Group. Blood 1994; 84:1361.
2. Gaidano G, Dalla-Favera R: Molecular pathogenesis of AIDS-related lymphomas. Adv Cancer Res 1995; 67:113.
3. Carbone A, Gloghini A, Vaccher E, et al: Kaposi's sarcoma–associated herpesvirus DNA sequences in AIDS-related and AIDS-unrelated lymphomatous effusions. Br J Haematol 1996; 94:533.
4. Cesarman E, Chang Y, Moore PS, et al: Kaposi's sarcoma–associated herpesvirus-like DNA sequences in AIDS-related body-cavity–based lymphomas. N Engl J Med 1995; 332:1186.
5. Mitelman F: Catalog of Chromosome Aberrations in Cancer, 4th ed. New York, Wiley-Liss, 1991.
6. Eshleman JR, Markowitz SD: Microsatellite instability in inherited and sporadic neoplasms. Curr Opin Oncol 1995; 7:83.
7. Gamberi B, Gaidano G, Parsa NZ, et al: Lack of microsatellite instability in non-Hodgkin lymphoma. Blood 1997; 89:975.
8. Look AT: Oncogenic role of "master" transcription factors in human leukemias and sarcomas: A developmental model. Adv Cancer Res 1995; 67:25.
9. Tycko B, Sklar J: Chromosomal translocations in lymphoid neoplasia: A reappraisal of the recombinase model. Cancer Cells 1990; 2:1.
10. Limpens J, de Jong D, van Krieken JHJM, et al: *Bcl-2/J*$_H$ rearrangements in benign lymphoid tissues with follicular hyperplasia. Oncogene 1991; 6:2271.
11. Liu Y, Hernandez AM, Shibata D, et al: *BCL2* translocations frequency rises with age in humans. Proc Natl Acad Sci U S A 1994; 991:8910.
12. Mller JR, Janz S, Goedert JJ, et al: Persistence of immunoglobulin heavy chain/c-*myc* recombination-positive lymphocyte clones in the blood of human immunodeficiency virus–infected homosexual men. Proc Natl Acad Sci U S A 1995; 92:6577.
13. Trümper L, Daus H, Bonin FV, et al: *NPM/ALK* fusion mRNA expression occurs in peripheral blood B lymphocytes of healthy donors as evidenced by reverse transcriptase polymerase chain reaction (RT-PCR). Blood 1996; 88(Suppl 1):225a.
14. Houldsworth J, Mathew S, Rao PH, et al: *REL* protooncogene is frequently amplified in extranodal diffuse large cell lymphoma. Blood 1996; 87:25.
15. Bhatia K, Huppi K, Spangler G, et al: Point mutations in the c-*MYC* transactivation domain are common in Burkitt's lymphoma and mouse plasmacytoma. Nature Genet 1993; 5:56.
16. Bhatia K, Spangler G, Gaidano G, et al: Mutations in the coding region of c-*myc* occur frequently in acquired immunodeficiency syndrome–associated lymphomas. Blood 1994; 84:883.
17. Hua C, Raffeld M, Ko HS, et al: Mechanism of *bcl2* activation in human follicular lymphoma. Oncogene 1990; 5:233.
18. Seto M, Jaeger U, Hockett RD, et al: Alternative promoters and exons, somatic mutation, and transcriptional deregulation of the *bcl-2*–Ig fusion gene in lymphoma. EMBO J 1988; 7:123.
19. Tanaka S, Louie DC, Kant JA, et al: Frequent incidence of somatic mutations in translocated *bcl2* oncogenes of non-Hodgkin's lymphomas. Blood 1992; 79:229.
20. Tanaka S, Louie D, Kant J, et al: Application of a PCR mismatch technique to the *bcl-2* gene: Detection of point mutations in *bcl-2* genes of malignancies with a t(14;18). Leukemia 1992; 6(Suppl 1):15S.
21. Cesarman E, Dalla-Favera R, Bentley D, et al: Mutations in the first exon are associated with altered transcription of c-*myc* in Burkitt lymphoma. Science 1987; 238:1272.
22. Migliazza A, Martinotti S, Chen W, et al: Frequent somatic hypermutation of the 5′ noncoding region of the *BCL-6* gene in B-cell lymphoma. Proc Natl Acad Sci U S A 1995; 92:12520.
23. Neri A, Knowles DM, Greco A, et al: Analysis of *RAS* oncogene mutations in human lymphoid malignancies. Proc Natl Acad Sci U S A 1988; 85:9268.
24. Gaidano G, Ballerini P, Gong JZ, et al: p53 mutations in human lymphoid malignancies: Association with Burkitt lymphoma and chronic lymphocytic leukemia. Proc Natl Acad Sci U S A 1991; 88:5413.
25. Hollstein M, Sidransky D, Vogelstein B, et al: p53 mutations in human cancers. Science 1991; 253:49.
26. Gaidano G, Hauptschein RS, Parsa NZ, et al: Deletions involving two distinct regions of 6q in B-cell non-Hodgkin's lymphoma. Blood 1992; 80:1781.
27. Offit K, Wong G, Filippa DA, et al: Cytogenetic analysis of 434 consecutively ascertained specimens of non-Hodgkin's lymphoma: Clinical correlations. Blood 1991; 77:1508.
28. Kieff E, Leibowitz D: Oncogenesis by herpesvirus. *In* Weinberg RA (ed): Oncogenes and the Molecular Origin of Cancer. Cold Spring Harbor, NY, Cold Spring Harbor Laboratory Press, 1989, p 259.
29. Chang Y, Cesarman E, Pessin MS, et al: Identification of herpesvirus-like DNA sequences in AIDS-associated Kaposi's sarcoma. Science 1994; 266:1865.
30. Ballerini P, Gaidano G, Gong JZ, et al: Multiple genetic lesions in acquired immunodeficiency syndrome–related non-Hodgkin's lymphoma. Blood 1993; 81:166.
31. Hamilton-Dutoit SJ, Pallesen G: A survey of Epstein-Barr virus gene expression in sporadic non-Hodgkin's lymphomas. Am J Pathol 1992; 140:1315.
32. Neri A, Barriga F, Inghirami G, et al: Epstein-Barr virus infection precedes clonal expansion in Burkitt's and acquired immunodeficiency–associated lymphoma. Blood 1991; 77:1092.
33. zur Hausen H, Schulte-Holthausen H, Klein G, et al: EBV DNA in biopsies of Burkitt tumors and anaplastic carcinomas of the nasopharynx. Nature 1970; 228:1056.
34. Raab-Traub N, Flynn K: The structure of the termini of the Epstein-Barr virus as a marker of clonal cellular proliferation. Cell 1986; 47:883.
35. Gratama JW, Ernberg I: Molecular epidemiology of Epstein-Barr virus infection. Adv Cancer Res 1995; 67:197.
36. Gaidano G, Pastore C, Gloghini A, et al: Distribution of human herpesvirus-8 sequences throughout the spectrum of AIDS-related neoplasia. AIDS 1996; 10:941.
37. Gaidano G, Pastore C, Gloghini A, et al: Human herpesvirus type 8 (HHV-8) in haematologic neoplasia. Leuk Lymphoma 1997; in press
38. Pastore C, Gloghini A, Volpe G, et al: Distribution of Kaposi's sarcoma–herpesvirus sequences among lymphoid malignancies in Italy and Spain. Br J Haematol 1995; 91:918.
39. Moore PS, Gao SJ, Dominguez G, et al: Primary characterization of a herpesvirus agent associated with Kaposi's sarcoma. J Virol 1996; 70:549.
40. Roizman B, Desrosiers RC, Fleckenstein B, et al: The family Herpesviridae: An update. Arch Virol 1992; 123:425.
41. Roizman B: The family Herpesviridae. *In* Roizman B, Whitley RJ, Lopez C (eds): The Human Herpesviruses. New York, Raven Press, 1993, p 1.
42. Cesarman E, Moore PS, Rao PH, et al: In vitro establishment and characterization of two acquired immunodeficiency syndrome–related lymphoma cell lines (BC-1 and BC-2) containing Kaposi's sarcoma–associated herpesvirus-like (KSHV) DNA sequences. Blood 1995; 86:2708.
43. Gaidano G, Cechova K, Chang Y, et al: Establishment of AIDS-related lymphoma cell lines from lymphomatous effusions. Leukemia 1996; 10:1237.
44. Renne R, Zhong W, Herndier B, et al: Lytic growth of Kaposi's sarcoma–associated herpesvirus (human herpesvirus-8) in culture. Nature Med 1996; 2:342.
45. Arvanitakis L, Geras-Raaka E, Gershengorn MC, et al: Kaposi's sarcoma–associated herpesvirus (KSHV-HHV-8) ORF-74 encodes a constitutively active G protein–coupled receptor that is expressed in Kaposi's sarcoma and primary effusion lymphoma. Blood 1996; 88(Suppl 1):205a.
46. Chang Y, Moore PS, Talbot SJ, et al: Cyclin encoded by KS herpesvirus. Nature 1996; 382:410.
47. Moore PS, Boshoff C, Weiss RA, et al: Molecular mimicry of human cytokine and cytokine response pathway genes by KSHV. Science 1996; 274:1739.
48. Nador RG, Arvanitakis L, Reed JA, et al: Expression of Kaposi's sarcoma–associated herpesvirus (KSHV/HHV-8) cyclin and G protein–coupled receptor genes during latent and lytic replication in primary effusion lymphoma (PEL) cell lines. Blood 1996; 88(Suppl 1):635a.

49. Weisenburger DD: Pathological classification of non-Hodgkin lymphoma for epidemiological studies. Cancer Res 1992; 52:5456.

50. Acker B, Hoppe RT, Colby TV, et al: Histologic conversion in the non-Hodgkin's lymphomas. J Clin Oncol 1983; 1:11.

51. Cullen MH, Lister TA, Brearley RL, et al: Histological transformation of non-Hodgkin's lymphoma: A prospective study. Cancer 1979; 44:645.

52. Ersboll J, Schultz HB, Pedersen-Bjergaard J, et al: Follicular low-grade non-Hodgkin's lymphoma: Long-term outcome with or without tumor progression. Eur J Haematol 1989; 42:155.

53. Garvin AJ, Simon RM, Osborne CK, et al: An autopsy study of histologic progression in non-Hodgkin's lymphoma: 192 cases from the National Cancer Institute. Cancer 1983; 52:393.

54. Hubbard SM, Chabner BA, De Vita VT Jr, et al: Histologic progression in non-Hodgkin's lymphoma. Blood 1982; 59:258.

55. Risdall R, Hoppe RT, Warnke R: Non-Hodgkin's lymphomas: A study of the evolution of the disease based upon 92 autopsied cases. Cancer 1979; 44:529.

56. Woda B, Knowles DM II: Nodular lymphocytic lymphoma eventuating into diffuse histiocytic lymphoma. Cancer 1979; 43:303.

57. Inghirami G, Knowles DM: The immune system: Structure and function. In Knowles DM (ed): Neoplastic Hematopathology. Baltimore, Williams & Wilkins, 1992, p 27.

58. Bastard C, Tilly H, Lenormand B, et al: Translocations involving band 3q27 and Ig gene regions in non-Hodgkin's lymphoma. Blood 1992; 79:2527.

59. Offit K, Jhanwar S, Ebrahim SAD, et al: t(3;22)(q27;q11), a novel translocation associated with diffuse non-Hodgkin's lymphoma. Blood 1989; 74:1876.

60. Baron BW, Nucifora G, McNabe N, et al: Identification of the gene associated with the recurring chromosomal translocations t(3;14)(q27;q32) and t(3;22)(q27;q11) in B-cell lymphomas. Proc Natl Acad Sci U S A 1993; 90:5262.

61. Kerckaert J-P, Deweindt C, Tilly H, et al: LAZ3, a novel zinc-finger encoding gene, is disrupted by recurring chromosome 3q27 translocations in human lymphoma. Nature Genet 1993; 5:66.

62. Miki T, Kawamata N, Arai A, et al: Molecular cloning of the breakpoint for 3q27 translocation in B-cell lymphomas and leukemias. Blood 1994; 83:217.

63. Ye BH, Lista F, Lo Coco F, et al: Alterations of BCL-6, a novel zinc-finger gene, in diffuse large cell lymphoma. Science 1993; 262:747.

64. Ye BH, Rao PH, Chaganti RSK, et al: Cloning of BCL-6, the locus involved in chromosome translocations affecting band 3q27 in B-cell lymphoma. Cancer Res 1993; 53:2732.

65. Chardin P, Courtois G, Mattei MG, et al: The KUP gene, located on human chromosome 14, encodes a protein with two distant zinc fingers. Nucleic Acid Res 1991; 19:1431.

66. Di Bello PR, Withers DA, Bayer CA, et al: The Drosophila broad complex encodes a family of related proteins containing zinc fingers. Genetics 1991; 129:385.

67. Harrison SD, Travers AA: The tramtrack gene encodes a Drosophila finger protein that interacts with the ftz transcriptional regulatory region and shows a novel embryonic expression pattern. EMBO J 1990; 9:207.

68. Numoto M, Niwa O, Kaplan J, et al: Transcriptional repressor ZF5 identifies a new conserved domain in zinc-finger proteins. Nucleic Acid Res 1993; 21:3767.

69. Bardwell VJ, Treisman R: The POZ domain: A conserved protein-protein interaction motif. Genes Dev 1994; 8:1664.

70. Chen Z, Brand NJ, Chen A, et al: Fusion between a novel Kruppel-like zinc-finger gene and the retinoic acid receptor-α locus due to a variant t(11;17) translocation associated with acute promyelocytic leukemia. EMBO J 1993; 12:1161.

71. Chang C-C, Ye B-H, Chaganti RSK, et al: BCL-6, a POZ/zinc-finger protein, is a sequence-specific transcriptional repressor. Proc Natl Acad Sci U S A 1996; 93:6947.

72. Cattoretti G, Chang C, Cechova K, et al: BCL-6 protein is expressed in germinal center B cells. Blood 1995; 86:45.

73. Ye B, Cattoretti G, Shen Q, et al: The BCL-6 proto-oncogene controls germinal center formation and the Th2-type inflammation. Nature Genetics, in press.

74. Bastard C, Deweindt C, Kerckaert JP, et al: LAZ3 rearrangements in non-Hodgkin's lymphoma: Correlation with histology, immunophenotype, karyotype, and clinical outcome in 217 patients. Blood 1994; 83:2423.

75. Dallery E, Galiegue-Zouitina S, Collyn-d'Hoohge M, et al: TTF, a gene encoding a novel small G protein, fuses to the lymphoma-associated LAZ3 gene by t(3;4) chromosome translocation. Oncogene 1995; 10:2171.

76. Ye BH, Chaganti S, Chang C-C, et al: Chromosomal translocations cause deregulated BCL6 expression by promoter substitution in B-cell lymphoma. EMBO J 1995; 14:6209.

77. Lo Coco F, Gaidano G, Louie DC, et al: p53 mutations are associated with histologic transformation of follicular lymphoma. Blood 1993; 82:2289.

78. Volpe G, Vitolo U, Carbone A, et al: Molecular heterogeneity of B-lineage diffuse large cell lymphoma. Genes Chromosom Cancer 1996; 16:21.

79. Lo Coco F, Ye BH, Lista F, et al: Rearrangements of the BCL-6 gene in diffuse large cell non-Hodgkin lymphoma. Blood 1994; 83:1757.

80. Offit K, Lo Coco F, Louie DC, et al: Rearrangements of the bcl-6 gene as a prognostic marker in diffuse large cell lymphoma. N Engl J Med 1994; 331:74.

81. Tang SC, Visser L, Hepperle B, et al: Clinical significance of bcl-2 MBR gene rearrangement and protein expression in diffuse large cell non-Hodgkin lymphoma: An analysis of 83 cases. J Clin Oncol 1994; 12:149.

82. Yunis JJ, Mayer MG, Arnesen MA, et al: BCL-2 and other genomic alterations in the prognosis of large cell lymphoma. N Engl J Med 1989; 320:1947.

83. Cleary ML, Galili N, Sklar J: Detection of a second t(14;18) breakpoint cluster region in human follicular lymphomas. J Exp Med 1986; 164:315.

84. Cleary ML, Sklar J: Nucleotide sequence of a t(14;18) chromosomal breakpoint in follicular lymphoma and demonstration of a breakpoint cluster region near a transcriptionally active locus on chromosome 18. Proc Natl Acad Sci U S A 1985; 82:7439.

85. Cleary ML, Smith SD, Sklar J: Cloning and structural analysis of cDNAs for bcl-2 and a hybrid bcl-2/immunoglobulin transcript resulting from the t(14;18) translocation. Cell 1986; 47:19.

86. Tsujimoto Y, Finger LR, Yunis J, et al: Cloning of the chromosome breakpoints of neoplastic B cells with the t(14;18) chromosomal translocation. Science 1984; 226:1097.

87. Ladanyi M, Offit K, Jhanwar SC, et al: MYC rearrangement and translocations involving band 8q24 in diffuse large cell lymphomas. Blood 1991; 77:1057.

88. Nagai M, Ikeda K, Tasaka T, et al: Genomic rearrangement of the c-myc proto-oncogene in non-AIDS–related lymphoma in Japan. Leukemia 1991; 5:462.

89. Raghoebier S, Kramer MHH, van Krieken JHJM, et al: Essential differences in oncogene involvement between primary nodal and extranodal large cell lymphoma. Blood 1991; 78:2680.

90. Yano T, Jaffe ES, Longo DL, et al: MYC rearrangements in histologically progressed follicular lymphomas. Blood 1992; 80:758.

91. Neri A, Chang C-C, Lombardi L, et al: B-cell lymphoma–associated chromosomal translocation involves candidate oncogene lyt-10, homologous to NF-kB p50. Cell 1991; 67:1075.

92. Chang C-C, Zhang, J, Lombardi L, et al: Rearranged NFKB-2 genes in lymphoid neoplasms code for constitutively active nuclear transactivators. Mol Cell Biol 1995; 15:5180.

93. Neri A, Fracchiolla NS, Roscetti E, et al: Molecular analysis of cutaneous B- and T-cell lymphomas. Blood 1995; 86:3160.

94. Sander CA, Yano T, Clark HM, et al: p53 mutation is associated with progression in follicular lymphomas. Blood 1993; 82:1994.

95. National Cancer Institute–Sponsored Study of Classifications of Non-Hodgkin's Lymphoma: Summary and description of a working formulation for clinical usage: The Non-Hodgkin's Lymphoma Pathologic Classification Project. Cancer 1982; 49:2112.

96. Dalla-Favera R, Ye BH, Lo Coco F, et al: Identification of genetic lesions associated with diffuse large cell lymphoma. Ann Oncol 1994; 5:S55.

97. Dalla-Favera R: Chromosomal translocations involving the c-myc oncogene in lymphoid neoplasia. In Kirsch IR (ed): The Causes and Consequences of Chromosomal Aberrations. Boca Raton, CRC Press, 1993, p 312.

98. Crews S, Barth R, Hood L, et al: Mouse c-myc oncogene is located on chromosome 15 and translocated to chromosome 12 in plasmacytomas. Science 1982; 218:1319.

99. Shen-Ong GL, Keath EJ, Piccoli SP, et al: Novel c-myc oncogene RNA from abortive immunoglobulin-gene recombination in mouse plasmacytomas. Cell 1982; 31:443.

100. Smegi J, Spira J, Bazin H, et al: Rat c-*myc* oncogene is located on chromosome 7 and rearranges in immunocytomas with t(6;7) chromosomal translocation. Nature 1983; 306:497.

101. Dalla-Favera R, Bregni M, Erickson J, et al: Human c-*myc* oncogene is located on the region of chromosome 8 that is translocated in Burkitt lymphoma cells. Proc Natl Acad Sci U S A 1982; 79:7824.

102. Dalla-Favera R, Martinotti S, Gallo RC, et al: Translocation and rearrangements of the c-*myc* oncogene in human undifferentiated B-cell lymphomas. Science 1983; 219:963.

103. Davis M, Malcolm S, Rabbits TH: Chromosome translocations can occur on either side of the c-*myc* oncogene in Burkitt lymphoma cells. Nature 1984; 30:286.

104. Hollis GF, Mitchell KF, Battey J, et al: A variant translocation places the lambda immunoglobulin genes 3′ to the c-*myc* oncogene in Burkitt's lymphoma. Nature 1984; 307:752.

105. Taub R, Kirsch I, Morton C: Translocation of c-*myc* gene into the immunoglobulin heavy-chain locus in human Burkitt lymphoma and murine plasmacytoma cells. Proc Natl Acad Sci U S A 1982; 79:7837.

106. Henriksson M, Lüscher B: Proteins of the Myc network: Essential regulators of cell growth and differentiation. Adv Cancer Res 1996; 68:109.

107. Bissonette RP, Echeverri F, Mahboubi A, et al: Apoptotic cell death induced by c-*myc* is inhibited by *bcl-2*. Nature 1992; 359:552.

108. Evan GI, Wyllie AH, Gilbert CS, et al: Induction of apoptosis in fibroblasts by c-*myc* protein. Cell 1992; 69:119.

109. Fanidi A, Harrington EA, Evan GI: Cooperative interaction between c-*myc* and *bcl-2* proto-oncogenes. Nature 1992; 359:554.

110. Shi Y, Glynn JM, Guilbert LJ, et al: Role for c-*myc* in activation-induced apoptotic cell death in T-cell hybridomas. Science 1992; 257:212.

111. Amati B, Brooks MW, Levy N, et al: Oncogenic activity of the c-*myc* protein requires dimerization with Max. Cell 1993; 72:233.

112. Amati B, Dalton S, Brooks MW, et al: Transcriptional activation by the human c-*myc* oncoprotein in yeast requires interaction with Max. Nature 1992; 359:423.

113. Blackwood EM, Eisenman RN: Max: A helix-loop-helix zipper protein that forms a sequence-specific DNA-binding complex with *myc*. Science 1991; 251:1211.

114. Blackwood EM, Lüscher B, Eisenman RN: Myc and Max associate in vivo. Genes Dev 1992; 6:71.

115. Gu W, Cechova K, Tassi V, et al: Differential regulation of target gene expression by Myc/Max ratio. Proc Natl Acad Sci U S A 1993; 90:2935.

116. Kretzner L, Blackwood EM, Eisenman RN: Myc and Max proteins possess distinct transcriptional activities. Nature 1992; 359:426.

117. Ayer DE, Kretzner L, Eisenman RN: Mad: A heterodimeric partner for Max that antagonizes Myc transcriptional activity. Cell 1993; 72:211.

118. Zervos AS, Gyuris J, Brent R: MXI-1, a protein that specifically interacts with Max to bind Myc-Max recognition sites. Cell 1993; 72:223.

119. Neri A, Barriga F, Knowles DM, et al: Different regions of the immunoglobulin heavy-chain locus are involved in chromosomal translocations in distinct pathogenetic forms of Burkitt lymphoma. Proc Natl Acad Sci U S A 1988; 85:27.

120. Pelicci PG, Knowles DM, Magrath I, et al: Chromosomal breakpoints and structural alterations of the c-*myc* locus differ in endemic and sporadic forms of Burkitt lymphoma. Proc Natl Acad Sci U S A 1986; 83:2984.

121. ar-Rushdi A, Nishikura K, Erikson J, et al: Differential expression of the translocated and untranslocated c-*myc* oncogene in Burkitt's lymphoma. Science 1983; 222:390.

122. Hayday AC, Gillies SD, Saito H, et al: Activation of a translocated human c-*myc* gene by an enhancer in the immunoglobulin heavy-chain locus. Nature 1984; 307:334.

123. Rabbits TH, Forster A, Baer R, et al: Transcriptional enhancer identified where the human C immunoglobulin heavy-chain gene is unavailable to the translocated c-*myc* gene in a Burkitt's lymphoma. Nature 1983; 306:806.

124. Cory S: Activation of cellular oncogenes in hematopoietic cells by chromosome translocation. Adv Cancer Res 1986; 47:189.

125. Lieberson R, Ong J, Shi X, et al: Immunoglobulin gene transcription ceases upon deletion of a distant enhancer. EMBO J 1995; 14: 6229.

126. Bentley DL, Groudine M: A block to elongation is largely responsible for decreased transcription of c-*myc* in differentiated HL-60 cells. Nature 1986; 321:702.

127. Eick D, Bornkamm GW: Transcriptional arrest within the first exon is a fast-control mechanism in c-*myc* gene expression. Nucl Acid Res 1986; 14:8331.

128. Zajac-Kaye M, Gelmann EP, Levens D: A point mutation in the c-*myc* locus of a Burkitt lymphoma abolishes binding of a nuclear protein. Science 1988; 240:1776.

129. Papas T, Lautenberg J: Sequence curiosity in v-*myc* oncogene. Nature 1995; 318:237.

130. Beijersbergen RL, Hijmans EM, Zhu L, et al: Interaction of c-*myc* with the pRb-related protein p107 results in inhibition of c-*myc*–mediated transactivation. EMBO J 1994; 13:4080.

131. Gu W, Bhatia K, Magrath IT, et al: Binding and suppression of the c-*myc* transcriptional activation domain by p107. Science 1994; 264:251.

132. Hoang AT, Lutterbach B, Lewis BC, et al: A link between increased transforming activity of lymphoma-derived *MYC* mutant alleles, their effective regulation by p107, and altered phosphorylation of the c-*MYC* transactivation domain. Mol Cell Biol 1995; 15:4031.

133. Lombardi L, Newcomb EW, Dalla-Favera R: Pathogenesis of Burkitt lymphoma: Expression of an activated c-*myc* oncogene causes the tumorigenic conversion of EBV-infected human B lymphoblasts. Cell 1987; 49:161.

134. Loke SL, Stein C, Zhang Z, et al: Delivery of c-*myc* antisense phosphorothioate oligodeoxynucleotides to hematopoietic cells in culture by liposome fusion: Specific reduction in c-*myc* protein expression correlates with inhibition of cell growth and DNA synthesis. Curr Top Microbiol Immunol 1988; 141:282.

135. Magrath IT: Prospects for the therapeutic use of antisense oligonucleotides in malignant lymphomas. Ann Oncol 1994; 5:S67.

136. McManaway ME, Neckers LM, Loke SL, et al: Tumor-specific inhibition of lymphoma growth by an antisense oligodeoxynucleotide. Lancet 1990; 335:808.

137. Adams JM, Harris AW, Pinkert CA, et al: The c-*myc* oncogene driven by immunoglobulin enhancers induces lymphoid malignancy in transgenic mice. Nature 1985; 318:533.

138. Pelicci P-G, Knowles DM II, Arlin ZA, et al: Multiple monoclonal B-cell expansions and c-*myc* oncogene rearrangements in acquired immunodeficiency syndrome–related lymphoproliferative disorders: Implications for lymphomagenesis. J Exp Med 1986; 164:2049.

139. Gaidano G, Lo Coco F, Ye BH, et al: Rearrangements of the *BCL-6* gene in acquired immunodeficiency syndrome–associated non-Hodgkin's lymphoma: Association with diffuse large cell subtype. Blood 1994; 84:397.

140. Carbone A, Gaidano G, Gloghini A, et al: *BCL-6* protein expression in AIDS-related non-Hodgkin's lymphomas: Inverse relationship with Epstein-Barr virus–encoded latent membrane protein-1 expression. Am J Pathol 1997; 150:155.

141. Gaidano G, Capello D, Pastore C, et al: Analysis of HHV-8 infection in AIDS-related and AIDS-unrelated primary central nervous system lymphoma. J Infect Dis 1997; 175:1193.

142. Luppi M, Barozzi P, Marasca R, et al: HHV-8–associated primary cerebral B-cell lymphoma in HIV-negative patient after long-term steroids [Letter]. Lancet 1996; 347:980.

143. Nador RG, Cesarman E, Chadburn A, et al: Primary effusion lymphoma: A distinct clinicopathologic entity associated with Kaposi's sarcoma–associated herpesvirus. Blood 1996; 88:645.

144. Morris SW, Kirstein MN, Valentine MB, et al: Fusion of a kinase gene, *ALK*, to a nucleolar protein gene, *NPM*, in non-Hodgkin's lymphoma. Science 1994; 263:1281.

145. Shiota M, Fujimoto J, Semba T, et al: Hyperphosphorylation of a novel 80-kDa protein-tyrosine kinase similar to Ltk in a human Ki-1 lymphoma cell line, AMS3. Oncogene 1994; 9:1567.

146. Hunter T: Oncogene products in the cytoplasm. *In* Weinberg RA (ed): Oncogenes and the Molecular Origins of Cancer. Cold Spring Harbor, NY, Cold Spring Harbor Laboratory Press, 1989, p 147.

147. Fujimoto J, Shiota M, Iwahara T, et al: Characterization of the transforming activity of p80, a hyperphosphorylated protein in a Ki-1 lymphoma cell line with chromosomal translocation t(2;5). Proc Natl Acad Sci U S A 1996; 93:4181.

148. Kuefer MU, Look AT, Tripp R, et al: Retrovirus-mediated gene

transfer of *NPM/ALK* causes lymphoid malignancy in mice. Blood 1996; 88(Suppl 1):450a.

149. Lamant L, Meggetto F, al Saati T, et al: High incidence of the t(2;5)(p23;q35) translocation in anaplastic large cell lymphoma and its lack of detection in Hodgkin's disease: Comparison of cytogenetic analysis, reverse transcriptase-polymerase chain reaction, and p-80 immunostaining. Blood 1996; 87:284.

150. Sarris AH, Luthra L, Papadimitracopoulou V, et al: Amplification of genomic DNA demonstrates the presence of the t(2;5)(p23;q35) in anaplastic large cell lymphoma, but not in other non-Hodgkin's lymphomas, Hodgkin's disease, or lymphomatoid papulosis. Blood 1996; 88:1771.

151. Ye HT, Ponzoni M, Merson A, et al: Molecular characterization of the t(2;5)(p23;q35) translocation in anaplastic large cell lymphoma (Ki-1) and Hodgkin's disease. Blood 1996; 87:1081.

152. Shiota M, Fujimoto J, Takenaga M, et al: Diagnosis of t(2;5)(p23; q35)-associated Ki-1 lymphoma with immunohistochemistry. Blood 1994; 84:3648.

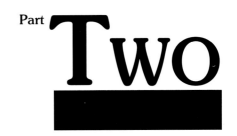

Part

TWO

CLINICAL ASPECTS

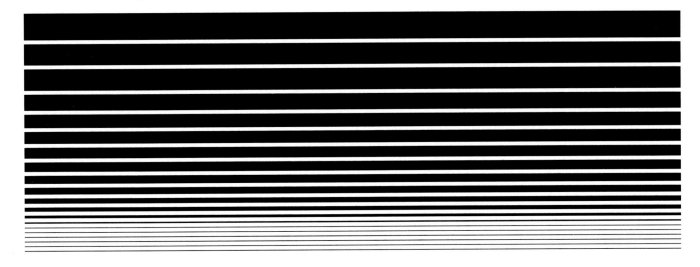

Chapter Nineteen

Follicular Lymphoma

Ama Rohatiner
T. Andrew Lister

BACKGROUND

Follicular lymphoma is the most common of the low-grade B-cell lymphomas identified in currently used and proposed classifications,[1–3] occurring with a frequency of 4 in 100,000 per year in the Western world.[4] Its etiology is unknown, although much has been discovered recently about the molecular events related to its development.

Follicular lymphoma may be regarded as the paradigm for the other low-grade B-cell lymphomas. In all respects there are similarities between them; however, in terms of prognosis, measured as frequency of response, freedom from progression, and survival, follicular lymphoma is best—or least bad!

It is both a rewarding and tantalizing illness to manage, taxing all the resources of the physician. The initial decision is whether to intervene; later options range from modest chemotherapy via high-dose therapy and hematopoietic cell rescue to antibody-targeted irradiation and the prospect of DNA vaccine therapy. Regression of lymphadenopathy usually occurs; subsequent progression is the rule rather than the exception. The disease itself is by far the most common cause of death, transformation to an aggressive lymphoma often being the terminal event. There is much room for refining conventional therapy and for developing novel approaches.

PATHOLOGY

Follicular lymphoma is a relatively easy diagnosis to establish, most of the time.[5–7] Routine hematoxylin and eosin staining reveals a characteristic pattern of disruption of the normal nodal architecture by follicular aggregates, composed of small and large follicular center cells (centrocytes and centroblasts).[8–11] The *degree* of follicularity may vary, as may the *relative proportion* of smaller to larger cells in the follicles, although usually there is a preponderance of small cells. The prognostic significance of these differences has been debated; however, there is no doubt that transformation (over time) from an obviously follicular pattern with a low proportion of large cells to a diffuse pattern with mostly large cells is a grave event.[12–16] Infiltration of the bone marrow, which is common, is usually paratrabecular and patchy.[17] Immunologically, the abnormal follicular center cells are invariably of B-cell origin, expressing CD19, CD20,[18–20] and (monoclonal) surface immunoglobulin. CD10 is usually expressed, whereas CD5 is not.[19, 20]

A nonrandom cytogenetic translocation t(14;18) occurs in most cases of follicular lymphoma before and after transformation.[21–25] Cloning of the t(14;18) breakpoint led to the identification of the B-cell leukemia/lymphoma-2 (*BCL2*) gene.[26] This was followed by elucidation of the consequences of the gene's becoming juxtaposed to the immunoglobulin heavy chain gene.[27–29] More recently it has been shown that *BCL2* induces apoptosis,[30] providing a potential role for the hyperexpression of the gene seen[31] in follicular lymphoma. Although a role for this translocation in follicular lymphoma is hardly doubted, it has been detected at the molecular level in the bone marrow of patients who have been in clinical remission of the disease for many years.[23, 32–34] It has also been detected at a very low frequency in hyperplastic tonsils[35] and the peripheral blood; no case of lymphoma has yet been reported in a patient in whom this occurred. All this notwithstanding, it is not overly simplistic to suggest, when the translocation is found in the context of lymphoma, that the chances of long survival would be enhanced were the clone of cells bearing it eliminated.

NATURAL HISTORY, PRESENTATION, AND CLINICAL COURSE

Sporadic case reports of patients presenting with lymphadenopathy and splenomegaly that regressed partially and temporarily following irradiation appeared in the literature during the first quarter of the century. The clinicopathologic syndrome, Brill-Symmers disease, (at least as worthy of an eponymous title as Hodgkin's disease), was graphically described by Symmers in 1938.[36] All the features recognized today are to be found in this series of case histories. Many patients had had a period of asymptomatic lymphadenopathy before developing systemic symptoms. Multiple sites were often involved; splenomegaly was common. The illness followed a course in which repeated episodes of lymphadenopathy continued to reveal "giant follicular hyperplasia" or "sarcomatous change," or a leukemic picture appeared. Occasionally, Hodgkin's disease was reported. Local irradiation resulted in regression of palpable disease for variable periods. The median survival (not reported, but calculated by the authors) was about 5 years.

What has happened since? In the intervening years, one of the few constant features of the histologic classifications of lymphoma has been follicular (sometimes called "nodular") lymphoma. Techniques for determining the distribu-

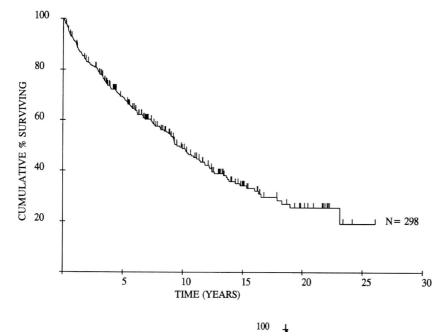

Figure 19–1. Overall survival of newly diagnosed follicular lymphoma at St. Bartholomew's Hospital.

Figure 19–2. Duration of first and subsequent remissions of stage III-IV follicular lymphoma at St. Bartholomew's Hospital.

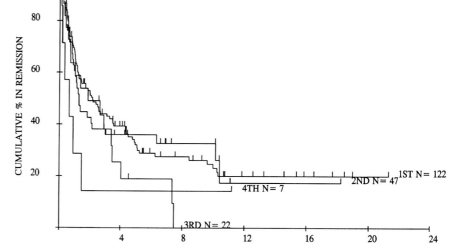

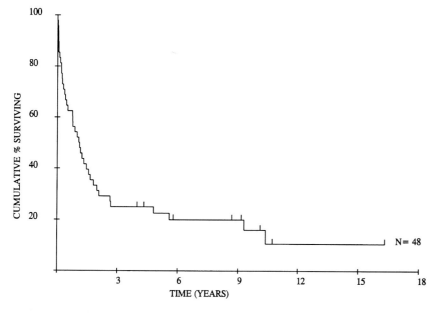

Figure 19–3. Survival following histologic transformation in patients at St. Bartholomew's Hospital not receiving high-dose therapy.

Table 19–1. Clinical Stage of 299 Patients with Follicular Lymphoma

Stage	No. of Patients°	Percentage
I	44 (2)	15
II	40 (8)	14
III	40 (8)	17
IV	161(57)	54

°The no. of patients with B symptoms is shown in parentheses.

Table 19–3. Extranodal Sites of Disease in 299 Patients with Follicular Lymphoma°

Site	Percentage of Total
Bone marrow	45
Liver	8
Skin	5
Lung	4†
"Nasopharyngeal"	3
Nervous system	1
All other	9

°Includes I[E].
†Excluding pleural effusions (8%).

tion and volume of disease have improved. The number of therapeutic options has increased. Radiation therapy has largely been supplanted by chemotherapy of many types and intensity. Concurrent with these advances, the median survival appears to have been increased to about 10 years (Fig. 19–1).[37–40] However, the *pattern* of the illness has not yet convincingly been demonstrated to have been altered; repeated regressions (Fig. 19–2), usually incomplete, are the rule rather than the exception. Transformation is the most ominous prognostic factor[40] and is frequently, although not always,[41] a terminal event (Fig. 19–3). This change in the pathology may occur early in the course of the illness, after several recurrences many years after the diagnosis of follicular lymphoma has been made, or never.[14–18, 42] The frequency with which it occurs is independent of whether treatment is started at the time of diagnosis or later.[15] Patients may also present with centroblastic lymphoma (Kiel classification) but with evidence of a residual follicular pattern, suggesting that the tumor arose from follicular lymphoma. Alternatively, there may be discordance between a peripheral lymph node that shows *follicular* histology and, for example, an abdominal mass that on biopsy reveals diffuse *centroblastic* lymphoma. There are also patients who are found to have centroblastic lymphoma in large tumor masses and, concurrently, paratrabecular infiltration typical of follicular lymphoma in the marrow.

Regardless of the pattern of evolution, however, most people who develop follicular lymphoma die of it, with it, or because of its treatment.

The characteristics of 299 consecutive patients newly diagnosed with follicular lymphoma at St. Bartholomew's Hospital and investigated according to convention at the time may be used to illustrate the common findings at presentation (Tables 19–1 to 19–3). The numbers of men and women were approximately equal (52% to 48%), and the median age was 55 years (ranging from 20 to 90). Only 25% had constitutional B symptoms, but despite this, 82% proceeded to therapy immediately. This may be a reflection of an enthusiastic intervention policy in place for several years. The frequency of peripheral blood involvement is not

recorded but is well known to be reasonably common even at the morphologic level.[43, 44]

MANAGEMENT

INVESTIGATION

Management of the patient with follicular lymphoma begins with confirmation of the diagnosis by a pathologist well versed in lymphoma. This is usually based on an excision biopsy of an easily accessible peripheral lymph node; however, this may be misleading. In the light of the prognostic significance of transformation, it is essential that the most suspicious (i.e., rapidly enlarging) node be sampled. Not infrequently this may be intraabdominal. In the past this might have entailed laparotomy, but this is no longer necessarily the case. Tru-Cut needle biopsy, as opposed to fine-needle aspiration or biopsy, has been shown convincingly to yield diagnostic tissue in a high proportion of cases.[45] If doubt exists, repeat biopsy should be performed. Fresh and frozen tissue may be invaluable for tests beyond morphology and phenotype. The proliferative index may be demonstrated, and molecular studies may be undertaken. In addition, the tissue may be essential if immunotherapy is to be considered. Finally, the research potential of the tissue bank cannot be overestimated. Obviously the patient must be apprised of the reasons for *considering* extra biopsies.

Further investigation depends on the overall circumstances of the patient and the enthusiasm of the physician. It is influenced by the therapeutic options and whether the patient presents de novo or later in the course of the illness. Once again, the rationale for the tests must be made clear to the patient. Provided that intervention is anticipated, a full history and clinical examination are usually complemented by computed tomographic (CT) scan, peripheral blood count and film, bone marrow biopsy, and biochemical tests of liver and kidney function. Other tests, for example, serum lactate dehydrogenase (LDH) and β_2-microglobulin, may be valuable in assessing the prognosis.

At the completion of investigation, ideally within 2 weeks of presentation, it should be possible to give the patient a reasonable outline of what to expect, not only immediately but in the future, and advice about therapy.

THERAPY
Strategy

The basic tenet of lymphoma therapy is that resolution of lymphadenopathy and other sites of involvement results in

Table 19–2. Distribution of Lymphadenopathy in 34 Patients with Stage I Nodal Follicular Lymphoma

Site	No. of Patients	Percentage of Total
Neck	14	5
Axilla	6	2
Groin	14	5

the patient feeling better (at least) and living longer. In addition, it has been shown specifically that patients with follicular lymphoma in whom remissions are achieved live longer than those in whom they are not,[40] and longer than expected without therapy. However, the decision of whether to treat or not is complicated by the fact that many patients present with lumps that are not too large and are not causing any immediate trouble beyond anxiety and being unsightly. Spontaneous regressions, rarely complete, may occur.[46] Furthermore, there is no evidence that early intervention in "fit" patients improves the prognosis,[47] despite the fact that progression demanding therapy occurs within a median of 1 to 2 years. Thus, based on these findings, extensively reported predominantly from Stanford University Medical Center, it is conventional for the management of follicular lymphoma to be expectant unless the patient has one of the following:

1. Constitutional symptoms
2. Embarrassment of a vital organ by compression or infiltration, particularly of the bone marrow
3. Bulky adenopathy
4. Obvious progression
5. Evidence of transformation

Some consider that small-volume, localized lymphadenopathy may be a valid exception to this, based on the fact that local irradiation results in prolonged freedom from progression and possibly cure. It has not been proven that this is any more than a reflection of the natural history of the disease following excision biopsy.

The decision about intervention is essentially the same at recurrence as at re-presentation following apparently successful therapy, provided transformation has not supervened. Clearly both the persuasion of the patient and the philosophy of the physicians are highly relevant. The fact that an expectant approach can be accepted for a malignant disease afflicting middle-aged people is a disappointing reflection of our inability to convert a treatment-sensitive disease into a curable one. There is no room for complacency.

Once the criteria for therapy have been fulfilled, the important questions to be answered are (1) which specific treatment(s) should be used and (2) for how long treatment should be continued. Statements about one treatment being "better than" or "as good as" another are almost invariably based on phase II or III trials of only the *first* treatment the patient receives. Since this is a repeatedly responsive illness for most people, it is not surprising that *survival* advantages of one therapy over another have rarely been reported. Thus, statements frequently made such as "nothing is better than chlorambucil" must be interpreted within the limitations of the data. For example, the fact that retrospective analyses of open studies suggest no survival advantage for CHOP (cyclophosphamide, hydroxydaunomycin, Oncovin, prednisone) as initial therapy over other therapies[48] does *not* imply that it may not be better, or effective later in the disease, or when alkylating agents alone have failed. Data about the *relative* efficacy of the many different options available at the time of progression or recurrence are rarely based on randomized trials. In contrast, there is no evidence that prolonged conventional-dose cytotoxic therapy carries any advantage. This may not be the same for interferon (see later).

Radiation Therapy

Involved-field irradiation almost invariably causes complete clinical regression of follicular lymphoma confined to one (or two) sites, provided that the lymphadenopathy is not too bulky. A dose-response curve has been reported, "within-field" recurrence following doses of greater than 45 Gy being rare.[49] Disease-free survival after 10 years is on the order of 70%.[50–58] In contrast with the situation for patients with advanced follicular lymphoma, it is customary to recommend irradiation in this context at the initial presentation in the anticipation of cure for a relatively high proportion of patients. No randomized trial of early intervention compared with expectant management has been published. Adjuvant therapy, in the form of chlorambucil, or CVP (cyclophosphamide, vincristine, prednisone) has not been shown unequivocally to be beneficial, although trials comparing irradiation alone with irradiation and CHOP were promising.[56, 57]

Both total-nodal[59] and low-dose total-body irradiation[60–64] yield similar results to chlorambucil in stage III follicular lymphoma; however, they are usually not used alone. Provocative open phase II data have suggested that combined-modality therapy may be curative.[65]

Total-body irradiation and cyclophosphamide have recently been used with increasing frequency as consolidation therapy, but it must be emphasized that this is a highly experimental approach. Similarly, targeted irradiation has yielded high response rates with relatively little toxicity. (Both these approaches are reviewed later.)

Finally, irradiation has an important role to play in the palliative treatment of solitary lesions or when chemotherapy either has failed or is inappropriate. Thus, radiation therapy has a limited but important role in the treatment of follicular lymphoma. It may be the treatment of choice at the initial presentation if it is highly localized, and it is an occasional invaluable palliative measure. Its role in other contexts is the subject of clinical trials.

Single-Agent Chemotherapy

Most patients with follicular lymphoma are treated with chemotherapy, usually several times. Expectant management from the time of presentation does not mean *no* therapy. A small proportion may escape treatment for many years, but the *median* time to treatment in the larger series at Stanford was between 1 and 2 years.[46] Moderately modest therapy usually induces remission, if incomplete, repeatedly, *prior* to transformation; it is almost always irrelevant after this has happened. Thus, the next best thing after curing follicular lymphoma would be the prevention of transformation.

Alkylating Agents. Chlorambucil (and subsequently cyclophosphamide) has been an almost invariable component of therapy for follicular lymphoma since the efficacy of the drug was first reported. The earliest studies using relatively low doses continuously yielded reduction in lymphadenopathy that was generally obvious within the first 6 weeks.[66, 67] These findings have been amply confirmed over the past half century, as illustrated in Table 19–4. Data from other studies, either open phase II or randomized phase III trials, support this, the response rate exceeding 75% and complete remissions being achieved in approximately

30%.[60, 69–71] The addition of prednisolone makes no apparent difference.[72, 73]

The time until recurrence or progression correlates positively with the amount of therapy and also the closeness of surveillance. Recurrence or progression may be expected in most, the reported median duration of remission being between 1 and 4 years.[40] The ease of administration of the oral preparation of these drugs and their infrequent and minimal side effects, coupled with their "effectiveness," made them an obvious first choice of treatment for follicular lymphoma. The fact that, given intermittently, provided transformation has not occurred, they are repeatedly effective lends further support to their role. It is reasonable to assert that the alkylating agents have made a significant impact on the natural history of follicular lymphoma; this must not be allowed to divert attention from the disappointing observation that for most people, given alone, they only "control" or "contain" the illness.

Vinca Alkaloids, Corticosteroids, and Anthracycline Antibiotics. These three groups of drugs are by far the most frequent partners for alkylating agents in combination chemotherapy for follicular lymphoma. At the same time that alkylating agents were emerging as the cornerstone of therapy for lymphoma, vincristine and prednisolone were being shown to be spectacularly successful in inducing remission in childhood lymphoblastic leukemia. Less impressive but undoubtedly relevant responses were also achieved with vincristine in lymphosarcoma, follicular lymphoma rarely being cited separately (Table 19–5).[74–77] In 1996, vincristine was used only anecdotally alone. Corticosteroids were first tested in lymphoma in 1949.[78] The largest single series in lymphosarcoma reported a response rate of 68% (see Table 19–5).[79] Prednisolone is often used to improve bone marrow function, particularly in patients with thrombocytopenia and obviously in those with hemolytic anemia; occasionally it is used in refractory disease in high doses. Much more often, steroids are used in combination with an alkylating agent because of their complementary activity and bone marrow sparing.

Single-agent data about the anthracycline antibiotics, particularly doxorubicin (Adriamycin), in the treatment of follicular lymphoma are remarkably sparse.[80–82] Inevitably, having been discovered later, they took second or third place to other therapies for lymphoma; hence, the available data are likely to weigh against them since the patients who received them may have been heavily pretreated. The same applies to similar drugs, such as mitoxantrone. In addition, they are myelotoxic and cardiotoxic, and they cause mucositis. Not surprisingly, they have no established

role outside combination chemotherapy for follicular lymphoma.

Purine Analogues. Fludarabine and 2-chloro-2′-deoxyadenosine (CdA; now cladribine) are being increasingly used in the treatment of follicular lymphoma refractory to or recurrent after prior treatment with alkylating agents or combination chemotherapy. More is known about fludarabine[83–90] than about cladribine,[91, 92] and little is known about 2′-deoxycoformycin. It is likely that there will be relatively little difference between them. It is quite clear that the treatment is extremely well tolerated, causing little nausea and vomiting and no alopecia. Response rates in previously treated patients are in the 40% range, most being incomplete.[83–89] In the only study undertaken in newly diagnosed patients, the response rate is superficially higher, with 37% entering complete remission.[90] These results are summarized in Table 19–6. It seems most likely that this group of drugs will establish a role in the treatment of follicular lymphoma, although it is not yet clear what it will be. Limitation on their use may be imposed by their specific anti-T-cell effects and the risk of "unexpected" infection,[93] some concern over hemotoxicity, even at low doses, and hemolytic anemia. If its role is to be an alternative "containment" like chlorambucil, the oral formulation will constitute a further advance.

Combination Chemotherapy

The availability of several different compounds that separately yielded regression of all types of lymphoma inevitably led to the testing of cyclic combination therapy in follicular lymphoma. Highly effective in Hodgkin's disease and somewhat effective in aggressive non-Hodgkin's lymphoma, this approach has been least impressive in follicular lymphoma.

Clinical trials in the late 1960s and early 1970s, more open phase II than III, suggested that the complete remission rate, *as defined at the time*, was higher with the combination of cyclophosphamide, vincristine, and prednisolone[94–96] than with alkylating agents alone. Some later phase III trials[69, 71] supported this, and longer freedom from progression was observed. However, *overall* response rates were the same, and no overall survival advantage was demonstrated

Table 19–5. Vincristine and Prednisolone for Lymphosarcoma

Drug	Response Rate	Percentage	References
Vincristine	43/76	57	74–77
Prednisolone	15/22	68	79

Table 19–4. Alkylating Agent Therapy for Follicular Lymphoma

Institute	Year	Response Rate	Percentage	Reference
Royal Marsden Hospital/Winnipeg General	1958	9/12	75	67
Stanford	1972	36/42	86	68
St. Bartholomew's	1996	99/115	86*	206

*31 (27%) had complete remission.

Table 19–6. Fludarabine for Follicular Lymphoma

Circumstances	Response Rate		Overall (%)	References
	CR	PR		
Prior therapy	79/167	55/167	74/167 (44)	83–89
No prior therapy	24/49	18/49	32/49 (65)	90

CR, complete response; PR, partial response.

(Fig. 19–4).[60, 69–71] Despite this, and the necessity of intravenous therapy and inevitable alopecia, it is regarded by many as the treatment of (first) choice. In Europe it has been selected as the control arm of a randomized trial comparing it with fludarabine.

Data from other trials testing other combinations usually based on CVP show the same results. Most open study data relate to the use of CVP with doxorubicin (CHOP), sometimes with bleomycin. This combination has not been shown to give a significantly higher complete remission rate in either open label or randomized trials (56% to 79%) than other combinations,[97–104] and a retrospective analysis of a large series of patients lends no support to this combination *curing* any more patients when given as initial therapy than any other treatment.[48] Although it has not been proven, it is considered by some authors that patients with certain presentation features may benefit from this more intensive approach.

Other alternative combinations and sequences of combinations are being tested. A very intensive program ("alternating triple therapy" [ATT]) has been reported to give a high complete response rate; only preliminary data are available concerning freedom from recurrence.[105] However, the therapy may eliminate the t(14;18)-bearing clone from the bone marrow. The long-term significance of this is not absolutely clear, but no other nonmyeloablative therapy has been said to do this. An alternative combination of fludarabine, mitoxantrone, and dexamethasone similarly produces an impressive response rate in high-risk patients.[106]

High-Dose Therapy Requiring Hematopoietic Stem Cell Support

There is approximately 10 years' experience with the use of myeloablative therapy for all types of low-grade B-cell lymphoma. Virtually all the data come from phase II studies testing the treatment in patients who are in remission or certainly responsive. Most patients have received cyclophosphamide and total-body irradiation (Cy + TBI).[107–110] Support has primarily been with autologous bone marrow; in some cases it has been treated in vitro to deplete residual lymphoma cells.[107–109, 111] CD34+ selection has been tested as an alternative.[112] More recently, peripheral blood progenitor cells (PBPCs) have been used to support the high-dose treatment.[113, 114]

There is striking similarity in the results of the reasonably mature studies. At St. Bartholomew's Hospital, patients have been treated in second or subsequent remission that was either complete or nearly complete. Remission having been induced, marrow was harvested and the mononuclear cell fraction treated in vitro with, initially, a single antibody (anti-CD20) and, subsequently, multiple antibodies and complement. The early mortality was approximately 5%, with patients being admitted to the hospital for about 6 weeks. Freedom from progression for patients with Cy + TBI in second remission was significantly better than for a historical control group (Fig. 19–5), but no survival advantage has been shown.[108] This may be explained partly by the early mortality and the occurrence of a disturbing incidence of myelodysplasia[108, 115, 116] in addition to recurrence. It may, of course be the case that there will be no survival advantage because this treatment is not good enough.

The results from the Dana-Farber Cancer Institute (DFCI) for similar patients superficially look the same.[107] A potentially important difference, however, has emerged in relation to the importance of in vitro treatment of the bone marrow prior to reinfusion. At DFCI, multiple antibody and complement manipulation resulted in t(14;18)-negative marrow (as measured by polymerase chain reaction [PCR] analysis) being reinfused in half the patients. The recurrence rate was strikingly worse in patients receiving "contaminated" marrow.[117] This finding is supported by data at the University of Nebraska.[118] At St. Bartholomew's Hospital, it has only rarely been possible to achieve PCR negativity with either single or multiple antibodies.[119] However, the *overall* freedom from progression pattern is the same at both centers, the St. Bartholomew's curve (all PCR-positive)lying between the DFCI PCR-positive and PCR-negative curves.

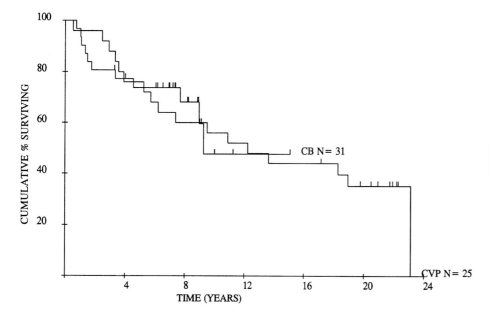

Figure 19–4. Survival following chorambucil or CVP as initial therapy for follicular lymphoma: update from St. Bartholomew's Hospital trial, 1987.[71] $\chi^2_1 = 0.0006$; $P = .98$.

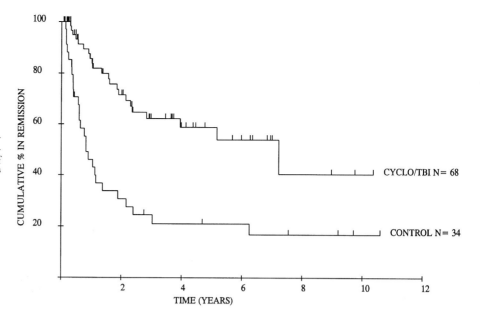

Figure 19–5. Duration of remission of follicular lymphoma following cyclophosphamide and total-body irradiation: update of St. Bartholomew's Hospital trial, 1994.[108] $\chi^2_1 = 17.17$; $P < .001$.

Various explanations for this apparent discrepancy may be made. It seems impossible to escape the interpretation that the results show that elimination or reduction of the t(14;18) clone is an intelligent goal, even though in the conventional therapy setting the relevance of the presence of t(14;18)-bearing cells is unclear.[32, 120]

Much less and almost no published data are available about the use of this treatment early in the course of the disease. Relatively small numbers of patients have been treated in first remission. Long followup will be required to allow wise interpretation of the results.

It has by no means been shown that this approach has a proven role in the treatment of follicular lymphoma, even though it may be the "best bet" for some patients in 1997. A randomized trial is in progress in Europe testing its use in patients for whom conventional therapy has failed and who are responding to CHOP. The study also investigates the value of in vitro treatment of the marrow. Another randomized trial is comparing a combination of doxorubicin and interferon with the same chemotherapy, followed by cy + TBI with PBPC support. Whatever the result of these trials, which will not be known for several years, two things are already clear: (1) a significant proportion of patients will not be cured and (2) the therapy is toxic and costly. Both of these issues can be addressed. The efficacy of the treatment might be increased, for example, by substituting targeted irradiation for total-body irradiation. Better methods of depleting the hematopoietic stem cell collection of lymphoma cells might reduce recurrence risk, although proving this without gene marking studies will be difficult. Alternatively, the myeloablative therapy might be followed by immunotherapy. Provided that the patients' immune systems were able to respond, or be augmented, this is the ultimate "minimal residual disease" situation in which to test such a strategy. The fact that this type of therapy may not be appropriate for a large number of patients with follicular lymphoma by virtue of their age or concomitant problems should not impede its investigation. As far as reducing the toxicity is concerned, the use of PBPC rescue should limit the risk of infection in the postreinfusion phase; the synthesis of thrombopoietin will reduce the risk of hemorrhage even further.

Recent data suggest that allogeneic transplantation may offer an alternative for younger patients with resistant disease.[120a] More experience is needed.

Biologic Therapy

Nonspecific Immunotherapy

Interferon. Interferon therapy was introduced into clinical trials for the treatment of malignant lymphoma more than 20 years ago following preclinical studies with L1210 leukemia and lymphoma in AKR mice.[121, 122] Regrettably, its role in follicular lymphoma remains uncertain. There is no doubt that given alone to patients with either previously treated or newly diagnosed disease, interferon causes regression of lymphadenopathy in about 50% of cases with doses that are reasonably compatible with an ambulatory existence.[123–130] The response rate (usually partial) is the same regardless of whether there has been previous therapy or the source of interferon. Responsiveness is usually slow, there being possibly several months before maximal response is achieved. Despite this, the drug is almost never used alone to induce remission, probably for a variety of reasons ranging from the perceived risk of slow responsiveness, through the undoubted toxicity experienced by as many as 25% of patients, to the high cost. Much interest has, however, been focused on its use in combination with chemotherapy and also as continuation therapy.

Enthusiasm for combining interferon with chemotherapy arose from the demonstration of synergy between alkylating agents and interferon in the treatment of murine lymphoma[131, 132] and from similar synergy in human breast cancer xenografts in nude mouse models.[133] The rationale for continuation therapy lay in the length of time needed to induce remission when active disease was present and from extrapolation of the findings in hairy cell leukemia and chronic myeloid leukemia.

Five randomized trials have accrued more than 1000 patients over the past 10 years; followup continues. One trial, conducted in France, compared a doxorubicin-containing regimen with the same regimen and interferon as induction therapy, followed, in responding patients, with the same therapy on alternative months for 1 year. Patients eligible for entry were considered to be at high risk on the basis of a large tumor burden. Response rate, event-free survival, and overall survival were all significantly better for the group randomized to receive interferon.[134] This is the only study to have been positive in terms of overall survival and indeed is the only trial that has shown any novel approach to prolong survival as well as freedom from progression. Data from the other studies, with relatively similar criteria for entry, are variously positive in some respects but less impressive. In two, one combining interferon with an alkylating agent alone,[135] the other combining it with a doxorubicin-containing regimen,[136] there was no difference in response rate. In these studies, freedom from progression for patients entering complete remission was better for patients randomized to receive interferon as maintenance therapy[135–137]; in another study, it was noncontributory.[138] In none was an overall survival advantage demonstrated.

It has to be asked how different these results are, and whether the single study revealing a survival advantage for patients receiving interferon from the outset, with a reasonably modest doxorubicin-containing combination throughout, means it should be *standard* therapy.

Certainly, interferon should be discarded only after serious consideration in the light of the survival advantage reported. On the other hand, it may be wise to conduct a meta-analysis to see whether all the data together support its use.

Interleukin-2. This is the cytokine that has been investigated most as nonspecific immunotherapy as an alternative to interferon-α.[139–141] The results are reviewed in Chapter 14. There is limited enthusiasm for it in light of the alternatives.

Specific Immunotherapy. The development of techniques allowing the large-scale production of monoclonal antibodies to cell surface determinants on malignant cells has made the investigation of antibody therapy feasible.

Passive Serotherapy. A clonal proliferation of B cells makes follicular lymphoma an ideal disease in which to test immunotherapy. Studies in animals and humans, both in vitro, first reported more than 20 years ago showed that the specific idiotypic determinants of the variable regions of the heavy and light chains of the immunoglobulin molecule were potential targets. Clinical trials subsequently showed that administration of the antiidiotype resulted in regression of lymphadenopathy and that this could be long lasting.[142] At least as important pragmatically is the fact that the process of preparing the (murine) antiidiotypic antibodies is substantial, raising serious questions about the practicality of widespread use of antiidiotype therapy, unless cure was likely.

The normal differentiation antigens also expressed on the surface of follicular lymphoma cells have also been explored as targets for immunotherapy, the difficulties of production of large amounts potentially not being a problem. Generally, the experience with murine antibodies has been disappointing.[143–149] Failure has been ascribed to a variety of causes, particularly antigen modulation and uptake by normal tissue. The treatment has also been restricted by the development of human antimouse antibodies (HAMAs).

Great store, therefore, was set on the potential of the first "humanized" monoclonal antibody, CAMPATH-1H, a pan-B-cell antibody.[150, 151] This proved too toxic to be used in the doses required to achieve clinical regression of overt lymphoma. Whether lower, less toxic dose schedules would have been effective in patients with a low tumor burden remains unanswered.

More recently a humanized (primatized) antibody to the CD20 determinant has been produced. Phase I and II trials have been conducted, and high response rates have been reported with minimal toxicity, following four injections of antibody delivered at weekly intervals.[152, 153] Phase III trials were beginning at the time of writing, mostly in patients who have received prior therapy. Their outcome is awaited with interest. It will need to be determined whether such treatment is relevant at all, an *alternative* to cytotoxic chemotherapy, or an adjuvant to cytotoxic therapy. It may be argued that phase III studies should be conducted in the chemotherapy-naive setting, in a disease such as follicular lymphoma. It seems most unlikely that 4 weeks' exposure to an antibody would compromise the outcome of subsequent treatment; it might just avert the necessity for it.

It is encouraging that antibody therapy has been shown to be active in a dose and schedule that are feasible. It remains to be determined at which point in the illness its role might be best exploited.

Antibody-Delivered Therapy. The "magic bullet" concept has been further tested with irradiation[154–161] and toxins conjugated to antibody.[162–165] Phase I studies suggest that the use of irradiation is substantially less toxic, although antibody-blocked ricin has entered phase II trials as consolidation of remission. Phase II studies of anti-CD20-^{131}I in both low and high doses following determination of the feasibility of therapy by biodistribution assessment have already yielded most intriguing results. In the first, conducted at the University of Michigan, which tested a relatively low dose of irradiation given after unlabeled anti-CD20, responses were seen in almost all of the patients with follicular lymphoma.[159, 160] Almost 50 patients have now been treated; the response rate in patients with refractory or recurrent disease exceeds 75%, many patients continuing free from progression, although the followup period is still quite brief.

An alternative approach has been taken in Seattle, where bone marrow–ablative doses of ^{131}I have been delivered either by anti-CD20 or anti-CD37. Complete remission was achieved in 16 of 19 patients who finally received the therapy, 43 having originally been considered.[157, 160, 161] Long-term followup will determine which, if either, of these treatments is better, and, as important, how broadly applicable they are. Both are exciting; both have limitations. The low-dose therapy currently is preceded by large doses of unlabeled antibody that is expensive: the bone marrow support required for the high-dose therapy makes it appropriate only for younger patients. Both are restricted in terms of repeated use by the antibodies being murine and the risk of HAMA development. Perhaps "low-dose" therapy might be *complementary* to conventional chemotherapy and "high dose" might replace total-body irradiation. Phase III trials will help define the role of these treatments, provided they are conducted in the right population of patients and it is clear whether cure or control is being sought.

Active Immunotherapy. Following murine studies in which it was demonstrated that injection of idiotype with an immune adjuvant resulted in humoral response,[166] trials have been conducted in patients who have been induced into clinical remission. Immune responses were observed in more than half the patients, some of whom had received myeloablative therapy.[167] Subsequent freedom from progression was significantly better for patients in whom immune responses were observed than for those in whom they were not.[168] Even considered in isolation, these results are most exciting. Within the context of the possibility of achieving remissions with chemotherapy in which the only reasonable persistent abnormality is the molecular detection of cells bearing the t(14;18), they are even more so.

There remain major caveats about this treatment for follicular lymphoma in general. At the practical level, the logistics of producing idiotype for vaccination are daunting, from the processing of a lymph node of at least 2 cm in diameter prior to therapy from each patient to creating and maintaining the cell lines until the appropriate time for vaccination arrives. At the theoretical level, even in the clinical trial, humoral responses were not seen in all the patients, so the patients' immune system may not be able to respond adequately. Methods enabling the extraction of DNA from as many as 10^6 cells and transferring it to a vector for DNA vaccination may well obviate the practical problem, or at least alleviate it. Phase I trials are in progress to test the toxicity of this treatment given by intramuscular injection and to measure the immune response.

With regard to the effectiveness of the treatment in eliciting a clinically meaningful response, the murine data suggest that antigen is not enough, even with a nonspecific adjuvant. More recent studies suggest that certain growth factors, particularly granulocyte-macrophage colony-stimulating factor (GM-CSF), enhance the response.[169] It may also be helpful to ensure a cellular response by increasing or inducing costimulatory molecules that are not usually expressed in follicular lymphoma but may be induced to do so under appropriate culture conditions. Studies may be envisaged to test the effect of immunizing with autologous lymphoma cells on which costimulatory molecules have been induced; in the first instance the endpoint would have to be cellular responsiveness. In the longer term, DNA vaccination with idiotype, GM-CSF, and costimulatory molecules might result in a maximal response.

Although it is clear from the human studies that at least a proportion of patients can mount a humoral response, albeit possibly inadequate, there are few in vitro data yet to suggest that the T-cell system in the patient is able to respond adequately. Limited in vitro data show that a blastogenic response is achieved when autologous T lymphocytes are cultured with (autologous) follicular lymphoma cells induced to express B7.[170] This is a far cry from proving that anergy will not be a complete stumbling block to this approach. Time will tell, provided that the appropriate laboratory and clinical studies can be conducted within the restraints imposed by our redeveloping health care systems. Perhaps the dendritic cell holds the answer.[171]

Antisense Therapy. It is possible to synthesize antisense oligonucleotides to the region of DNA spanned by the t(14;18) translocation.[172, 173] A lymphoma cell line bearing the t(14;18) has been induced in mice and the mice subsequently treated with antisense, with reduction of tumor cell burden.[174] These experiments have led to phase I studies of antisense therapy in humans.

Other experiments have shown that mutations occur within the BCL2 protein in the cells of patients with follicular lymphoma bearing the t(14;18).[175–178] These mutations might interfere with heterodimerization between BCL-2 and other related proteins concerned with apoptosis, or antiapoptosis. The increasing complexity surrounding the process suggests that these changes might be important in the development of transformation, but exploiting them therapeutically may be difficult.

THE REAL CHOICES

PHILOSOPHICAL ISSUES

Earlier discussions reflect the spectrum of alternatives that exist for the treatment of follicular lymphoma. They range from the conventional with a predictable outcome, which is progressively less satisfactory with the passage of time, to the highly experimental, with the enthusiasts' aspiration but no promise of cure. The hackneyed adage that "all patients should be entered into a clinical trial" (preferably conducted at a referral center) does not relieve the physician of the responsibility of choosing the most intelligent options at any one time in the illness.

Regardless of whether treatment is being recommended in the context of a clinical trial, the number of serious options will be reasonably limited. This will be because the informed physician should be able to discard some, or because the criteria for entry into a trial will have been tailored to certain circumstances. At the most elementary level, regardless of other prognostic factors, that which is appropriate for the aged and infirm may not be so for the otherwise young and fit.

PROGNOSTIC FACTORS AND PROGNOSTIC INDICES

Most studies reporting the outcome of clinical trials have incorporated analyses of the correlation between various pretreatment variables and outcome of the treatment being tested, using response to therapy, freedom from progression (or duration of remission), and survival as endpoints. Many retrospective analyses have been performed, using univariate and multivariate analyses; most are concerned with patients who have received no prior therapy. Little data are available concerning the relevance of the findings at the time of recurrence (or indeed the relevance of the features at initial presentation or outcome of treatment). Inevitably, such analyses concentrate on relatively simple features about which data can be drawn from the case records, such as age, number, and distribution of lymph nodes and bone marrow involvement. With successive treatments, unless patients are being entered into a trial with particularly rigid criteria, the amount of information may be expected to diminish. Studies assessing the prognostic significance of factors that cannot be routinely measured are likely to involve highly selected groups of patients and must be interpreted cautiously.

Nevertheless, provided the data are seen in perspective, they may be useful for broadly predicting the risk of treatment failure, and forming the basis of selection criteria either for a specific therapy or entry into a clinical trial. Prognostic indices have been constructed on the basis of several features allowing potentially more sophisticated grouping of patients. Needless to say, extrapolating from the group to the individual, when none of the factors is highly discriminating, is fallible.

Although the differences in overall survival by stage are not great, apart for a significant advantage for stage I disease, most analyses have been conducted for patients with either localized disease (stages I and II) treated initially with irradiation alone or advanced disease treated with chemotherapy.

Localized Disease

The most cited analysis for patients with localized disease, which is a relatively small proportion of all the patients with follicular lymphoma, was conducted at the Princess Margaret Hospital, Toronto.[179] On the basis of the demonstration that age, stage, B symptoms, and the size of the largest lymph node mass were independent predictors of survival, a prognostic factor index was proposed with these groups:

Group I—younger patients (<70 years of age); maximum lymph node size 5 cm, regardless of stage I or II (disease-free survival of 75% at 10 years)

Group II—stage II with a nodal mass larger than 5 cm in diameter (disease-free survival 58% at 10 years)

Group III—patients older than 70 years of age (disease-free survival <20% at 10 years)

Advanced Disease

Many studies of advanced follicular lymphoma have involved a range of prognostic factors, as discussed in the following sections.

Pathology

Histology. There is widespread agreement that the small group of patients with follicular lymphoma in whom all the malignant cells are large has a more aggressive course than the rest. Treatment is customarily with anthracycline-containing combination chemotherapy. Much less agreement exists about the possible differences between cases with differing proportions of smaller to larger cells. This is due at least in part to the issue of how the different proportions are calculated and presented. It has been variously reported that patients with a higher proportion of large cells (nodular mixed lymphocytic and histiocytic lymphoma in the Rappaport classification) benefit from combination chemotherapy,[180] possibly including an anthracycline antibiotic, and certainly in terms of first remission duration.[181, 182] This is not a universal finding, and the survival data are not convincing. No distinction is made between the two categories in the Kiel classification, but the latter have been distinguished in the proposed Revised European-American Lymphoma (REAL) classification. Similarly, some studies have indicated that the degree of follicularity may correlate with prognosis.[183–185] Although this may be the case, once again the stumbling block of such information lies in the definition of what constitutes follicularity.

Determinants of Proliferation (in the Lymph Node). Conflicting data have been reported about the prognostic significance of the mitotoxic index.[186–188] An alternative measure of proliferation, Ki67 on the cell surface, has been investigated.[189–191] Although there is no doubt that the Ki67 score is higher in more aggressive rather than less aggressive lymphomas, it has not been proved convincingly to predict for outcome within follicular lymphoma, largely because the range of results is narrow.

Cytogenetics and Molecular Genetics. The presence or absence of the t(14;18) translocation, identified at the molecular level, has not been shown to be prognostically significant at the initial presentation.[192, 193]

Clinical Features. Advanced age,[194–199] the presence of B symptoms,[196–198] general debility (manifest by a poor Karnofsky score), and advanced stage[196–200] all have been reported to correlate with a worse outcome. A high tumor burden recorded differently by different groups in terms of the number of lymph nodes, the estimated size of the liver and spleen, and peripheral blood involvement almost invariably predict for a poor outcome.[196–200] Increases in LDH level[196–200] and possibly β_2-microglobulin[201] may be surrogate markers for high tumor burden; they have been shown to be adverse prognostic factors. Anemia, sometimes a reflection of extensive bone marrow involvement, also correlates with shorter survival.[40, 198]

Outcome of Therapy. The best predictor of prolonged survival is the quality of the response to therapy. It can therefore be considered as a prognostic factor only from the time of assessment of *response*. It should not be considered alongside pretreatment variables, although the actual treatment (not outcome) could be. In follicular lymphoma (as in other lymphomas) the achievement of complete or good partial remission confers an equal and highly statistically significant survival advantage.

Response to treatment at second and subsequent recurrence has not been so accurately documented. However, again responders fair significantly better than nonresponders.[40]

Prognostic Indices. Several prognostic indices have been proposed, broadly based on the general state of the patient and an assessment of the bulk (or state of advancement of the disease), dividing the patients into two or three groups. Leonard and associates[198] used age, gender, hemoglobin level, stage, and performance status, whereas Romaguera and colleagues[199] used only gender, the size of the enlarged nodes, and the number of extranodal sites. Others have exploited the same parameters as have been investigated for prognostic significance in aggressive lymphoma. In Lyon, the LNH-84 index divides patients into three groups according to stage, number of extranodal sites, presence or absence of a lymph node mass exceeding 10 cm in diameter, and the LDH level (increased or not).[202] Similarly, the International Index has three groups based on a score calculated according to age, stage, Karnofsky score, and serum LDH.[203] Both of these have been applied to patients with follicular lymphoma[204] and have been reported to define groups with prognoses different enough to allow them to be considered as the basis for entry criteria into clinical trials. Validation is necessary, and it must be reemphasized that in this illness, extrapolation from the group to the individual may not be correct.

Prognostic Factors After First Treatment Failure. Few studies have addressed this issue systematically. The introduction of the use of high-dose therapy with its much higher morbidity and mortality rates (and cost) has concentrated efforts on the critical issue of determining in which patient population such an approach is warranted. It has also belatedly been recognized that the interpretation of any clinical trial of novel therapy needs such data to justify entry criteria.

Both group and single-center data define the number of previous treatment failures as the most important factor.[205, 206] Age and treatment failure were significant for survival from recurrence and from the time of second remission.[206] LDH has also been found to be important.[207] These observations are helpful in a broad sense and may give some feel for the expectations of novel approaches to treatment failure. Their retrospective nature and the small number of conclusions that can be drawn limit their contribution. They emphasize the necessity of prospective observation and recording.

THE ACTUALITY

Following the establishment of the diagnosis, and presuming that the overall circumstances warrant further intervention, investigation should be completed to determine the anatomic stage of disease and allow an approximate determination of tumor bulk. The extent of this investigation, as previously indicated, is determined by the intentions of the physician and whether a clinical trial is being entered. They may well not influence long-term outcome.

AT THE TIME OF DIAGNOSIS

Management should be expectant unless the history gives a clear indication of progression, B symptoms are present, or there is organ impairment. Followup is regular every 3 months in the first instance: investigation may be limited to routine inquiry, clinical examination, and further relatively crude assessment of progression. In 1997 this approach is almost entirely unchallenged for those with advanced disease. Hitherto conventionally, patients with limited localized disease were usually advised to have involved-field irradiation. Recent studies suggest surgery with observation may result in identical survival.

There is little leeway for any clinical trial to be undertaken at this point that would have the possibility of demonstrating a novel approach improving survival. A surrogate endpoint could be the need for cytotoxic therapy: Evaluation of a biologic approach, providing toxicity was low, would be acceptable.

AT THE TIME THERAPY IS INDICATED

Localized Disease (Stage I, Small Volume; Stage II). Involved-field irradiation is the therapy of choice. Achievement of complete remission (very much the rule) is followed by observation.

Advanced Disease. Cytotoxic therapy of known efficacy, limited toxicity, and duration should be prescribed. Equivalent alternatives include chlorambucil or cyclophosphamide alone, or CVP. Assessment of response is by clinical examination, CT scanning, and morphology or bone marrow biopsy. The achievement of complete or near complete response should be followed by observation. Management of a lesser response depends on the circumstances: the age and general health of the patient are the prime considerations. Observation may well be appropriate; in the younger patient in whom the outcome is anticipated to be poor, further therapy with alternative chemotherapy, such as a doxorubicin-containing combination or fludarabine, may be indicated. Some consider that the "hard-to-achieve remission" should be consolidated with high-dose therapy, although no overall survival advantage has been proved.

AT THE TIME OF FIRST PROGRESSION

It is always wise to document the histology at the time of progression since this will influence treatment selection. Progression of follicular low-grade lymphoma is treated with the same method that was effective initially, unless the first remission was shorter than 1 year. Under these circumstances, an alternative, for example, a purine analogue given alone or CHOP, should be used (assuming there to be no overriding contraindication). Achievement of second (or subsequent) remission may be managed expectantly, although many now consider consolidation with high-dose therapy "indicated," despite no proof of survival advantage. Failure to achieve clinical remission with whichever therapy is selected is probably an indication for second-line follicular lymphoma therapy and a greater incentive for consolidating this remission, if achieved, with high-dose therapy. Progression with transformation is treated whenever feasible with intensive therapy followed, if complete response is achieved, by high-dose therapy. Failure to achieve complete response is an indication for consideration of high-dose therapy.

AT THE TIME OF SECOND OR SUBSEQUENT PROGRESSION

Repeated progression, or recurrence, is quite sensibly managed in the same way as the first, with much the same likelihood of success as earlier, at least on the first three occasions. Inevitably, however, the chance of long survival declines, as the justification for pursuing experimental therapy increases, particularly if previous remissions have been short.

TRANSFORMATION

Transformation must always be considered a grave prognostic factor, treatment for untransformed follicular lymphoma being entirely inappropriate. Management should be for aggressive non-Hodgkin's lymphoma, with CHOP or a variant being the least intensive alternative. If prolonged survival is seen as a realistic goal, complete remission must be achieved. Hence, if this is not apparent after a maximum of four cycles of CHOP, attempts should be made to induce remission with a second-line treatment. At St. Bartholomew's Hospital, this is VP-16 with intermediate-dose ara-C (cytosine arabinoside); different preferences are exercised elsewhere. Complete remission, as conventionally defined, may be perceived for the large majority to be only a means to an end. Those who are "fit enough" should then proceed to high-dose therapy. Data about the outcome of the latter approach appear conflicting.[208, 209] However, this almost certainly reflects the extent of disease at the time of therapy. The outcome for patients receiving Cy + TBI in *remission* of transformed follicular lymphoma is similar to that of other types of aggressive lymphoma, with approaching 50% being alive and well 3 years later. This goal may be unattainable because of the underlying state of the patient or poor responsiveness to conventional dose therapy.

This conventional approach represents the least invasive way of achieving a median survival of 8 to 10 years, made up for the *average* patient with follicular lymphoma of three episodes of disease, treated with an expectation of response of about 75%, every 3 years, with eventual death the result of the disease or its therapy. Hospital admission will have been infrequent, as will outpatient visits, and quality of life perceived by the physicians as "pretty good."

The prognosis of follicular lymphoma will only be improved by the incorporation of newer therapies if the attitude toward it among physicians is changed. Specifically, in this multiple-responsive illness, the testing of novel strategies, obviously providing that they are no more toxic in preclinical and phase I human trials, must be undertaken much earlier in the disease. There is *no* evidence that the testing of a treatment with toxicity no greater than chlorambucil would, if it failed, compromise subsequent responsiveness to conventional therapy. It follows logically that efforts must be made to increase accrual into therapeutic trials.

ASPIRATIONS FOR THE MILLENNIUM

The accumulating data about the molecular basis of follicular lymphoma, and the results of early clinical trials of novel treatments outlined earlier, make it possible to plan an overall strategy for the future that might lead to a better outcome. Such a strategy inevitably depends on close collaboration between many groups and the conducting of potentially long-term clinical trials. The disease is not rare, however, and the opportunity is great. The hypothesis should be that the disease is curable, but its proof must depend on the potential of the molecular detection of the t(14:18) as a surrogate marker of success or failure (by no means certain). This might be valuable only in a negative sense, but the length of the clinical course of the disease at present demands it. The strategy and its testing depend on the fact that approximately 4 in 100,000 new cases are diagnosed each year in the Western world, and that today there are thousands of patients at later points in the illness, with first, second, or third recurrence, or remission in whom certain treatments may appropriately be tested.

The following paradigm is proposed:

1. *At initial presentation,* manage expectantly. In 10 years this might be superseded by a trial of biologic therapy aimed at preventing or postponing cytotoxic therapy.
2. *At first indication for therapy,* conduct a randomized trial comparing humanized monoclonal antibody therapy with chlorambucil, with second randomization to further antibody therapy or observation. The endpoints of this trial would be clinical remission rate and freedom from recurrence (and survival), coupled with molecular response data. Management of remission would be expectant.
3. *At failure* (first, second, or third), which might never occur prospectively but has already occurred in many.

Option 1—Compare chemotherapy program reported to induce molecular remission with conventional therapy. Endpoints would be clinical and molecular response rates and duration. Further management of success would be expectant.

Option 2—Induce remission with conventional therapy. If successful (clinically), compare consolidation with antibody-targeted irradiation with no further therapy. Endpoints would be molecular remission and survival.

Option 3—Induce remission with conventional therapy or ATT and test immunotherapy (with vaccination or co-stimulation). Endpoints would be induction of molecular remission and freedom from recurrence and would be supported by immune responsiveness.

Option 4—Induce remission with conventional therapy and compare consolidation with high-dose chemoradio-therapy (targeted radiation therapy, not total-body irradiation) with observation. At the same time test novel in vitro manipulation of autologous support, for example, antisense oligonucleotide therapy.

The sequence in which these options might be tested should be dictated by anticipated toxicity as well as efficacy. Cost may be an issue.

A nontrial "best bet" sequence, possibly unwisely ignoring interferon, might be as shown in Figure 19–6, failure of previous therapy being the indication for the next step.

It is fortunate that there are so many options and opportunities for testing them. The practicalities of conducting trials and the conflicting interests that may interfere with them should not be allowed to prevent their urgent consideration.

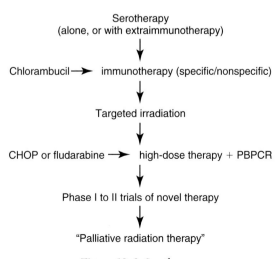

Serotherapy
(alone, or with extraimmunotherapy)
↓
Chlorambucil → immunotherapy (specific/nonspecific)
↓
Targeted irradiation
↓
CHOP or fludarabine → high-dose therapy + PBPCR
↓
Phase I to II trials of novel therapy
↓
"Palliative radiation therapy"

Figure 19–6. Serotherapy.

CONCLUSION

The natural history and clinical course of follicular lymphoma have been presented, and the current treatment options have been reviewed. It is to be hoped that the next edition of this book will see the answers to some of the questions posed.

Acknowledgments

We are very grateful to Stephanie Thomas for typing the manuscript and checking and changing the references again and again.

REFERENCES

1. Gerard-Marchant R, Hamlin I, Lennert K, et al: Classification of non-Hodgkin's lymphomas. Lancet 1974; 2:406.
2. Non-Hodgkin's Lymphoma Pathologic Classification Project: National Cancer Institute–sponsored study of classifications of non-Hodgkin's lymphomas: Summary and description of a Working Formulation for clinical usage. Cancer 1982; 49:2112.
3. Harris NL, Jaffe ES, Stein H, et al: A revised European-American classification of lymphoid neoplasms: A proposal from the International Lymphoma Study Group. Blood 1994; 84:1361.
4. Devesa SS, Fears T: Non Hodgkin's lymphoma time trends: United States and International Data. Cancer Res 1992; 52:5465s.
5. Gall EA, Morrison HR, Scott AT: The follicular type of malignant lymphoma: a survey of 63 cases. Ann Intern Med 1941; 14:2073.
6. Gall EA, Mallory TB: Malignant lymphoma: A clinicopathological survey of 618 cases. Am J Pathol 1942; 18:381.
7. Rappaport H, Winter HJ, Hicks EB: Follicular lymphoma: A re-evaluation of its place in the scheme of malignant lymphoma based on a survey of 253 cases. Cancer 1956; 9:792.
8. Rappaport H: Malignant Lymphomas in Tumors of Hematopoietic System. Washington, DC, Armed Forces Institute of Pathology, 1966, p 91.
9. Mann RB, Berard CW: Criteria for the cytologic subclassification of follicular lymphomas: A proposed alternative method. Hematol Oncol 1983; 1:187.
10. Metter GE, Nathwani BN, Burke JS, et al: Morphological subclassification of follicular lymphoma: Variability of diagnoses among hematopathologists, a collaborative study between the Repository Center and Pathology Panel for Lymphoma Clinical Studies. J Clin Oncol 1985; 3:25.
11. Nathwani BN, Metter GE, Miller TP, et al: What should be the morphologic criteria for the subdivision of follicular lymphomas? Blood 1986; 68:837.
12. Cullen MH, Lister TA, Brearley RL, et al: Histological transformation of non-Hodgkin's lymphoma: A prospective study. Cancer 1979; 44:645.
13. Armitage JO, Dick FR, Corder MP: Diffuse histiocytic lymphoma after histologic conversion: A poor prognostic variant. Cancer Treat Rep 1981; 65:413.
14. Ostrow SS, Diggs CH, Sutherland JC, et al: Nodular poorly differentiated lymphocytic lymphoma: Changes in histology and survival. Cancer Treat Rep 1981; 65:929.
15. Hubbard SM, Chabner BA, DeVita VJ Jr, et al: Histologic progression in non-Hodgkin's lymphoma. Blood 1982; 59:258.
16. Ersboll J, Schultz HB, Pedersen-Bjergaard J, et al: Follicular low-grade non-Hodgkin's lymphoma: Long-term outcome with or without tumor progression. Eur J Haematol 1989; 42:155.
17. Dick F, Bloomfield CD, Brunning RD: Incidence, cytology, and histopathology of non-Hodgkin's lymphoma of the bone marrow. Cancer 1972; 33:1382.
18. Harris NL, Nadler LM, Bhan AK: Immunohistologic characterization of two malignant lymphomas of germinal center type (centroblastic/centrocytic and centrocytic) with monoclonal antibodies: Follicular and diffuse lymphomas of small cleaved cell type are related but distinct entities. Am J Pathol 1984; 117:262.
19. Picker LJ, Weiss LM, Medeiros LJ, et al: Immunophenotypic criteria for the diagnosis of non-Hodgkin's lymphoma. Am J Pathol 1987; 128:181.
20. Jaffe ES: The role of immunophenotypic markers in the classification of non-Hodgkin's lymphomas. Semin Oncol 1990; 17:11.
21. Fukuhara S, Rowley JD: Chromosome 14 translocations in non-Burkitt lymphomas. Int J Cancer 1978; 22:14.
22. Weiss LM, Warnke RA, Sklar J, et al: Molecular analysis of the t(14;18) chromosomal translocation in malignant lymphomas. N Engl J Med 1987; 317:1185.
23. Lee MS, Blick MB, Pathak S, et al: The gene located at chromosome 18 bank q21 is rearranged in uncultured diffuse lymphomas as well as follicular lymphomas. Blood 1987; 70:90.
24. Fifth International Workshop on Chromosomes in Leukemia-Lymphoma: Correlation of chromosome abnormalities with histologic and immunologic characteristics in non-Hodgkin's lymphoma and adult T-cell leukemia-lymphoma. Blood 1987; 70:1554.
25. Yunis JJ, Oken MM, Kaplan ME, et al: Distinctive chromosomal abnormalities in histologic subtypes of non-Hodgkin's lymphoma. N Engl J Med 1982; 307:1231.
26. Tsujimoto Y, Finger LR, Yunis JJ, et al: Cloning of the chromosome breakpoint of neoplastic B cells with the t(14;18) translocation. Science 1986; 226:1097.
27. Cleary ML, Smith SD, Sklar J: Cloning and structural analysis of c-DNAs for *bcl*-2 and a hybrid *bcl*-2/immunoglobulin transcript resulting from the t(14;18) translocation. Cell 1986; 47:19.
28. Tsujimoto Y, Croce CM: Analysis of the structure, transcripts, and protein products of *bcl*-2, the gene involved in human follicular lymphoma. Proc Natl Acad Sci U S A 1986; 83:5214.
29. Chen LZ, Nourse J, Cleary ML: The *bcl*-2 candidate protooncogene product is a 24-kilodalton integral-membrane protein highly expressed in lymphoid cell lines and lymphomas carrying the t(14;18) translocation. Mol Cell Biol 1989; 9:315.
30. Hockenberry D, Nunez G, Milliman C, et al: *Bcl*-2 is an inner mitochondrial membrane protein that blocks programmed cell death. Nature 1990; 348:334.
31. Reed JC, Cuddy M, Slabiak T: Oncogenic potential of *bcl*-2 demonstrated by gene transfer. Nature 1988; 336:259.
32. Price CGA, Meerabux J, Murtagh S, et al: The significance of circulating cells carrying t(14;18) in long remission from follicular lymphoma. J Clin Oncol 1991; 9:1527.
33. Finke J, Slannina J, Lange W, et al: Persistence of circulating t(14;18) cells in long-term remission after radiation therapy for localized-stage follicular lymphoma. J Clin Oncol 1993; 11:1668.
34. Lambrechts AC, Hupkes PE, Dorssers LCJ, et al: Translocation t(14;18) positive cells are present in the circulation of the majority of patients with localized (stage I + II) follicular non-Hodgkin's lymphoma. Blood 1993; 82:2510.
35. Limpens J, De Jong D, Van Krieken JH, et al: *Bcl*-2/JH rearrangements in benign lymphoid tissues with follicular hyperplasia. Oncogene 1991; 6:2271.
36. Symmers D: Giant follicular lymphadenopathy with or without splenomegaly. Arch Pathol 1938; 26:603.
37. Jones SE, Fuks Z, Bull M, et al: Non-Hodgkin's lymphoma: IV. Clinicopathologic correlation in 405 cases. Cancer 1973; 31:806.
38. Anderson T, De Vita V, Simon R, et al: Malignant lymphoma: II. Prognostic factors and response to treatment of 473 patients at the National Cancer Institute. Cancer 1982; 50:2708.
39. Brittinger G, Bartels H, Common H, et al: Clinical and prognostic relevance of the Kiel classification of non-Hodgkin's lymphomas: Results of a prospective multicentre study by the Kiel lymphoma study group. Hematol Oncol 1984; 2:269.
40. Gallagher CJ, Gregory WM, Jones AE, et al: Follicular lymphoma: Prognostic factors for response and survival. J Clin Oncol 1986; 4:1470.
41. Yuen AR, Kamel OW, Halpern J, et al: Long-term survival after histologic transformation of low-grade follicular lymphoma. J Clin Oncol 1995; 13:1726.
42. Acker B, Hoppe RT, Colby TV, et al: Histologic conversion in the non-Hodgkin's lymphomas. J Clin Oncol 1983; 1:11.
43. Schnitzer B, Loesel LS, Reed RE: Lymphosarcoma cell leukemia: A clinicopathologic study. Cancer 1970; 26:1082.
44. Melo JV, Robinson DSF, de Oliveira MP, et al: Morphology and immunology of circulating cells in leukaemic phase of follicular lymphoma. J Clin Pathol 1988; 41:951.

45. Pappa VI, Hussain HK, Reznek RH, et al: The role of image-guided core needle biopsy in the management of patients with lymphoma. J Clin Oncol 1996; 14:2427.

46. Horning SJ, Rosenberg SA: The natural history of initially untreated low-grade non-Hodgkin's lymphomas. N Engl J Med 1984; 311:1471.

47. Young RC, Longo DL, Glatstein E, et al: The treatment of indolent lymphomas: Watchful waiting versus aggressive combined modality treatment. Semin Hematol 1988; 25(Suppl):11.

48. Dana BW, Dahlberg S, Nathwani BN, et al: Long-term follow-up of patients with low-grade malignant lymphomas treated with doxorubicin-based chemotherapy or chemoimmunotherapy. J Clin Oncol 1993; 11:644.

49. Fuks Z, Kaplan HS: Recurrence rates following radiation therapy of nodular and diffuse malignant lymphomas. Radiology 1973; 108:675.

50. Chen MG, Prosnitz LR, Gonzales-Serva A, et al: Results of radiotherapy in control of stage I and II non-Hodgkin's lymphoma. Cancer 1979; 43:1245.

51. Gomez GA, Barlos M, Krishnamsetty RM, et al: Treatment of early—stage I and II—nodular poorly differentiated lymphocytic lymphoma. Am J Clin Oncol 1986; 9:40.

52. Gospodarowicz MG, Bush RS, Brown TC, et al: Prognostic factors in nodular lymphomas: A multivariate analysis based on the Princess Margaret Hospital experience. Int J Radiat Oncol Biol Phys 1984; 10:489.

53. Paryani SB, Hoppe RT, Cox RS: Analysis of non-Hodgkin's lymphomas with nodular and favourable histologies, stages I and II. Cancer 1983; 52:2300.

54. Reddy S, Saxema VS, Pelletiere EV, Hendrickson FR: Stage I and II non-Hodgkin's lymphomas: Long-term results of radiation therapy. Int J Radiat Oncol Biol Phys 1989; 16:687.

55. Carde P, Burgers JMV, Van Glabbeke M, et al: Combined radiotherapy-chemotherapy for early stages in non-Hodgkin's lymphoma: The EORTC controlled lymphoma trial. Radiother Oncol 1984; 2:301.

56. McLaughlin P, Fuller LM, Velasquez WS, et al: Stage I-II follicular lymphoma: Treatment results of 76 patients. Cancer 1986; 58:1596.

57. Monfardini S, Banfi A, Bonadonna G, et al: Improved five-year survival after combined radiotherapy-chemotherapy for stage I and II non-Hodgkin's lymphoma. Int J Radiat Oncol Biol Phys 1980; 6:125.

58. Richards MA, Gregory WM, Hall PA, et al: Management of localised non-Hodgkin's lymphoma: The experience at St. Bartholomew's Hospital, 1972–1985. Hematol Oncol 1989; 7:1.

59. Glatstein E, Fuks Z, Goffinet DR, et al: Non-Hodgkin's lymphoma of stage III extent. Cancer 1976; 37:2806.

60. Hoppe RT, Kushlan P, Kaplan HS, et al: The treatment of advanced-stage favorable histology non-Hodgkin's lymphoma: A preliminary report of a randomized trial comparing single-agent chemotherapy, combination chemotherapy, and whole-body irradiation. Blood 1981; 58:592.

61. Mendenhall NP, Noyes WD, Million RR: Total-body irradiation for stage II-IV non-Hodgkin's lymphoma: Ten-year follow-up. J Clin Oncol 1989; 7:67.

62. Lybeert MLM, Meerwaldt JH, Deneve W: Long-term results of low-dose total-body irradiation for advanced non-Hodgkin lymphoma. Int J Radiat Oncol Biol Phys 1987; 13:1167.

63. Chaffey JT, Hellman S, Rosenthal DS, et al: Total-body irradiation in the treatment of lymphocytic lymphoma. Cancer Treat Rep 1977; 61:1149.

64. Choi CH, Timothy AR, Kaufman SD, et al: Low-dose fractionated total-body irradiation in the treatment of non-Hodgkin's lymphoma. Cancer 1979; 43:1636.

65. McLaughlin P, Fuller LM, Velasquez WS, et al: Stage III follicular lymphoma: Durable remissions with combined chemotherapy-radiotherapy regimen. J Clin Oncol 1987; 5:867.

66. Galton DAG, Israels LG, Nabarro JDN, et al: Clinical trial of *p*(di-chloroethylamino) phenylbutyric acid (CB 1348) in malignant lymphoma. Br Med J 1955; 2:1172.

67. Israels LG, Galton DAG, Till M, et al: Clinical evaluation of CB 1348 in malignant lymphoma and related diseases. Ann NY Acad Sci 1958; 68:915.

68. Jones SE, Rosenberg SA, Kaplan HS: Non-Hodgkin's lymphomas: II. Single-agent therapy. Cancer 1972; 30:31.

69. Kennedy BJ, Bloomfield CD, Kiang DT, et al: Combination versus successive single-agent chemotherapy in lymphocytic lymphoma. Cancer 1978; 41:23.

70. Portlock CS, Rosenberg SA, Glatstein E, et al: Treatment of advanced non-Hodgkin's lymphomas with favorable histology: Preliminary results of a prospective trial. Blood 1976; 47:747.

71. Lister TA, Cullen MH, Beard MEJ, et al: Comparison of combined and single-agent chemotherapy in non-Hodgkin's lymphoma of favourable histological sub-type. Br Med J 1978; 1(6112):533.

72. Cavallin-Stahl E, Moller TA, With the Swedish Lymphoma Group: Predimustines: Cyclophosphamide-vincristine-prednisolone in the treatment of non-Hodgkin's lymphoma with favourable histology: Results of a national cancer care program in Sweden. Semin Oncol 1986; 13:19.

73. Ezdinli EZ, Anderson JR, Melvin F, et al: Moderate versus aggressive chemotherapy of nodular lymphocytic poorly differentiated lymphoma. J Clin Oncol 1985; 3:769.

74. Carbone PP, Bono V, Frei E, et al: Clinical studies with vincristine. Blood 1963; 21:640.

75. Whitelaw DM, Kim HS: Vincristine in the treatment of neoplastic disease. Can Med Assoc J 1964; 90:1385.

76. Carbone PP, Spurr C: Management of patients with malignant lymphoma. A comparative study with cyclophosphamide and vinca alkaloids. Cancer Res 1968; 28:811.

77. Desal DV, Ezdinli EZ, Stutzman L: Vincristine therapy of lymphomas and chronic lymphatic leukaemia. Cancer 1970; 26:352.

78. Pearson OH, Eliel LP, Rawson RW, et al: ACTH and cortisone-induced regression of lymphoid tumours in man. Cancer 1949; 2:943.

79. Kofman S, Perlia CP, Boesen E, et al: The role of corticosteroids in the treatment of malignant lymphomas. Cancer 1962; 2:338.

80. Bonadonna G, Monfardini S, De Lena M, et al: Clinical trials with Adriamycin: Results of a three-year study. In Carter SK, di Marco A, Ghione M, et al (eds): International Symposium in Adriamycin. New York, Springer-Verlag, 1972; p 139.

81. Blum RH, Carter SK: Adriamycin: A new anticancer drug with significant activity. Ann Intern Med 1974; 80:249.

82. O'Bryan RM, Luce JK, Talley TW, et al: Phase II evaluation of Adriamycin in human neoplasia. Cancer 1973; 32:1.

83. Leiby JM, Snider KM, Kraut EH, et al: Phase II trial of 9-b-D-arabinofuranosyl-2-fluoroadenine 5'-monophosphate in non-Hodgkin's lymphoma: Prospective comparison of response with deoxycytidine kinase activity. Cancer Res 1987; 47:2719.

84. Hochster H, Cassileth P: Fludarabine phosphate therapy of non-Hodgkin's lymphoma. Semin Oncol 1990; 17:63.

85. Whelan JS, Davis CL, Rule S, et al: Fludarabine phosphate for the treatment of low-grade lymphoid malignancy. Br J Cancer 1991; 64:120.

86. Redman JR, Cabanillas F, Velasquez WS, et al: Phase II trial of fludarabine phosphate in lymphoma: An effective new agent in low-grade lymphoma. J Clin Oncol 1992; 10:790.

87. Hiddeman W, Unterhalt M, Pott C, et al: Fludarabine single-agent therapy for relapsed low-grade non-Hodgkin's lymphomas—a phase II study of the German Low-Grade Non-Hodgkin's Lymphoma Study Group. Semin Oncol 1993; 20(Suppl 7):28.

88. Zinzani PL, Lauria F, Rondelli D, et al: Fludarabine—an active agent in the treatment of previously treated and untreated low-grade non-Hodgkin's lymphoma. Ann Oncol 1993; 4:575.

89. Pigaditou A, Rohatiner AZS, Whelan JS, et al: Fludarabine in low-grade lymphoma. Semin Oncol 1993; 20(Suppl 7):24.

90. Solal-Céligny P, Brice P, Brousse N, et al: Phase II trial of fludarabine monophosphate as first-line therapy in patients with advanced follicular lymphoma: A multicenter study by the Groupe d'Etude des Lymphomes de l'Adult. J Clin Oncol 1996; 14:514.

91. Kay AC, Saven A, Carrera CJ, et al: 2-Chlorodeoxy-adenosine treatment of low-grade lymphomas. J Clin Oncol 1992; 10:371.

92. Hickish T, Serafinowski P, Cunningham D, et al: 2-Chlorodeoxyadenosine: Evaluation of a novel predominantly lymphocyte selective agent in lymphoid malignancies. Br J Cancer 1993; 6:139.

93. Schilling PJ, Vadhan-Raj S: Concurrent cytomegalovirus and *Pneumocystis* pneumonia after fludarabine therapy for chronic lymphocytic leukemia [Letter]. N Engl J Med 1990; 323:833.

94. Hoogstraten B, Owens AH, Lenhard RE, et al: Combination chemotherapy in lymphosarcoma and reticulum cell sarcoma. Blood 1969; 33:370.

95. Luce JK, Gamble JF, Wilson HE, et al: Combined cyclophosphamide, vincristine, and prednisolone therapy of malignant lymphoma. Cancer 1971; 28:306.

96. Bagley CM, De Vita VT, Berrard CW, et al: Advanced lymphosarcoma: Intensive cyclical combination chemotherapy with cyclophosphamide, vincristine, and prednisolone. Ann Intern Med 1972; 76:227.

97. Rodriguez V, Cabanillas F, Burgess MA, et al: Combination chemotherapy ("CHOP-bleo") in advanced non-Hodgkin's lymphoma. Blood 1977; 49:325.

98. McKelvey EM, Gottlieb JA, Wilson HE, et al: Hydroxydaunomycin (Adriamycin) in malignant lymphoma. Cancer 1976; 38:1434.

99. Jones SE, Grozea PN, Metz EN, et al: Superiority of Adriamycin-containing combination chemotherapy in the treatment of diffuse lymphoma: A Southwest Oncology Group study. Cancer 1979; 43:417.

100. Kalter S, Holmes L, Cabanillas F: Long-term results of treatment of patients with follicular lymphomas. Hematol Oncol 1987; 5:127.

101. Peterson BA, Anderson JR, Frizzera G, et al: Nodular mixed lymphoma: A comparative trial of cyclophosphamide and cyclophosphamide, Adriamycin, vincristine, prednisone, and bleomycin [Abstract]. Blood 1985; 66:216a.

102. Sullivan M, Netman PR, Kadin ME: Combined-modality therapy of advanced non-Hodgkin's lymphoma: An analysis of remission duration and survival in 95 patients. Blood 1983; 62:1.

103. Anderson KC, Skarin AT, Rosenthal DS, et al: Combination chemotherapy for advanced non-Hodgkin's lymphomas other than diffuse histiocytic or undifferentiated histologies. Cancer Treat Rep 1984; 68:1343.

104. Lepage E, Sebban D, Gisselbrecht C, et al: Treatment of low-grade non-Hodgkin's lymphomas: Assessment of doxorubicin in a controlled trial. Hematol Oncol 1990; 8:31.

105. McLaughlin P, Hagenmeister FB, Swan F, et al: Intensive conventional-dose chemotherapy for stage IV low-grade lymphoma: High remission rates and reversion to negative of peripheral blood *bcl*-2 rearrangement. Ann Oncol 1994; 5(Suppl 2):73.

106. McLaughlin P, Hagenmeister FB, Romguera JE, et al: Fludarabine, mitoxantrone, and dexamethasone: An effective new regimen for indolent lymphoma. J Clin Oncol 1996; 14:1262.

107. Freedman AS, Ritz J, Neuberg D, et al: Autologous bone marrow transplantation in 69 patients with a history of low-grade B-cell non-Hodgkin's lymphoma. Blood 1991; 77:2524.

108. Rohatiner AZS, Johnson PWM, Price CGA, et al: Myeloablative therapy with autologous bone marrow transplantation as consolidation therapy for recurrent follicular lymphoma. J Clin Oncol 1994; 12:117.

109. Bierman P, Vose J, Anderson J, et al: High dose with autologous hematopoietic rescue for follicular non-Hodgkin's lymphoma [Abstract]. Proc Am Soc Clin Oncol 1996; 15:317.

110. Colombat P, Binet CH, Linassier C, et al: High-dose chemotherapy with autologous marrow transplantation in follicular lymphoma. Leuk Lymphoma 1992; 7:3.

111. Fouillard L, Gorin NC, Laporte JP, et al: Feasibility of autologous bone marrow transplantation for early consolidation of follicular non-Hodgkin's lymphoma. Eur J Haematol 1991; 6:279.

112. Gorin NC, Lopez M, Laporte JP, et al: Preparation and successful engraftment of purified CD34+ bone marrow progenitor cells in patients with non-Hodgkin's lymphoma. Blood 1995; 85:1647.

113. Bastion Y, Brice P, Haioun C, et al: Intensive therapy with peripheral blood progenitor transplantation in 60 patients with poor prognosed follicular lymphoma. Blood 1995; 86:3257.

114. Haas R, Moos M, Karcher A, et al: Sequential high-dose therapy with peripheral blood progenitor cell support in low-grade non-Hodgkin's lymphoma. J Clin Oncol 1994; 12:1685.

115. Darrington DL, Vose JM, Anderson JR: Incidence and characterization of secondary myelodysplastic syndrome following high-dose chemoradiotherapy and autologous stem cell transplantation for lymphoid malignancies. J Clin Oncol 1994; 12:2527.

116. Soiffier R, Takvorian T, Whelan M: Myelodysplastic syndrome as a latter complication following autologous bone marrow transplantation for non-Hodgkin's lymphoma. J Clin Oncol 1994; 12:2535.

117. Gribben JG, Freedman AS, Neuberg D, et al: Immunologic purging of marrow assessed by PCR before autologous bone marrow transplantation for B-cell lymphoma. N Engl J Med 1991; 325:1525.

118. Sharp JG, Kessinger A, Mann S, et al: Outcome of high-dose therapy and autologous transplantation in non-Hodgkin's lymphoma based on the presence of tumor in the marrow or infused hematopoietic harvest. J Clin Oncol 1996; 14:214.

119. Johnson PWM, Price CGA, Smith T, et al: Detection of cells bearing the t(14;18) translocation following myeloablative treatment and autologous bone marrow transplantation for follicular lymphoma. J Clin Oncol 1994; 12:798.

120. Lambrechts AC, Hupkes PE, Dorssers LCJ, et al: Clinical significance of t(14;18) positive cells in the circulation of patients with stage III or IV follicular lymphoma during first remission. J Clin Oncol 1994; 12:1541.

120a. Van Besien KW, Khouri IS, Giralt AS, et al: Allogeneic bone marrow transplantation for refractory and recurrent low-grade lymphoma: The case for aggressive management. J Clin Oncol 1995; 13:1096.

121. Gresser I, Brouty-Boye D, Thomas M-T, et al: Interferon and cell division: I. Inhibition of the multiplication of mouse leukaemia L1210 cells in vitro by an interferon preparation. Proc Natl Acad Sci U S A 1970; 66:1052.

122. Gresser I, Maury C, Tovey MG: Interferon and murine leukaemia: VII. Therapeutic effect of interferon preparations after diagnosis of lymphoma in AKR mice. Int J Cancer 1976; 7:647.

123. Gutterman JU, Blumenschein GR, Alexanian R: Leukocyte interferon-induced tumor regression in human metastatic breast cancer, multiple myeloma, and malignant lymphoma. Ann Intern Med 1980; 93:399.

124. Horning SJ, Merigan TC, Krown SE: Human interferon alpha in malignant lymphoma and Hodgkin's disease. Cancer 1985; 56:1305.

125. Louie AC, Gallagher JC, Sikora K, et al: Follow-up observations on the effect of human leukocyte interferon in non-Hodgkin's lymphoma. Blood 1981; 58:712.

126. Quesada JR, Hawkins M, Horning S, et al: Collaborative phase I-II study of recombinant DNA-produced leukocyte Interferon (clone A) in metastatic breast cancer, malignant lymphoma, and multiple myeloma. Am J Med 1984; 77:427.

127. O'Connell MJ, Colgan JP, Oken MM, et al: Clinical trial of recombinant leukocyte A interferon as initial therapy for favorable histology non-Hodgkin's lymphomas and chronic lymphocytic leukaemia. J Clin Oncol 1986; 4:128.

128. Wagstaff J, Loynds P, Crowther D: A phase II study of human rDNA α-2 interferon in patients with low-grade non-Hodgkin's lymphoma. Cancer Chemother Pharmacol 1986; 18:54.

129. Leavitt J, Ratanathathorn V, Ozer H, et al: Alfa-2b interferon in the treatment of Hodgkin's disease and non-Hodgkin's lymphoma. Semin Oncol 1987; 14(Suppl 2):18.

130. Foon KA, Roth MS, Bunn PA: Interferon therapy of non-Hodgkin's lymphoma. Cancer 1987; 59:601.

131. Gresser I, Maury C, Tovey M: Efficacy of combined interferon cyclophosphamide therapy after diagnosis of lymphoma in AKR mice. Eur J Cancer 1978; 14:97.

132. Chirigos MA, Pearson JW: Cure of murine leukaemia with drugs and interferon treatment. J Natl Cancer Inst 1973; 51:1367.

133. Balkwill FR, Moodie EM: Positive interactions between human interferon and cyclophosphamide or Adriamycin in a human tumor model system. Cancer Res 1984; 44:904.

134. Solal-Celigny P, Lepage E, Brousse N, et al: Recombinant interferon alfa-2b combined with a regimen containing doxorubicin in patients with advanced follicular lymphoma. N Engl J Med 1993; 329:1608.

135. Rohatiner AZS, Crowther D, Radford J, et al: The role of interferon in follicular lymphoma. Proc ASCO 1996; 15:416.

136. Smalley RV, Andersen JW, Hawkins MJ, et al: Interferon alpha combined with cytotoxic chemotherapy for patients with non-Hodgkin's lymphoma. N Engl J Med 1992; 327:1336.

137. Hagenbeek A, Carde P, Somers R, et al: Maintenance of remission with human recombinant alpha-2 interferon (Roferon-A) in patients with stages III and IV follicular malignant non-Hodgkin's lymphoma: Results from a prospective, randomized phase III clinical trial in 331 patients [Abstract]. Blood 1992; 80(Suppl 1):288.

138. Peterson BA, Petrioni G, Oken MM: Cyclophosphamide versus cyclophosphamide + interferon-α-2b in follicular low-grade lymphomas: A preliminary report of an intergroup trial (CALGB 8691 and EST 7486) [Abstract]. Proc Am Soc Clin Oncol 1993; 12:1240.

139. Benyunes MC, Fefer A: Interleukin-2 in the treatment of hematologic malignancies. In Atkins MB, Mier JW (eds): Therapeutic Applications of Interleukin-2. New York, Marcel Dekker, 1993, p 163.

140. Margolin K: The clinical toxicities of high-dose interleukin-2. In Atkins MB, Mier JW (eds): Therapeutic Applications of Interleukin-2. New York, Marcel Dekker, 1993, p 331.

141. Weber JS, Yang JC, Topalian SL, et al: The use of interleukin-2 and lymphokine-activated killer cells for the treatment of patients with non-Hodgkin's lymphoma. J Clin Oncol 1992; 10:33.

142. Brown SL, Miller RA, Horning SJ, et al: Treatment of B-cell lymphomas with anti-idiotype antibodies alone and in combination with alpha interferon. Blood 1989; 73:651.

143. Dyer MJS, Hale G, Hayhoe FGJ, et al: Effects of CAM-PATH-1 antibodies in vivo in patients with lymphoid malignancies: Influence of antibody isotype. Blood 1989; 73:1431.

144. Grossbard ML, Press OW, Appelbaum FR, et al: Monoclonal antibody–based therapies of leukemia and lymphoma. Blood 1992; 80:863.

145. Nadler LM, Stashenko P, Hardy R, et al: Serotherapy of a patient with a monoclonal antibody directed against a human lymphoma–associated antigen. Cancer Res 1980; 40:3147.

146. Press OW, Appelbaum F, Ledbetter JA, et al: Monoclonal antibody IF5(anti-CD20) serotherapy of human B cell lymphomas. Blood 1987; 69:584.

147. Hu E, Epstein AL, Naeve GS, et al: A phase 1a clinical trial of LYM-1 monoclonal antibody serotherapy in patients with refractory B cell malignancies. Hematol Oncol 1989; 7:155.

148. Scheinberg DA, Straus DJ, Yeh SD, et al: A phase I toxicity, pharmacology, and dosimetry trial of monoclonal antibody OKB7 in patients with non-Hodgkin's lymphoma: Effects of tumor burden and antigen expression. J Clin Oncol 1990; 8:792.

149. Rankin EM, Hekman A, Somers R, et al: Treatment of two patients with B cell lymphoma with monoclonal anti-idiotypic antibodies. Blood 1985; 65:1373.

150. Hale G, Dyer MJS, Clark MR, et al: Remission induction in non-Hodgkin lymphoma with reshaped human monoclonal antibody CAMPATH-1H. Lancet 1988; 2:1394.

151. Clendeninn NJ, Nethersell ABW, Scott JE, et al: Phase I/II trials of CAMPATH-1H, a humanized anti-lymphocyte monoclonal antibody (MoAb), in non-Hodgkin's lymphoma (NHL) and chronic lymphocytic leukemia (CLL) [Abstract]. Blood 1992; 80(Suppl):158a.

152. Maloney DG, Liles TM, Czerwinski CK, et al: Phase I clinical trial using escalating single-dose infusion of chimeric anti-CD20 monoclonal antibody (IDEC C2 B8) in patients with recurrent B-cell lymphoma. Blood 1994; 84:8457.

153. Maloney DG, Bodkin D, Grillo-Lopez A, et al: Final report of a phase II trial in relapsed non-Hodgkin's lymphoma [Abstract]. Blood 1994; 84:169a.

154. Parker BA, Vassos AB, Halpern SE, et al: Radioimmunotherapy of human B-cell lymphoma with ^{90}Y-conjugated anti-idiotype monoclonal antibody. Cancer Res 1990; 50(Suppl):1022s.

155. Kaminski MS, Fig LM, Zasadny KR, et al: Imaging, dosimetry, and radioimmunotherapy with iodine-131–labeled anti-CD37 antibody in B-cell lymphoma. J Clin Oncol 1992; 10:1696.

156. Goldenberg DM, Horowitz JA, Sharkey RM, et al: Targeting, dosimetry, and radioimmunotherapy of B-cell lymphomas with iodine-131–labeled LL2 monoclonal antibody. J Clin Oncol 1991; 9:548.

157. Press OW, Eary JF, Badger CC, et al: Treatment of refractory non-Hodgkin's lymphoma with radiolabeled MB-1 (anti-CD37) antibody. J Clin Oncol 1989; 7:1027.

158. DeNardo SJ, DeNardo GL, O'Grady LF, et al: Pilot study of radioimmunotherapy of B-cell lymphoma and leukemia using ^{131}I Lym-1 monoclonal antibody. Antibody Immunoconj Radiopharmacol 1988; 1:17.

159. Kaminski MS, Zasadny KR, Francis IR, et al: Radioimmunotherapy of B-cell lymphoma with ^{131}I anti-B1 (anti-CD20) antibody. N Engl J Med 1993; 329:459.

160. Kaminski MS, Zasadny KR, Francis IR, et al: Iodine–131-anti-B1 radioimmunotherapy for B-cell lymphoma. J Clin Oncol 1996; 14:1974.

161. Press OW, Eary JF, Frederick R, et al: Radiolabeled-antibody therapy of B-cell lymphoma with autologous bone marrow support. N Engl J Med 1993; 329:1219.

162. Amlot PL, Stone MJ, Cunningham D, et al: A phase I study of an anti-CD22-deglycosylated ricin A chain immunotoxin in the treatment of B-cell lymphomas resistant to conventional therapy. Blood 1993; 82:2624.

163. Vitetta ES, Stone M, Amlot P, et al: Phase I immunotoxin trial in patients with B-cell lymphoma. Cancer Res 1991; 51:4052.

164. Grossbard ML, Freedman AS, Ritz J, et al: Serotherapy of B-cell neoplasms with anti-B4–blocked ricin: A phase I trial of daily bolus infusion. Blood 1992; 79:576.

165. Grossbard ML, Lambert JM, Goldmacher VS, et al: Anti-B4–blocked ricin: A phase I trial of 7-day continuous infusion in patients with B-cell neoplasms. J Clin Oncol 1993; 11:726.

166. Campbell MJ, Esserman L, Byers NE, et al: Idiotype vaccination against murine B cell lymphoma: Humoral and cellular requirements for the full expression of anti-tumor immunity. J Immunol 1990; 145:1029.

167. Kwak LW, Campbell MJ, Czerwinski BS, et al: Induction of immune responses in patients with B-cell lymphoma against the surface-immunoglobulin idiotype expressed by their tumors. N Engl J Med 1992; 327:1209.

168. Hsu FJ, Caspar CB, Kwak LW, et al: Results of a trial of idiotype-specific vaccine therapy for B-cell lymphoma [Abstract]. Blood 1986; 10:273a.

169. Tao MH, Levy R: Idiotype/granulocyte colony-stimulating factor fusion protein as a vaccine for B cell lymphoma. Nature 1993; 362:755.

170. Shamash J, Davies DC, Salam A, et al: Induction of CD80 expression in low-grade B cell lymphoma: A potential immunotherapeutic target. Leukemia 1995; 9:1349.

171. Hsu FJ, Benika C, Fangoni F, et al: Vaccination of patients with B-cell lymphoma using autologous pulsed dendritic cells. Nature Med 1996; 2:52.

172. Reed J, Cuddy M, Maldars S, et al: *Bcl*-2 mediated tumorigenicity of a human T-lymphoid cell line: Synergy with *Myc* and inhibition by *bcl*-2 antisense. Proc Natl Acad Sci U S A 1990; 87:3660.

173. Cotter F, Johnson P, Hall P, et al: Antisense oligonucleotides suppress B-cell lymphoma growth in a SCID-hn mouse model. Oncogene 1994; 9:3049.

174. Cotter FE, Pocock CFE: In vitro modelling and antisense therapy in malignancy. *In* Thomas NS (ed): Apoptosis and Cell Cycle Control in Cancer. Oxford, Bios Scientific, 1995, p 161.

175. Seto M, Jaeger V, Hockett RD, et al: Alternative promotors and exons, someric mutation, and deregulation of the *bcl*-2 Ig fusion gene in lymphoma. EMBO J 1988; 7:123.

176. Tanaka S, Kant J, Reed J: G to A polymorphism in the second exon of the *bcl*-2 gene. Nucleic Acid Res 1991; 19:1964.

177. Reed JC, Tanaka S: Somatic point mutations in the translocated *bcl*-2 genes of non-Hodgkin's lymphomas and lymphocytic implications for mechanisms of tumor progression. Leuk Lymphoma 1993; 10:1571.

178. Pappa V, Wilkes S, Rohatiner AZS, et al: Detection of somatic mutations of the *bcl*-2 oncogene in follicular non-Hodgkin's lymphoma [Abstract]. Blood 1994; 84:444a.

179. Sutcliffe SB, Gospodarowicz MK, Bush RS, et al: Role of radiation therapy in localized non-Hodgkin's lymphoma. Radiother Oncol 1985; 4:211.

180. Longo DL, Young RC, Hubbard SM, et al: Prolonged initial remission in patients with nodular mixed lymphomas. Ann Intern Med 1984; 100:651.

181. Peterson BA, Anderson JR, Frizzera G, et al: Combination chemotherapy prolongs survival in follicular mixed lymphoma (FML) [Abstract]. Proc Am Soc Clin Oncol 1990; 9:259.

182. Glick JH, Barnes JM, Ezdinli EZ: Nodular mixed lymphoma: Results of a randomized trial failing to confirm prolonged disease-free survival with COPP chemotherapy. Blood 1981; 58:920.

183. Warnke RA, Kim H, Fuks Z, et al: The coexistence of nodular and diffuse patterns in nodular non-Hodgkin's lymphomas: Significance and clinicopathologic correlation. Cancer 1977; 40:1229.

184. Ezdinli EZ, Costello WG, Kucuk O, et al: Effect of the degree of nodularity on the survival of patients with nodular lymphomas. J Clin Oncol 1987; 5:413.

185. Hu E, Weiss LM, Hoppe RT, et al: Follicular and diffuse mixed small cleaved and large cell lymphoma: A clinicopathologic study. J Clin Oncol 1985; 3:1183.

186. Ackerman M, Brandt L, Johnson A, et al: Mitotic activity in non-Hodgkin's lymphoma: Relation to the Kiel classification and to prognosis. Br J Cancer 1987; 55:219.

187. Bastion Y, Berger F, Bryon PA, et al: Follicular lymphomas: Assessment of prognostic factors in 127 patients followed for 10 years. Ann Oncol 1991; 2(Suppl 2):123.

188. Ellison DJ, Nathwani BN, Metter GE, et al: Mitotic counts in follicular lymphomas. Hum Pathol 1987; 18:502.

189. Macartney JC, Camplejohn RS, Morris R, et al: DNA flow cytometry of follicular non-Hodgkin's lymphoma. J Clin Pathol 1991; 44:215.

190. Rehn S, Glimelius B, Strang P, et al: Prognostic significance of flow cytometry studies in B-cell non-Hodgkin lymphoma. Hematol Oncol 1990; 8:1.
191. Holte H, de Lange Davies C, Beiske K, et al: Ki67 and 4F2 antigen expression as well as DNA synthesis predict survival at relapse/tumour progression in low-grade B-cell lymphoma. Int J Cancer 1989; 44:975.
192. Levine EG, Arthur DC, Frizzera G, et al: Cytogenetic abnormalities predict clinical outcome in non-Hodgkin's lymphoma. Ann Intern Med 1988; 108:14.
193. Pezzella F, Jones M, Ralfkiaer E, et al: Evaluation of *bcl*-2 protein expression and 14;18 translocation as prognostic markers in follicular lymphoma. Br J Cancer 1992; 65:87.
194. Rudders RA, Kaddis M, DeLellis RA, et al: Nodular non-Hodgkin's lymphoma: Factors influencing prognosis and indications for aggressive treatment. Cancer 1979; 43:1643.
195. Soubeyran P, Eghbali H, Bonichon F, et al: Low-grade follicular lymphomas: Analysis of prognosis in a series of 281 patients. Eur J Cancer 1991; 27:1606.
196. Gospodarowicz MK, Bush RS, Brown TC, et al: Prognostic factors in nodular lymphomas: A multivariate analysis based on the Princess Margaret Hospital experience. Int J Radiat Oncol Biol Phys 1984; 10:489.
197. Lepage E, Sebban D, Gisselbrecht C, et al: Treatment of low-grade non-Hodgkin's lymphomas: Assessment of doxorubicin in a controlled trial. Hematol Oncol 1990; 8:31.
198. Leonard RCF, Hayward RL, Prescott RJ, et al: The identification of discrete prognostic groups in low grade non-Hodgkin's lymphoma. Ann Oncol 1991; 2:655.
199. Romaguera JE, McLaughlin P, North L, et al: Multivariate analysis of prognostic factors in stage IV follicular low-grade lymphoma: A risk model. J Clin Oncol 1991; 9:762.
200. Steward WP, Crowther D, McWilliam LJ, et al: Maintenance chlorambucil after CVP in the management of advanced stage, low-grade histologic type non-Hodgkin's lymphoma: A randomized prospective study with an assessment of prognostic factors. Cancer 1988; 61:441.
201. Litam P, Swan F, Cabanillas F, et al: Prognostic value of serum β_2 microglobulin in low-grade lymphoma. Ann Intern Med 1991; 114:855.
202. Coiffier B, Gisselbrecht C, Vose JM, et al: Prognostic factors in aggressive malignant lymphomas: Description and validation of a prognostic index that could identify patients requiring a more intensive chemotherapy. J Clin Oncol 1991; 9:211.
203. Shipp MA, Harrington D, Anderson J, et al: Development of a predictive model for aggressive lymphoma: The international NHL prognostic factors project. N Engl J Med 1993; 329:987.
204. Coiffier B, Bastion Y, Berger F, et al: Prognostic factors in follicular lymphomas. Semin Oncol 1993; 20(Suppl 5):89.
205. Weisdorf DJ, Anderson JW, Glick JH, et al: Survival after relapse of low-grade non-Hodgkin's lymphoma: Implications for marrow transplantation. J Clin Oncol 1992; 10:942.
206. Johnson PMW, Rohatiner AZS, Whelan JS, et al: Patterns of survival in patients with recurrent follicular lymphoma: A 20-year study from a single center. J Clin Oncol 1995; 13:140.
207. Spinolo JA, Cabanillas F, Dixon, et al: Therapy of relapsed or refractory low-grade follicular lymphoma: Factors associated with complete remission, survival, and time to treatment failure. Ann Oncol 1992; 3:227.
208. Freedman AS, Takvorian T, Anderson KC, et al: Autologous bone marrow transplantation in B-cell non-Hodgkin's lymphoma: Very low treatment-related mortality in 100 patients in sensitive relapse. J Clin Oncol 1990; 8:784.
209. Schouten HC, Bierman PJ, Baughan WP, et al: Autologous bone marrow transplantation in follicular non-Hodgkin's lymphoma before and after histologic transformation. Blood 1989; 74:2579.

Chapter Twenty

"Diffuse" Low-Grade B-Cell Lymphomas

Ama Rohatiner
T. Andrew Lister

BACKGROUND

The "diffuse" low-grade B-cell lymphomas are a heterogenous group in terms of biology, morphology, and clinical behavior. However, they share the following features: most patients present with advanced disease, at an older age. Conventional therapy is worthwhile in terms of palliative responses, but remissions are rarely complete and hardly ever more than temporary. Immunophenotypic analysis shows clear differences in antigen expression, and this, together with the differences in clinical features between the subgroups, confirms that they represent distinct biologic entities.

A study from Lyon, France, has described the clinical course of more than 200 patients with "nonfollicular" low-grade B-cell lymphoma.[1] According to this report, the incidence is increasing in comparison with a similar analysis performed at the same referral center 16 years earlier. However, it is difficult to be sure whether this represents a true increase or the fact that nonfollicular lymphomas are being recognized more frequently, which in turn may reflect changes in referral pattern.

In 1984, the Kiel Lymphoma Group analyzed the clinical course and prognostic relevance of the Kiel classification for more than 700 patients with low-grade lymphoma.[2] The results can be summarized as follows: the survival curves of patients with low-grade lymphoma show an inexorable decline in contrast with the plateau seen for patients with high-grade lymphoma. The results from St. Bartholomew's Hospital show the same pattern (Fig. 20–1). In terms of histologic subtype, in the Kiel study, the survival of patients with follicular lymphoma and small lymphocytic lymphoma was the most favorable, followed by that of patients with lymphoplasmacytoid lymphoma, whereas those with mantle cell lymphoma had the worst prognosis. Again, these results are paralleled by those from St. Bartholomew's Hospital.

Diffuse low-grade B-cell lymphomas characteristically involve the marrow; leukemic manifestations are therefore not uncommon. Before the advent of monoclonal antibodies, the term "lymphosarcoma cell leukemia" was used.[3] It is now clear that the cases in question were non-Hodgkin's lymphomas (NHLs) presenting in a leukemic phase, or lymphomas that had progressed to such a phase. The latter has been arbitrarily defined as a situation in which abnormal lymphocytes represent more than 5×10^9/L of the circulating white blood cell count. Both mantle cell and lymphoplasmacytoid lymphomas may present with or develop a leukemic phase, although not as commonly as does follicular lymphoma.

The main focus of this chapter is *treatment,* but incidence and pathology are alluded to briefly at the beginning of each section. The following subtypes are referred to, using the terminology of the proposed Revised European-American Lymphoma (REAL) classification[4]:

1. Small lymphocytic lymphoma
2. Lymphoplasmacytoid lymphoma
3. Mantle cell lymphoma
4. Nodal marginal zone lymphoma (extranodal marginal zone lymphomas, otherwise known as low-grade B-cell lymphomas of mucosa-associated lymphoid tissue [MALT] are described in Chapter 24)
5. Splenic marginal zone lymphoma

The relationship among the newly proposed REAL classification, the Kiel classification, and the Working Formulation is shown in Table 20–1.

SMALL LYMPHOCYTIC NHL

Background

Small lymphocytic lymphomas represent only 4% of adult NHL. The relationship between this entity and chronic lymphocytic leukemia (CLL) has long been the subject of debate and controversy. Richter, writing in 1928,[5] commented on "the relation of leukemia to tumor . . . when the cells in the blood are morphologically identical with those of the tumor, a genetic relationship between the blood picture and the organ changes is generally assumed." Some would go so far as to say that the distinction is purely semantic and merely a consequence of the way in which different terminologies have developed. Small lymphocytic lymphoma has featured in every lymphoma classification to date, albeit in various

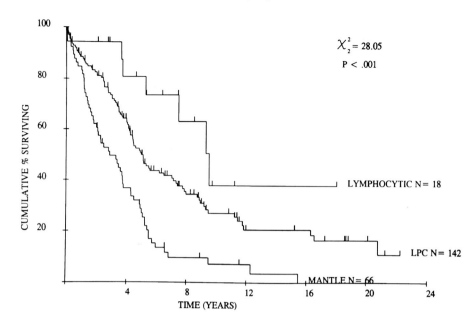

$$\chi^2_2 = 28.05$$
$$P < .001$$

Figure 20–1. Survival of patients with low-grade B-cell diffuse lymphoma.

guises. To some degree, the terminology probably reflects the clinical course of the illness, patients presenting with lymphocytosis generally being considered to have CLL, whereas those with lymph node masses without lymphocytosis are described as having small lymphocytic lymphoma, with or without bone marrow involvement. Thus, the latter term has often been considered to describe the nodal counterpart of CLL. However, it has been suggested that the reason for the difference in distribution relates to differences in adhesion molecules.[6]

The series of patients described by Pangalis and associates in 1977[7] confirmed that the two entities are histologically similar and probably represent different expressions of the same underlying process. However, the clinical and hematologic presentations differed sufficiently to justify their separation: the clinical course of 108 patients, diagnosed as having small lymphocytic lymphoma on the basis of lymph node biopsy, was reviewed. Fifty-nine patients did not have a peripheral blood lymphocytosis at all; furthermore, only 6 patients subsequently developed the hematologic picture of CLL. The contention that small lymphocytic lymphoma represents simply the tissue mani-

festation of CLL and that the development of leukemia is only a matter of time was therefore not substantiated. There was no difference in survival between patients with and without bone marrow involvement. A proportion of patients classified as having small lymphocytic lymphoma had monoclonal gammopathy, and it may well be that this group would now be described as having lymphoplasmacytoid lymphoma.

In a similar study from M. D. Anderson Hospital,[8] clinical and histopathologic data for 84 patients with small lymphocytic lymphoma were reviewed. Three groups of patients were identified: (1) those with "classic" CLL (56 patients); (2) those with a paraprotein (11 patients); and (3) those with neither a lymphocytosis nor a paraprotein (17 patients). All presented with generalized lymphadenopathy. The median survival overall was relatively short at 4½ years. In the past, the term "lymphocytic lymphoma" was probably also used to describe some T-cell and MALT lymphomas. In the proposed REAL classification it is suggested that henceforth the terminology be restricted to tumors that show the characteristic morphology and immunophenotype of B-cell chronic lymphocytic leukemia (B-CLL).

Table 20–1. Comparison of Three Lymphoma Classification Systems

Working Formulation	Kiel Classification	REAL Classification
Small lymphocytic (A)	B-CLL/PLL	Small lymphocytic
(A)	Lymphoplasmacytoid	Lymphocytic with plasmacellular differentiation
(A)	Lymphoplasmacytic	Lymphoplasmacytic
Not included	Not included	Marginal zone, low grade
Not included	Not included	Follicle center, follicular +/− diffuse
Follicular small cleaved (B)	Centroblastic/centrocytic, follicular	Follicle center, follicular, grade I
Follicular mixed (C)	Centroblastic/centrocytic, follicular	Follicle center, follicular, grade II
Follicular large cell (D)	Centroblastic, follicular	Follicle center, follicular, grade III
Diffuse mixed (F)	Centroblastic/centrocytic diffuse	Follicle center, diffuse, mixed
Diffuse small cleaved (E)	Centrocytic	Mantle cell
Not listed	Monocytoid B cell	Marginal zone, low grade (low-grade B-cell lymphoma of MALT, if extranodal)

REAL, Revised European-American Lymphoma; B-CLL, B-cell chronic lymphocytic leukemia; PLL, prolymphocytic leukemia; MALT, mucosa-associated lymphoid tissue.

As many as 15% of patients with small lymphocytic lymphoma develop high-grade lymphoma eventually.[2, 7–9] Such transformation to high-grade histology was called "Richter's syndrome,"[10] following the original case report in 1928 of a patient who presented with a 7-week history of lymph node enlargement and weight loss.[5] The patient's blood count was compatible with CLL. The course of the illness is succinctly described as "progressive, downward"; the patient died 3 weeks after admission to the hospital.[5] At autopsy, the lymph nodes showed two distinct populations of cells: small lymphocytes, identical to those in the blood but also much larger "endothelioid" cells. The consensus of opinion now is that the transformation represents the same clone, with cytogenetic and immunologic data to support this hypothesis.[11] However, cases have been described in which the high-grade lymphoma expresses either a different light-chain isotype or different immunoglobulin gene rearrangement from that of the original.[12]

Morphology

The enlarged lymph node is diffusely replaced by a monomorphic proliferation of cells that are equal in size to, or slightly larger than, normal peripheral blood lymphocytes. The characteristic features are a round nucleus with dense heterochromatin and very scanty cytoplasm.[2, 7–9] Scattered among the small lymphocytes there may be larger cells gathered together to form "proliferation centers," which are not dissimilar to follicles.

Immunocytochemistry

Ninety-five percent of small lymphocytic lymphomas are of B-cell origin, although reactive T cells may be present.[2, 13] The cells express low-density surface immunoglobulin, usually IgM, (or IgD) and are typically CD5+, CD23+, and CD43+.[13–15] They also express pan-B-cell antigens but are CD10–.[16] The proliferative rate in terms of Ki67 reactivity is usually very low.[17]

Cytogenetics

Thirty percent of cases have been shown to be associated with trisomy 12,[18] abnormalities of 13q involving the retinoblastoma gene locus being seen in as many as 25%. The translocation (11;14) and rearrangement of *BCL1* have also been reported,[19–21] but it is possible that these cases in fact represent mantle cell lymphoma.

Clinical Features

Small lymphocytic lymphoma is a disease of older people. Most patients present with peripheral lymphadenopathy or symptoms resulting from vital organ embarassment by lymph node masses. Generalized lymphadenopathy and hepatosplenomegaly are usually found. The bone marrow is usually involved, as may be the peripheral blood.

Treatment

The Older Person. Not all patients with the diagnosis of small lymphocytic lymphoma require treatment at presentation. As is often the case with CLL, the person with few symptoms other than generalized lymphadenopathy may be managed expectantly in the first instance, with careful followup and intervention only when symptoms supervene. When B symptoms appear, or if the lymph node enlargement becomes uncomfortable, treatment is indicated. Several options are available. Most patients are treated in the first instance with chlorambucil, given as a single agent. The obvious advantage of this treatment is that the drug can be given orally on an outpatient basis with little, if any, toxicity. Most patients have a useful response in terms of a reduction in the size of lymph nodes and spleen. The response is likely to last for a year or longer, and patients who respond to chlorambucil are likely to respond to the drug again at the time of subsequent recurrence or progression.[22, 23] There is no evidence that the use of more intensive treatment, for example, the combination CVP (cyclophosphamide, vincristine, prednisolone), or indeed an adriamycin-containing treatment such as CHOP (cyclophosphamide, hydroxydaunomycin, Oncovin, prednisone) is any better.[24] However, in a situation in which chlorambucil is no longer effective, such more intensive regimens can be useful.

The Younger Person. The treatment strategy outlined earlier is entirely appropriate in an illness with a median survival of approximately 10 years if the patient is older. However, in a person younger than 60 years of age, it would be wrong to accept that there is nothing better than such a palliative approach. The advent of the purine analogues has altered the philosophy of treatment in younger patients with this diagnosis, although to aim for cure may be contentious, and it is certainly experimental. The purine analogues, 2-deoxycoformycin 2-chlorodeoxyadenosine (2-CDA) and fludarabine monophosphate, have shown encouraging activity against lymphoproliferative malignancies. Fludarabine has been the most extensively investigated, particularly in CLL. There are few data for patients with small lymphocytic lymphoma as such, but the highly promising results in CLL certainly warrant its investigation in this disease, particularly if the aim is to achieve complete remission, to then proceed to myeloablative therapy with hematopoetic progenitor cell support.

The rationale for using fludarabine in lymphoid malignancies is based on preclinical studies that showed activity against L1210 and P388 leukemia[25] and against lymphoma in a human tumor-cloning system.[26] The activity of fludarabine in CLL was established in the initial phase I/II trial reported by Grever and colleagues in 1986.[27] Fludarabine, 20 mg/m[2] daily for 5 days by intravenous injection, was administered monthly. The largest clinical experience has been developed at the M. D. Anderson Cancer Center. High response rates have been seen in previously treated patients with advanced stage disease (39 of 68 in the original study reported by Keating and coworkers[28]). In a subsequent study, fludarabine was given in combination with prednisone.[29] Once more a high response rate (54%) was achieved, but the addition of prednisone was not shown to be associated with greater efficacy or better survival compared with that in patients receiving fludarabine alone. Fludarabine has also been evaluated in newly diagnosed patients with CLL, with a 79% response rate.[30]

The interest lies in the fact that *complete* remissions can be achieved, which is unusual with any other treatment for CLL or small lymphocytic lymphoma. Although such complete remissions are not durable, if the aim is to eventually proceed to myeloablative therapy, then they are useful. There are virtually no data for such treatment in patients with small lymphocytic lymphoma, mainly because of the age group involved. However, it may well become a realistic objective for the younger person. The use of peripheral blood progenitor cells as opposed to autologous bone marrow will make the treatment safer and therefore more applicable to a greater number of patients.

LYMPHOPLASMACYTOID LYMPHOMA AND WALDENSTRÖM'S MACROGLOBULINEMIA

In the past, this subtype of lymphoma has been variously categorized: in the updated Kiel classification,[31] it was termed "immunocytoma," and in turn subdivided into three categories: lymphoplasmacytic, lymphoplasmacytoid, and polymorphic. In the Working Formulation,[32] the latter was included as lymphoma of intermediate grade, whereas the other two were classified as subtype A, that is, among the lymphomas termed "low grade." The proposed REAL classification[4] recognizes that lymphoplasmacytoid lymphomas are not a single entity and that these tumors represent variable degrees of maturation toward the immunoglobulin-secreting plasma cell. The tumor cell proliferation is made up of a heterogenous population of lymphocytes, plasma cells, and lymphoplasmacytoid cells.[2, 33]

LYMPHOPLASMACYTOID LYMPHOMA

It has been variously suggested that lymphoplasmacytoid lymphoma represents 7% to 19% of NHLs.[2, 34, 35] These differences may relate to different practices with regard to performing lymph node biopsies in addition to bone marrow trephine biopsies. The diagnosis of lymphoplasmacytoid lymphoma is difficult to make without a lymph node section being available.

Immunocytochemistry

Lymphoplasmacytoid lymphomas are by definition of B-cell origin and are characterized by the presence of both surface and intracytoplasmic immunoglobulin, usually of IgM type.[36, 37] The spectrum of morphology is reflected in the immunocytochemistry: lymphoplasmacytoid cells may be HLA-DR, CD19+ and CD20+, but those tending toward the plasma cell phenotype do not express these three antigens but are instead CD38+.[33, 36] No specific chromosome abnormality has been demonstrated, but immunoglobulin heavy and light chain genes are rearranged.

Clinical Features

As in small lymphocytic lymphoma, the lymphoplasmacytoid subtype generally occurs in older people. Most patients present with lymphadenopathy, with or without splenomegaly. The bone marrow is often involved, and a proportion of patients have a serum paraprotein. In Waldenström's macroglobulinaemia (WM; see later), the paraprotein concentrations are greater than 20 g/L. In the Kiel study,[2] 29% of patients with lymphoplasmacytoid lymphoma had a monoclonal serum gammopathy (with a prevalence of IgM over IgG and IgA). A positive direct Coomb's test was found in 13% of patients (as compared with only 5% of patients with B-CLL), but this was not necessarily associated with overt autoimmune hemolytic anemia. Transformation to high-grade lymphoma may occur and is associated with a universally bad prognosis (Papamichael D, personal communication, 1997).

In a retrospective analysis from St. Bartholomew's Hospital,[38] the clinical characteristics and outcome for 62 patients treated at St. Bartholomew's Hospital over a 14-year period were reviewed. There was a male-to-female ratio of 2 : 1; the mean age was 61 years, with a range of 30 to 82 years. Most patients presented with stage IV disease, in almost all cases reflecting bone marrow infiltration. In terms of clinical features at presentation, most presented with lymph node enlargement, approximately half had splenomegaly and less than 50% had B symptoms. One third had hepatomegaly, and just under half had a serum paraprotein.

Treatment

Once more, most patients are older, and in general therefore the aim is to keep the person as well as possible for as long as possible. In practice, it is unusual to see a person with this diagnosis who does not have an indication for treatment from the outset. This may be manifest as lymphadenopathy or splenomegaly that is causing discomfort or as symptoms of anemia or infection as a consequence of bone marrow infiltration. Several treatment options are available; the choice depends on the person's age, whether or not the person is being treated in the context of a clinical trial, and the persuasion of the treating physician.

In the series from St. Bartholomew's Hospital described earlier,[38] the initial therapy was either chlorambucil or CVP. There was no difference in outcome, and subsequently patients received chlorambucil or chlorambucil with prednisolone. In terms of response to treatment, "clinical remission" (no evidence of disease on clinical examination) was achieved in 53% of patients, with an overall response rate of 79%. Complete remissions were rare (13%) as compared with partial remissions (34%), but the survival of patients achieving a remission of some sort was significantly longer than that of patients who had no response.

The question of whether achievement of complete response, as opposed to partial response, is of prognostic importance has been variously reported. In the prospective study from the Kiel group,[2] survival of patients in whom complete or partial response was achieved was significantly longer than that of patients who did not respond to treatment. However, after 3 years' followup, the survival curve of patients in complete remission was significantly better than that of those in partial remission. The median duration of response was 15 months for patients in whom complete or "good partial response" was achieved. For those in whom only a "poor partial response" was achieved, the median time to progression was only 4 months ($P = < 0.001$). The median survival overall was 14 months, with fewer than 20% of patients surviving more than 5 years. Multivariate regression analysis showed age to be the only pretreatment factor that independently predicted for response. The presence of an M band did not have prognostic significance. The results of this study and those of Nabholtz and associates[39] confirm that lymphoplasmacytoid lymphoma has a prognosis much worse than that of other patients included in subtype A of the Working Formulation. The two diseases should be considered as different entities, and they should be approached differently.

There are relatively few data for patients with lymphoplasmacytoid lymphoma treated with fludarabine. However, the experience at St. Bartholomew's Hospital shows that it can be useful, even in patients who have received several previous treatments.[40] In newly diagnosed patients, the response rate is approximately 50%, comparable with that of single akylating agents.[41] Thus, fludarabine may be a useful addition to the potential treatment options. Its precise role remains to be established.

There is a dearth of data for myeloablative therapy in this disease, mainly because patients tend to be older and because complete remission is rarely achieved. At St. Bartholomew's Hospital, 12 patients have received cyclophosphamide + total body irradiation + autologous bone marrow transplant the marrow mononuclear cell fraction being treated in vitro with the monoclonal antibody anti-CD20 and complement; 4 continue in remission between 2 and 8 years. Given the incurability of this disease with conventional treatment in younger patients, it would seem reasonable to therefore try to achieve complete remission with a view to proceeding to high-dose treatment.

WALDENSTRÖM'S MACROGLOBULINEMIA

Waldenström's original description in 1944[42] related to patients who had bone marrow infiltration by what would now be called lymphoplasmacytoid cells and a high level of circulating IgM. WM is part of the spectrum of illness covered by the term "lymphoplasmacytoid lymphoma"; however, it is somewhat different because the clinical picture may be dominated by the problems associated with circulating IgM.

Immunocytochemistry

The malignant cells always express monoclonal IgM of the same light chain type as is detected in the blood. Immunophenotyping may show surface Ig, or there may only be intracytoplasmic Ig.[43] The cells also express CD19, CD20, and CD22, with sometimes CD5 (a T-cell-associated antigen), CD10, CD21, and CD38.[43] There is thus a phenotypic relationship with both myeloma (which represents more differentiated cells) and CLL (representing less differentiated cells). It has recently been demonstrated that there are frequent somatic mutations in the D and/or J_H segments of the Ig gene in patients with WM and Richter's syndrome but not in CLL.[44] This suggests that WM and Richter's syndrome arise under the influence of antigenic stimulation and selection, whereas CLL may arise from a separate subpopulation of cells that have nonmutated Ig genes.[44] Depression of normal immunoglobulin levels is less frequently seen than in myeloma.

Clinical Features

Patients with WM present with lymph node enlargement and splenomegaly, together with bone marrow infiltration,

but these symptoms may be accompanied by those of hyperviscosity.[45–47] There may also be symptoms due to cryoglobulinemia and cold agglutinin anemia. In addition, a few patients develop peripheral neuropathy, renal disease, and amyloidosis. As for lymphoplasmacytoid lymphoma in general, most patients are older, and 55% are men.

Hyperviscosity presents with symptoms of dizziness, tiredness, and a propensity for bleeding from the mucous membranes.[48, 49] Symptoms do not usually become apparent until the plasma viscosity is at least four times that of normal serum.[48] Symptoms due to cryoglobulinemia are less common, but patients may complain of Raynaud's syndrome, joint pains, purpura, and peripheral neuropathy.[43] There may be renal impairment. Hemolytic anemia may also occur as a result of the abnormal IgM reacting with specific red blood cell antigens at temperatures lower than 37°C.[50]

Tissue deposition of IgM may also cause problems. Between 5% and 10% of patients with WM have a demyelinating peripheral neuropathy that can be sensory, motor, or both.[51–55] Renal involvement usually presents with nephrotic syndrome, which may be due to complicating amyloidosis or the result of precipitation of IgM on the endothelial side of the glomerular basement membrane.[45, 46] However, such renal complications are infrequent and usually less severe than those seen in myeloma, perhaps partly because of the lower frequency and severity of hypercalcemia in WM.

Treatment

The two components of WM need to be considered separately, as discussed in the following sections.

Treatment of IgM-Induced Complications. Plasmaphoresis rapidly reduces the level of IgM but is not an end in itself and needs to be given together with effective chemotherapy for the underlying lymphoma.

Treatment for Lymphoma. Until recently, standard treatment comprised chlorambucil and prednisolone. Approximately 50% of newly diagnosed patients would be expected to respond.[54–56] Treatment is generally continued to the point of maximum response. The median survival for patients treated in this way has been reported to be 5 years. CVP and CHOP have also been used but have not resulted in any improvement in survival.[57] Small numbers of patients have been treated with interferon-α or interferon-γ, given in conjunction with prednisolone, occasional responses being reported in patients resistant to conventional treatment.

Recently, the purine analogues fludarabine and 2-CDA have been shown to result in high response rates in patients in whom conventional treatment had failed.[58, 59] The results are even more impressive in newly diagnosed patients, with response rates approaching 80%.[60, 61] Most of these studies have been conducted at M. D. Anderson Cancer Center; with regard to 2-CDA, two cycles of treatment appeared to suffice when given to patients who had become resistant to a combination of an alkylating agent and prednisolone.[58] The drug was most effective in those patients in whom recurrence had occurred off treatment or during the first year of primary refractory disease. Little benefit was observed in patients with later phases of resistant disease.[58] In newly diagnosed patients, again two cycles of treatment were administered, resulting in responses of long duration.[61] It is clear that patients who respond once are likely to respond again at the time of subsequent recurrence.

MANTLE CELL LYMPHOMA

With the identification of a specific cytogenetic and associated molecular change, the subtype of mantle cell lymphoma has been the subject of much attention. Previously called "centrocytic lymphoma" and included among the low-grade lymphomas in the updated Kiel classification,[31] mantle cell lymphoma was classified as diffuse, small cleaved cell NHL in the intermediate grade of the Working Formulation[32] and has also previously been referred to as "diffuse, poorly differentiated lymphocytic lymphoma," "diffuse, intermediate lymphocytic lymphoma," and "mantle zone lymphoma."

Morphology

The tumor is characterized by expansion of the mantle zone that surrounds lymph node germinal centers by a homogenous population of small lymphoid cells that resemble the smaller cells of follicular lymphoma. Mitoses, however, are more numerous, and there are hardly any larger cells. Typically, the nuclei are irregular or "cleaved."[62, 63] As the disease progresses, the germinal centers become effaced by the neoplastic infiltrate, justifying the terminology "diffuse."

Immunocytochemistry

The tumor cells are monoclonal B cells that express surface immunoglobulin, most often IgM or IgD. The cells are characteristically CD5 + and pan B-cell antigen positive but lack expression of CD10 and CD23.[15, 63–66] There is overexpression of cyclin D1, which can be detected with appropriate antibodies.

Cytogenetics

Most cases of mantle cell lymphoma are associated with the chromosome translocation characterized as t(11;14)(q13;q32), which has confirmed this illness to be a discrete entity. The translocation involves the immunoglobulin heavy-chain gene on chromosome 14 and the *BCL1* locus on chromosome 11.[67, 68] The molecular consequence of the translocation is overexpression of the protein cyclin D1, coded by the *PRAD-1* gene,[67, 68] which is situated close to the breakpoint and is critical for progression of cells from the G_1 phase of the cell cycle to S phase. Using polymerase chain reaction analysis, the t(11;14) translocation has been described in approximately 60% of cases of mantle cell lymphoma. Deregulation of *PRAD-1* expression following translocation of the gene to a position near to the immunoglobulin heavy-chain locus suggests a role in the etiology of the disease.

Clinical Features

Like the other subtypes of diffuse low grade B-cell lymphoma, mantle cell lymphoma is typically an illness of older adults. The presentation is usually one of generalized lymphadenopathy, with or without hepatosplenomeg-aly. Bone marrow infiltration is almost invariably seen, with involvement of the peripheral blood in more than one third of patients.[2, 65, 69–75] Extranodal involvement is relatively common, particularly gastrointestinal tract infiltration.[2, 38] Elevated levels of lactate dehydrogenase (LDH) or β_2-microglobulin are seen in more than 50% of patients.[70, 72, 75] The median survival overall is between 30 and 40 months,[2, 65, 69–75] being shorter in patients with a high percentage of large cells[72] and longer in patients with localized disease.[70] Factors associated with a worse prognosis are similar to those described for other subtypes of lymphoma, namely older age, disseminated stage, poor performance status, the presence of splenomegaly, elevated LDH and β_2-microglobulin levels, and a low serum albumin.[70, 72, 75] In the original report by Brittinger and associates,[2] almost half the patients presented with *rapid* lymph node enlargement, and 41% complained of constitutional symptoms. The bone marrow was infiltrated in 64%. Rapid lymph node enlargement, a low performance status, involvement of the liver, and an elevated serum LDH were identified as poor prognostic factors.[2]

The difference in outcome between patients with follicular lymphoma and mantle cell lymphoma was clearly shown in an Eastern Cooperative Oncology Group (ECOG) study reported in 1978, patients with nodular, poorly differentiated lymphoma (follicular lymphoma) having a clearly better survival at 2 years than those with diffuse-PDL (mantle cell lymphoma).[8] Mantle cell lymphoma is a demonstrably incurable disease with conventional treatment. Patients die as a consequence of developing resistance to treatment; a proportion develop large cell lymphoma during the course of the illness.[72]

Treatment

With conventional therapy, the clinical course of the illness represents an inexorable pattern of progression, irrespective of which specific treatment is used and despite responsiveness to treatment in 50% to 90% of patients (Table 20–2). Responses are rarely complete, and the median time to treatment failure is less than 18 months in most series.[70] In the past, most patients have been treated with chlorambucil, the combination CVP or CHOP.[64, 69, 76] A randomized prospective comparison between CVP and CHOP showed no advantage for the addition of adriamycin, with similar response rates for the two groups of patients and survival being equally short in both arms,[76] confirming other reports.[69, 71] In contrast, one report does suggest an advantage for adriamycin-containing treatment in a subgroup of patients: a retrospective analysis was undertaken of 65 patients treated at two centers in Italy.[75] The median survival was only 3½ years, confirming the poor survival pattern described in other series. When the International Index[77] was applied, good performance status, a normal LDH, normal β_2-microglobulin, younger age (<65 years) and a favorable "prognostic risk category" (according to the International Index) were associated with a better outcome ($P < 0.5$). For patients with such favorable prognostic scores (low and low-intermediate risk disease), there was a suggestion of a survival advantage with anthracycline-containing regimens, but clearly these patients may already have had a better prognosis.

Table 20–2. Results of Treatment for Mantle Cell Lymphoma

No. of Patients	CR (%)	CR + PR (%)	Failure-Free Survival (mo)	Overall Survival (mo)	Reference No.
36	53	86	20	36	69
52	31	56	14	52	70
42	41	N/ST	N/ST	31	71
37	41	84	10	32	76 (COP group)
26	58	88	7	37	76 (CHOP group)
66	9	71	10	36	72
55	N/ST	N/ST	N/ST	32	73
29°	52°	83°	19°	45°	74
35	40	60	20	45	74
65	51	86	N/ST	42	75
14	29	N/ST	18	32	79

°Originally classified as intermediate grade in the Working Formulation.

N/ST, not stated; COP, cyclophosphamide, vincristine, prednisolone; CHOP, cyclophosphamide, adriamycin, vincristine, prednisolone; CR, complete response; PR, partial response.

A recent report from the European Organization for the Research and Treatment of Cancer (EORTC) has evaluated response to treatment in patients with mantle cell lymphoma, some of whom were included in a protocol for intermediate-grade lymphoma and the rest in a study for patients with low-grade lymphoma.[74] The first group received either CHVMP-VB (cyclophosphamide, doxorubicin, teniposide, prednisolone, vincristine, and bleomycin) or ProMace-MOPP (doxorubicin, cyclophosphamide, etoposide, mechlorethamine, vincristine, procarbazine, prednisone). In the low-grade study, patients were treated with CVP as remission induction and were then randomized between maintenance interferon or no further treatment. Overall survival and response rate were similar to those of patients with other subtypes of intermediate-grade lymphoma, but duration of response and progression-free survival were considerably shorter for patients with mantle cell lymphoma. In comparison with low-grade lymphoma, response rate, duration of response, and progression-free survival were the same for patients with mantle cell lymphoma as for those with other low-grade subtypes; however, the overall survival of patients with mantle cell lymphoma was only half as long (median 45 versus 84 months). Interferon did not confer any benefit. Overall, no treatment appeared to be superior to any other.[74]

A study from Germany has compared treatment comprising prednimustine and mitoxantrone with COP (cyclophosphamide, vincristine prednisolone) as induction therapy, followed by a second randomization (in responding patients) to maintenance interferon or to no further treatment. The study was conducted in patients with both follicular lymphoma and mantle cell lymphoma, the latter group numbering 37. As would be expected, in the mantle cell lymphoma group, only 19% of patients entered complete remission, and the median survival was extremely short at 2½ years. Data regarding outcome of the two treatments and the role of interferon are not yet available.[78]

At St. Bartholomew's Hospital, a stringent policy of rebiopsy at virtually each recurrence has been pursued. A retrospective analysis[72] reviewed the clinical course of 66 newly diagnosed patients. Serial biopsies had been per-formed in 50 patients. The median survival was only 3 years. Factors predictive for poor outcome were advanced stage, older age (>70 years), low sodium and albumin levels, and the presence of splenomegaly. "Blastic transformation" was identified in 32% of cases during the course of the illness and was found at autopsy in 70% of patients.

In view of the appalling prognosis of patients with this illness, experimental options are currently being evaluated. Myeloablative therapy supported by autologous bone marrow transplantation has been used in small numbers of patients, mainly because mantle cell lymphoma is essentially a disease of older people and, again, because complete remissions are rare. However, a preliminary report from the University of Nebraska suggests that this treatment may be useful, although longer followup is required.[79] Small numbers of patients with disease deemed refractory to conventional therapy have been treated with radiolabeled (iodine-131 conjugated) anti CD20 antibody with some success (Kaminski M, personal communication, 1997).

NODAL MARGINAL ZONE LYMPHOMA (MONOCYTOID B-CELL LYMPHOMA)

In the proposed REAL classification, lymphomas arising from the marginal zone are grouped together in view of their common origin. Thus, MALT lymphomas and monocytoid B-cell lymphomas are thought to be related. A study from the Massachusetts General Hospital[80] showed that although there were no differences in antigen expression among these two subtypes, there were clinical differences. Patients with MALT lymphomas generally had localized disease (78%), and their survival was considerably better than that of those with nodal marginal zone lymphoma who often had extranodal involvement. However, the relationship with MALT lymphomas is complex. They may occur in the context of extranodal MALT lymphomas,[81, 82] for example, lymph nodes secondarily involved by gastric or parotid MALT lymphomas have a histologic appearance identical to that of nodal marginal zone lymphomas. They are also known to occur in patients with Sjögren's syndrome and have rarely been described as involving lymph nodes (with or without bone marrow infiltration), in the absence of extranodal disease.[83–85]

Immunocytochemistry

Not surprisingly, nodal marginal zone lymphomas share the immunophenotypic features of MALT lymphomas. The cells are characteristically surface immunoglobulin positive (IgM). They are also CD19+, CD20+, and CD22+ but CD5–, CD10–, and CD23–.[81–83] These tumors are considered to be the neoplastic counterpart of monocytoid B cells, which are reactive cells that occur in the context of infectious diseases such as toxoplasmosis or in association with Hodgkin's disease and some types of NHL.

Clinical Features

Unusually, there is a female predominance in nodal marginal zone lymphoma, but again this is an illness of older people with a median age at diagnosis of 65 years.[82, 83] Most patients present with peripheral lymphadenopathy, most often in the neck, around the parotid gland. Transformation to high-grade lymphoma does occur. There is at present no consensus as to the best treatment, individual cases being managed according to site.

SPLENIC MARGINAL ZONE LYMPHOMA, WITH (OR WITHOUT) VILLOUS LYMPHOCYTES

Splenic marginal zone lymphoma is a rare and only recently described entity that was not listed in either the Kiel classification or the Working Formulation. The lymphoma characteristically involves the spleen and has been regarded as the splenic counterpart of the MALT lymphomas (see Chapter 5). The white blood cell count is usually increased, and the circulating cells have short villi on the surface, often situated at one pole of the cell, hence the name.[84, 85]

Immunochemistry

The immunophenotype is similar to that of MALT lymphomas, that is, the cells express surface immunoglobulin and a proportion also have cytoplasmic immunoglobulin. They express CD19, CD20, CD22, and CD79a but are typically CD5- and CD10-.[85, 86]

Clinical Features

Patients with splenic marginal zone lymphoma generally present with symptoms of an enlarged spleen.[84, 85] The bone marrow is usually involved, but lymph node enlargement is rare. There may be a paraprotein. Often the diagnosis is only made at splenectomy, performed when alternative attempts to establish the cause of the splenomegaly have failed.

Treatment

Since this subtype of low-grade B-cell lymphoma has been described only relatively recently, there are few data for the results of treatment. In addition, the number of patients recognized to have this illness is quite small. However, following splenectomy, the illness tends to present problems owing to bone marrow infiltration. Most patients have been treated with alkylating agents, given alone or with prednisolone, as for CLL.[84, 85]

CONCLUSION

The increasing sophistication of immunocytochemistry and molecular biology has led to the recognition of several different subtypes of low-grade B-cell lymphoma. The number of diseases appears to increase with each new lymphoma classification. Recognition of specific nonrandom chromosome translocations for some, and moreover, in the case of mantle cell lymphoma, the molecular consequences of the translocation have confirmed the different subtypes to be related but discrete entities. This rapid increase in understanding of the biology of the diseases has not been paralleled by much improvement in their outcome. Most patients with diffuse low-grade B-cell lymphoma die because of the illness. Some die as a consequence of treatment for the illness and a few, because these are diseases of older people, die of unrelated causes. Some progress has unquestionably been made, and the future does not look entirely bleak. Recognition of the different patterns of illness and evaluation of new approaches such as antibody therapy and targeted irradiation hopefully will identify the subtypes in which most benefit for a particular treatment may be gained.

Acknowledgments

The authors are most grateful to Dr. Andrew Norton for his helpful comments about the pathology and thank Mrs. Chris Sykes for typing the manuscript.

REFERENCES

1. Peuchmaur M, Scoazec JY, Gaulard P, et al: Analytical study of the different subtypes of non-Hodgkin's lymphoma: Clinical, histological, and immunohistochemical aspects. *In* Solal-Celigny P, Brousse N, Reyes F, et al (eds): Non-Hodgkin's Lymphomas, London, Manson, 1993, pp 107–155.
2. Brittinger G, Bartels H, Common H, et al: Clinical and prognostic relevance of the Kiel classification on non-Hodgkin's lymphomas: Results of a prospective multi-centre study by the Keil Lymphoma Study Group. Haematol Oncol 1984; 2:269.
3. Isaacs R: Lymphosarcoma cell leukaemia. Ann Intern Med 1937; 11:657.
4. Harris NL, Jaffe ES, Stein H, et al: A revised European-American classification of lymphoid neoplasms: A proposal from the International Lymphoma Study Group. Blood 1994;84:1361.
5. Richter MN: Generalized reticular cell sarcoma of lymph nodes associated with lymphatic leukemia. Am J Pathol 1928;4:285.
6. Inghirami G, Wieczorek R, Zhu B-Y, et al: Differential expression of LFA-1 molecules in non-Hodgkin's lymphoma and lymphoid leukemia. Blood 1988;72:1431.
7. Pangalis GA, Nathwani BN, Rappaport H: Malignant lymphoma, well-differentiated lymphocytic: Its relationship with chronic lymphocytic leukemia and macroglobulinemia of Waldenström. Cancer 1977;39:999.
8. Evans HL, Butler JJ, Youness EL: Malignant lymphoma, small lymphocytic type. Cancer 1978;41:1440.
9. Dick F, Maca R: The lymph node in chronic lymphocytic leukemia. Cancer 1978;41:283.

10. Long JC, Aisenberg AC: Richter's syndrome: A terminal complication of chronic lymphocytic leukemia with distinct clinicopathologic features. Am J Clin Pathol 1975;63:786.
11. Nowell P, Finan J, Glover D, Guerry D: Cytogenetic evidence for the clonal nature of Richter's syndrome. Blood 1981;58:183.
12. Van Dongen JJM, Hooijkaas H, Michiels JJ, et al: Richter's syndrome with different immunoglobulin light chains and different heavy chain rearrangements. Blood 1984;64:571.
13. Van der Reijden HJ, Van der Gag R, Pinkster J, et al: Chronic lymphocytic leukemia: Immunologic markers and functional properties of the leukemic cells. Cancer 1982;50:2826.
14. Aisenberg AC, Wilkes BM: Monoclonal antibody studies in B-cell chronic lymphocytic leukemias and allied disorders. Hematol Oncol 1983;1:13.
15. Stein H, Lennert K, Feller AC, Mason DY: Immunohistological analysis of human lymphoma: Correlation of histological and immunological categories. Adv Cancer Res 1984;42:67.
16. Burns BF, Warnke RA, Doggett RS, Rouse RV: Expression of a T-cell antigen (Leu-1) by B-cell lymphomas. Am J Pathol 1983;113:165–171.
17. Medeiros LJ, Strickler JG, Picker LJ, et al: "Well-differentiated" lymphocytic neoplasms: Immunologic findings correlated with clinical presentation and morphologic features. Am J Pathol 1987;129:523.
18. Knuutila S, Elonen E, Teerenhovi L, et al: Trisomy 12 in B cells of patients with B-cell chronic lymphocytic leukemia. N Engl J Med 1986;314:865.
19. Athan E, Foitl D, Knowles D: Bcl-1 rearrangement: Frequency and clinical significance among B-cell chronic lymphocytic leukemias and non-Hodgkin's lymphomas. Am J Pathol 1991;138:591.
20. Croce C, Tsujimoto Y, Erikson J, et al: Chromosome translocations and B-cell neoplasia. Lab Invest 1984;51:258.
21. Tsujimoto Y, Ynis J, Onorato-Showe L, et al: Molecular cloning of the chromosomal breakpoint of B-cell lymphomas and leukemias with the t(11;14) chromosome translation. Science 1984;224:14.
22. Han T, Ezdinli EZ, Shimaoka K, et al: Chlorambucil versus combined chlorambucil-corticosteroid therapy in chronic lymphocytic leukemia. Cancer 1973;31:502.
23. Idestrom K, Kimby E, Bjorkholm M, et al: Treatment of chronic lymphocytic leukaemia and well-differentiated lymphocytic lymphoma with continuous low or intermittent high-dose prednimustine versus chlorambucil/prednisolone. Eur J Cancer 1982;18:1117.
24. Liepman M, Votaw ML: The treatment of chronic lymphocytic leukemia with COP chemotherapy. Cancer 1978;41:1664.
25. Tavoussi M, Avramis VI: Pharmacodynamics of fludarabine phosphate (F-ara-AMP) in P388 leukaemia-bearing mice after toxic and non-toxic regimens. Proc Am Soc Clin Oncol 1986;5:45.
26. Lathan B, Diehl V, Clark GM, et al: Cytotoxic activity of 9-b-D-arabinofuranosyl-2-fluoroadenine 5-monophosphate (fludarabine, NSC 312887) in a human tumor cloning system. Eur J Cancer Clin Oncol 1988;24:1891.
27. Grever MR, Coltman CA, Files JL, et al: Fludarabine monophosphate in chronic lymphocytic leukemia. Blood 1986;68:223a.
28. Keating MJ, Kantarjian H, Talpaz M, et al: Fludarabine: A new agent with major activity against chronic lymphocytic leukemia. Blood 1989;74:19.
29. Keating MJ, Kantarjian HM, O'Brien S, et al: Fludarabine (FLU)-prednisolone (PRED)—a safe, effective combination in refractory chronic lymphocytic leukemia. Proc Am Soc Clin Oncol 1989;8:201.
30. Keating M, Kantarjian H, O'Brien S: Fludarabine: A new agent with marked cytoreductive activity in untreated chronic lymphocytic leukemia. J Clin Oncol 1991;9:44.
31. Stansfeld AG, Diebold J, Kapanci Y, et al: Updated Kiel classification for lymphomas. Lancet 1988;1:292.
32. Non-Hodgkin's Lymphoma Pathologic Classification Project: National Cancer Institute–sponsored study of classifications of non-Hodgkin's lymphomas: Summary and description of a Working Formulation for clinical usage. Cancer 1982;49:2112.
33. Harris NL, Bhan AK: B-cell neoplasms of the lymphocytic, lymphoplasmacytoid, and plasma cell types: Immunologic analysis and clinical correlation. Hum Pathol 1985;16:829.
34. Glimelius B, Hagberg H, Sundstrom C: Morphological classification of non-Hodgkin malignant lymphoma. Scand J Haematol 1983;30:13.
35. Leonard RCF, Cuzick J, MacLennan ICM, et al: Prognostic factors in non-Hodgkin's lymphoma: The importance of symptomatic stage as an adjunct to the Kiel histopathological classification. Br J Cancer 1983;47:91.
36. Stein H, Bonk A, Tolksdorf G, et al: Immunohistologic analysis of the organization of normal lymphoid tissue and non-Hodgkin's lymphomas. J Histochem Cytochem 1980;28:746.
37. Habeshaw JA, Bailey D, Stansfeld AG, Greaves MF: The cellular content of non-Hodgkin's lymphomas: A comprehensive analysis using monoclonal antibodies and other surface marker techniques. Br J Cancer 1983;47:327.
38. Richards MA, Hall PA, Gregory WM, et al: Lymphoplasmacytoid and small cell centrocytic non-Hodgkin's lymphoma—a retrospective analysis from St. Bartholomew's Hospital, 1972–1986. Haematol Oncol 1989;7:19.
39. Nabholtz J-M, Friedman S, Collin F, et al: Modification of Kiel and Working Formulation classification for improved survival in non-Hodgkin's lymphoma. J Clin Oncol 1987;5:1634.
40. Rohatiner AZS, Tirovola E, Pigaditou A, et al: Fludarabine in low-grade lymphoma—the SBH experience. Haematol Blood Transfus (In Press).
41. Rohatiner A, Foran J, Coiffier B, et al: Fludarabine in newly diagnosed diffuse low-grade non-Hodgkin's lymphoma. Proc Am Soc Clin Oncol 1996;15:419.
42. Waldenström J: Incipient myelomatosis or essential hyperglobulinemia with fibrinogenopenia—a new syndrome? Acta Med Scand 1944;117:216.
43. Dimopoulos MA, Alexanian R: Waldenström's macroglobulinemia. Blood 1994;83:1452.
44. Aoki H, Takishita M, Kosaka M, et al: Frequent somatic mutations in D and/or JH segments of Ig gene in Waldenström's macroglobulinemia and chronic lymphocytic leukemia (CLL) with Richter's syndrome but not in common CLL. Blood 1995;85:1913.
45. Krajny M, Pruzanski W: Waldenström's macroglobulinemia: Review of 45 cases. Can Med Assoc J 1976;114:899.
46. Kyle RA, Garton JP: The spectrum of IgM monoclonal gammopathy in 430 cases. Mayo Clin Proc 1987;62:719.
47. Facon T, Brouillard M, Duhamel A, et al: Prognostic factors in Waldenström's macroglobulinemia. J Clin Oncol 1993;11:1553.
48. Alexanian R: Blood volume in monoclonal gammopathy. Blood 1977;49:301.
49. Crawford J, Cox EB, Cohen HJ: Evaluation of hyperviscosity in monoclonal gammopathies. Am J Med 1985;79:13.
50. Rosse WF, Adams J, Logue G: Hemolysis by complement and cold reaction antibody. Am J Hematol 1977;2:259.
51. Dellagi K, Dupouey P, Brouet JC, et al: Waldenström's macroglobulinemia and peripheral neuropathy: A clinical and immunologic study of 25 patients. Blood 1983;62:280.
52. Nobile-Orazio E, Marmireli P, Baldini L, et al: Peripheral neuropathy in macroglobulinemia. Neurology 1987;37:1506.
53. Kelly JJ, Adelman LS, Berkman E, et al: Polyneuropathies associated with IgM monoclonal gammopathies. Arch Neurol 1988;45:1355.
54. Petrucci MT, Avvisati G, Tribalto M, et al: Waldenström's macroglobulinemia: Results of a combined oral treatment in 34 newly diagnosed patients. J Intern Med 1989;226:443.
55. Foerster J: Waldenström's macroglobulinemia. In Lee GR, Bithel TC, Foerster J, et al (eds): Wintrobe's Clinical Hematology. Philadelphia, Lea & Febiger, 1993, p 2250.
56. MacKenzie MR, Fudenberg HH: Macroglobulinemia: An analysis of forty patients. Blood 1972;39:874.
57. McCallister BD, Bayrd ED, Harrison EG, et al: Primary macroglobulinemia. Am J Med 1967;43:394.
58. Dimopoulos MA, Weber D, Delasalle KB, et al: Treatment of Waldenström's macroglobulinemia resistant to standard therapy with 2-chlorodeoxyadenosine: Identification of prognostic factors. Ann Oncol 1995;6:49.
59. Kantarjian HM, Alexanian R, Koller CA, et al: Fludarabine therapy in macroglobulinemic lymphoma. Blood 1990;75:1928.
60. Dimopoulos MA, O'Brien S, Kantarjian H, et al: Fludarabine therapy in Waldenström's macroglobulinemia. Am J Med 1993;95:49.
61. Dimopoulos MA, Kantarjian HM, Estey EH, et al: Treatment of Waldenström macroglobulinemia with 2-chlorodeoxyadenosine. Ann Intern Med 1993;118:195.
62. Banks P, Chan J, Cleary M, et al: Mantle cell lymphoma: A proposal for unification of morphologic, immunologic, and molecular data. Am J Surg Pathol 1992;16:637.
63. Tolksdorf G, Stein H, Lennert K: Morphological and immunological definition of a malignant lymphoma derived from germinal centre cells with cleaved nuclei (centrocytes). Br J Cancer 1980;41:168.

64. Zukerberg L, Medeiros L, Ferry J, et al: Diffuse low-grade B-cell lymphomas: Four clinically distinct subtypes defined by a combination of morphologic and immunophenotypic features. Am J Clin Pathol 1993;100:373.

65. Swerdlow SH, Habeshaw JA, Dhaliwal HS, et al: Centrocytic lymphoma: A distinct clinicopathologic and immunologic entity. Am J Pathol 1983;113:181.

66. Harris N, Nadler L, Bhan A: Immunohistologic characterization of two malignant lymphomas of germinal center type (centroblastic/centrocytic and centrocytic) with monoclonal antibodies: Follicular and diffuse lymphomas of small cleaved cell types are related but distinct entities. Am J Pathol 1984;117:262.

67. Athan E, Foitl D, Knowles D: *Bcl-1* rearrangement: Frequency and clinical significance among B-cell chronic lymphocytic leukemias and non-Hodgkin's lymphomas. Am J Pathol 1991;138:591.

68. Williams ME, Westermann CD, Swerdlow SH: Genotypic characterization of centrocytic lymphoma: Frequent rearrangement of the chromosome 11 *bcl-1* locus. Blood 1990;76:1387.

69. Fisher RI, Dahlberg S, Nathwani BN, et al: A clinical analysis of two indolent lymphoma entities: Mantle cell lymphoma and marginal zone lymphoma: A Southwest Oncology Group study. Blood 1995;85:1075.

70. Berger F, Felman P, Sonet A, et al: Nonfollicular small B-cell lymphomas: A heterogeneous group of patients with distinct clinical features and outcome. Blood 1994;83:2829.

71. Weisenburger DD, Nathwani BN, Diamond LW, et al: Malignant lymphoma, intermediate lymphocytic type: A clinicopathologic study of 42 cases. Cancer 1981;48:1415.

72. Norton AJ, Matthews J, Pappa V, et al: Mantle cell lymphoma: Natural history defined in a serially biopsied population over a 20-year period. Ann Oncol 1995;6:249.

73. Pittaluga S, Wlodarska I, Stul MS, et al: Mantle cell lymphoma: A clinicopathological study of 55 cases. Histopathology 1995;26:17.

74. Teodorovic I, Pittaluga S, Kluin-Nelemans JC, et al for the European Organization for the Research and Treatment of Cancer Lymphoma Cooperative Group: Efficacy of four different regimens in 64 mantle cell lymphoma cases: Clinicopathologic comparison with 498 other non-Hodgkin's lymphoma subtypes. J Clin Oncol 1995;13:2819.

75. Zucca E, Roggero E, Pinotti G, et al: Patterns of survival in mantle cell lymphoma. Ann Oncol 1995;6:257.

76. Meusers P, Engelhard M, Bartels H, et al: Multicentre randomized therapeutic trial for advanced centrocytic lymphoma: Anthracycline does not improve the prognosis. Hematol Oncol 1989;7:365.

77. Shipp MA, Harrington D, Anderson J, et al: A predictive model for aggressive non-Hodgkin's lymphoma: The international NHL prognostic factors project. N Engl J Med 1993;329:987.

78. Hiddemann W, Unterhalt M, Thiemann M: Characteristics and clinical course of follicle center lymphomas and mantle cell lymphomas: A study on the clinical relevance of the REAL classification. Blood 1994;84(Suppl 1):449a.

79. Stewart DA, Vose JM, Weisenburger, et al: The role of high-dose therapy and autologous hematopoietic stem cell transplantation for mantle cell lymphoma. Ann Oncol 1995;6:263.

80. Ngan B-Y, Warnke R, Wilson M, et al: Monocytoid B-cell lymphoma: A study of 36 cases. Hum Pathol 1991;22:409.

81. Shin S, Sheibani K, Fishleder A, et al: Monocytoid B-cell lymphoma in patients with Sjögren's syndrome: A clinicopathologic study of 13 patients. Hum Pathol 1991;22:422.

82. Sheibani K, Burke JS, Swartz WG, et al: Monocytoid B-cell lymphoma: Clinicopathologic study of 21 cases of a unique type of low-grade lymphoma. Cancer 1988;62:1531.

83. Cogliatti S, Lennert K, Hansmann M, et al: Monocytoid B-cell lymphoma: Clinical and prognostic features of 21 patients. J Clin Pathol 1990;43:619.

84. Melo JV, Hegde U, Parreira A, et al: Splenic B-cell lymphoma with circulating villous lymphocytes: Differential diagnosis of B-cell leukaemias with large spleens. J Clin Pathol 1987;40:642.

85. Schmid C, Kirkham N, Diss T, et al: Splenic marginal zone cell lymphoma. Am J Surg Pathol 1992;16:455.

86. Jadayel D, Matutes E, Dyer MJ, et al: Splenic lymphoma with villous lymphocytes: Analysis of *BCL-1* rearrangements and expression of the cyclin D1 gene. Blood 1994;83:3664.

Twenty-One

━━ Diffuse Large Cell and ━━ Immunoblastic Lymphomas

Ellen R. Gaynor
Richard I. Fisher

The non-Hodgkin's lymphomas (NHLs) are a diverse group of diseases with varying presentations, natural histories, and responses to therapy. The Working Formulation provides a conceptual framework in which the lymphomas are grouped as low (indolent), intermediate, or high grade with respect to their natural histories.[1] As seen in Table 21–1, diffuse large cell lymphoma is classified in the intermediate category, whereas large cell immunoblastic lymphoma is considered to be a more aggressive lymphoma and thus is classified in the high-grade category. From a clinical standpoint, these lymphomas can be considered as a single group because they share similar clinical presentations and natural histories and because they require similar treatment approaches.

DIFFUSE LARGE CELL LYMPHOMA

As a group diffuse large cell lymphomas account for approximately one third of all NHLs. They are biologically diverse with respect to their cell of origin. However, most are derived from lymphocytes: 75% are of B-cell origin, and 25% are of T-cell origin. The prognostic significance of T-cell or B-cell origin has been and continues to be debated in the literature. It appears that with intensive chemotherapeutic regimens, the cell of origin impacts little, if at all, on potential curability.

Approximately one third of patients present with early-stage disease (stage I or II), with the remainder having clinically disseminated disease at diagnosis. Extralymphatic sites of disease involvement are common. The natural history of the disease is aggressive, with a median survival of less than 1 year in untreated patients.

DIFFUSE LARGE CELL IMMUNOBLASTIC LYMPHOMA

With the use of older, less aggressive combination chemotherapy regimens, it appeared that diffuse immunoblastic lymphoma had a slightly worse prognosis than diffuse large cell lymphoma, thus accounting for its classification as high grade in the Working Formulation. With newer treatment approaches, this prognostic difference is less apparent. As seen in Table 21–1, the Working Formulation

further subdivides the immunoblastic lymphomas into three types: plasmacytoid, clear cell, and polymorphous. Although these descriptors imply a particular cell of origin, immunologic studies have shown that T-cell or B-cell origin cannot be accurately predicted based on morphology. Hence, the subclassification of immunoblastic lymphoma has little clinical usefulness. Those immunoblastic lymphomas of B-cell origin may be associated with circulating monoclonal immunoglobulins. They are frequently found in the gastrointestinal tract, and they are the type of lymphoma found in association with Sjögren's syndrome.

Like diffuse large cell lymphoma, immunoblastic lymphoma is an aggressive malignancy that is rapidly fatal if untreated. Like all the diffuse aggressive lymphomas, it is frequently curable with intensive chemotherapy.

SUMMARY

It is important to appreciate the fact that the morphologic distinction between diffuse large cell and immunoblastic lymphoma does not provide significant information about prognosis. Statistically significant prognostic factors for these lymphomas relate to their clinical presentation, such as stage of disease, tumor burden, and sites of disease involvement. The virulence of their behavior, their tendency to early and widespread dissemination, and their potential for cure with aggressive therapy support their being grouped together from a therapeutic perspective.

CLINICAL FEATURES AND STAGING

Although diffuse large cell and immunoblastic lymphomas can occur at any age, they are, in general, diseases of middle-aged and older adults. Unlike indolent lymphomas that are almost always widely disseminated at diagnosis, diffuse large cell and diffuse immunoblastic lymphomas present as early-stage disease in approximately 30% of cases. Because they are potentially curable and because the best and frequently only chance of cure resides in the initial therapeutic choice, it is essential that the patient be

Table 21–1. Working Formulation of Non-Hodgkin's Lymphomas

I. Low grade
Small lymphocytic
Follicular, predominantly small cleaved cell
Follicular, mixed small cleaved and large cell
II. Intermediate grade
Follicular, predominantly large cell
Diffuse, small cleaved cell
Diffuse, mixed small cleaved and large cell
Diffuse, large cell
Cleaved cell
Noncleaved cell
Sclerosis
III. High grade
Large cell, immunoblastic
Plasmacytoid
Clear cell
Polymorphous
Epithelioid component
Lymphoblastic
Small noncleaved cell

accurately and completely staged at the time of diagnosis. It is imperative that the expertise of an experienced hematopathologist be sought in every case to establish the diagnosis and to ensure that the patient's lymphoma is accurately classified.

The staging system used for these lymphomas is the Ann Arbor staging system (Table 21–2), which was originally proposed as a staging system for Hodgkin's disease.[2] Although it is used extensively, the four-stage system has serious limitations when applied to NHL. For example, in Hodgkin's disease, the distinction between stages III and IV has definite prognostic and therapeutic implications, with the former being curable in some instances with radiation therapy while the latter requires treatment with systemic chemotherapy. In contrast, stages III and IV NHL are treated with systemic chemotherapy, and the difference in prognosis between the two stages becomes less distinct with the use of aggressive chemotherapy. Furthermore, although the Ann Arbor system clearly separates patients by extent of disease, it does not address the issue of disease bulk. Bulk of disease has both prognostic and therapeutic importance in NHL. For example, patients with stage II disease that is

Table 21–2. Ann Arbor Staging Classification

Stage	Criteria
I	Involvement of a single lymph node region or of a single extranodal organ or site (I$_E$)
II	Involvement of ≥2 lymph node regions on the same side of the diaphragm, or localized involvement of an extranodal site or organ (II$_E$) and of ≥1 lymph node regions on the same side of the diaphragm
III	Involvement of lymph node regions on both sides of the diaphragm, which may also be accompanied by localized involvement of an extranodal organ or site (III$_E$) or spleen (III$_S$) or both (III$_{SE}$).
IV	Diffuse or disseminated involvement of ≥1 distant extranodal organs with or without associated lymph node involvement

Fever >38°, night sweats, and/or weight loss >10% of body weight in the 6 months preceding admission are defined as systemic symptoms, and denoted by the suffix B. Asymptomatic patients are denoted by the suffix A.

nonbulky have a better prognosis than do patients with bulky stage II disease (bulk being defined as a tumor mass >10 cm in diameter in one location or a mediastinal mass >⅓ of the thoracic diameter). Although patients with and without bulky disease both may be classified as having stage II disease according to the Ann Arbor system, the optimal therapy for each would be quite different.

Several other pretreatment prognostic factors have been identified for NHL, including patient age, presence or absence of B symptoms, serum lactose dehydrogenase (LDH), tumor size as discussed earlier, number of nodal and extranodal sites of disease, and stage of disease at diagnosis.[3–8] Each of these clinical characteristics has been identified in one or more series of patients with aggressive lymphoma to be of prognostic importance with regard to patient outcome.

Recently, the International Non-Hodgkin's Lymphoma Prognostic Factors Project used pretreatment prognostic factors in a sample of several thousand patients with aggressive lymphomas treated with doxorubicin-based combination chemotherapy to develop a predictive model of outcome for aggressive NHL.[9] Five pretreatment characteristics were found to be independently statistically significant: age in years (≤60 versus >60); tumor stage I or II (localized) versus III or IV (advanced); number of extranodal sites of involvement (≤1 versus >1); patient performance status (0 or 1 versus >2); and serum LDH level (normal versus abnormal).

With the use of these five pretreatment risk factors, patients could be assigned to one of four risk groups based on the number of presenting risk factors: low (0 or 1); low intermediate (2); high intermediate (3); and high (4 or 5). When patients were analyzed by risk factors, they were found to have very different outcomes with regard to complete response (CR), relapse-free survival (RFS), and overall survival (OS) rates. For example, low-risk patients had an 87% CR rate and an OS rate of 73% at 5 years. This is in contrast with a 44% CR rate and 26% 5-year survival in patients classified in the high-risk group.

The value of any staging system is its ability to predict the likelihood of response to a proposed treatment. It is hoped that the use of a predictive model such as that proposed by Shipp and associates[8] will allow clinicians to predict, prior to therapy, the patient's likelihood of responding adequately to the proposed treatment. Those whose outcome is predicted to be favorable with conventional therapy should be spared the added toxicity that is often associated with more aggressive experimental therapy. On the other hand, those in whom a CR is unlikely with conventional therapy would be identified as candidates for more aggressive treatment.

It is assumed that prognostic factors are surrogate markers of the biologic heterogeneity of the lymphomas. Their biologic diversity is only beginning to be understood. For example, the expression of the nuclear Ki-67 antigen, which is an index of cell proliferation, appears to identify a subset of patients whose lymphomas exhibit a very virulent course. Miller and colleagues recently demonstrated that the OS rate of patients with a high Ki-67 proliferative index was significantly reduced compared with patients whose lymphomas had a low proliferative index.[10] One-year survival estimates among 60 patients studied was 82% for those with a low proliferative index versus 18% for those with a high proliferative index. Using a multivariate regression analysis incorporating commonly used clinical prognostic features, the authors confirmed the independent effect of proliferation on survival. Based on these data, it thus appears that the Ki-67 monoclonal antibody identifies a group of patients with rapidly fatal NHL for whom currently used chemotherapy regimens appear to be inadequate.

Cytogenetic studies and molecular analysis of protooncogenes and tumor suppressor genes are providing insights into the pathogenesis of NHL. Unlike the case with the indolent lymphomas, no single genetic abnormality has been consistently found to be associated with diffuse large cell lymphoma, but rearrangement of *bcl*-2 has been observed to occur in 20% to 30% of patients. A high level of *bcl*-2 protein confers a survival advantage on the B cell that may be an important factor in the pathogenesis of some B-cell malignancies. Yunis and colleagues found that 23 patients with immunoblastic or follicular lymphoma who had a *bcl*-2 oncogene rearrangement had a poor response to therapy, with only 7 achieving a CR as compared with 21 of 26 patients without this rearrangement who achieved a CR.[11]

Offit and coworkers have recently reported on the incidence of rearrangement of the *bcl*-6 gene in patients with diffuse large cell lymphoma.[12] This gene is known to have structural similarities to a class of transcription factors that participate in the control of cell proliferation and differentiation. The authors studied the incidence of *bcl*-6 gene rearrangement in 102 patients with diffuse large cell lymphoma. Presence of the rearrangement was found in 23 patients, 19 of whom had extranodal disease. Rearrangement of *bcl*-6 appeared to correlate with a favorable clinical outcome, with the 3-year freedom from progression being estimated to be 82% as compared with 56% for patients without this rearrangement.

Studies of biologic and karyotypic diversity among these lymphomas are in their infancy. It seems quite likely, however, that such studies will enable clinicians to more precisely predict a given patient's likelihood of response to a proposed therapy. Such studies hold out the promise of allowing clinicians to tailor therapy to the individual patient based on pretreatment assessment of the patient's prognosis.

A proposed pretreatment staging evaluation is outlined in Table 21–3. As a minimum, all patients should have a (1) complete blood count and chemistry survey; (2) chest radiograph and computed tomographic (CT) scan of the thorax; (3) CT scan of the abdomen and pelvis; and (4) bilateral iliac crest bone marrow biopsies. Because bone marrow involvement increases the likelihood of lymphomatous involvement of the meninges, many clinicians would recommend that a lumbar puncture be performed in these patients for cytologic and chemical analyses of the cerebrospinal fluid. Patients who present with lymphomatous involvement of the meninges should receive a course of intrathecal chemotherapy; many investigators would also give cranial radiation therapy in addition to the chemotherapy.

In certain situations additional studies may be indicated. For example, patients who have unexplained bone pain or elevation of the alkaline phosphatase level should be evaluated with a bone scan. Plain radiographs of any abnormal area on the bone scan should be obtained to look for lymphomatous involvement of the skeleton. Gallium

Table 21–3. Pretreatment Staging Evaluation

1. History and physical examination
2. Complete blood count and chemistry survey
3. Chest radiograph
4. CT scan of chest, abdomen, and pelvis
5. Bilateral iliac crest bone marrow biopsies
6. Other, as indicated by results of 1–5 (see text)

scanning is of limited usefulness in the staging of lymphomas. Although it is useful for detecting disease above the diaphragm, its utility below the diaphragm is limited by the frequent fecal uptake of gallium. It may be effective, however, in detecting active disease in those situations in which CT scan abnormalities remain after therapy.

Although the staging procedures closely parallel those employed in the staging of Hodgkin's disease, there is one important difference. Staging laparotomy is used routinely in patients with Hodgkin's disease who present with stage I or II disease. Detection of disease in the abdomen in these situations not only upstages the disease but also may dictate a change in therapeutic strategy. Since all patients with diffuse large cell lymphoma or immunoblastic lymphoma are treated with systemic chemotherapy, the staging laparotomy is unnecessary.

One further difference between the staging of Hodgkin's disease and the staging of NHL relates to the evaluation of the lymphoid tissue of Waldeyer's ring. This lymph node region is rarely involved in Hodgkin's disease but is often involved in NHL. Because there is a high correlation between the involvement of Waldeyer's ring and the involvement of the gastrointestinal tract, the finding of disease in Waldeyer's ring necessitates studies of the gastrointestinal tract to document the presence or absence of disease.

TREATMENT

Diffuse large cell lymphoma and immunoblastic lymphoma are systemic diseases at the time of diagnosis; therefore, chemotherapy is the mainstay of treatment. A variety of chemotherapy regimens have been developed over the past 25 years. Those most commonly used today and many of those discussed in this chapter are shown in Table 21–4.

EARLY-STAGE DISEASE (STAGES I AND II NONBULKY)
Phase II Trials

Until about 15 years ago, irradiation as a sole modality of treatment was the therapy employed in the management of early-stage diffuse large cell lymphoma. Results with radiation therapy alone have varied widely, with better results being achieved in those series employing vigorous pretreatment staging procedures, including staging laparotomy.[13]

In patients treated with radiation therapy alone, relapses were observed in nodal sites both within and outside the irradiated field.[14] In addition, relapses occurred in bone marrow and other parenchymal organs, suggesting the presence of microscopic disease in these organs at the time

Table 21–4. Chemotherapeutic Regimens

Regimens	Dose and Route	Day	Frequency
CHOP			
C = cyclophosphamide	750 mg/m² IV	1	Repeat every 21 days
H = hydroxydaunomycin	50 mg/m² IV	1	
O = Oncovin	1.4 mg/m² IV (maximum 2 mg)	1	
P = prednisone	100 mg PO	1–5	
M-BACOD			
M = methotrexate°	3000 mg/m² IV	15	Repeat every 21 days
B = bleomycin	4 mg/m² IV	1	
A = Adriamycin	45 mg/m² IV	1	
C = cyclophosphamide	600 mg/m² IV	1	
O = Oncovin	1 mg/m² IV	1	
D = dexamethasone	6 mg/m² PO	1–5	
m-BACOD			
m = methotrexate°	200 mg/m² IV	8, 15	Repeat every 21 days
B = bleomycin	4 mg/m² IV	1	
A = Adriamycin	45 mg/m² IV	1	
C = cyclophosphamide	600 mg/m² IV	1	
O = Oncovin	1.4 mg/m² IV	1	
D = Decadron	6 mg/m² PO	1–5	
ProMACE-MOPP			
Pro = prednisone	60 mg/m² PO	1–14	Repeat every 28 days
M = methotrexate	1500 mg/m² IV	15	
A = Adriamycin	25 mg/m² IV	1, 8	
C = cyclophosphamide	650 mg/m² IV	1, 8	
E = etoposide	120 mg/m² IV	1, 8	
Followed by MOPP after maximal response			
M = mechlorethamine	6 mg/m² IV	1, 8	Repeat every 28 days
O = Oncovin	1.4 mg/m² IV	1, 8	
P = procarbazine	100 mg/m² PO	1–14	
P = prednisone	40 mg/m² PO	1–14	
ProMACE/CytaBOM			
Pro = prednisone	60 mg/m² PO	1–14	Repeat every 21 dyas
M = methotrexate°	1500mg/m² Iv	15	
A = Adriamycin	25 mg/m² IV	1	
C = cyclophosphamide	650 mg/m² IV	1	
E = etoposide	120 mg/m² IV	1	
Cyta = cytarabine	300 mg/m² IV	8	
B = bleomycin	5 mg/m² IV	8	
O = Oncovin	1.4 mg/m² IV	8	
M = methotrexate	120 mg/m² IV	8	
MACOP-B			
M = methotrexate°	400 mg/m² IV	8, 36, 64	
A = Adriamycin	50 mg/m² IV	1, 15, 29, 43, 57, 71	
C = cyclophosphamide	350 mg/m² IV	1, 15, 29, 43, 57, 71	
O = Oncovin	1.4 mg/m² IV (maximum 2 mg)	8, 22, 36, 50, 64, 78	
P = predisone	75 mg/m² PO	1–84	
B = bleomycin	10 mg/m² IV	22, 50, 78	

°Leucovorin rescue is given 24 hours after each methotrexate dose.

of diagnosis. The size of the irradiated field did not correlate with treatment outcome, suggesting that the use of larger ports would not have contributed to improved treatment outcome.

Radiation therapy as the sole modality of treatment for early-stage aggressive lymphoma is mainly of historical interest. Several series have now shown excellent results with the use of combined modality therapy (CMT). Hence, given the morbidity associated with the use of staging laparotomy to identify those patients who might be candidates for treatment with radiation therapy alone, standard treatment now consists of chemotherapy alone or, more commonly, radiation therapy in combination with chemotherapy.

When it had been established that the CHOP (cyclophosphamide, hydroxydaunomycin, Oncovin, prednisone) regimen was effective therapy for advanced-stage disease, several investigators pursued the use of this regimen in patients with early-stage disease either alone or in combination with radiation therapy. The rationale for the use of CMT in the setting of early-stage disease is that, although apparently clinically localized, these lymphomas have a propensity to systemic spread early in the course of the disease. Using chemotherapy (frequently as an abbreviated treatment course compared with the treatment of advanced disease, in combination with radiation therapy) should address the problem of failure due to undetected microscopic spread that was evident when radiation therapy as the sole modality was employed.

Miller and Jones were among the earliest investigators to use the CHOP regimen in the treatment of localized aggressive lymphomas.[15] Forty-five patients with localized disease were treated with CHOP chemotherapy alone (28 patients) or with initial CHOP followed by involved-field radiation therapy (IFRT). All patients were clinically staged: 15 patients had clinical stage I disease and 30 patients had clinical stage II disease. In this nonrandomized study, patients were assigned treatment with chemotherapy alone or chemotherapy and radiation therapy on the basis of bone marrow reserve and tumor response to initial chemotherapy. Patients who required a reduction in chemotherapy dose, who were usually those older than 65 years, or those who failed to achieve a CR after three courses of initial chemotherapy were treated with CMT. Patients receiving chemotherapy alone received between 6 and 11 cycles of CHOP. Patients receiving CMT received between two and eight courses of CHOP followed by IFRT.

With a median follow-up of 41 months at the time of reporting, 42 patients (92%) were alive, and 38 (84%) were continually free of disease. Survival and RFS were not statistically different for patients receiving chemotherapy alone or chemotherapy plus radiation therapy. The clinical stage at the time of initial treatment did not impact in a statistically significant manner on survival or RFS.

Of seven patients who failed therapy, relapses were seen at initially involved as well as distant sites. Of 11 patients older than 65 years, only 1 (9%) relapsed. These elderly patients had, in general, received less intensive chemotherapy, with CHOP being given at reduced doses initially. They were also more likely to have received fewer courses of therapy.

The results obtained by Miller and Jones thus suggested that initial systemic therapy with a doxorubicin (Adriamycin)-containing drug regimen is an effective treatment strategy for patients with clinically localized disease.[15] The use of systemic therapy with or without radiation therapy obviated the need for extensive surgical staging of these patients. Furthermore, the results obtained in the elderly patients suggested that clinically undetected disease may be eliminated with relatively few courses of effective chemotherapy, although the minimum number of courses needed to achieve a successful outcome was not determined by this study.

Connors and associates conducted a prospective study employing an abbreviated course of CHOP chemotherapy (three cycles) followed by IFRT in 78 consecutive patients.[16] Thus, they attempted to build on the knowledge gained from previous studies by designing a prospective study that intentionally omitted staging laparotomy, employed a fixed brief and tolerable course of doxorubicin-based chemotherapy, and administered IFRT to all patients. The patients enrolled in the study ranged in age from 21 to 82 years, with a median age of 64 years. Patients had either clinical stage I or II disease with favorable characteristics defined as absence of B symptoms and absence of bulky disease.

Treatment was administered in two phases: Initially, three cycles of CHOP chemotherapy were given. After a 3- to 4-week rest period, patients received IFRT. The radiation therapy port was designed to encompass the entire original site of disease in as small a volume as possible. Draining lymph nodes were usually included in the port in the case of extranodal disease. Three patients who had a pathologically confirmed complete resection of a gastrointestinal lymphoma prior to the initiation of therapy did not receive radiation therapy following the prescribed course of chemotherapy.

Seventy-seven of seventy-eight patients (99%) had achieved a CR and 66 (86%) had remained free of disease with a median followup off therapy of 30 months at the time of reporting. The one patient who progressed on therapy and 10 of 11 who relapsed after therapy died of their disease. The actuarial survival rate for the entire group was thus 84%.

The authors reported a detailed failure analysis.[16] Of 11 patients who relapsed, 4 relapses were believed to be potentially preventable by improved staging or by the use of central nervous system (CNS) prophylaxis in patients presenting with sinus involvement. Nine of 11 patients who relapsed did so within the first 9 months after therapy, and in each case, the histopathology was the same as that at the time of initial diagnosis. In contrast, 2 patients relapsed late at 20 and 35 months after therapy. In both cases, relapsed disease contained an indolent component. Hence, the authors advised careful histologic review in cases of late relapse following this treatment program. In 9 cases, relapse was at distant sites; in 2 cases, relapse involved the treated port and an area contiguous to it.

The results obtained by Connors and associates thus support the use of a brief chemotherapy program followed by IFRT as a successful approach to the management of patients with localized diffuse aggressive lymphomas.[16] The study did include elderly patients, and therefore the results are probably more widely applicable than those in studies that exclude the elderly.

Employing a slightly more prolonged treatment program, Tondini and colleagues recently reported similar results in a larger series of patients.[17] Between 1985 and 1990, 183 consecutive patients with stage I or II diffuse aggressive lymphomas with no more than three sites of disease were treated with four to six cycles of CHOP chemotherapy followed by extended-field radiation therapy (EFRT). Treatment was begun with chemotherapy. Patients who did not achieve a CR before the fourth cycle of CHOP were given an additional two cycles. After a rest period of 4 weeks, patients received radiation therapy to areas involved with disease and to proximal uninvolved nodal areas.

The CR rate was 98% at the end of the combined therapy. Diagnostic excision of all measurable disease was performed prior to therapy in 33% of the patients. Of the remaining patients, 87% achieved a CR with chemotherapy alone and 11% with the addition of radiation therapy. Three patients failed to achieve a CR.

After a median followup of 51 months, 26 patients have relapsed, and of these, 25 have died. Hence the 5-year RFS and OS rates were 83%. There was a trend toward a higher relapse rate for patients achieving CR at the time of radiation therapy (31%) as compared with patients achieving a CR with chemotherapy (15%) or initial surgery (10%), but this result was not statistically significant.

Allowing for differences in patient selection, length and dose of chemotherapy, and radiation therapy dosage and ports, the results of the three series cited earlier[15–17] are similar and support the efficacy of CHOP chemotherapy in this setting. Prior to publication of results of the Intergroup study in advanced-stage disease (see later) in which CHOP was found to be equivalent to newer regimens, there was an interest in investigating the value of using newer and more aggressive chemotherapy regimens in the treatment of early-stage disease. Longo and colleagues reported on the use of an abbreviated course of the ProMACE-MOPP (Pro = prednisone; MACE = methotrexate, Adriamycin, cyclophosphamide, etoposide; MOPP = mechlorethamine, Oncovin, procarbazine, prednisone regimen followed by IFRT).[18] Forty-seven patients with clinical stage I or I$_E$ aggressive lymphomas were treated with four cycles of ProMACE-MOPP followed by IFRT. The median age of the patients was 45 years, with a range of 19 to 82 years. The doses of the myelotoxic drugs were reduced to 75% of that given to patients with advanced disease.

Forty-five patients (96%) achieved a CR, and no patient had relapsed at the time of reporting, with a median follow-up of 42 months. Forty-four of 45 responding patients received radiation therapy at a time when the primary lesion was either not detectable or was believed to have been stable for two cycles of chemotherapy.

Only 10% of the patients were older than 60 years of age, older patients generally required more dose reductions in chemotherapy than did younger patients. The authors pointed out that among 18 patients older than 50 years of age, only 2 received the treatment on time and at full dose.[18]

Although the data support this treatment approach as a successful one, it does not appear to have wide applicability to the elderly. Only patients with stage I disease were included in this study. Given the results obtained with the CHOP regimen, it is probably unnecessary to use such aggressive therapy in early-stage disease.

Randomized Trials

No randomized, prospective trials employing doxorubicin-based chemotherapy in patients who have been uniformly staged have yet been reported. Two randomized trials are being conducted currently by the cooperative groups.

Whether there is a need for radiation therapy in addition to full-course chemotherapy is addressed in a study being conducted by the Eastern Cooperative Oncology Group (ECOG). Patients are randomized to receive eight cycles of CHOP alone or the same chemotherapy followed by IFRT. The data from Connors and coworkers[16] and Longo and associates[18] would suggest that radiation therapy adds to chemotherapy by allowing fewer cycles of therapy to be given with equivalent results, by reducing the toxicity of chemotherapy, and by allowing the use of less chemotherapy, which is of particular importance in the treatment of the elderly, although the long-term toxicity of this approach is unknown.

The Southwest Oncology Group (SWOG) is currently conducting a randomized trial comparing chemotherapy alone (eight cycles of CHOP) versus short-course chemotherapy (three cycles of CHOP) followed by IFRT. The main objective of this study is to compare two curative approaches with respect to differences in survival, time to treatment failure, and toxicity.

Summary

The best approach to the management of a patient with early-stage disease remains to be defined; therefore, if possible, patients should be encouraged to participate in a clinical trial. If this is not possible, the currently available data would suggest that either eight cycles of CHOP or three cycles of CHOP followed by IFRT is a reasonable approach to treatment.

ADVANCED-STAGE DISEASE (STAGES II BULKY, III, AND IV)

Phase II Trials

Investigators at the National Cancer Institute (NCI) were among the first to demonstrate that some patients with advanced-stage disease are curable. Using combination chemotherapy regimens, they were able to achieve complete remissions in 45% of treated patients, with approximately 70% to 80% of these being durable remissions.[19, 20] In the early studies relapses beyond 2 years after therapy were rare, and therefore a disease-free survival (DFS) of 2 years was tantamount to cure. Based on these observations subsequent trials focused on achieving higher numbers of CRs, with the assumption being that this would translate into increased numbers of patients cured of their disease.

The CHOP regimen was one of the first combination therapy programs to use doxorubicin. Between 1974 and 1981 the SWOG conducted a series of trials to compare CHOP with CHOP-bleomycin or with CHOP plus either bacille Calmette-Guérin or levamisole.[21–23] The CR rates for patients with clinical stage III or IV aggressive histologies of NHL varied from 44% to 61%. The CR rates for patients with diffuse large cell lymphoma varied from 58% to 62%. More recently, Coltman and coworkers have updated these results with up to 14 years of followup, demonstrating that CHOP is curative for 32% of patients with advanced diffuse large cell lymphoma.[24] This analysis provided an important benchmark for future comparison of pilot studies and demonstrated that patients continue to relapse following CHOP chemotherapy for up to 7 years, thereby challenging the widely held tenet that a 2-year DFS was tantamount to cure. This finding has obvious implications with regard to followup of these patients as well as to the interpretation of study results published after only a short period of followup.

With the recognition of the need to improve on the results achieved with the CHOP regimen, new and more complex regimens were developed in the 1970s and 1980s. These regimens are frequently referred to as the second- and third-generation regimens to distinguish them from the earlier regimens such as CHOP.

One of the second-generation regimens, M-BACOD (M = methotrexate; BACOD = bleomycin, Adriamycin, cyclophosphamide, Oncovin, Decadran) was developed in 1975 to incorporate the relatively nonmyelotoxic high-dose methotrexate with leucovorin rescue in midcycle following myelotoxic therapy that was delivered at the beginning of the cycle.[25] The design of this regimen therefore attempted to address the problem of midcycle tumor regrowth that had been observed with regimens such as CHOP, which was given every 21 days. The third-generation regimens such as ProMACE-MOPP, ProMACE-CytaBOM (Cyta = cytarabine; BOM = bleomycin, Oncovin, mechlorethamine), and MACOP-B (methotrexate, Adriamycin, cyclophosphamide, Oncovin, prednisone, bleomycin) were planned to implement two dominant hypotheses: the Goldie-Coldman hypothesis of drug resistance and the

Hyrniuk hypothesis of dose intensity. To achieve these aims, they were designed in such a fashion that more noncross-resistant agents were delivered as frequently as possible.

Many phase II studies of second- and third-generation regimens have been reported in the literature. This chapter reviews results from phase II trials of those regimens that subsequently were employed in randomized phase III trials in aggressive lymphoma.

m-BACOD

As noted earlier, the initial M-BACOD regimen employed high-dose methotrexate with leucovorin rescue. This approach was effective; however, it was costly and required hospitalization. Studies showed that moderate-dose methotrexate had significant activity as a single agent as well, as when employed as part of a combination chemotherapy regimen. Thus, investigators at the Dana-Farber Cancer Institute piloted the m-BACOD regimen, treating 134 patients with diffuse histiocytic or undifferentiated lymphoma between 1981 and 1986.[26] The median age of the patients was rather young at 49 years; 76% of the patients had stage III or IV disease.

Eighty-two (61%) of 134 patients achieved a CR, and 62 (76%) of these patients remained in CR with a median followup of 3.6 years. The predicted survival at 1, 3, and 5 years was 80%, 63%, and 60%, respectively, with a 5-year DFS rate of 74% for those patients achieving a CR. Pulmonary toxicity caused therapy to be discontinued in 18% of treated patients; this toxicity was fatal in one patient. Mucositis occurred more frequently with the m-BACOD regimen (44% of patients) as compared with the earlier M-BACOD regimen (12% of patients).

As noted earlier, it has been observed previously that bone marrow involvement in aggressive lymphomas appears to increase the risk of CNS relapse. Only 1 of 10 M-BACOD and none of 13 m-BACOD patients with bone marrow involvement subsequently developed CNS lymphoma. This relapse rate (4.3%) was found to be identical to the rest of the group (4.3%), suggesting that marrow-positive large cell lymphoma patients may not be at increased risk for subsequent CNS relapse when systemic therapy employed high or moderate doses of methotrexate.

As had been observed in the CHOP studies, late relapses beyond 24 months were observed in patients treated with m-BACOD. Thirteen of 19 relapses occurred within 24 months of therapy; an additional 6 patients relapsed after 24 months. The data suggest that approximately 40% of advanced-stage patients may relapse with sufficient followup.

SWOG conducted a confirmatory phase II trial of the m-BACOD regimen[27]; 106 eligible patients participated in the study. By study design, patients were stratified at registration as having either normal or impaired bone marrow reserve status. Twenty-eight patients (26%) were judged to have impaired status, and these patients received decreased doses of cyclophosphamide and doxorubicin, beginning with the first cycle of therapy. Of the eligible patients, 76% had diffuse large cell histology, 75% had stage III or IV disease, and 46% had B symptoms.

The overall CR rate was 56%, with a marked difference in CR rates for the normal reserve and impaired marrow

groups. With a median followup of 41 months, 64% of the patients with normal marrow reserve were free of disease at 3 years. In contrast, only 3 (38%) of 8 in the marrow reserve group remained free of disease at 36 months. The 3-year survival rate of patients with normal marrow reserve was 61% as compared with 29% of patients with impaired marrow reserve.

The toxicity experienced by both treatment groups was severe. Overall, severe or greater toxicity occurred in 97% of the patients in the normal marrow group and in 89% of the marrow impaired group. Hence, despite decreased dosage, the marrow-impaired group experienced toxicity similar to those treated with full doses, and thus it is not certain how much more chemotherapy these patients would have received and whether full-dose chemotherapy would have resulted in improved outcome.

Fatal toxicity occurred in nine patients (8%). Eight deaths were due to overwhelming sepsis in association with profound granulocytopenia. The other death was due to progressive pulmonary fibrosis, which was believed to be secondary to bleomycin.

ProMACE REGIMENS

The ProMACE regimens were developed and piloted at the NCI. The ProMACE-MOPP flexitherapy program was designed to alternate two treatment regimens based on an individual patient's rate of tumor response.[28] At the time of initial reporting, the median followup was 31 months, and at that time the projected 4-year survival rate was 65%. These patients have now been followed for more than 9 years and, excluding deaths unrelated to lymphoma or its treatment, the actual survival is only 50%. The difference between the projected and the actual survival is attributed to a number of relapses and lymphoma-related deaths that occurred after the initial report.

ProMACE-MOPP (day 1, day 8) is a modification of the flexitherapy program. This modification was designed to address the Goldie-Coldman hypothesis, which states that the emergence of clinical drug resistance may be minimized by using the greatest number of active agents as soon as possible in the treatment of the tumor.[29] In the flexitherapy program, MOPP was introduced after the third or fourth month of therapy. In the modified regimen, all eight drugs were given during each monthly cycle. A phase II study of this regimen was not reported, but it was used as one arm of a two-arm randomized trial (see later).

A third ProMACE regimen developed at the NCI was ProMACE-CytaBOM.[29] The rationale for this regimen was to use several nonmyelotoxic agents with antitumor activity in lymphoma on day 8 to allow recovery from the myelosuppressive effects of the drugs given on day 1 so that each cycle could be given every 3 weeks rather than every 4 weeks, as had been done with the ProMACE-MOPP regimen. This scheduling would allow a 25% increase in dose intensity of this regimen as compared with ProMACE-MOPP. The NCI did not conduct a phase II trial of this regimen but rather used it as one arm of a two-arm randomized study (see later).

SWOG conducted a phase II trial of ProMACE-CytaBOM based on initial reports from the NCI in which the regimen produced an 84% CR rate with an RFS rate of approximately 80%.[30] Seventy-eight eligible patients took part in the SWOG study. The median age of the patients was 54 years, with 61% of patients having stage III or IV disease and 49% having B symptoms. Sixty percent of patients had diffuse large cell histology.

CRs were observed in 51 patients (65%), with 50% of these patients alive and free of disease at 3 years. Fifty-seven percent of the entire group was alive at 3 years. Patients with stage II disease had a better OS and RFS as compared with patients with more advanced disease.

Five patients (6%) died as a result of treatment, and another 18 patients experienced life-threatening toxicity, the most serious being related to myelosuppression. Deep venous thrombosis was an unusual and unexplained toxicity that occurred in 9 patients (12%) while they were receiving therapy.

MACOP-B

The MACOP-B regimen, designed by investigators at the NCI of Canada, is a 12-week treatment program of continuous weekly therapy with doxorubicin and cyclophosphamide given during odd-numbered weeks and vincristine given during even-numbered weeks with either bleomycin or moderate-dose methotrexate with folinic acid rescue.[31] Oral prednisone is given daily throughout, and all patients are treated with cimetidine or ranitidine to minimize gastritis.

One hundred twenty-six patients with diffuse large cell lymphoma (which by the investigators' definition included some patients with diffuse mixed cell lymphoma), stages I and II if bulky or associated with B symptoms, and stage III or IV were eligible if they had had no prior therapy. Patients ranged in age from 16 to 71 years, with a median age of 55 years.

In a recent update of the original report, the authors reported an 84% CR rate with a 3-year survival of 67%.[32] The actuarial 8-year survival is projected to be 62%, and failure-free survival at 8 years is projected to be 52%. The median followup of patients is 76 months.

One of the practical difficulties with the regimen is that 50% of patients developed severe mucositis, which was believed to be caused by the methotrexate component of the treatment. Eleven percent of patients experienced major infectious complications, and 6% died as a result of treatment.

The authors examined prognostic factors associated with outcome in treated patients. Factors found to be of prognostic import include age older than 60 years, the presence of B symptoms, and the presence of more than one extranodal site of disease involvement. There was a clear difference in outcome for patients according to the number of adverse prognostic factors present.

Schneider and associates at Memorial Sloan-Kettering Cancer Center subsequently performed a phase II confirmatory trial of the MACOP-B regimen.[33] Previously untreated patients with stages II, III, and IV intermediate and high-grade lymphoma were eligible. High-risk patients were randomized to a study of MACOP-B versus autologous bone marrow transplantation (ABMT) as first-line therapy if they were younger than 50 years of age with a good performance status and had no bone marrow involvement by lymphoma. Patients with acquired immunodeficiency syndrome (AIDS), AIDS-related complex (ARC), or who were positive for human immunodeficiency virus (HIV) were not eligible for ABMT and thus were treated with MACOP-B. Seventy patients were enrolled on the study.

The percentage of CRs was quite low compared with the Vancouver experience, being 52% for diffuse large cell lymphoma and 58% for all other histologies. Eight patients who were HIV positive had a similar CR rate to their HIV negative counterparts but had a much higher mortality (75% versus 49%) secondary to causes other than lymphoma. Excluding the HIV-positive patients, the CR duration of patients with diffuse large cell lymphoma was 54% at 25 months.

Mucositis was the most common nonhematologic toxicity, being seen in 48 of 64 patients (75%). Fifty percent of patients required hospitalization during therapy, usually for neutropenic fever or severe mucositis. There were five deaths (7%) attributable to treatment.

SWOG also conducted a confirmatory phase II trial of the MACOP-B regimen.[34] One hundred nine eligible patients with stage II, III, and IV intermediate or high-grade lymphoma were treated. The median age of the patients was 53.5 years. Sixty-three percent of patients had diffuse large cell histology, and 70% had stage III or IV disease.

As had been observed in the study by Schneider and colleagues, the CR rate was low compared with results obtained in the Vancouver study.[33] Fifty-four percent of patients achieved a CR; there were no significant differences in response among histologic subtypes when patients were analyzed by stage or symptom status. With a median followup of 46 months at the time of reporting, the 3-year survival was 51%, and 63% of patients achieving CR were alive and disease free at 3 years. Patients with stage II disease had a significantly better survival than did patients with stage III or IV disease; the 3-year estimates of survival for stages II, III, and IV were 67%, 57%, and 37%, respectively.

The toxicity encountered was more severe than that originally reported. Severe granulocytopenia occurred in 51% of patients; severe mucositis occurred in 25% of patients. The primary determinant of treatment tolerance was age, with life-threatening toxicity seen in 47% of patients older than 60 years of age and 13% of those younger than 60. Five patients (5%) died as a result of treatment.

Randomized Trials

Initial single-institution studies of the second- and third-generation regimens appeared promising and suggested that the number of patients cured of their disease might be double that which had been achieved with the CHOP regimen. These results were not surprising because many patients treated in the single-institution studies had less advanced-stage disease and were younger than the patients treated in the cooperative group trials of CHOP. As is obvious, confirmatory trials of the second- and third-generation studies failed to attain the excellent results initially reported. The results obtained in the SWOG confirmatory trials were, in fact, very similar to those which had been achieved with CHOP.

Because of the selection bias inherent in single-institution studies, it is important that not only confirmatory studies be performed but also that randomized comparisons be done, either comparing the newer regimens to each other or, perhaps more appropriately, comparing the newer regimens with the standard first-generation regimen, CHOP. The following sections review the results of several randomized studies performed in the treatment of diffuse aggressive lymphomas.

ProMACE-MOPP Versus ProMACE-CytaBOM

In a single-institution study using ProMACE-MOPP versus ProMACE-CytaBOM, 193 patients with stages II, III, and IV follicular large cell, diffuse large cell, diffuse mixed, immunoblastic, and diffuse small noncleaved cell (non-Burkitt's) lymphomas were randomized to receive either ProMACE-MOPP or ProMACE-CytaBOM.[29] Responding patients received at least six cycles of therapy or two cycles after a maximum clinical response. Patients with evidence of continued response between cycles 4 and 6 received two additional cycles of therapy until the sites of presumed residual disease appeared unchanged for two cycles. Patients with initial bone marrow involvement who achieved a CR were treated with 2400 cGy prophylactic cranial irradiation. Ninety-nine patients were randomized to ProMACE-MOPP, and 94 were randomized to ProMACE-CytaBOM.

The median followup of patients in this study was 5 years at the time of reporting. Seventy-three (74%) of 99 patients treated with ProMACE-MOPP achieved a CR, and 30 (41%) of these have relapsed. Forty-five patients (45%) treated with this regimen died: 42 from uncontrolled lymphoma, 2 from treatment-related causes, and 1 unrelated to lymphoma or its treatment.

By comparison, 81 of 94 patients (86%) randomized to ProMACE-CytaBOM achieved a CR, and 22 (27%) of the complete responders have relapsed. Thirty-one (33%) patients have died: 22 from uncontrolled lymphoma, 6 related to treatment (all from *Pneumocystis carinii* pneumonia), and 3 from causes unrelated to lymphoma.

The CR rate for ProMACE-CytaBOM is significantly higher than that achieved with ProMACE-MOPP, with a *P* value of .048. The plateau of the DFS curve is at 54% for ProMACE-MOPP and 69% for ProMACE-CytaBOM (*P* = .082). The plateau of the survival curve is at 53% for ProMACE-MOPP and at 69% for ProMACE-CytaBOM (*P* = .046). If four patients are included in the survival analysis who died of intercurrent causes, the *P* value for the difference in survival between the two treatments is .082, because three of these deaths occurred on the ProMACE-CytaBOM arm.

MACOP-B Versus ProMACE-MOPP

In a prospective, randomized, multicenter trial conducted by the Italian NHL Cooperative Study Group, 221 patients were randomized to receive either MACOP-B or six cycles of ProMACE-MOPP.[35] The purpose of the study was to compare the third-generation regimen MACOP-B with the second-generation regimen ProMACE-MOPP. Patients eligible for the study included those with diffuse intermediate to high-grade NHL, with stages II bulky, III, and IV disease. The median age of the patients on the MACOP-B arm was 46 years, and the median age on the ProMACE-MOPP arm was 50 years. No prior therapy was allowed, and patients with AIDS were excluded. Patients with bone marrow involvement and/or bulky disease received CNS prophylaxis with intrathecal methotrexate. One hundred four patients were assessable for response on the ProMACE-MOPP arm, and 93 were on the MACOP-B arm; results are reported based on intention to treat 114 patients on the ProMACE-MOPP arm and 107 patients on the MACOP-B arm.

Fifty-six (49.1%) of 114 patients randomized to ProMACE-MOPP achieved a CR compared with 56 (52.3%) of 107 of those randomized to MACOP-B. With a median followup of 41 months, the 3-year OS rates were 45.2% for ProMACE-MOPP and 52.3% for MACOP-B. Progression-free survival at 3 years was 36.4% for the ProMACE-treated patients and 36.1% for the MACOP-B patients. DFS at 3 years in the responding patients was 52.3% on the ProMACE arm and 50.3% on the MACOP-B arm. None of the differences in CR rate, 3-year survival, progression-free survival, or DFS was statistically significant.

Toxicities observed were not statistically significantly different on the two treatment arms. The most important grade 3 to 4 toxicities in both arms were leukopenia and granulocytopenia, followed by infection and mucositis, which were higher in the MACOP-B arm. The incidence of fatal toxicity was 4.3% on the ProMACE arm and 9.3% on the MACOP-B arm (*P* = .1).

Hence, the authors in this study were unable to show any difference in outcome between a third- and a second-generation regimen.[35] The results obtained with these two regimens were worse than those reported in the original single-institution trials of these regimens.

CHVmP Versus CHVmP + VB

The study conducted by the European Organization for the Research and Treatment of Cancer was a randomized, prospective trial designed to compare a first-generation to a second-generation regimen.[36] CHVmP (cyclophosphamide, hydroxydaunomycin, VM-26, prednisone) is considered a first-generation regimen. CHVmP+VB (CHVmP + vincristine, bleomycin) employs the same drugs, and in addition vincristine and bleomycin are given on day 15 of a 21-day cycle. In both arms of the study, adjuvant radiation therapy (3000 cGy) was given in instances of bulky disease or residual disease. In addition, patients achieving a CR were further randomized to maintenance therapy with cyclophosphamide, vincristine, and prednisone versus no further therapy. One hundred forty-one patients were enrolled in the study, 70 on the CHVmP arm and 71 on the CHVmP + VB arm. Patients were allowed to have no prior treatment, were stage III or IV, and had aggressive histology lymphoma.

A higher CR rate was achieved in the second-generation regimen compared with the first-generation regimen, 74% versus 49% (*P* = .001). Freedom from progression rates were 43% with CHVmP + VB versus 26% for CHVmP at 5 years (*P* = .006), and survival was also superior on the CHVmP + VB arm (48%) versus 28% on the CHVmP arm (*P* = .01).

Toxicity was similar on both arms except for a nonsignificant increase in grade 4 hematologic and grade 1 neurologic toxicity on the CHVmP + VB arm. No toxic deaths occurred on either arm during induction therapy.

Although this study does show a statistically significant improvement in outcome for a second-generation regimen as compared with a first-generation regimen, the study involved small numbers of patients and is not truly a test of the merits of the induction regimen alone because of the provision for adjuvant radiation and maintenance therapy. Interpretation of results is difficult because of the use of maintenance therapy in some of the complete responders. The study is reviewed in this chapter not because of its inherent worth but rather to present the reader with the results of one of the randomized, prospective trials reported to show a benefit from a newer regimen compared with standard therapy.

m-BACOD Versus CHOP

ECOG performed a prospective, randomized trial to compare prospectively standard therapy CHOP with m-BACOD.[37] Three hundred ninety-two patients were enrolled, of whom 325 were eligible for the study. Patients with stages III and IV diffuse mixed or diffuse large cell lymphoma with no prior treatment were eligible.

The CHOP regimen was administered as had been previously described, except that from 1984 to 1986 patients older than 60 years of age received a 25% dose reduction in the calculated doses of doxorubicin and cyclophosphamide. After 1986 all patients received full-dose therapy from the time of initiation of treatment. m-BACOD as given in this study differed from that originally reported in that only 8 cycles of therapy were given, whereas 10 had been given in the original report.

Eighty-eight (51%) of 174 patients treated with CHOP and 85 (56%) of 151 patients treated with m-BACOD achieved a CR ($P = .32$). With a median followup of 4 years, 91 patients treated with CHOP and 71 treated with m-BACOD have died. After 2 and 5 years, survival rates were 59% and 48%, respectively, for CHOP and 62% and 49%, respectively, for m-BACOD. There was no significant difference in OS between the two treatments ($P = .49$), and there was no significant difference between the two treatments with respect to time to treatment failure. There also was no difference in CR duration between the CHOP and m-BACOD arms.

The two arms did differ with regard to toxicity. Patients treated with m-BACOD had significantly more toxic reactions than did those treated with CHOP. This was true with respect to grades 2 to 4 hematologic toxicity, infections, and pulmonary toxicity. Most notable were the differences between treatment with regard to moderate, severe, and life-threatening pulmonary toxicity (CHOP 3% versus m-BACOD 23%), infections (CHOP 13% versus m-BACOD 35%), thrombocytopenia (CHOP 2% versus m-BACOD 37%), and stomatitis (CHOP 2% versus m-BACOD 37%). There were eight treatment-related deaths among patients treated with CHOP versus nine treatment-related deaths on the m-BACOD arm.

It is thus clear from the results obtained in this study that there was no advantage in terms of CR rate or outcome with the use of the m-BACOD regimen compared with CHOP. There clearly is more associated toxicity with m-BACOD, and because of this, CHOP would have to be considered the preferable therapy, given a choice between these two regimens.

MACOP-B Versus CHOP

The New Zealand Lymphoma Study Group reported results of a prospective, randomized trial comparing the third-generation regimen MACOP-B with the CHOP regimen.[38] Three hundred four patients were enrolled in the study, of whom 236 were eligible. Patients with bulky stage I and stages II, III, and IV disease were eligible. Eligible histologies included diffuse small cleaved cell, diffuse mixed small and large cell, follicular large cell, diffuse large cell, and immunoblastic lymphomas. The dose modifications and schedule of the MACOP-B and CHOP regimens were as originally described. Responding patients received at least six cycles of CHOP or two cycles after achieving a CR. MACOP-B was administered over the prescribed 12-week period. Median age of patients was 54 years for the MACOP-B arm and 53 years for the CHOP arm.

One hundred twenty-five patients (53%) were randomized to MACOP-B and 111 (47%) to CHOP. Sixty-four (51%) of 125 patients treated with MACOP-B achieved a CR as compared with 65 (59%) of 111 patients treated with CHOP ($P = .3$). CR rates for patients with diffuse mixed, diffuse large cell, and large cell immunoblastic lymphomas were 54% with MACOP-B and 59% with CHOP. Estimated failure-free survival at 4 years is 44% for MACOP-B and 32% for CHOP. Fifty-two patients on each arm have died. Estimated survival at 4 years was 56% for MACOP-B and 51% for CHOP ($P = .69$). Hence, there was no significant difference in rates of CR, failure-free survival, or OS between the CHOP and MACOP-B arms.

There was a difference in toxicity between the treatment arms. Patients who received MACOP-B experienced significantly more grade 3 or 4 hematologic toxicity ($P = .04$), stomatitis ($P < .0001$), and gastrointestinal ulceration ($P = .03$) as compared with the CHOP patients. The excess toxicity of the MACOP-B regimen was reflected in the greater percentage of patients being taken off protocol treatment owing to toxicity (18% of the MACOP-B patients compared with 2% of the CHOP patients). There were six fatal toxicities on the MACOP-B arm and five on the CHOP arm; hence, fatal toxicity occurred at a rate of 5% on both treatment arms.

Hence, as was seen in the ECOG trial, the efficacy of a newer, more complex chemotherapy regimen was equivalent to that of standard therapy with CHOP. Toxicity was significantly greater, however, with MACOP-B, and thus it cannot be considered, based on this study, to offer any advantage over CHOP therapy for patients with diffuse aggressive lymphomas.

CHOP Versus m-BACOD Versus ProMACE = CytaBOM Versus MACOP-B

In an Intergroup trial conducted by SWOG and ECOG, 1138 previously untreated patients with stages II bulky, III, and IV disease with intermediate or high-grade histology were randomized to one of four treatment arms: CHOP, m-BACOD, ProMACE-CytaBOM, or MACOP-B.[39] Eight hundred ninety-nine patients were eligible for the study. Each of the regimens was administered exactly as had been described in the prior phase II studies. The median age of patients was 54 years, with 25% of the patients being older than 64.

With a median followup of 49 months at the time of publication, no differences were observed among the four treatment arms with respect to CR or overall response rates: CR rates were 44% for CHOP, 48% for m-BACOD, 56% for ProMACE-CytaBOM, and 51% for MACOP-B. Because assessment of CR is difficult owing to persistent abnormalities on CT scans after treatment, the time to treatment failure, which is a measure of time to progression, relapse, or death from any cause, was analyzed as a more accurate estimate of the fraction of patients cured by the initial therapy. Forty-three percent of all eligible patients were estimated to be alive without disease at 3 years. By treatment arm, 43% on the CHOP arm, 43% on the m-BACOD arm, 44% on the ProMACE-CytaBOM arm, and 40% on the MACOP-B arm are projected to be alive without disease at 3 years (P = .35). Projected OS at 3 years for all eligible patients is 52%; 49% on the MACOP-B arm, 51% on the m-BACOD arm, 53% on the ProMACE-CytaBOM arm, and 55% on the CHOP arm (P = .90).

Toxicity observed in this trial was similar to that reported in phase II trials of the same regimens. Severe toxic reactions were related to granulocytopenia and subsequent infection. Grade 4 or life-threatening toxicity occurred in 31% of patients on the CHOP arm, 54% on the m-BACOD arm, 29% on the ProMACE-CytaBOM arm, and 43% on the MACOP-B arm. The incidence of grade 5 or fatal toxicity was 1% in the CHOP patients, 3% in the ProMACE-CytaBOM patients, 5% in the m-BACOD patients, and 6% in the MACOP-B patients. The difference in the fatality rates were not statistically different (P = .09). However, when fatal and life-threatening reactions were combined, significant differences were found between regimens, with CHOP and ProMACE-CytaBOM being less toxic than m-BACOD and MACOP-B (P = .001).

Hence, in this large prospective, randomized study, once again the efficacy of the CHOP regimen was found to be equivalent to the newer chemotherapy regimens. The toxicity profile as well as cost would also favor the use of CHOP over any of the three regimens with which it was compared.

Summary

Based on the available data from randomized, prospective studies, CHOP remains the standard therapy for advanced-stage diffuse large cell and immunoblastic lymphoma. With a projected DFS rate of 43%, it is obvious that it is far from ideal therapy, and there is clearly a need for better treatment approaches. We strongly advocate participation in a clinical trial, which is, in fact, the best available treatment. Outside of a clinical trial, CHOP remains standard therapy for these lymphomas.

New Therapeutic Approaches

Newer therapeutic approaches include (1) increasing the dose intensity of drugs used in standard regimens; (2) using strategies to overcome drug resistance; and (3) providing ABMT and peripheral stem cell support as rescue from marrow-ablative chemotherapy.

Dose Intensification

The concept of dose intensity may be an important determinant of treatment outcome; simply stated, it argues that increasing the drug dose per unit time will increase its effectiveness. It does appear that treatment-related variables such as the dose intensity of drug delivered play a role in determining outcome. What is not clear is the independence of treatment-related variables from pretreatment characteristics.

The third-generation regimens focused on the delivery of six to eight active drugs given at the highest possible dose intensity. As noted earlier, this approach did not seem to impact on improved results as compared with older regimens such as CHOP. With the availability of colony-stimulating factors (CSFs), the ability to maximize dose intensity has been improved as compared with dosages that can be delivered without CSF support. Hence, one rational approach to maximizing the efficacy of therapy is to dose-escalate the drugs given in standard regimens with CSF support. SWOG is about to undertake a randomized phase II study of dose-intensified CHOP and dose-intensified ProMACE-CytaBOM with granulocyte-CSF support. In both arms the doses of cyclophosphamide and doxorubicin will be escalated to determine in a pilot study if the results appear better than those seen in prior studies employing these drugs given at conventional doses.

Strategies to Overcome Drug Resistance

Multidrug resistance (MDR) is the phenomenon of cross resistance to a group of natural products (structurally and functionally distinct) that occurs following exposure to one member of this group. MDR is believed to result from reduced intracellular drug concentration that follows active efflux of the drug by p-glycoprotein, which is a membrane-bound protein. This protein is encoded by the *mdr*-1 gene. The normal physiologic function of this protein is unknown. One proposed function is that of inhibition of absorption and facilitation of excretion of toxic natural products.

There are various patterns of p-glycoprotein expression in tumors in humans. Some tumors, such as lymphomas, are derived from normal cell types where p-glycoprotein is not found. As Miller and colleagues have demonstrated, p-glycoprotein is rarely present in untreated lymphomas but is commonly found in lymphomas that have recurred following exposure to chemotherapy.[40] Although these data suggest a role for p-glycoprotein as a determinant of treatment outcome, clinical trials using p-glycoprotein inhibitors, such as verapamil and quinine, to restore sensitivity provide further evidence that this is the case. When verapamil was given with CVAD (cyclophosamide, vincristine, Adriamycin, dexamethasone), as shown by Miller and colleagues, responses were observed in patients with relapsed intermediate-grade lymphomas.[40]

Based on the data from treatment of patients with relapsed lymphoma, SWOG recently conducted a trial of verapamil and quinine given concurrently with the CVAD regimen in previously untreated patients with intermediate-grade lymphomas. The goal of this approach is to suppress MDR development and to overcome any low-level p-glycoprotein that may be present but undetected. Results of this trial are pending. Toxicity attributable to verapamil and quinine has been minimal, however.

Autologous Bone Marrow Transplantation

High-dose chemotherapy with autologous bone marrow support has established itself as effective salvage therapy for selected patients with refractory or relapsed diffuse aggressive lymphoma. In several series, 20% to 25% of treated patients have achieved prolonged DFS employing this approach.[41–44] Although there has been considerable variability in the selection criteria of these studies, several consistent findings have been observed. The patients who are likely to achieve a complete remission and possible cure are those who responded well to initial therapy, who respond well to salvage therapy pretransplant, and who enter transplant with no or minimal residual disease. Patients progressing on salvage therapy as well as those who responded poorly to initial therapy are unlikely to benefit. A variety of regimens have been used and shown to be effective.

The role of ABMT as initial therapy for patients judged to be at high risk of treatment failure with conventional therapy remains to be defined. Few randomized studies comparing ABMT with conventional therapy have been completed.

In a trial conducted by Gianni and coworkers, 75 patients with poor-risk aggressive NHL were randomized to treatment with MACOP-B or with a novel high-dose chemotherapy regimen requiring hematopoietic progenitor cell autotransplantation.[45] By using a crossover design, the authors sought to determine not only which was the most effective therapy but also which was the best therapeutic strategy; that is, does upfront versus salvage high-dose therapy result in better overall patient survival? The toxic death rate on the high-dose arm of the study was initially high (16%) but has decreased with modification of the treatment regimen. Thirty-eight patients were randomized to the high-dose therapy, and 37 patients were randomized to MACOP-B. After a median followup of 43 months, there is a statistically significant improvement in RFS (93% versus 68%, $P = .05$) and freedom from progression (88% versus 41%, $P = .0001$) in favor of the high-dose therapy arm. OS was not statistically improved, however, being 73% on the high-dose arm versus 62% on the MACOP-B arm.

The Groupe d'Etudes des Lymphomes des l'Adulte reported on a subset of 727 patients treated with the LNH87 protocol.[46] Three hundred seventy patients were randomized after achieving a CR with induction therapy to a consolidation phase in which patients were randomized to sequential chemotherapy or ABMT. Only one patient died of transplant-related complications. With a median followup of 21 months, the 2-year OS was 62% and DFS was 58%. OS and DFS did not differ between the consolidation arms ($P = .089$).

Finally, the Italian Cooperative Group compared the DHAP (dexamethasone, ara-C, Platinol) regimen to ABMT following very aggressive initial chemotherapy.[47] Patients identified as partial responders to induction therapy were eligible for randomization. Twenty-five patients were ran-

domized to receive DHAP, and 22 were to undergo ABMT. A CR was subsequently achieved in 4 (14%) of the patients in the DHAP arm and 3 (13.6%) of the patients on the ABMT arm. Stable clinical status was observed in 10 (40%) of the DHAP patients but only 1 (4.5%) of the ABMT patients. The probability of progression-free survival at 40 months was 74% for patients undergoing ABMT versus 22% for patients treated with DHAP.

The recommendations of a Consensus Conference on Intensive Chemotherapy plus Hematopoietic Stem Cell Transplantation in Malignancies were recently published.[48] Although some authors believe that their recommendations regarding the use of this approach in malignant lymphomas are too conservative, they include the following: High-dose chemotherapy should not be considered standard care in malignant lymphomas because no definitive study has established that it is either superior to or significantly worse than conventional combination chemotherapy in any stage of NHL. Although retrospective studies suggest that high-dose chemotherapy improves survival in relapsed aggressive NHL, the panel members believe that randomized trials are needed to confirm these data. Hence, they have recommended that for high-grade or intermediate-grade NHL, a randomized trial of conventional therapy versus high-dose therapy with bone marrow and/or peripheral stem cell support should be developed for those patients defined to be in poor prognostic groups.

SUMMARY

Most patients with advanced-stage large cell or immunoblastic lymphoma are not cured with conventional therapy. Hence, each treating physician must recognize the inadequacy of current therapy and urge all eligible patients to participate in well-designed clinical trials. The best therapy remains to be defined, and therefore the best approach for the patient is an experimental approach designed to improve our ability to cure the disease. If a patient is not eligible or does not wish to participate in a clinical trial, CHOP—as inadequate as it is—remains the gold standard against which all new therapy must be compared.

REFERENCES

1. The Non-Hodgkin's Lymphoma Pathologic Classification Project: National Cancer Institute sponsored study of classifications of non-Hodgkin's lymphomas: Summary and description of a working formulation for clinical usage. Cancer 1982; 49:2112.
2. Carbone PP, Kaplan HS, Musshoff K, et al: Report of the Committee on Hodgkin's Disease Staging Classification. Cancer Res 1971; 31: 1860.
3. Armitage JO, Dick FR, Corder MP, et al: Predicting therapeutic outcome in patients with diffuse histiocytic lymphoma treated with cyclophosphamide, Adriamycin, vincristine, and prednisone (CHOP). Cancer 1982; 50:1695.
4. Coiffier B, Lepage E: Prognosis of aggressive lymphomas: A study of five prognostic models with patients included in LNH-84 regimen. Blood 1989; 74:558.
5. Danieu L, Wong G, Koziner B, Clarkson B: Predictive model for prognosis in advanced diffuse histiocytic lymphoma. Cancer Res 1986; 46:5372.
6. Fisher RI, DeVita VT, Johnson BL, et al: Prognostic factors for advanced diffuse histiocytic lymphoma following treatment with combination chemotherapy. Am J Med 1977; 63:177.

7. Fisher RI, Hubbard SM, DeVita VT, et al: Factors predicting long-term survival in diffuse mixed, histiocytic, or undifferentiated lymphoma. Blood 1981; 58:45.

8. Shipp MA, Harrington DP, Klatt MM, et al: Identification of major prognostic subgroups of patients with large cell lymphoma treated with m-BACOD or M-BACOD. Ann Intern Med 1986; 104:757.

9. The International Non-Hodgkin's Lymphoma Prognostic Factors Project: A predictive model for aggressive non-Hodgkin's lymphoma. N Engl J Med 1993; 329:987.

10. Miller TP, Grogan TM, Dahlberg S, et al: Prognostic significance of the Ki-67–associated proliferative antigen in aggressive non-Hodgkin's lymphomas: A prospective Southwest Oncology Group trial. Blood 1994; 83:1460.

11. Yunis JJ, Mayer MG, Arnesen MA, et al: bcl-2 and other genomic alterations in the prognosis of large cell lymphoma. N Engl J Med 1989; 320:1047.

12. Offit K, LoCoco F, Louie DC, et al: Rearrangement of the bcl-6 gene as a prognostic marker in diffuse large cell lymphoma. N Engl J Med 1994; 331:74.

13. Vokes EE, Ultmann JE, Golomb HM, et al: Long-term survival of patients with localized diffuse histiocytic lymphoma. J Clin Oncol 1985; 3:1309-1317.

14. Hallahan DE, Farah R, Vokes EE, et al: The patterns of failure in patients with pathological stage I and II diffuse histiocytic lymphoma treated with radiation therapy alone. Int J Radiat Oncol Biol Phys 1989; 17:767.

15. Miller TP, Jones SE: Initial chemotherapy for clinically localized lymphomas of unfavorable histology. Blood 1983; 62:413.

16. Connors JM, Klimo P, Fairey RN, Voss N: Brief chemotherapy and involved field radiation therapy for limited-stage histologically aggressive lymphoma. Ann Intern Med 1987; 107:25.

17. Tondini C, Zanini M, Lombardi F, et al: Combined modality treatment with primary CHOP chemotherapy followed by locoregional irradiation in stage I or II histologically aggressive non-Hodgkin's lymphomas. J Clin Oncol 1993; 11:720.

18. Longo DL, Glatstein E, Duffey PL, et al: Treatment of localized aggressive lymphomas with combination chemotherapy followed by involved-field radiation therapy. J Clin Oncol 1989; 7:1295.

19. DeVita VT, Canellos GP, Chabner B, et al: Advanced diffuse histiocytic lymphoma, a potentially curable disease. Lancet 1975; 1:248.

20. Schein PS, DeVita VT, Hubbard S, et al: Bleomycin, Adriamycin, cyclophosphamide, vincristine, and prednisone (BACOP) combination chemotherapy in the treatment of advanced diffuse histiocytic lymphoma. Ann Intern Med 1976; 85:417.

21. Jones SE, Grozea PN, Metz EN, et al: Superiority of Adriamycin-containing combination chemotherapy in the treatment of diffuse lymphoma: A Southwest Oncology Group study. Cancer 1979; 43:417.

22. Jones SE, Grozea PN, Metz EN, et al: Improved complete remission rates and survival for patients with large cell lymphoma treated with chemoimmunotherapy: A Southwest Oncology Group study. Cancer 1983; 51:1083.

23. Jones SE, Grozea PN, Miller TP, et al: Chemotherapy with cyclophosphamide, doxorubicin, vincristine, and prednisone alone or with levamisole or with levamisole plus BCG for malignant lymphoma: A Southwest Oncology Group study. J Clin Oncol 1985; 3:1318.

24. Coltman CA, Dahlberg S, Jones SE, et al: Southwest Oncology Group studies in diffuse large cell lymphoma: A subset analysis. In Kimura K (ed): Cancer Chemotherapy: Challenges for the Future. Tokyo, Excerpta Medica, 1988, pp 194–202.

25. Skarin AT, Canellos GP, Rosenthal DS, et al: Improved prognosis of diffuse histiocytic and undifferentiated lymphoma by use of high-dose methotrexate alternating with standard agents (M-BACOD). J Clin Oncol 1983; 1:91.

26. Shipp MA, Yeap BY, Harrington DP, et al: The m-BACOD combination chemotherapy regimen in large cell lymphoma: Analysis of the completed trial and comparison with the M-BACOD regimen. J Clin Oncol 1990; 8:84.

27. Dana BW, Dahlberg S, Miller TP, et al: m-BACOD treatment for intermediate and high-grade malignant lymphomas: A Southwest Oncology Group phase II trial. J Clin Oncol 1990; 8:1155.

28. Fisher RI, DeVita VT, Hubbard SM, et al: Diffuse aggressive lymphomas: Increased survival after alternating flexible sequences of ProMACE and MOPP chemotherapy. Ann Intern Med 1983; 98:304.

29. Longo DL, DeVita VT, Duffey PL, et al: Superiority of ProMACE-CytaBOM over ProMACE-MOPP in the treatment of advanced diffuse aggressive lymphoma: Results of a prospective randomized trial. J Clin Oncol 1991; 9:25.

30. Miller TP, Dahlberg S, Jones SE, et al: ProMACE-CytaBOM is active with acceptable toxicity in patients with unfavorable non-Hodgkin's lymphomas: A Group Wide SWOG study. Proc Am Soc Clin Oncol 1987; 6:197a.

31. Connors JM, Klimo P: MACOP-B chemotherapy for malignant lymphomas and related conditions: 1987 update and additional observations. Semin Hematol 1988; 25:41.

32. O'Reilly SE, Hoskins P, Klimo P, Connors JM. MACOP-B and VACOP-B in diffuse large cell lymphomas and MOPP/ABV in Hodgkin's disease. Ann Oncol 1991; 2:17.

33. Schneider AM, Straus DJ, Schluger AE, et al: Treatment results with an aggressive chemotherapeutic regimen (MACOP-B) for intermediate and some high-grade non-Hodgkin's lymphomas. J Clin Oncol 1990; 8:94.

34. Weick JK, Dahlberg S, Fisher RI, et al: Combination chemotherapy of intermediate-grade and high-grade non-Hodgkin's lymphoma with MACOP-B: A Southwest Oncology Group study. J Clin Oncol 1991; 9:748.

35. Sertoli MR, Santini G, Chisesi T, et al: MACOP-B versus ProMACE-MOPP in the treatment of advanced diffuse non-Hodgkin's lymphoma: Results of a prospective randomized trial by the non-Hodgkin's lymphoma Cooperative Study Group. J Clin Oncol 1994; 12:1366.

36. Carde P, Meerwaldt JH, van Glabbeke M, et al: Superiority of second-over first-generation chemotherapy in a randomized trial for stage III-IV intermediate and high-grade non-Hodgkin's lymphoma (NHL): The 1980–1985 EORTC Trial. Ann Oncol 1991; 2:431.

37. Gordon LI, Harrington D, Andersen J, et al: Comparison of a second-generation combination chemotherapeutic regimen (m-BACOD) with a standard regimen (CHOP) for advanced diffuse non-Hodgkin's lymphoma. N Engl J Med 1992; 327:1342.

38. Cooper IA, Wolf MM, Robertson TI, et al: Randomized comparison of MACOP-B and CHOP in patients with intermediate grade non-Hodgkin's lymphoma. J Clin Oncol 1994; 12:769.

39. Fisher RI, Gaynor ER, Dahlberg S, et al: Comparison of a standard regimen (CHOP) with three intensive chemotherapy regimens for advanced non-Hodgkin's lymphoma. N Engl J Med 1993; 328:1002.

40. Miller TP, Grogan TM, Dalton WS, et al: P-glycoprotein expression in malignant lymphoma and reversal of clinical drug resistance with chemotherapy plus high-dose verapamil [Abstract]. J Clin Oncol 1991; 9:17–24.

41. Armitage JO: Bone marrow transplantation in the treatment of patients with lymphoma. Blood 1989; 73:1749.

42. Gribben JG, Goldstone AH, Linch DC, et al: Effectiveness of high-dose combination chemotherapy and autologous bone marrow transplantation for patients with non-Hodgkin's lymphomas who are still responsive to conventional-dose therapy. J Clin Oncol 1989; 7:1621.

43. Carey PJ, Proctor SJ, Taylor P, Hamilton PJ: Autologous bone marrow transplantation for high-grade lymphoid malignancy using melphalan/irradiation conditioning without marrow purging or cryopreservation. Blood 1991; 77:1593.

44. Philip T, Chauvin F, Armitage J, et al: Parma International Protocol—pilot study of DHAP followed by involved-field radiotherapy and BEAC with autologous bone marrow transplantation. Blood 1991; 77:1587.

45. Gianni AM, Bregni M, Siena S, et al: 5-year update of the Milan Cancer Institute Randomized Trial of High-Dose Sequential (HDS) vs MACOP-B Therapy for Diffuse Large Cell Lymphomas [Abstract]. Proc Am Soc Clin Oncol 1994; 13:373.

46. Haioun C, Lepage E, Gisselbrecht C, et al: Autologous bone marrow transplantation (ABMT) versus sequential chemotherapy in first complete remission aggressive non-Hodgkin's lymphoma (NHL): 1st interim analysis on 370 patients (LNH87 protocol) [Abstract]. Proc Am Soc Clin Oncol 1992; 11:316.

47. Tura S, Zinzani PL, Mazza P, et al: ABMT vs. DHAP in residual disease following third-generation regimens for aggressive non-Hodgkin's lymphomas [Abstract]. Blood 1992; 80:157.

48. Coiffier B, Philip T, Burnett AK, Symann ML: Consensus Conference on Intensive Chemotherapy Plus Hematopoietic Stem-Cell Transplantation in Malignancies: Lyon, France, June 4–6, 1993. J Clin Oncol 1994; 12:226.

Twenty-Two

Lymphoblastic Lymphoma

Tak Takvorian

Lymphoblastic lymphoma as a disease entity may have been first recognized in a 1905 article by Sternberg in which a lymphoma of the mediastinum was described which subsequently evolved into acute leukemia.[1, 2] Cooke[3] in 1932 reviewed the world's literature of 74 cases of the so-called Sternberg sarcoma and identified 9 new cases of males who presented with a mediastinal mass and leukemia, all of whom died within 6 months of diagnosis. Long before our current understanding of T and B lymphocyte subsets, an association was noted between this disease syndrome and the thymus gland,[4] in part because of the anatomic contiguity. In 1973 Smith and associates[5] reported that the malignant cell in a case of Sternberg sarcoma was a T cell and suggested a thymic origin for these lymphomas. Lukes and Collins[6] emphasized the "convoluted" configuration of the nuclei. The phrase "convoluted T-cell lymphoma," which has been used interchangeably with "lymphoblastic lymphoma," was proposed by Barcos and Lukes[7] in 1975. They described morphologically the nuclear convolutions, noting the histologic similarity of the appearance of lymphoblasts and prolymphocytes in acute lymphoblastic leukemia (ALL) and the cells in the mediastinal lymphoma. The next year Nathwani and colleagues[8] noted convoluted and nonconvoluted cell types and proposed the terminology "lymphoblastic lymphoma," describing in more detail the natural history of lymphoblastic lymphoma. In 16 patients they noted the clinical and pathologic hallmarks of lymphoblastic lymphoma: presentation in young males with a mediastinal mass, frequent concomitant bone marrow and central nervous system (CNS) involvement, and morphologic features similar to T-cell ALL. These observations[9] were subsequently extended, also noting that this was not just a disease of children; almost 50% of patients were older than 30 years of age, but mediastinal masses and leukemic presentation both were of decreased incidence in the older age group.

Lymphoblastic lymphoma was associated with a poor prognosis in the early studies. However, with more aggressive therapy, CNS prophylaxis, and attention to prognostic features, a subgroup of lymphoblastic lymphoma now ranks among the most curable of lymphomas. Lymphoblastic lymphoma is rare among adult lymphomas, constituting approximately 4% in the original Working Classification series,[10, 11] in which it is classified as a high-grade lymphoma, subtype I. However, it represents approximately one third to one half of lymphomas[12] within the pediatric age group,

50% of which occur after the age of 10 years.[13] The etiology remains unknown.

T-cell ALL and lymphoblastic lymphoma demonstrate considerable histologic, immunophenotypic, cytogenetic, and clinical similarities. They are clearly biologically related, and the distinction between the two is somewhat arbitrary and definitional. The analogy is often made to the relationship between chronic lymphocytic leukemia (CLL) and well-differentiated, B-cell, small cell lymphocytic lymphoma. This bias has often led to consideration of them as one entity.

However, lymphadenopathy predominates in lymphoblastic lymphoma, and peripheral blood involvement predominates in ALL. This has often led to treatment strategies that are modeled after lymphoma therapies for nodal dominant disease versus strategies that are bone marrow ablative in leukemic presentations. Weinstein and coworkers[14] defined greater than 10% lymphoblasts in the bone marrow as ALL, whereas the St. Jude staging system prescribed by Murphy[12, 15] and Bernard and associates[16] defined this breakpoint as greater than 25% lymphoblasts in the marrow or circulating in the peripheral blood. T-cell ALL is usually characterized by a more immature thymic phenotype compared with a more mature level of intrathymic T-cell differentiation for most lymphoblastic lymphomas. Nonetheless, the distinction between the two entities appears somewhat arbitrary, and sometimes it is difficult to distinguish between a leukemic conversion of lymphoblastic lymphoma and de novo ALL.

PATHOLOGY

By histologic evaluation alone, the morphology of lymphoblastic lymphoma is indistinguishable from ALL. The cells are homogeneous, immature lymphoid cells with scant cytoplasm and are somewhat larger than the mature cells of CLL.

On lymph node biopsy, the cells are diffusely infiltrative, obliterating the lymph node architecture, and invading capsular and pericapsular tissues. In approximately one third of cases the interfollicular and paracortical T-cell zones are uniquely involved, leaving residual islands of normal lymphoid tissue, including intact germinal centers. A starry-sky pattern of interspersed macrophages may be present focally but is infrequent. Crush artifact is characteristic,[17] mitoses are numerous, and there is single-file necrosis, suggestive of a high-grade process.

Rarely, lymphoblastic lymphoma may have a pseudo-follicular pattern of growth caused by the confinement of lymphoblasts by connective tissue planes. These pseudofollicles can be confused with a small cleaved cell lymphocytic lymphoma,[18, 19] although close attention to nuclear histologic detail and mitotic rate can usually distinguish the two.

The terminology "malignant lymphoma, lymphoblastic" focuses attention on the essential identity of this tumor, according to Jaffe and Berard.[20] The nuclei have a "blastic" appearance with finely distributed chromatin, containing multiple, small, inconspicuous nucleoli. The nuclei are round or oval and are variably convoluted (but the convolutions are minimal to absent in as many as 50% of cases). There is a high nuclear-to-cytoplasmic ratio.

Histochemically, these cells are terminal deoxynucleotidyl transferase (TdT) positive,[21–25] uniquely expressing intranuclear TdT, whereas essentially all B-cell and T-cell non-Hodgkin's lymphomas are TdT negative.[22, 26] McCaffrey[23, 27] and Kung[24] and coworkers, noting that both lymphoblastic lymphoma and T-cell ALL consistently expressed TdT, a marker of immature (thymic) T cells, suggested a thymic origin to these tumors. This is the immunologic marker that is most useful in confirming the diagnosis of lymphoblastic lymphoma.

Convoluted and nonconvoluted subtypes exist, distinguished only by convolutions of the nuclei in anywhere from less than 10% to more than 85% of the cells. Most lymphoblasts in the nonconvoluted subtype correspond in appearance to the L_1 ALL category of the Fab classification.

A third morphologic subtype has been described, variously termed "atypical," "large cell," "pleomorphic," or "L2 variant," constituting approximately 10% of lymphoblastic lymphomas.[13, 28] Morphologically, these lymphoblasts more closely resemble the L2 ALL category of the Fab classification. The cells are larger, with more abundant cytoplasm, and frequently have convoluted nuclei with one or two relatively prominent nucleoli.[17]

The morphologic subdivision of lymphoblastic lymphoma into these three subcategories does not yet appear to have prognostic significance. There are no readily apparent clinical syndromes associated with the three subtypes such as age or sex distribution, clinical presentation, incidence of leukemic conversion, or response to therapy. In addition, there are not corresponding unique immunophenotypes correlating with the histologic appearance.

IMMUNOLOGY

Because of the rarity of lymphoblastic lymphoma, the immunologic features have been better studied in ALL. Approximately 80% of lymphoblastic lymphomas are of T-cell origin, and the remaining 20% are derived from precursor B cells.[16, 29–33] T-cell phenotypes are disparate and correspond to prethymic and intrathymic stages of normal T-cell differentiation.[30] B-cell phenotypes only rarely express mature B-cell antigens.[31, 34, 35]

Childhood ALL can be classified as having an early pre-B, pre-B, B-cell[36] or T-cell origin, and each immunophenotypic group has diverse presenting clinical and biologic features that have prognostic significance. Approximately 15% to 25% of cases of childhood ALL are classified as T-cell ALL.[25, 29, 31, 37–40] They, too, are male patients presenting with a mediastinal mass and are generally older than B-cell ALL patients. They present with more advanced disease, including organomegaly, peripheral adenopathy, and hyperleukocytosis (white blood cell count >100 K). The T-cell leukemias have a poorer prognosis than those of B-cell origin, except for one recent trial.[41]

In contrast, although attempts have been made to identify immunologic subgroups of clinical and prognostic significance in patients with lymphoblastic lymphoma, these have not been reproducibly successful. Attempts to distinguish "lymphomatous" presentation from "leukemic" presentation by immunophenotype have similarly been unsuccessful.[42] Although morphologic features are homogenous, lymphoblastic lymphomas are immunologically diverse. Usually they are of early (stage I cortical) phenotype. Most express CD7, even those with immature phenotypes. In addition, most express CD5, CD2, and CD3+ or CD3− (surface or cytoplasmic), and many express CD1, CD4, and CD8+ or CD8−. Coexpression of two or more thymocyte differentiation antigens has been observed.

In one study in children with T-cell leukemia-lymphoma Crist and coworkers[43] demonstrated a correlation among the presenting clinical features, outcome, and the maturational stage of thymocytes. For example, patients with mature-stage T-cell lymphoma were less likely to have a mediastinal mass, but they concluded that these developmental subdivisions were not critical determinants of outcome once remission was achieved.

Innumerable other phenotypes have also been reported including pre-B-cell (less aggressive biology),[30, 44] "common" ALL (CALLA),[30, 45] and even biphenotypic.[29, 46] The latter has been reported in as many as 20% of patients with lymphoblastic lymphoma. Sheibani and associates[31] noted that the frequency of mediastinal masses was highest in the T-cell phenotype patients. Lineage switch[47] has been reported,[48–50] in which a T-cell lymphoblastic lymphoma underwent phenotypic alteration, changing to an acute myeloid leukemia. This may represent phenotypic conversion of cells derived from a pluripotent leukemic cell.[51] Natural killer cell phenotypes have been noted, and some have suggested that they may have a more aggressive course.[31, 52, 53] The patients are usually female and nonwhite and respond poorly and briefly to therapy.

Ten percent to 20% of cases express CALLA (CD10),[30] and this has sometimes been believed to be associated with the "good" prognosis of ALL. The B-cell phenotype, however, is only rarely seen in pediatric patients and CD10 positivity in T-cell lymphoblastic lymphoma has no obvious prognostic significance.[31] An unusually aggressive B-cell variant has been reported in which patients present without a mediastinal mass, but the disease invades bone and bone marrow.[30, 54, 55] Mediastinal masses may be less common in the non-T-cell phenotypes, and others have also noted the absence of mediastinal mass presentation in B-cell phenotypes.[29]

In the study by Cossman and colleagues,[30] 8 of the 11 cases presented had a T-cell phenotype, although only 8 cases had less than 25% lymphoblasts in the bone marrow. The other 3 cases demonstrated B-cell phenotypes and yet were morphologically indistinguishable from the T-cell cases and were TdT positive. A high percentage (45%) had helper or cytotoxic/suppressor phenotype, but none had expression of both, as some have reported.[56] Some have suggested that T-cell ALL is derived from the helper/inducer subset of T lymphocytes and lymphoblastic lymphoma from the suppressor subset.[57] Intratumor heterogeneity has also been observed,[30] and this may reflect growth or differentiation differences between subpopulations of individual neoplastic clones. Also, loss, and less commonly, gain of antigens have been reported in ALL and lymphoblastic lymphoma and may suggest a shift in differentiation of the neoplastic cells.[56] There is a more frequent expression of T-cell receptor α-β rather than γ-δ in lymphoblastic lymphoma,[58] the proportion of which is reversed in T-cell ALL. These data support the contention that fundamental biologic differences exist between T-cell lymphoblastic lymphoma and ALL.

Despite their T-cell lineage, lymphoblastic lymphomas are phenotypically distinct from cutaneous T-cell lymphomas and mycosis fungoides.[29] Lymphoblastic lymphoma also has a greater tendency to retain pan-T-cell antigens than the peripheral T-cell lymphomas.

CYTOGENETICS[42, 59–61]

The overall frequency of chromosome abnormalities in ALL/lymphoblastic lymphoma ranges from 50% to 90% and can be broadly divided into abnormalities involving chromosome number and structure.[61] In B-cell ALL karyotypic abnormalities have prognostic significance and define clinical, pathologic, and immunologically distinct subgroups.

T-cell ALL may also have unique, nonrandom cytogenetic patterns as compared with common ALL, and they are of prognostic significance. A characteristic translocation t(1;14) (p32;q11) has been noted in children with T-cell ALL,[62] with an incidence of 3% to 7%. These children present with a high circulating white blood cell count and a mediastinal mass and are older and male. The repeated observation of specific breakpoints on chromosomes 1, 14, and 7 suggests that genes near or at these sites play an important role in the malignant transformation/proliferation of thymocytes. Band q11 on chromosome 14 is involved in several translocations that seem specific for T-cell ALL, occurring in as many as 20% of cases.

In contrast, cytogenetics studies in lymphoblastic lymphoma and attempts to cytogenetically distinguish the two disorders have been few. A study by Kaneko and colleagues[42] found that T-cell ALL and lymphoblastic lymphoma share the same karyotypic abnormalities to a substantial degree, especially translocations involving the loci of T-cell receptor genes. Abnormal karyotypes were seen in 73% and 94% of T-cell ALL and lymphoblastic lymphoma, respectively, and in 30% to 50% included a breakpoint at 14q11, 7q34-36, or 7p15. They concluded, therefore, that in a large proportion of patients the two diseases are different manifestations of the same lymphoblastic disorder.

However, certain translocations were observed only in lymphoblastic lymphoma. In particular patients with t(9;17) presented with an anterior mediastinal mass without involvement of the bone marrow, and these patients had a rapidly progressive course.[63] This suggests that there may be subsets of lymphoblastic lymphoma distinct from T-cell ALL, which allow for a lymphomatous rather than a leukemic presentation of disease. Karyotypes have not yet consistently been shown to be of prognostic significance in contrast with ALL studies.[64–66]

NATURAL HISTORY

Although lymphoblastic lymphoma is uncommon in adults, constituting less than 5% of the non-Hodgkin's lymphomas, it represents a major subgroup of childhood and young adult lymphomatous disease. Although in the Working Formulation study[10] the median age at presentation was 16 years, its incidence appears bimodal, with a second peak incidence beyond age 40 years (7th decade, according to Nathwani and coworkers[9]). In females the distribution of incidence is more even. There is no known racial predilection.

In children the differential diagnosis, in addition to ALL, includes primarily other lymphomas including the diffuse small, noncleaved cell lymphomas (Burkitt's, non-Burkitt's, and undifferentiated) and diffuse large cell lymphoma. In adults, one must also consider small cleaved cell lymphoma, thymoma, neuroendocrine tumors such as oat cell tumors and cutaneous Merkel's cell tumors, and, more rarely, germ cell neoplasms and sarcomas. However, morphologic features, histochemical markers, and clinical presentation often can help distinguish these possibilities.

Most commonly patients are male (10:1), in their third decade of life, and they present with a large mediastinal mass and/or supradiaphragmatic adenopathy in the cervical, supraclavicular, or axillary regions.[54, 59] The mediastinal masses are usually bulky, greater than 10 cm in transverse diameter, and anterior in location. They occur in 40% to 60% of cases and are associated with pleural effusions. In contrast with other lymphomas, the mediastinal mass is often symptomatic with associated pressure symptoms, including superior vena caval syndrome, tracheal obstruction, and/or a pericardial effusion that can lead to tamponade.

Although predominant abdominal involvement is unusual as a primary manifestation (<5%), involvement of the liver or spleen is not uncommon, and more than 90% of patients present with advanced stage III or IV disease. Patients commonly present with B symptoms. Bone marrow may be apparently normal at presentation but a subsequent leukemic phase rapidly develops in most patients, indistinguishable from T-cell ALL.[67] The bone marrow is involved at presentation in at least 50% of cases. There is a strong correlation between bone marrow involvement and the incidence of CNS disease, thereby necessitating CNS assessment at the time of diagnosis. CNS involvement is more commonly leptomeningeal than parenchymal, and lymphoblastic lymphoma has the highest incidence of CNS involvement of all the lymphomas. The CNS is involved at presentation in 20% of cases and is often the initial site of

Table 22–1. Poor Prognostic Factors at Diagnosis in Relation to Survival

Series	Factors
Slater et al[67]	Age >30 years PR or late CR WBC >50 × 10⁹ CNS involvement
Coleman et al[70]	High LDH level (>1.5 times normal) BM involvement CNS involvement
Morel et al[71]	PR Age >40 years B symptoms LDH more than twice normal level Hgb <100 g/L (anemia)

PR, partial response; CR, complete response; WBC, white blood cell count; LDH, lactate dehydrogenase; BM, bone marrow; CNS, central nervous system; Hgb, hemoglobin.

relapse. Gonadal, breast, and skin involvement have also been reported.[7, 8, 68, 69] Primarily, cutaneous lymphoblastic lymphoma differs from the more usual variety by affecting very young children (<6 years of age), lack of male predominance, absence of a mediastinal mass, primary skin involvement, B-cell phenotype, and a less aggressive course.[44]

ALL and lymphoblastic lymphoma differ in a number of clinical features. Peripheral adenopathy and a mediastinal mass are distinctly unusual as presenting features in ALL; whereas splenomegaly, high circulating blast count and thrombocytopenia are more commonly evident at presentation in ALL. However, it nonetheless remains difficult in many circumstances to differentiate accurately between de novo ALL and a leukemic phase, or conversion, of lymphoblastic lymphoma.

An unusually aggressive B-cell variant has been noted. The bone marrow and bone (lytic lesions) are commonly involved rather than presentation with a mediastinal mass.[30, 54, 55]

Until recently, lymphoblastic lymphoma in the adult was associated with few long-term survivors and a poor prognosis. Certain prognostic factors have now been identified (Table 22–1).[67, 70, 71] Coleman and associates assigned patients to low- or high-risk prognostic groups based on the presence of extranodal involvement in the bone marrow or CNS or a baseline elevation in the LDH.[70] High complete remission rates and long-term disease-free survival are now accomplished with the use of intensive chemotherapy regimens in good-prognosis patients and of CNS prophylaxis.[54, 55, 67]

STAGING

The Ann Arbor staging system is most commonly used in the adult population and literature. Most patients present with stage III or IV disease and with B symptoms. In the pediatric population the staging system proposed by Murphy at St. Jude's is most commonly used.[15] Both classifications

emphasize the presence and importance of extranodal disease involvement, primarily in the bone marrow or CNS.

In addition to routine staging tests such as chest radiograph and laboratory screening (blood counts and chemistry profile), measurement of the serum lactate dehydrogenase (LDH) is an important prognostic determinant prior to the initiation of therapy. Assessment of the bone marrow by aspiration and biopsy and of the CNS by lumbar puncture is essential. Gallium scanning has taken on increased importance, particularly in the followup of residual masses. High-dose, late-imaged studies should be obtained.

PROGNOSTIC FACTORS

In the pediatric population, age 15 years and older, Fab L2 morphology, abnormal leukemic cell karyotype, and blast cell CD3 expression predicted a poor outcome of therapy in children with T-cell ALL.[72] In other series, a large leukemic burden as manifested by hyperleukocytosis,[73] high serum LDH, or massive organomegaly portended poor prognosis.

The definition of poor prognostic features in ALL remains controversial. Slater and coworkers[67] in the Memorial series focused on prognostic factors common to acute leukemia and found no differences in survival for ALL, leukemic lymphoblastic lymphoma, or nonleukemic lymphoblastic lymphoma. However, age older than 30 years, failure to attain a complete response or a late attainment of a complete remission during induction, white blood cell count higher than 50 10⁹/L, or CNS involvement were important poor prognostic determinants. (Age influenced the complete remission rate rather than relapse probability.) Leukemia at presentation, T-cell phenotype, and the presence of a mediastinal mass did not adversely affect outcome.

High LDH level and bone marrow and CNS involvement were identified by Coleman and associates[70] and are the most widely accepted poor risk features. In a retrospective analysis, patients were assigned to low- and high-risk groups as indicated by multivariant analysis of pretreatment prognostic factors. Ann Arbor stage IV disease with bone marrow or CNS involvement or initial LDH determination higher than 1.5 times normal defined a high-risk group. Freedom from release of low- and high-risk groups at 5 years were 94% and 19%, respectively (P = 1.0006), but these data have not been vigorously further substantiated.

In contrast, however, Morel and colleagues[71] did not report any survival advantage for patients without bone marrow involvement. In their series of 80 patients treated on a variety of induction protocols, including autologous bone marrow transplantation (ABMT) for some patients in first remission, an 82% complete response rate was observed. Actuarial overall survival at 30 months was 51%. The actuarial freedom from relapse rate was 46% at 30 months in patients achieving a complete remission. The small number of patients in each treatment group did not allow for any definitive conclusion regarding the prognostic value of Ann Arbor staging. Bernasconi and associates in Pavia[74] failed to demonstrate a significant correlation between pretreatment characteristics and outcome, except for Ann Arbor stage I disease (but the numbers were small).

TREATMENT

Treatment approaches have been disparate, and reported series are small owing to the rarity of this lymphoma, particularly in adults. Furthermore, because of the heterogeneous nature of presentation, direct comparison among various studies has not been possible, and protocol entry requirements differ widely. The disease has been approached both by marrow ablative and cyclical therapy, as modeled after ALL treatment and lymphoma treatment, respectively. Furthermore, alternating cyclical therapy with noncross-resistant regimens, such has been used in ALL, has also been effective.[74] Results of protocols using either treatment strategy are not significantly different. Rather, the recent combination of accurate prognostication, aggressive combination chemotherapy, and CNS prophylaxis has dramatically improved the response rate and disease-free survival of patients with lymphoblastic lymphoma (Table 22–2).

The early treatment of lymphoblastic lymphoma in children and adults using conventional therapy and radiation was dismal. The 5-year survival in children with localized disease before 1970 was approximately 10%, and in adults there were only rare survivors beyond 2 years.

In the 1970s there were some reports in children[76, 77] of long-term, disease-free survival. There was no similar success reported in adults until the early 1980s when Coleman and coworkers reported first a pilot study[78] and then a subsequent series of 44 adult patients treated at Stanford University Medical Center.[70] Their strategy involved initial CHOP (cyclophosphamide, hydroxydaunomycin, Oncovin, prednisone)-based therapy that was intensive and included L-asparaginase, CNS prophylaxis with radiation therapy and intrathecal chemotherapy, and maintenance chemotherapy with methotrexate and 6-mercaptopurine. The total duration of therapy was 1 year. The overall response rate was 100% (95% complete response), and at the time of publication in November 1986, there was a 26-month median followup with a 56% actuarial freedom from relapse at 3 years. Retrospectively, patients were assigned to low- and high-risk groups as indicated by a multivariant analysis of pretreatment prognostic factors. Ann Arbor stage IV disease with bone marrow or CNS involvement, or initial serum LDH concentration greater than one and a half times normal, defined a high-risk group. Freedom from relapse rates of low- and high-risk groups at 5 years were 94% and 19%, respectively ($P = .0006$). Both of these articles documented an apparent cure in certain cases with aggressive treatment. However, these results have not been updated, and at least one group has published failure in reproducing these results.[79]

CNS involvement, primarily meningeal, was a frequent site of disease progression or recurrence prior to the institution of CNS prophylaxis.[68, 78, 80] CNS prophylaxis and relapse have been treated with intrathecal and/or systemic methotrexate or ara-C and/or radiation therapy.[70, 81] In the pilot series[78] reported by Coleman and colleagues, 4 patients of 14 relapsed in the CNS, but prophylactic treatment with intrathecal methotrexate was delayed in the original schedule until week 8 or 9 following induction therapy and systemic methotrexate was administered as a single dose of 1 g/m^2 at that time. However, the subsequent use of intrathecal methotrexate earlier during the induction period and cranial radiation therapy decreased the incidence of CNS relapse (3% in the subsequent Coleman series[70]). However, despite a decrease in CNS recurrence, patient survival was not improved. Sweetenham and associates[79] could not reproduce these results and had 4 relapses in the CNS of 12 patients, and only 4 patients remain in complete remission.

Toxicity in the Stanford series was severe, with 3 (7%) of 44 patients succumbing to neutropenic sepsis. A complete response was achieved in most patients within two cycles of therapy, whereas two of three patients who achieved a complete response more slowly, relapsed. Finally, the relapse patterns were of note. Most patients relapsed in disseminated sites, especially in the bone marrow. This implied little role for consolidative mediastinal radiation therapy. Relapses occurred early (during or shortly after consolidation therapy) or more than 18 months beyond treatment.

Because of the clinical, histologic, immunologic, and biochemical similarities of lymphoblastic lymphoma and ALL, patients with lymphoblastic lymphoma have been included on ALL protocols at Memorial Sloan-Kettering Cancer Center since 1970. Slater and colleagues[67] reported the MSKCC series of 51 patients treated with one of five successive intensive protocols (L2 and L10/17). This consisted of a complex schedule of induction, consolidation, and maintenance therapy, including CNS prophylaxis. The full course of therapy ran approximately 3 years on the L2 protocol. The complete remission rate was 78%. In subset analysis there was no difference in survival at 2 years between patients with lymphoblastic lymphoma and ALL.

Table 22–2. Results of Combination Chemotherapy in Adult Lymphoblastic Lymphoma

Series	Regimen	Total No. of Patients	Outcome	Complete Response (%)
Coleman et al[70] (Stanford)	CHOP, asparaginase, maintenance to 1 yr	44	56% at 3 yr	95
Slater et al[67] (MSKCC)	Five protocols L10/17	51	45% survival at 4 yr	78
Bernasconi et al[74] (Pavia)	CHOP, intensification, maintenance for 3 yr	31	59% survival at 3 yr	77
Morel et al[71] (French multicenter)	Variety of ALL-like regimens, 2 yr maintenance	80	51% survival at 30 mo	82
Levine et al[75] (USC)	LSA2-L2	15	28.3-mo median overall survival	73

The projected 5-year survival rate for all patients treated with the L2 and L10/17 protocols was 45% for both the leukemic and nonleukemic lymphoblastic lymphomas. Poor prognostic factors included age older than 30 years (actuarial survival at 5 years was 40% for patients <30 years of age versus 20% for patients >30 years of age), a white blood cell count at presentation higher than 50,000/mL, and failure to achieve a complete response or the achievement of a complete response late into therapy. However, a leukemic phase at presentation, T-cell phenotype, and the presence of a mediastinal mass did not adversely affect survival.

Levine and coworkers[75] used a modification of the LSA2-L2 protocol (for childhood lymphoma) in 15 adult patients. The complex schedule had induction, consolidation, and maintenance phases, emphasized the use of ara-C and L-asparaginase and included CNS prophylaxis, with treatment extending over 3 years. Maintenance consisted of cyclical chemotherapy and intrathecal methotrexate. Mediastinal radiation therapy (2000 cGy) was also given. A complete response was achieved in 11 patients. Nine patients had bone marrow involvement at presentation, and six patients remained without evidence of disease 8 to 71 months or longer at the time of publication. The lower complete remission rate (73%) and median overall survival (28.3 months) compared with the Coleman series were attributed to less intensive induction therapy and the lower number of complete responders, respectively. However, median survival in partial or nonresponders was only 10 months. No prognostic factors were identified, but bone marrow involvement might have been a poor-prognosis indicator. There was one late relapse at 3.5 years despite 3 years of treatment.

Bernasconi and associates[74] reported in 31 patients the use of two consecutive multidrug programs, analogous to those used in ALL. In the first program induction therapy was followed by 3 years of continuous maintenance chemotherapy. The second program contained postremission intensification with alternating courses of noncross-resistant agents in a cyclical 8-month program. CNS prophylaxis was incorporated into both protocols. The complete remission rate was the same (77%), with a median overall and relapse-free survival of 18 and 29 months, respectively. The 3-year overall survival of complete responders was 59%. (The two programs were not compared owing to small numbers and sequential chronologic activation.) The authors failed to demonstrate a significant correlation between pretreatment characteristics and outcome.

Morel and coworkers[71] reported an important study of 80 adults patients with lymphoblastic lymphoma comparing various regimens including CHOP, the LNH-84 protocol, and two ALL regimens: FRALLE and LALA. Sixty-six patients (82%) achieved a complete remission with disease-free survival and overall survival rates of 46% and 51%, respectively, at 30 months (median followup, 55 months). The chemotherapy protocol did not appear to influence complete response rate, duration of complete response, or survival. The authors suggested that the choice of regimen does not appear to influence the outcome if it is sufficiently intensive and includes CNS prophylaxis. The value of long-term ALL-like maintenance was explored but uncertain. In this study, age and LDH were important pretreatment prognostic factors. Bone marrow involvement had no

prognostic value, even when analysis was restricted to patients receiving the ALL protocols.

There has been little role for radiation therapy outside the setting of CNS prophylaxis. Despite CNS radiation therapy prophylaxis,[79] relapses also occur within this site. In series using mediastinal radiation therapy, most patients nonetheless relapse in disseminated disease sites, particularly in the bone marrow, implying no benefit to mediastinal radiation therapy. However, at postmortem examination the mediastinum remained free of disease. Systemic relapse in part may be related to the rapid growth of lymphoblastic lymphoma and the lack of systemic protection while delivering focal radiation therapy.

Mott and associates,[82] however, reported a significant advantage for children with T-cell leukemia/lymphoma randomized to receive low-dose mediastinal radiation (1500 cGy): a 66% 4-year event-free survival for those children with lymphoma receiving radiation therapy versus 18% (P = .006) in those who did not. Starke and Wiltshaw[83] reported a significantly increased incidence of mediastinal relapse in patients not receiving mediastinal irradiation (although the patients were treated aggressively). Vecchi and coworkers[84] in a series of pediatric Sternberg's sarcoma (of whom 12 patients had T-cell disease) noted that the incidence of mediastinal relapse was significantly increased when mediastinal irradiation was omitted, but this was fraction size dependent. Weinstein[14] and Camitta and coworkers,[85] however, concluded that mediastinal radiation might be toxic in conjunction with doxorubicin and was not required for cure. In three cases in the Weinstein series, however, radiation therapy was used to help attain a complete remission or to treat initial respiratory distress in five patients.

The use of interferon has been reported with limited or no success. Ara-C, including high dosage levels, has been utilized[86, 87] as consolidative therapy.

PEDIATRIC EXPERIENCE

Prior to 1970 treatment for mediastinal lymphoma was primarily radiation therapy, and the 5-year survival rate in children, even with apparently localized disease, was approximately 10%. Because this disease predictably progressed to a leukemic phase with leptomeningeal involvement, treatment strategies were modeled after those used against ALL. Murphy in 1978, however, reported substantial improvement, with an 85% disease-free survival in stages I and II, but this decreased to 35% in stages III and IV in children treated with ALL-like regimens.[15]

In 1971 Aur and associates[77] published encouraging results in the treatment of childhood lymphoblastic lymphosarcoma with intensive chemotherapy and local radiation therapy. Wollner and colleagues[76] confirmed that these lymphomas respond to intensive multidrug therapy as used successfully for leukemia patients. In a followup study[88] they treated 43 children on a modified 10-drug LSA2-L2 protocol, 17 of whom had advanced disease and lymphoblastic histology, with an 88% actuarial survival at 40 months for the whole group. There was a 61% relapse-free survival at 5 years, and they were the first to show improved survival. Their strategy involved a complex induction phase, CNS prophylaxis with intrathecal methotrexate, and prolonged cyclical maintenance chemotherapy for a total of 3 years. Dahl and coworkers,[86] using a leukemia-derived protocol with intermittent pulses of teniposide (VM-26) and cytarabine, achieved a 73% 4-year event-free survival in advanced stage T-cell lymphomas. Although 2 of 19 patients had local mediastinal recurrence without radiation, they did not recommend its universal use since most patients' disease did not recur locally.

Weinstein and associates[89] published improved prognosis for pediatric patients with a long-term disease-free interval, stressing the use of CNS prophylaxis and the need for aggressive systemic therapy (APO [Adriamycin, prednisone, Oncovin]) even in situations presenting with localized disease. Treatment consisted of 2 years of therapy including CNS radiation and intrathecal methotrexate. Eighty-six percent of 11 patients who achieved complete remission remained disease free with a median followup of 41 months, with 1 relapse, in the CNS. Anderson and colleagues[90] reported and updated[91] an analysis of lymphoblastic lymphoma treated with a modified LSA2-L2 program, demonstrating a 76% disease-free survival at 24 months. This was superior to COMP (CCNU, Oncovin, methotrexate, prednisone) in this randomized study (confirmed by others[92]) and to ACOP (Adriamycin, cyclophosphamide, Oncovin, prednisone).[93]

Weinstein and coworkers[14] updated their prior study[89] and reported a 55% relapse-free survival at 3 years with the APO regimen in a predominantly pediatric population (median age 13 years, range from 2 to 22 years). The APO protocol however excluded patients with bone marrow involvement greater than 10%. The 5-year actuarial survival was 69% in the 21 patients. Six patients relapsed, including two with primary relapse in the CNS despite prophylaxis, and one in the CNS and testicle. No one relapsed in the bone marrow.

The United Kingdom Children's Cancer Study Group[94] treated an unselected series of 95 children with advanced-stage disease with an intensive ALL-like regimen consisting of an intensive 5-week induction followed by intensification at the 5-week and 20-week time points. This was followed by continuous oral daily 6-mercaptopurine, weekly oral methotrexate, and every-4-week vincristine/prednisone for 2 years. CNS prophylaxis with radiation therapy and intrathecal methotrexate was included. The 4-year event-free survival of 65%, with no significant difference between stage III and stage IV cases, was better than their previous series.[82]

BONE MARROW TRANSPLANTATION

Patients with poor prognosis lymphoblastic lymphoma have been candidates for protocols using intensified treatment with bone marrow transplantation as consolidation of primary therapy, since the median survival in relapsed or noncomplete response patients is less than 10 months. Initial reports were case studies of patients with multiple adverse prognostic features.[95] Early studies of disparate poor-prognosis lymphoma patients, with the breakout of analysis of lymphoblastic lymphoma patients, suggested a prolongation of overall survival and disease-free survival in poor-prognosis patients when transplanted (allogeneic or autologous source of bone marrow) in complete remission.[96-101] More recently, more homogenous studies of lymphoblastic lymphoma patients have substantiated these early encouraging results.[102-104] With the identification of poor prognostic features, patients have been selected for transplant study on the basis of these features in whom less than 20% survival is expected at 5 years with conventional therapy alone.

Limited pilot series of autologous or allogeneic bone marrow transplantation were performed in patients considered to have high-risk features, usually as determined by the criteria of Coleman. The Verdonck,[105] Milpied,[102, 106] Santini,[103, 107] and Baro[108] data (Table 22–3) presents the results of bone marrow transplantation in 74 patients, most of whom were in complete remission at the time of transplantation. At reportage, there was a 2- to 4-year disease-free survival that varied from 66% to 85%. There was no difference in outcome for autologous versus allogeneic sources of bone marrow, most patients did not undergo ex vivo bone marrow purging, and most patients had CNS prophylaxis.

In these limited series, the efficacy of bone marrow transplantation was apparently not influenced by the prior involvement of the bone marrow with lymphoma. Efficacy was also not diminished for patients with poor-risk features as defined by Coleman. Bone marrow transplantation had its greatest success in patients in first complete remission compared with relapsed or subsequent remission patients, but the studies are small and not controlled, prognostic factors are variable, and followup is short.

More recently, the European Bone Marrow Transplantation Group (EBMTG) reported a retrospective series of 214 patients[104] who underwent ABMT between 1981 and 1992. This is the largest published series of adults undergoing that type of transplantation for lymphoblastic lym-

Table 22–3. Pilot Bone Marrow Transplantation Trials in Lymphoblastic Lymphoma

Series	No. of Patients	Median Age (yr)	Preparation (No. of Patients)	Remission Status	BM Type	Results
Verdonck et al[105]	9	22	CHOP (6) ALL regimens (3)	CR (1)	Autologous	Relapse at 4, 8 mo; 1 patient with AML at 7 mo
Milpied et al[102, 106]	25	23	ALL regimens (19) NHL regimens (6)	CR (1)	Autologous (13) Allogeneic (12)	DFS 68% at 4 yr (median followup 20 mo)
Santini et al[103, 107]	18	22	LSA2-L2	CR (1)	Autologous	14 NED at 1–60+ mo
Baro et al[108]	22	25	ALL regimens (16) NHL regimens (8)	CR (14) PR (8)	Autologous	85% at 2 yr (median followup 19 mo)

PR, partial remission; CR, complete remission; BM, bone marrow; AML, acute mylogenous leukemia; DFS, disease-free survival; NED, no evidence of disease.

phoma and included 105 patients in first complete remission. The actuarial overall survival rate at 6 years for the entire group was 42%.

The major predictor of outcome was disease status at the time of ABMT. The 6-year actuarial overall survival was 63% for patients transplanted in first complete remission compared with 15% for those with refractory/resistant disease at ABMT (which is still better than conventional salvage therapy). Transplantation in second complete remission resulted in a 31% rate of actuarial overall survival at 6 years.

Univariate analysis did not identify any factor that predicted outcome for first remission patients (although information on LDH was not available). Involvement of the CNS or bone marrow at presentation did not adversely affect survival following ABMT. Five-year actuarial overall survival was 48% in this group. However, according to the data of Coleman and associates, it is not necessarily clear that patients with less than stage IV disease would have done poorly without transplantation. The authors conclude that ABMT is effective therapy for adults with lymphoblastic lymphoma, even in patients resistant to conventional dose therapy. Results for patients transplanted in second complete remission are superior to conventional dose salvage, but a prospective, randomized study (which is currently underway between the EBMTG and the United Kingdom Lymphoma Group) is suggested for first-remission patients.

FUTURE DIRECTIONS

In summary, lymphoblastic lymphoma is a rare but aggressive form of lymphoma, affecting primarily young people but potentially curable with rapid recognition of the diagnosis and institution of appropriate, aggressive therapy. It shares many features with T-cell ALL, and the distinction between the two diseases is somewhat arbitrary. Success can be accomplished with either a cyclical lymphomatous approach or marrow ablative leukemic approach without apparent advantage as long as the dosage is intense and the CNS is prophylaxed. Risk groups have been defined for which specific therapy can be targeted. However, poor-prognostic factors need to be further studied for substantiation of risk and appropriate protocols designed. Early intensification in patients identified to have poor-prognostic features, the setting in which bone marrow transplantation has had its early success, is an obvious way to proceed at present. Efforts aimed at decreasing the toxicity of therapy, determining the length of treatment, and detection of minimal disease remain to be determined and will require cooperative studies because of the rarity of this tumor at any single institution.

REFERENCES

1. Sternberg C: Leukosarkomatose and Myeloblasten leukaamie. Beitr Pathol 1916; 61:75.
2. Sternberg C: Zur Kenntnis des Chloroms (Chloromyelosarkom): Ziegler's Beitrage zur Pathologischen Anatomie und zur Allgemeinen Pathologie. Jena 1905; 36:437.
3. Cooke JV: Mediastinal tumor in acute leukemia: A clinical and roentgenologic study. Am J Dis Child 1932; 44:1153.
4. Webster R: Lymphosarcoma of the thymus: Its relation to acute lymphatic leukemia. Med J Aust 1961; 48:582.
5. Smith JL, Barker CR, Clein GP, et al: Characterization of malignant mediastinal lymphoid neoplasm (Sternberg sarcoma) as thymic in origin. Lancet 1973; 1:74.
6. Lukes RJ, Collins RD: Immunologic characterization of human malignant lymphomas. Cancer 1974; 34(suppl):1488.
7. Barcos MP, Lukes RJ: Malignant lymphoma of convoluted lymphocytes—a new entity of possible T-cell type. *In* Sinks LF, Godden JO (eds): Conflicts in Childhood Cancer: An Evaluation of Current Management, Vol 4. New York, Alan Liss, 1975, pp 147–148.
8. Nathwani BN, Kim H, Rappaport H: Malignant lymphoma, lymphoblastic. Cancer 1976; 38:964.
9. Nathwani BN, Diamond LW, Winberg CD, et al: Lymphoblastic lymphoma: A clinicopathologic study of 95 patients. Cancer 1981; 48:2347.
10. Rosenberg SA: The non-Hodgkin's lymphoma pathologic classification project: The National Cancer Institute–sponsored study of classifications of non-Hodgkin's lymphomas. Cancer 1982; 49:2112.
11. Simon R, Durrleman S, Hoppe, RT, et al: The Non-Hodgkin's Lymphoma Classification Project: Long-term follow-up of 1153 patients with non-Hodgkin's lymphoma. Ann Intern Med 1988; 109:939.
12. Murphy SB: Classification, staging, and end results of treatment of childhood non-Hodgkin's lymphomas: Dissimilarities from lymphomas in adults. Semin Oncol 1980; 7:332.
13. Kjeldsberg CR, Wilson JF, Berard CW: Non-Hodgkin's lymphoma in children. Hematol Pathol 1983; 14:612.
14. Weinstein MJ, Cassidy JR, Levey R: Long-term results of the APO protocol for treatment of mediastinal lymphoblastic lymphoma. J Clin Oncol 1983; 1:537.
15. Murphy SB: Childhood non-Hodgkin's lymphoma. N Engl J Med 1978; 299:1446.
16. Bernard A, Boumsell L, Reinherz EL, et al: Cell surface characterization of malignant T cells from lymphoblastic lymphoma using monoclonal antibodies: Evidence for phenotypic differences between malignant T cells from patients with acute lymphoblastic leukemia and lymphoblastic lymphoma. Blood 1981; 57:1105.
17. Knowles DM: Lymphoblastic lymphoma. *In* Knowles D (ed): Textbook of Neoplastic Hematopathology. Baltimore, Williams & Wilkins, 1992, pp 715–747.
18. Ioachim HL, Finkbeiner JA: Pseudonodular pattern of T-cell lymphoma. Cancer 1980; 45:1370.
19. Schwartz JE, Grogan TM, Hicks MJ, et al: Pseudonodular T-cell lymphoblastic lymphoma. Am J Med 1984; 77:947.
20. Jaffe ES, Berard CW: Lymphoblastic lymphoma—a term rekindled with new precision. Ann Intern Med 1978; 89:415.
21. Koziner B, Mertelsmann R, Filippa DA, et al: Adult lymphoid neoplasia of T and N cell types: Differentiation of normal and neoplastic hematopoietic cells. Cold Spring Harbor Symp Quant Biol 1978; 843.
22. Braziel RM, Keneklis T, Donlan JA, et al: Terminal deoxynucleotide transferase in non-Hodgkin's lymphomas. Am J Clin Pathol 1983; 80:655.
23. McCaffrey R, Harrison TA, Parkman R, et al: Terminal deoxynucleotidyl transferase activity in human leukemic cells and in normal human thymocytes. N Engl J Med 1975; 292:775.
24. Kung PC, Long JC, McCaffrey RP, et al: Terminal deoxynucleotidyl transferase in the diagnosis of leukemia and malignant lymphoma. Am J Med 1978; 64:788.
25. Murphy S, Jaffe ES: Terminal transferase activity and lymphoblastic neoplasms. N Engl J Med 1984; 311:1373.
26. Bearman RM, Winberg CD, Maslow WC, et al: Terminal deoxynucleotidyl transferase activity in neoplastic and non-neoplastic hematopoietic cells. Am J Clin Pathol 1981; 75:794.
27. McCaffrey R, Smoler DF, Baltimore D: Terminal deoxynucleotidyl transferase in a case of childhood acute lymphoblastic leukemia. Proc Natl Acad Sci U S A 1973; 70:521.
28. Griffith RC, Kelly DR, Nathwani BN, et al: A morphologic study of childhood lymphoma of the lymphoblastic type: The Pediatric Oncology Group experience. Cancer 1987; 59:1126.
29. Weiss LM, Bindl JM, Picozzi VJ, et al: Lymphoblastic lymphoma: An immunophenotypic study of 26 cases in comparison with T-cell acute lymphoblastic leukemia. Blood 1986; 67:464.
30. Cossman J, Chused T, Fisher R, et al: Diversity of immunologic phenotypes of lymphoblastic lymphoma. Cancer Res 1983; 43:4486.

31. Sheibani K, Nathwani BN, Winberg CD, et al: Antigenically defined subgroups of lymphoblastic lymphoma: Relationship to clinical presentation and biologic behavior. Cancer 1987; 60:183.

32. Grogan T, Spier C, Wirt DP, et al: Immunologic complexity of lymphoblastic lymphoma. Diagn Immunol 1986; 4:81.

33. Salloum E, Henry-Amar M, Caillou B, et al: Lymphoblastic lymphoma in adults: A clinicopathologic study of 34 cases treated at the Institute Gustave-Roussy. Cancer Clin Oncol 1988; 24:1609.

34. Anderson KC, Bates MP, Slaughenhoupt BL, et al: Expression of human B-cell-associated antigens on leukemias and lymphomas: A model of human B-cell differentiation. Blood 1984; 63:1424.

35. Foon KA, Todd RF: Immunologic classification of leukemia and lymphoma. Blood 1986; 68:1.

36. Crist WM, Grossi CE, Pullen J, et al: Immunologic markers in childhood acute lymphocytic leukemia. Semin Oncol 1985; 12:105.

37. Borella L, Sen L: T-cell surface markers on lymphoblasts from acute lymphocytic leukemia. J Immunol 1973; 111:1257.

38. Sen L, Borella L: Clinical importance of lymphoblasts with T markers in childhood acute leukemia. N Engl J Med 1975; 292:828.

39. Tsukimoto I, Wong KY, Lampkin BC: Surface markers and prognostic factors in acute lymphocytic leukemia. N Engl J Med 1976; 294:245.

40. Dow LW, Borella L, Sen L, et al: Initial prognostic factors and lymphoblast-erythrocyte rosette formation in 109 children with acute lymphoblastic leukemia. Blood 1977; 50:671.

41. Clavell LA, Gelber RD, Cohen HJ, et al: Four-agent induction and intensive asparaginase therapy for treatment of childhood acute lymphoblastic leukemia. N Engl J Med 1986; 315:657.

42. Kaneko Y, Frizzera G, Shikano T, et al: Chromosomal and immunophenotypic patterns in T-cell acute lymphoblastic leukemia and lymphoblastic lymphoma. Leukemia 1989; 3:886.

43. Crist WM, Shuster JJ, Falletta J, et al: Clinical features and outcome in childhood T-cell leukemia-lymphoma according to a stage of thymocyte differentiation: A Pediatric Oncology Group study. Blood 1988; 72:1891.

44. Link MP, Roper M, Dorfman RF, et al: Cutaneous lymphoblastic lymphoma with pre-B markers. Blood 1983; 61:838.

45. Borowitz MJ, Croker BP, Metzgar RS: Lymphoblastic lymphoma with the phenotype of common acute lymphoblastic leukemia. Am J Clin Pathol 1983; 79:387.

46. Childs CC, Chrystal GS, Strauchen, et al: Biphenotypic lymphoblastic lymphoma: An unusual tumor with lymphocytic and granulocytic differentiation. Cancer 1986; 57:1019.

47. Stass S, Mirro J, Melvin S, et al: Lineage switch in acute leukemia. Blood 1984; 64:701.

48. Kjeldsberg CR, Nathwani BN, Rappaport H: Acute myeloblastic leukemia developing in patients with mediastinal lymphoblastic lymphoma. Cancer 1979; 44:2316.

49. Hermann R, Han T, Barcos MP, et al: Malignant lymphoma of pre-T-cell type terminating in acute myelocytic leukemia: A case report with enzymic and immunologic marker studies. Cancer 1980; 46:1383.

50. Posner MR, Said J, Pinkus GS, et al: T-cell lymphoblastic lymphoma with subsequent acute non-lymphocytic leukemia: A case report. Cancer 1982; 50:118.

51. Nosaka T, Ohno H, Doi S, et al: Phenotypic conversion of T-lymphoblastic lymphoma to acute biphenotypic leukemia composed of lymphoblasts and myeloblasts: Molecular genetic evidence of the same clonal origin. J Clin Invest 1988; 81:1824.

52. Swerdlow SH, Habeshaw JA, Richards MA, et al: T lymphoblastic lymphoma with Leu-7 positive phenotype and unusual clinical course: A multiparameter study. Leuk Res 1985; 9:167.

53. Sheibani K, Winberg CD, Burke JS, et al: Lymphoblastic lymphoma expressing natural killer cell–associated antigens: A clinicopathologic study of six cases. Leuk Res 1987; 11:371.

54. Picozzi VJ, Coleman CN: Lymphoblastic lymphoma. Semin Oncol 1990; 17:96.

55. Rosen PJ, Feinstein DI, Pattengale PK, et al: Convoluted lymphocytic lymphomas in adults: A clinicopathologic entity. Ann Intern Med 1978; 89:319.

56. Roper M, Crist WM, Metzgar R, et al: Monoclonal antibody characterization of surface antigens in childhood T-cell lymphoid malignancies. Blood 1983; 61:830.

57. Nadler LM, Reinherz EL, Weinstein HJ, et al: Heterogeneity of T-cell lymphoblastic malignancies. Blood 1980; 55:806.

58. Gouttefangeas C, Bensussan A, Boumsell L: Study of the CD3-associated T-cell receptors reveals further differences between T-cell acute lymphoblastic lymphoma and leukemia. Blood 1990; 75:931.

59. Streuli RA, Kaneko Y, Variakojis D, et al: Lymphoblastic lymphoma in adults. Cancer 1981; 47:2510.

60. Smith SD, Morgan R, Gemmel R, et al: Clinical and biological characterization of T-cell neoplasias with rearrangements of chromosome 7 band q34. Blood 1988; 71:395.

61. Third International Workshop on Chromosomes in Leukemia. Cancer Genet Cytogenet 1981; 4:95.

62. Carroll AJ, Crist WM, Link MP, et al: The t(1;14)(p34;q11) is nonrandom and restricted to T-cell acute lymphoblastic leukemia: A Pediatric Oncology Group study. Blood 1990; 76:1220.

63. Kaneko Y, Frizzera G. Maseki N, et al: A novel translocation, t(9;17)(q34;q23), in aggressive childhood lymphoblastic lymphoma. Leukemia 1988; 2:745.

64. Kaneko Y, Rowley JD, Variakojis D, et al: Correlation of karyotype with clinical features in acute lymphoblastic leukemia. Cancer Res 1982; 42:2918.

65. Williams DL, Tsiatis A, Brodeur GM, et al: Prognostic importance of chromosome number in 136 untreated children with acute lymphoblastic leukemia. Blood 1982; 60:864.

66. Bloomfield CD, Goldman AI, Alimena G, et al: Chromosomal abnormalities identify high-risk and low-risk patients with acute lymphoblastic leukemia. Blood 1986; 67:415.

67. Slater DE, Mertelsmann R, Koziner, et al: Lymphoblastic lymphoma in adults. J Clin Oncol 1986; 4:57.

68. Herman TS, Hammond N, Jones SE, et al: Involvement of the central nervous system of non-Hodgkin's lymphoma: The Southwest Oncology Group experience. Cancer 1979; 43:390.

69. Bernard A, Murphy SB, Melvin S, et al: Non-T, non-B lymphomas are rare in childhood and associated with cutaneous tumor. Blood 1982; 59:549.

70. Coleman CN, Picozzi VJ, Cox RS, et al: Treatment of lymphoblastic lymphoma in adults. J Clin Oncol 1986, 4:1628.

71. Morel P, Lepage E, Brice P, et al: Prognosis and treatment of lymphoblastic lymphoma in adults: A report on 80 patients. J Clin Oncol 1992; 10:1078.

72. Pui CH, Behm FG, Singh B, et al: Heterogeneity of presenting features and their relation to treatment outcome in 120 children with T-cell acute lymphoblastic leukemia. Blood 1990; 75:174.

73. Pullen DJ, Sullivan MP, Falletta JM, et al: Modified LSA$_2$-L$_2$ treatment in 53 children with E-rosette–positive T-cell leukemia: Results and prognostic factors (a Pediatric Oncology Group study). Blood 1982; 60:1159.

74. Bernasconi C, Brusamolino E, Lazzarino M, et al: Lymphoblastic lymphoma in adult patients: Clinicopathological features and response to intensive multiagent chemotherapy analogous to that used in acute lymphoblastic leukemia. Ann Oncol 1990; 1:141.

75. Levine AM, Forman ST, Meyer DR, et al: Successful therapy of convoluted T-lymphocyte lymphoma in the adult. Blood 1983; 61:92.

76. Wollner N, Burchenal JH, Lieberman PH, et al: Non-Hodgkin's lymphoma in children. Cancer 1976; 37:123.

77. Aur RJA, Hustu HU, Simone JV, et al: Therapy of localized and regional lymphosarcoma of childhood cancer. Cancer 1971; 27:1328.

78. Coleman CN, Cohen JR, Burke JS, et al: Lymphoblastic lymphoma in adults: Results of a pilot protocol. Blood 1981; 52:679.

79. Sweetenham JW, Mead GM, Whitehouse JMA: Adult lymphoblastic lymphoma: High incidence of central nervous system relapse in patients treated with the Stanford University protocol. Ann Oncol 1992; 3:839.

80. Mackintosh RD, Colby TV, Podolsky WJ, et al: Central nervous system involvement in non-Hodgkin's lymphoma: An analysis of 105 cases. Cancer 1982; 49:586.

81. Morra E, Lazzarino M, Inveradi D, et al: Systemic high-dose ara-C treatment of meningeal leukemia in acute lymphoblastic leukemia and non-Hodgkin's lymphoma. J Clin Oncol 1986; 4:1207.

82. Mott MG, Chessells JM, Willoughby ML, et al: Report from the United Kingdom Children's Cancer Study Group: Adjuvant low-dose radiation in childhood T-cell leukemia/lymphoma. Br J Cancer 1984; 50:457.

83. Starke ID, Wiltshaw E: Sternberg's lymphoma: Effect of treatment regimen upon prognosis in 38 cases. Br J Haematol 1980; 46:351.

84. Vecchi V, Serra L, Pession A, et al: Childhood non-Hodgkin's lymphoma and "leukemia-lymphoma" syndrome: Long-term results with the modified LSA$_2$-L$_2$ protocol. Pediatr Hematol Oncol 1986; 3:217.

85. Camitta BM, Lauer SJ, Casper JT, et al: Effectiveness of a six-drug regimen (APO) without local irradiation for treatment of mediastinal lymphoblastic lymphoma in children. Cancer 1985; 56:738.

86. Dahl GV, Rivera G, Pui CH, et al: A novel treatment of childhood lymphoblastic leukemia and non-Hodgkin's lymphoma: Early and intermittent use of teniposide plus cytarabine. Blood 1985; 66:1110.

87. Peters W, Willemze R, Colly L: Intermediate- and high-dose cytosine arabinoside containing regimens for induction and consolidation therapy for patients with acute lymphocytic leukemia and lymphoblastic non-Hodgkin's lymphoma: The Leyden experience and review of the literature. Semin Oncol 1987; 14:86.

88. Wollner N, Exelby R, Lieberman PH: Non-Hodgkin's lymphoma in children: A progress report on the original patients treated with LSA₂-L₂ protocol. Cancer 1979; 44:1990.

89. Weinstein JH, Vance ZB, Jaffe N, et al: Improved prognosis for patients with mediastinal lymphoblastic lymphoma. Blood 1979; 53:687.

90. Anderson JR, Wilson JF, Jenkin ET, et al: Childhood non-Hodgkin's lymphoma: The results of a randomized therapeutic trial comparing a 4-drug regimen (COMP) with a 10-drug regimen (LSA₂-L₂). N Engl J Med 1983; 308:559.

91. Anderson JR, Jenkin RDT, Wilson JF, et al: Long-term follow-up of patients treated with COMP or LSA₂-L₂ therapy for childhood non-Hodgkin's lymphoma: A report of CCG-551 from Children's Cancer Group. J Clin Oncol 1993; 11:1024.

92. Sullivan MP, Boyett J, Pullen J, et al: Pediatric Oncology Group experience with modified LSA₂-L₂ therapy in 107 children with non-Hodgkin's lymphoma (Burkitt's lymphoma excluded). Cancer 1985; 55:323.

93. Hvizdala EV, Berard C, Callihan BT, et al: Lymphoblastic lymphoma in children—a randomized trial comparing LSA₂-L₂ with the A-COP+ therapeutic regimen: a Pediatric Oncology Group study. J Clin Oncol 1988; 6:26.

94. Eden OB, Hann I, Imeson J, et al: Treatment of advanced-stage T-cell lymphoblastic lymphoma: Results of the United Kingdom Children's Cancer Study Group (UK CCSG) Protocol 8503. Br J Haematol 1992; 82:310.

95. Garrett TJ, Grossbard E, Hopfan S, et al: Bone marrow transplantation for the therapy of refractory adult T-cell acute lymphoblastic lymphoma. Cancer 1980; 45:2006.

96. Ernst P, Maraninchi D, Jacobsen N, et al: Marrow transplantation for non-Hodgkin's lymphoma: A multicentre study from the European Cooperative Bone Marrow Transplant Group. Bone Marrow Transplant 1986; 1:81.

97. Phillips GL, Herzig RH, Lazarus HM, et al: High-dose chemotherapy, fractionated total-body irradiation, and allogeneic marrow transplantation for malignant lymphoma. J Clin Oncol 1986; 4:480.

98. Nademanee AP, Forman SJ, Schmidt GM, et al: Allogeneic bone marrow transplantation for high risk non-Hodgkin's lymphoma during first complete remission. Blut 1987; 55:11.

99. Verdonck LF, Dekker ML, Kempen ML, et al: Intensive cytotoxic therapy followed by autologous bone marrow transplantation for non-Hodgkin's lymphoma of high-grade malignancy. Blood 1985; 65:984.

100. Braine HG, Santos GW, Kaizer H, et al: Treatment of poor-prognosis non-Hodgkin's lymphoma using cyclophosphamide and total-body irradiation regimens with autologous bone marrow rescue. Bone Marrow Transplant 1987; 2:7.

101. Goldstone AH, Singer CRJ, Gribben JG, et al: Fifth report of EBMTG experience of ABMT in malignant lymphoma. Bone Marrow Transplant 1988; 3(Suppl 1):33.

102. Milpied N, Ifrah N, Kuentz M, et al: Bone marrow transplantation for adult poor-prognosis lymphoblastic lymphoma in first complete remission. Br J Haematol 1989; 73:82.

103. Santini G, Coser P, Chisesi T, et al: Autologous bone marrow transplantation for advanced-stage adult lymphoblastic lymphoma in first complete remission: A pilot study of the non-Hodgkin's Lymphoma Cooperative Study Group. Bone Marrow Transplant 1989; 4:399.

104. Sweetenham JW, Liberti G, Pearce R, et al: High-dose therapy and autologous bone marrow transplantation for adult patients with lymphoblastic lymphoma: Results of the European Group for Bone Marrow Transplantation. J Clin Oncol 1994; 12:1358.

105. Verdonck LF, Dekker AW, de Gast GC, et al: Autologous bone marrow transplantation for adult poor-risk lymphoblastic lymphoma in first remission. J Clin Oncol 1992; 10:644.

106. Milpied N, Ifrah N, Kuentz M, et al: Treatment of lymphoblastic lymphoma: Beneficial effect of bone marrow transplantation in first complete remission. Blood 1987; 70:297a.

107. Santini G, Coser P, Chisesi T, et al: Autologous bone marrow transplantation for advanced-stage adult lymphoblastic lymphoma in first complete remission: Report of the Non-Hodgkin's Lymphoma Co-operative Study Group. Ann Oncol 1991; 29(Suppl 2):181.

108. Baro J, Richard C, Sierra J, et al: Autologous bone marrow transplantation in 22 adult patients with lymphoblastic lymphoma responsive to conventional dose chemotherapy. Bone Marrow Transplant 1992; 10:33.

Chapter

Twenty-Three

Burkitt's Lymphoma

The Small Noncleaved Cell Lymphomas

Ian T. Magrath

"Small noncleaved cell lymphoma" (SNCL) is a term originally coined by Lukes and Collins and was based on their morphologic classification of cells of the normal germinal center.[1] This term was used in the National Cancer Institute (NCI) Working Formulation[2] and essentially replaces the Rappaport term "undifferentiated lymphoma."[3] Neither term is a satisfactory designation for the tumor, or set of tumors that they have come to be associated with, since the cells of these lymphomas are significantly larger than those of the "small cell lymphomas" and are not "undifferentiated" insofar that they express the phenotypic characteristics of lymphocytes of the B-cell lineage. The designation "small noncleaved cell" was given to these lymphomas to differentiate them from the "large, noncleaved cell lymphomas" that arise from germinal centers, but many pathologists consider that there is a continuous morphologic spectrum between these two "entities"—a continuum that is present also at a cytogenetic level, since a fraction of large cell lymphomas bear the same chromosomal translocations present in SNCLs. Although Lukes based his terminology on his belief that similarly small, noncleaved lymphoid cells could be observed in normal germinal follicles, SNCLs differ from lymphomas of germinal center cell origin in that they never have a follicular (nodular) morphology, and occur predominantly in the first two decades of life. These tumors may, however, occasionally selectively involve germinal follicles, for example in mesenteric lymph nodes,[4] whereas cell lines derived from Burkitt's lymphomas—one of the two morphologic subtypes of SNCLs—express many of the surface characteristics of normal germinal center lymphocytes.[5] Interestingly, a fraction of SNCLs occurring in adults bear the same chromosomal translocation (14;18) that is observed in the majority of follicular lymphomas and some 20% to 30% of large cell lymphomas in adults. There can be little doubt, therefore, that morphology does not necessarily reflect the cellular origins of these tumors, and in the most recent lymphoma classification (the Revised European-American Lymphoma classification) it has been proposed that the term "SNCL" be abandoned in favor of the eponymous designations, Burkitt's and Burkitt-like lymphomas.[6]

Morphologically, SNCLs are divided into Burkitt's lymphomas, which account for the major fraction of these tumors in children, and non-Burkitt's lymphomas (Burkitt-like lymphomas), which account for the major fraction of SNCLs in adults. This subdivision is based largely on the degree of cellular pleomorphism, being greater in the non-Burkitt's lymphomas. It is not clear that such a separation has prognostic significance,[7] nor has any biologic correlate with morphology been established, although the non-Burkitt's lymphomas in adults appear to be more heterogeneous at a molecular level than SNCLs in children, and it is tumors in this morphologic subset that sometimes contain 14;18 translocations.[8] This biologic heterogeneity is perhaps explained by the recognition that the SNCLs of non-Burkitt's type have a histologic appearance intermediate between that of Burkitt's lymphoma and that of large cell lymphomas of B-cell origin—that is, there is a gradual morphologic transition between these two entities.[6, 9] Not surprisingly, there is also overlap between cytogenetic findings.[10] Whether large cell lymphomas with 8;14 translocations represent the same "biologic" entity as Burkitt's lymphoma, and would have the same prognosis when treated with the same therapy, remains unknown.

In equatorial Africa, where Burkitt's lymphoma occurs at particularly high incidence (5 to 15 per 100,000 children per year, as opposed to 2 to 3 per million in the United States), such that it is often referred to as "endemic" Burkitt's lymphoma, the tumor frequently presents with involvement of the jaw, and the distribution of the tumor is climatically determined.[11] Elsewhere in the world, the vast majority of patients present with abdominal tumor, jaw involvement is uncommon, and distribution is not related to climate. Most SNCLs bear an 8;14 chromosomal translocation, which juxtaposes the c-*myc* oncogene to heavy-chain immunoglobulin sequences, but some 15% to 20% of lymphomas have a "variant" translocation in which c-*myc* is juxtaposed to light-chain sequences.[12] Structural abnormalities in the c-*myc* gene, whether gross rearrangement or point mutation, are a hallmark of (but not exclusive to) the SNCL—presumably a consequence of the morphologic and biologic overlap between the SNCL and large cell lymphomas discussed previously. Interestingly, the chromosomal breakpoint locations, with respect to 8;14 translocations, differ in various world regions, an observation that has been interpreted as indicating etiologic differences.[13] Mutations in *p53*

423

are present in some 37% of SNCLs regardless of geography,[14] and the SNCLs are variably associated with Epstein-Barr virus (EBV), ranging from 20% to 30% in North American SNCL (whether or not human immunodeficiency virus–associated) to 95% in equatorial African SNCL.[15]

The SNCLs are tumors of the B-cell lineage and thus express surface IgM, B-cell markers such as CD19, CD20, and CD22, and (although usually not in the non-Burkitt's subtype) CD10, the common acute lymphoblastic leukemia (ALL) antigen.[6] They have a high growth fraction and very short doubling time (measured at 3 days in skin tumors in African children).[16] At a molecular level, translocations involving chromosome 8 result in deregulation of the c-*myc* gene—perhaps this should be accepted as the defining lesion in these tumors. If this definition were to be used, the SNCL of adults that bears a 14;18 translocation would have to be considered a separate pathologic entity. It would be of considerable interest to determine whether the latter have a different prognosis when treated with the same therapy as SNCL with a c-*myc* deregulation.

Burkitt's lymphoma was originally recognized in Africa. Jaw tumors in African children were first observed by a missionary physician, Sir Albert Cook, who reached Uganda in 1897.[17] However, Burkitt's lymphoma was brought into prominence by an Irish surgeon, Dennis Burkitt, who observed malignant tumors (he initially believed them to be sarcomas) with a predilection for the jaw in East African children.[18] The histologic appearance of these tumors was described in 1960 by O'Conor, who also recognized them to be of lymphoid origin.[19] Several reports of histologically identical tumors in Europe and the United States were published soon after these initial descriptions.[20–22] The association of EBV with Burkitt's lymphoma was recognized in 1964, after isolation of the virus from a cell line derived from Burkitt's lymphoma.[23]

The overall survival of children with non-Hodgkin's lymphoma (NHL) before the 1970s was very poor (5% to 30%).[24] Almost all patients who did survive were those who had presented with localized disease that was treated by surgery or radiation with or without chemotherapy.[25, 26] Relapses were common, usually occurring at sites distant from the primary site,[25] suggesting that the cause was failure to treat occult disease. Encouraging therapeutic results, however, were obtained in the treatment of African Burkitt's lymphoma. Burkitt, seeing that surgery of jaw lesions was both disfiguring and unsuccessful, and having no access to radiation, turned to chemotherapy. Long-term remissions were observed in patients (usually with very limited disease) who were treated with only one or two doses of cyclophosphamide.[27] Some long-term survivors were also observed in patients treated with cyclophosphamide as a single agent in the United States.[28] The success of the MOPP (nitrogen mustard, vincristine, procarbazine, and prednisone) combination drug regimen developed for Hodgkin's disease in the 1960s had an impact on the development of combination chemotherapy for the treatment of NHL and led to the introduction of combinations of cyclophosphamide, methotrexate, and vincristine in patients with African and North American Burkitt's lymphoma.[29] In children with NHL, regimens based on those normally used for ALL were initially used by pediatric oncologists because of the clinical

and morphologic similarity between these two "entities," along with the marked tendency of patients with NHLs to relapse in the bone marrow.[30, 31] To resolve the issue as to which of these approaches was better, the Children's Cancer Study Group (CCSG) conducted a randomized study in all childhood histologic subtypes of NHL in which the LSA$_2$L$_2$ regimen, a treatment protocol derived from a treatment approach used for ALL, was compared with pulse chemotherapy consisting of cyclophosphamide, Oncovin, methotrexate, and prednisone (COMP).[32] Both regimens had a total duration of 18 months. LSA$_2$L$_2$ was found to provide inferior therapy for the treatment of SNCL, even though the latter gave only an approximately 50% disease-free survival. Since that time, improvements in chemotherapy have resulted in steady improvements in the fraction of long-term survivors.

There is now broad agreement that the primary therapy of the SNCL is combination chemotherapy, whereas radiation is of minimal value. The most recent results suggest that 80% to 90% of all children and a similar fraction of adults with SNCL can be cured with intensive, short-duration chemotherapy.[33–35] As we become more familiar with the biology of the malignant lymphomas, new approaches that stem from a knowledge of the biochemical changes that give rise to neoplasia, and thus may be made tumor-specific, are likely to be developed.

CLINICAL PRESENTATIONS AND ANATOMIC DISTRIBUTION OF TUMOR

The SNCLs usually present with extranodal disease. Presentation with peripheral lymphadenopathy, particularly generalized lymphadenopathy, is uncommon. Although almost any organ of the body may be involved, the abdomen is the most common site of involvement in SNCLs of the sporadic variety of small noncleaved lymphomas (i.e., those occurring in the United States and Europe), being present in almost 90% of patients. Patients usually present with abdominal pain or swelling, a change in bowel habits, nausea and vomiting, gastrointestinal bleeding, a syndrome consistent with acute appendicitis or intussusception, or, rarely, intestinal perforation. Presentation with a right iliac fossa mass is common, occurring in 25% of patients in the NCI series (some 40% of patients overall had tumor at this site).[36] At surgery, bowel (small or large) and regional lymph nodes are the most frequent sites of disease. However, not infrequently, many of the enlarged lymph nodes in the lymphatic drainage area of a bowel mass prove not to be involved with tumor. The peritoneum may be invaded by adjacent visceral tumor or involved by multiple plaques of tumor, in which case there will usually be ascites. Retroperitoneal structures, including kidneys and pancreas, may be primarily or secondarily involved. Occasionally liver (rarely in the absence of bowel involvement) and/or spleen are sites of disease. Ovarian involvement is quite common in females. Abdominal involvement is present in about 50% of African patients, but the tumor less often arises in bowel wall (retroperitoneal and omental tumor are common), and involvement of the right iliac fossa (appendiceal/cecal region) is rather uncommon.[37]

In equatorial Africa, the maxilla and mandible are the most common sites of tumor, although jaw involvement is age-dependent, occurring particularly in young children in association with the developing molar teeth (suggesting a role for growth factors in the predilection for this site). In fact, 70% of children below 5 years of age with Burkitt's lymphoma have jaw involvement compared with 25% of patients above 14 years.[38] Maxillary tumors are twice as common as mandibular tumors, but multiple quadrant involvement is the rule rather than the exception. In very young children, orbital involvement is often present in patients who do not have jaw tumors, although at least some of these orbital tumors arise in the maxilla. Jaw involvement in SNCL in the United States occurs in about 15% to 20% of patients at presentation, is not age-related, more often involves the mandible, and frequently affects only a single jaw quadrant.[39]

Patients with SNCLs in North Africa, the Middle East, and South America appear to have a spectrum of organ involvement similar to that seen in the sporadic variety, most patients presenting with abdominal disease, and jaw involvement being uncommon.[40] However, more frequent jaw involvement has been reported in several world regions, including some Asian countries, South Africa (where both whites and nonwhites appear to have as high a frequency of jaw tumors as in the endemic form of the disease), Turkey, Japan, and the Middle East.[41–46] These data should be interpreted cautiously, since because of the prominence of jaw involvement in the first reports of Burkitt's lymphoma from Uganda, in some countries the diagnosis of Burkitt's lymphoma may have been more likely to be made in the presence of jaw tumor. Interestingly, in the endemic region of Africa itself, the percentage of patients with jaw tumors appears to be inversely proportional to the incidence of the disease (i.e., jaw tumors occur more commonly in lowland regions where the incidence is higher, than in highland regions.[47, 48] This probably reflects the tendency for the median age of patients with Burkitt's tumor to be higher in lower-incidence areas.

In the sporadic variety of SNCL, bone marrow involvement at presentation occurs in some 20% of patients,[49] but there is evidence from in vitro culture and karyotyping of microscopically normal bone marrow that occult involvement occurs in approximately another 20% of patients.[50] Some patients may present with a clinical syndrome consistent with leukemia without any solid lymphomatous masses, apart from lymphadenopathy and hepatosplenomegaly—a disease usually referred to as "L3" type of ALL (after the French-American-British classification), Burkitt's cell leukemia, and, more recently, acute B-cell leukemia. Not all leukemias that conform to the criteria of L3 morphology express surface immunoglobulin and have 8;14 translocations.[51] The L3 morphologic subtype constitutes 2% to 5% of most large series of patients with ALL, and since ALL has a much higher incidence than SNCL in children (some 20-fold), L3 leukemia contributes significantly to the overall incidence of the SNCL.

In African patients with Burkitt's lymphoma, bone marrow involvement occurs in only about 8% of patients at presentation, but the proportion of patients who have occult bone marrow involvement,[37, 49] and the proportion of patients presenting with ALL (uncommon in equatorial Africa) who have L3 ALL, are not known. Even after multiple relapses, marrow involvement is rarely seen in African patients, whereas in North America, until recently, approximately 90% of patients who died from chemotherapy-resistant tumor had had bone marrow involvement either at presentation or at relapse.[49]

Involvement of the central nervous system (CNS) sometimes occurs at presentation in patients with SNCL. It is commonly seen in the presence of bone marrow disease—approximately two thirds of patients with bone marrow disease present with CNS involvement.[52, 53] Meningeal infiltration is the commonest manifestation of CNS involvement, but cranial nerve infiltration, intracerebral disease, paraspinal involvement, or some combination of these may also be present.[52, 53] The most frequently observed combination is meningeal and cranial nerve involvement. The ophthalmic nerves and the facial nerve are more often affected, although any cranial nerve may be involved, including the optic nerve, with resultant visual impairment. CNS involvement, particularly paraspinal, is distinctly more common in patients with endemic Burkitt's lymphoma (where it usually occurs in the absence of bone marrow involvement). Paraplegia occurs in some 15% of equatorial African patients at presentation, while cerebrospinal fluid (CSF) malignant pleocytosis or cranial nerve involvement occurs in approximately one third of patients.[37] Intracerebral infiltration is distinctly rare and usually, but not invariably, associated with recurrent tumor—particularly in the setting of previous involvement of the meninges.[53, 54] Severe pain or limb paralysis can result from involvement of peripheral nerves or the brachial or sacral plexi.

Other sites that may be involved include peripheral lymph nodes, pleurae, endocrine and salivary glands, pharynx, bones, pericardium, breast, testis, skin, and, rarely, mediastinum. Fever, weight loss, and night sweats are uncommonly caused by the tumor itself.

DIAGNOSIS

The diagnosis of SNCL must be made by biopsy, which, in view of the high frequency of abdominal involvement, frequently entails laparotomy. Cytogenetics, immunophenotyping, and genotyping provide confirmation of the diagnosis and are particularly helpful in patients with a purely leukemic presentation. Acute B-cell leukemia expresses surface immunoglobulin and is TdT negative, whereas all other ALLs are TdT positive and do not express surface immunoglobulin. TdT-positive cells are normally found only in the bone marrow, where they are present in very small numbers.

Serum lactate dehydrogenase levels, although nonspecific, usually correlate with tumor burden and are often useful in the recognition of relapse, or as an indicator of more widespread disease (e.g., in the bone marrow) than is apparent from clinical examination.[55–57] Other such correlates include soluble interleukin II receptor (SIL2-R)[58] and β_2-microglobulin (β_2-m).[59]

Table 23–1. St. Jude Staging Scheme Used for Childhood Non-Hodgkin's Lymphoma

Stage	Definition
I	Single tumor (extranodal) Single anatomic area (nodal) Excluding mediastinum or abdomen
II	Single tumor (extranodal) with regional node involvement Primary gastrointestinal tumor with or without involvement of associated mesenteric nodes only, grossly completely resected On same side of diaphragm: a) Two or more nodal areas b) Two single (extranodal) tumors with or without regional node involvement
III	On both sides of the diaphragm: a) Two single tumors (extranodal) b) Two or more nodal areas All primary intrathoracic tumors (mediastinal, pleural, thymic) All extensive primary intra-abdominal disease All primary paraspinal or epidural tumors regardless of other sites
IV	Any of the above with initial central nervous system or bone marrow involvement (<25%)

Patients with more than 25% of blast cells in the bone marrow are considered to have acute B-cell leukemia.

STAGING SYSTEMS AND STAGING PROCEDURES

There are several staging systems commonly used for the SNCL, but the most widely used are those of St. Jude, for children (Table 23–1), and the Ann Arbor scheme, which is generally used in adults with this disease. Another scheme, designed originally in Uganda, is suitable for African patients with Burkitt's lymphoma. The St. Jude system is used for all histologic types of childhood lymphoma and separates patients with limited-stage disease (stage I or II, with one or two masses on one side of the diaphragm or resected intraabdominal disease) from those with extensive intrathoracic or intraabdominal disease (stage III). Patients with bone marrow infiltration greater than 5% and less than 25% on aspirate, and patients with involvement of the CNS, are classified as stage IV. Patients with marrow involvement of 25% or more are considered to have B-cell ALL but should receive therapy according to protocols for SNCL. The staging system for African patients with Burkitt's lymphoma includes a separate stage, AR, for patients with essentially completely resected (at least 90%) intraabdominal disease and does not separate patients with bone marrow involvement or CNS disease into a separate category because involvement of these sites of disease does not appear to be associated with a worse prognosis in African patients.[37] The Ann Arbor system, designed for nodal lymphomas (originally, of course, Hodgkin's disease), is not well suited to patients with SNCL, which is predominantly extranodal. For treatment purposes, many childhood cooperative groups separate patients into two or three risk groups. The French Society of Pediatric Oncology, for example, categorizes children with SNCL into groups A (localized or resected abdominal disease), C, patients with CNS disease or greater than 70% of tumor cells in the bone marrow, and B, all other

patients, whereas others use only low- and high-risk categories.[60, 61]

Staging procedures should be done expeditiously (within 24 to 48 hours) because of the rapidity of tumor growth. Even patients in whom all intraabdominal tumor has been resected may have regrowth within days, necessitating more intensive therapy. A detailed history and physical examination are essential, and peripheral blood, bone marrow, and cerebrospinal fluid examination must always be performed because of the propensity for tumor to involve these sites. Bilateral bone marrow aspirates and biopsies rather than a single aspirate are highly recommended because of the frequent discrepancies between aspirates and biopsies.[62] Abnormal liver function tests may suggest hepatic involvement, and renal function tests (including assessment of urine output) and measurement of the serum uric acid level are essential for determining the presence of uric acid nephropathy as well as the likelihood of the development of a tumor lysis syndrome (see later). Special procedures such as endoscopic examinations may be useful to determine the extent of pharyngeal tumor or upper gastrointestinal bleeding, and to obtain a biopsy. Imaging studies should normally include a gallium scan, which in the SNCLs provides an excellent whole-body image and may reveal previously unsuspected sites of tumor.[63] Spectrophotometry is frequently used to more precisely localize regions of abnormal gallium uptake. Computerized tomography (CT) provides excellent images of the abdomen and chest, although in young people a lack of intraabdominal fat can make interpretation of abdominal CT scans difficult, while adequate filling of the bowel with contrast medium is essential for distinction between bowel loops and tumor.[64] Ultrasonography is most useful when retroperitoneal fat is minimal (e.g., in small children) or sufficient oral contrast material cannot be swallowed, and to delineate testicular masses.[65] Ultrasonography may also be used to evaluate questionable findings on abdominal CT scans. Head CT provides valuable documentation of the extent of disease in patients with head and neck involvement, especially where there is pharyngeal or sinus involvement, but is otherwise not normally indicated, although a baseline study of the brain is often obtained in view of the potential for neurotoxicity of many treatment regimens presently in use. Magnetic resonance imaging (MRI) of the head and neck, chest, abdomen, skeleton, and CNS may be indicated in some circumstances but is not used routinely. Focal bone marrow involvement may be detected by MRI of the axial skeleton, but there is no evidence that this is of importance to the choice of treatment or outcome. Lymphangiography is not routinely recommended because of the predominantly extranodal sites of disease, and bone scan usually adds little to the gallium scan in detecting bone involvement. Radionuclide liver and spleen scans also appear to add little to modern computerized tomograms and ultrasonographic images, while positron emission tomography, although of theoretical value in confirming the presence of viable tumor (e.g., after therapy), is not widely available and has been little studied in SNCL. Contrast radiography is not a routine staging study but is sometimes used in the evaluation of a patient with abdominal pain. Plain radiographs are useful in evaluating potential sites of bony disease or sinus involvement, but like contrast radiography, have largely been superseded by CT.

Lactate dehydrogenase and interleukin-2 levels provide objective correlates of tumor volume[55-58] and are particularly valuable in comparing the mean tumor burdens of one series of patients with those of another. Such measurements should generally be included in the evaluation of the patient at initial presentation. Staging laparotomy is not performed in patients with SNCL, but information derived from a diagnostic laparotomy may provide valuable information.

MANAGEMENT

GENERAL CONSIDERATIONS

Because of the extremely rapid growth rate of SNCL, patients may present with a variety of life-threatening complications arising from the physical encroachment of tumor masses on vital structures, or from the large volume of tumor present. Such complications include airway obstruction, cardiac tamponade or arrhythmias, paraplegia, gastrointestinal bleeding, obstruction or perforation of the bowel, renal outflow tract obstruction, superior (rare) or inferior vena caval obstruction, and raised intracranial pressure. Patients may present with oliguric renal failure from uric acid nephropathy related to a large tumor burden, sometimes complicated by renal outflow tract obstruction. If uncorrected before chemotherapy, uricosemic renal failure may lead to fatal electrolyte disturbances (Fig. 23–1).

Although immediate interventionary measures may be required in some circumstances, for example, tracheotomy

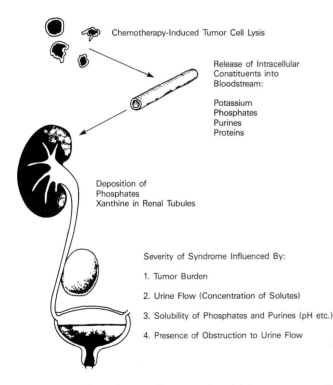

Figure 23–1. Schema depicting the causes of renal failure in patients with a high tumor burden.

Chemotherapy-Induced Tumor Cell Lysis

Release of Intracellular Constituents into Bloodstream:

Potassium
Phosphates
Purines
Proteins

Deposition of Phosphates Xanthine in Renal Tubules

Severity of Syndrome Influenced By:

1. Tumor Burden

2. Urine Flow (Concentration of Solutes)

3. Solubility of Phosphates and Purines (pH etc.)

4. Presence of Obstruction to Urine Flow

or hemodialysis, reduction of tumor bulk must be accomplished as rapidly as possible, and specific therapy should be instituted at the earliest possible time. Surgical intervention should be considered in patients with serious gastrointestinal bleeding before specific treatment to control bleeding, but in patients with widely disseminated or massive tumor, surgical control of bleeding may be extremely difficult to establish. Fortunately, this complication is uncommon. Rarely, enteroenteric or enterovesical fistula may be present or may supervene after chemotherapy-induced tumor lysis. Surgical correction, in such cases, may be best delayed until chemotherapeutic control of tumor has been established and the patient is in a recovery phase from myelosuppression. Ureteric obstruction (rarely, urethral obstruction) is best managed by hemodialysis (to normalize serum electrolyte, uric acid, urea, and creatinine levels) followed by appropriate chemotherapy. The use of ureteral stents or nephrostomy tubes is not recommended unless there is no alternative, because of the risk of ureteric perforation or urinary leakage.

Venous compression within the abdomen secondary to massive intraabdominal tumor may give rise to several complications. Intraluminal thrombosis may result, necessitating consideration of anticoagulation or physical containment of thrombus (e.g., an inferior vena cava filter) to prevent pulmonary embolus. Anticoagulation can be hazardous because of the accompanying risk of gastrointestinal bleeding from involvement of bowel, or the presence of thrombocytopenia from bone marrow involvement or chemotherapy. In addition, anticoagulation by oral drugs is difficult to control when potentially hepatotoxic chemotherapeutic agents, for example, methotrexate, are to be administered, and less rapidly reversible, so that heparin is the drug of choice if anticoagulation is necessary. Apart from the risk of embolus, major venous or lymphatic obstruction may lead to marked edema or ascites and difficulty in establishing an adequate diuresis before and during the initial chemotherapy (see later).

HYPERURICEMIA AND THE ACUTE TUMOR LYSIS SYNDROME

The extremely high growth fraction and cell turnover rate of the SNCL has the potential for the development of renal complications resulting from the increased solute burden on the kidneys. The likelihood that uric acid nephropathy will occur before or immediately after institution of chemotherapy, leading ultimately to renal failure (the so-called "acute tumor lysis syndrome") (see Fig. 23–1), correlates directly with the tumor burden.[66, 67] This syndrome, which was originally recognized as sudden death from acute hyperkalemia in patients undergoing induction therapy,[68] does not occur in patients with completely resected disease or low tumor burdens.

Whereas it is important to initiate specific therapy as soon as possible, starting chemotherapy in the presence of hyperuricemia and impaired urinary output is likely to result in the death of the patient, probably from a sudden increase in serum potassium levels, because potassium released from tumor cells cannot be excreted efficiently in the absence of an adequate urine flow. Therefore, the biochemical abnormalities must be corrected and a good urine flow established (or hemodialysis instituted) before the initiation of specific therapy. This period of biochemical correction should not exceed 24 to 48 hours at most. Reduction of serum uric acid levels to normal can usually be accomplished within this time by alkaline diuresis and allopurinol administration (uricase is an alternative to allopurinol in Europe) in all patients except those with additional renal compromise due to ureteric obstruction, or rarely, massive involvement of the kidneys by tumor. In such circumstances hemodialysis may be required before chemotherapy. In this case, chemotherapy should be commenced after the completion of a period of hemodialysis, when biochemical parameters are close to normal.

In all patients with a high tumor burden it is imperative to maintain a high urine flow (200 to 250 mL/m^2/hr in patients at highest risk) for the first few days after the initiation of chemotherapy to ensure that the high solute burden created by tumor lysis can be accommodated without the intratubular deposition of oxypurines and phosphates, a consequence of exceeding their solubility in urine. Because of relatively poor solubility of phosphates in alkaline urine, it is preferable to maintain the urine pH at about 7 and to not administer bicarbonate during chemotherapy. At this pH, uric acid is some 10 to 12 times more soluble (solubility is some 150 mg/L at pH 5) and xanthine more than twice as soluble (solubility at pH 5 is some 50 mg/L) than at pH 5. The solubility of hypoxanthine differs little at either pH (140 to 150 mg/L). Allopurinol should be given at high dosage, for example, 10 mg/kg, a dose that will ensure that a significant proportion of purine metabolites is excreted as xanthine and hypoxanthine. It is not advisable to completely prevent uric acid production, because of its much greater solubility than the other oxypurines at pH 7. The objective of allopurinol therapy is to increase the total amount of oxypurine that can be excreted in a given volume of urine rather than to prevent uric acid formation. Clearly, the establishment of a high urine flow is imperative in patients with a high tumor burden to decrease the risk of deposition of xanthine and oxyxanthines in the renal tubules.

Because acute hyperkalemia may occur within hours of starting therapy, potassium supplements should be avoided shortly before and during the first few days of therapy unless there is significant hypokalemia. Ideally the patient should be mildly hypokalemic before the commencement of chemotherapy. Hyperkalemia, however, is most unlikely to occur in the presence of a high urine output. Hypocalcemia, a consequence of hyperphosphatemia, should not be treated unless symptomatic, and intravenous calcium chloride should be given with great caution, if at all, because of the risk of extraosseous calcification in the presence of a high serum phosphate level. Systemic alkalinity increases the possibility of symptomatic hypocalcemia, including tetany and cardiac arrhythmias—an additional reason for limiting bicarbonate administration to the period immediately before specific therapy. Rarely, hemodialysis may be required for symptomatic hypocalcemia.

Clearly, maintaining a high urine flow in order to permit excretion of the solute burden and avoidance of major electrolyte disturbances and purine deposition in the kidney is the key to the management of the tumor lysis syndrome. If this cannot be accomplished, rapid progression of biochemical abnormalities will occur, necessitating urgent hemodialysis. However, the presence of serous effusions (ascites, and sometimes pleural effusions) or even limb edema from venous and/or lymphatic obstruction may complicate the management of the acute tumor lysis syndrome. In such patients vigorous hydration is complicated by weight gain and an inappropriately low urine flow. This situation can usually be managed by the judicious use of diuretics (furosemide alone or in combination with chlorothiazides) and careful monitoring of the central venous pressure or, better, pulmonary wedge venous pressure. However, if an acceptable urine output cannot be maintained, hemodialysis should be instituted. Patients at high risk for the acute tumor lysis syndrome or who require intensive monitoring for any reason are much better managed in a critical care unit.

In addition to hydration, the French and German cooperative group protocols call for the use of a "prephase," that is, low-dose chemotherapy given a week before initiation of the major induction regimen in the hope that tumor lysis will be more controlled. No objective data exist that demonstrate the superiority of this approach over hyperhydration, nor have data been presented that demonstrate that the rate of tumor lysis is slower when low-dose chemotherapy is administered, but this approach is clearly effective in the overall management of patients.

MANAGEMENT OF NEUROLOGIC EMERGENCIES

The primary neurologic emergencies encountered in patients with SNCLs include paraplegia, cranial nerve or nerve plexus palsies, meningeal infiltration, and intracerebral tumor. Radiation is no longer considered appropriate therapy for any of these problems (with the possible exception of intracerebral tumor), since there is no evidence that this approach is superior to chemotherapy in rapidly reversing the acute problem. In fact radiation is probably an inferior modality for the treatment of the SNCLs and carries an attendant risk of additional toxicities. Reversal of neurologic complications (including paraplegia) has been observed frequently in African Burkitt's lymphoma with chemotherapy alone,[37] and the tradition of emergency irradiation is being less and less adhered to in the United States and Europe.

CHOICE OF THERAPEUTIC MODALITY

The primary therapeutic modality for the SNCLs is chemotherapy, regardless of stage or sites of disease. Radiation may be considered in patients with testicular or intracerebral disease, but even in these circumstances, there is no evidence (when optimal chemotherapy is used) that radiation adds therapeutic benefit, although it certainly adds toxicity. With the most effective regimens available today, 90% to 100% of patients with limited disease and 80% to 90% of patients with more extensive disease can be expected to be cured. Patients with CNS disease may have a slightly worse prognosis. Surgery appeared, in an earlier era, to have a role in the treatment of patients with completely resectable abdominal tumors,[36, 69] although in recent years, the improvements in survival have confused this issue; since patients with extensive, unresectable intra-abdominal disease enjoy an 80% to 90% cure rate with the best available therapy, the advantage of attempting to resect intraabdominal disease is not clear. There can be no doubt that the majority of patients with resectable disease have a somewhat lower tumor burden than those with unresectable disease, making it difficult to demonstrate that resection itself provides a survival advantage. In practice, resection of small tumors in the abdomen is usually performed at the time of the diagnostic procedure. The decision whether to resect tumors of relatively large size, but of such distribution as to be resectable (e.g., a large mass arising from bowel or ovary), is more difficult. Such a decision may have to be made at the diagnostic laparotomy before a definitive diagnosis has been made, and resection is then more likely to be undertaken. If a diagnosis of SNCL is highly likely, then a decision to resect disease must be made on the basis of the extent of surgery required and the potential immediate and late surgical risks. Once the diagnosis has been made, attempts to resect intraabdominal disease are not usually made when a treatment protocol of known high efficacy is to be used. There are several reasons for this. Resectability is usually not possible to judge on the basis of imaging studies alone, so that the patient may undergo a futile major surgical procedure immediately before chemotherapy with a consequent delay in the initiation of therapy (although this should rarely be more than a few days) and its potential for increasing morbidity in the first cycle of therapy. Indeed, because of the rapid growth rate of SNCL, unless chemotherapy is instituted within a very few days of surgery, there is a significant possibility of tumor regrowth, again rendering the procedure pointless. There are also theoretical considerations that mitigate against a high degree of enthusiasm for attempting to resect large tumors even if technically feasible; if the reason that patients with a large tumor burden have a worse prognosis (or at least, did so in the recent past) is that there is a greater likelihood that chemotherapy-resistant cells (resulting from mutation) will be present, such resistant cells may also be present in microscopic residual disease. If risk-adapted therapy is used such that patients with resected disease are treated with less therapy, gross resection of tumor would mean that the patient would be treated as a low-risk patient and therefore actually be put at higher risk of recurrence than if he or she were treated with a more intensive regimen designed for high-risk patients. The latter consideration leads to the recommendation that even if a large tumor mass is completely resected, in the absence of new information, patients should be treated with a regimen designed for patients with a high tumor burden.

GENERAL PRINCIPLES OF CHEMOTHERAPY OF THE SMALL NONCLEAVED CELL LYMPHOMAS

The significantly lower response rates and very low cure rates achieved in the 1960s with single agents dictates that all patients should be treated with drug combinations. Although the earliest combination treatment regimens used in African patients were of short duration,[70, 71] and some patients in the United States were treated with regimens based on these results,[72] most treatment protocols—extrapolated, presumably, from the need for long-duration therapy in ALL—were of much longer duration (in excess of a year).[73, 74] More recently, there has been a powerful

movement to return to short-duration regimens, although for high-risk patients these are much more intensive than those used in an earlier era. In addition to greater efficacy, such regimens have many advantages—the patient is sooner able to return to a normal lifestyle, and, since cumulative doses of individual drugs are low, the risk of late effects, including infertility and second malignancies, is likely to be less. It will be some years, however, before the true toxic cost of such regimens can be accurately assessed. The financial cost of short-duration, intensive therapy remains high, because during therapy a high proportion of patients develop febrile episodes that necessitate additional in-hospital time and the use of expensive antibiotics. Nonetheless, the total cost of therapy is likely to be lower than that of long-duration regimens, particularly if colony-stimulating factors can be demonstrated to lessen the incidence of febrile episodes, documented infections, and the time in hospital.

Because the SNCLs are very rapidly growing tumors, successive treatment cycles should be begun as soon as possible. CNS prophylaxis is an essential component of therapy, the only possible exception to this being patients with minimal disease, for example, stage I disease or completely resected intraabdominal disease, in whom CNS spread rarely occurs. Intrathecal therapy with methotrexate and cytarabine (ara-C) is used, supplemented, particularly in patients with extensive disease, by intravenous infusions of high doses of S-phase-specific agents such as methotrexate and ara-C. Radiation of the cranium or craniospinal axis has not been shown to have an advantage over chemotherapeutic CNS prophylactic therapy, although it has been associated with significant intellectual impairment and other late effects. In some studies cranial radiation has not provided adequate CNS prophylaxis—indeed, recurrence in the CNS has been observed during or shortly after CNS radiation,[75] whereas a combination of intrathecal therapy and high-dose S-phase-specific agents is highly effective.[33–35, 75] Thus, there is no justification for using cranial irradiation as prophylaxis against CNS spread. Whether intraventricular therapy, while clearly not necessary for CNS prophylaxis, may have a role in the treatment of overt CNS disease remains unknown.

It has repeatedly been demonstrated that treatment protocols based on the principles used for treatment of ALL, such as the LSA_2L_2 and BFM (Berlin-Frankfurt-Münster) 75/81 protocols are suboptimal for the treatment of SNCLs.[32, 76] Combination chemotherapy regimens designed for children with SNCL, consisting of intensive doses of alkylating agents (cyclophosphamide, sometimes alternating with ifosfamide) given in combination with other active agents (especially methotrexate, vincristine, anthracyclines, epipodophyllotoxins, and ara-C (Figs. 23–2 and 23–3), have been shown to be highly effective for patients with SNCL, whether adults or children. With these protocols, overall survival rates of 80% to 90% have been reported.[33–35] Protocols designed for adults with diffuse aggressive lymphomas appear to be inferior to such treatment regimens.[77, 78] Most protocols include cyclophosphamide in doses of at least 1 g/m² and either high (3 to 8 g/m²) or intermediate-dose methotrexate as well as intrathecal methotrexate and often, intrathecal Ara-C. Most also include an anthracycline, although a recent CCSG study was unable to demonstrate any advantage to the inclusion of daunomycin

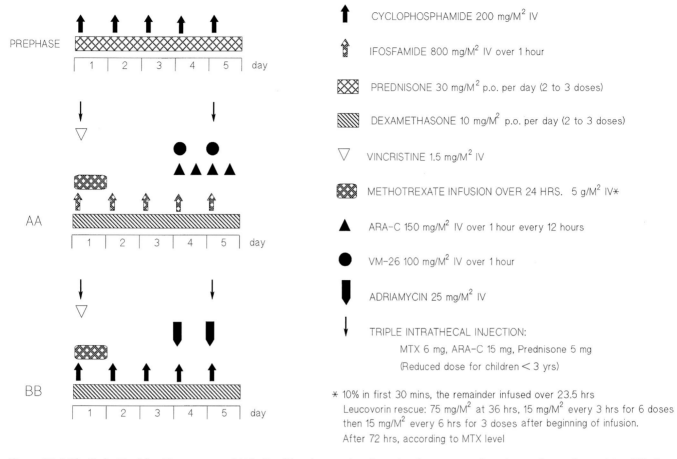

PREPHASE

AA

BB

CYCLOPHOSPHAMIDE 200 mg/M² IV

IFOSFAMIDE 800 mg/M² IV over 1 hour

PREDNISONE 30 mg/M² p.o. per day (2 to 3 doses)

DEXAMETHASONE 10 mg/M² p.o. per day (2 to 3 doses)

VINCRISTINE 1.5 mg/M² IV

METHOTREXATE INFUSION OVER 24 HRS. 5 g/M² IV✱

ARA–C 150 mg/M² IV over 1 hour every 12 hours

VM–26 100 mg/M² IV over 1 hour

ADRIAMYCIN 25 mg/M² IV

TRIPLE INTRATHECAL INJECTION:
MTX 6 mg, ARA–C 15 mg, Prednisone 5 mg
(Reduced dose for children < 3 yrs)

✱ 10% in first 30 mins, the remainder infused over 23.5 hrs
Leucovorin rescue: 75 mg/M² at 36 hrs, 15 mg/M² every 3 hrs for 6 doses
then 15 mg/M² every 6 hrs for 3 doses after beginning of infusion.
After 72 hrs, according to MTX level

Figure 23–2. The Berlin-Frankfurt-Münster protocol 86 for B-cell lymphomas. The schema for administration of initial cytoreductive therapy (V) and blocks AA and BB for patients with bone marrow involvement are shown. A total of four therapy cycles—two each of AA and BB are administered after the prephase (V). Patients with all other stages were treated with a slightly modified protocol in which intermediate-dose (500 mg/m²) instead of high-dose methotrexate was given, vincristine was not included, and intrathecal drug doses were twice as high. MTX, methotrexate. (Adapted from Reiter A, Schrappe M, Parwaresch R, et al: Non-Hodgkin's lymphomas of childhood and adolescence: Results of a treatment stratified for biological subtypes and stage. A report of the BFM group. J Clin Oncol 1995; 13:359; and Reiter A, Schrappe M, Ludwig W-D, et al: Favorable outcome of B-cell acute lymphoblastic leukemia in childhood: A report of three consecutive studies of the BFM group. Blood 1992; 80:2471.)

in the COMP protocol.[79] Additional drugs currently being used in Société Française d'Oncologie Pédiatrique (SFOP), BFM, and NCI protocols for high-risk patients include etoposide (VP-16), high-dose Ara-C, and ifosfamide.[33–35] Although most treatment protocols incorporate a corticosteroid, this practice is based more on tradition and their lack of myelotoxicity than on either theoretical considerations or empirical experience. Corticosteroids are not very effective agents for B-cell tumors, and the additional immunosuppressive effect they have is not to be taken lightly in the context of the very intensive and immunosuppressive regimens now being used for patients with SNCL. Indeed, the degree of immunosuppression encountered in these protocols may not be much less than that experienced by patients undergoing the massive therapy preceding bone marrow transplantation.[80]

In fact, bone marrow transplantation per primum (i.e., in first remission) has been considered as an option for patients with very extensive disease—largely because of the earlier poor results obtained. The disadvantages of this approach are the limited availability of matched allogeneic donors, the theoretical risk of reinfusion of the patients' own tumor cells

if autologous marrow is used, and the specialized facilities and staff required to conduct such an intensive and potentially toxic treatment approach optimally (mortality rates in the region of 10% can be expected from the treatment alone). A pilot study of marrow transplantation in children with high-risk SNCL[81] and a recent retrospective analysis of adult patients treated with this approach in France[82] do not indicate any advantage to this approach and indeed, suggest that the survival rate in patients treated with bone marrow transplantation in first remission may actually be worse. This suggests that the chemotherapy regimens used immediately before transplantation, even though of very high dose, are inferior, in terms of tumor cell kill, to those used in patients not subjected to transplantation.

USE OF COLONY-STIMULATING FACTORS IN THERAPY

The use of very intensive treatment regimens in which successive cycles of therapy are rapidly administered suggests that colony-stimulating factors (CSFs) should have an important role in ameliorating toxicity and increasing received dose intensity. Although this could well be the case, it should not be assumed that this will be so. Granulocyte colony-stimulating factor (G-CSF) and granulocyte/macrophage colony-stimulating factor (GM-CSF), for example, do not increase the rate of platelet recovery, and GM-CSF, in particular, may even impair recovery from thrombocytopenia.[83] In addition, nonmyeloid toxicities may not have recovered fully by the time of granulocyte recovery. Thus, depending upon the policies adopted with regard to initiation of each successive treatment cycle, more rapid recovery of the granulocyte count does not necessarily translate into the more rapid commencement of the next cycle of therapy. Indeed, in a recent randomized study at the NCI, there was no difference in the duration of cycles in which GM-CSF was administered compared with those in which it was not.[35] To a degree, the value of colony-stimulating factors may prove to be protocol-dependent, and there is a need for more controlled clinical trials to assess their role in the treatment of SNCL.

RELAPSE PATTERN AND PREDICTION OF OUTCOME

The relapse pattern of patients with SNCL has remained remarkably constant over time in spite of marked differences in the duration and intensity of therapy; relapse occurs within some 8 months from the commencement of therapy or does not occur at all. Exceptions to this exist only in African patients,[37] in whom a very small number of relapses occur later than a year from the onset of treatment—relapses as late as 5 years have been reported—and in occasional patients with underlying human immunodeficiency virus (HIV) infection (few survive long enough to experience late relapse). Both sets of patients belong to populations at high risk for the development of SNCL, and it is possible that such late relapses represent the reinduction of a second SNCL. Indeed, in one HIV patient an apparent recurrent tumor occurring 3 years after the first was shown, on the basis of molecular findings, to be of different clonal origin

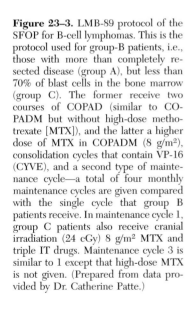

Figure 23–3. LMB-89 protocol of the SFOP for B-cell lymphomas. This is the protocol used for group-B patients, i.e., those with more than completely resected disease (group A), but less than 70% of blast cells in the bone marrow (group C). The former receive two courses of COPAD (similar to COPADM but without high-dose methotrexate [MTX]), and the latter a higher dose of MTX in COPADM (8 g/m²), consolidation cycles that contain VP-16 (CYVE), and a second type of maintenance cycle—a total of four monthly maintenance cycles are given compared with the single cycle that group B patients receive. In maintenance cycle 1, group C patients also receive cranial irradiation (24 cGy) 8 g/m² MTX and triple IT drugs. Maintenance cycle 3 is similar to 1 except that high-dose MTX is not given. (Prepared from data provided by Dr. Catherine Patte.)

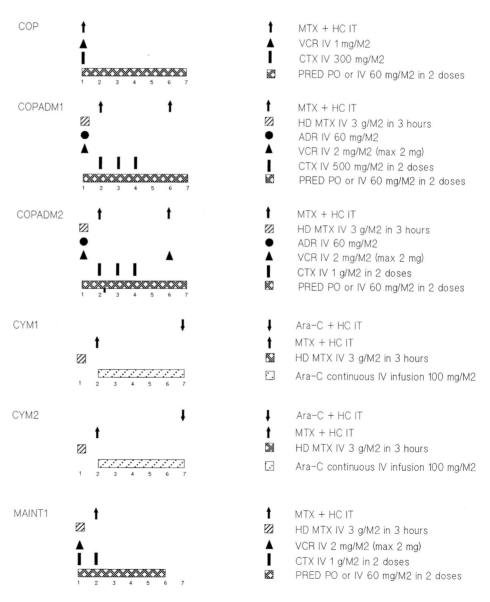

from the first lymphoma.[84] Similarly, in African patients, some late relapses have also been shown, on the basis of glucose phosphate dehydrogenase isoenzymes in heterozygous females, to be of separate clonal origin.[85] The biologic basis for the uniformly early relapse pattern in patients who do not belong to the high-risk groups is unknown, but it would seem probable that the 8-month time period represents that required for a drug-resistant cell clone to become clinically apparent. This is consistent with the potential doubling time of African Burkitt's lymphoma, which is approximately 24 hours (the measured doubling time of skin lesions is about 3 days), and the very high growth fraction, which approaches 100%.[16] This suggests that tumor cannot lie "dormant." If a cell clone were to double every 24 hours, a single cell would give rise to more than 10^6 cells in less than 3 weeks, and to more than 10^{12} cells in less than 6 weeks. Thus, even if the average actual doubling time were significantly greater than 3 days, it would still be feasible for a lymphoma cell clone resistant to primary therapy to become apparent as recurrent tumor within a few months. Regardless of the biologic considerations, patients with SNCL can be considered cured if they have not relapsed within a period of some 8 to 10 months from the time of presentation. This means that quite accurate assessment of the results of clinical studies can be made in a much shorter time than is the case for most other neoplasms.

CHEMOTHERAPY REGIMENS AND RESULTS OF TREATMENT

Patients with Limited Disease. Patients with limited disease, that is, localized or completely resected intraabdominal disease (stages I and II, St. Jude, and A and AR, NCI) have an excellent prognosis (90% to 100% cure rate) and require less intensive therapy than patients with more extensive disease. Most protocols use drug combinations that include cyclophosphamide, vincristine, methotrexate, and sometimes doxorubicin (Adriamycin), with or without prednisone. A randomized clinical trial conducted by the CCSG demonstrated that 6 months is not inferior to 18 months of therapy,[86] but recent protocols conducted in France, Germany, and the United States are achieving as good results as those obtained in this CCSG study with only two or three cycles of therapy and a treatment duration of 2 to 3 months.[33–35] In the BFM protocols 81/83 and 83/86, for example, patients with limited disease received only 8 and 6 weeks of therapy, respectively, yet achieved survival in excess of 90%,[34] whereas almost 100% of patients achieved disease-free survival with the SFOP LMB 89 protocol for limited disease, which includes two cycles of therapy without CNS prophylaxis.[33] Similarly, 100% of a smaller number of early-stage patients treated with the current NCI protocol remain disease-free with a median followup of some 24 months.[35] Current U.S. childhood cooperative group protocols are also moving to very short duration therapies for patients with limited disease.

Radiation therapy does not play a role in the treatment of localized disease. A randomized study conducted by the Pediatric Oncology Group (POG) in which the role of radiation, in addition to chemotherapy, in patients with localized tumor was examined showed no difference in outcome,[87] while limited-stage patients treated without radiation therapy on a number of single-arm studies conducted in the last decade have also enjoyed excellent disease-free survival rates.[34, 35, 57, 88, 89]

Patients with Extensive Disease. Recent intensive short-duration treatment protocols applied to patients with unresectable abdominal disease without bone marrow or CNS involvement (the majority of patients) have resulted in cure rates between 80% and 90%.[33–35, 89] Although patients with bone marrow involvement used to have a significantly worse prognosis,[33, 57, 88, 90] the results in this group of patients are now similar to those in patients with stage III disease (Table 23–2).[33–35] Several clinical trials attest to the lack of a need for prolonged therapy. For example, the SFOP compared 4 months of therapy with 7 months of therapy and found no difference in outcome.[33] The BFM 83/86 protocol, in which even high-risk patients received 12 weeks of therapy, achieved better results than longer-duration therapy provided by earlier CCSG,[32, 74] NCI,[57] and SFOP [89] protocols (see Fig. 23–3). In the United States, the preliminary results of the HiC-COM protocol of the Dana Farber Cancer Center,[91] which has a 2-month therapy duration, appear to be similar to the earlier SFOP (LMB-0281) results,[89] whereas the results of the current NCI protocol,[33] which comprises a total of four cycles of two alternating regimens, lasting approximately 3 months, are similar to those of the more recent SFOP (LMB-89) protocol.[33, 60] In the SFOP's LMB-0281 protocol, 16 of 21 (76%) patients with bone marrow disease (but without CNS involvement) achieved long-term survival.[89] No difference was apparent between patients with less than or more than 25% of tumor cells in the bone marrow, but patients with CNS disease had a poor prognosis (19% disease free at 2 years). Using the same protocol, investigators in Lyon also obtained excellent results but noted that patients with extensive, multiorgan involvement in the abdomen (often with additional disease outside the abdomen) had a poor outcome—less than 40% achieved long-term disease-free survival.[92] In the more recent SFOP LMB-89 protocol (see Fig. 23–3), this result appears to have been significantly improved—80% to 90% of patients with extensive (>70%) bone marrow involvement are disease-free at 2 years.[60]

Table 23–2. Results of Various Protocols Used in the Treatment of Patients (Adults and Children) with Small Noncleaved Cell Lymphoma

Protocol	No. of Patients	Stage III (%)	Stage IV (%)	Reference
HiC-COM	20	92	50	Schwann et al[91]
SFOP LMB-84°	201	80	68	Patte et al[33]
BFM 81, 84, 86	150	74	68, 78†	Reiter et al[34]
SFOP 89	181	87	85, 87†	Patte et al[110]
89-C-41	42	97‡	80	Magrath et al[35]
81-01 and 84-30§	26	91‡	24	Lopez et al[77]
L-2, L-10, and L-17§	29	69‡	41	Straw et al[111]
Vanderbilt§	20	—	60°°	McMaster et al[94]

°Excludes patients with central nervous system disease at presentation.
†Stage IV and acute B-cell leukemia provided separately.
‡Includes stages I and II.
§Ann Arbor staging system.
°°Includes all stages, although 16 were stage IV.
SFOP, Société Française d'Oncologie Pédiatrique; BFM, Berlin-Frankfurt-Münster.

Adult patients with SNCLs have, in general, been treated with regimens designed primarily for intermediate-grade lymphomas, and in these patient groups they represent very much a minority, such that it has usually been difficult or impossible to obtain a clear idea of their prognosis. In general, the consensus has been that these patients do poorly. However, identical results (50% to 60% long-term survival) were obtained in adults and children with the NCI protocol 77-04,[57] a result that has been confirmed with more recent analysis of these same patients, and by use of a modified version of this protocol at Stanford University.[93] Similar results were obtained with a protocol designed specifically for patients with poor-prognosis NHL, used in adult patients with SNCL at Vanderbilt University.[94] That there is no difference in the prognosis of adults and children when treated with the same regimens has been confirmed by the recent excellent results achieved in both adults and children with the SFOP and recent NCI (89-C-41) protocols (overall survival approximately 90%).[35, 82]

All major protocols currently in use for the treatment of patients with SNCL include cyclophosphamide, vincristine, and high-dose methotrexate. Such protocols also usually include an anthracycline, but often at a very low cumulative dose. These drugs are complemented by a several other drugs, depending on the protocol in question. Ifosfamide, high-dose ara-C, and an epipodophyllotoxin are included in BFM and NCI protocols, and the value of these agents, which have been shown to be effective in patients with recurrent tumor,[95–97] in primary therapy is presently the subject of a POG trial. Occasionally, protocols include cisplatin.[98] Although the role of each agent is difficult to evaluate in combination regimens, the most important considerations are outcome and toxicity. Thus, in a maximally effective regimen, unless untoward toxicity (whether short term or long term) that can be assigned to a particular drug is encountered, there may be little point in conducting numerous randomized studies to address this issue.

The prognosis of patients with CNS disease, the patient group with the worst outcome, has also improved markedly in recent years. Although CNS disease has been considered, in the past, to be an obstacle to cure,[99] the relatively good survival of African patients with CNS disease, at both presentation and at relapse, when treated with intrathecal and systemic chemotherapy, has always argued against this dogma.[37] It seems likely that the differences in prognosis between African patients and patients in Europe and the United States relate more to differences in the associated disease sites than to the CNS disease per se.[53] In African patients, CNS disease is frequently associated with limited systemic disease, for example, jaw tumor only.[37] In Europe and the United States, on the other hand, CNS disease is almost always associated with extensive systemic disease, particularly bone marrow involvement.[53] This suggests that increased intensity of systemic therapy may be at least as important as improved CNS-directed therapy in the treatment of these patients. Indeed, the recent trend toward adding high-dose ara-C and increasing the dose of high-dose methotrexate administered in otherwise standard protocols, thus providing both improved CNS and systemic therapy, has been associated with markedly improved results. In the current SFOP protocol (LMB-89), for example, in patients with the highest tumor burdens (with or without CNS

disease), who are treated with high-dose ara-C and high-dose MTX (8 g/m²) followed by cranial irradiation, an event-free survival of 72% has been achieved.[60] It must be stated that there is no evidence that the addition of radiation had any role in the production of this result, and the combination of these drugs along with radiation could prove to be quite neurotoxic. Even without radiation, the use of intensive intrathecal therapy and high-dose systemic ara-C and methotrexate increases the risk of neurotoxicity, as exemplified by the results of a recent POG protocol.[100] It may be better to reserve CNS irradiation for the rare patient with intraparenchymal brain disease, although even then an important role of radiation in overall therapy is assumed rather than demonstrated (an assumption that could be incorrect, given the relative radioresistance of the SNCLs).

CNS prophylaxis is indicated in almost all patients with SNCLs and usually includes a combination of intrathecal ara-C and methotrexate, coupled with intermediate- or high-dose methotrexate. Patients with totally resected abdominal disease and stage I patients, who rarely develop CNS disease, are sometimes not given CNS prophylaxis—as for example in the current SFOP protocol (LMB-89). To date, the excellent outcome of this group of patients justifies this policy. Although occasional patients with early-stage disease do develop CNS recurrence, the risk of patients with very limited stage disease may be no greater than the very small risk of developing a major CNS toxicity (necrotizing encephalomyelitis, blindness, or paraplegia) from intrathecal therapy, and it may prove possible to salvage rare cases of CNS recurrence in patients treated with such minimal therapy.

TREATMENT OF RECURRENT SMALL NONCLEAVED CELL LYMPHOMA

In general, patients with recurrent disease after modern, intensive chemotherapy have a low chance of survival, but, remarkably, some patients whose tumors recur do achieve long-term survival after a salvage regimen. Most patients are currently treated with a different chemotherapy regimen, often including cisplatin, since they have usually not been exposed to this agent. Patients who have a significant response are usually then treated with very high dose chemotherapy followed by autologous bone marrow transplantation.[101, 102] There is no doubt that a successful outcome of intensive salvage therapy can be predicted according to the previous response to treatment. Patients with relapse responsive to conventional approaches have a much better prognosis with high-dose therapy, and a relapse-free survival in this patient group of close to 50% has been reported, although these patients were selected on the basis of the lack of marrow involvement. Patients with recurrent tumor that is resistant to conventional therapy have an extremely poor prognosis—no survivors after 9 months were observed in the Lyon study.[101, 102] Patients with a partial response to primary treatment (i.e., with residual disease, but no progressive disease) appear to have a good prognosis with very high-dose regimens.

Interestingly, the results of the Parma study, in which

patients with recurrent NHL who achieve a marked response to a salvage regimen (DHAP, consisting of dexamethazone, high dose ara-C, and Platinol) were randomized to receive an autologous marrow transplant or to continue with the same salvage regimen, did not, when first reported, show a significant difference between the two arms of the study, although followup at that time was very short.[103] All patients included in this study were selected both by virtue of the absence of bone marrow involvement at relapse and by their response to the salvage regimen (DHAP). Recent results have demonstrated that in this group of patients (most of whom had diffuse large cell lymphoma), bone marrow transplantation was superior to conventional therapy. Certainly, long-term survival in patients with relapsed Burkitt's lymphoma treated with high-dose therapy and an autologous bone marrow transplant have been described.[104] Major responses to DHAP in patients with SNCL who relapse after an intensive regimen such as those discussed earlier, however, is unlikely, such that few patients would be eligible for autologous transplantation. Moreover, in considering options for patients with SNCL, one must take into consideration the fact that the Parma regimen includes patients with several different types of lymphoma.

A group of patients that appears to do well with high-dose salvage therapy, including marrow transplantation, is that in which CNS relapse occurs. In one series of 10 such patients, 5 patients were reported to achieve long-term survival.[105] However, a similar fraction of patients with isolated CNS relapse have also achieved long-term survival when treated with conventional systemic therapy and intrathecal chemotherapy.[53]

Although very high dose therapies have resulted in the survival of a fraction of patients who relapse, it remains unclear whether this represents the best approach to the treatment of recurrent disease. Autologous bone marrow transplantation carries the theoretical risk of reinfusion of malignant cells, and although considerable effort has been put into purging bone marrow with drugs or monoclonal antibodies, a definite advantage to such procedures has not yet been demonstrated. Allogeneic transplantation has the theoretical advantage of a graft-versus-tumor effect, but the disadvantage of a higher rate of toxic complications, including graft-versus-host disease, and overall, it appears that the outcome is similar with either source of hematopoietic rescue.[106, 107] Further, the latter is hindered by the limited availability of suitable donors. In addition, the results of bone marrow transplantation programs are artificially boosted by patient selection. Perhaps the most telling argument that the role of bone marrow transplantation needs to be reassessed is the findings of both a recent retrospective study and prospective studies that patients who are treated by such an approach during the first remission do not appear to have as good a survival rate as patients treated with the best conventional regimens.[82, 108] Although it may be appropriate to explore potentially better conditioning regimens, it could also be argued that improving conventional salvage regimens is as valid an approach to the treatment of the now rather small fraction of patients who relapse.

Limited information exists with respect to the efficacy of biologic response modifiers in patients with SNCL who relapse.[109] In general, such patients have a very short anticipated life span—particularly if they have not responded to a salvage regimen—such that they are relatively uncommonly entered into either phase I and phase II clinical trials or into trials that are exploring the efficacy of biologic response modifiers.

FUTURE CONSIDERATIONS

The treatment of NHLs—in both children and adults—has improved greatly in the last 15 years. The best reported results indicate that today 80% to 90% of all such patients can be cured when treated optimally. This result has largely been achieved by the use of intensive combination drug therapy and prophylactic therapy directed against the development of CNS involvement. Yet there is an ever-present challenge to improve the results of treatment even further, and to lessen its toxicity and inconvenience. In this regard, we are likely to see the increasing use of cloned CSFs, particularly combinations of factors, although, as discussed previously, their role in the therapy of the SNCL is presently unclear.

Targeted therapy, for example, with anti-idiotypic or other monoclonal antibodies, perhaps coupled to drug, toxin, or radionuclide, has been under study for a number of years, yet, although some responses have been seen, this approach is still in its infancy. The role of such approaches in the therapy of the NHLs in general, and the SNCLs in particular, is likely to take years to define.

Particularly exciting is the new knowledge of the molecular genetic and resultant biochemical abnormalities that underlie the pathogenesis of the lymphoid neoplasms—an area of research that is particularly advanced with respect to the SNCL (see Chapter 18). This information will soon be utilized in the development of improved diagnostic techniques and identification of prognostic subgroups. It may even prove possible to develop highly specific treatment approaches directed against those very abnormalities that are responsible for the manifestation of the disease as a neoplastic process. Such therapy will, therefore, be truly tumor-specific with promise of minimal toxicity.[110]

REFERENCES

1. Lukes RJ, Collins RD: New approaches to the classification of the lymphomata. Br J Cancer 1975; 31(suppl II):1.
2. National Cancer Institute sponsored study of classifications of non-Hodgkin's lymphoma: Summary and description of a working formulation for clinical usage. Cancer 1982; 49:2112.
3. Rappaport H: Tumors of the Hematopoietic System. Atlas of Tumor Pathology, Section III, Fasc 8. Washington DC, Armed Forces Institute of Pathology, 1966, pp 97–161.
4. Mann RB, Jaffe ES, Braylan RC, et al: Non-endemic Burkitt's lymphoma. N Engl J Med 1976; 295:685.
5. Mclennan ICM, Gray D: Antigen driven selection of virgin and memory B cells. Immunol Rev 1986; 91:61.
6. Harris N, Jaffe E, Stein H, et al: A proposal for an international consensus on the classification of lymphoid neoplasms. Blood 1994; 84:1361.
7. Wilson JF, Kjeldsberg CR, Sposto R, et al: The pathology of non-Hodgkin's lymphoma of childhood: II. Reproducibility and relevance of the histologic classification of "undifferentiated" lymphomas (Burkitt's versus non-Burkitt's). Hum Pathol 1987; 18:1008.

8. Yano T, Van Krieken J, Magrath I, et al: Histogenetic correlations between subcategories of small non-cleaved cell lymphomas. Blood 1992; 79:1282.
9. Sigaux F, Berger R, Bernheim A, et al: Malignant lymphomas with band 8q24 chromosome abnormality: A morphologic continuum extending from Burkitt's to immunoblastic lymphoma. Br J Haematol 1984; 57:393.
10. Bloomfield CD, Arthur DC, Frizzera G, et al: Nonrandom chromosome abnormalities in lymphoma. Cancer Res 1983; 43:2975.
11. Burkitt DP: Geographical distribution. In Burkitt DP, Wright DH (eds): Burkitt's Lymphoma. Edinburgh, Churchill Livingstone, 1970, pp 186–197.
12. Magrath IT: The pathogenesis of Burkitt's lymphoma. Recent Adv Cancer Res 1990; 55:133.
13. Shiramizu B, Barriga F, Neequaye J, et al: Patterns of chromosomal breakpoint location in Burkitt's lymphoma: Relevance to geography and EBV association. Blood 1991; 77:1516.
14. Bhatia K, Gutierrez MI, Huppi K, et al: The pattern of p53 mutations in Burkitt's lymphoma differs from that of solid tumors. Cancer Res 1992; 52:1.
15. Magrath IT, Jain V, Bhatia K: Epstein Barr virus and Burkitt's lymphoma. Semin Cancer Biol 1992; 3:285.
16. Iverson UIOH, Ziegler JL, et al: Cell kinetics of African cases of Burkitt's lymphoma. A preliminary report. Eur J Cancer 1972, 8:305.
17. Davies JNP, Elmes S, Hutt MSR, et al: Cancer in an African Community, 1897–1956. An analysis of the records of Mengo Hospital, Kampala, Uganda: Part 1. Br Med J 1964; 1:259.
18. Burkitt D: A sarcoma involving the jaws in African Children. Br J Surg 1958; 46:218.
19. O'Conor G: Malignant lymphoma in African children: II. A pathological entity. Cancer 1961; 14:270.
20. O'Conor GRH, Smith EB: Childhood lymphoma resembling Burkitt's lymphoma in the United States. Cancer 1965; 18:411.
21. Dorfman RF: Childhood lymphosarcoma in St Louis, Missouri, clinically and histologically resembling Burkitt's lymphoma. Cancer 1965; 18:418.
22. Wright DH: Burkitt's tumor in England. A comparison with childhood lymphosarcoma. Int J Cancer 1966; 1:503–514.
23. Epstein MA, Achong BG, Barr YM: Virus particles in cultured lymphoblasts from Burkitt's lymphoma Burkitt-type lymphoma. Lancet 1964; 1:702.
24. Rosenberg S, Diamond HD, Dargeon HW, Craver LF: Lymphosarcoma in childhood. N Engl J Med 1958; 259:505.
25. Jenkin RDT, Sonley MJ: The management of malignant lymphoma in childhood. In Neoplasia in Childhood. Chicago, Year Book Medical, pp 305–319, 1969.
26. Glatstein E, Kim H, Donaldson S, et al: Non-Hodgkin's lymphoma: VI. Results of treatment in childhood. Cancer 1974; 34:204.
27. Burkitt D: Long term remissions following one and two dose chemotherapy for African lymphoma. Cancer 1967; 20:756.
28. Arseneau JC, Canellos GP, Banks PM, et al: American Burkitt's lymphoma—A clinicopathological study of 30 cases: I. Clinical factors relating to long term survival. Am J Med 1975; 58:314.
29. Olweny, CLM, Katongole-Mbidde E, Otim D, et al: Long-term experience with Burkitt's lymphoma in Uganda. Int J Cancer 1980; 26:261.
30. Wanatabe A, Sullivan MP, Sutow WW, Wilbur JR: Undifferentiated lymphoma, non-Burkitt's type: Meningeal and bone marrow involvement in children. Am J Dis Child 1973; 125:57.
31. Hutter JJ, Favara BE, Nelson M, Holton CP: Non-Hodgkin's lymphoma in children. Correlation of CNS disease with initial presentation. Cancer 1975; 36:2132.
32. Anderson JR, Jenkin DT, Wilson JF, et al: Long-term follow-up of patients treated with COMP or LSA₂L₂ therapy for childhood non-Hodgkin's lymphoma: A report of CCG-551 from the Childrens Cancer Group. J Clin Oncol 1993; 11:1024.
33. Patte C, Philip T, Rodary C, et al: High survival rate in advanced-stage B-cell lymphomas and leukemias without CNS involvement with a short intensive polychemotherapy: Results from the French Pediatric Oncology Society of a randomized trial of 216 children. J Clin Oncol 1991; 9:123.
34. Reiter A, Schrappe M, Parwaresch R, et al: Non-Hodgkin's lymphomas of childhood and adolescence: Results of a treatment stratified for biological subtypes and stage. A report of the BFM group. J Clin Oncol, 1995; 13:359.
35. Magrath IT, Adde M, Shad A, et al: Adults and children with small

noncleaved cell lymphoma have a similar excellent outcome when treated with the same chemotherapy regimen. J Clin Oncol 1996; 14:925.
36. Janus CE, Brennan M, Sariban E, Magrath IT: Surgical resection and limited chemotherapy for abdominal undifferentiated lymphomas. Cancer Treat Rep 1984; 68:599.
37. Magrath IT: African Burkitt's lymphoma: History, biology, clinical features, and treatment. Am J Pediatr Hematol Oncol 1991; 13(2):222.
38. Burkitt DP: General features and facial tumours. In Lymphoma. Burkitt DP, Wright DH (eds): Burkitt's Lymphoma. Edinburgh, Churchill Livingstone, 1970, pp 6–15.
39. Sariban EDA, Magrath IT: Jaw involvement in American Burkitt's lymphoma. Cancer 1984; 53:141.
40. Ladjadj Y, Philip T, Lenoir GM, et al: Abdominal Burkitt-type lymphomas in Algeria. Br J Cancer 1984; 49:503.
41. Hesseling P, Wood RE, Nortje CJ, Mouton S: African Burkitt's lymphoma in the Cape province of South Africa and Namibia. Oral Surg Oral Med Oral Pathol 1989; 68:162.
42. Yagi KI, Rahman El Sheikh A, El Din Abbas K, Prabhu SR: Burkitt's lymphoma in the Sudan. Int J Oral Surg 1984; 13:517.
43. Miyoshi I: Japanese Burkitt's lymphoma. Clinicopathological review of 14 cases. Jpn J Clin Oncol 1983; 13:489.
44. Anaissie E, Geha S, Allam C, et al: Burkitt's lymphoma in the Middle East. A study of 34 cases. Cancer 1985; 56:2539.
45. Suvatte V, Mahasandana C, Tanphaichitr VS, et al: Burkitt's lymphoma in Thai children: An analysis of 25 cases. Southeast Asian J Trop Med Public Health 1983; 14:385.
46. Cavdar CO, Gozdasoglu S, Yavuz G, et al: Burkitt's lymphoma between African and American types in Turkish children in clinical, viral (EBV) and molecular studies. Med Pediatr Oncol 1993; 21:36.
47. Kamunvi F, Njino MJ: Epidemiology of jaw tumours in Nyanza province with special reference to Burkitt's lymphoma: Report of preliminary findings in the Nyanza general hospital, Kisumu, Kenya. East Afr Med J 1985; 62:122.
48. Kitinya JN, Lauren PA: Burkitt's lymphoma on mount Kilimanjaro and in the inland regions of northern Tanzania. East Afr Med J 1982; 59:256.
49. Magrath IT, Ziegler JL: Bone marrow involvement in Burkitt's lymphoma and its relationship to acute B-cell leukemia. Leuk Res 1980; 4:33.
50. Benjamin D, Magrath IT, Douglass EC, Corash LM: Derivation of lymphoma cell lines from microscopically normal bone marrow in patients with undifferentiated lymphomas; evidence of occult bone marrow involvement. Blood 1983; 61:1017.
51. Mangan KF, Rauch AE, Bishop M, et al: Acute lymphoblastic leukemia of Burkitt's type (L-3 ALL) lacking surface immunoglobulin and the 8;14 translocation. Am J Clin Pathol 1985; 83:121.
52. Sariban E, Janus C, Edwards B, Magrath IT: Central nervous system involvement in American Burkitt's lymphoma. J Clin Oncol 1983; 11:677.
53. Haddy TB, Adde MA, Magrath IT: Central nervous system involvement in small non-cleaved cell lymphoma: Is CNS disease per se a poor prognostic sign? J Clin Oncol 1991; 9:1973.
54. Magrath IT, Mugerwa J, Bailey I, et al: Intracerebral Burkitt's lymphoma: Pathology, clinical features and treatment. Q J Med 1974; 43:489.
55. Csako G, Magrath I, Elin R: Serum total and isoenzyme lactate dehydrogenase activity in American Burkitt's lymphoma. Am J Clin Pathol 1982; 78:712.
56. Magrath IT, Lee YJ, Anderson T, et al: Prognostic factors in Burkitt's lymphoma: Importance of total tumor burden. Cancer 1980; 45:1507.
57. Magrath IT, Janus C, Edwards BK, et al: An effective therapy for both undifferentiated (including Burkitt's) lymphomas and lymphoblastic lymphomas in children and young adults. Blood 1984; 63:1102.
58. Wagner DK, Kiwanuka J, Edwards BK, et al: Soluble interleukin-2 receptor level in patients with undifferentiated and lymphoblastic lymphomas: Correlation with survival. J Clin Oncol 1987; 5:1262.
59. Hagberg HKA, Simonsson B: Serum β₂-microglobulin in malignant lymphoma. Cancer 1983; 51:2220.
60. Patte C, Leverger G, Rubie H, et al: High cure rate in B-cell (Burkitt's) leukemia in the LMB 89 protocol of the SFOP (French Pediatric Oncology Society) [Abstract]. Proc Am Soc Clin Oncol 1993; 12:1050.
61. Shad A, Jain V, Magrath I: Small non-cleaved cell lymphomas. In Brian MC, Carbone PP (eds): Current Therapy in Hematology-Oncology, 5th ed. Philadelphia, Decker, 1994, pp 351–359.

62. Haddy TB, Parker RI, Magrath IT: Bone marrow involvement in young patients with non-Hodgkin's lymphoma: The importance of multiple bone marrow samples for accurate staging. Med Pediatr Oncol 1989; 17:418.

63. Sandrock D, Lastoria S, Magrath IT, Neumann RD: The role of gallium scintigraphy in patients with small non-cleaved cell lymphoma. Eur J Nucl Med 1993; 20:119.

64. Krudy AD, Dunnick N, Magrath IT, et al: CT of American Burkitt's lymphoma. Am J Radiol 1981; 136:747.

65. Shawker TH, Dunnick N, Head GL, Magrath IT: Ultrasound evaluation of American Burkitt's lymphoma. J Clin Ultrasound 1979; 7:279.

66. Cohen LF, Balow J, Magrath IT, et al: Acute tumor lysis syndrome: A review of 37 patients with Burkitt's lymphoma. Am J Med 1980; 68:486.

67. Tsokos G, Balow J, Spiegel RJ, Magrath IT: Renal and metabolic complications of undifferentiated and lymphoblastic lymphomas. Medicine 1981; 60:218.

68. Arseneau JC, Bagley CM, Anderson T, Canellos GP: Hyperkalemia, a sequel to chemotherapy of Burkitt's lymphoma. Lancet 1973; 1:10.

69. Magrath IT, Lwanga S, Carswell W, Harrison N: Surgical reduction of tumour bulk in management of abdominal Burkitt's lymphoma. Br Med J 1974; 2:308.

70. Olweny CLM, Katongole-Mbidde E, Kaddu-Mukasa A, et al: Treatment of Burkitt's lymphoma: Randomized clinical trials of single-agent versus combination chemotherapy. Int J Cancer 1976; 17:436.

71. Ziegler J, Magrath IT, Olweny CLM: Cure of Burkitt's lymphoma: 10 year follow-up of 157 Ugandan patients. Lancet 1979; 2:936.

72. Ziegler JL: Treatment results of 54 American patients with Burkitt's lymphoma are similar to the African experience. N Engl J Med 1977; 297:75.

73. Wollner N, Burchenal JH, Lieberman PH, et al: Non-Hodgkin's lymphoma in children. A comparative study of two modalities of therapy. Cancer 1976; 37:123.

74. Anderson JR, Wilson JF, Jenkin DT, et al: Childhood non-Hodgkin's lymphoma. The results of a randomized therapeutic trial comparing a 4-drug regimen (COMP) with a 10-drug regimen (LSA₂L₂). N Engl J Med 1983; 308:559.

75. Reiter A, Schrappe M, Ludwig W-D, et al: Favorable outcome of B-cell acute lymphoblastic leukemia in childhood: A report of three consecutive studies of the BFM group. Blood 1992; 80:2471.

76. Müller-Weihrich S, Henze G, Jobke A, et al: BFM-Studie 1975–81 zur Behandlung der Non-Hodgkin-Lymphoma hoher Malignität bei Kinder und Jugendlichen. Klin Pädiatr 1982; 194:219.

77. Lopez TM, Hagemeister FB, McLaughlin P, et al: Small non-cleaved cell lymphoma in adults: Superior results for stages I–III. J Clin Oncol 1990; 8:615.

78. McMaster ML, Greer JP, Greco A, et al: Effective treatment of small non-cleaved-cell lymphomas with high-intensity, brief-duration chemotherapy. J Clin Oncol 1991; 9:941.

79. Chilcote M, Krailo C, Kjeldsberg C, et al: Daunomycin plus COMP vs COMP therapy in childhood non-lymphoblastic lymphomas. Proc Am Soc Clin Oncol 1991; 10:289(1011A).

80. Mackall CL, Fleisher RA, Brown MR, et al: Lymphocyte depletion during treatment with intensive chemotherapy for cancer. Blood 1994; 84:2221.

81. O'Leary M, Ramsay NK, Nesbit ME Jr, et al: Bone marrow transplantation for non-Hodgkin's lymphoma in children and young adults. A pilot study. Am J Med 1983; 74:497.

82. Soussain C, Patte C, Ostronoff M, et al: Small non-cleaved cell lymphoma and leukemia in adults. A retrospective study of 65 adults treated with the LMB pediatric protocols. Blood 1995; 85:664.

83. Magrath IT, Adde M, Shad A, et al: Preliminary results of an intensive protocol including GM-CSF for patients with small noncleaved cell and immunoblastic lymphomas. Blood 1991; 10(suppl 1):114A.

84. Barriga F, Lee J, Whang-Peng C, Morrow E, Jaffe J, Cossman I and Magrath I. Development of a second clonally discrete Burkitt's lymphoma in a human immunodeficiency virus (HIV) positive homosexual patient. Blood 1988; 72:792.

85. Biggar RJ, Nkrumah FK, Henle W, et al: Very late relapses in patients with Burkitt's lymphoma; clinical and serological studies. J Natl Cancer Inst 1981; 66:439.

86. Meadows AT, Sposto R, Jenkin RDT, et al: Similar efficacy of 6 and 18 months of therapy with four drugs (COMP) for localized non-Hodgkin's lymphoma of children: A report from the Children's Cancer Study Group. J Clin Oncol 1989; 17:92.

87. Link MP, Donaldson SS, Berard CW, et al: Results of treatment of childhood localized non-Hodgkin's lymphoma with combination chemotherapy with or without radiotherapy. N Engl J Med 1990; 322:1169.

88. Müller-Weihrich S, Beck J, Henze G, et al: BFM-Studie 1981/83 zur Behandlung hochmaligner Non-Hodgkin-Lymphoma bei Kindern: Ergebnisse einer nach histologisch-immunologischem Typ und aus breitungsstadium stratefizierten Therapie. Klin Pädiatr 1984; 196:135.

89. Patte C, Philip T, Rodary C, et al: Improved survival rate in children with stage III and IV B cell non-Hodgkin's lymphoma and leukemia using multi-agent chemotherapy: Results of a study of 114 children from the French Pediatric Oncology Society. J Clin Oncol 1986; 4:1219.

90. Murphy S, Bowman W, Abromowitch M, et al: Results of treatment of advanced stage Burkitt's lymphoma and B-cell, (SIg+) acute lymphoblastic leukemia with high-dose fractionated cyclophosphamide and coordinated high-dose methotrexate and cytarabine. J Clin Oncol 1986; 4:1732.

91. Schwann M, Blattner SR, Lynch E, Weinstein HJ: HiC-COM: A 2 month intensive chemotherapy regimen for children with stage III and IV Burkitt's lymphoma and B-cell acute lymphoblastic leukemia. J Clin Oncol 1991; 9:133.

92. Philip T, Pinkerton R, Biron P, et al: Effective multiagent chemotherapy in children with advanced B-cell lymphoma: Who remains the high risk patient? Br J Haematol 1987; 65:159.

93. Berstein JI, Coleman CN, Strickler JG, et al: Combined modality therapy for adults with small non-cleaved cell lymphoma (Burkitt's and non-Burkitt's types). J Clin Oncol 1988; 4:847.

94. McMaster ML, Greer JP, Greco FA, et al: Effective treatment of small-noncleaved-cell lymphoma with high-intensity, brief-duration chemotherapy. J Clin Oncol 1991; 9:941.

95. Gentet JC, Patte C, Quintana E, et al: Phase II study of cytarabine and etoposide in children with refractory or relapsed non-Hodgkin's lymphoma: A study of the French Society of Pediatric Oncology. J Clin Oncol 1990; 8:661.

96. Magrath I, Adde M, Sandlund J, Jain V: Ifosfamide in the treatment of high-grade recurrent non-Hodgkin's lymphomas. Hematol Oncol 1991; 9:267.

97. Jones GR, Ettinger LJ: Continuous infusion of high-dose cytosine arabinoside for treatment of childhood acute leukemia and non-Hodgkin's lymphoma in relapse. Semin Oncol 1985; 12:150.

98. Gasparini M, Rottoli L, Massimino M, et al: Curability of advanced Burkitt's lymphoma in children by intensive short-term chemotherapy. Eur J Cancer 1993; 29A:692.

99. Murphy SB: Prognostic features and obstacles to cure of childhood non-Hodgkin's lymphoma. Semin Oncol 1977; 4:265.

100. Murphy S, Magrath IT: Workshop on pediatric lymphomas: Current results and prospects. Ann Oncol 1991; 2(suppl):219.

101. Philip T, Pinkerton R, Hartmann O, et al: The role of massive therapy with autologous bone marrow transplantation in Burkitt's lymphoma. Clin Haematol 1986; 15:205.

102. Philip T, Biron P, Philip I, et al: Massive therapy and autologous bone marrow transplantation in pediatric and young adults Burkitt's lymphoma (30 courses in 28 patients: A 5-year experience). Eur J Cancer Clin Oncol 1986; 22:1015.

103. Philip T, Chaivin F, Bron D, et al: PARMA international protocol: Pilot study on 50 patients and preliminary analysis of the ongoing randomized study (62 patients). Ann Oncol 1991; 2(suppl):57.

104. Appelbaum FR, Deisseroth A, Graw RG Jr, et al: Prolonged complete remission following high dose chemotherapy of Burkitt's lymphoma in relapse. Cancer 1978; 41:1059.

105. Philip T, Biron P, Maraninchi D, et al: Massive chemotherapy with ABMT in 50 cases of bad prognosis non-Hodgkin's lymphoma. Br J Hematol 1985; 60:599.

106. Appelbaum FR, Sullivan KM, Buckner CD, et al: Treatment of malignant lymphoma in 100 patients with chemotherapy, total body irradiation and marrow transplantation. J Clin Oncol 1987; 5:1440.

107. Chopra R, Goldstone AH, Pearce R, et al: Autologous versus allogeneic bone marrow transplantation for non-Hodgkin's lymphoma: A case controlled analysis of the European bone marrow transplant group registry data. J Clin Oncol 1992; 10:1690.

108. Sweetenham JW, Proctor SJ, Blaise D, et al: High-dose therapy and autologous bone marrow transplantation in first complete remission

for adult patients with high grade non-Hodgkin's lymphoma: The EBMT experience. Ann Oncol 1994; 5(suppl 2):155.

109. Ochs J, Abromowitch M, Rudnick S, et al: Phase I-II study of recombinant alpha-2 interferon against advanced leukemia and lymphoma in children. J Clin Oncol 1986; 4:883.

110. Magrath IT, Bhatia K, Huber B: Genetic intervention in the control of neoplasia. *In* Developmental Biology and Cancer. Boca Raton, FL, CRC Press, 1992, pp 479–523.

111. Patte C, Michon J, Leverger G, et al: High survival rate of childhood B-cell lymphoma and leukemia (ALL) as result of the LMB 89 protocol of the SFOP. Med Pediatr Oncol 1993; 21:2(A).

112. Straus DJ, Wong GY, Liu J, et al: Small non-cleaved-cell lymphoma (undifferentiated lymphoma, Burkitt's type) in American adults: Results with treatment designed for acute lymphoblastic leukemia. Am J Med 1991; 90:328.

Chapter Twenty-Four

— Peripheral T-Cell Lymphoma —

James O. Armitage

Clinicians often find the phrase "peripheral T-cell lymphoma" to be confusing. The name has nothing to do with the site of involvement by the lymphoma. Rather, it refers to lymphomas of a mature, rather than an immature, T-cell immunophenotype. Thus, the distinction is between immature, central, or thymic lymphomas (i.e., lymphoblastic lymphomas) and T-cell lymphomas with a more mature immunophenotype. Peripheral T-cell lymphomas make up the great majority of T-cell non-Hodgkin's lymphomas found in adults.

For the purposes of this chapter, peripheral T-cell lymphoma refers to non-Hodgkin's lymphomas with a T-cell immunophenotype that are not lymphoblastic lymphomas, not cutaneous T-cell lymphomas (i.e., mycosis fungoides), and not adult T-cell leukemia/lymphoma associated with infection by human T-cell lymphotropic virus, type I (HTLV-I). Although the latter two conditions are subtypes of peripheral T-cell lymphoma, they are dealt with individually in chapters elsewhere in this book. Also, most clinicians do not consider cutaneous T-cell lymphoma and adult T-cell leukemia/lymphoma when they refer to peripheral T-cell lymphoma.

One of the problems in caring for these patients is determining when a patient with an atypical T-cell proliferative process actually has lymphoma. With B-cell proliferations, this process is somewhat easier. B-cell proliferations can be more easily identified as being clonal (i.e., κ λ light-chain restricted), and B-cell lymphoma seems more likely to grow as a tumorous mass or to infiltrate the bone marrow and peripheral blood. There are several T-cell proliferations that can be difficult to classify. For example, the entity often referred to as "angioimmunoblastic lymphadenopathy with dysproteinemia" has been a source of controversy.[1] Although this has often been referred to as a "benign" proliferation of a mixture of cell types, it is now clear using T-cell gene rearrangement studies that these processes often have a clonal T-cell proliferation, and they certainly often have a rapidly fatal course.[2] A number of angiocentric T-cell proliferations have also caused confusion. Processes that in the past might have been called "lethal midline granuloma" and "lymphomatoid granulomatosis" now are frequently recognized as representing peripheral T-cell lymphomas.[3] Once again, this is based on a proliferation of atypical T-cells, demonstration of a monoclonal T-cell population using T-cell receptor gene rearrangement stud-

ies, and a rapidly fatal natural history that can be modified with chemotherapy. Finally, there are patients who present with a systemic illness and organ infiltration by atypical T lymphocytes.[4] With the same criteria, some of these patients can be identified as having peripheral T-cell lymphoma. The broader spectrum of illness seen with peripheral T-cell lymphomas than with the more common B-cell lymphomas has made these malignancies frequently challenging clinical problems for clinicians.

A useful way to consider the spectrum of peripheral T-cell lymphoma is to recognize the numerous clinical "syndromes" with which they can present. Several of these are listed in Table 24–1. The most common presentation of both peripheral T-cell lymphoma and B-cell lymphoma is as a nodal or extranodal tumor. With peripheral T-cell lymphomas, biopsy reveals the tumor to represent a proliferation of atypical lymphoid cells that have a T-cell immunophenotype. The only distinction between B-cell and T-cell lymphomas with this presentation is documentation of the immunophenotype or finding characteristic gene rearrangements. However, there are a number of more unusual presentations that are highly associated with the peripheral T-cell lymphomas. One of these is the hemophagocytic syndrome.[5] This process can be seen with viral infections but is also frequently associated with the presence of a peripheral T-cell lymphoma. In fact, some have suggested that the recognition of the hemophagocytic syndrome (i.e., in the past often referred to as "malignant histiocytosis") should lead to a search for peripheral T-cell lymphoma.

The clinical syndrome of pulmonary infiltrates and/or central nervous system findings, frequently associated with systemic symptoms, is characteristic of lymphomatoid granulomatosis.[6] Patients presenting with destructive and often necrotic facial and/or sinus tumors represent another clinical syndrome often associated with a malignant, angiocentric proliferation of T cells.[7] The latter syndrome seems to be quite variable in its geographic frequency. Finally, patients occasionally present with an obscure, systemic illness, and the diagnosis of T-cell lymphoma may be possible after extensive studies of biopsy specimens showing infiltration by atypical T cells.[4]

Peripheral T-cell lymphomas can present with a wide spectrum of clinical and histopathologic features. However, because available treatments can modify the natural history of these disorders in a way favorable to the patient, it is

Table 24–1. Presenting Clinical Syndromes of Peripheral T-Cell Lymphoma

Typical nodal or extranodal lymphoma
Hemophagocytic syndrome
Pulmonary syndrome
Facial/sinus syndrome
Systemic illness with atypical organ infiltration

important to recognize this variety of appearances so that a diagnosis can be reached quickly.

HISTOPATHOLOGIC SUBTYPES

A variety of classification schemes for non-Hodgkin's lymphomas have been applied to the peripheral T-cell lymphomas.[8–13] Unfortunately, none of them are perfectly applicable. Peripheral T-cell lymphomas can be made up predominately of small lymphocytes, a mixture of small lymphocytes and large transformed lymphocytes, and predominately large cells. A wide variety of diagnostic terms have been used to describe entities that we know sometimes represent peripheral T-cell lymphomas. A number of these are listed in Table 24–2.

A study of 134 patients with peripheral T-cell lymphoma from Nashville, Los Angeles, and Omaha found that 17% of the lymphomas were small cell, 40% were mixed cell, and 43% were made up predominately of large cells.[14] Thus, when the Working Formulation is used for classification, most peripheral T-cell lymphomas are considered aggressive lymphomas, and most are assigned to the diffuse mixed, diffuse large cell, and immunoblastic categories.[15] The small cell peripheral T-cell lymphomas are more difficult to classify and might be called "small lymphocytic" or "diffuse small cleaved cell lymphoma," or they might be unclassified with the Working Formulation.

Data from Stanford University are also available for 50 peripheral T-cell lymphomas that were classified histologically based on the size of the cells in the tumor.[16] These investigators found that 62% of the tumors were made up of predominately large cells. Of these, more than half were classified as immunoblastic. The authors found 22% of the lymphomas to be diffuse proliferations of mixed large and small cells, and 16% were what they referred to as "monomorphic medium-sized cells" but presumably would correspond to the small cell lymphomas in the other series.

The Kiel classification has also been used to classify patients with peripheral T-cell lymphoma. A study from Spain

Table 24–2. Histopathologic Terms Used to Describe Entities That Often or Sometimes Represent Peripheral T-Cell Lymphomas

Angioimmunoblastic lymphadenopathy
Lethal midline granuloma
Malignant midline reticulosis
Lymphomatoid granulomatosis
Polymorphic reticulosis
Angiocentric immunoproliferative lesion
Malignant histiocytosis
Histiocytic medullary reticulosis

classified 41 patients with noncutaneous peripheral T-cell lymphoma using a modification of the Kiel classification.[10] They found that 20 patients belonged to the low-grade group and 21 to the high-grade group. Low-grade lymphomas included three T-cell chronic lymphocytic leukemias, five lymphoepithelioid (i.e., Lennert's) lymphomas, four angioimmunoblastic lymphadenopathy–type T-cell lymphomas, and eight pleomorphic small cell lymphomas. The most common high-grade subclassification was pleomorphic medium and large cell, with 11 cases. There were seven anaplastic (Ki-1–positive) large cell lymphomas, and three immunoblastic lymphomas. Seventy percent of the cases were of T-helper phenotype. The classification was not useful in predicting outcome in that there was no difference in survival between the low-grade and the high-grade groups.

Because peripheral T-cell lymphomas do not fit easily into the most commonly used classification schemes, specific histopathologic classification systems have been proposed. One system was proposed by Japanese, German, and English pathologists.[9] They divided the tumors into those of low-grade or high-grade malignancy, analogous to the Kiel classification.[17] To the low-grade category they assigned lymphomas with cells that were characteristic of chronic lymphocytic leukemia, mycosis fungoides/Sézary syndrome, lymphoepithelioid lymphomas (i.e., also called Lennert's lymphoma), lymphomas with the characteristics of angioimmunoblastic lymphadenopathy, a subtype they classified as "T-zone lymphoma," and a lymphoma with small but pleomorphic T cells. Although this classification system might be useful to pathologists in identifying specific types of lymphoma, many of these so-called low-grade malignancies are associated with a fairly short life span.

The Japanese, German, and English classification system identified three types of peripheral T-cell lymphomas with a high grade of malignancy.[9] These were mixed pleomorphic medium and large cell lymphomas, immunoblastic lymphomas, and large cell anaplastic lymphomas. The latter tumor is unusual in that it is associated with a particular immunologic characteristic—that is, staining for the Hodgkin's disease–associated, or Ki-1, antigen. The authors recognized that even with their scheme, all peripheral T-cell lymphomas could not be easily classified, and they provided a categorization for unclassified low-grade and high-grade peripheral T-cell lymphomas, apparently with the distinction between the two being based largely on the number of large transformed cells in the tumor.

An important histologic subgroup of peripheral T-cell lymphomas that does not always fit easily into other classification systems is represented by the angiocentric lesions. In these cases, the tumor cells surround and invade vessel walls, often causing necrosis. These lesions have been variously called "lymphomatoid granulomatosis,"[6] "polymorphic reticulosis,"[18] "midline malignant reticulosis,"[18] "angiocentric immunoproliferative lesions,"[19] and "angiocentric lymphoma."[19] It may be that these lesions represent a spectrum from benign-appearing angioimmunoblastic lymphadenopathy with dysproteinemia and immunoblastic lymphoma. That is, the more benign appearing lesions might represent an early (possibly premalignant) phase of the disease that progresses to a high-grade peripheral T-cell lymphoma. The diagnosis reached by the pathologist might vary based on the time in the course of the illness that the biopsy was performed and, perhaps, the site of the biopsy. However, it seems likely that all these tumors represent a neoplastic disorder of T cells.

This spectrum of histopathologic findings seen in the angiocentric lesions and in the angioimmunoblastic lymphadenopathy with dysproteinemia–like lesions might be thought of as the T-cell counterpart to the spectrum of illnesses that one sees in the follicular B-cell lymphomas. In these disorders a comparative "benign" proliferation of atypical lymphoid follicles on the one extreme progresses to an aggressive B-cell large cell lymphoma.

The spectrum of appearance of peripheral T-cell lymphomas might represent, in part, a result of cytokine production as often documented in these tumors.[9] The production of cytokines might affect the histologic appearance and the clinical spectrum of these disorders.

IMMUNOLOGIC AND GENETIC CHARACTERISTICS

For a patient to be diagnosed as having a peripheral T-cell lymphoma, immunophenotyping must identify the tumor cells as having a mature T-cell immunophenotype. Certain histologic subtypes are more likely to type as peripheral T-cell lymphomas than others. For example, lymphomas classified as diffuse mixed and immunoblastic in the Working Formulation have a fairly high frequency of being found to be peripheral T-cell lymphomas. In the Omaha experience, approximately 40% of the patients classified as diffuse mixed lymphoma typed as peripheral T cell. However, it is difficult to predict which patients with diffuse mixed lymphoma, immunoblastic lymphoma, or other types will be proved to be of T-cell immunophenotype. In one study at the National Cancer Institute, peripheral T-cell lymphoma could be identified morphologically only 61% of the time.[20]

Identification of peripheral T-cell lymphomas is more complicated than with B-cell lymphomas. With B-cell lymphomas, monoclonal antibodies can prove not only B-cell origin but also clonality because of light-chain restriction (i.e., the tumor stains with only κ λ light chains). No equivalent studies exist for peripheral T-cell lymphomas. It is possible to confuse a diffuse large cell B-cell lymphoma that has a high degree of infiltration by reactive T-lymphocytes with a peripheral T-cell lymphoma because of this problem.[21, 22] Proving clonality requires analysis of the T-cell receptor genes to look for a monoclonal rearrangement. Although it might not be necessary to perform such studies in a patient with an obvious lymphoma in which the tumor cells unequivocally stain as T cells with a mature immunophenotype, this approach can be necessary to resolve difficult cases.[23]

The specific immunophenotype of peripheral T-cell lymphomas can vary considerably.[12, 24–27] Most cases have a helper/inducer phenotype (i.e., stain with CD4). Approximately 10% to 30% of the tumors are of the cytotoxic/suppressor immunophenotype (i.e., stain with CD8). The remainder of the tumors stain for a T-cell antigen (e.g., CD3) and both or neither of the helper/suppressor and cytotoxic/suppressor antigens. Unusual immunophenotypes occur

frequently and can help confirm the diagnosis of lymphoma.[12, 24, 25] Antibodies are available that can identify T cells in paraffin sections, sometimes obviating the need for a second biopsy.[28, 29]

The importance of immunophenotype in prognosis has been suggested, but the results have been contradictory. One study from France found a better survival for patients with the helper/inducer immunophenotype.[30] Another study has shown that the presence of HLA-DR and of the transferrin receptor on the surface of peripheral T-cell lymphomas predicts a good outcome.[31] However, the complex immunophenotypes often seen in these patients, and the preliminary nature of these studies, suggest that the information should be used cautiously until more data are available.

Two studies have identified unusual immunophenotypes with a particular clinical syndrome and adverse clinical outcome. Patients with lymphomas that expressed the neural cell adhesion molecule (NCAM), identified by reacting with the monoclonal antibody CD56, have been found to have unusual sites of involvement.[32] In one series of 46 patients with peripheral T-cell lymphoma, 11 (24%) reacted with CD56. These patients had involvement of the central nervous system (36%), gastrointestinal tract (27%), nasopharynx (27%), and muscle (18%). Less frequently, tumors involved the pituitary, thyroid, parathyroids, adrenals, and pancreas. Thus, peripheral T-cell lymphomas that express NCAM seem to have a predisposition for unusual sites of extranodal involvement. Another group of patients with peripheral T-cell lymphoma have been shown to express cytoplasmic S100 B protein.[33] Only a small percentage of normal circulating T lymphocytes are S100 positive. They usually have a suppressor immunophenotype. Hanson and associates described four patients with a chronic T-cell lymphoproliferative disorder that was S100 positive in all the cases.[33] The patients presented with prominent hepatosplenomegaly but not lymphadenopathy. Three patients had apparent central nervous involvement, and all four had circulating tumor cells. Three of the four patents died within 8 months of diagnosis.

Cytogenetic abnormalities have been identified in most patients with peripheral T-cell lymphoma in whom studies have been successfully completed.[26, 34, 35] It is now clear that there is an association between Ki-1–positive anaplastic large cell lymphomas and the specific chromosomal translocation t(2;5) (p23;q35). This translocation is seen in patients with anaplastic large cell lymphoma regardless of the immunophenotype and has been seen in patients with B-cell anaplastic large cell lymphoma. A number of other specific chromosomal abnormalities have been identified in patients with T-cell malignancies. These include inv(14) (q11;q32), t(8;14) (q24;q11), t(11;14) (p13;q11), and t(11;14) (p15;q11). Most of these rearrangements occur at a site of a known oncogene, and the suggestion has been made that the chromosomal abnormality activates the oncogene in a way that contributes to the development or progression of the lymphoma.

A recent evaluation of lymph node cytogenetic material from the University of Nebraska Medical Center found 16 cases of peripheral T-cell lymphoma with chromosomal abnormalities.[34, 35] Fifteen of the 16 patients had abnormal clones characterized by at least one structural abnormality, and the other patient had only a numerical abnormality.

Chromosomes involved in structural abnormalities in three or more cases included chromosomes 1 and 6 (six patients), chromosome 2 (five patients), and chromosomes 4, 11, 14, and 17 (three patients each). All the cases with structural abnormalities included at least one clone with a breakpoint at or near a previously described oncogene. The case with only the numerical abnormality was a monosomy 14 with a small marker chromosome that might have been a derivative chromosome 14 with a q11 breakpoint. The most frequently observed breakpoint was at chromosome 6q23, the locus of the *myb* oncogene.

EPSTEIN-BARR VIRUS

Epstein-Barr virus has been associated with a number of malignancies, including Burkitt's lymphoma, nasopharyngeal carcinoma, Hodgkin's disease, posttransplant immunoproliferative disease and lymphoma, and peripheral T-cell lymphoma. The association of this virus with peripheral T-cell lymphoma has fairly recently been recognized.

Although Epstein-Barr virus is widely known to infect B cells, it is also capable of infecting certain T lymphocytes.[36] Three patients who developed an illness characterized by fever, pneumonia, abnormal immunoglobulins, hematologic abnormalities, and extraordinarily high titers of antibody to components of the Epstein-Barr virus were described in 1988.[36] Each of these patients was identified as having peripheral T-cell lymphoma of the helper T-cell phenotype. The Epstein-Barr virus genome was found by in situ hybridization in the tumors of each patient. The tumor in each patient had an aggressive course and led to the patient's death.

Subsequent reports have confirmed the association of Epstein-Barr virus infection and peripheral T-cell lymphoma.[37–45] Peripheral T-cell lymphomas that have been demonstrated to have evidence of tumor cell infection by Epstein-Barr virus include those with the angioimmunoblastic lymphadenopathy and dysproteinemia type;[39] lethal midline granuloma with angiocentric lesions;[40, 43] pleomorphic cell type;[42] and a tumor presenting like malignant histiocytosis with the hemophagocytic syndrome that was shown to be peripheral T-cell lymphoma.[45] The peripheral T-cell lymphomas have been shown to be both of helper and suppressor phenotype.

The chances that a peripheral T-cell lymphoma might be associated with infection of the tumor cells by the Epstein-Barr virus seems to vary according to the site of origin of the lymphoma. One study from Holland demonstrated that peripheral T-cell lymphomas originating in the nose or nasal sinuses (100%) and lung (33%) were more likely to be associated with Epstein-Barr virus then lymphomas of the skin (0%) or gastrointestinal tract (8%).[37] The association of infection seemed to be by site of origin of the lymphoma rather than by the presence or absence of an angiocentric tumor growth pattern.

Infection by Epstein-Barr virus is frequently associated with lymphomas that occur in immunosuppressed patients. The occurrence of such high-grade B-cell lymphomas has been a major problem in patients after organ transplantation. T-cell lymphomas have been rarely reported in this setting.

However, posttransplant peripheral T-cell lymphomas have been reported.[41] In at least 5 of 22 reported cases there was an association with Epstein-Barr virus in the tumor cells.[41]

Infection by the Epstein-Barr virus is associated with a few cases of peripheral T-cell lymphoma. A small percentage of posttransplant peripheral T-cell lymphomas may be associated with infection by Epstein-Barr virus, but this association is much stronger for nasal and sinus lymphomas.

CLINICAL CHARACTERISTICS

Patients with peripheral T-cell lymphoma can present with an extraordinarily wide variety of clinical syndromes. When one sees an unusual condition such as the hemophagocytic syndrome or necrotic nasal/facial lesions, one should consider the possibility that the underlying condition might be a peripheral T-cell lymphoma. However, most patients with peripheral T-cell lymphomas present with nodal or extranodal masses in a manner analogous to that of patients with B-cell lymphomas.

A series of 134 patients with peripheral T-cell lymphoma was collected from Tennessee, Southern California, and Nebraska.[14] The clinical characteristics of these patients are summarized in Table 24–3. The median age was 57 years,

Table 24–3. Peripheral T-Cell Lymphoma Series[14]: Patient Characteristics°

Characteristic	No. (%) of Patients
Total no. of patients	134
Male/female	79:55
Preceding disorder of the immune system	36 (27)
Other lymphoproliferative disorders	15 (11)
Angioimmunoblastic lymphadenopathy	6
Atypical dermatitis	4
Mononucleosis	2
Lymphomatoid papulosis	2
Lymphomatoid granulomatosis	1
Different lymphoma	11 (8)
"Autoimmune" arthritis	6 (4)
Preceding nonhematologic malignancy	4 (3)
Stage	
I	10 (7)
II	28 (21)
II	29 (22)
IV	67 (50)
Symptom status	
A	58 (43)
B	76 (57)
Histologic group	
Large cell	58 (43)
Mixed	53 (40)
Small cell	23 (17)
Hypercalcemia (Ca²⁺ measured in 122 patients)	3 (2)
HTLV-I positive (measured in 24 patients)	1 (4)
Elevated LDH level (measured in 113 patients)	98 (87)
Bone marrow involvement†	41 (35)
Large cell	12 (24)
Mixed	16 (33)
Small cell	13 (68)

°Median age is 57 years (range of 4–97 years).
†Includes only patients who had bone marrow biopsy.
HTLV-I, human T-cell lymphotropic virus, type I; LDH, lactate dehydrogenase.

with an age range of 4 to 97 years. Fifty-nine percent of the patients were male. Twenty-seven percent of the patients had previously been diagnosed as having some other disorder of the immune system. Eleven percent had had another lymphoproliferative disorder (e.g., angioimmunoblastic lymphadenopathy), which might have represented an early phase of the lymphoma, previously diagnosed. Some patients had previously been diagnosed as having B-cell lymphoma or Hodgkin's disease. Four percent of the patients had been diagnosed as having an autoimmune arthritis before the appearance of the lymphoma. The occurrence of a peripheral T-cell lymphoma as a complication of other immune disorders is a real phenomenon that seems to occur at a higher than expected incidence.

Patients with peripheral T-cell lymphoma not associated with HTLV-I infection are not likely to present with hypercalcemia.[14] However, a number of adverse factors were frequent in these patients. For example, 87% had an elevated level of lactate dehydrogenase (LDH) at the time of diagnosis, and 57% of the patients had B symptoms. Fifty percent were stage IV. Bone marrow involvement was seen in 31% and skin involvement in 13%. Whether or not skin involvement occurs more frequently in patients with peripheral T-cell lymphomas than in those with B-cell lymphomas is unclear. Because it has been widely believed that patients with peripheral T-cell lymphomas are more likely to have cutaneous involvement, it may be that the frequent incidence of skin involvement in some reports relates to more patients with skin involvement having tumors immunotyped.

Peripheral T-cell lymphomas seem to share the same characteristics as B-cell lymphomas in the frequency of bone marrow involvement.[14] However, one report has suggested a very high incidence of marrow involvement when immunohistochemical studies were performed.[46, 47] Patients with predominantly large cells are less likely to have bone marrow involvement (24% in the series) than those with mixed small and large cells (33%) or those with small cells (68%). However, unlike patients with B-cell lymphomas, the patients with large cell peripheral T-cell lymphoma did not have a worse prognosis than those with predominately small cells.

KI-1–Positive Anaplastic Large Cell Lymphoma. The ability to perform immunophenotyping on paraffin-embedded specimens has led to the recognition that a significant number of patients with extranodal anaplastic lesions that were believed to represent undifferentiated carcinomas in fact had anaplastic large cell lymphoma. It was subsequently demonstrated that most of these patients had T-cell lymphomas that were Ki-1, or CD30, positive.[48] Ki-1 is an antigen that was originally recognized on Hodgkin's disease tumor cells.[49] It can be found occasionally on all types of non-Hodgkin's lymphomas but is especially likely to be present on anaplastic large cell lymphomas.[50–52]

It has become apparent that patients with Ki-1–positive anaplastic large cell lymphoma represent many of the cases that were formerly called "malignant histiocytosis."[53] A characteristic chromosomal abnormality, t(2;5), is frequently associated with this subtype of lymphoma.[54] Although often presenting in an extranodal site, this subtype can also present primarily in lymph nodes. The tumor has a response rate to combination chemotherapy that is no worse, and some have

suggested better than that of other large cell lymphomas when age, stage, and symptom status are taken into account.[55–58]

Facial/Nasal Lymphomas. It has become apparent that most non-Hodgkin's lymphomas with facial or nasopharyngeal presentations are peripheral T-cell lymphomas.[59] These lymphomas do not seem to have an even geographic distribution and have been reported more frequently in Latin America and Asia.[7, 60] As noted previously, there seems to be an association with infection by Epstein-Barr virus.[40, 43]

Patients who in the past would have been diagnosed as having lethal midline granuloma also appear to be examples of extranodal presentations of peripheral T-cell lymphoma.[61] These tumors are usually angiocentric; whether there is a premalignant phase that degenerates into lymphoma or the patients have lymphoma from the outset is unclear. These patients can respond to effective combination chemotherapy regimens with or without radiation therapy.

Hemophagocytic Syndrome. Peripheral T-cell lymphomas are highly associated with a clinical syndrome manifested by fever, hepatosplenomegaly, liver function abnormalities, thrombocytopenia, and erythrophagocytosis seen on bone marrow biopsy and, occasionally, biopsy of other organs. The association is sufficiently strong that some have suggested that any patient presenting with the hemophagocytic syndrome should undergo an evaluation aimed at finding a peripheral T-cell lymphoma.[5, 62] As with other presentations of peripheral T-cell lymphoma, combination chemotherapy can be effective.

Peripheral T-Cell Lymphoma Occurring in a Setting of Immunodeficiency. Peripheral T-cell lymphomas have been reported in patients with a variety of immunologic abnormalities. As described earlier, peripheral T-cell lymphoma can occur in patients who are immunosuppressed after solid organ transplantation.[63] Peripheral T-cell lymphomas have been reported with unusual extranodal localizations in patients infected by human immunodeficiency virus.[64] There are also reports of peripheral T-cell lymphoma developing in patients with hypogammaglobulinemia[65] and Chédiak-Higashi syndrome.[66]

Unusual Presentations. Patients who presented with a clinical syndrome of systemic illness, liver dysfunction, and unusual organ infiltration by postthymic T cells have been described.[67] Documentation of the clonal origin of the T cells and their atypical characteristics led to the diagnosis of peripheral T-cell lymphoma. These patients have had a poor clinical outcome despite combination chemotherapy.

Patients with adult celiac disease seem to be at increased risk for developing intestinal peripheral T-cell lymphoma.[68] Peripheral T-cell lymphoma has been reported presenting with profound eosinophilia.[69] This syndrome has been found in patients who present with what appears to be systemic vasculitis.[70] Peripheral T-cell lymphomas have been diagnosed in patients who initially appeared to have dysmyelopoietic syndrome.[71] Peripheral T-cell lymphomas have been reported masquerading as hairy cell leukemia.[72] Other unusual presentations include peripheral neuropathy, granulomatous liver disease, and angioedema with diffuse pulmonary infiltrates.[73–75] Peripheral T-cell lymphomas have been reported to involve essentially all organs, including the central nervous system.[76]

PRIMARY THERAPY

Once diagnosed as having peripheral T-cell lymphoma, the patient should undergo an evaluation similar to that of any other subgroup of patients with non-Hodgkin's lymphoma. This should include, in addition to a careful history and physical examination, a complete blood count, a chemistry profile, a chest radiograph, computed tomograms of the abdomen and pelvis, and a bone marrow biopsy. Careful attention should be directed to any historical or physical finding suggesting unusual sites of extranodal involvement.

There is no doubt that combination chemotherapy can be curative in patients with peripheral T-cell lymphoma. In a series of 110 patients, physicians participating in the Nebraska Lymphoma Study Group followed a uniform treatment protocol using radiation therapy for patients with minimal, nonbulky, localized lymphoma (7 patients) or a six-drug combination-chemotherapy regimen (103 patients).[77] The six-drug chemotherapy regimen included cyclophosphamide, doxorubicin (Adriamycin), procarbazine, bleomycin, vincristine, and prednisone. Eighty-three percent of these patients had B-cell lymphoma and 19% had T-cell lymphoma. The overall complete remission rate was slightly higher in the patients with B-cell lymphoma (75% versus 53%, *P* = NS). However, complete remissions were equally durable, with 70% or more of the complete responders in both groups remaining in remission after 3 years of followup. Patients with stage I/III peripheral T-cell lymphoma had an excellent outlook with this treatment approach. The 3-year overall survival was 73%, and the 3-year event-free survival was 66%. However, none of the patients with stage IV peripheral T-cell lymphoma achieved a complete remission, and none survived as long as 2 years. This is in contrast with a 44% 3-year survival in stage IV patients with B-cell lymphoma.

Numerous other studies have demonstrated the curative potential of combination chemotherapy in patients with peripheral T-cell lymphoma.[30, 78–81] There is little evidence that any particular combination chemotherapy is superior to the others as long as an effective regimen is used. A series from Hong Kong demonstrated that patients who received combination-chemotherapy regimens such as BACOP (bleomycin, Adriamycin, cyclophosphamide, Oncovin, prednisone) (i.e., regimens that have been demonstrated to cure other types of non-Hodgkin's lymphoma) had a better survival than when much less intensive regimens were used.[78] The authors found a higher complete response rate (84% versus 19%, *P* < .01) and a superior disease-free survival (80% versus 0% at 18 months) in patients who received more aggressive regimens.

Another study, from France, found similar results using an aggressive combination-chemotherapy regimen (LNH-80 or LNH-84).[30] The authors found a 77% complete remission rate with only 23% of the complete responders eventually relapsing. Once again, these patients had a superior survival when compared with others treated with less aggressive regimens.

Patients with the angioimmunoblastic lymphadenopathy type of peripheral T-cell lymphoma have sometimes been felt to have a lower-grade neoplasm. However, the median survival of these patients has been poor. Sixty-seven such

patients were treated in a German study.[79] Patients were treated with a combination-chemotherapy regimen named COP-BLAM/IMVP-16 (cyclophosphamide, Oncovin, prednisone, bleomycin, Adriamycin, Matulane/etoposide). To be participants in the study, the patients were initially treated with prednisone, and if they went into a durable complete remission they received no further therapy. Patients were treated with combination chemotherapy at the outset if they were believed to have life-threatening manifestations of the disease. The complete response rate with primary prednisone therapy was 29% in contrast with 64% with primary chemotherapy. The authors concluded that primary chemotherapy was a more effective treatment approach.

PROGNOSTIC FACTORS

A number of studies have tried to identify those factors predictive of outcome when patients are treated for peripheral T-cell lymphomas.[8, 14, 30, 77, 78–88] These include histopathologic, immunologic, and clinical characteristics. Investigators who have tried to identify immunologic characteristics (e.g., helper versus suppressor immunophenotype) as predictors of outcome have generally found negative results, although there are exceptions.[30] Unlike B-cell lymphomas, small cell peripheral T-cell lymphomas do not necessarily have an excellent outlook.[8]

The clinical characteristics of patients with peripheral T-cell lymphomas, like those in patients with B-cell lymphomas, are predictive of outcome. Localized versus disseminated disease, tumor mass size, and LDH levels have all been found to be important predictors of treatment outcome.[14, 30, 86] As in other types of non-Hodgkin's lymphomas, older patients are probably less likely to have a good treatment outcome. Some authors have found a high tumor proliferative fraction[82, 88] or bone marrow involvement[82, 83] to predict poor outcome. Currently, there is probably no reason to approach patients with peripheral T-cell lymphoma in a different way from those with B-cell lymphoma. It is likely that the International Prognostic Index will be equally applicable to patients with T-cell as to those with B-cell lymphoma.[89]

IS THERE A PROGNOSTIC DIFFERENCE BETWEEN B-CELL AND T-CELL LYMPHOMAS?

There has been a disagreement in the literature on the prognostic significance of a particular lymphoma's having a B-cell or a T-cell immunophenotype. Some authors have found that peripheral T-cell lymphomas have a worse outlook than corresponding B-cell lymphomas, whereas others have found no difference. These results are summarized in Table 24–4. At least eight studies have contrasted the results between patients with B-cell lymphomas and those with peripheral T-cell lymphomas.[47, 77, 90–95] Six studies found T-cell lymphomas to have a worse prognosis,[77, 90–93, 95] whereas two studies found no difference.[47, 94] No studies have found B-cell lymphoma to have a poorer prognosis than T-cell lymphoma.

One large study from Japan compared 449 patients with B-cell lymphoma to 92 patients with peripheral T-cell

Table 24–4. Comparative Prognosis for Patients with T-Cell and B-Cell Lymphomas

Reference	No. of Patients	Factors Favoring Patients with B-Cell NHL	T-Cell NHL
Shimoyama et al[90]	552	Survival	—
Coiffier et al[91]	361	Freedom from relapse	—
Armitage et al[77]	110	Survival and progression-free survival	—
Lippman et al[92]	103	Disease-free survival	—
Kwak et al[47]	98	—	—
Shimizu et al[93]	48	Complete remission rate survival	—
Cheng et al[94]	70	—	—
Brown et al[95]	51	Survival	—

NHL, non-Hodgkin's lymphoma.

lymphoma; cases of adult T-cell leukemia/lymphoma were excluded.[90] The authors found that B-cell lymphomas were more likely to present with low and intermediate histologic grades, whereas patients with peripheral T-cell lymphoma were more likely to have a higher histologic grade, B symptoms, and poor performance status. The overall survival of the patients with the B-cell lymphoma was superior.

A study from France reported 361 patients with aggressive non-Hodgkin's lymphoma who were immunophenotyped and who all received treatment with the LNH-84 regimen.[43] More than 90% of the patients had diffuse mixed cell, diffuse large cell, or immunoblastic lymphoma using the Working Formulation classification. Seventy percent of the patients had a B-cell immunophenotype and 30% a T-cell immunophenotype. Patients with peripheral T-cell lymphoma were more likely to present with an advanced stage (P = .0002) and to have B symptoms (P > .01). Although there was no difference in response rate to the chemotherapy regimen, patients with peripheral T-cell lymphoma were more likely to relapse from remission (43% versus 29%, P<.001). Patients with peripheral T-cell lymphoma had a shorter overall survival (42 versus 50 months, P < .05). A multivariate analysis showed that the T-cell immunophenotype was a significant adverse prognostic factor, independent of other adverse risk factors.

One hundred ten patients treated by physicians participating in the Nebraska Lymphoma Study Group had a diffuse mixed, diffuse large cell, or immunoblastic lymphoma, and all patients were prospectively immunophenotyped.[77] All patients received the same six-drug chemotherapy regimen. Patients with peripheral T-cell lymphoma had a significantly worse survival and progression-free survival. However, this poorer outlook was a result of the especially poor outcome seen in patients with stage IV disease. Patients with less extensive lymphomas did equally well whether they had a B-cell or a T-cell immunophenotype.

An Arizona study of 103 consecutively accrued patients with diffuse large cell lymphoma found 83 to have a B-cell immunophenotype and 20 a T-cell immunophenotype.[92] Patients with B-cell lymphoma were more likely to have bulky disease, and patients with T-cell lymphoma were more likely to have skin involvement. Eight-three per-

cent of the patients with each immunophenotype received a doxorubicin-containing combination-chemotherapy regimen. Disease-free survival was significantly shorter in the patients with T-cell lymphoma (median 11 months versus 43 months, P = .01). In fact, no patient with peripheral T-cell lymphoma remained disease-free for longer than 2 years, in contrast with 55% of the patients with B-cell lymphoma. However, the actuarial overall survival did not vary significantly between the two groups (P = .23).

The prognostic significance of having a peripheral T-cell lymphoma rather than a B-cell lymphoma remains somewhat controversial. However, most studies have shown a poorer progression-free survival in patients with peripheral T-cell lymphoma, and several have shown a worse overall survival.

SALVAGE THERAPY

As with all types of non-Hodgkin's lymphoma, patients with peripheral T-cell lymphoma who fail to be cured with a primary combination-chemotherapy regimen have an extremely poor outlook. In general, the approach to salvage chemotherapy in these patients should not vary from that for patients with B-cell lymphoma.

A variety of unusual salvage approaches have been reported for patients with relapsed peripheral T-cell lymphoma. A recent report suggested that patients with peripheral T-cell lymphoma, in contrast with patients with B-cell lymphoma, could respond to treatment with retinoic acids.[96] The authors used 13-*cis*-retinoic acid in a selected group of 18 patients with relapsed refractory lymphoma. Five complete remissions and one partial remission were noted in 12 patients with peripheral T-cell lymphoma, whereas none of the six patients with B-cell lymphoma responded. Five patients with relapsed peripheral T-cell lymphoma treated with cyclosporine have been reported.[97] None responded. There is a single report of a patient with a suppressor T-cell mediastinal lymphoma treated with a thymic humoral factor.[98] This patient's disease may have been better classified as lymphoblastic lymphoma than peripheral T-cell lymphoma.

Several patients with relapsed peripheral T-cell lymphoma have undergone autologous bone marrow transplantation. One report described 41 patients who underwent autologous bone marrow transplantation for relapsed, recurrent non-Hodgkin's lymphoma and who were immunophenotyped before transplant.[99] Seventeen of these patients were found to have peripheral T-cell lymphoma, and 24 had B-cell lymphoma. All had histologically aggressive lymphomas. The complete response rate to transplant slightly favored patients with peripheral T-cell lymphoma (59% versus 42%), and the actuarial 2-year survival was comparable (35% versus 30%). Twenty-eight percent of the peripheral T-cell lymphoma patients had a 2-year event-free survival.

Thirteen children and adolescents with peripheral T-cell lymphoma who underwent bone marrow transplantation have been reported. Some of these patients were included in the previous series.[100] Ten patients received autologous and three allogeneic transplants. Six of the 13 patients were disease free for 6 to 37 months at the time of the report. One of the patients who relapsed after an autologous transplant subsequently had long-term disease-free survival following an allogeneic transplant.

SUMMARY

Peripheral T-cell lymphomas represent a broad spectrum of disease. These tumors are more likely than B-cell lymphomas to pursue an aggressive clinical course. Most patients with peripheral T-cell lymphoma have a mixture of large and small lymphocytes or predominately large transformed cells composing most of the tumor. Combination-chemotherapy regimens or, in patients with localized disease, a combination of chemotherapy and radiation therapy can produce a significant number of disease-free survivors. Whether the chances for prolonged disease-free survival are worse in patients with peripheral T-cell lymphoma remains a point of controversy. However, most studies that have looked at this factor have found that patients with peripheral T-cell lymphoma do significantly less well than corresponding patients with B-cell lymphomas.

Although immunophenotyping of newly diagnosed non-Hodgkin's lymphomas is a useful undertaking, it is unusual for the treatment to be based on the immunophenotype. The same regimens that seem to be effective in B-cell aggressive non-Hodgkin's lymphomas are active in peripheral T-cell lymphomas. However, results of therapy in all types of non-Hodgkin's lymphoma are suboptimal. Patients who fail to be cured with a primary combination-chemotherapy regimen can sometimes be salvaged with high doses of therapy and bone marrow transplantation.

The geographic variation in the frequency of peripheral T-cell and B-cell lymphomas almost certainly represents a difference in etiologic factors. Identification of etiologic factors of these and other types of non-Hodgkin's lymphomas remains the most important area for research if overall mortality is to be significantly altered. Unless an extremely effective new therapy is found, identification of the cause of peripheral T-cell and B-cell lymphomas, and using that information to reduce the incidence of the disease, would be the best way to alter mortality from these aggressive neoplasms.

REFERENCES

1. Frizzera G, Moran EM, Rappaport H: Angioimmunoblastic lymphadenopathy with dysproteinemia. Lancet 1974; 1:1070.
2. Tobinai K, Minato K, Ohtsu T, et al: Clinicopathologic, immunophenotypic, and immunogenotypic analyses of immunoblastic lymphadenopathy–like T-cell lymphoma. Blood 1988; 72:1000.
3. Lippman S, Grogan T, Spier C, et al: Lethal midline granuloma with a novel T-cell phenotype as found in peripheral T-cell lymphoma. Cancer 1987; 59:936.
4. Farcet JP, Gaulard P, Marolleau JP, et al: Hepatosplenic T-cell lymphoma: Sinusal/sinusoidal localization of malignant cells expressing the T-cell receptor. Blood 1990; 75(11):2213.
5. Chan E, Chan G, Todd D, et al: Peripheral T-cell lymphoma presenting as hemophagocytic syndrome. Hematol Oncol 1989; 7:275.
6. Fauci AS, Haynes BF, Costa J, et al: Lymphomatoid granulomatosis: Prospective clinical and therapeutic experience over ten years. N Engl J Med 1983; 306:68.
7. Aviles A, Rodriguez L, Guzman R, et al: Angiocentric T-cell lymphoma of the nose, paranasal sinuses and hard palate. Hematol Oncol 1992; 10:141.
8. Weisenburger D, Linder J, Armitage JO: Peripheral T-cell lymphoma: A clinicopathologic study of 42 cases. Hematol Oncol 1987; 5:175.
9. Suchi T, Lennert K, Tu L-Y, et al: Histopathology and immunohistochemistry of peripheral T-cell lymphomas: A proposal for their classification. J Clin Pathol 1987; 40:995.
10. Montalban C, Obeso G, Gallego A, et al: Peripheral T-cell lymphoma: A clinicopathological study of 41 cases and evaluation of the prognostic significance of the updated Kiel classification. Histopathology 1993; 22:303.
11. Weis J, Winter M, Phyliky R, et al: Peripheral T-cell lymphomas: Histologic, immunohistologic, and clinical characterization. Mayo Clin Proc 1986; 61:411.
12. Watanabe S: Pathology of peripheral T-cell lymphomas and leukemias. Hematol Oncol 1986; 4:45.
13. Nakamura S, Suchi T: A clinicopathologic study of node-based, low-grade, peripheral T-cell lymphoma. Cancer 1991; 67:2565.
14. Armitage JO, Greer JP, Levine, AM, et al: Peripheral T-cell lymphoma. Cancer 1989; 63:158.
15. The Non-Hodgkin's Lymphoma Pathologic Classification Project. Cancer 1982; 49:2112
16. Weiss LM, Crabtree GS, Rouse RV, Warnke RA: Morphologic and immunologic characterization of 50 peripheral T-cell lymphomas. Am J Pathol 1985; 118:316.
17. Lennert K, Mohri N, Stein H, Kaiserling E: The histopathology of malignant lymphoma. Br J Haemotol 1975; 31(Suppl):193.
18. Jaffe E: Pathologic and clinical spectrum of post-thymic T-cell malignancies. Cancer Invest 1984; 2(5):413.
19. Lipford E, Margolick J, Longo D, et al: Angiocentric immunoproliferative lesions: A clinicopathologic spectrum of post-thymic T-cell proliferations. Blood 1988; 72:1674.
20. Jaffe E, Strauchen J, Berard C: Predictability of immunologic phenotype by morphologic criteria in diffuse aggressive non-Hodgkin's lymphomas. Am J Clin Pathol 1982; 77:46.
21. Ramsay A, Smith W, Isaacson P: T-cell–rich B-cell lymphoma. Am J Surg Pathol 1988; 12:433.
22. Rodriguez J, Pugh W, Cabanillas F: T-cell–rich B-cell lymphoma. Blood 1993; 82:1586.
23. Bertness V, Kirsch I, Hollis G, et al: T-cell receptor gene rearrangements as clinical markers of human T-cell lymphomas. N Engl J Med 1985; 313:534.
24. Grogan T, Fielder K, Rangel C, et al: Peripheral T-cell lymphoma: Aggressive disease with heterogeneous immunotypes. J Clin Pathol 1985; 83:279.
25. Borowitz M, Reichert T, Brynes R, et al: The phenotypic diversity of peripheral T-cell lymphomas: The Southeastern Cancer Study Group experience. Hum Pathol 1986; 17:567.
26. Ebrahim S, Ladanyi M, Desai S, et al: Immunohistochemical, molecular, and cytogenetic analysis of a consecutive series of 20 peripheral T-cell lymphomas and lymphomas of uncertain lineage, including 12 Ki-1 positive lymphomas. Genes Chromosom Cancer 1990; 2:27.
27. Oertel J, Oertal B, Lobeck, et al: Cytologic and immunocytologic studies of peripheral T-cell lymphomas. Acta Cytol 1991; 35:3.
28. Linder J, Ye Y, Harrington D, et al: Monoclonal antibodies marking T lymphocytes in paraffin-embedded tissue. Am J Pathol 1987; 127:1.
29. Linder J, Ye Y, Armitage JO, Weisenburger D: Monoclonal antibodies marking B-cell non-Hodgkin's lymphomas in paraffin-embedded tissue. Mod Pathol 1988; 1:29.
30. Coiffier B, Berger F, Byron PA, et al: T-cell lymphomas: Immunologic, histologic, clinical, and therapeutic analysis of 63 cases. J Clin Oncol 1988; 6:1584.
31. Harrington D, Linder J, Weisenburger D, et al: Peripheral T-cell lymphoma (PTCL): An immunophenotypic and clinical analysis. Lab Invest 1987; 56:29A.
32. Kern WF, Spier CM, Hanneman EH, et al: Neural cell adhesion molecule–positive peripheral T-cell lymphoma: A rare variant with a propensity for unusual sites of involvement. Blood 1992; 79:2432.
33. Hanson C, Bockenstedt P, Schnitzer B, et al: S100-positive, T-cell chronic lymphoproliferative disease: An aggressive disorder of an uncommon T-cell subset. Blood 1991; 78:1803.
34. Vose J, Weisenburger D, Sanger W, et al: Peripheral T-cell lymphoma—a brief review. Leuk Lymphoma 1990; 3:77.
35. Schouten HC, Sanger WG, Weisenburger DD, Armitage JO, for the Nebraska Lymphoma Study Group: Chromosomal abnormalities in patients with non-cutaneous T-cell non-Hodgkin's lymphoma. Eur J Cancer 1990; 26:618.

36. Jones JF, Shurin S, Abramowsky C, et al: T-cell lymphomas containing Epstein-Barr viral DNA in patients with chronic Epstein-Barr virus infections. N Engl J Med 1988; 318:733.

37. DeBruin PC, Jiwa M, Oudejans J, et al: Presence of Epstein-Barr virus in extranodal T-cell lymphomas: Differences in relation to site. Blood 1994; 83:1612.

38. Richel D, Lepoutre J, Kapsenberg J, et al: Epstein-Barr virus in a CD8-positive T-cell lymphoma. Am J Pathol 1990; 136:1093.

39. Anagnostopoulos I, Hummel M, Finn T, et al: Heterogeneous Epstein-Barr virus patterns in peripheral T-cell lymphoma of angio-immunoblastic lymphadenopathy type. Blood 1992; 80:1804.

40. Harabuchi Y, Yamanaka N, Kataura A, et al: Epstein-Barr virus in nasal T-cell lymphomas in patients with lethal midline granuloma. Lancet 1990; 335:128.

41. Van Gorp J, Doornewaard H, Verdonck L, et al: Posttransplant T-cell lymphoma. Cancer 1994; 73:3064.

42. Korbjuhn P, Anagnostopoulos I, Hummel M, et al: Frequent latent Epstein-Barr virus infection of neoplastic T cells and bystander B cells in human immunodeficiency virus–negative European peripheral pleomorphic T-cell lymphomas. Blood 1993; 82:217.

43. Mishima K, Horiuchi K, Kojya S, et al: Epstein-Barr virus in patients with polymorphic reticulosis (lethal midline granuloma) from China and Japan. Cancer 1994; 73:3041.

44. Cheng AL, Su IJ, Chen YC, et al: Characteristic clinicopathologic features of Epstein-Barr virus–associated peripheral T-cell lymphoma. Cancer 1993; 72:909.

45. Su IJ, Hsu YH, Lin MT, et al: Epstein-Barr virus–containing T-cell lymphoma presents with hemophagocytic syndrome mimicking malignant histiocytosis. Cancer 1993; 72:2019.

46. Gaulard P, Kanavaros P, Farcet JP, et al: Bone marrow histologic and immunohistochemical findings in peripheral T-cell lymphoma: A study of 38 cases. Hum Pathol 1991; 22:331.

47. Kwak L, Wilson M, Weiss L, et al: Similar outcome of treatment of B-cell and T-cell diffuse large-cell lymphomas: The Stanford experience. J Clin Oncol 1991; 9:1426.

48. Stein H, Mason DY, Gerdes J, et al: The expression of the Hodgkin's disease–associated antigen Ki-1 in reactive and neoplastic lymphoid tissue: Evidence that Reed-Sternberg cells and histiocytic malignancies are derived from activated lymphoid cells. Blood 1985; 66:848.

49. Schwab U, Stein H, Gerdes J, et al: Production of a monoclonal antibody specific for Hodgkin and Sternberg-Reed cells of Hodgkin's disease and a subset of normal lymphoid cells. Nature 1982; 299:65.

50. Sandlund JT, Pui CH, Santana VM, et al: Clinical features and treatment outcome for children with CD30+ large cell non-Hodgkin's Lymphoma. J Clin Oncol 1994; 12:895.

51. Penny RJ, Blaustein JC, Longtine JA, et al: Ki-1–positive large cell lymphomas—a heterogeneous group of neoplasms: Morphologic, immunophenotypic, genotypic, and clinical features of 24 cases. Cancer 1991; 68:362.

52. Piris M, Brown DC, Gatter KC, Mason DY: CD30 expression in non-Hodgkin's lymphoma. Histopathology 1990; 17:211.

53. Delsol G, Al Saati T, Gatter KC, et al: Coexpression of epithelial membrane antigen (EMA), Ki-1, and interleukin-2 receptor by anaplastic large cell lymphomas: Diagnostic value in so-called malignant histiocytosis. Am J Pathol 1988; 130:59.

54. Bitter MA, Franklin WA, Larson RA, et al: Morphology in Ki-1 (CD30)–positive non-Hodgkin's lymphoma is correlated with clinical features and the presence of a unique chromosomal abnormality, t(2;5)(p23;q35). Am J Surg Pathol 1990; 14:305.

55. Shulman L, Frisard B, Antin J, et al: Primary Ki-1 anaplastic large cell lymphoma in adults: Clinical characteristics and therapeutic outcome. J Clin Oncol 1993; 11:937.

56. Reiter A, Schrappe M, Tiemann M, et al: Successful treatment strategy for Ki-1 anaplastic large cell lymphoma of childhood: A prospective analysis of 62 patients enrolled in three consecutive Berlin-Frankfurt-Munster group studies. J Clin Oncol 1994; 12:899.

57. Greer J, Kinney M, Collins R, et al: Clinical features of 31 patients with Ki-1 anaplastic large-cell lymphoma. J Clin Oncol 1991; 9:539.

58. Offit K, Ladanyi M, Gangi MD, et al: Ki-1 antigen expression defines a favorable clinical subset on non-B cell non-Hodgkin's lymphoma. Leukemia 1990; 4:625.

59. Chan JKC, Lau WH, Lo STH: Most nasal/nasopharyngeal lymphomas are peripheral T-cell neoplasms. Am J Surg Pathol 1987; 11:418.

60. Weiss L: Primary nasal T-cell lymphoma [Abstract]. Fifth International Conference on Malignant Lymphoma, Lugano Vol 72, 1993, p 57.

61. Chott A, Rappersberger K, Schlossarek W, Radaszkiewicz T: Peripheral T-cell lymphoma presenting primarily as lethal midline granuloma. Hum Pathol 1988; 19:1093.

62. Falini B, Pileri S, DeSolas I, et al: Peripheral T-cell lymphoma associated with hemophagocytic syndrome. Blood 1990; 75(2):434.

63. Garvin AJ, Self S, Sahovic EA, et al: The occurrence of a peripheral T-cell lymphoma in a chronically immunosuppressed renal transplant patient. Am J Surg Pathol 1988; 12:64.

64. Lum GH, Cosgriff TM, Byrne R, Reddy V: Primary T-cell lymphoma of muscle in a patient infected with human immunodeficiency virus. Am J Med 1993; 95:545.

65. Durham JC, Stephens DS, Rimland D, et al: Common variable hypogammaglobulinemia complicated by an unusual T-suppressor/cytotoxic cell lymphoma. Cancer 1987; 59:271.

66. Argyle JC, Kjeldsberg CR, Marty J, et al: T-cell lymphoma and the Chédiak-Higashi syndrome. Blood 1982; 60:672.

67. Diez-Martin JL, Lust JA, Witzig TE, et al: Unusual presentation of extranodal peripheral T-cell lymphomas with multiple paraneoplastic features. Cancer 1991; 68:834.

68. Alegre VA, Winkelmann RK, Diez-Martin JL, Banks PM: Adult celiac disease, small- and medium-vessel cutaneous necrotizing vasculitis, and T-cell lymphoma. J Am Acad Dermatol 1988; 19:973.

69. O'Shea JJ, Jaffee ES, Lane HC, et al: Peripheral T-cell lymphoma presenting as hypereosinophilia with vasculitis. Am J Med 1987; 82:539.

70. Foley JF, Linder J, Koh J, et al: Cutaneous necrotizing granulomatous vasculitis with evolution to T-cell lymphoma. Am J Med 1987; 82:839.

71. Auger MJ, Nash JRG, Mackie MJ: Marrow involvement with T-cell lymphoma initially presenting as abnormal myelopoiesis. J Clin Pathol 1986; 39:134.

72. Greenberg BR, Grogan TM, Takasugi BJ, et al: A unique malignant T-cell lymphoproliferative disorder with neutropenia simulating hairy cell leukemia. Cancer 1985; 56:2823.

73. Gherardi R, Gaulard P, Prost C, et al: T-cell lymphoma revealed by a peripheral neuropathy. Cancer 1986; 58:2710.

74. Saito K, Nakanuma Y, Ogawa S, et al: Extensive hepatic granulomas associated with peripheral T-cell lymphoma. Am J Gastroenterol 1991; 86:1243.

75. Harrison NK, Twelves C, Addis BJ, et al: Peripheral T-cell lymphoma presenting with angioedema and diffuse pulmonary infiltrates. Am Rev Respir Dis 1988; 138:976.

76. Morgello S, Maiese K, Petito CK: T-cell lymphoma in the CNS: Clinical and pathologic features. Neurology 1989; 39:1190.

77. Armitage JO, Vose JM, Linder J, et al: Clinical significance of immunophenotyping in diffuse aggressive non-Hodgkin's lymphoma. J Clin Oncol 1989; 7:1783.

78. Liang R, Todd D, Chan TK, et al: Intensive chemotherapy for peripheral T-cell lymphomas. Hematol Oncol 1992; 10:155.

79. Siegert W, Agthe A, Griesser H: Treatment of angioimmunoblastic lymphadenopathy (AILD)–type T-cell lymphoma using prednisone with or without the COPBLAM/IMVP-16 regimen. Ann Intern Med 1992; 117:364.

80. Greer JP, York JC, Cousar JB, et al: Peripheral T-cell lymphoma: A clinicopathologic study of 42 cases. J Clin Oncol 1984; 2:788.

81. Haioun C, Gaulard P, Bourquelot P, et al: Clinical and biological analysis of peripheral T-cell lymphomas: A single-institution study. Leuk Lymphoma 1992; 7:449.

82. Chott A, Augustin I, Wrba F, et al: Peripheral T-cell lymphomas: A clinicopathologic study of 75 cases. Hum Pathol 1990; 21:1117.

83. Caulet S, Delmer A, Audouin J, et al: Histopathological study of bone marrow biopsies in 30 cases of T-cell lymphoma with clinical, biological, and survival correlations. Hematol Oncol 1990; 8:155.

84. Nakamura S, Suchi T, Koshikawa T, et al: Clinicopathologic study of 212 cases of peripheral T-cell lymphoma among the Japanese. Cancer 1993; 72:1762.

85. Pinkus GS, O'Hara CJ, Said JW: Peripheral/post-thymic T-cell lymphomas: A spectrum of disease. Cancer 1990; 65:971.

86. Noorduyn LA, Van Der Valk P, Van Heerde P, et al: Stage is a better prognostic indicator than morphologic subtype in primary noncutaneous T-cell lymphoma. Am J Clin Pathol 1990; 93:49.

87. Remotti D, Perscarmona E, Burgio VL, et al: Prognostic value of histologic classification of peripheral T-cell lymphoma: A clinicopathologic study of 71 HTLV-I negative cases. Leuk Lymphoma 1992; 8:371.

88. Grierson HL, Wooldridge TN, Purtilo DT, et al: Low proliferative activity is associated with a favorable prognosis in peripheral T-cell lymphoma. Cancer Res 1990; 50:4845.

89. Shipp MA, Harrington DP, Anderson JR, et al: Development of a predictive model for aggressive lymphoma: The International Non-Hodgkin's Lymphoma Pfactors Project. N Engl J Med 1993; 329:987.

90. Shimoyama M, Oyama A, Tajima K, et al: Differences in clinicopathological characteristics and major prognostic factors between B-lymphoma and peripheral T-lymphoma excluding adult T-cell leukemia/lymphoma. Leuk Lymphoma 1993; 10:335.

91. Coiffier B, Brousse N, Peuchmaur M, et al: Peripheral T-cell lymphomas have a worse prognosis than B-cell lymphomas: A prospective study of 361 immunophenotyped patients treated with the LNH-84 regimen. The GELA (Groupe d'Etude des Lymphomes Agressives). Ann Oncol 1990; 1:45.

92. Lippman SM, Miller TP, Spier CM, et al: The prognostic significance of the immunotype in diffuse large-cell lymphoma: A comparative study of the T-cell and B-cell phenotype. Blood 1988; 72:436.

93. Shimizu K, Hamajima N, Ohnishi K, et al: T-cell phenotype is associated with decreased survival in non-Hodgkin's lymphoma. Jpn J Cancer Res 1989; 80:720.

94. Cheng AL, Chen YC, Wang CH, et al: Direct comparisons of peripheral T-cell lymphoma with diffuse B-cell lymphoma of comparable histological grades—should peripheral T-cell lymphoma be considered separately? J Clin Oncol 1989; 7:725.

95. Brown DC, Heryet A, Gatter KC, Mason DY: The prognostic significance of immunophenotype in high-grade non-Hodgkin's lymphoma. Histopathology 1989; 14:621.

96. Cheng AL, Su IJ, Chen CC, et al: Use of retinoic acids in the treatment of peripheral T-cell lymphoma: A pilot study. J Clin Oncol 1994; 12:1185.

97. Cooper DL, Braverman IM, Sarris AH, et al: Cyclosporine treatment of refractory T-cell lymphomas. Cancer 1993; 71:2335.

98. Shohat D, Shaklai M, Nemes L, Trainin N: Immune modulation of a T-suppressor cell lymphoma by thymic humoral factor, a thymic hormone. Cancer 1984; 54:2122.

99. Vose JM, Peterson C, Bierman PJ, et al: Comparison of high-dose therapy and autologous bone marrow transplantation for T-cell and B-cell non-Hodgkin's lymphomas. Blood 1990; 76:424.

100. Gordon BG, Weisenburger DD, Warkentin PI, et al: Peripheral T-cell lymphoma in childhood and adolescence. Cancer 1993; 71:257.

Chapter **Twenty-Five**

Primary Extranodal Lymphomas

Simon B. Sutcliffe
Mary K. Gospodarowicz

The term "malignant lymphoma" refers to cancer of the lymphatic/reticuloendothelial system and comprises two major categories of malignant disease—Hodgkin's disease and non-Hodgkin's lymphoma. Both Hodgkin's disease and non-Hodgkin's lymphoma share the commonalities of frequent presentation with lymphadenopathy; a common symptomatology of fever, night sweats, and weight loss; a common staging classification; and a therapeutic approach using radiation and/or chemotherapy. They also have important distinguishing features in terms of age spectrum, histologic and cytologic appearances, prognosis, and the frequency with which non-Hodgkin's lymphomas present as primary extranodal tumors—a circumstance of extreme rarity in Hodgkin's disease.

"Primary extranodal lymphoma" refers to a localized presentation of lymphoma arising within an extranodal tissue and deemed to be the site of origin of the lymphoma even though regional lymphadenopathy may be present. The term implies that disseminated disease is not clinically evident, thus distinguishing extranodal presentation with or without lymphadenopathy (stages I to IIE) from disseminated or stage IV disease. The term also has more relevance when applied to the tissue of origin, for example, tonsil, paranasal sinus, or thyroid lymphoma, than to an anatomic region of the body, for example, head and neck lymphoma.

This chapter addresses primary extranodal lymphomas other than those arising in skin or the central nervous system (CNS). Although it is not known whether mediastinal large cell lymphoma arises from nodal or extranodal (thymic) tissue, it is included as a characteristic clinic entity distinguishable from nodal lymphoma of equivalent stage presenting in nonmediastinal sites.

Whereas Hodgkin's disease virtually always arises in nodal tissue and relatively less commonly involves extranodal tissues by extension from nodal tissue or by dissemination, non-Hodgkin's lymphomas have a much greater propensity to disseminate early through systemic circulation of lymphoma cells. In principle, therefore, it is not really surprising that extranodal lymphomas have been recorded in virtually every tissue of the body, as either primary or metastatic lesions. It is also clear, however, that certain tissues are much more commonly the site of primary extranodal lymphoma, for example, gastrointestinal (GI) tract and tonsil, and that there are factors that determine preferential patterns of

spread of lymphoma and the receptiveness of certain tissues or organs to accommodate metastatic growth.

The following three principal issues are considered with respect to primary extranodal lymphoma:

- *Does the presentation of localized disease in an extranodal site confer a different prognosis than a presentation of similar stage in a nodal site?* The data presented in Figure 25–1 suggest that when analyzed by stage alone, there is no difference in survival for patients presenting with nodal or extranodal lymphoma. This is somewhat surprising given that primary extranodal lymphomas are much more commonly of diffuse large cell type (or more aggressive histologic types) than nodal lymphomas, despite otherwise comparable prognostic attributes. Thus, the distinction between nodal versus extranodal lymphoma does not constitute a prognostically relevant distinction without further analysis of the subcategories of extranodal disease.

- *Do all primary extranodal lymphomas have a similar natural history and prognosis?* A more detailed review of the natural history and prognosis of extranodal lymphoma reveals a wide diversity that largely reflects the frequency with which low-grade, indolent tumors constitute a substantial proportion of presentations, conferring a "favorable" prognosis (≥60% 5-year survival rate)—for example, GI tract, Waldeyer's ring, orbit, salivary gland, and lungs—as opposed to sites or tissues where intermediate- and high-grade histologic types constitute the dominant proportion—for example, testis or ovary, bone, breast, or primary CNS. Even with certain sites or tissues, the histologic spectrum and prognosis can be extremely heterogeneous, for example, primary cutaneous lymphoma with T-cell and B-cell representation through low-grade to high-grade malignancies (see Chapter 27). An important concept in primary extranodal lymphoma is mucosa-associated lymphoid tissue (MALT) and its subsequent relationship to low-grade malignancy. The possible etiologic association with antigenic stimulation and favorable natural history with low metastatic potential are features of MALT lymphomas. This contrasts with the more fulminant presentation and early

449

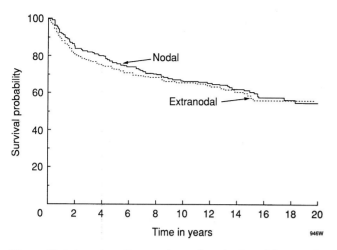

Figure 25–1. Cause-specific survival rates from the date of diagnosis for extranodal and nodal presentations of stages I and II non-Hodgkin's lymphoma. (From Sutcliffe SB, Gospodarowicz MK: Localized extranodal lymphomas. *In* Keating A, Armitage J, Burnett A, Newland A [eds]: Haematological Oncology. Cambridge, Cambridge Medical Reviews, 1992, pp 189–222.)

and widespread dissemination of disease in sites or tissues characterized by intermediate- or high-grade tumors, for example, bone or testis. Primary CNS lymphomas also present characteristic features related to the histologic type, the growth pattern (largely confined to the nervous system), the probability of local recurrence (high), and the etiologic role of immunodeficiency, particularly acquired immunodeficiency syndrome (AIDS) and post–organ transplantation (see Chapter 27).

- Do the same management principles apply to localized nodal and extranodal lymphoma? Both nodal and extranodal non-Hodgkin's lymphomas share a number of common prognostic determinants, for example, stage, symptoms, tumor bulk, and histologic type. These attributes define the survival probability, largely as a measure of the likelihood of primary tumor control with therapy, either as a function of recurrence after radiation or complete response after chemotherapy or combined-modality therapy. The site of extranodal disease provides the additional dimensions of histologic characteristics, preferential organ localization, and patterns of relapse or dissemination that may be factored into the initial management plan.

GENERAL ASPECTS OF EXTRANODAL LYMPHOMA

INCIDENCE AND DISTRIBUTION

Non-Hodgkin's lymphomas account for approximately 5% of human cancers, with an age-standardized incidence of around 17 per 100,000 persons. They occur more commonly with advancing age (Fig. 25–2) and do not show the bimodal adult age distribution characteristic of Hodgkin's disease.

The frequency of occurrence of primary extranodal lymphoma has been reported as

- 24% of all nondisseminated lymphomas in the U.S. Surveillance, Epidemiology, and End Results group of cancer registries, 1950 to 1964 data[1]
- 41% of all patients with non-Hodgkin's lymphoma (stages I–IV) from a population-based registry in the Netherlands[2]
- 37% of all patients with non-Hodgkin's lymphoma (stages I–IV) from a contemporary population-based registry of all new cases in western Denmark[3]
- 50% of patients with stages I and II non-Hodgkin's lymphoma or 31.5% of all patients (stages I–IV) seen at Princess Margaret Hospital (PMH) from 1967 to 1988[4]

The distribution of primary extranodal presentation (stages I and IIE) in the PMH series is shown in Figure 25–3 and in comparison with the series of Freeman and associates[1] and Otter and colleagues in Tables 25–1 and 25–2.[2]

PATHOLOGY

Traditional classifications of non-Hodgkin's lymphoma derive from morphologic observations stressing architectural change in relation to normal tissue anatomy (usually lymph node) and cytologic appearances of infiltrating malignant cells. Subsequently, concepts emphasizing lineage, function, and differentiation using phenotypic and molecular techniques have been introduced. Morphologic classifications are more suited to lymph node interpretation. The four classic classifications, which formed the basis for clinical studies, are as follows:

- Rappaport—nodular versus diffuse; variable differentiation of lymphocytes; histiocytic cells; mixed lymphocytic and histiocytic populations[5]
- Lukes and Collins—B cell versus T cell; small lymphocyte, plasmacytoid lymphocyte, follicular center cell—small and large, cleaved and noncleaved; T-cell tumors—small lymphocytes, convoluted or cerebriform cells, lymphoepithelial, immunoblastic lesions[6]

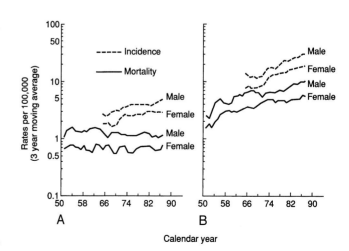

Figure 25–2. Incidence and mortality rates expressed per 100,000 of the population for non-Hodgkin's lymphoma (ICD 9: 200,202) for patients younger (A) or older (B) than 50 years of age for the Province of Ontario. Age is adjusted to the world standard population. ICD, International Classification of Diseases. Data from the Division of Epidemiology and Statistics, Ontario Cancer Treatment and Research Foundation.)

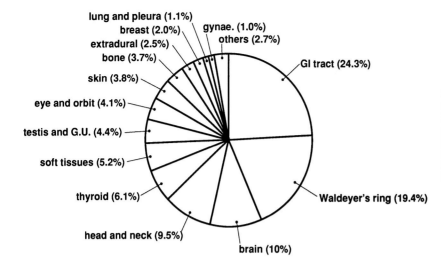

Figure 25–3. Distribution of extranodal presentations of stages I and II non-Hodgkin's lymphoma by site—Princess Margaret Hospital series, 1967–1988. GU, genitourinary; GI, gastrointestinal; gynae., gynecologic. (From Sutcliffe SB, Gospodarowicz MK: Localized extranodal lymphomas. *In* Keating A, Armitage J, Burnett A, Newland A [eds]: Haematological Oncology. Cambridge, Cambridge Medical Reviews, 1992, pp 189–222.)

- Kiel—lymphocytic, immunocytic, and centrocytic tumors; centroblastic/centrocytic tumors; centroblastic, immunoblastic, and lymphoblastic tumors[7]; subsequent additional distinction of B-cell and T-cell lineage[8]
- Working Formulation prognostic categories—low, intermediate, and high grade, characterized predominately by Rappaport groupings but applicable to other classifications[9]

When applied to the characterization of primary extranodal lymphoma, limitations of these classifications become apparent.

- The extranodal site architecture does not necessarily align itself with nodal architecture, displaying a clear distinction of nodular (follicular) and diffuse effacement of tissue.
- Extranodal tissue biopsies are frequently small and often crushed or distorted. Issues relating to sample size, adequacy of material for interpretation, and representativeness of tissue involved by lymphoma arise. There are also issues related to preservation and handling of small fragments or biopsy specimens and the adequacy of material for phenotypic and molecular analysis.
- Distinction of normal physiologic lymphoid aggregates from localized involvement of tissue by lymphoma, for example, Askanazy nodules in bone marrow biopsy specimens and periportal lymphocytic infiltrates in liver

biopsy specimens can be difficult. In certain sites, there has historically been controversy as to the nature of lymphoid pseudotumors, for example, orbital, pulmonary, and GI pseudotumors, and their distinction from low-grade malignant lymphoma.

- Although these histologic classifications applied satisfactorily to nodal and B-cell lymphoma, the histologic classification of T-cell disease in nodal and extranodal sites posed difficulties. Additionally, the classification as a guide to prognostication is often limited in various categories of T-cell disease, for example, angioimmunoblastic lymphadenopathy, lymphomatoid granulomatosis, and peripheral T-cell lymphomas.

A recently proposed Revised European-American Lymphoma (REAL) classification for malignant lymphomas addresses some of these issues by including all the lymphoproliferative disorders.[10] The REAL classification identifies a number of distinct disease entities not represented in previous classifications (Table 25–3). It is based on the premise that B-cell malignancies are distinct from T-cell malignancies and attempts to describe a number of clinical entities, while treating the grade of disease as a variable within a given disease rather than the basis for classification, as does the Working Formulation.

Several of the histopathologic and clinical entities are of particular importance to the primary extranodal lymphomas. The most common is MALT lymphoma (discussed in the following section).

Table 25–1. Distribution of Patients with Non-Hodgkin's Lymphoma°

Series	Period	Total Number	Stages I and II (No.)	Primary Extranodal (No.)	Percentage Extranodal
Freeman et al[1] (1972)	1950–1964	1467	—	1467†	24
Otter et al[2] (1989)	1981–1986	580	242	236	40.7
Sutcliffe and Gospodarowicz[4] (1992)	1967–1988	2254‡	1391	708§	31.4

°Number of patients
†Refers to nondisseminated lymphoma.
‡Excludes 79 patients with primary brain lymphoma.
§Clinical stages IE and IIE.

Table 25–2. Sites of Primary Extranodal Non-Hodgkin's Lymphoma*

	Series		
	Freeman et al[1] (1972): Nondisseminated Lymphoma	*Otter et al[2] (1989): Stages I–IV*	*Sutcliffe and Gospodarowicz[3] (1992): Stages I and IIE*
Gastrointestinal	36.7	16.6	24.3
Waldeyer's	13.6		19.4
Other head and neck	4.7		9.5
Thyroid	2.5		6.1
Eye and orbit	—		4.1
Genitourinary	0.16		4.4
Gynecologic	—		1.0
Breast	2.2		2.0
Bone	4.7		3.7
Extradural	—		2.5
Lung and pleura	3.6		1.1
Soft tissue	8.6		5.2
Skin	7.5		3.8
Brain	—		10
Others	14.7		2.7
No. of patients	1467	580	787

*Expressed as a percentage of total.

Mucosal-Associated Lymphoid Tissue Lymphoma

MALT lymphomas deserve special attention. These are low-grade B-cell tumors of MALT predominantly in the GI tract, pharynx, salivary glands, lung, and thyroid. They are characterized by a prolonged clinical course and persistent disease at the site of origin. They have a characteristic lymphoepithelial lesion consisting of centrocyte-like cells lying within the lamina propria and infiltrating the glandular epithelium of the mucosa. Tumors arising from MALT tissues demonstrate a clonal origin, and there is evidence of malignancy in otherwise "benign" lymphoepithelial lesions within MALT tissues.[11, 12] There has also been demonstration of clonality within the otherwise apparently benign lymphoepithelial lesion and subsequent malignancy within another MALT-tissue epithelial system in archival material over a long natural history of illness.[13]

MALT lymphomas are usually associated with preexisting chronic immune system stimulation. Most MALT lymphomas arise in the stomach, but they may involve other known MALT sites such as thyroid and salivary glands as well as other less well-described situations, including breast and bladder tissue. The cause of this disease has now been linked to infection with *Helicobacter pylori*. Although typical MALT lymphomas are low-grade small B-cell neoplasms, they may transform into intermediate-grade large cell lymphomas. Current experience with these neoplasms suggests that MALT lymphomas tend to remain localized and may be cured with local therapy, even when transformed.[14]

Immunoproliferative small intestinal disease (IPSID) is an indolent lymphoma, probably of MALT origin, involving upper small intestine with associated malabsorption and α-heavy-chain disease.[15] Large cell transformation may occur. Some early clonal IPSID lesions have been noted to regress after antibiotic therapy, suggesting that immune stimulation is involved in their pathogenesis.

Peripheral T-Cell Lymphomas

Peripheral T-cell lymphomas are a heterogeneous group of T-cell neoplasms, more common in Asia, usually affecting adults and commonly generalized at presentation. Eosinophilia and pruritus are common. An aggressive clinical course is typical, and although the disease is potentially curable, some are resistant to current chemotherapeutic regimens. Specific subtypes of peripheral T-cell lymphoma should be considered because of their importance in primary extranodal lymphomas.

Intestinal T-Cell Lymphoma (With or Without Enteropathy)

Intestinal T-cell lymphoma, previously called "malignant histiocytosis of the intestine" is uncommon.[15–17] It commonly involves the jejunum, is associated with a previous history of gluten-sensitive enteropathy in approximately 50% of cases, and is referred to as "enteropathy-associated T-cell lymphoma (EATL)." Most EATLs are high-grade pleomorphic large cell lymphomas and are associated with a poor prognosis. They are usually CD3+, CD7+, CD4–, and CD8– peripheral T-cell lymphomas. They express HML-1, supporting an origin from the intraepithelial T cells of MALT. Non-EATL T-cell lymphomas can occur anywhere in the GI tract. Most are CD4+. Some are classified as Ki-1–positive anaplastic large cell lymphomas.

Angiocentric Lymphoma

Angiocentric lymphoma includes disorders previously known as "lethal midline granuloma," "nasal T-cell lymphoma," "lymphomatoid granulomatosis," and so forth. It is characterized by an angiocentric and angioinvasive infiltrate.[18] The most typical example of this disease includes angiocentric T-cell sinonasal lymphoma. Although less common in Western countries, sinonasal lymphomas are the second most common group of extranodal lymphomas in patients in China. Many are angioinvasive T-cell lymphomas,

Table 25–3. International Lymphoma Study Group REAL Classification

B-Cell Neoplasms

I. Precursor B-cell neoplasm
  Precursor B-lymphoblastic leukemia/lymphoma
II. Peripheral B-cell neoplasms
  • B-cell CLL/prolymphocytic lymphoma/small lymphocytic lymphoma
  • Lymphoplasmacytoid lymphoma/immunocytoma
  • Mantle cell lymphoma
  • Follicle center lymphoma, follicular
    Provisional cytologic grades: I, small cell; II, mixed small and large cell; III, large cell
    Provisional subtype: diffuse, predominantly small cell type
  • Marginal zone B-cell lymphoma
    Extranodal (MALT type ± monocytoid B cell)
    Provisional subtype: Nodal (± monocytoid B cell)
  • Provisional entity: Splenic marginal zone lymphoma (± villous lymphocytes)
  • Hair cell leukemia
  • Plasmacytoma/plasma cell myeloma
  • Diffuse large B-cell lymphoma; subtype: primary mediastinal (thymic) B-cell lymphoma
  • Burkitt's lymphoma
  • Provisional entity: High-grade B-cell lymphoma, Burkitt-like

T Cell and Putative NK-Cell Neoplasms

I. Precursor T-cell neoplasm
  Precursor T-lymphoblastic lymphoma/leukemia
II. Peripheral T-cell and NK-cell neoplasms
  • T-cell CLL/prolymphocytic leukemia
  • Large granular lymphocyte leukemia (LGL)
    T-cell type, NK-cell type
  • Mycosis fungoides/Sézary syndrome
  • Peripheral T-cell lymphomas, unspecified
    Provisional cytologic categories: Medium-sized cell, mixed medium and large cell, large cell, lymphoepitheliod cell
    Provisional subtype: Hepatosplenic γδ T-cell lymphoma
    Provisional subtype: Subcutaneous panniculitic T-cell lymphoma
  • Angioimmunoblastic T-cell lymphoma (AILD)
  • Angiocentric lymphoma
  • Intestinal T-cell lymphoma (± enteropathy-associated)
  • Adult T-cell lymphoma/leukemia (ATL/L)
  • Anaplastic large cell lymphoma, CD30+, T– and null cell type
    Provisional entity: Anaplastic large cell lymphoma, Hodgkin-like

REAL, Revised European-American Lymphoma; CLL, chronic lymphocytic leukemia; MALT, mucosal-associated lymphoid tissue; NK, natural killer.

express the CD4+ immunophenotype, and may have clonal T-cell receptor gene rearrangements. Sinonasal T-cell lymphomas usually follow an aggressive course. Other sites of angiocentric lymphoma include the skin, lung, and CNS. Recent studies suggest that some pulmonary cases may be associated with B-cell proliferation and may represent a distinct disease entity.[19]

Anaplastic Large Cell (CD30+) Lymphoma

Anaplastic large cell (CD30+) lymphoma is a distinct entity with a predilection for skin involvement and generalized disease.[20] The prognosis ranges from *indolent* for disease involving skin only to *aggressive* for patients with generalized disease. Two forms of the disease have been recognized: (1) a systemic form (CD30+, epithelial membrane antigen [EMA] positive) with nodal and extranodal involvement including skin, and (2) a primary cutaneous form (EMA-negative CLA-positive) with involvement limited to the skin. Primary cutaneous tumors occur predominantly in adults, may spontaneously regress, and are indolent but incurable. The systemic form appears to behave similarly to other large cell lymphomas and is aggressive but potentially curable.

Certain studies have indicated that there may be a different genetic origin to large cell tumors arising in nodal versus extranodal sites. Raghoebier and colleagues[21] have demonstrated that *BCL2* rearrangement occurs much more commonly in nodal and cleaved large cell lymphoma compared with its infrequent occurrence and more common demonstration of c-*myc* arrangement in extranodal and noncleaved large cell lymphomas, implying that the fundamental changes at the genomic level between nodal and extranodal lymphomas may be different. This is also supported by the finding of a high frequency of *BCL6* rearrangement in diffuse large cell lymphoma involving extranodal sites. Furthermore, the presence of *BCL6* in diffuse large cell lymphoma has been associated with a favorable outcome independent of other recognized prognostic factors.[22]

ETIOLOGY

Despite increasingly detailed knowledge of genomic events underlying the progression and expression of malignant lymphoma, information on causative agents is lacking for both nodal and extranodal lymphoma. Tentative evidence for a role for environmental factors has been reviewed.[23, 24] An expanding literature is evolving for a potential causal relationship between immunodeficiency, prolonged antigenic stimulation, and the development of lymphoma. Thus, in cases of organ transplantation,[25] AIDS,[26] X-linked lymphoproliferative syndrome,[27] and primary immunodeficiency states,[28] there is an excess risk that the patient will develop malignant lymphoma. Such tumors are usually of B-cell, intermediate- or high-grade histologic type, commonly involving or presenting in extranodal sites such as the CNS, the GI tract, liver, and bone marrow. Although extranodal lymphoma is more common with conventional immunosuppression for organ transplantation, the more recent experience with cyclosporine has demonstrated equivalence of nodal and extranodal presentations.[25] A potential role for Epstein-Barr virus (EBV) has been intimated for lymphomagenesis in association with immunodeficiency.

Lymphomas also occur in excess after therapy for Hodgkin's disease.[29] Both B- and T-cell tumors are recorded, and they are of intermediate- or high-grade type. There is no clear relationship to EBV. In this setting, both cellular immunodeficiency from disease and from treatment-related processes and the carcinogenic impacts of cytotoxic chemotherapy and/or radiation may be etiologically relevant. A potential role for infectious agents in the etiology of GI lymphoma (GIL) has derived from two separate observations. In IPSID, or α-chain disease, a common small bowel lymphoma occurring in the circumstance of economic deprivation and poor sanitation in the Middle East and Mediterranean, Ben Ayed and associates reported complete remission in two of six patients treated with antibiotics alone for stage A disease.[30] Various intestinal organisms in the context of intestinal bacterial overgrowth were noted in this report. More substantial is the evidence relating to *H. pylori* as an etiologic factor for low-grade MALT lymphoma of the stomach. As outlined by Isaacson,[31] *H. pylori* is present in the stomach of persons with gastric lymphoma, the prevalence of infection is related to the development of gastric lymphoma, the presence or absence of infection correlates with lymphoma, and infection precedes the development of lymphoma.[31, 32] In the absence of organized lymphoid tissue in the stomach, *H. pylori* is believed to stimulate an accumulation of lymphoid tissue, which, in the presence of persisting infection, antigenic stimulation, and activation of lymphoid cells, results in the evolution of a clonal, low-grade B-cell MALT lymphoma.[33] Such tumors are cytokine sensitive and potentially reversible.[34] The cytokine dependence is lost with histologic progression of the low-grade lesion to a large cell lymphoma.

Although an infectious organism has not been defined for Sjögren's syndrome or Hashimoto's disease, both disorders are characterized by lymphocytic infiltration at sites (salivary gland and thyroid gland) normally lacking organized lymphoid tissue. In both circumstances, the evolution of a lymphoepithelial lesion to a clonal low-grade B-cell MALT lymphoma is recognized[35, 36]; also recognized is a relationship to the development of MALT lymphoma in other organ systems.[13]

CLINICAL ASSESSMENT AND STAGING INVESTIGATIONS

The clinical assessment of patients with primary extranodal lymphoma follows the principles established for assessment of patients with nodal presentations. However, patients with primary extranodal lymphoma, unlike those with nodal or generalized lymphoma, may present to specialists not accustomed to dealing with malignant lymphoma. In such cases, assessment of the local disease extent may be excellent, but the assessment to exclude disseminated disease may be deferred until after treatment of the local problem. In some situations this approach may be appropriate, but in others it may lead to inappropriately extensive surgical resection. The initial assessment should elucidate symptoms related to the presenting site of disease and, in addition, symptoms related to generalized disease and specifically to lymphoma.

The assessment of the extent of disease is one of the most important steps in selecting appropriate therapy. Routine staging investigations include a full physical examination; a complete blood cell count; tests for erythrocyte sedimentation rate (ESR), liver function, and lactic dehydrogenase (LDH) levels; imaging tests; and a bone marrow biopsy. The minimal imaging investigations include a chest radiograph and computed tomography (CT) of the abdomen and pelvis. Appropriate imaging tests should be performed to delineate the extent of extranodal disease and its size, invasiveness, and effect on other organs. In uncertain cases, a cytologic examination of an effusion, or a needle biopsy of a suspicious

lesion, may help clarify the extent of disease. Traditionally, bipedal lymphangiography has been useful in assessing pelvic and paraaortic lymph nodes. The specificity and sensitivity of lymphangiography in expert hands have been reported to exceed that of CT.[37] However, with improvements in CT technology and the increased use of chemotherapy in early-stage disease, the overall value of lymphangiography has diminished.[38] In addition, the value of lymphangiography in other cancers has been disappointing, resulting in a marked decline in its use and also, therefore, a decrease in the number of specialists with expertise in interpretation of the test. Magnetic resonance imaging (MRI) is useful to delineate the extent of disease in soft tissues, but it is especially useful in illustrating the extent of bone, extradural, and brain involvement. The use of gadolinium enhances MRI imaging in the CNS. Gallium scanning, especially high-dose gallium (10 mCi), is a useful general screening tool for malignant lymphoma. In addition to its use in staging, it is also valuable in assessing the response to therapy.[39, 40] The presence of asymptomatic GIL should be excluded in patients with primary lymphoma of Waldeyer's ring or the thyroid gland. Traditionally, imaging of the upper GI tract has been performed, but endoscopy with biopsy is now preferred.

STAGING CLASSIFICATION

The Ann Arbor staging classification originally developed for staging of Hodgkin's disease has been used for non-Hodgkin's lymphoma for approximately 20 years.[41–43] Supradiaphragmatic lymphoid regions in the Ann Arbor classification include the cervical lymph nodes (including cervical, supraclavicular, occipital, and preauricular nodes); infraclavicular; right and left axillary; epitrochlear/brachial; mediastinal; and hilar lymph nodes. Infradiaphragmatic lymph node regions include the paraaortic, mesenteric, iliac, inguinofemoral, and popliteal lymph nodes. In the Ann Arbor classification, Waldeyer's ring, thymus, spleen, appendix, and Peyer's patches of the small intestine are considered lymphatic tissues, and involvement of these areas does not constitute an "E" lesion, which was defined originally as "extralymphatic" involvement. However, most clinicians recognize the unique pathologic and clinical characteristics of primary lymphoma affecting these organs and consider them as separate entities. Therefore, in this chapter all sites of extranodal lymphoma are considered to be in the E category, even if they are not, by definition, extralymphatic.

Although the Ann Arbor classification has been widely accepted, its limitations have been known for many years. In the spectrum of non-Hodgkin's lymphoma, the Ann Arbor classification differentiates locoregional disease from widespread lymphoma and documents the anatomic extent of disease and presence or absence of B symptoms. However, the classification is not optimal for describing the extent of local disease, invasion of adjacent organs, or tumor bulk—the latter is one of several important prognostic factors in lymphoma. The extent of extranodal involvement is not documented, and associated lymphatic involvement is poorly represented by the Ann Arbor lymph node regions. For example, a patient presenting with two skin nodules located only centimeters apart may be classified as stage I or stage IV. Similarly, extensive extranodal lymphoma involving the hard palate, maxillary sinus, nose, and orbit may be classified as stage I or stage IV. These differences in the interpretation of the Ann Arbor classification create confusion in understanding treatment recommendations and confound comparisons of treatment results. The recently published TNM Supplement recommends classification of the involvement of paired extranodal organs as stage I disease.[44] Although this may be prognostically valid in patients with bilateral involvement of tonsils, it does not accurately reflect the prognosis of stage I disease when applied to involvement of both lungs or two kidneys. Several modifications to the Ann Arbor classification have been proposed. In primary head and neck lymphoma, the size of the primary tumor may be classified according to the TNM classification for squamous cell carcinoma of that region. In gastric lymphoma, substaging of stage I to reflect the depth of the stomach wall penetration has been suggested.[45] In stage II disease, distinction of involvement of the immediate nodal region versus more extensive regional lymph node involvement has been found to be of prognostic significance.[46, 47] However, until the biology of lymphomas is better delineated, the Ann Arbor classification, supplemented by a description of tumor bulk, the sites of involvement, and the pathologic appearance, remains the foundation of the assessment of patients with non-Hodgkin's lymphoma.

The assessment of an extranodal site involved by non-Hodgkin's lymphoma should determine the anatomic extent of involvement, any extension of the disease beyond the organ of interest, invasion of neighboring organs or structures, and tumor bulk. For example, the assessment of gastric lymphoma should document the proportion of the stomach involved by tumor; the maximal depth of penetration of the stomach wall; the presence of extension into the perigastric fat or omentum; invasion of the pancreas, spleen, or diaphragm; and the largest tumor diameter. The assessment of lymphoma involving paranasal sinuses should document each involved site, for example, right maxillary sinus, nasal cavity, ethmoid sinus, right orbit, and nasopharynx. In addition, invasion of the soft tissues of the face, bone erosion, and, more specifically, erosion of the base of the skull should also be recorded.

PROGNOSTIC FACTORS AND PATTERNS OF FAILURE

Although the anatomic extent of disease indexed by the Ann Arbor stage is an important prognostic factor, other factors are known to influence the outcome in patients with non-Hodgkin's lymphomas. These include the histologic type, phenotype, tumor bulk, number of involved sites, and proliferation indices[48] as well as age, gender, and performance status.[3] Additional prognostic factors, likely related to tumor bulk and extent of disease, include the hemoglobin and albumin levels, LDH levels, ESR, and β_2-microglobulin.[49–53]

In addition to these factors, the site of extranodal lymphoma has further prognostic implications, for example, lymphoma presenting in testis, ovary, eye, CNS, and liver has a particularly adverse prognosis. Prognostic factors are of special importance in primary extranodal lymphomas, in which the stage, although important, may play a lesser role than the histologic type, tumor bulk, or anatomic extent of

disease. For example, in gastric lymphoma, stage I disease may represent a 2-cm gastric ulcer or a massive unresectable tumor invading the pancreas, posterior abdominal wall, and diaphragm. Stage I lymphoma of the nasopharynx may present as a small nasopharyngeal lesion or may involve the ethmoid and sphenoid sinuses, the orbit, and the base of the skull. The differences in outcome in such cases are substantial.

Knowledge of the pattern of relapse after therapy has additional impact on the management of extranodal lymphoma. It is known that lymphomas presenting in the testis are associated with relapse in the brain or meninges. The association of CNS relapse with lymphoma involving paranasal sinuses and other parameningeal sites, such as the extradural space, is less clear. CNS relapse from lymphoma involving these sites may be due to previously unrecognized direct tumor extension into the CNS. The use of combined-modality therapy and CNS prophylaxis in lymphomas involving these high-risk sites has reduced, but not eliminated, the risk of relapse in the CNS. In low-grade lymphoma involving MALT sites, especially the gut-associated lymphoid tissue (GALT), the recognition of the association of GI, thyroid, and Waldeyer's ring involvement has led to a more appropriate patient assessment. This is particularly important since most of these patients, many of whom have a low-grade lymphoma, are treated with surgery and irradiation rather than systemic chemotherapy. Recent advances in understanding the causes of MALT lymphomas and their association with *H. pylori* infection in gastric lymphoma and with Hashimoto's thyroiditis in thyroid lymphomas have had an immediate impact on therapeutic approaches. Efforts to eradicate treatable causes of the inflammatory process may improve the outcome in MALT lymphomas. Primary head and neck lymphomas, thyroid lymphomas, and GILs may present with massive, locally extensive tumors invading adjacent organs and compromising vital functions such as vision, respiration, and renal function. An aggressive combined-modality approach is required, and achievement of local control is essential, since local failure is the most common pattern of relapse in such cases and is largely unsalvageable with additional therapy.

PRINCIPLES OF TREATMENT

In most situations patients with primary extranodal non-Hodgkin's lymphoma and localized disease are treated with curative intent. A palliative approach is used in situations in which, because of the condition of the patient or the extent and/or location of the disease, a radical treatment carries no chance of cure. The perception that low-grade lymphomas are usually generalized at presentation and are associated with prolonged survival has limited the use of curative treatment strategies in some patients with primary extranodal lymphoma. Knowledge of the histologic type, extent, and pattern of disease is essential to select the appropriate treatment strategy. Local therapy is routinely used for cure and local control. However, the recognition of occult distant disease mandates the use of systemic chemotherapy in a large proportion of patients. The main modalities used in treatment programs for non-Hodgkin's lymphoma are radiation therapy and chemotherapy, although surgery is used in the diagnosis and management of selected extranodal sites. The initial decision for patients treated with curative intent is the use of local treatment alone—surgery, irradiation, or both—versus a local and systemic approach—surgery and chemotherapy or chemotherapy and irradiation. The choice is pragmatic and predicated on the recognition of the potential for local control, inherent risk of occult distant disease, and availability of curative chemotherapy. All these factors are based on clinical observations and past experience rather than the knowledge of basic genetic or biologic factors.

Local Treatment Methods

The role of surgery in the management of primary non-Hodgkin's lymphoma is poorly defined. Many case series include few patients with stage I primary extranodal lymphoma cured with surgery alone. In general, the cure with surgery alone is infrequent, but a resection of the primary tumor may be helpful.[54–56] For example, resection of the segment of bowel involved by lymphoma relieves obstruction and facilitates subsequent chemotherapy, irradiation, and assessment of response to treatment. Indeed most reports of GIL suggest improved outcome in cases where surgical resection of the primary tumor was performed.[47, 54, 57, 58] Unfortunately, there are no studies comparing the management of localized extranodal non-Hodgkin's lymphoma with and without surgical resection. The situations in which a resection of the primary tumor is helpful include GIL, especially localized intestinal disease, and testicular lymphoma. However, since treatment also involves radiation therapy and chemotherapy, aggressive surgical approaches requiring sacrifice of cosmesis or function are not indicated. There is no indication for amputation in primary bone lymphoma, mastectomy in breast lymphoma, or cystectomy in bladder lymphoma. Accordingly, preoperative or intraoperative diagnosis is essential. For example, in the approach to treatment of parotid tumors, where radical surgical resection carries a risk of nerve injury, early diagnosis of lymphoma may prevent unnecessary sacrifice of the facial nerve.

The principles of radiation therapy are to deliver an adequate dose of radiation to the target volume—the full extent of disease with appropriate margins. The proper design of radiation treatment plans takes into consideration all staging data, awareness of normal anatomy, familiarity with common routes of lymphatic spread, and appreciation of the radiation tolerance of normal organs and tissues. The correct application of dose and fractionation schedule should ensure local control with acceptable acute toxicity and minimize the potential for late complications. The technique should guarantee reproducibility of treatment on a daily basis. Current radiation techniques employ custom-designed fields that conform to an individual patient's anatomy and tumor location. The common terms used to describe the extent of radiation therapy are "involved field," "extended field," and "total lymphoid irradiation." Involved-field radiation is most commonly used in localized lymphomas and implies treatment to the extranodal site and its immediate lymph node drainage area. A treatment plan including irradiation to the adjacent, second-echelon lymph nodes would be considered extended-field radiation. However, the use of these terms in the literature varies

considerably. "Total lymphoid irradiation" implies treatment to all the major lymphoid regions, and its use at present is uncommon. The application of radiation fields varies from parallel opposed fields to three- or four-field techniques with the intent of providing a homogeneous distribution of radiation dose within the target area. This frequently requires the use of radiation beam–modifying devices such as shields and compensators. Patient-immobilizing devices are used to ensure day-to-day reproducibility of therapy.

The dose of radiation required to achieve local control varies depending on the histologic type and tumor bulk.[50, 52] Low-grade lymphomas are more responsive to radiation, and doses of 20 to 35 Gy delivered in 10 to 20 fractions over 2 to 4 weeks result in local control rates in excess of 95%. Lower doses have been reported to produce local control, especially in low-bulk disease. There are no prospective, randomized trials designed to determine the optimal radiation dose and, with current excellent results and few complications, it is unlikely that such trials will be undertaken. Large cell lymphomas are said to be less sensitive to radiation. However, their response is dependent on the tumor bulk. In the setting of combined-modality therapy, excellent local control has been obtained with doses of 30 to 35 Gy delivered in 1.75- to 3-Gy fractions.

Systemic and Combined-Modality Therapy

There are many reasons to consider chemotherapy in the management of primary extranodal non-Hodgkin's lymphoma. The experience in treating extranodal lymphomas with local therapy alone has documented a high risk of distant failure, especially in patients with intermediate- or high-grade lymphoma, older patients, and those with bulky disease.[50, 52, 59] The risk of occult disease in distant sites is high in patients with non-MALT-related lymphoma.[60–62] Chemotherapy, especially combinations based on doxorubicin (Adriamycin) such as CHOP (cyclophosphamide, hydroxy-daunomycin, Oncovin, prednisone), ProMACE (prednisone, methotrexate, Adriamycin, cyclophosphamide, etoposide), MACOP-B (methotrexate, Adriamycin, cyclophosphamide, Oncovin, prednisone, bleomycin), M-BACOD (methotrexate, bleomycin, Adriamycin, cyclophosphamide, Oncovin, dexamethasone), and so forth, has been documented to cure patients with malignant lymphoma, principally those with diffuse large cell lymphoma.[63] The choice of a chemotherapy regimen is based on histologic type, irrespective of the site of disease. In most instances in which chemotherapy and radiation are combined, chemotherapy is given first. This makes possible an assessment of the response to chemotherapy and the reduction of disease bulk, thereby allowing the use of a lower radiation dose. Such an approach has been shown to improve local control over that obtained with radiation alone and to reduce distant relapse rates.

The use of a combined-modality approach in presentations with high distant failure rates has resulted in improved relapse-free and overall survival.[61, 62, 64–66] Currently, patients with stage I and II extranodal lymphoma without poor prognostic features, such as large tumor bulk (>10 cm), high LDH levels, a high-grade histologic type, or a T-cell phenotype, who are able to complete therapy achieve 80%

to 90% 5-year survival. The use of chemotherapy in MALT-related lymphomas, in which the primary tumor can be controlled with local treatment methods, is less well defined. The relative morbidity and long-term effects of each approach should be considered.

In summary, the principles of therapy for primary extranodal non-Hodgkin's lymphoma are similar to those of localized nodal lymphoma. The choice of local versus systemic therapy is established by considering the histologic type and tumor characteristics, including disease extent and bulk. In general, low-grade lymphomas are treated with radiation therapy alone, and intermediate- and high-grade lymphomas are treated with chemotherapy followed by radiation therapy. The choice of brief chemotherapy followed by radiation, a full curative course of chemotherapy followed by adjuvant radiation, or chemotherapy alone is based chiefly on tumor bulk, the presence of adverse prognostic factors such as B symptoms and high LDH levels, and the anatomic extent of disease. Intestinal and testicular lymphoma may be an exception to that approach, given the potential for complete surgical excision. Special consideration has to be given to organs in which curative doses of radiation compromise function, such as lungs and kidneys. CNS prophylaxis with intrathecal methotrexate or cytosine arabinoside should be given to patients with high-grade lymphomas and considered in patients with testicular lymphoma and tumor involving parameningeal sites. These principles are most important in cases of primary extranodal lymphomas involving rare sites, where the available literature may not reflect the optimal approach.

ASSESSMENT OF RESPONSE AND FOLLOWUP

In non-Hodgkin's lymphoma, the key determinant of cure is the ability to eradicate disease—the attainment of complete remission. In patients treated with radiation alone, response is usually assessed 4 to 6 weeks after the completion of therapy. Since the fractionation schedule for the radiation dose is determined before treatment and is usually based on information regarding the dose-response relationship and tolerance of tissues within the treatment volume, the presence of residual disease at the end of the treatment course is not an indication for additional radiation therapy. The assessment of response includes examination of the organ of presentation and followup general examination to rule out disease progression. In patients treated with chemotherapy or combined-modality therapy, when chemotherapy is used first, the response is assessed after one or two courses of chemotherapy and every 1 to 2 months thereafter. Chemotherapy is complete after two further courses after attainment of clinical remission. A gallium scan 1 to 2 months after completion of chemotherapy is useful in determining the completeness of response of a previously gallium-avid tumor.[40]

Remission assessment for patients with primary extranodal lymphoma comprises the demonstration of disease-free status on general assessment and also at an organ-specific level. Issues that require special consideration include the following:

- Knowledge of the pattern of relapse, which is helpful in planning followup procedures. In situations in which

local relapse is uncommon, as in orbital lymphoma, completely resected gastric lymphoma, or small-bulk Waldeyer's ring lymphoma, long-term repeated imaging or endoscopic examination of the presenting site is not indicated. However, followup should include a complete physical examination with particular attention to any new adenopathy or unusual symptoms. Patients with low-grade lymphomas, especially non-MALT-associated diseases, are at prolonged risk of relapse. Although most recurrences in patients with intermediate-grade lymphoma occur within 2 to 3 years after the diagnosis, late relapse occurs especially in patients presenting with stages I and II disease. Therefore prolonged followup is indicated in all patients with primary extranodal lymphomas.

- Evaluation of an organ or tissue that is anatomically or architecturally abnormal as a result of prior involvement by lymphoma, for example, CNS lymphoma.
- Primary bone lymphoma presenting persisting radiologic and MRI abnormalities after treatment. Radioisotope bone scan almost certainly identifies changes that cannot distinguish active disease from bone healing and remodeling. Resolution of gallium activity may be helpful in such cases.
- The evaluation of paired organs or sites, for example, testis, kidney, salivary and lacrimal glands, eye and orbit, lung, ovary, particularly when one organ has been the primary site of disease and may have been removed as part of initial therapy. The increased risk of disease recurrence or progression in the paired "normal" organ is well established.
- The evaluation of a site or organ where a substantial component has been removed surgically, for example, stomach, and small or large bowel. Residual imaging abnormalities reflecting the surgical procedure and/or persistence or progression of lymphoma may be apparent. Endoscopic evaluation with biopsies may be desirable. In MALT lesions of the GI tract, the presence of persisting *H. pylori* infection may well constitute appropriate grounds for antibiotic use.

The role of tissue biopsy to establish control of disease at the primary site should be considered individually relative to the degree of clinical uncertainty about remission evaluation and the morbidity of acquiring tissue either by guided fine-needle aspiration or core biopsy. If biopsy is pursued, sufficient tissue for phenotypic and molecular analysis should be acquired.

After establishment of complete remission, the schedule of followup assessment will reflect the expectation of events and their time course. Consideration must be directed to the following:

- Histologic type—recurrence risk is expressed in most patients with intermediate- and high-grade lymphoma within 3 years after therapy. For patients with localized low-grade lymphoma, there is probably no period when there is no risk of relapse; there is also no strong predictive probability of relapse related to the period of observation, although the frequency of relapse becomes less after 8 to 10 years.
- Organ of presentation—certain primary extranodal lymphomas recur locally or within the tissues of origin

with a much higher probability than at remote sites, such as primary CNS lymphoma; GIL and MALT sites; paired organ sites such as salivary or lacrimal gland, testes, orbit, and eye.

- Whether the primary extranodal lesion was resected or remains in situ—although the risk of relapse in the excised organ is abolished through resection, the risk within the tissues of origin must be considered, for example, the GI tract. If the organ of origin remains in situ, it will remain the principal focus of local recurrence, especially if bulky at presentation and if not subsequently irradiated.

- Bulk of disease at the presentation site and the use of locoregional irradiation in the treatment plan. Tumor bulk in a nonresected organ predicts local and distant relapse. Local disease control in a site receiving a tumoricidal dose of radiation therapy is expected unless substantial tumor bulk was present at the time of radiation.

Management of relapse usually involves systemic chemotherapy. However, in patients who relapse with localized disease, repeat combined chemotherapy and radiation may offer a higher chance of prolonged disease control. In selected circumstances of low-grade lymphoma recurring with localized small-bulk disease, involved-field radiation alone may offer lengthy disease control.

TREATMENT COMPLICATIONS

Complications of therapy are summarized in Table 25–4. Complications may be considered generally, for example, risks of surgical procedures and anesthetic risk; or non-specific effects of radiation therapy and chemotherapy, for example, fatigue, nausea, emesis, blood count effects, and so forth; however, the more significant treatment effects, particularly in the long term, are more specific to the organ involved or to the anatomic site receiving therapy. In principle, the impacts of surgery relate to functional consequences to the remainder of the organ, the system involved, or adjacent structures related to the excised tissue; radiation impacts are dose- and volume-related and apply to all tissues and their respective tolerances within the irradiated volume. Chemotherapy effects relate mainly to drug and organ-specific impacts, for example, vinca neuropathy, anthracycline cardiotoxicity, bleomycin pulmonary effects, and hematologic and gonadal impacts. The induction of second malignancies is a recognized low-probability event in survivors of therapy for non-Hodgkin's lymphoma. Cutaneous and hematologic malignancies have been the most commonly characterized second malignant tumors.[67, 68]

SPECIFIC ASPECTS OF PRIMARY EXTRANODAL LYMPHOMA

GASTROINTESTINAL LYMPHOMA

Demographics. Non-Hodgkin's lymphoma of the GI tract is one of the most common lymphomas and accounts for 4% to 20% of all non-Hodgkin's lymphomas and for 30% to 45% of extranodal presentations.[1, 47, 59] It has been suggested that the incidence of GIL has increased in the last two decades.[69] However, in the spectrum of malignancies, it is rare and accounts for 1% to 10% of all GI tract

Table 25–4. Treatment Complications

	Surgery	Radiation	Chemotherapy ± Radiation Therapy
General Area- or Organ-Specific	Complications of anesthesia and surgical morbidity	Fatigue Anorexia Decreased white blood cells, platelets	Fatigue Decreased white blood cells, platelets Drug-specific side effects Nausea or emesis Alopecia Gonadal function Second neoplasia
Stomach and bowel	Small stomach B_{12} absorption Adhesions Malabsorption Diarrhea Colostomy or ileostomy	Nausea, emesis, diarrhea Peptic ulcer Stricture Proctitis	? Risk of perforation through nonexcised lesion Drug-related constipation
Waldeyer's ring and paranasal sinuses		Radiation pharyngitis Xerostomia Dental caries	Mucositis Neutropenic infection
Thyroid	Laryngeal nerve injury Hypoparathyroidism	Radiation esophagitis Hypothyroidism	Hypothyroidism
Testis		Nausea and diarrhea Groin skin reaction Infertility and hypogonadism/	Infertility (recovery variable) ? Hypogonadism
Orbit or eye		Cataract Retinal neovascularization	
Bone	Pathologic fracture		
Breast	Cosmetic effects	Acute skin reaction	
Extradural	Paralysis	Radiation myelitis	
Skin or brain	See Chapters 26 and 27		
Kidney		Radiation nephritis	Nephropathy
Lung		Radiation pneumonitis	Pulmonary fibrosis

malignancies.[1, 70–72] The lymphoid tissue in the GI tract, known as GALT, differs structurally and functionally from peripheral lymph nodes. These differences have also been noted in lymphoid tissue associated with other mucosae, giving rise to the term "MALT." The unique immunophysiologic characteristics of MALT have been defined in the last decade mainly by Isaacson and his collaborators.[15, 45, 73–76] The lymphoid tissue of MALT may be a normal tissue component, as in the intestine, or it may be acquired as a consequence of an autoimmune or inflammatory disorder, as in the stomach. Therefore, lymphomas of the GI tract have a distinct pattern of disease from that of non-MALT-associated lymphomas—they tend to remain localized for long periods, seldom disseminate to bone marrow, and hence respond favorably to local therapy. Studies of these lymphomas have demonstrated that they are monoclonal, capable of disseminating, and, like other low-grade lymphomas, may transform into more aggressive higher-grade lymphomas.[77] Gastric lymphoma has been associated with gastritis induced by *H. pylori*.[78] A large nested case-control study demonstrated that patients with gastric lymphomas have a substantially higher rate of immunologic evidence of prior infection with *H. pylori* than matched controls.[32] Understanding the etiology of gastric lymphoma has far-reaching implications with respect to the etiology of other extranodal lymphomas, especially those occurring in tissues normally devoid of lymphocytes, and to the prevention and treatment of these disorders.

Within the spectrum of primary GILs, those involving the stomach are the most common, accounting for 55% to 70% of cases; followed by intestinal lymphoma, usually involving the ileum (20% to 35%); and colorectal lymphomas (5% to 10% of all cases).[3, 71, 79–81] Primary lymphomas of the esophagus, duodenum, and ampulla of Vater are distinctly uncommon but have been described.[82–86] The rationale for the approach to disease presenting in these uncommon sites is based on experience gained in other GI sites and is predicated on the histologic findings, bulk, and anatomic extent of disease.

Three distinct lymphomas arise in the intestine.[15] First, intestinal B-cell lymphoma is seen in older patients in Western countries and resembles gastric lymphoma. Second, a distinct lymphoma also seen in the West is intestinal T-cell lymphoma, an EATL first described in patients with celiac disease (gluten-sensitive enteropathy). Patients with celiac disease have a 200-fold increased risk of developing primary intestinal T-cell lymphoma.[16, 87, 88] A third lymphoma, an IPSID, occurs mainly in the Middle East and North Africa but has also been described in South Africa, India, the Far East, and Central America.[89–91] The pathogenesis of this process remains unknown. It is believed that the disease involves the clonal proliferation of immunoglobulin A (IgA) heavy-chain-producing B lymphocytes. IPSID occurs most frequently during adolescence and young adulthood in the second and third decades of life and affects men more often than women. Patients present with symptoms of malabsorption. The disease affects the whole length of the intestine, with predominant involvement in the jejunum and duodenum.

Clinical Features, Diagnosis, and Staging. There are considerable differences in presentation of Mediterranean B-cell lymphoma (IPSID) and Western B-cell intestinal lymphoma. Western B-cell lymphoma affects mainly older patients, whereas IPSID commonly presents earlier. IPSID preferentially presents with diffuse involvement of jejunum and duodenum, whereas Western B-cell lymphoma presents with focal involvement of the lower ileum or colon. Presenting symptoms vary depending on the site and the extent of involvement. Anorexia, pain, upper GI bleeding, and nausea are more common with upper GI involvement, although abdominal distention, nausea, vomiting, diarrhea, and lower intestinal bleeding are typical signs of intestinal involvement. Symptoms of small bowel obstruction are common in ileal B-cell lymphomas, although symptoms of malabsorption are the main presenting features of intestinal T-cell lymphoma and IPSID. B symptoms such as fever and night sweats are uncommon; however, weight loss associated with anorexia, pain, or obstructive symptoms is frequent and is often related to the primary presentation rather than a symptom of lymphoma per se.

Radiologic procedures commonly identify the site and nature of disease. Within the stomach, lymphoma is most common at the pyloric antrum, followed by the body, then the cardia. Lesions may appear polypoid, ulcerative, or as diffuse thickening of the stomach wall, giving rise to both rigidity and alteration of mucosal texture. Although CT is not well suited to imaging of the intraluminal component of lymphoma, visualization of wall thickening and regional node size is possible. Imaging of small bowel lymphoma more commonly illustrates luminal narrowing or obstruction, with the more gross impact of mass size and mesenteric node status being defined by CT. In both the large and the small bowel, lesions may be annular, ulcerative, proliferative, or polypoid. Diagnosis is made by examination of an adequate tissue sample, most commonly obtained by endoscopy or exploratory surgery. With access to fresh, frozen, and fixed material and immunophenotyping or genotypic studies, a preoperative diagnosis should be achievable on most patients with gastric lymphoma.

The basic Ann Arbor staging classification is used to describe the extent of GIL. However, within the stage II category, the distinction between local (first-echelon lymph nodes—paragastric or paraintestinal) and distant (other regional lymph nodes—celiac, paraaortic, or iliac) nodal involvement is of prognostic significance.[46, 47, 58, 92] At the 1993 Workshop on GILs, a modification to the Ann Arbor classification was adopted to reflect the extent of the primary tumor and that of regional lymph node involvement (Table 25–5).[46]

Pathology and Prognostic Factors. Published reports on experience with GIL have been mainly based on the Rappaport and Kiel classifications. These classifications are well suited to nodal lymphomas but fail to represent the unique histologic types and special features associated with GILs. Developments in the understanding of these diseases have led to a proposal by Isaacson and colleagues for a new classification of GIL.[93] This proposal with revision of the name "centrocytic lymphoma" after Banks and associates[94] has been endorsed by the 1993 Workshop on GIL as a preferred pathologic classification for GIL (Table 25–6).[46] Sufficient data are available to support the adoption of this classification, and it is in total agreement with the subsequently published REAL classification. Morton and associates illustrated the prognostic value of histology in the

Table 25–5. Primary Gastrointestinal Lymphoma: Staging Classification

Stage I—Tumor confined to GI tract
 Single primary site
 Multiple, noncontiguous lesions
Stage II—Tumor extending into abdomen from primary GI site
 Nodal involvement
  Stage II$_1$—Local, i.e., paragastric in cases of gastric lymphoma and
   paraintestinal in cases of intestinal lymphoma
  Stage II$_2$—Distant, i.e., mesenteric in cases of intestinal primary,
   otherwise: paraaortic, paracaval, pelvic, inguinal
Stage IIE
 Extension outside primary site to involve adjacent organs or tissues
  Enumerate actual site of involvement, e.g., IIE (pancreas), IIE
  (posterior abdominal wall). When there is both nodal involvement
  and penetration to involve adjacent organs, stage should be denoted
  using both a subscript ($_1$ or $_2$) and E, e.g., for stomach lymphoma
  with involvement of paragastric lymph nodes and direct extension
  into the pancreas, correct designation would read II$_1$E (pancreas).
Stage IV—Disseminated extranodal involvement or a GI tract lesion
 with supradiaphragmatic nodal involvement

GI, gastrointestinal.
 Adapted from Rohatiner A, d'Amore F, Coiffier B, et al: Report on a workshop
convened to discuss the pathological and staging classifications of gastrointestinal tract
lymphoma. Ann Oncol 1994; 5:397; with kind permission from Kluwer Academic
Publishers.

retrospective study of the GILs in the British National Lymphoma Investigation (BNLI) Group.[95] In the BNLI experience, the stage and MALT status, irrespective of grade, were the most significant factors identified in a multivariate analysis of gastric lymphoma; the stage and the presence of T-cell histology were the most significant factors in intestinal lymphoma.[95] The prognostic value of the revised classification has been also supported by d'Amore and colleagues in the Danish study of GIL.[47]

The most frequently identified prognostic factors affecting the outcome in GILs include the anatomic extent of disease measured by stage, tumor size, depth of bowel wall invasion, and extent of nodal involvement (substage II$_1$ and II$_2$); the histologic type, including both phenotype B cell versus T cell and grade; the site of involvement; and age.[14, 47, 58, 81, 95, 96] Other prognostic factors include B symptoms, the performance status, the ESR, LDH levels, and β$_2$-microglobulin levels.[47, 97]

Treatment and Outcome. The treatment of GIL remains controversial. The impact of various prognostic

Table 25–6. Gastrointestinal Lymphoma: Pathologic Classification

B-cell lymphomas
 Low-grade B-cell lymphoma of MALT
 High-grade B-cell lymphoma of MALT, with or without evidence of
  low-grade component
 Immunoproliferative small intestinal disease (IPSID), low-grade,
  mixed, or high-grade
 Mantle cell lymphoma
 Burkitt-like lymphoma
 Other types of low- or high-grade lymphoma corresponding to periph-
  eral node equivalent
T-cell lymphomas
 Enteropathy-associated T-cell lymphoma (EATCL)
 Other types not associated with enteropathy

MALT, mucosal-associated lymphoid tissue.
 Adapted from Rohatiner A, d'Amore F, Coiffier B, et al: Report on a workshop
convened to discuss the pathological and staging classifications of gastrointestinal tract
lymphoma. Ann Oncol 1994; 5:397; with kind permission from Kluwer Academic
Publishers.

factors cannot be separated from treatment results. Many reports include only patients who have had surgical resection of the tumor. There are no randomized studies to assess the impact of therapy, and published reports frequently include patients treated over a 20- to 30-year period. Accordingly, in an unselected population of patients with GIL, the results of one particular treatment policy are difficult to compare with those of another.

Gastric Lymphoma. The traditional therapeutic strategies in gastric lymphoma include a complete surgical resection with postoperative radiation therapy, postoperative chemotherapy, or both. Surgery alone employing partial or total gastrectomy has been reported to cure a small proportion of patients.[55] Such treatment is commonly offered to patients with a low-grade lymphoma.[56] However, surgery alone requires careful followup since low-grade MALT-associated lymphoma is a multifocal disease.[98] Most studies with long-term followup report relapse-free rates and survivals inferior to those found when adjuvant therapy has been used. D'Amore, in a retrospective review of the Danish Lymphoma Study Group experience, found that patients with gastric lymphoma who received radiation as part of their therapy had a relative risk of relapse reduced to 0.3.[47] In the PMH experience, patients with stages IA and IIA gastric lymphoma treated with complete gross surgical resection and low-dose (20 to 25 Gy) postoperative radiation had an 86% 10-year relapse-free survival.[14, 58] In this favorable group of patients, the depth of stomach wall invasion did not affect the outcome. Others have shown good results in patients with complete resection of the tumor followed by chemotherapy alone or combined-modality therapy.[57] It is uncertain whether the favorable outcome in these reports was the effect of surgery or low tumor bulk allowing complete surgical resection. Surgical resection is associated with significant morbidity and mortality, and its use in an unselected patient population may have an adverse effect on outcome.

Recently, several reports have suggested that treatment with chemotherapy alone or chemotherapy followed by radiation may produce similar results. Maor and associates reported a series of 34 patients treated with chemotherapy and radiation without gastrectomy.[99] Six patients died of recurrent disease and two of treatment toxicity. Of the 26 surviving patients, 24 did not require gastrectomy. Taal and Burgers reported from Amsterdam a 64% disease-free survival at 4 years in patients treated with radiation therapy alone without prior tumor resection.[100] The updated Amsterdam experience treating gastric lymphoma with chemotherapy and radiation or radiation therapy alone, without an attempt at surgical resection, revealed a 5-year relapse-free survival of 85% in stage I and 58% in stage II patients. Although these reports suggest that a successful therapeutic approach does not have to include surgical resection of the primary tumor, they have to be interpreted with caution. Chemotherapy alone is curative in only a proportion of patients with diffuse large cell lymphoma, and there is no evidence for cure of low-grade lymphoma. The use of radiation therapy in lieu of surgical resection has to be considered in the context of its toxicity. Although moderate-dose radiation therapy (35 to 45 Gy) produces high local control rates, the dose required to control unresected disease is higher than that used in an adjuvant setting

(25 Gy). In most instances in which radiation therapy is used to treat gastric lymphoma, the left kidney is exposed to a radiation dose in excess of tolerance levels. The long-term morbidity of strategies including chemotherapy alone or radiation and chemotherapy without surgical resection has not been compared with those including resection. When resection of the primary tumor is not feasible, combined-modality including doxorubicin-based (e.g., CHOP) chemotherapy followed by radiation is recommended. However, the reported ultimate local control and survival rates in such cases have been lower.

Regression of primary low-grade B-cell gastric MALT lymphoma after treatment with antibiotics, including ampicillin with either metronidazole and tripotassium dicitrobismuthate or omeprazole, has raised the possibility that eradication of *H. pylori* may be sufficient therapy for selected patients with early low-grade lymphoma of the stomach.[34] However, the data are limited, and further followup is needed before such a treatment strategy can be recommended.

Intestinal Lymphoma. The treatment of primary intestinal lymphoma is less controversial than that of gastric lymphoma. In most cases the tumor is diagnosed at laparotomy, and surgical resection is standard. In advanced disease, in which resection is not technically feasible, treatment comprises doxorubicin-based chemotherapy followed, in some patients, by irradiation. Our policy has been to treat low-grade intestinal lymphoma with surgical resection followed by adjuvant whole abdominal radiation (20 to 25 Gy in 1- to 1.25-Gy daily fractions). In intermediate-grade lymphoma we recommend surgery followed by chemotherapy. If a short course of chemotherapy is used, whole abdominal radiation is added. In patients in whom complete tumor resection is not feasible, chemotherapy followed by radiation therapy is recommended.[14, 58] However, in the absence of randomized trials, the optimal treatment strategy is not known. The outcome reported in the literature varies depending on the extent of disease and histologic type. In a large series of intestinal lymphomas, Domizio and associates documented a 75% 5-year survival for patients with low-grade B-cell lymphomas and only a 25% 5-year survival for those with T-cell tumors.[101] The poor outcome of patients with intestinal T-cell lymphoma has also been documented in the BNLI[95] and Danish experience.[47] The site of involvement was also of prognostic significance, with lesions in the terminal ileum having the best survival. Other prognostic factors in primary intestinal lymphoma include age, performance status, B symptoms, and mesenteric lymph node involvement (stage II disease).[47, 95]

The terms "IPSID," "α heavy-chain disease," and "Mediterranean lymphoma" all refer to various manifestations of B-cell lymphoma affecting the small intestine.[102] Patients present with poor performance status and severe malabsorption and frequently cannot tolerate standard therapy. Overall survival is poor. Several authors have reported that treatment with the tetracycline group of antibiotics can produce clinical, histologic, and immunologic remissions.[89, 91, 103, 104] Remissions have also been described after chemotherapy.[89, 91, 103, 105] The role of radiation therapy and surgical resection remains to be defined. Despite several available treatments, in general IPSID is a highly lethal

disease, with survival rates being as low as 23% at 5 years.[103] Patients with resectable stage I and II$_1$ disease have a 5-year survival of 40% to 47% compared with 0% to 25% for unresectable or stage II$_2$ disease.[79, 89, 103]

Rectal Lymphoma. Rectal presentations are less common than presentations at other sites in the lower intestinal tract. Diffuse small noncleaved cell lymphoma is the most common, although diffuse large cell lymphomas also occur.[106, 107] Treatment usually includes chemotherapy and irradiation (30 to 40 Gy in 1.5 to 2 Gy daily fractions) for patients presenting with bulky lesions and/or intermediate-grade lymphoma. Involved-field radiation therapy alone (30 to 35 Gy in 1.5 to 1.75 Gy daily fractions) has been successful in providing long-term disease control for MALT lymphoma of the rectum. Abdominoperineal resection should be discouraged because there is no evidence that it improves local control or survival.[107]

Patterns of Failure. The pattern of relapse in GIL is closely related to the extent of primary tumor and treatment. However, in general, local relapse is predominant. This is especially seen in bulky unresectable tumors with direct extension to other intraabdominal organs. When local disease is controlled, either by complete surgical resection or multimodality therapy, extraabdominal relapse becomes more common. Disease dissemination is also a function of the histologic type. Systemic involvement is uncommon in MALT lymphomas but is usual in high-grade disease such as Burkitt's lymphoma, with CNS relapse constituting part of the disease spectrum. Extraabdominal relapse is more common in intestinal lymphoma, especially when mesenteric involvement is present.

HEAD AND NECK LYMPHOMA

The term "lymphoma of the head and neck" is somewhat misleading inasmuch as it has relatively little meaning if applied to those tissues or organs present within the anatomic region of the head and neck, for example, the brain, thyroid, orbit, skin, neck nodes, and so forth. The term is more appropriately applied to lymphomas arising in Waldeyer's ring, the nasal fossa, paranasal sinuses, and the oral cavity and adnexa (most commonly the salivary glands). The proportionate representation of sites at PMH is shown in Table 25–7.

Table 25–7. Distribution of Sites of Stage I-II Extranodal Non-Hodgkin's Lymphoma of Head and Neck, Princess Margaret Hospital, 1967–1988 (204 patients)

	Percentage
Tonsil	35.0
Nasopharynx	17.5
Base of tongue	5.2
Larynx and hypopharynx	1.3
Oral cavity	16.0
Salivary glands	9.6
Paranasal sinuses	8.0
Nasal cavity	2.2

From Sutcliffe SB, Gospodarowicz MK: Localized extranodal lymphomas. *In* Keating A, Armitage J, Burnett A, Newland A (eds): Haematological Oncology. Cambridge, Cambridge Medical Review, pp 189–222.

Waldeyer's Ring Lymphoma (Tonsil, Base of Tongue, and Nasopharynx)

Demographics, Clinical Features, and Diagnosis. Characteristically, men are affected with Waldeyer's ring lymphoma more than women (1.5 to 2.0:1), and the disease occurs most frequently after 50 years of age. Dysphagia, airway obstruction, eustachian tube blockage, a mass lesion, and neck adenopathy are the common modes of presentation, depending on the principal site of the tumor. B symptoms are uncommon with early-stage disease. Frequently, the lesion may be visible by examination and may be effectively imaged for site, size, local extension, and neck adenopathy by CT or MRI. Multiple sites of involvement may be apparent within the tissues of Waldeyer's ring.

Diagnosis is achieved by tissue biopsy, and although surgery may debulk the primary lesion, resection is never a curative procedure for lymphoma arising in Waldeyer's ring. Full staging evaluation is mandatory, given estimates of 30% of patients with tonsillar lymphoma having advanced disease, and should include investigation of the GI tract with imaging or endoscopy, given a clear pattern of a failure relationship between Waldeyer's ring lesions and the GI tract, and vice versa.

Pathology and Prognostic Factors. Most tumors are of diffuse, large cell type (intermediate grade) with low- and high-grade lesions relatively uncommon. B-cell tumors predominate. Prognostic factors influencing tumor control include the histologic type, tumor bulk, and stage (IE versus IIE or IIE localized nodal versus IIE extensive nodal disease). These prognostic factors principally influence overall survival through their relationship to primary tumor control (local tumor bulk) or to the risk of occult, more extensive systemic disease (stage and extent of nodal disease).

Treatment, Patterns of Failure, and Outcome. Traditionally, most experience has reflected the use of local radiation therapy with high local control rates using involved-field techniques (primary tumor plus draining neck nodes) and moderate radiation doses (35 to 50 Gy). Overall survival rates of 50% to 60% for stage IE lesions and 25% to 50% for IIE lesions have been recorded.[108–115] After radiation therapy, most failures occur distant to the radiation field, indicating a high risk of occult systemic disease with apparently localized Waldeyer's ring presentations. Clear patterns of relapse involving disseminated nodal failure, bone marrow, and GI tract have been identified, but no apparent predilection for CNS failure has been defined to warrant consideration of CNS prophylaxis.

The overall relapse rate and the pattern of failure after radiation therapy strongly indicate the need for effective therapy for both local tumor and occult systemic disease. A combined-modality approach using an anthracycline-based chemotherapy regimen to achieve complete remission with adjuvant radiation therapy to the primary tumor and neck nodes (35 to 40 Gy) would be common current practice. For patients with stages I to IIE disease, there is no indication for CNS prophylaxis. With such therapy, local control rates in excess of 80% and overall survival rates of 60% to 75% should be achieved depending on the bulk and nodal extent of the presenting lesion.[116–118]

Paranasal Sinus and Nasal Cavity Lymphoma

Demographics, Clinical Features, and Diagnosis. Paranasal sinus and nasal cavity lymphomas occur more commonly in men and in those older than 50 years of age. Important differences in clinical features, phenotypic and genotypic characteristics, and prognosis are apparent between Western and Asian populations presenting with nasal fossa and midline sinus lymphomas.[119, 120] Common presenting features include painless nasal obstruction, nasal discharge, nasal hemorrhage, "tearing" of the eyes, facial swelling, or palatal lesions with dental impacts. In Asian patients, a destructive, erosive lesion (polymorphic reticulosis/lethal midline granuloma) may be a more characteristic presentation. Examination may define the lesion by anterior or posterior rhinoscopy. Lesions within the maxillary sinus may affect the nasal fossa, orbit, palate/buccogingival recess, or anterior facial integrity (facial swelling, asymmetry, and loss of nasolabial fold) (Fig. 25–4).

Diagnosis is achieved by tissue biopsy. Surgical procedures are never curative. Tumor extent is most effectively documented by CT or MRI evaluation, taking account of soft tissue swelling and bone destruction. Evaluation of opacified sinuses as an indication of tumor bulk presents difficulties in the distinction of tumor from retained mucus. Full staging evaluation indicates that most tumors are stage I-IIE and rarely have coexistent B symptoms (fever, night sweats, and weight loss).

Pathology and Prognostic Factors. Tumors are most commonly of diffuse, large cell type including immunoblastic lesions.[121, 122] Both B-cell and T-cell tumors are seen—B-cell tumors are more common in Western populations, although the T:B ratio is higher than for nodal lymphoma; in Asian populations, T-cell tumors predominate

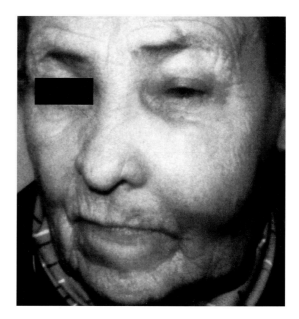

Figure 25–4. Malignant lymphoma of the left maxillary anterior sinus is bulging through the anterior wall with loss of the nasolabial fold and encroachment on the floor of the left orbit.

and show the characteristic features of angioinvasion, necrosis, and epitheliotropism within the spectrum of angiocentric, immunoproliferative disease.[123] Low-grade tumors are rare.

Given the limited histologic diversity of paranasal sinus tumors, the principal prognostic factors are bulk and stage. Bulk is difficult to characterize in terms of mass lesion dimension because of the problem of interpretation of opacified sinuses. In this context, the American Joint Committee on Cancer classification for head and neck cancers, which stresses the local extent of the primary lesion, nodal disease, and distant metastases (TNM classification), may be more descriptive of the extent of disease than the Ann Arbor classification. Stage IE lesions (Ann Arbor) have a better prognosis than stage IIE tumors. It is not yet clear whether all T-cell tumors have a worse prognosis than B-cell lesions, although patterns of failure would seem to imply a greater difficulty in achieving local control of T-cell lesions.[124] Further interpretation of T-cell lesions through characterization of genomic and late membrane protein expression of EBV may also provide prognostic usefulness.[125]

Treatment and Outcome. With radiation therapy, using involved-field techniques and moderate dosage (35 to 45 Gy), high local control rates and overall 5-year survival rates of 30% to 50% have been reported.[112, 118, 126] Recent reports of radiation therapy in T-cell lymphoma in Asian populations have indicated that failure of local control may be substantial. The systemic failure rate is also significant, with patterns characteristic of angiocentric, immunoproliferative T-cell disease, for example, skin and lung.[124] In Western populations, although the systemic failure rate is substantial after radiation alone (≥50%), no clear pattern is apparent, and no predilection for GI tract or CNS recurrence has been reported.

The high systemic failure rate after local radiation has established the current practice of combined-modality therapy (anthracycline-based chemotherapy with adjuvant radiation) for lymphoma presenting in the nasal fossa and paranasal sinuses. For Western populations, overall 5-year survival rates of 60% to 70% should be achieved. Further information is required to characterize optimal therapy and prognosis for patients with T-cell lymphoma of nasal fossa and sinuses.

Salivary Gland Lymphoma

Demographics and Clinical Features. Lymphoma of the salivary gland affects women more than men and occurs more commonly in people older than 50 years of age. The parotid gland is the site of occurrence in approximately 80% of cases, followed by the submandibular salivary gland. Sublingual or minor salivary glands are rarely the presentation site of clinically manifest lymphoma. Presentation is usually with an asymptomatic salivary gland mass. An antecedent history of Sjögren's syndrome or connective tissue disorder should be actively elicited.[127]

Pathology. Tumors are most commonly of low-grade type and B-cell lineage.[128] It is important to distinguish lymphoma arising within a lymph node within the salivary gland from lymphoma originating in the salivary gland. Typically,

the low-grade lesion of the salivary gland is characterized by myoepithelial sialadenitis—a "benign" myoepithelial or lymphoepithelial lesion demonstrating lymphoid infiltration of the salivary gland with acinar atrophy and proliferation of ductal cells. This latter lesion is characteristic of the relationship to Sjögren's syndrome and is also considered to be part of the spectrum of MALT lymphoma/monocytoid B-cell lesion. Molecular studies have indicated the clonal identity between the lymphoepithelial salivary gland lesion and subsequent MALT lymphoma of the GI tract over a 13-year clinical history.[13] In the evolution of a "benign" salivary gland infiltrate to a monoclonal malignant lymphoma, the role of chronic autoantigenic stimulation has been questioned.

Treatment and Outcome. Radiation offers excellent local control for limited-stage salivary gland lymphoma. Overall survival at 5 years approaches 70% to 80%, but there is a continuing relapse risk distal to the radiation field characteristic of the natural history of low-grade lymphoma. There is no role for chemotherapy in the management of low-grade tumors, although a combined-modality approach using anthracycline-based chemotherapy and radiation is standard therapy for transformed intermediate- or high-grade lesions.

THYROID LYMPHOMA

Demographics, Clinical Features, and Diagnosis. Lymphomas of the thyroid gland constitute 2.5% to 3% of all non-Hodgkin's lymphomas and 5% of thyroid malignancies. Women are affected more commonly than men, and the modal age of presentation is over 60 years. Patients usually present with a rapidly enlarging neck mass causing local obstructive and infiltrative symptoms. Tumors are often bulky, and neck adenopathy is common.

Diagnosis is by biopsy. Surgical resection is rarely complete and is not indicated beyond achieving a satisfactory tissue sample. Most thyroid lymphomas (about 80%) present with stage I or II disease. The predictive association of preexisting chronic lymphocytic thyroiditis (Hashimoto's disease) and subsequent lymphoma of the thyroid gland is well established.[36]

Pathology and Prognostic Factors. In excess of 80% of thyroid lymphomas are of diffuse large cell type (intermediate-grade lesions). Low-grade tumors are relatively uncommon. B-cell tumors are typical. Despite the association of lymphocytic thyroiditis and lymphoma, no conclusive evidence of clonality has been established in lymphocytic thyroiditis.[129] Given that most patients are older than 60 years of age and have diffuse, large cell tumors, the other important prognostic variables are tumor bulk—assessed by size, fixation, invasion or adenopathy, stage IE versus IIE, and retrosternal adenopathy. MALT-related thyroid lymphomas have a better prognosis than non-MALT lymphomas.[130]

Treatment, Patterns of Failure, and Outcome. Surgery is a diagnostic procedure, not a definitive intervention for clinically evident thyroid lymphoma. With locoregional radiation fields and moderate-dose radiation (35 to 45 Gy), local control is achieved in more than 75% of patients. Overall, survival rates at 5 years range from 40% to 75% with relapse-free rates of 38% to 64% depending on the admixture of prognostic attributes.[131–136] Given the high relapse rates distal to the radiation field, chemotherapy alone [137] and, more commonly, combined-modality therapy have become the standard treatment approach. Local failure is uncommon with radiation therapy. Systemic progression after radiation is noted in the GI tract, liver, and spleen. Tonsillar recurrence and also lung and bone progression are recorded. The linkage between the GI tract and Waldeyer's ring progression accords with the categorization of thyroid lymphoma within the MALT system.[138] CNS involvement is rare.

Localized thyroid lymphoma of intermediate-grade type is generally treated with combined-modality therapy. Radiation therapy alone may still be considered appropriate therapy for patients with limited, small-bulk disease confined to the thyroid gland. With combined-modality therapy, local control, overall survival, and relapse-free proportions should exceed 70%.[133, 134, 136]

ORBITAL LYMPHOMA

Demographics and Clinical Features. Primary malignant lymphomas account for approximately 10% of orbital tumors. Primary lymphomas of the orbit and eye account for about 4% of all primary extranodal stages I and II non-Hodgkin's lymphoma and 2.0% of all stages I and II lymphoma in the PMH experience. Lymphoma of the extraocular orbital space is considerably more common than lymphoma of the eye (intraocular lymphoma), and the two types of presentation should be distinguished by virtue of their clearly different natural history. The tumors are commonly seen in the elderly, with a median age in the sixth decade.

Topographically, these tumors arise in superficial tissues including the conjunctiva and eyelids (Fig. 25–5A), or in deep tissues including the lacrimal gland and retrobulbar tissues (Fig. 25–5B). Typically the superficial conjunctival tumors present as salmon-pink mass lesions in the fornices. Symptoms include ptosis, blurred vision, chemosis, and epiphora. Tumors of the retrobulbar region present with swelling and proptosis with disturbance of ocular movement. Vision is not usually impaired unless papilledema or optic nerve dysfunction is apparent. Bilateral involvement occurs in approximately 10% to 15% of cases. Involvement of the skin of the orbit is uncommon.

Diagnosis and Staging. It is not possible to differentiate benign and malignant lymphoid lesions of the orbit by clinical criteria; therefore, a biopsy of the lesion is mandatory for diagnosis. Distinction between malignant tumors and benign lymphoid hyperplasia can be difficult, and examination of fresh tissue using flow cytometric and molecular techniques is helpful.

Imaging techniques, including ultrasonography, CT, and MRI, may yield information regarding the site, extent, and invasion of orbital lymphoma. The delineation of local disease extent is as important as staging evaluation performed to rule out generalized lymphoma. Imaging of the orbit is essential for planning the target volume in a manner allowing minimal radiation damage. As with all lymphomas presenting in extranodal sites, assessment to rule out generalized lymphoma is required.

Pathology and Prognostic Factors. Most orbital lymphomas are B-cell neoplasms. Although the histologic type of lesion may vary, the characteristic histologic type is a small cell lymphocytic lymphoma of low grade. Most superficial conjunctival lesions present with a small lymphocytic, follicular, or diffuse small cleaved cell histologic appearance. Although large cell lymphomas of follicular or diffuse type do occur, they are less common and tend to involve the lacrimal gland or present as retro-orbital masses.[139]

Most patients present with stage I disease and small-bulk tumors. The main prognostic factor is the histologic subtype. The large cell lymphomas are associated with lower local control and survival rates than the small cell lymphocytic lymphomas. Patients with diffuse small cleaved or noncleaved cell lymphoma have a higher risk of distant relapse than those presenting with small lymphocytic or follicular small cleaved cell lymphomas.[140, 141] The risk of distant relapse is less in patients presenting with conjunctival

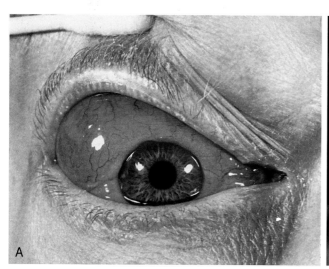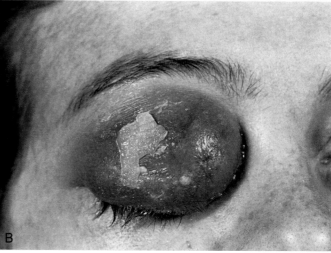

Figure 25–5. Primary orbital lymphoma presenting as a typical "salmon-pink" conjunctival infiltrate demonstrable by eversion of the eyelid (*A*) and as a gross lesion protruding through the orbit, involving the upper eyelid and causing unilateral occlusion of vision (*B*).

lymphoma than in those presenting with orbital lesions. This may represent an increased risk of distant failure with increasing tumor bulk or, alternatively, may reflect the effect of the histologic type, since conjunctival tumors are commonly low-grade lymphomas.[48, 142] Bilateral lesions do not have the unfavorable prognosis of generalized lymphoma, and in some series the incidence of distant relapse is reported to be similar for unilateral (30%) and bilateral (25%) cases.[143]

Treatment, Patterns of Failure, and Outcome. Treatment should be directed to cure while preserving vision and the integrity of the orbit. Extensive surgery should therefore be avoided. Orbital lesions are typically easily controlled with low to moderate doses of radiation. Conjunctival lesions may be treated with direct orthovoltage (250 kV) or 5 to 10 MV photon beams. Treatment with an anterior orthovoltage x-ray field or electron beam provides satisfactory therapy for anterior lesions limited to the eyelid or bulbar conjunctiva, with the advantage of sparing orbital structures compared with the use of a megavoltage photon beam. If an anterior orthovoltage field is used, a small lead eye shield suspended in the beam to shield the lens can result in a lens dose of less than 5% to 10%.[141, 144] For unilateral retrobulbar tumors, a two-field technique using megavoltage photon beams (4 to 6 MV) or a cobalt 60 beam is appropriate, with a corneal shield placed in the anterior field and the lateral field angled posteriorly to spare the lens in both eyes.[145] An alternative arrangement employs an isocentric technique with two oblique (wedged) fields with a shield inserted in both fields, with the patient looking at the shield for each treatment field.[146]

The results of radiation therapy (20 to 30 Gy in 10 to 20 daily fractions) document a local control rate in excess of 95% for patients with low-grade orbital and conjunctival lymphomas. Higher radiation doses are not required, and their use results in higher acute and long-term morbidity. Fewer data are available for intermediate- and high-grade lymphomas. However, the dose-control data for lymphoma in general suggest that for patients with small-bulk tumors (≤2.5 cm), a dose of 35 Gy in 1.75- to 2-Gy fractions provides excellent local control. For patients with larger intermediate- and high-grade tumors, short-duration doxorubicin-based (e.g., CHOP) chemotherapy (three courses) followed by radiation to a dose of 30 to 35 Gy in 1.5- to 1.75-Gy daily fractions is recommended. The complications of radiation therapy, commonly seen when doses of 40 Gy or more are used, include cataract formation, keratitis, and sicca syndrome. The tolerance dose of the lacrimal gland is 40 Gy in 20 daily fractions.[145] Damage to the optic nerve and retina should not be seen with a radiation dose of 40 Gy or less.

The overall actuarial 10-year survival rates reported in the literature are 75% to 80%. These excellent survival rates are likely due to an excess of tumors of a low-grade histologic type. Complete response rates to radiation therapy reported in the literature are 90% to 95%.[142, 144, 145, 147–149] After a complete response has been achieved, the risk of locoregional failure is extremely low. The common sites of relapse are the contralateral orbit and the development of generalized lymphoma. Distant failure rates vary from 20% to 50%, but as in other cases of low-grade lymphoma, failures can be successfully managed and prolonged survival is common. In

patients presenting with large cell lymphoma, particularly with bulky orbital lesions, the risk of distant failure is 30% to 60%. Failures may not be salvaged with further radiation therapy; therefore, a combined-modality approach is recommended for such patients. Occasionally, in patients with bulky tumors, in whom the cornea cannot be protected, the use of radiation therapy alone may result in severe radiation complications. In such patients, the use of chemotherapy alone or combined-modality therapy is preferable.

OCULAR LYMPHOMA

Primary ocular lymphoma together with primary meningeal and spinal cord lymphomas is part of the spectrum of the primary CNS lymphomas. Unlike primary lymphoma of the brain, this disease is rare but is associated with a poor prognosis. Although systemic dissemination is rare, involvement of the CNS is common and ultimately results in death.[150]

Demographics and Clinical Features. Primary intraocular lymphoma is well documented in the literature. The peak incidence is in the sixth to seventh decade of life, although the age range of reported cases is from 27 to 81 years.[151] Two patterns of intraocular involvement tend to occur.[152–154] Lymphoma involving the optic nerve, retina, and vitreous is commonly associated with involvement of the CNS. Lymphoma involving the uveal tract (choroid, ciliary body, and iris) may be associated with visceral involvement. Symptoms include slow and gradual loss of vision. The eye usually shows no external signs of inflammation. Cellular opacities ("flare") are commonly seen in vitreous or anteriorly. The diagnosis is commonly confused with an inflammatory syndrome of uveitis and vitritis or glaucoma.[155] CNS involvement usually occurs late.[156, 157] Bilateral involvement is common, although symptoms usually affect one eye earlier than the other.

Diagnosis. The correct diagnosis can be established after vitreous aspiration biopsy and cytologic examination using appropriate immunocytochemical and molecular techniques. In addition to systemic evaluation, cytologic examination of the cerebrospinal fluid and imaging of both eyes and brain with MRI or CT is required to delineate the extent of local disease.

Pathology. There is little information on the histologic type of these tumors. In the older literature, most cases were classified as reticulum cell sarcoma, suggesting that diffuse large cell type is the most frequent histologic type. Both B-cell and T-cell phenotypes have been reported.[153, 158] In patients with AIDS, ocular involvement is associated with a high-grade histologic type.

Treatment and Outcome. The results of treatment are poor, with rare long-term control and usually only temporary palliation after radiation therapy to the orbit. The reported survivals range from 6 to 18 months. There are also reports of complete response with high-dose intravenous cytosine arabinoside.[159] The optimal management of this rare disease has not been defined; however, with recognition of the pattern of failure, the presence of bilateral involvement, extension to the CNS, and a significant risk of systemic disease, it is apparent that the therapy should include irradiation to both orbits and the whole brain, and systemic and intrathecal chemotherapy.[151, 153, 160, 161]

GENITOURINARY TRACT LYMPHOMA

Primary non-Hodgkin's lymphoma of the genitourinary tract is uncommon. Testicular lymphoma, a disease occurring in older men, with a distinct clinical course, is the most common presenting type. Until recently, it was associated with poor survival. Presentations in other genitourinary tract sites are less common, although series of patients with primary lymphoma of the bladder, kidney, female urethra, and prostate have been described. Localized lymphoma may also present in the epididymis, spermatic cord, and ureter, but only isolated case reports are available for review.[162, 163, 164]

Testicular Lymphoma

Demographics and Clinical Features. Testicular lymphoma accounted for 2.3% of high-grade (Kiel classification) non-Hodgkin's lymphomas registered with the BNLI.[165] Most patients with primary testicular lymphoma are older than 50 years of age at presentation, whereas most germ cell tumors of the testis, except for spermatocytic seminoma, occur in patients younger than 50 years of age. Lymphoma accounts for 25% to 50% of primary testicular tumors in men older than 50 years of age, and it is the most common testicular tumor in patients older than 60 years of age; there is no racial predilection.[60] There is no known association of testicular lymphoma with any previous testicular abnormality. A number of series have documented synchronous or metachronous involvement of the contralateral testis. The incidence of bilateral involvement has been reported to be as high as 18% to 20%.[166] This is in contrast with germ cell testicular tumors, in which the incidence of bilateral involvement is 3% to 5%. Successive involvement of the opposite testis may occur months to years after orchiectomy and may be with a different histologic subtype of lymphoma.

Most patients present with painless swelling of the testis. The swelling may be present for weeks to a few months, but occasionally it may be of several years' duration. An antecedent history of orchitis and trauma has been described, but in contrast with the situation with germ cell tumors, a history of maldescent is rare.

Diagnosis. Diagnosis is most frequently obtained after pathologic assessment of the excised primary tumor. The staging assessment is focused on identification of regional lymph node spread in the paraaortic area and distant spread in Waldeyer's ring, lungs, bone, pleura, skin, and CNS. A careful physical examination, imaging of the retroperitoneum and chest, and assessment of the bone marrow and cerebrospinal fluid are required.

Pathology and Prognostic Factors. Lymphomas of the testis vary considerably in size but are frequently large. Involvement of the epididymis and spermatic cord is common, and vascular invasion is frequent. Involvement of the tunica vaginalis or scrotal skin is rare. Essentially all primary lymphomas of the testis have diffuse architecture, and almost all reported cases are of intermediate- or high-grade histologic type, with diffuse large cell lymphoma the most common. The unwary pathologist can mistake primary testicular lymphoma for seminoma, and a high index of suspicion is required when testicular tumors are examined in older patients. The anatomic extent of

disease is the most important prognostic factor. The presence of lymph node metastases (stage II disease), especially bulky adenopathy, is associated with a poorer outcome.[167, 168] Other prognostic factors include the size of the primary tumor (>9 cm), the presence of systemic symptoms, and age older than 65 years.[60, 169]

Treatment, Patterns of Failure, and Outcome. The initial therapy invariably involves a radical inguinal orchiectomy. Indeed, some patients with truly localized disease have been cured with orchiectomy alone.[60, 167, 170] Primary testicular lymphoma has been recognized as a lethal disease, with only primary brain lymphoma having a worse survival. The historical overall 5-year survival rates range from 16% to 50%, with a median survival of 12 to 24 months. Distant failures were commonly observed in the past. The traditional postorchiectomy therapy for stages I and II testicular lymphoma involved irradiation (35 Gy) of the paraaortic and ipsilateral pelvic lymph nodes. With this approach, the cure rates were 40% to 50% for stage I and 20% to 30% for stage II. There is little evidence that radiation therapy to the retroperitoneal lymph nodes affects survival, although it does improve disease control in retroperitoneal lymph nodes. Reports documenting long-term results of treatment with doxorubicin-based chemotherapy are infrequent. The best results have been obtained by Connors and associates, who reported 15 stage I and II patients treated with three courses of CHOP chemotherapy and radiation to scrotum alone in patients with stage I disease, or scrotum and pelvic and paraaortic lymph nodes in patients with stage II disease.[65] They observed a 93% actuarial relapse-free survival at 4 years. No CNS prophylaxis was used, and no CNS relapses were observed in this study. Other studies, however, have documented CNS relapse despite a treatment approach that included CHOP chemotherapy.[165]

The pattern of failure after orchiectomy alone or orchiectomy and radiation therapy is well documented. Disease progression occurs mainly in extranodal sites, including less commonly involved sites such as skin, pleura, and Waldeyer's ring, as well as the usual sites of systemic involvement of lymphoma such as lung, liver, spleen, bone, and bone marrow. CNS progression with intracerebral and leptomeningeal involvement has been noted in as many as 30% of patients. Failures usually become manifest within 1 to 2 years after the initial therapy, but late relapse, especially isolated late CNS relapse, has been observed. Failure in the contralateral testis is well documented and occurs in 5% to 35% of patients.[171]

In summary, it appears that doxorubicin-based systemic chemotherapy improves the survival of patients with localized testicular lymphoma.[65, 172] The role of radiation therapy is less clear, especially if a full course of doxorubicin-based chemotherapy (such as CHOP, six to eight courses) is used. Regional lymph node irradiation (paraaortic and ipsilateral pelvic–35 Gy in 20 daily fractions) is used in stage I and II disease, although excellent results have been obtained without irradiation of the regional lymph nodes in stage I disease.[65] Low-dose radiation (25 to 30 Gy in 10 to 15 daily fractions) to the contralateral testis eliminates the risk of failure at this site, carries little morbidity in this elderly patient population, and is recommended for all patients with primary testicular lymphoma. The role of CNS prophylaxis is controversial.[65, 173] Connors and associates did not observe failure in the CNS in patients treated with combined-modality therapy,[65] whereas Moller and colleagues observed that systemic chemotherapy did not prevent CNS relapse.[173] Although commonly used, intrathecal chemotherapy may be ineffective, since the pattern of failure includes parenchymal brain involvement. Prophylaxis with intrathecal chemotherapy and cranial irradiation (20 to 24 Gy in 1.8- to 2-Gy daily fractions) is associated with a considerable toxicity and may be hazardous in elderly patients.[65, 165, 172]

Bladder Lymphoma

Demographics and Clinical Features. Primary non-Hodgkin's lymphoma of the urinary bladder is extremely uncommon. It accounts for 0.15% to 0.2% of primary lymphoma cases.[1] The relative rarity of this condition has limited most publications to individual case reports.[174–179] Published reports indicate that primary lymphoma of the bladder occurs in the sixth and seventh decades of life and is more common in women. Patients present with hematuria, frequency, and dysuria. A history of cystitis is a preceding feature in many cases.[174, 175, 180, 181]

Diagnosis and Pathology. The diagnosis is made on cystoscopic biopsy of the tumor. Cystoscopic appearances reveal a submucosal mass with an edematous and friable mucosa and frequent displacement of the bladder wall. Frequently, the tumor mass is large and extends through the bladder wall into the perivesical tissues. Tumors are usually of small cell or lymphocytic type. Large cell lymphomas have been described but are less common. Low-grade and MALT lymphomas have been described.[182, 183] The occurrence of MALT lymphoma is supported by reports of long-term survival after local therapy alone in patients with bulky primary bladder lymphoma.

Treatment and Outcome. Treatment has traditionally involved partial cystectomy and/or radiation therapy to the pelvis. The prognosis is related to the histologic type and extent of the tumor.[184] As in other extranodal lymphomas, low-grade lesions may be managed with radiation therapy alone, but intermediate-grade lymphomas should be treated with doxorubicin-based chemotherapy followed by local irradiation. There are limited data regarding the optimal dose and technique of radiation, but there is no reason to suggest that the sensitivity of the tumor would be different from that of other extranodal lymphomas. Several reports suggest that primary lymphoma of the bladder is associated with a favorable prognosis.[180, 181] Long-term survival has been observed in about 40% to 50% of patients.

Renal Lymphoma

Demographics and Clinical Features. The kidney is one of the most common sites of lymphomatous spread in disseminated disease. However, because the kidney does not normally contain lymphoid tissue, primary renal lymphoma is rare and not generally part of the differential diagnosis of renal masses. Primary renal lymphoma is rarely clinically appreciated. Nonspecific symptoms such as vague abdominal pain, fever, night sweats, weight loss, anemia, and hematuria may be the only presenting symptoms. Physical signs may include hypertension, abdominal masses, and signs of disseminated lymphoma.

Treatment and Outcome. Primary renal lymphoma is

rare, and only individual cases have been described.[185, 186, 187] In our experience, one patient with stage IE follicular large cell lymphoma of the kidney was alive without evidence of recurrent disease 15 years after nephrectomy and postoperative radiation to the renal fossa. Similar case reports support primary renal lymphoma as a separate clinical entity.[187, 188] However, because of the rarity of such cases, no comment can be made regarding the pattern of disease and treatment results other than as directed according to general principles of management recognizing important prognostic factors, especially the histologic appearance.

Prostatic Lymphoma

Demographics, Clinical Features, and Pathology. Primary non-Hodgkin's lymphoma of the prostate is extremely rare. There were no cases of localized prostate lymphoma in the series of carefully assessed patients evaluated and treated at PMH between 1967 and 1988 or in several other modern series of patients with localized extranodal lymphoma.[3, 48, 52, 59] When reported, disease tends to affect men in the sixth to seventh decades of life, although an occasional report includes a younger patient. Patients commonly present with obstructive or irritative urinary symptoms, and the diagnosis is obtained after transurethral resection or biopsy of the prostate gland.[189, 190] The most common histologic type is diffuse lymphoma of intermediate or high grade, although low-grade lymphoma has also been reported.[189, 191] Most reported cases have not been staged rigorously, and it is questionable how many had truly localized disease.

Treatment and Outcome. Survival in published cases is uniformly poor, with rapid systemic dissemination of the disease.[189] This further raises doubt about the existence of primary lymphoma of the prostate as opposed to prostatic presentation of generalized lymphoma. Accordingly, a careful staging assessment of patients presenting with involvement of the prostate gland is mandatory, and treatment with chemotherapy followed by radiation to the pelvis is appropriate in cases without evidence of generalized disease.

Ureteral Lymphoma

Primary lymphoma of the ureter is rare, probably related to the absence of lymphoid tissue in the ureteral wall. Most reported cases are due to extrinsic ureteral compression. Periureteral and peripelvic involvement in the absence of renal involvement is unusual. There are only a few documented cases of primary lymphoma of the ureter.[164, 192, 193] In the absence of published experience, treatment is directed according to the histologic type, tumor bulk, and anatomic extent of disease.

Urethral Lymphoma

Primary lymphoma of the urethra is rare.[194–197] All cases of primary urethral lymphoma have been reported in women. Most patients are older than 60 years of age, present with a firm urethral mass, and may complain of hematuria or vaginal spotting. The lesion frequently arises in the submucosa, and cystourethroscopy reveals normal urothelium. The tumor may present on the meatal epithelium and resemble a urethral caruncle or polyp. The pathologic finding is usually a B-cell lymphoma of intermediate grade, although a case of T-cell lymphoma has been reported.[196] Long-term disease control in patients managed with radiation therapy alone, excision of tumor, and radiation or chemotherapy has been reported.[194–196, 198, 199] As in other cases of intermediate-grade lymphoma, a short course of doxorubicin-based chemotherapy followed by involved-field radiation represents a logical treatment approach.

FEMALE GENITAL TRACT LYMPHOMA

Lymphoma of the Ovary

Demographics, Clinical Features, and Diagnosis. Lymphoma of the ovary is rare as a primary presentation, although ovarian involvement in advanced, systemic lymphoma is not uncommon, particularly in those with high-grade disease.[200–202] Osborne and Robboy cited lymphoma of the ovary as accounting for less than 0.2% of all primary presentations of lymphoma.[200] The usual modes of presentation are by mass lesion in the abdomen and pelvis, abdominopelvic pain, or an unexpected finding during the course of investigation of other gynecologic complaints.

The preoperative assessment of a solid ovarian lesion commonly leads to a surgical oophorectomy with or without surgical resection of disease extension to the Fallopian tubes, omentum, parametrium, or lymph nodes. The disease is commonly bilateral and often of fairly bulky size (median size, 8 cm).[203] The disease is less frequently confined to the ovary, and for most it is often unclear whether the ovary is the primary site or is involved secondarily to extensive systemic spread. In the series of 39 patients reported by Monterroso and colleagues, only 10% of lesions were believed to have arisen primarily in the ovary after staging and followup assessment.[203]

Pathology and Prognostic Factors. Although all histologic types have been observed, Osborne and Robboy reported age-related differences in the pathologic findings in ovarian lymphoma.[200] All lesions occurring in patients younger than 20 years of age (14 of 40 cases) were high-grade lymphomas, whereas those occurring in older women comprised both intermediate- and occasionally low-grade tumors. Frequent initial misdiagnosis as granulosa cell tumors or dysgerminoma was noted in the series of Monterroso and associates,[203] the histologic representation comprising diffuse small noncleaved cell (Burkitt's-like), 54%; diffuse large cell, 31%; diffuse mixed, 8%; large cell immunoblastic, 5%; and follicular and diffuse small cleaved cell lymphoma, 2%. Most tumors were of B-cell type. Important factors influencing outcome are stage, unilaterality versus bilaterality, and histologic type. Insufficient data prevent more definitive statements.

Treatment and Outcome. In the small series reported over long periods, various forms of treatment have been used singly or in combination. A 2- and 5-year overall survival of 42% and 24%, respectively, has been cited.[200] Because lymphomas of the ovary are most commonly of intermediate- or high-grade type and clearly are most commonly associated with extensive dissemination, the initial treatment approach should comprise chemotherapy. Considerations should include the intensity of therapy, the need for CNS prophylaxis, and the role of treatment intensification with marrow or stem cell support for those with high-grade lesions. Radiation therapy may be appropriate in the circumstance of a localized presentation with residual disease after surgery or after definitive chemotherapy. Local control is, however, a lesser issue given the usual resection of the presentation lesion and the common pattern of failure being one of systemic disease progression.

Lymphoma of the Uterus, Uterine Cervix, and Vagina

Demographics and Clinical Features. Non-Hodgkin's lymphomas of the uterus and vagina occur most commonly around the age of 50 years,[204, 205] with a range of 20 to 80 years; three fourths of patients are postmenopausal.[206] Lesions of the uterine cervix are more common than endometrial or vaginal lesions and may present as an asymptomatic, unexpected finding after hysterectomy for other reasons, or may present with bleeding, pain, dyspareunia, and/or postcoital bleeding. Clinically apparent lesions are typically large (50% exceeding 4 cm) and are usually endophytic with local invasion into paracervical tissues, giving rise to a barrel-shaped lesion. Occasionally tumors arise from a cervical polyp. Vaginal lymphoma presents with vaginal bleeding. The lesion is commonly indurated or nodular and rarely ulcerative.[205]

Diagnosis and Pathology. Uterine lymphoma is commonly diagnosed after hysterectomy. Exfoliative cytologic findings are rarely diagnostic as the tumor does not usually breach the mucosal surface. In Harris and Scully's series, 75% of lesions were localized (stage IE) and 25% were more advanced (stages IIE and IV).[204] In the series of Muntz and associates, the stage representation of cervical lesions was IE, 44%; IIE, 42%; III, 12%; and IV, 2%.[206] Of the vaginal lesions reported by Prevot, 12 were stage IE; 2, stage IIE; and 2, stage IV.[205]

Diffuse large cell lymphoma constitutes the majority of lesions of the cervix, endometrium, and vagina (about 70%). Low- and high-grade lesions also occur. When studied, tumors are almost always of B-cell lineage, although rare T-cell angiocentric pleomorphic tumors have been described.[205] Although there is no clinical indication of a MALT origin for female genital tract tumors in humans, the female genital tract is part of a common mucosal immunologic system in mice.[207]

Treatment, Patterns of Failure, and Outcome. The standard therapy for patients with stage IE lesions has usually been radiation therapy with or without antecedent surgery. There is no evidence that radical gynecologic surgery is necessary, and, indeed, there is no strong indication for more than a diagnostic biopsy with subsequent detailed staging evaluation. Radiation alone for localized low-grade tumors offers a high probability of local control. Combined-modality therapy for intermediate- or high-grade tumors is appropriate, and, given the impact of radiation on ovarian function in those in the reproductive age range, the use of chemotherapy alone has been recommended with some clinical justification.[208, 209] A 5-year overall survival rate of 73% is quoted by Harris and Scully, comprising an 89% 5-year rate for patients with stage IE disease and 20% for those with stages IIE to IV.[204] Important prognostic factors include the stage and histologic type.

Local failure is uncommon after surgery and radiation for endometrial, cervical, or vaginal lymphoma. Disease progression may be anticipated in approximately 20% of patients with stage IE lesions, particularly in those with intermediate- or high-grade lesions, and it is usually systemic in nature. CNS failure is rarely recorded. No clear pattern of failure has been identified. Vaginal lesions have been characterized on progression in subcutaneous tissues of the abdominal wall, intraabdominal nodes, lung, and inguinal nodes.[205]

BREAST LYMPHOMA

Demographics and Clinical Features. Primary non-Hodgkin's lymphoma of the breast is rare. It comprises approximately 2% of localized extranodal presentations. In addition, primary breast lymphoma accounts for only 0.04% to 0.5% of all malignant breast tumors. The median age is in the sixth decade of life, but the disease may affect very young and very old women as well. Hugh and associates[210] confirmed the previous observation by Adair and Hermann[211] of the bimodal pattern of presentation of primary breast lymphoma. Breast lymphoma affecting young women tends to be associated with pregnancy and lactation and is a high-grade lymphoma commonly presenting with bilateral disease diffusely involving both breasts.[212, 213] In contrast, the disease affecting older women tends to present with discrete masses and is commonly unilateral.[214] Reports in the literature suggest synchronous bilateral involvement in up to 13% of cases and metachronous contralateral involvement in 7% of cases occurring up to 10 years after the first lesion.[212, 215–219] The diffuse bilateral lymphoma may disseminate rapidly to the CNS.

The disease usually presents as a distinct mass in the breast with or without axillary adenopathy. Many series report an unexplained right-sided preponderance, but this does not appear to affect the outcome. The upper outer quadrant is the most common presenting site; however, a mass in that location may represent nodal disease in the axillary tail rather than primary lymphoma of the breast. Because primary lymphoma of the breast is so rare, most patients are believed to have carcinoma of the breast after biopsy. The bilateral diffuse breast lymphoma affecting young women may clinically mimic inflammatory carcinoma of the breast.[219, 220] Breast engorgement, tenderness, and heaviness may be clinically misleading, especially in pregnant or lactating women.

Diagnosis, Pathology, and Prognostic Factors. The diagnosis is usually obtained by breast biopsy. The mammographic appearances simulate carcinoma, although calcifications are not usually seen. Staging assessment should include assessment of the contralateral breast in addition to the usual staging investigations. Cerebrospinal fluid examination should be performed in patients with high-grade tumors.

The most commonly reported histologic type is diffuse large cell lymphoma. In younger women, high-grade lesions, either immunoblastic or undifferentiated lymphoma, indistinguishable from the classic Burkitt's lymphoma, may occur.[212] High-grade lymphomas are more common in younger women and frequently occur in association with pregnancy.[213, 221] Low-grade lymphomas are less common,

although cases of MALT lymphoma affecting the breast have been reported.[214, 217] Vascular invasion is frequently noted. Prognostic factors are difficult to evaluate in this rare disease. In most series the stage of disease is the most important prognostic factor; other reports identify a high-grade histologic type and bilateral involvement as ominous prognostic factors.

Treatment, Patterns of Failure, and Outcome. Traditionally, patients with localized breast lymphoma have been treated with surgery, surgery followed by radiation therapy, or biopsy followed by radiation. Most reports are based on patients treated without the systematic use of doxorubicin-based chemotherapy. The completeness of surgical excision does not appear to affect local control. Thus, mastectomy is not recommended and breast preservation is possible in most patients. Properly planned and delivered radiation therapy results in excellent local control, especially in patients presenting without bulky disease or those with a low-grade histologic type. The radiation volume should include the whole breast and the ipsilateral axillary lymph nodes. As in other lymphomas, a tumor dose of 35 Gy in 1.75- to 2-Gy fractions over 4 weeks achieves excellent local control. Local failures commonly occur in patients treated with surgery alone or with chemotherapy; however, no reports include patients treated with modern chemotherapy alone. Distant failures are common when surgery and radiotherapy are the only modalities employed. The most common sites of failure include lungs, brain, liver, spleen, and distant nodal sites. Isolated CNS relapses have been reported. Similarly, late failure in the contralateral breast may occur after therapy of unilateral primary breast lymphoma. The overall survival of patients treated with local treatment methods ranges from 40% to 66% at 5 to 10 years.[210, 218, 222–224] The local control rates in patients treated with radiation therapy range from 75% to 78%.[222, 223] The risk of distant relapse is higher in patients with stage II disease, and their survival has been reported to be as low as 20%.

Current recommendations for treatment include the use of combined-modality therapy in all patients with intermediate- and high-grade lymphoma. Patients with low-grade lymphoma may be successfully treated with radiation therapy alone. CNS prophylaxis with intrathecal chemotherapy should be given to all patients with a high-grade histologic type, especially those with bulky or bilateral disease.

BONE LYMPHOMA

Demographics and Clinical Features. Non-Hodgkin's lymphoma involving bone is not uncommon in advanced disease but constitutes less than 5% of localized extranodal presentations.[1, 62] The male to female ratio is 1.6:1, and the mean age at presentation is 46 years.

Patients commonly present with local bone pain, soft tissue swelling, and a mass lesion or a pathologic fracture. In the Mayo clinic analysis,[225] 60% of patients had lymphoma restricted to bone (one third to two or more bones, and two thirds confined to one bone), 25% had bone and soft tissue disease, and 15% had secondary bone involvement from soft tissue. Long bones are the most common presentation site—in the series of Bacci and colleagues, the sites of involvement in 26 cases were femur (6), tibia (6), spine (6), ilium (4), humerus (1), scapula (2), and ulna (1).[226] Presentation sites in the PMH series were femur (7), humerus (2), scapula (2), ilium (2), tarsus (2), sternum (2), clavicle (2), and ribs (2), with single cases presenting in vertebrae, fibula, maxilla, and mandible.[62]

Diagnosis and Staging. Radiologic examination may reveal blastic, lytic, or mixed lytic and sclerotic features with medullary and/or cortical changes. Periosteal erosion may be apparent. MRI has added substantially to the evaluation of bone lymphoma, contributing both to the evaluation of the primary lesion in terms of medullary, cortical, and soft tissue extent (of particular importance in radiation therapy planning) and to the identification of other sites of involvement in the skeleton.[227] The diagnosis is established by bone biopsy, and radical surgery, including amputation, is not required as a part of successful therapy. Surgical consideration, appropriate to alleviation of the risk of pathologic fracture, is appropriate in the context of continuing combined-modality therapy. Full staging evaluation reveals approximately 60% of presentations to be primary (stage IE) and 40% to be advanced (stage IV). Nodal involvement is uncommon.

Pathology and Prognostic Factors. In the large Mayo clinic series, 75% of all classifiable bone lymphomas were of intermediate grade (diffuse mixed or large cell lesions).[225] The remainder were low- or high-grade lesions. In the PMH series, 21 of 27 cases of primary bone lymphoma were diffuse large cell lesions.[62] Prognostic factors determining outcome include the stage, site of bone presentation, solitary lesion versus multifocality, tumor bulk, and histologic type.

Treatment, Patterns of Failure, and Outcome. Cure of lymphoma of bone by surgery alone has been recorded, although this would no longer be considered appropriate therapy. With radical radiation therapy, 5- and 10-year overall survival rates of 58% and 53% are reported for solitary bone lesions, 42% and 35% for multifocal osseous lesions, and 22% and 13% for patients with prior soft tissue disease. The outcome is also influenced by the site of solitary presentation, with 10-year overall survival rates of 78% for femoral lesions, 59% for mandible and maxillary lesions, 36% for pelvic presentations, and 24% for lymphoma presenting in the vertebral body. Key issues relating to radiation control are the intramedullary and soft tissue extent of disease in relation to the radiation volume. MRI has been particularly important in this circumstance, revealing a heretofore unrecognized extension of disease beyond that visualized by radiologic imaging or radionuclide scanning. Previous treatment approaches using radiation alone have indicated high levels of local control within the radiation field (approximately 85%); unacceptable rates of locomarginal failure (20%), probably related to underestimation of the tumor extent and bulk; and a systemic failure rate approaching 50%. There is no clear preponderant risk of failure in the CNS or bone, although both are recorded. There is no increased incidence of second tumor, either bone or soft tissue, as a result of primary therapy.

Patients with localized lymphoma of bone should be treated with combined-modality therapy comprising initial anthracycline-based combination chemotherapy and subsequent radiation therapy to the whole bone to a minimal dose of 35 Gy. There is no indication for CNS prophylaxis. With current combined-modality therapy, overall survival and relapse-free rates should exceed 70% at 5 years.

EXTRADURAL LYMPHOMA

Demographics and Clinical Features. Extradural spinal cord compression occurs in 0.1% to 6.5% of patients with non-Hodgkin's lymphoma, either as the first presentation or as recurrent disease.[228, 229] Non-Hodgkin's lymphoma accounts for approximately 11% of cases of spinal extradural compression, but in radiation therapy series it may account for as many as 35% of cases.[230, 231] Extradural compression may arise either as a result of direct extension of the tumor in the vertebral body, paraspinal soft tissue mass, or retroperitoneal lymph nodes or as a result of an isolated deposit within the spinal canal. In retrospective studies it is difficult to differentiate primary extradural lymphomas from primary lymphoma of bone presenting with extradural compression. Primary extradural lymphoma may occur at any age but is most common between the ages of 40 and 70 years.[61, 232–234] In the PMH experience, all patients with primary extradural lymphoma presented with stage I disease; however, patients presenting with extradural involvement and regional lymph nodes have been described by others.[61, 233, 234] The etiology of primary extradural lymphoma has not been defined.

The clinical presentation of extradural lymphoma is no different from that of any other malignancy at the same site. A history of back pain is usually followed by the development of leg weakness, sensory loss, and impairment of sphincter function. The diagnosis is made late, since back pain is common and malignancy in a younger age group is not suspected. Symptoms are frequently attributed to injury or arthritis, given normal conventional imaging of the spine. The thoracic region is consistently the most common site of extradural lymphoma.[61, 228, 235]

Diagnosis, Pathology, and Prognostic Factors. Historically, the clinical diagnosis of extradural lymphoma was established by myelography. Currently, CT-myelography and MRI provide much better definition of disease extent. Patients usually present as an emergency, and the management of spinal cord compression should be undertaken before the usual staging procedures are contemplated. After the initial biopsy and decompression, the presence of systemic lymphoma should be excluded by investigations including bone scan and cytologic examination of the cerebrospinal fluid. Intermediate-grade lymphoma, usually diffuse large cell lymphoma, is the most common histologic type. Low-grade lymphoma has also been reported but is less common.

The outcome in primary extradural lymphoma is measured not only by the local control, relapse-free rate, and survival but also by the functional outcome, with mobility and the neurologic status being equally important outcome measures. The most important prognostic factor for preservation of neurologic function is the extent and duration of symptoms after diagnosis and the degree of neurologic deficit at presentation. The prognostic factors for survival are the same as in other localized lymphomas and include age, the histologic type, and the tumor bulk.

Treatment, Patterns of Failure, and Outcome. The presence of spinal cord compression constitutes a medical emergency. Histologic diagnosis is imperative, and surgical biopsy and decompression are the first steps in management. Complete tumor removal is unnecessary, since further therapy is always required. The main objectives of surgery include adequate decompression of the spinal cord and removal of tissue appropriate for histologic diagnosis. Postoperative therapy has historically involved radiation therapy to the affected area of the spine. Megavoltage photon therapy is used, with the dose to the tumor limited to 35 to 40 Gy in 1.75- to 2-Gy fractions. Doses in excess of 40 Gy are discouraged to avoid the risk of radiation myelitis. The radiation fields should take into account the presence of any paraspinal mass or regional lymph node involvement. Radiation results in excellent local disease control but, as with other localized intermediate-grade lymphomas, is associated with a 40% to 50% distant failure rate at sites including mediastinum, pleura, bone, bone marrow, and CNS. The use of doxorubicin-based chemotherapy after surgery and irradiation is associated with a reduced distant failure rate and an improved survival. In the PMH experience the survival of patients treated with radiation alone was 33% compared with 86% at 5 years for those treated with combined-modality therapy.[61] Although the traditional approach is to deliver radiation before chemotherapy, this may not be the most optimal sequence. Eeles and colleagues documented that chemotherapy followed by radiation does not compromise neurologic function compared with that achieved when radiation is followed by chemotherapy.[233] A controversial aspect of the management of primary extradural lymphoma surrounds the issue of the CNS prophylaxis. Although some have demonstrated extradural involvement as a risk factor for meningeal relapse,[236] the PMH experience has not documented isolated CNS relapse in patients treated without CNS prophylaxis. Accordingly, the necessity for routine intrathecal chemotherapy in patients with localized extradural lymphoma and no evidence of dural invasion has been questioned.[61]

LUNG LYMPHOMA

Demographics. Lung involvement is uncommon as a primary manifestation of lymphoma, occurring in less than 4% of all extranodal presentations and less than 1% of primary localized extranodal presentations. It is rare as a primary lung neoplasm. The most common primary lung lymphoma is the small B-cell low-grade bronchus-associated lymphoid tissue (BALT) lymphoma. BALT is inconspicuous in adults, but the tissue undergoes hyperplasia in patients with chronic immune-mediated diseases such as chronic infections, connective tissue diseases, rheumatoid arthritis, and Sjögren's syndrome. Low-grade B-cell lymphomas represent 50% to 90% of all primary lung lymphomas. Three broad categories of lymphoma of the lung require recognition: (1) the previously mentioned low-grade B-cell tumor (BALT/MALT lymphoma) previously considered benign, reactive, or pseudolymphoma; (2) a much less common intermediate- or high-grade tumor usually of diffuse, large cell B-cell type; and (3) rare T-cell lymphomas usually occurring as part of a more widespread angiocentric and angiodestructive systemic process such as lymphomatoid granulomatosis or peripheral T-cell lymphoma. Patients are commonly older than 50 years of age with an equal male to female ratio.

Clinical Features, Diagnosis, and Staging. Clinical and radiologic features correlate to a large extent with the type of lymphoma.[237] In a series of 70 patients with primary lymphoma of lung, 61 (87%) had low-grade disease. Almost half these patients were asymptomatic and were defined by routine chest radiographs. In the remainder, symptoms comprised cough (39%), dyspnea (21%), hemoptysis (10%), chest pain (10%), and vasculitis with cryoglobulinemia (31%). Chest radiology indicated a localized opacity (87%) consisting of an alveolar mass or pneumonia-like consolidation with an air bronchogram (51%), occasional cavitation, and bilateral lesions (21%). Nine patients (13%) had intermediate- or high-grade lesions. All were symptomatic, and none were identified on routine chest radiographs. Radiologic changes included localized opacities (6), diffuse infiltration (2), and pleural effusion (2).

Bronchoscopy may be diagnostic. Endobronchial lymphoma may be present with airway compromise or obstruction, although, more commonly, diffuse submucosal tumor is present in association with intrathoracic lymphoma.[238] Abnormal features include inflammatory change in the mucosa with luminal stenosis. Such changes were present in almost half the cases with low-grade tumor, and in seven with intermediate- or high-grade lesions in the series of Cordier and colleagues.[237] Biopsy was commonly positive, and bronchoalveolar lavage was successful in identifying cells for diagnosis and phenotyping. Percutaneous lung biopsy or open-lung biopsy is required if noninvasive techniques are nondiagnostic. Low-grade tumors are commonly confined to the lung or mediastinal/hilar nodes; intermediate- and high-grade lesions and T-cell tumors are commonly found to be systemic on full evaluation.

Pathology. Satzstein introduced the concept of pseudolymphoma to characterize lymphocytic tumors (mature-appearing small lymphocytic tumors often demonstrating lymphoplasmacytoid differentiation) with an 80% 5-year overall survival.[239] The concept of pseudolymphoma has now been replaced; such tumors are monoclonal B-cell tumors with lymphoplasmacytic/cytoid or immunocytic differentiation. Clinical features comprising multifocality within the lung with organ localization over very protracted periods, recurrence in the lung, and, more rarely, progression in the GI tract have identified this lesion as being related to the MALT lymphomas. Rarely, the tumor is associated with Sjögren's syndrome and/or dysproteinemia. Less commonly, diffuse large cell lesions of centrocytic/centroblastic, centroblastic, or immunoblastic type occur. These lesions are also of B-cell type. The rare T-cell lymphomas affecting lung demonstrate the characteristic features of angiocentricity, angiodestruction, and necrosis and are commonly systemic involving skin, kidney, and CNS.

In the report of Cordier and colleagues, monoclonal serum immunoglobulin was demonstrated in 30% of patients with low-grade lymphoma, including 2 of 61 patients with cryoglobulinemia, and in 2 of 9 patients with large cell tumors, 1 with cryoglobulinemia.[237]

Treatment, Prognostic Factors, and Outcome. The initial treatment has commonly been surgical resection; however, given current less invasive alternatives to achieve a secure diagnosis, there is no strong indication that resection contributes to the outcome. Low-grade lymphoma has been treated by chemotherapy, usually of a single alkylating or nonanthracycline-combination type. Lesions are commonly chemoresponsive and are also radioresponsive, although tolerance issues limit the applicability of radiation to limited regions of the lung. There is no indication that such treatments are curative, although prolonged survival is common—94% overall survival at 5 years with a median survival not reached at 10 years and no clear impact of type of therapy on outcome.[237, 240] The prognosis is clearly substantially worse for intermediate- and high-grade lesions even when they are treated with chemotherapy or combined-modality therapy, with a survival expectancy of 47% at 5 years[241] and a median survival of 3 years, with 6 of 9 patients dying of lymphoma in the series of Cordier and associates.[237] Major prognostic factors for pulmonary lymphoma include the histologic type and stage.

Low-grade lesions may be managed conservatively to achieve symptom control using surgical resection, modest chemotherapy, or limited-field, low-dose radiation therapy. The natural history is indolent, and disease progression is usually confined to the lung over long periods. Extrathoracic disease occurs in a minority and may involve the lung, bone marrow, liver, or, rarely, multiple extranodal sites. Intermediate- and high-grade lesions are aggressive and require chemotherapy or combined-modality therapy. Despite such therapy, systemic progression is common, and relapse-free rates of approximately 40% to 50% are expected. T-cell lymphomas have a poor prognosis, with a 50% mortality at 2 years despite combination or combined-modality treatment.

MEDIASTINAL LARGE CELL LYMPHOMA

Demographics and Clinical Features. There has been controversy about whether mediastinal large cell lymphoma should be considered a separate entity, but the clinicopathologic features have certain characteristics distinguishing this tumor from nodal lymphoma. There is a predominant female to male ratio, and patients are commonly in the 25- to 40-year age group.[242–244]

The tumor presents as a rapidly growing invasive tumor with contiguous spread within mediastinal tissues. Chest pain, cough, and dyspnea are common, B symptoms are frequently present, and 30% to 40% of patients have superior vena caval obstruction. Pleural and pericardial invasion with effusion are common. The lesion is frequently bulky (65% are >10 cm in diameter) and involves the thymus.

Diagnosis and Pathology. Diagnosis is by biopsy through mediastinoscopy, mediastinotomy, or thoracotomy/thoracoscopy approaches. Sufficient tissue for phenotypic and genotypic studies is mandatory because the differential diagnosis includes Hodgkin's disease, lymphoblastic lymphoma, thymoma, germinoma/teratoma, and Castleman's disease. Mediastinal large cell lymphoma is confined to the thorax in three quarters of patients but is commonly extensive.

Tumors are diffuse, with moderate to marked sclerosis and some necrosis, and with a large cell malignant infiltrate demonstrating some pleomorphism. Malignant cells are of B lineage (CD19+, CD20+, CD45+, and HLA-DR+). Clonal surface and cytoplasmic immunoglobulin expression are uncommon. Fifty percent of cases demonstrate c-*myc* gene

alteration, and immunoglobulin gene rearrangement can usually be detected. The cell of origin is considered to be a terminally differentiated B cell or thymic B cell. Occasional T-cell tumors are recognized.

Treatment, Prognostic Factors, and Outcome. Although this tumor was originally believed to have a particularly adverse prognosis, the outcome for patients treated by chemotherapy or combined-modality therapy is now considered equivalent to that of other large cell lesions of equivalent stage, that is, complete remission rates of 70% to 80% and overall 5-year survival of 50%. Factors determining the outcome include bulk (>10 cm), the use of chemotherapy as opposed to radiation alone, stage (extrathoracic versus localized), and achievement of complete remission. With radiation therapy after chemotherapy to optimize local control, disease progression is most commonly systemic and frequently involves the upper abdomen, kidneys (either focal or diffuse), and liver. CNS involvement is not characteristic.

UNCOMMON SITES OF PRIMARY EXTRANODAL LYMPHOMA

Lymphoma of the Spleen

Primary splenic lymphoma accounts for approximately 1% of non-Hodgkin's lymphomas, usually arising in those older than 60 years of age, and has a female to male ratio of 2:1. Commonly, primary splenic lymphoma presents as splenomegaly or as unexplained hypersplenism with an abnormal peripheral blood count. Lymphoma symptoms are rare other than in a subset of patients who present a more fulminant picture of fever, weight loss, left upper quadrant pain, and extensive splenic infarction.[245–249] Primary splenic lymphoma is diagnosed by splenectomy. In the more fulminant presentations, there may be adherence or invasion to the diaphragm, stomach, or pancreas. Hilar and abdominal node sampling and liver biopsies should be undertaken if a preoperative diagnosis of splenic lymphoma is considered or if percutaneous needle aspiration cytologic examination suggests this diagnosis. Cytopenias commonly respond to splenectomy. The disease commonly affects the white pulp and consists of either a small cell tumor—usually a well or poorly differentiated lymphocytic type and with a nodular or diffuse architecture—or a large cell tumor of diffuse histiocytic or mixed cell type. Special stains, detailed morphologic examination, and red pulp localization distinguish small cell lymphoma from hairy cell leukemia.

Treatment usually involves splenectomy. Additional therapy might comprise local radiation therapy for low-grade disease if any residuum remained in the left upper quadrant after surgery. For patients with large cell lymphoma, adjuvant chemotherapy would be an appropriate recommendation, although the disease is sufficiently rare that patterns of failure cannot be used to direct therapy after splenectomy.

Lymphoma of the Pancreas

Primary pancreatic lymphoma is rare. It accounts for 1% to 3% of all pancreatic malignancies and is rarely considered in the differential diagnosis of pancreatic mass lesions. Patients are usually older than 60 years of age[250] and present as with pancreatic carcinoma, that is, nausea and emesis, epigastric pain, anorexia, jaundice, malaise and fatigue, fever, and night sweats. The history is usually short, and a mass lesion may be palpable. The lesion is defined by CT and is commonly a sizable (3 to 12 cm, median 8 cm) lesion in the head of the pancreas. Diagnosis may be achieved by preoperative percutaneous guided-needle biopsy or trans-duodenal needle biopsy.[251, 252] More frequently a laparotomy with wedge biopsy permits a secure diagnosis and allows bypass procedures to be performed to relieve biliary obstruction. Tumors are most commonly of large cell, "histiocytic," or mixed cell type. Low-grade tumors are relatively uncommon. Access to phenotypic, cell cycle, and genotypic analysis is important when guided-needle biopsy material forms the basis for diagnosis.

There is no indication for radical surgery for primary pancreatic lymphoma. Biliary obstruction may be relieved surgically, although such obstruction is usually managed effectively with systemic chemotherapy.[251] Radiation may have a role in the uncommon low-grade lymphoma or for palliation. Combined-modality therapy is the appropriate therapy for intermediate-grade, mixed, and large cell tumors with particular consideration to the choice of agents and schedule in patients with obstructive jaundice.

Lymphoma of the Liver

Primary non-Hodgkin's lymphoma of the liver is exceptionally rare. A recent report cited 68 cases in the literature, including five new cases.[253] The authors described an age range of 7 to 87 years (median 55 years), a male to female ratio of 3.1:1, and no differences in disease pattern between Eastern and Western populations. A relationship of primary lymphoma of the liver to preexisting immunologic disease states, for example, systemic lupus erythematosus, AIDS, cyclosporine/transplantation, and hepatitis-B–induced chronic active hepatitis, has been proposed, with a role for continuous antigen stimulation and autoantibody production. Presenting features include epigastric and right upper quadrant pain, fatigue, hemorrhagic diathesis, anorexia, nausea, and vomiting. Fifty percent of patients have B symptoms, most commonly weight loss. Hepatomegaly may be present. Stigmata of other disease states may be apparent. Jaundice is uncommon.[254–256] Liver enzyme levels are usually abnormally elevated, with normal α-fetoprotein and carcinoembryonic antigen levels. Hypoechogenic and homogeneous masses may be present on ultrasonography, and hypodense, nonenhancing mass lesions are characteristic on CT imaging. Hepatitis B surface antigen is present in approximately 25% of patients. Primary liver lymphoma arises as a solitary mass in 61% of patients, as multiple masses in 33%, and as a diffuse lesion in 4%. Those with preexisting AIDS or chronic liver disease usually have multiple lesions. When recorded, 60% of tumors are of diffuse, large cell type; 17% are high-grade tumors; and 4% are of follicular type. Eighty percent of tumors are of B-cell type. T-cell lesions are rarely recorded.

Treatment-related data to direct therapy are limited. Partial hepatectomy has been advocated for solitary lesions. There is no rationale for more extensive surgery and no role for radiation given that tumors are commonly multiple and of large cell type, and liver tolerance for radiation is limited.

Multiagent, anthracycline-based chemotherapy, with allowance for any related liver dysfunction, particularly if preexistent to lymphoma, would appear to be the most appropriate recommendation.

Lymphoma Affecting Soft Tissues

Primary extranodal non-Hodgkin's lymphomas of the soft tissues are extremely rare.[257–259] In the Mayo Clinic experience, primary extranodal soft tissue lymphoma of the extremities represented 0.11% of all lymphomas.[257] Patients present with soft tissue swelling. The swelling is usually painless, but in cases the tumor mass may be tender. Diagnosis is obtained after biopsy or resection of the lesion and demonstration of the absence of disseminated lymphoma. In some patients it may be difficult to distinguish extranodal soft tissue presentations from the total effacement of an aberrant lymph node by a malignant lymphoma. These cases may also be confused with primary lymphoma of the skin presenting with extensive subcutaneous soft tissue involvement.

All histologic grades have been reported. Tumors may be confined to the subcutaneous connective tissue or may involve muscle. Presentations in extremities, chest, or abdominal wall have been reported. There is little information on which to base treatment recommendations. However, there is no reason to think that the principles that apply to the management of other localized lymphomas are not appropriate for primary lymphoma of soft tissues. Thus, the use of involved-field radiation for low-grade lymphomas and combined-modality therapy for intermediate- and high-grade lymphomas is recommended.

Other Sites (Heart, Pleura, and Adrenal Gland)

Primary lymphoma of the heart, defined as lymphoma involving only heart and pericardium, is highly unusual in patients without known immune compromise.[260, 261] Most cases have been described in patients with human immunodeficiency virus or after organ transplantation.[25, 26, 262, 263] In a few reported cases the diagnosis has been made premortem.[264, 265] Presenting symptoms are usually congestive heart failure, pericardial effusion, and occasionally complete heart block. The pathologic lesion is usually B-cell lymphoma of large cell type. The clinical course is characteristically acute in onset and short in duration with a high rate of early death. Prolonged survival has been reported after chemotherapy.[266]

Primary lymphoma of the pleura arising in association with chronic tuberculous pyothorax has been reported in Japan.[267, 268] A few cases have been reported in Western countries as a complication of chronic empyema. Most cases are B-cell lymphomas. The outcome in reported cases treated with chemotherapy was poor, with a median survival of 9 months and a 2-year survival of 31.4%.[267] Poor performance status was the main adverse prognostic factor.

Few cases of primary adrenal lymphoma has been reported in the literature.[193, 269, 270] The disease was most common in elderly men. Presenting symptoms were usually secondary to the mass effect of the tumor. A number of cases had bilateral involvement of adrenal glands. Both B-cell and

T-cell lymphomas have been reported. Diagnosis was usually made after a biopsy or resection of the suprarenal mass with or without nephrectomy. Many cases have been managed with surgery and chemotherapy, but survival was poor.[269, 270]

SUMMARY

The term "primary extranodal non-Hodgkin's lymphoma" encompasses a heterogeneous group of diseases that may affect any organ or body part. Traditionally, an attempt to rationalize this heterogeneity has been made through the histologic classification, anatomic stage, and other conventionally derived prognostic factors remitting from analysis of the treatment outcome of nodal and extranodal low-grade and diffuse large cell lymphoma. The basis for the heterogeneity of presentation, behavior, response to therapy, and pattern of failure has remained elusive.

Several novel lines of inquiry suggest that the combination of conventional prognostic determinants to management strategy of primary extranodal lymphoma are of limited value. The concept of innate or acquired lymphoid tissue in extranodal organs and the role of chronic antigenic stimulation, autoimmunity, and immune dysregulation as an important component of the etiology and pathogenesis of lymphoma is becoming increasingly recognized through observations relating to congenital and acquired immunodeficiency states, Hashimoto's and Sjögren's syndrome, Crohn's disease, IPSID, and MALT lymphomas of the GI tract. The role of surface determinants and tissue microenvironments as a basis of preferential determination of spread patterns of lymphoma, and the potential molecular basis for preferential organ localization, is being actively explored.[22, 271] In addition, current classifications are attempting to define specific disease entities that may have their basis in unique etiologic or pathogenetic mechanisms, within which the roles of histologic type, stage, and other determinants may have differing prognostic and management usefulness.

The experience available to guide the management of patients with primary extranodal lymphomas is limited. Large retrospective studies are available in commonly encountered lymphomas (GIL, Waldeyer's ring, bone, orbital, and thyroid lymphoma), whereas only infrequent case reports are available in uncommon presenting sites (such as the adrenal gland, liver, and spleen). In this chapter, an attempt has been made to summarize the principles of lymphoma management that allow an appropriate treatment strategy for lymphoma presenting in any organ or site. However, further refinements in the management of these diseases are required to maximize cure rates and to reduce immediate and long-term morbidity of the disease and its treatment. Gains in our understanding of the genetic and molecular basis of non-Hodgkin's lymphoma have to be translated into medical practice to benefit patients. This may require a complete reevaluation of our interpretation of existing treatment modalities in the context of newly acquired information, relating to etiology, pathogenesis, and classification, particularly as it applies to primary extranodal lymphoma. Because of the infrequent occurrence of primary extranodal lymphomas, such gains in the interpretation of treatment approaches will be achieved only through collaborative prospective clinical trials designed around commonly agreed classification and investigation.

REFERENCES

1. Freeman C, Berg JW, Cutler SJ: Occurrence and prognosis of extranodal lymphomas. Cancer 1972; 29:252.
2. Otter R, Gerrits WB, Sandt MM, et al: Primary extranodal and nodal non-Hodgkin's lymphoma: A survey of population-based registry. Eur J Cancer 1989; 25:1203.
3. D'Amore F, Christensen BE, Brincker H, et al: Clinicopathological features and prognostic factors in extranodal non-Hodgkin lymphomas: Danish LYFO Study Group. Eur J Cancer 1991; 27(10):1201.
4. Sutcliffe SB, Gospodarowicz MK: Localized extranodal lymphomas. *In* Keating A, Armitage J, Burnett A, et al (eds): Haematological Oncology. Cambridge, Cambridge University Press, 1992, pp 189–222.
5. Rappaport H: Tumors of the hematopoietic system. *In* Atlas of Tumor Pathology, Sec III, Fasc 8. Washington, DC, Armed Forces Institute of Pathology, 1966, pp 97–161.
6. Lukes LJ, Collins RD: Immunologic characterization of human malignant lymphomas. Cancer 1974; 34:1448.
7. Lennert K, Stern H, Kaiserling E: Cytological and functional criteria for the classification of malignant lymphomata. Br J Cancer 1975; 31(Suppl 2):29.
8. Stansfeld AG, Diebold J, Noel H, et al: Updated Kiel classification for lymphomas. Lancet 1988; 1:292.
9. National Cancer Institute–sponsored study of classifications of Non-Hodgkin's lymphoma: Summary and description of a working formulation for clinical usage. Cancer 1982; 49:2112.
10. Harris NL, Jaffe ES, Stein H, et al: A revised European-American classification of lymphoid neoplasms: A proposal from the International Lymphoma Study Group [see comments]. Blood 1994; 84:1361.
11. Falzon M, Isaacson PG: The natural history of benign lymphoepithelial lesion of the salivary gland in which there is a monoclonal population of B cells: A report of two cases. Am J Surg Pathol 1991; 15:59.
12. Fishleder A, Tubbs R, Hesse B, et al: Uniform detection of immunoglobulin gene rearrangement in benign lymphoepithelial lesions. N Engl J Med 1987; 316:1118.
13. Diss TC, Peng H, Wotherspoon AC, et al: Brief report: A single neoplastic clone in sequential biopsy specimens from a patient with primary gastric-mucosa–associated lymphoid-tissue lymphoma and Sjögren's syndrome. N Engl J Med 1993; 329:172.
14. Gospodarowicz MK, Sutcliffe SB, Clark RM, et al: Outcome analysis of localized gastrointestinal lymphoma treated with surgery and postoperative radiation. Int J Radiat Oncol Biol Phys 1990; 19:1351.
15. Isaacson PG: Gastrointestinal lymphoma. Hum Pathol 1994; 25:1020.
16. Spencer J, Cerf-Bensussan N, Jarry A, et al: Enteropathy associated T-cell lymphoma (malignant histiocytosis of the intestine) is recognized by a monoclonal antibody (HML-1) that defines a membrane molecule on mucosal lymphocytes. Am J Pathol 1988; 132:1.
17. Isaacson PG, O'Connor NTJ, Spencer JEA: Malignant histiocytosis of the intestine: A T-cell lymphoma. Lancet 1985; 2:688.
18. Ferry J, Sklar J, Zukerberg L, et al: Nasal lymphoma: A clinicopathologic study with immunophenotypic and genotypic analysis. Am J Surg Pathol 1991; 15:268.
19. Guinee D, Kingma D, Fishback N, et al: Pulmonary lesions with features of lymphomatoid granulomatosis/angiocentric immunoproliferative lesion (LYG/AIL); evidence for Epstein-Barr virus within B lymphocytes [Abstract]. Mod Pathol 1994; 7:151.
20. Beljaards RC, Kaudewitz P, Berti E, et al: Primary cutaneous CD30-positive large cell lymphoma: Definition of a new type of cutaneous lymphoma with a favorable prognosis. A European Multicenter Study of 47 patients. Cancer 1993; 71:2097.
21. Raghoebier S, Kramer MHH, van Kruker JHJM, et al: Essential differences in oncogene involvement between primary nodal and extranodal large cell lymphoma. Blood 1991; 78:2680.
22. Offit K, Lo Coco F, Louie D, et al: Rearrangement of the *bcl-6* gene as a prognostic marker in diffuse large cell lymphoma. N Engl J Med 1994; 331:74.
23. Greene MH. Non-Hodgkin's lymphoma and mycosis fungoides. *In*

Schottenfeld D, Fraumeni JFJ (eds): Cancer Epidemiology and Prevention. Philadelphia, WB Saunders, 1982, pp 754–778.

24. Weisenburger DD: Epidemiology of non-Hodgkin's lymphoma: Recent findings regarding an emerging epidemic. Ann Oncol 1994; 5(Suppl):19.

25. Penn I: Tumors in the immunocompromised patient. Ann Rev Med 1988; 39:63.

26. Kaplan LD: AIDS-associated lymphoma. *In* Sande MA, Volberding PA (eds): The Medical Management of AIDS. Philadelphia, WB Saunders, 1988, pp 307–315.

27. Grierson H, Purtilo DT: Epstein-Barr virus infections in males with the X-linked lymphoproliferative syndrome. Ann Intern Med 1987; 106:538.

28. Filipovich AH, Heinitz KJ, Robison LL, et al: The immunodeficiency cancer registry. Am J Pediatr Hematol Oncol 1987; 9:183.

29. Jacquillat C, Khayat D, Desprez-Curaly JP, et al: Non-Hodgkin's lymphoma occurring after Hodgkin's disease: Four new cases and a review of the literatures. Cancer 1984; 53:459.

30. Ben Ayed F, Halphen M, Najjar T, et al: Treatment of alpha chain disease: Results of a prospective study in 21 Tunisian patients by the Tunisian-French Intestinal Lymphoma Study Group. Cancer 1989; 63:1251.

31. Isaacson PG: Gastric lymphoma and *Helicobacter pylori*. N Engl J Med 1994; 330:1310.

32. Parsonnet J, Hansen S, Rodriguez L, et al: *Helicobacter pylori* infection and gastric lymphoma. N Engl J Med 1994; 330:1267.

33. Hussel T, Isaacson PG, Crabtree JE, et al: The response of cells from low-grade B-cell gastric of mucosa-associated lymphoid tissue to *Helicobacter pylori*. Lancet 1993; 342:571.

34. Wotherspoon AC, Doglioni C, Diss C, et al: Regression of primary low-grade B-cell gastric lymphoma of mucosa-associated lymphoid tissue type after eradication of *Helicobacter pylori*. Lancet 1993; 342:575.

35. Zulman J, Jaffe R, Talal N: Evidence that the malignant lymphoma of Sjögren's syndrome is a monoclonal B-cell neoplasm. N Engl J Med 1978; 299:1215.

36. Holm LE, Blomgren H, Lowhagen T: Cancer risks in patients with chronic lymphocytic thyroiditis. N Engl J Med 1985; 312:601.

37. Castellino RA: Diagnostic imaging evaluation of Hodgkin's disease and non-Hodgkin's lymphoma. Cancer 1991; 67:1177.

38. North LB, Wallace S, Lindell M Jr, et al: Lymphography for staging lymphomas: Is it still a useful procedure? Am J Roentgenol 1993; 161:867.

39. Tumeh SS, Rosenthal DS, Kaplan WD, et al: Evaluation with Ga-67 SPECT. Radiology 1987; 164:111.

40. Kaplan WD, Jochelson MS, Herman TS, et al: Gallium-67 imaging: A predictor of residual tumor viability and clinical outcome in patients with diffuse large-cell lymphoma. J Clin Oncol 1990; 8:1966.

41. Beahrs OH, Henson DE, Hutter RV, et al: American Joint Committee on Cancer: Manual for Staging of Cancer, 4th ed. Philadelphia, JB Lippincott, 1992.

42. Carbone PP, Kaplan HS, Mushoff K, et al: Report of the Committee on Hodgkin's Disease Staging Classification. Cancer Res 1971; 31:1860.

43. Hermanek P, Sobin LH: UICC International Union Against Cancer, TNM Classification of Malignant Tumors, 4th ed, 2nd Rev. Berlin, Springer-Verlag, 1992.

44. Hermanek P, Henson DE, Hutter RVP, et al: Hodgkin disease and non-Hodgkin lymphoma. Berlin, Springer-Verlag, 1993, pp 45–46.

45. Radaszkiewicz T, Dragosics B, Bauer P: Gastrointestinal malignant lymphomas of the mucosa-associated lymphoid tissue: Factors relevant to prognosis. Gastroenterology 1992; 102:1628.

46. Rohatiner A, d'Amore F, Coiffier B, et al: Report on a workshop convened to discuss the pathological and staging classifications of gastrointestinal tract lymphoma. Ann Oncol 1994; 5:397.

47. D'Amore F, Brincker M, Gronbaek K, et al: Non-Hodgkin's lymphoma of the gastrointestinal tract: A population-based analysis of incidence, geographic distribution, clinicopathologic presentation features, and prognosis. J Clin Oncol 1994; 12:1673.

48. Tsutsui K, Shibamoto Y, Yamabe H, et al: A radiotherapeutic experience for localized extranodal non-Hodgkin's lymphoma: Prognostic factors and re-evaluation of treatment modality. Radiother Oncol 1991; 21:83.

49. The International non-Hodgkin's Lymphoma Prognostic Factors Project: A predictive model for aggressive Non-Hodgkin's lymphoma. N Engl J Med 1993; 329:987.

50. Bush RS, Gospodarowicz MK: The place of radiation therapy in the management of patients with localized non-Hodgkin's lymphoma. *In* Malignant Lymphomas. Bristol Myers Cancer Symposia Series, No 3. Orlando, FL, Academic Press, 1982, pp 485–502.

51. Velasquez WS, Fuller LM, Jagannath S, et al: Stages I and II diffuse large cell lymphomas: Prognostic factors and long-term results with CHOP-bleo and radiotherapy. Blood 1991; 77:942.

52. Sutcliffe SB, Gospodarowicz MK, Bush RS, et al: Role of radiation therapy in localized non-Hodgkin's lymphoma. Radiother Oncol 1985; 4:211.

53. Mackintosh JF, Cowan RA, Jones M, et al: Prognostic factors in stage I and II high- and intermediate-grade non-Hodgkin's lymphoma. Eur J Cancer Clin Oncol 1988; 24:1617.

54. Romaguera JE, Velasquez WS, Silvermintz KB, et al: Surgical debulking is associated with improved survival in stage I-II diffuse large cell lymphoma. Cancer 1990; 66:267.

55. Thirlby RC: Gastrointestinal lymphoma: A surgical perspective. Oncology 1993; 7:29.

56. Seifert E, Schulte SE, Stolte M: Long-term results of treatment of malignant non-Hodgkin's lymphoma of the stomach. Z Gastroenterol 1992; 30:505.

57. Shepherd FA, Evans WK, Kutas G, et al: Chemotherapy following surgery for stages IE and IIE non-Hodgkin's lymphoma of the gastrointestinal tract. J Clin Oncol 1988; 6:253.

58. Gospodarowicz M, Bush R, Brown T, et al: Curability of gastrointestinal lymphoma with combined surgery and radiation. Int J Radiat Oncol Biol Phys 1983; 9:3.

59. Gospodarowicz MK, Sutcliffe SB, Brown TC, et al: Patterns of disease in localized extranodal lymphomas. J Clin Oncol 1987; 5:875.

60. Doll DC, Weiss RB: Malignant lymphoma of the testis. Am J Med 1986; 81:515.

61. Rathmell AJ, Gospodarowicz MK, Sutcliffe SB, et al: Localized extradural lymphoma: Survival, relapse pattern, and functional outcome. The Princess Margaret Hospital Lymphoma Group. Radiother Oncol 1992; 24:14.

62. Rathmell AJ, Gospodarowicz MK, Sutcliffe SB, et al: Localised lymphoma of bone: Prognostic factors and treatment recommendations. The Princess Margaret Hospital Lymphoma Group. Br J Cancer 1992; 66:603.

63. Longo DL, Hathorn J: Current therapy for diffuse large cell lymphoma. Prog Hematol 1987; 15:115.

64. Connors JM, Klimo P, Fairey RN, et al: Brief chemotherapy and involved field radiation therapy for limited stage, histologically aggressive lymphoma. Ann Intern Med 1987; 107:25.

65. Connors JM, Klimo P, Voss N, et al: Testicular lymphoma: Improved outcome with early brief chemotherapy. J Clin Oncol 1988; 6:776.

66. Prestidge BR, Horning SJ, Hoppe RT: Combined modality therapy for stage I-II large cell lymphoma. Int J Radiat Oncol Biol Phys 1988; 15:633.

67. Lishner M, Slingerland J, Barr J, et al: Second malignant neoplasms in patients with non-Hodgkin's lymphoma. Hematol Oncol 1991; 9:169.

68. Travis LB, Curtis RE, Glimelius B, et al: Second cancers among long-term survivors of non-Hodgkin's lymphoma. J Natl Cancer Inst 1993; 85:1932.

69. Devesa SS, Fears T: Non-Hodgkin's lymphoma time trends: United States and International data. Cancer Res 1992; 52:5432.

70. Gupta S, Pant G, Gupta S: A clinicopathological study of primary gastrointestinal lymphoma. J Surg Oncol 1981; 16:49.

71. Contreary K, Nance F, Becker W: Primary lymphoma of the gastrointestinal tract. Ann Surg 1980; 191:593.

72. Hermann R, Panahon AM, Barcos MP, et al: Gastrointestinal involvement in non-Hodgkin's lymphoma. Cancer 1980; 46:215.

73. Isaacson P, Wright DH: Malignant lymphoma of mucosa-associated lymphoid tissue. Cancer 1983; 52:1410.

74. Isaacson P, Wright DH: Extranodal malignant lymphoma arising from mucosa-associated lymphoid tissue. Cancer 1984; 53:2515.

75. Isaacson PG, Spencer J: Malignant lymphoma of mucosa-associated lymphoid tissue. Histopathology 1987; 11:445.

76. Isaacson PG: Extranodal lymphomas: The MALT concept. Verh Dtsch Ges Rheumatol 1992; 76:14.

77. Chan J, Ng C, Isaacson P: Relationship between high-grade lymphoma and low-grade B-cell mucosa-associated lymphoid tissue lymphoma (MALToma) of the stomach. Am J Pathol 1990; 136:1153.

78. Wotherspoon AC, Ortiz HC, Falzon MR, et al: *Helicobacter pylori*–associated gastritis and primary B-cell gastric lymphoma [see comments]. Lancet 1991; 338:1175.

79. Weingrad DN, Decosse JJ, Sherlock P, et al: Primary gastrointestinal lymphoma: A 30-year review. Cancer 1982; 49:1258.

80. Lewin KJ, Ranchod M, Dorfman RF: Lymphomas of the gastrointestinal tract: A study of 117 cases presenting with gastrointestinal disease. Cancer 1978; 42:693.

81. Azab MB, Henry AM, Rougier P, et al: Prognostic factors in primary gastrointestinal non-Hodgkin's lymphoma: A multivariate analysis, report of 106 cases, and review of the literature. Cancer 1989; 64:1208.

82. Cirillo M, Federico M, Curci G, et al: Primary gastrointestinal lymphoma: A clinicopathological study of 58 cases. Haematologica 1992; 77:156.

83. Bolondi L, De Giorgio R, Santi V, et al: Primary non-Hodgkin's T-cell lymphoma of the esophagus: A case with peculiar endoscopic ultrasonographic pattern. Dig Dis Sci 1990; 35:1426.

84. Pawade J, Soon Lee C, Ellis D, et al: Primary lymphoma of the ampulla of Vater. Cancer 1994; 73:2083.

85. Nagrani M, Lavigne B, Siskind B, et al: Primary non-Hodgkin's lymphoma of the esophagus. Arch Intern Med 1989; 149:193.

86. Najem AZ, Porcaro JL, Rush BF Jr: Primary non-Hodgkin's lymphoma of the duodenum. Cancer 1984; 54:895.

87. Swinson CM, Slavin G, Coles EC, et al: Coeliac disease and malignancy. Lancet 1983; 1:111.

88. Chott A, Dragosics B, Radaszkiewicz T: Peripheral T-cell lymphomas of the intestine. Am J Pathol 1992; 141:1361.

89. Al-Mondhiry H: Primary lymphomas of the small intestine: East-West contrast. Am J Hematol 1986; 22:89.

90. Alpha-chain disease and related small-intestinal lymphoma: A memorandum. Bull WHO 1976; 54:615.

91. Khojasteh A, Haghshenass M, Haghighi P: Immunoproliferative small intestinal disease: A "Third World" lesion. N Engl J Med 1983; 308:1401.

92. Blackledge G, Bush H, Dodge O, et al: A study of gastrointestinal lymphoma. Clin Oncol 1979; 5:209.

93. Isaacson PG, Spencer J, Wright DH: Classifying primary gut lymphomas [Letter]. Lancet 1988; 2:1148.

94. Banks P, Chan J, Cleary M, et al: Mantle cell lymphoma: A proposal for unification of morphologic, immunologic and molecular data. Am J Surg Pathol 1992; 16:637.

95. Morton JE, Leyland MJ, Vaughan Hudson G, et al: Primary gastrointestinal non-Hodgkin's lymphoma: A review of 175 British National Lymphoma Investigation cases. Br J Cancer 1993; 67:776.

96. Valicenti RK, Wasserman TH, Kucik NA: Analysis of prognostic factors in localized gastric lymphoma: The importance of bulk of disease. Int J Radiat Oncol Biol Phys 1993; 27:591.

97. Aviles A, Diaz MJ, Rodriguez L, et al: Prognostic value of serum beta$_2$ microglobulin in primary gastric lymphoma. Hematol Oncol 1991; 9:115.

98. Wotherspoon AC, Doglioni C, Isaacson PG: Low-grade gastric B-cell lymphoma of mucosa-associated lymphoid tissue (MALT): A multifocal disease. Histopathology 1992; 20:29.

99. Maor MH, Velasquez WS, Fuller LM, et al: Stomach conservation in stages IE and IIE gastric non-Hodgkin's lymphoma [see comments]. J Clin Oncol 1990; 8:266.

100. Taal BG, Burgers JM: Primary non-Hodgkin's lymphoma of the stomach: Endoscopic diagnosis and the role of surgery. Scand J Gastroenterol 1991;188(Suppl 33):33.

101. Domizio P, Owen RA, Shepherd NA, et al: Primary lymphoma of the small intestine: A clinicopathological study of 119 cases. Am J Surg Pathol 1993; 17:429.

102. Haber DA, Mayer RJ: Primary gastrointestinal lymphoma. Semin Oncol 1988; 15:154.

103. Al-Bahrani Z, Al-Mohindry H, Bakir F, et al: Clinical and pathologic subtypes of primary intestinal lymphoma: Experience with 132 patients over a 14-year period. Cancer 1983; 52:1666.

104. Seligmann M, Ranbaud JC: Alpha-chain disease: A possible model for pathogenesis of human lymphomas. *In* Twomey JJ, Good RA (eds): Immunopathology of Lymphoreticular Neoplasms. New York, Plenum Press, 1978, pp 425–447.

105. Salem PA, Nassas VH, Shahid MJ, et al: "Mediterranean abdominal lymphoma" or immunoproliferative small intestinal disease: I. Clinical aspects. Cancer 1977; 40:2941.

106. Aosaza K, Ohsawa M, Soma T, et al: Malignant lymphoma of the rectum. Jpn J Clin Oncol 1990; 20:380.

107. Heule BV, Taylor CR, Terry R, et al: Presentation of malignant lymphoma in the rectum. Cancer 1982; 49:2602.

108. Brugere J, Schlienger M, Gerard-Marchant R, et al: Non-Hodgkin's malignant lymphoma of upper digestive and respiratory tract: Natural history and results of radiotherapy. Br J Cancer 1975; 31:435.

109. Teshima T, Chatani M, Inoue T, et al: Radiation therapy for primary non-Hodgkin's lymphoma of the head and neck in stage I-II. Strahlenther Onkol 1986; 162:478.

110. De Pena CA, Van Tassel P, Lee Y-Y: Lymphoma of the head and neck. Radiol Clin North Am 1990; 28:723.

111. Banfi A, Bonadonna G, Ricci SB, et al: Malignant lymphoma of Waldeyer's ring: Natural history and survival after radiotherapy. Br Med J 1972; 3:140.

112. Wang CC: Primary malignant lymphoma of the oral cavity and paranasal sinuses. Radiology 1971; 100:151.

113. Hoppe RT, Burke JS, Glatstein E, et al: Non-Hodgkin's lymphoma: Involvement of Waldeyer's ring. Cancer 1978; 42:1096.

114. Conley SF, Staszak C, Clamon GH, et al: Non-Hodgkin's lymphoma of the head and neck: The University of Iowa experience. Laryngoscope 1987; 97:291.

115. Wulfrank D, Speelman T, Pauwels C, et al: Extranodal non-Hodgkin's lymphoma of the head and neck. Radiother Oncol 1987; 8:199.

116. Ossenkoppele GJ, Mol JJ, Snow GB, et al: Radiotherapy versus radiotherapy plus chemotherapy in stages I and II non-Hodgkin's lymphoma of the upper digestive and respiratory tract. Cancer 1987; 60:1505.

117. Liang R, Ng RP, Todd D, et al: Management of stage I-II diffuse aggressive non-Hodgkin's lymphoma of the Waldeyer's ring: Combined-modality therapy versus radiotherapy alone. Hematol Oncol 1987; 5:223.

118. Fuller LM, Hagemeister FB, Sullivan MP, et al: Hodgkin's Disease and Non-Hodgkin's Lymphomas in Adults and Children. New York, Raven Press, 1988.

119. Su IJ, Hsieh HC, Lin KH, et al: Aggressive peripheral T-cell lymphomas containing Epstein-Barr viral DNA: A clinicopathologic and molecular analysis. Blood 1991; 77:799.

120. Liang R, Todd D, Chau TK, et al: Nasal lymphoma: A retrospective analysis of 60 cases. Cancer 1990; 66:2205.

121. Fellbaum C, Hansmann ML, Lennett K: Malignant lymphomas of the nasal and paranasal sinuses. Virchows Arch A Pathol Anat Histopathol 1989; 414:399.

122. Campo E, Cardesa A, Alos K, et al: Non-Hodgkin's lymphomas of nasal cavity and paranasal sinuses. Am J Clin Pathol 1991; 96:184.

123. Weiss LM, Arber DA, Simckler JC: Nasal T-cell lymphoma. Ann Oncol 1994; 5(Suppl 1):39.

124. Itami J, Itami M, Mikata A, et al: Non-Hodgkin's lymphoma confined to the nasal cavity: Its relationship to the polymorphic reticulosis and results of radiation therapy. Int J Radiat Oncol Biol Phys 1991; 20:797.

125. Kanavaros P, Lescs M-C, Briere J, et al: Nasal T-cell lymphoma: A clinicopathologic entity associated with peculiar phenotype and with Epstein-Barr virus. Blood 1993; 81:2688.

126. Robbins KT, Kong JS, Fuller LM, et al: A comparative analysis of lymphomas involving Waldeyer's ring and the nasal cavity and paranasal sinuses. J Otolaryngol 1985; 14:7.

127. Kassan SS, Thomas TL, Moutsopoulos HM, et al: Increased risk of lymphoma in sicca syndrome. Ann Intern Med 1978; 89:888.

128. Gleeson MJ, Bennett MH, Cawson RA: Lymphomas of salivary glands. Cancer 1986; 58:699.

129. Hyjek E, Smith WJ, Isaacson PG: Primary B cell lymphoma of salivary glands and its relationship to myoepithelial sialadenitis. Hum Pathol 1988; 19:766.

130. Laing RW, Hoskin P, Vaughan Hudson V, et al: The significance of MALT histology in thyroid lymphoma: A review of patients from the BNLI and Royal Marsden Hospital. Clin Oncol 1994; 6:300.

131. Makepeace AR, Fermont DC, Bennett MH: Non-Hodgkin's lymphoma of the tonsil: Experience of treatment over a 27-year period. J Laryngol Otol 1987; 101:1151.

132. Blair TJ, Evans RG, Buskirk SJ, et al: Radiotherapeutic management of primary lymphoid lymphoma. Int J Radiat Oncol Biol Phys 1985; 11:365.

133. Tupchong L, Hughes F, Harmer CL: Primary lymphoma of the thyroid: Clinical features, prognostic factors, and results of treatment. Int J Radiat Oncol Biol Phys 1986; 12:1813.

134. Vigliotti A, Kong JS, Fuller LM, et al: Thyroid lymphomas stages IE and IIE: Comparative results for radiotherapy only, combination

chemotherapy only, and multimodality treatment. Int J Radiat Oncol Biol Phys 1986; 12:1807.

135. Makepeace AR, Fermont DC, Bennett MH: Non-Hodgkin's lymphoma of the thyroid. Clin Radiol 1987; 38:277.

136. Tsang R, Gospodarowicz MK, Sutcliffe SB, et al: Non-Hodgkin's lymphoma of the thyroid gland: Prognostic factors and treatment outcome. Int J Radiat Oncol Biol Phys 1993; 27:599.

137. Leedman PJ, Sheridan WP, Downey WF, et al: Combination chemotherapy as single modality therapy for stage IE and IIE thyroid lymphoma. Med J Aust 1990; 152:40.

138. Anscombe AM, Wright DH: Primary malignant lymphoma of the thyroid—a tumour of mucosa-associated lymphoid tissue: Review of seventy-six cases. Histopathology 1985; 9:81.

139. Letschert JG, Gonzalez GD, Oskam J, et al: Results of radiotherapy in patients with stage I orbital non-Hodgkin's lymphoma. Radiother Oncol 1991; 22:36.

140. Kim JH, Fayos JV: Primary orbital lymphoma: A radiotherapeutic experience. Int J Radiat Oncol Biol Phys 1976; 1:1099.

141. Dunbar SF, Linggood RM, Doppke KP, et al: Conjunctival lymphoma: Results and treatment with a single anterior electron field—a lens-sparing approach [see comments]. Int J Radiat Oncol Biol Phys 1990; 19:249.

142. Fitzpatrick PJ, Macko SM: Lymphoreticular tumors of the orbit. Int J Radiat Oncol Biol Phys 1984; 10:333.

143. Sigelman J, Jakobiec FA: Lymphoid lesions of the conjunctiva: Relation of histopathology to clinical outcome. Ophthalmology 1978; 85:371.

144. Jereb B, Lee H, Jakobiec FA, et al: Radiation therapy of conjunctival and orbital lymphoid tumors. Int J Radiat Oncol Biol Phys 1984; 10:1013.

145. Bessell EM, Henk JM, Wright JE, et al: Orbital and conjunctival lymphoma treatment and prognosis. Radiother Oncol 1988; 13:237.

146. Donaldson S, McDougall I, Egbert PR, et al: Treatment of orbital pseudotumor (idiopathic orbital inflammation) by radiation therapy. Int J Radiat Oncol Biol Phys 1980; 10:79.

147. Minehan KJ, Martenson J Jr, Garrity JA, et al: Local control and complications after radiation therapy for primary orbital lymphoma: A case for low-dose treatment. Int J Radiat Oncol Biol Phys 1991; 20:791.

148. Mittal BB, Deutsch M, Kennerdell J, et al: Paraocular lymphoid tumors. Radiology 1986; 159:793.

149. Reddy EK, Bhatia P, Evans RG: Primary orbital lymphomas. Int J Radiat Oncol Biol Phys 1988; 15:1239.

150. Buettner H, Bolling JP: Intravitreal large cell lymphoma. Mayo Clin Proc 1993; 68:1011.

151. Trudeau M, Shepherd FA, Blackstein ME, et al: Intraocular lymphoma: Report of three cases and review of the literature. Am J Clin Oncol 1988; 11:126.

152. Char DH, Ljungl B-M, Miller T, et al: Primary intraocular lymphoma (ocular reticulum cell sarcoma): Diagnosis and management. Ophthalmology 1988; 95:625.

153. Qualman SJ, Mendelsohn G, B MR, et al: Intraocular lymphoma: Natural history based on a clinicopathologic study of eight cases and review of the literature. Cancer 1983; 52:878.

154. Vogel MH, Font RL, Zimmerman LE, et al: Reticulum cell sarcoma of the retina and uvea: Report of six cases and review of the literature. Am J Opthalmol 1968; 66:205.

155. Corriveau C, Easterbrook M, Payne DG: Intraocular lymphoma and the masquerade syndrome. Can J Ophthalmol 1986; 21:144.

156. Freeman LN, Schachat AP, Knox DL, et al: Clinical features, laboratory investigations, and survival in ocular reticulum cell sarcoma. Ophthalmology 1987; 94:1631.

157. Rosenbaum TJ, MacCarty CS, Buettner H: Uveitis and cerebral reticulum cell sarcoma (large cell lymphoma): Case report. J Neurosurg 1979; 50:660.

158. Michelson JB, Michelson PE, Borden GM, et al: Ocular reticulum cell sarcoma. Arch Ophthalmol 1981; 99:1409.

159. Strauchen JA, Dalton J, Friedman AH: Chemotherapy in the management of intraocular lymphoma. Cancer 1989; 63:1918.

160. Margolis L, Fraser R, Lichter A, et al: The role of radiation therapy in the management of ocular reticulum cell sarcoma. Cancer 1980; 45:688.

161. Simon JW, Friedman AH: Ocular reticulum cell sarcoma. Br J Ophthalmol 1980; 64:793.

162. Salem Y, Miller H: Lymphoma of the genitourinary tract. J Urol 1994; 151:1162.

163. Schned AR, Variakojis D, Straus FH, et al: Primary histiocytic lymphoma of the epididymis. Cancer 1979; 43:1156.

164. Buck DS, Peterson MS, Borochovitz D, et al: Non-Hodgkin lymphoma of the ureter: CT demonstration with pathologic correlation. Urol Radiol 1992; 14:183.

165. Crellin AM, Hudson BV, Bennett MH, et al: Non-Hodgkin's lymphoma of the testis. Radiother Oncol 1993; 27:99.

166. Gowing NFC: Malignant lymphoma of the testis. *In* Pugh RCB (ed): Pathology of the Testis. London, Blackwell Scientific, 1976, pp 334–355.

167. Duncan PR, Checa F, Gowing NFC, et al: Extranodal non-Hodgkin's lymphoma presenting in the testicle. Cancer 1980; 45:1578.

168. Read R: Lymphoma of the testis: Results of treatment, 1960–1977. Clin Radiol 1981; 32:687.

169. Buskirk SJ, Evans RG, Banks PM, et al: Primary lymphoma of the testis. Int J Radiat Oncol Biol Phys 1982; 8:1699.

170. Jackson SM, Montessori GA: Malignant lymphoma of the testis: Review of 17 patients in British Columbia with survival related to pathological subclassification. J Urol 1980; 123:881.

171. Turner RR, Colby TV, MacKintosh FR: Testicular lymphomas: A clinicopathologic study of 35 cases. Cancer 1977; 48:2095.

172. Martenson JA Jr, Buskirk SJ, Ilstrup DM, et al: Patterns of failure in primary testicular non-Hodgkin's lymphoma. J Clin Oncol 1988; 6:297.

173. Moller MB, d'Amore F, Christensen BE: Testicular lymphoma: A population-based study of incidence, clinicopathological correlations, and prognosis. Eur J Cancer 1994; 30a:1760.

174. Aigen AB, Phillips M: Primary malignant lymphoma of the urinary bladder. Urology 1986; 28:235.

175. Guthman DA, Malek RS, Chapman WR, et al: Primary malignant lymphoma of the bladder. J Urol 1990; 144:1367.

176. Gupta DR, Gilmore AM, Ward JP: Primary malignant lymphoma of the bladder. Br J Urol 1985; 57:238.

177. Pontius EE, Nourse MH, Paz L, et al: Primary malignant lymphoma of the bladder. J Urol 1963; 90:58.

178. Santino AM, Shumaker EJ, Garces J: Primary malignant lymphoma of the bladder. J Urol 1970; 103:310.

179. Wang CC, Scully RE, Leadbetter WF: Primary malignant lymphoma of the urinary bladder. Cancer 1969; 24:772.

180. Ohsawa M, Aozasa K, Horiuchi K, et al: Malignant lymphoma: Report of three cases and review of the literature. Cancer 1993; 72:1969.

181. Heaney JA, Dellellis RA, Rudders RA: Non-Hodgkin's lymphoma arising in the lower urinary tract. Urology 1985; 25:479.

182. Abraham N Jr, Maher TJ, Hutchison RE: Extranodal monocytoid B cell lymphoma of the urinary bladder. Mod Pathol 1993; 6:145.

183. Pawade J, Banerjee SS, Harris M, et al: Lymphomas of mucosa-associated lymphoid tissue arising in the urinary bladder. Histopathology 1993; 23:147.

184. Melekos MD, Matsouka P, Fokaefs E, et al: Primary non-Hodgkin's lymphoma of the urinary bladder. Eur Urol 1992; 21:85.

185. Dobkin SF, Brem AS, Caldamone AA: Primary renal lymphoma. J Urol 1991; 146:1588.

186. Harris GJ, Lager DJ: Primary renal lymphoma. J Surg Oncol 1991; 46:273.

187. Poulios C: Primary renal non-Hodgkin lymphoma. Scand J Urol Nephrol 1990; 24:227.

188. Parveen T, Navarro-Roman L, Medeiros LJ, et al: Low-grade B-cell lymphoma of mucosa-associated lymphoid tissue arising in the kidney [see comments]. Arch Pathol Lab Med 1993; 117:780.

189. Bostwick DG, Mann RB: Malignant lymphomas involving the prostate: A study of 13 cases. Cancer 1985; 56:2932.

190. Patel DR, Gomez GA, Henderson ES, et al: Primary prostatic involvement in non-Hodgkin lymphoma. Urology 1988; 32:96.

191. Franco V, Florena AM, Quintini G, et al: Monocytoid B cell lymphoma of the prostate. Pathologica 1992; 84:411.

192. Chen HH, Panella JS, Rochester D, et al: Non-Hodgkin lymphoma of ureteral wall: CT findings. J Comput Assist Tomogr 1988; 12:157.

193. Curry NS, Chung CJ, Potts W, et al: Isolated lymphoma of genitourinary tract and adrenals. Urology 1993; 41:494.

194. Nabholtz JM, Friedman S, Tremeaux JC, et al: Non-Hodgkin's lymphoma of the urethra: A rare extranodal entity. Gynecol Oncol 1989; 35:110.

195. Touhami H, Brahimi S, Kubisz P, et al: Non-Hodgkin's lymphoma of the female urethra. J Urol 1987; 137:991.

196. Selch MT, Mark RJ, Fu YS, et al: Primary lymphoma of female urethra: Long-term control by radiation therapy. Urology 1993; 42:343.
197. Vogeli T, Engstfeld EJ: Non-Hodgkin lymphoma of the female urethra. Scand J Urol Nephrol 1992; 26:111.
198. Vapnek JM, Turzan CW: Primary malignant lymphoma of the female urethra: Report of a case and review of the literature. J Urol 1992; 147:701.
199. Simpson RH, Bridger JE, Anthony PP, et al: Malignant lymphoma of the lower urinary tract: A clinicopathological study with review of the literature. Br J Urol 1990; 65:254.
200. Osborne BM, Robboy SJ: Lymphomas or leukemia presenting as ovarian tumors: An analysis of 42 cases. Cancer 1983; 52:1933.
201. Paladugu RR, Bearman RM, Rappaport H: Malignant lymphoma with primary manifestation in the gonad: A clinicopathologic study of 38 patients. Cancer 1980; 45:561.
202. Woodruff JD, Castillord RD, Novak ER: Lymphoma of the ovary: A study of 35 cases from the ovarian tumour registry of the American Gynecological Society. Am J Obstet Gynecol 1963; 85:912.
203. Monterroso V, Jaffe ES, Merino MJ, et al: Malignant lymphomas involving the ovary: A clinicopathologic analysis of 39 cases. Am J Surg Pathol 1993; 17:154.
204. Harris NL, Scully RE: Malignant lymphoma and granulocytic sarcoma of the uterus and vagina: A clinicopathologic analysis of 27 cases. Cancer 1984; 53:2530.
205. Prevot S, Hugol D, Audouin J, et al: Primary non-Hodgkin's malignant lymphoma of the vagina: Report of three cases with review of the literature. Pathol Res Pract 1992; 188:78.
206. Muntz HG, Ferry JA, Flynn D, et al: Stage IE primary malignant lymphomas of the uterine cervix. Cancer 1991; 68:2023.
207. McDermott MR, Bienenstock J: Evidence for a common mucosal immunologic system: I. Migration of B immunoblasts to intestinal, respiratory, and genital tissues. J Immunol 1979; 122:1892.
208. Johnston C, Senekjian E, Ratain M, et al: Conservative management of primary cervical lymphoma using combination chemotherapy: A case report. Gynecol Oncol 1989; 35:391.
209. Sandvei R, Loke K, Svendson E, et al: Case report: Successful pregnancy following treatment of primary malignant lymphoma of the uterine cervix. Gynecol Oncol 1990; 38:128.
210. Hugh JC, Jackson FI, Hanson J, et al: Primary breast lymphoma: An immunohistologic study of 20 new cases. Cancer 1990; 66:2602.
211. Adair FE, Hermann JB: Primary lymphosarcoma of the breast. Surgery 1944; 16:836.
212. Mambo NC, Burke JS, Butler JJ: Primary malignant lymphoma of the breast. Cancer 1977; 39:2033.
213. Shepherd JJ, Wright DH: Burkitt's tumour presenting as bilateral swelling of the breasts in women of child-bearing age. Br J Surg 1967; 54:776.
214. Mattia AR, Ferry JA, Harris NL: Breast lymphoma: A B-cell spectrum including the low-grade B-cell lymphoma of the mucosa-associated lymphoid tissue. Am J Surg Pathol 1991; 17:574.
215. Brustein S, Filippa DA, Kummel M, et al: Malignant lymphoma of the breast: A study of 53 patients. Ann Surg 1987; 205:144.
216. Dixon JM, Lumsden AB, Krajewski A, et al: Primary lymphoma of the breast. Br J Surg 1987; 74:214.
217. Lamovec J, Jaucar J: Primary malignant lymphoma of the breast: Lymphoma of the mucosa-associated lymphoid tissue. Cancer 1987; 60:3033.
218. Giardini R, Piccolo C, Rilke F: Primary non-Hodgkin's lymphomas of the female breast. Cancer 1992; 69:725.
219. Wiseman C, Liao KT: Primary lymphoma of the breast. Cancer 1972; 29:1705.
220. Schouten JT, Weese JL, Carbone PP: Lymphoma of the breast. Ann Surg 1981; 194:749.
221. Armitage JD, Feagler JR: Burkitt lymphoma during pregnancy with bilateral breast involvement. JAMA 1976; 237:247.
222. DeBlasio D, McCormick B, Straus D, et al: Definitive irradiation for localized non-Hodgkin's lymphoma of breast. Int J Radiat Oncol Biol Phys 1989; 17:843.
223. Liu FF, Clark RM: Primary lymphoma of the breast. Clin Radiol 1986; 37:567.
224. Jeon HJ, Akagi T, Hoshida Y, et al: Primary non-Hodgkin malignant lymphoma of the breast: An immunohistochemical study of seven patients and literature review of 152 patients with breast lymphoma in Japan. Cancer 1992; 70:2451.
225. Ostrowski ML, Unni KK, Banks PM, et al: Malignant lymphoma of bone. Cancer 1986; 58:2646.
226. Bacci G, Ferraro A, Casadei R, et al: Primary lymphoma of bone: Long-term results in patients treated with vincristine–Adriamycin–cyclophosphamide and local radiation. J Chemother 1991; 3:189.
227. Salter M, Sollaccio RJ, Bernreuter WK, et al: Primary lymphoma of bone: The use of MRI in pretreatment evaluation. Am J Clin Oncol 1989; 12:101.
228. Friedman M, Kim TH, Panahon AM: Spinal cord compression in malignant lymphoma: Treatment and results. Cancer 1976; 37:1485.
229. Herman TS, Hammond N, Jones SE, et al: Involvement of the central nervous system by non-Hodgkin's lymphoma: The Southwest Oncology Group experience. Cancer 1979; 43:390.
230. Gilbert R, Kim J, Posner J: Epidural spinal cord compression from metastatic tumour: Diagnosis and treatment. Ann Neurol 1978; 3:40.
231. Khan FR, Glicksman AS, Chu FCH, et al: Treatment by radiotherapy of spinal cord compression due to extradural metastases. Radiology 1967; 89:495.
232. Cappellani G, Giuffre F, Tropea R, et al: Primary spinal epidural lymphomas: Report of ten cases. J Neurosurg Sci 1986; 30:147.
233. Eeles RA, O'Brien P, Horwich A, et al: Non-Hodgkin's lymphoma presenting with extradural spinal cord compression: Functional outcome and survival. Br J Cancer 1991; 63:126.
234. Epelbaum R, Haim N, Ben-Shahar M, et al: Non-Hodgkin's lymphoma presenting with spinal epidural involvement. Cancer 1986; 58:2120.
235. Haddad P, Thaell JF, Kiely JM, et al: Lymphoma of the spinal extradural space. Cancer 1976; 38:1862.
236. MacKintosh FR, Colby TV, Podolsky WJ, et al: Central nervous system involvement in non-Hodgkin's lymphoma: An analysis of 105 cases. Cancer 1982; 49:586.
237. Cordier JF, Chailleux E, Lauque D, et al: Primary pulmonary lymphomas: A clinical study of 70 cases in nonimmunocompromised patients. Chest 1993; 103:201.
238. Eng J, Sabanathan S: Endobronchial non-Hodgkin's lymphoma. J Cardiovasc Surg 1993; 34:351.
239. Satzstein SL: Pulmonary malignant lymphoma and pseudolymphomas: Classification, therapy, and prognosis. Cancer 1963; 16:928.
240. L'Hoste RJ Jr, Filippa DA, Lieberman PH: Primary pulmonary lymphomas: A clinicopathologic analysis of 36 cases. Cancer 1984; 54:1397.
241. Kennedy JL, Nathwani BN, Burke JS, et al: Pulmonary lymphomas and their pulmonary lymphoid lesions: A clinicopathologic and immunologic study of 64 patients. Cancer 1985; 56:539.
242. Lamarre L, Jacobson JO, Arsenberg AC, et al: Primary large cell lymphoma of the mediastinum: A histologic and immunophenotypic study of 29 cases. Am J Surg Pathol 1989; 13:730.
243. Todeschini G, Ambrosetti A, Meneghini V: Mediastinal large B-cell lymphoma with sclerosis: A clinical study of 21 patients. J Clin Oncol 1990; 8:804.
244. Sutcliffe SB: Primary mediastinal malignant lymphoma. Semin Thorac Cardiovasc Surg 1992; 4:55.
245. Ahmann DL, Kiely JM, Harrison EG Jr, et al: Malignant lymphoma of the spleen: A review of 49 cases in which the diagnosis was made at splenectomy. Cancer 1966; 19:461.
246. Kehoe J, Straus DJ: Primary lymphoma of the spleen: Clinical features and outcome after splenectomy. Cancer 1988; 62:1433.
247. Kraemer BB, Osborne BM, Butler JJ: Primary splenic presentation of malignant lymphomas and related disorders: A study of 49 cases. Cancer 1984; 54:1606.
248. Harris NL, Aisenberg AC, Meyer JE, et al: Diffuse large cell (histiocytic) lymphoma of the spleen: Clinical and pathologic characteristics of ten cases. Cancer 1984; 54:2460.
249. Narang S, Wolf BC, Neiman RS: Malignant lymphoma presenting with prominent splenomegaly: A clinicopathologic study with special reference to intermediate cell lymphoma. Cancer 1985; 55:1948.
250. Fischer MA, Kabakow B: Lymphoma of the pancreas. Mt Sinai J Med 1987; 54:423.
251. Webb TH, Lillemoe KD, Pitt HA, et al: Pancreatic lymphoma: Is surgery mandatory for diagnosis or treatment? Ann Surg 1989; 209:25.
252. Tuchak JM, DeJong SA, Pickleman J: Diagnosis, surgical intervention, and prognosis of primary pancreatic lymphoma. Am Surg 1993; 59:513.

253. Ohsawa M, Aozasa K, Horiuchi K, et al: Malignant lymphoma of the liver: Report of five cases and review of the literature. Dig Dis Sci 1992; 37:1105.

254. Dement SH, Mann RB, Staal SP, et al: Primary lymphoma of the liver: Report of six cases and review of the literature. Am J Clin Pathol 1987; 88:255.

255. Osborne BM, Butler JJ, Guarda LA: Primary lymphoma of the liver: Ten cases and review of the literature. Cancer 1985; 56: 2902.

256. Anthony PP, Sarsfield P, Clarke T: Primary lymphoma of the liver: Clinical and pathologic features of ten patients. J Clin Pathol 1990; 43:1007.

257. Travis WD, Banks PM, Reiman HM: Primary extranodal soft tissue lymphoma of the extremities. Am J Surg Pathol 1987; 11:359.

258. Scally J, Garrett A: Primary extranodal lymphoma in muscle. Br J Radiol 1989; 62:81.

259. Rosenberg SA, Diamond HB, Jaslowitz B, et al: Lymphosarcoma: A review of 1269 cases. Medicine (Baltimore) 1961; 40:31.

260. Chou S-T, Arkles LB, Gill GD, et al: Primary lymphoma of the heart: A case report. Cancer 1983; 52:744.

261. Zaharia L, Gill PS: Primary cardiac lymphoma. Am J Clin Oncol 1991; 14:142.

262. Kaplan LD, Abrams DI, Feigal E, et al: AIDS-associated non-Hodgkin's lymphoma in San Francisco. JAMA 1989; 261:719.

263. Penn I: Cancer after cyclosporine therapy. Transplant Proc 1988; 20(Suppl 1):276.

264. Pozniak AL, Thomas RD, Hobbs CB, et al: Primary malignant lymphoma of the heart: Antemortem cytologic diagnosis. Acta Cytologica 1986; 30:662.

265. Dorsay TA, Ho VB, Rovira MJ, et al: Primary cardiac lymphoma: CT and MR findings. J Comput Assist Tomogr 1993; 17:978.

266. Nand S, Mullen GM, Lonchyna VA, et al: Primary lymphoma of the heart: Prolonged survival with early systemic therapy in a patient. Cancer 1991; 68:2289.

267. Aozasa K, Ohsawa M, Iuchi K, et al: Prognostic factors for pleural lymphoma patients. Jpn J Clin Oncol 1991; 21:417.

268. Aozasa K, Ohsawa M, Iuchi K, et al: Artificial pneumothorax as a risk factor for development of pleural lymphoma. Jpn J Cancer Res 1993; 84:55.

269. Choi CH, Durishin M, Garbadawala ST, et al: Non-Hodgkin's lymphoma of the adrenal gland. Arch Pathol Lab Med 1990; 114:883.

270. Harris GJ, Tio FO, Von Hoff DD: Primary adrenal lymphoma. Cancer 1989; 63:799.

271. Kluin, PM: *Bcl*-6 in lymphoma—sorting out a wastebasket [Editorial]. N Engl J Med 1994; 331:116.

Twenty-Six

Primary Central Nervous System Lymphoma

Howard A. Fine
Jay S. Loeffler

Primary central nervous system lymphoma (PCNSL) is defined as a non-Hodgkin's lymphoma that is confined to the craniospinal axis without systemic involvement. PCNSL is not to be confused with established systemic lymphoma with secondary spread to the central nervous system (CNS), which occurs in 5% to 29% of patients with systemic lymphoma.[1] Historically, this entity was referred to as "reticulum cell sarcoma," "microglioma," or "perivascular sarcoma," but it has now been well established that the cell of origin is a malignant lymphocyte.[2–5] This chapter discusses the epidemiology, pathology, clinical diagnosis, and results of therapy, as well as the current recommendations and future directions for PCNSL in immunocompetent and immunocompromised patients.

EPIDEMIOLOGY

IMMUNOCOMPROMISED PATIENTS

In the past, PCNSL was considered a rare tumor, accounting for 1% to 2% of all lymphomas and less than 5% of all primary CNS tumors.[6–8] Although most patients with PCNSL are immunocompetent, patients with both acquired and congenital immunodeficiencies are at significant risk for the development of this tumor. The two congenital immunodeficiency states that are most commonly associated with PCNSL are severe combined immunodeficiency and the Wiskott-Aldrich syndromes.[9, 10] PCNSL has also been reported in immunoglobulin A deficiency syndrome.[11] Not all congenital immunodeficiency syndromes, however, are associated with an increased risk of PCNSL. For example, although ataxia-telangiectasia is clearly associated with an increased risk of systemic lymphomas, there have been no reported cases of PCNSL.[12]

Iatrogenic immunodeficiency also predisposes to the development of this tumor. The largest group of these patients consists of organ allograft recipients. In particular, kidney recipients have a significantly increased risk of lymphomas, presumable secondary to chronic iatrogenic immunosuppression. Penn reported that the risk of developing lymphoma in a large group of renal allograft recipients

was 350 times that of the immunocompetent population.[13] As many as 50% of these lymphomas were PCNSL. Recent data suggest that cardiac allograft recipients may be at even greater risk for the development of PCNSL.[14] In a series of 182 heart allograft recipients, Weintraub and Warnke reported three cases of PCNSL, a rate that appears higher than that in the renal transplant population.[14] Why this should be true is unclear, although it is possible that this apparent increase in PCNSL in heart transplant patients may reflect a greater degree of immunosuppression currently used in transplant protocols (in particular the use of cyclosporine), compared with regimens used over a decade ago when Penn first reported the experience with the kidney allograft recipient.

Other disease conditions, particularly those believed to involve autoimmune mechanisms, such as systemic lupus erythematosus, rheumatoid arthritis, and sarcoidosis, have been associated with the development of PCNSL.[15–17] Whether there is truly an increased risk of PCNSL in this patient population is not known. Furthermore, even if there is an increased risk of the development of this tumor in this patient population, it is difficult to know whether the risk factor is the disease itself or the immunosuppressive therapy (such as glucocorticoids) used to treat many of these patients.

The largest group of immunodeficient patients who are at risk for the development of PCNSL are those infected with the human immunodeficiency virus (HIV). In particular, patients with the diagnosis of acquired immunodeficiency syndrome (AIDS) are at particularly high risk of PCNSL: the reported incidence is 2% to 6%.[18] The marked increase in the incidence of PCNSL as a whole can be largely, although not exclusively (see later), attributed to the outbreak of the AIDS epidemic. The AIDS Cooperative Group recently reported the development of 8 cases of lymphoma in 55 patients being treated in trials of antiviral drugs (azidothymidine), 5 of whom developed PCNSL.[19] Although this represents a relatively small patient population, it does suggest a higher than expected number of PCNSL cases. Thus, it appears probable that as supportive care improves for patients with AIDS, the incidence of PCNSL will continue to rise in this patient population.

481

IMMUNOCOMPETENT PATIENTS

Of just as much concern as the rise of PCNSL in immunocompromised patients is the apparent increase in the incidence of this disease in otherwise normal, immunocompetent patients. In 1988 Eby and coworkers, using data from the National Cancer Institute's Surveillance, Epidemiology, and End Results (SEER) program, compared the incidence of PCNSL from 1973 to 1975 to the incidence from 1982 to 1984.[20] They excluded from their analysis young, never-married men, a group previously believed to be at risk for AIDS. These investigators found that the incidence of PCNSL increased from 2.7 to 7.5 cases per 10 million population from the study period in the 1970s to that in the 1980s. It could be argued that this apparent increase in the incidence of PCNSL is an artifact of the inclusion of undiagnosed AIDS patients and/or better screening techniques (such as computed tomography [CT] scans, magnetic resonance imaging [MRI] scans, and stereotaxic surgery). The fact, however, that the observed increase occurred, for the most part, before the AIDS epidemic and before the advent of these more sensitive screening techniques, argues for a true increase in the incidence of PCNSL. Supportive of these observations, investigators at Memorial Sloan-Kettering Cancer Center in New York have reported a 17-fold increase in PCNSL in the 5 years between 1985 and 1990 compared with the prior 20 years.[21] The etiologic factors responsible for this increase in PCNSL in non-AIDS patients are unknown at this time. Some have speculated that if the incidence of this disease continues to rise at the present rate, it will be the most common primary tumor of the CNS by the year 2000. Before such sweeping conclusions can be drawn, however, it should be realized that not every institution has seen the same dramatic increase in the frequency of this tumor. In our own experience, we have witnessed a threefold increase in PCNSL in non-AIDS patients from 1987 to 1992 compared with the rate from 1981 to 1986. Since 1992, however, the number of patients diagnosed with PCNSL has remained constant, and PCNSL (in non-AIDS patients) represented only 1.2% of all primary brain tumors undergoing biopsy at our institution.

BIOLOGY

IMMUNOCOMPETENT PATIENTS

The etiology of the neoplastic lymphocyte clone in immunocompetent patients with PCNSL remains speculative. Several hypotheses concerning the pathophysiology exist, the most simple of which is that the neoplastic transformation occurs in clones of lymphocytes that routinely inhabit the CNS. Alternatively, neoplastic transformation may occur in a systemic population of lymphocytes that possess specific tropism for the CNS (i.e., through expression of specific cell surface adhesion molecules), or develop such a tropism after the transformation events. In support of the latter hypothesis, Bashir and colleagues examined immunophenotypic markers in 18 cases of CNS lymphoma (14 primary and 4 secondary).[22] As had been previously reported, all lymphoma cells were of B-cell origin. Although most tumors were positive for pan-B-cell markers, most

CNS lymphoma cells were negative for various B-cell-restricted activation markers such as B5, Blast 2, and BB1. This is in contrast to systemic lymphomas, which are almost always positive for these antigens. There were no significant immunophenotypic differences between primary and secondary CNS lymphomas. The total number of CNS lymphomas examined in this study was small; however, if these data can be confirmed in a larger series, the hypothesis that PCNSL represents a clonal proliferation of lymphoma cells with a predilection for the CNS will be supported. The reason for this is that if PCNSL was the result of transformation of a naturally occurring CNS lymphocyte population, one would expect different phenotypes between primary and secondary CNS lymphomas.

A third hypothesis for the etiology of PCNSL is based on the idea that the CNS is a immunologic sanctuary. Neoplastic lymphocytes may be eradicated systemically by an intact immune system but find relative protection within the CNS. This could explain the curious observation that systemic dissemination of PCNSL is unusual, even in advanced stages of disease. This hypothesis is based on the premise that the CNS has a "privileged" status relative to the immune system. Although this concept is still evolving, the original concept was first proposed many years ago with the discovery of the blood-brain barrier (BBB). The anatomic substrate for the BBB is the continuous sealing of interendothelial spaces by tight junctions and the lack of fenestrations or pores normally found in capillaries in other parts of the body.[23, 24] Thus, the BBB effectively limits the movement of macromolecules into or out of the brain parenchyma.[24] Relative to immunologic reactions, these physiologic restraints imparted by the BBB may effectively limit the exposure of foreign antigens within the CNS to the cellular and humoral immune system. This "hiding" of foreign antigen effectively isolates the CNS from the immune system, making the CNS a so-called immunologically privileged site.

Experimental evidence confirming the immunologic privileged status of the CNS comes from experiments in the 1920s by Murphy and Sturm, who demonstrated that mouse sarcoma could survive in rat brain.[25] Alternately, the tumor failed to grow if an autograft of rat splenic tissue was cotransplanted with the mouse sarcoma, demonstrating the animals' immunocompetence to destroy the xenograft if antigen-presenting and effector cells could "see" the foreign antigens in the correct context. Since these initial experiments, many types of incompatible tissue types have been transplanted into animal and human brains with little or no graft rejection.[26, 27] Other examples of diminished immune responses to foreign antigens within the CNS are the so-called slow viruses, in which the virus causes progressive tissue destruction over years with little or no inflammatory response.

In addition to the growing data demonstrating diminished antigen presentation within the CNS, some investigators have suggested that the BBB may limit the movement of immune effector cells into the CNS. Neither experimental nor clinical evidence support this conclusion, however. Animal models of autoimmune diseases such as experimental allergic encephalitis (EAE) and clinical disease states such as multiple sclerosis demonstrate the potential ability of immune effector cells to invade the CNS.[28] Thus, the difficulty of the intact immune system to see foreign antigens within the CNS may be the principal determinant of the presumed immunologic privileged status of the CNS. Although much has yet to be learned, these data clearly suggest that some type of immunologic sanctuary for tumor cells may exist within the CNS. Thus, regardless of how and where PCNSL malignant lymphocytes develop, once these cells gain access to the CNS they appear to proliferate rapidly within the subarachnoid space and disseminate throughout the craniospinal axis without significant impedance from the immune system.

IMMUNOCOMPROMISED PATIENTS

As mentioned, the high incidence of PCNSL in the AIDS population resembles that in other immunosuppressed patients, implicating the immune system in the pathogenesis of this disease. There are many biologic similarities between AIDS patients and the congenital or iatrogenic immunosuppressed populations who develop PCNSL. The malignant lymphocytes in these two groups of immunocompromised patients tend to be oligoclonal or polyclonal and usually high grade (immunoblastic and small-noncleaved), in contrast with the monoclonal tumors found in PCNSLs of immunocompetent patients, which are often low- to intermediate-grade tumors.[29] Another similarity between these two groups of immunocompromised patients is the tendency for the degree of immunosuppression to be related to the risk of developing PCNSL. For example, the risk of PCNSL in transplant patients is related to the dose and number of immunosuppressive agents as well as the duration of treatment. An analogous situation appears to occur in patients with AIDS, in whom the risk of developing PCNSL increases with declining CD4 lymphocyte counts (and thus more immunosuppression).[30]

Epstein-Barr virus (EBV) appears to play a role in the pathogenesis of PCNSL in the immunosuppressed population. In contrast with immunocompetent patients with PCNSL, immunosuppressed patients with PCNSL consistently have EBV genomic DNA found within their malignant lymphocytes.[31–34] This relationship is intriguing since EBV is known to induce B-lymphocyte proliferation in vitro. Furthermore, there is strong epidemiologic evidence linking EBV to endemic Burkitt's lymphoma.[35, 36] It is believed that EBV infects certain B lymphocytes, causing a clonal expansion that in an immunocompetent patient is limited by immune mechanisms, particularly cellular immune responses. In the immunocompromised hosts, the T-lymphocyte population is quantitatively (AIDS) and/or qualitatively (cyclosporine-treated/T-cell depletion for allogeneic bone marrow transplantation) abnormal, allowing EBV-induced B-lymphocyte proliferation to proceed unrestrained. This, along with the possibly decreased immunologic surveillance within the CNS may contribute to the development of PCNSL in this patient population. Consistent with this hypothesis is a recent report from Memorial Sloan-Kettering Cancer Center that demonstrated that EBV-associated lymphoma occurring after allogeneic bone marrow transplantation was associated with T-cell depletion of the donor marrow.[28] The importance of an intact cellular response was suggested by the observation that five of these transplant patients with EBV-related lymphomas were successfully treated with unirradiated donor leukocytes, achieving either clinical or pathologic complete responses.

CLINICAL AND RADIOGRAPHIC PRESENTATION

More than 70 manuscripts have appeared in the literature reporting the clinical characteristics of small series of patients with either AIDS- or non-AIDS-associated PCNSL. We recently reviewed 40 reports of non-AIDS-associated PCNSL[37–74] and 32 reports of AIDS-associated PCNSL[12, 19, 75–104] and synthesized the data for these 1100 patients to determine general clinical characteristics and treatment outcomes in this patient population. Most of the remaining data in this chapter are abstracted from this data base.[29]

IMMUNOCOMPETENT AND IMMUNOCOMPROMISED PATIENTS

The median age of diagnosis of PCNSL is 55 years for immunocompetent patients and 31 years for AIDS patients, although PCNSL has been described in patients of all ages (Table 26–1). A male-to-female ratio of 3:2 is seen in the immunocompetent patients, whereas 90% of AIDS patients are males. This preponderance of male over female AIDS patients with PCNSL almost certainly represents the early epidemiology of the AIDS epidemic. Now, as an increasing number of women are being infected with HIV, it is quite likely that we will see an increasing number of immunocompromised women developing PCNSL.

Most patients present with symptoms suggestive of an intracranial mass lesion. As with any primary or metastatic lesion of the CNS, symptoms are related to tumor size and location. However, there are some neurologic symptoms that are more typical of this patient population compared with populations with other intracranial tumors. Since 50% of these lesions develop in the frontal lobes and the lesions are often multifocal, personality changes, headaches, and lethargy are common symptoms. Seizures are less commonly

Table 26–1. Patient Characteristics at Diagnosis

Characteristics	Immunocompetent Group	AIDS Group
Total no. of patients	792	315
Male/female ratio	442/328 (1.35:1)	118/16 (7.38:1)
Mean age (yr)	55.2	30.8
History of opportunistic infection or Kaposi's sarcoma	Not available	115/143 (80%)
Symptoms:		
Average duration before diagnosis (mo)	2.77	1.81
Types: Neurologic (%)	56.4	51.0
Deficits: Mental status (%)	34.6	53.3
Changes:		
Seizures (%)	11.2	26.7
Increased intracranial pressure (%)	32.4	14.2

AIDS, acquired immunodeficiency syndrome.

seen in patients with PCNSL than in patients with gliomas, meningiomas, or metastatic disease, probably because these lesions less commonly involve the seizure-prone cerebral cortex at the time of diagnosis. The duration of symptoms is usually only a few weeks or months, but the range can be up to many months.

Patients with AIDS-associated PCNSL can present with clinical signs and symptoms slightly different from those of their immunocompetent counterparts. AIDS patients more often present with an encephalopathic picture, characterized by significant changes in mental status. The global neurologic deficits associated with AIDS-associated PCNSL are probably a result of a number of factors including the multifocal nature of the disease, associated infectious processes such as viral encephalitis and/or toxoplasmosis, and progressive multifocal leukoencephalopathy. It has been demonstrated at autopsy that most AIDS patients with PCNSL have at least one (and often more) additional active pathologic CNS processes.[105]

It can be assumed that most patients with PCNSL have disseminated disease throughout the CNS at the time of diagnosis. Radiographically, however, only 25% of immunocompetent patients and 50% of AIDS patients have multifocal lesions at diagnosis (Table 26–2). When a multifocal radiographic picture is seen in an otherwise healthy person, the diagnosis of systemic metastatic cancer is often entertained. Since the treatment of metastatic cancer is quite different from the treatment of PCNSL in the immunocompetent host (see later), the importance of a histologic diagnosis cannot be overstated.

Ocular involvement by lymphoma is another manifestation of the multifocal nature of PCNSL. The retro-orbital area is the most common site of eye metastases from systemic lymphoma, whereas malignant cells more commonly infiltrate the vitreous, retina, and/or choroid in PCNSL patients.[106–108] Diagnosis is usually made by the demonstration of a pleocytosis within the aqueous humor by

slit-lamp examination. The prevalence of ocular involvement in PCNSL at the time of diagnosis remains unclear. Some reports claim it to be as high as 20%; however, our review of the literature suggests that it is found in only 5%, although one must question whether most patients are eventually evaluated for ocular involvement. Although some patients may complain of blurred vision or vitreous floaters, most patients are unaware of ocular involvement. If a deliberate effort to screen patients for ocular involvement is not made, many cases will undoubtedly be missed. Thus, a careful neurophthalmologic examination including the use of slit-lamp examination of the vitreous and indirect ophthalmoscopy for retinal or choroidal disease is recommended for all patients before the initiation of therapy.

Whatever the true incidence of ocular involvement by PCNSL, it has been well documented that the disease process occasionally begins in the eye as a nonspecific, unilateral uveitis. The uveitis typically does not respond to conventional therapy and usually becomes bilateral. As many as 80% of patients with ocular lymphoma progress to PCNSL.[107, 108] Thus, any patient with ocular lymphoma should undergo enhanced MRI of the brain as part of the initial evaluation.

Rarely, PCNSL can arise from the leptomeninges and spinal cord (<10% of all PCNSL) in isolation of brain disease. PCNSL of the spinal cord presents usually with bilateral lower limb weakness in the absence of back pain. Pain and sensory symptoms can follow, but the cerebrospinal fluid is usually normal. Prognosis is poor, with survival averaging only a few months. Leptomeningeal presentation, like carcinomatous or lymphomatous meningitis, is associated with cranial neuropathies, progressive lumbosacral root syndrome, and often signs and symptoms of increased intracranial pressure. This is in contrast with more common presentations of PCNSL, in which clinical signs or symptoms of leptomeningeal disease (e.g., cranial neuropathies, hydrocephalus, cervical and lumbosacral radiculopathies) are uncommon despite the relatively high incidence of a malignant pleocytosis at presentation. Diagnosis of PCNSL presenting as leptomeningeal disease is established by a meningeal biopsy and/or the finding of malignant lymphocytes within the CNS. These patients often have hydrocephalus with no obvious parenchymal disease. Our experience suggests that these patients have a prognosis as poor as those presenting with spinal cord disease.

Radiographic imaging studies may be suggestive of the diagnosis of PCNSL (see Table 26–2). Angiographic studies have shown that most of these lesions are avascular or hypovascular in nature. Brain scanning with or without single photon emission computed tomography (SPECT) capabilities using technetium 99m demonstrates increased uptake in almost all patients with PCNSL. These observations are, however, mainly of historical interest, for modern imaging with CT and/or MRI has replaced angiography and nuclear brain scanning. Ninety percent of patients with PCNSL have an isodense or hyperdense lesion on nonenhanced CT scan. This corresponds to an intense signal on the nonenhanced T_1 MRI image. This appearance differs from that of other primary brain tumors (gliomas and meningiomas) and most metastatic lesions, which tend to be hypodense. The hyperdense radiographic appearance of PCNSL probably represents both the close packing of the

Table 26–2. Radiographic Findings at Presentation

Radiographic Finding	Immunocompetent Group	AIDS Group
Angiography	60 avascular, 13 vascular	No data
Brain scan	8 of 8 positive for technetium 99m	No data
CT scan		
Noncontrast	201	67
Hypodense	21 (10.4%)	6 (9.0%)
Iso- or hyperdense	180 (89.6%)	61 (91.0%)
Contrast		
Any enhancement	245 (97.2%)	91 (90.1%)
No enhancement	7 (2.8%)	10 (9.9%)
Pattern of enhancement		
Irregular	86 (45.0%)	25 (39.1%)
Homogeneous	105 (55.0%)	39 (60.9%)
Ring	0 (0.0%)	47 (52.0%) for all enhanced scans
Distribution		
Solitary	290 (72.0%)	87 (48.0%)
Multiple	100 (25.0%)	94 (52.0%)
Diffuse	14 (3.0%)	No data

AIDS, acquired immunodeficiency syndrome.

small lymphocytic cells (which generally have high nuclear-to-cytoplasmic ratios) and the fact that PCNSL tends to have less associated cerebral edema than gliomas and most metastatic tumors.

After the administration of contrast material, more than 90% of PCNSLs enhance on CT and MRI; half of them do so homogeneously. A T_1-weighted MRI scan with gadolinium often demonstrates a greater number of lesions than are seen on CT. The lesions are most often (75%) located adjacent to cortical convexities or ventricular surfaces with indistinct borders and a variable amount of cerebral edema. Thus, an angiographically avascular lesion that is isohyperdense in relation to the normal cortex, enhances homogeneously, and is located adjacent to the ventricular surface is highly suggestive of PCNSL.

A special note should be made concerning those rare PCNSL lesions that do not enhance on CT and/or MRI. DeAngelis recently reported that 10 of 85 (12%) immunocompetent patients with PCNSL had nonenhancing lesions.[21] This group of patients was not treated with corticosteroids before scanning and had nonenhancing lesions at diagnosis or at relapse. In a few patients with multifocal disease, some lesions enhanced whereas others did not on the same scan. Nonenhancing tumors cause significant diagnostic problems and present therapeutic implications, suggesting that the tumor resides behind an intact BBB (see Treatment).

Although AIDS- and non-AIDS-associated PCNSL have similar radiographic findings, there are some important differences. The most important difference is the incidence of radiographic multifocal disease, which is twice as common in AIDS patients compared with their non-AIDS-associated PCNSL counterparts (50% versus 25%, respectively). Additionally, ring enhancement, a pattern rarely seen in non-AIDS PCNSL patients, is seen in 50% of AIDS patients.

DIAGNOSIS

IMMUNOCOMPETENT PATIENTS

Although the diagnosis of PCNSL usually requires histologic verification, the diagnostic algorithm differs for the immunocompetent versus the AIDS patient (Fig. 26–1A). In the immunocompetent patient who is found to have an intracranial mass with radiographic criteria suggestive of PCNSL (as described previously), a tissue diagnosis should be made immediately. Corticosteroids should be withheld until diagnostic tissue is obtained unless the patient is in immediate danger of herniation. The reason for this is that corticosteroids appear to have significant cytotoxic activity against PCNSL such that two thirds of patients have some radiographic response to steroids alone, with some patients achieving a complete radiographic remission. Even for patients not experiencing a radiographic complete response, the lymphotoxic effects of corticosteroids can disrupt cellular morphology, making histologic diagnosis from biopsied material impossible. If the patient requires the immediate use of corticosteroids or if PCNSL was not considered and the patient was placed on corticosteroids, repeat CT and/or MRI should be performed before a diagnosis is made. If the tumor is smaller or resolved

completely, the diagnosis of PCNSL is quite likely. Nevertheless, nonneoplastic contrast-enhancing lesions such as multiple sclerosis and sarcoidosis can also resolve after corticosteroid administration, and thus a tissue diagnosis should still be obtained. If the lesion has completely resolved on the corticosteroid therapy, the patient should be slowly weaned from the drug and followed closely for recurrence of the abnormality on CT and/or MRI. If it recurs, the patient should have a tissue diagnosis made immediately.

Our recommendation is to try to establish the diagnosis without neurosurgical intervention whenever possible. Therefore, if a lumbar puncture can be safely performed (no evidence of obstruction or increased intracranial pressure) cerebrospinal fluid should be obtained for both routine studies and cytologic examination. Although previous reports have suggested that the incidence of positive cerebrospinal fluid cytologic tests at the diagnosis of PCNSL is small, our review of the literature suggests that a malignant pleocytosis may be found in nearly one third of all patients. Markers of clonogenicity such as κ and λ light-chain immunohistochemistry and polymerase chain reaction (PCR) amplification of B-cell immunoglobulin gene rearrangement may be helpful in distinguishing between a clonal proliferation of lymphocytes in the cerebrospinal fluid from a reactive pleocytosis.[109–111] Even with these additional studies, however, most patients require a biopsy of the intracranial mass to establish the pathologic diagnosis.

When a tissue diagnosis is required, several neurosurgical techniques are appropriate. The easiest and safest procedure is a stereotactic biopsy. In the hands of an experienced neurosurgeon, stereotactic biopsy can be performed in almost any region of the brain without significant risks. A potential problem with samples obtained from stereotactic biopsies is the small amount of tissue, potentially making it difficult to differentiate lymphoma from inflammatory cells. With the use of immunohistochemical staining and molecular analysis (i.e., PCR), however, a definitive diagnosis can usually be made. If a definitive diagnosis cannot be obtained via a stereotactic biopsy, an open biopsy for additional tissue is recommended. No data are available to suggest that an extended craniotomy and major resection of tumor are beneficial to these patients, probably because radiation and chemotherapy offer such an effective means of cytoreduction.

After histologic confirmation of PCNSL, patients should undergo a full evaluation of the craniospinal axis, if this was not done before surgery. This includes examination of the cerebrospinal fluid, enhanced MRI of the spinal axis, and a neurophthalmologic examination as described previously. The extent of staging that is necessary to evaluate the possibility of systemic disease should be kept to a minimum. From our experience, as well as that in the literature, a thorough physical examination, routine blood studies, and a chest radiograph are sufficient for screening for systemic involvement. If these procedures are unrevealing, it is unlikely that more extensive studies (gallium scans, body CT scans, bone marrow aspirate, and biopsy) will disclose an occult systemic lymphoma.

IMMUNOCOMPROMISED PATIENTS

The diagnostic decision algorithm in AIDS patients is more difficult because of the higher probability of another

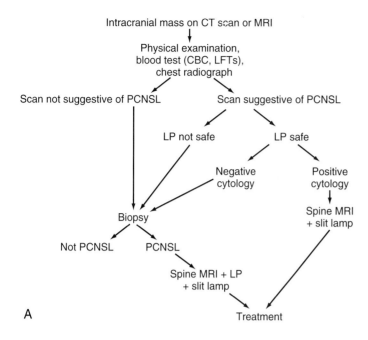

A

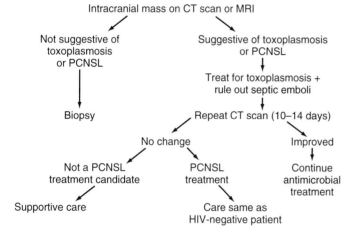

B

Figure 26–1. Diagnostic algorithms for patients found to have head computed tomographic (CT) or magnetic resonance imaging (MRI) scans demonstrating lesions consistent with primary central nervous system lymphoma. *A,* Diagnostic algorithm for immunocompetent human immunodeficiency virus (HIV) seronegative patients. *B,* Diagnostic algorithm for HIV-seropositive patients. CBC, complete blood count; LFT, liver function test; PCNSL, primary central nervous system lymphoma; LP, lumbar puncture.

CNS abnormality such as toxoplasmosis or multifocal leukoencephalopathy.[18, 112] The multiple small, ring-enhancing lesions characteristic of cerebral toxoplasmosis, in particular, can appear identical to PCNSL on CT and/or MRI scans. The decision process is further complicated by the poor survival of AIDS patients with PCNSL (see later), leading many physicians to conclude that these patients should not be subjected to an invasive procedure but rather treated empirically. A reasonable strategy for an AIDS patient with presumed PCNSL (enhancing, periventricular lesion or lesions) is to empirically treat the patient with antitoxoplasmosis drugs, during which time the patient can be evaluated for bacteremia, fungemia, or other sources of septic emboli (Fig. 26–1*B*). This strategy is probably only valid for patients who have positive serologic tests for toxoplasmosis. For the rare HIV-positive patient who is negative for toxoplasmosis antibodies, the likelihood of

cerebral toxoplasmosis is small. Luft and colleagues recently reported a prospective trial using this approach in 49 AIDS patients with enhancing CNS lesions.[113] Thirty-five (71%) of 49 patients responded to clindamycin and pyrimethamine therapy, and 30 (86%) of these had clinical improvement by day 7. Thirty-two (91%) of those with a response improved by day 14. Two of the patients in whom therapy failed underwent a stereotactic biopsy and were found to have PCNSL. Therefore, if an AIDS patient has not improved clinically or radiographically after 10 to 14 days of empiric antitoxoplasmosis therapy, a stereotactic biopsy should be considered. Needless to say, a biopsy should be considered only for a patient in whom there is no intent to treat should the diagnosis of PCNSL be made.

Since structural imaging studies such as CT and MRI cannot accurately differentiate infectious from malignant cerebral lesions in patients with AIDS, there is a growing interest in evaluating the role of functional imaging such as SPECT and positron emission tomography (PET) for these patients. Hoffman and associates recently reported results using [^{18}F]fluoro-2-deoxyglucose (FDG) and PET in 11 AIDS patients with cerebral lesions.[114] FDG-PET was able to accurately differentiate between PCNSL and abnormalities with an infectious cause in all patients. Both qualitative visual inspection of the images and semiquantitative analysis using count ratios were performed and revealed similar results. Thus, it appears from this pilot that FDG-PET may be useful in the management of AIDS patients with CNS lesions since high FDG uptake most likely represents a PCNSL.

We believe that all other non-AIDS immunocompromised patients who present with an enhancing periventricular lesion (or lesions) require a histologic confirmation of PCNSL before any therapy is initiated.

PATHOLOGY

IMMUNOCOMPETENT PATIENTS

Histologically, PCNSL grows in sheets of cells, infiltrating the brain parenchyma between blood vessels in a characteristic vasocentric pattern. Tumor margins are poorly defined and usually extend a substantial distance from the borders of the mass lesion seen on radiographic studies. Neither necrosis nor hemorrhage is a common histologic feature; however, as is true for any large intracerebral mass, necrosis can occasionally be found. In our 792 immunocompetent patients with PCNSL, pathologic examination was available in 539 patients (Table 26–3). When immunophenotyping was performed, almost all PCNSLs were of B-lymphocyte origin. According to the Working Formulation definitions, 50% of the PCNSLs in immunocompetent patients were large cell, with the next most common histologic type being immunoblastic (18%) (Fig. 26–2; see

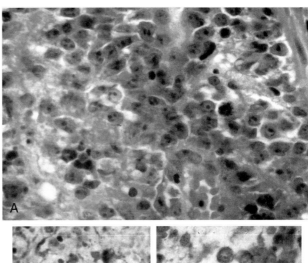

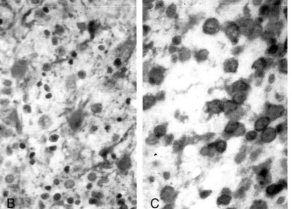

Figure 26–2. Histologic sections of a large cell primary central nervous system lymphoma. *A,* The tumor is characterized by angiocentricity (tendency to aggregate around small blood vessels), as well as clumped, peripherally located nuclear chromatin, and prominent nucleoli (hematoxylin and eosin, ×400). *B,* Glial fibrillary acidic protein (GFAP) immunoperoxidase staining of the tumor. GFAP is a known intermediate filament found exclusively in cells of astrocytic origin. The darkly staining cells with the elongated processes are reactive astrocytes, often found in areas of abnormality within the cerebrum (tumor, infection, ischemia). *C,* Leukocyte common antigen (LCA) immunoperoxidase staining of the tumor. LCA is a protein found on the surface of almost all cells of lymphocytic origin. The darkly staining cells are the tumor cells, proving the lymphocytic nature of this neoplasm. (See also color section.)

Table 26–3. Method of Tissue Diagnosis and Histologic Type

	Immunocompetent	AIDS
Positive cerebrospinal fluid cytologic tests	79/255 (31%)	3/13 (23%)
Surgery		
Biopsy (only)	170 (38%)	78 (70%)
Resection	277 (62%)	33 (30%)
Histologic type		
Large cell	268 (50%)	61 (37%)
Immunoblastic	96 (18%)	57 (35%)
Centroblastic	38 (7%)	—
Lymphoblastic	37 (7%)	—
Lymphocytic	23 (4%)	1
Small noncleaved	21 (4%)	42 (25%)
Small cleaved	20 (4%)	—
Mixed	19 (4%)	3 (2%)
Not otherwise specified	17 (3%)	0
Total	**539 patients** (68% of all patients)	**164 patients** (52% of all patients)

AIDS, acquired immunodeficiency syndrome.

also color section). There was an equal distribution of other histologic types. T-cell lymphomas are relatively rare and tend to present with leptomeningeal disease. Although there is a suggestion that the incidence of T-cell PCNSL is rising, many believe this is an artifact owing to the increasing use of newer immunohistochemical stains that might be detecting reactive T lymphocytes. This is an important point since for unclear reasons many PCNSLs are associated with a reactive lymphocytosis.

IMMUNOCOMPROMISED PATIENTS

There does appear to be a difference between the frequency of specific histologic subtypes in AIDS-associated PCNSL and that in immunocompetent patients. In our review of 315 AIDS patients, pathologic examination was available in 164 patients. Sixty percent of the AIDS patients had a high-grade histologic type (compared with 22% of immunocompetent patients), with large cell (37%), immunoblastic (35%), and small noncleaved (25%) the three most predominate subtypes. When reported, almost all AIDS-associated PCNSLs contained EBV genomic DNA, a finding quite rare in immunocompetent patients.

TREATMENT

IMMUNOCOMPETENT PATIENTS
Radiation Therapy

The literature is replete with anecdotal experiences with either surgery, radiation therapy, chemotherapy, or some combination of these. As discussed in the previous section on diagnosis, the only role of surgery in this disease is to establish a diagnosis and to offer ventricular shunting in the rare case of persistent hydrocephalus. Unlike the situation in patients with malignant gliomas, the extent of surgery has little role in prolonging survival or improving the quality of life for patients with PCNSL. The reasons for this are related to the diffuse infiltrative and multifocal nature of PCNSL and the effectiveness of corticosteroids, radiation therapy, and chemotherapy.

Postoperative whole-brain radiation therapy has been the conventional therapy for patients with PCNSL, with median survivals of 8 to 18 months in most series. A review of 308 patients with PCNSL treated with radiation therapy and corticosteroids alone reported only 21 survivors at 5 years.[57]

Early studies documented improved survival of patients with PCNSL treated with surgery and radiation therapy compared with surgery alone. Henry and colleagues reported a median survival of 4.6 months after surgical excision alone and 15.2 months after surgery and radiation therapy.[115] It was also noted that most patients improved neurologically during the first few weeks of therapy, and complete responses were seen in most patients at the completion of radiation therapy. Uncontrolled, retrospective studies suggested that a dose-response relationship existed for PCNSL. This was first reported in 1967 by Sagerman and associates, who noted near-100% treatment failures at doses below 30 Gy but observed some prolonged survivors at higher doses.[116] Later studies confirmed that the only 2-year survivors were patients treated with doses of whole-brain radiation at or above 45 Gy. Murray and colleagues' analysis of 198 patients included 54 patients who received 50 Gy or greater, with the remainder receiving lower doses.[46] Actuarial survival (life table) at 5 years was 42.3% for patients treated with greater than 50 Gy compared with 12.8% for those receiving lower doses ($P<.05$).

Some authors have suggested the use of craniospinal radiation in the initial treatment of patients with PCNSL. This recommendation was based on the relatively high incidence of leptomeningeal dissemination at the time of relapse. There are no convincing data, however, that craniospinal radiation therapy is superior to whole-brain therapy in prolonging disease-free survival. This is because in most patients whose disease recurs in the leptomeninges, it also recurs in the brain at the site of original presentation. Furthermore, craniospinal radiation fields significantly affect large amounts of bone marrow in the vertebral bodies and the pelvis. This can make subsequent administration of systemic chemotherapy more difficult secondary to diminished bone marrow reserve. Therefore, we do not recommend the routine use of spinal axis radiation therapy except in the rare cases of PCNSL presenting as an intramedullary mass.

In the absence of a prospective randomized study, the Radiation Therapy Oncology Group (RTOG) evaluated a high-dose regimen of radiation therapy in a single-arm prospective study conducted from 1983 to 1987.[117] Forty-one immunocompetent patients received 40 Gy to the whole brain and meninges followed by a boost of 20 Gy to the original enhancing tumor volume and a 2-cm margin in all directions. The median survival for the entire group was 11.6 months, with 48% of the patients alive at 1 year and 28% at 2 years. A univariate analysis showed improved survival for patients with a better preradiation Karnofsky performance status (KPS), a lower age, and male sex. Patients with a KPS of 70% or greater survived 21.1 months (median) compared with 5.6 months (median) for KPS of less than 70 ($P = .001$). Below the age of 60 years, patients survived a median of 23.1 months compared with 7.6 months for older patients ($P = .001$). A multivariate analysis using the Cox regression model indicated that KPS was the most significant prognostic variable ($P<.01$). Survival according to sex was also statistically significant ($P<.01$), with the median survival for men 19.8 months compared with 6.8 months for women. Although the Cox regression analysis indicated that sex was the second most important prognostic factor, closer inspection showed that the women were older and tended to have a worse KPS. Therefore, the selection of sex in the model may have masked the true prognostic significance of age. In fact, when the investigators excluded sex from the regression model, age became significant ($P<.05$). The actuarial survival curves from all subsets showed a continuous downward force of mortality, suggesting that radiation therapy alone was not a curative therapy for patients with PCNSL. Based on these disappointing results, the RTOG concluded that further studies should include some form of chemotherapy.

Careful analysis of patterns of failure after radiation therapy can provide direction for future therapy. Although initial clinical and radiographic responses to radiation therapy are gratifying, failure to achieve durable local control remains the major therapeutic challenge in the treatment of PCNSL. In the recent RTOG study discussed previously, in only 3 of 41 patients did therapy fail outside the nervous system, and in 1 patient it failed in the eye. Overall, therapy failed in 92% of patients within the radiation therapy volume, 83% suffered only local relapse, and 9% had both local and distant failure. Most "in-field" failures, however, were outside the original site of disease. Loeffler and associates reviewed the patterns of failure of 254 patients in the literature and found documentation of sites of failure in 204.[57] Relapse within the radiation therapy volume occurred in 78% of patients, with only 8% failing outside the CNS.

Since most patients with relapsed PCNSL have received prior high doses of radiation therapy, further conventional radiation therapy cannot be safely administered. However, there is a growing interest in the use of stereotactic radiosurgery for small, focally recurrent PCNSL. Radiosurgery is the delivery of a single dose of highly accurate and precise small-field irradiation using stereotactically directed, highly collimated, narrow beams of radiation. Since 1988, we have treated 11 PCNSL lesions in 7 patients. Eight of the 11 lesions completely responded to radiosurgery by 6 months. However, in all patients the therapy subsequently failed in new cranial or spinal sites. The median survival from radiosurgery was 9 months. This single-day outpatient procedure is an excellent source of palliation for relapsed PCNSL, but because of the highly infiltrative nature of this disease, it should not be considered as a potentially curative therapy.

In summary, even with the use of the highest tolerable doses (60 Gy) of radiation therapy, prolonged disease-free survival is rare when radiation is used alone. Ultimately, in the vast majority of patients the disease will recur within the radiation therapy volume (whole brain). Why is PCNSL so resistant to radiation therapy when histologically identical local (stage I, IE) extraneural lymphomas are readily curable? Some have suggested that the microenvironment of the brain alters the radiosensitivity of PCNSL, and others have argued that PCNSL is truly a systemic disease and that CNS "reseeding" occurs, thus preventing any local therapy from being effective. Whatever the explanation, the growing data suggest that surgery and radiation therapy alone are not sufficient to eradicate PCNSL.

Chemotherapy

With both the recognition that radiation therapy alone is not curative of PCNSL and the successful use of chemotherapy in systemic lymphomas, there has come a growing interest in systemic therapy to treat patients with PCNSL. Along with all the difficulties of drug therapy for systemic lymphomas, PCNSL presents several unique challenges to the effective use of chemotherapy. Probably the largest challenge is problematic drug delivery secondary to variable penetration of different chemotherapeutic agents into the brain parenchyma. The limiting factor here is the unique microarchitecture of the cerebral vasculature, the BBB. What makes the BBB unique compared with other vascular beds is the presence of tight junctions between cells rather than the usual fenestrations found between endothelial cells in most other parts of the body.[23] This effectively eliminates any passive diffusion of large water-soluble molecules from the blood to the CNS.[24] In addition, endothelial cells that make up the BBB tend to have few cytoplasmic vacuoles, thus limiting the transfer of material into the CNS through passive endocytosis. Finally, it has been shown that endothelial cells that constitute the BBB have an extraordinary number of mitochondria, suggesting that these cells are quite metabolically active. It has been suggested that this metabolic activity is geared toward keeping potentially toxic substances out of the CNS. Consistent with this hypothesis is the observation that cerebral endothelium expresses high levels of the multidrug-resistant (MDR) p-glycoprotein.[118] Thus, the cerebral endothelium is an effective barrier to the entry of many potentially toxic substances, including chemotherapy.

Despite the limitations of variable drug penetration through the BBB, it has been known for more than a decade that a number of chemotherapeutic agents are capable of inducing responses in patients with recurrent PCNSL (Figs. 26–3 and 26–4). This is because some lipid-soluble and/or very small-molecular-weight drugs are capable of penetrating the BBB. These include drugs such as the nitrosoureas, methotrexate, cytarabine, procarbazine, and 5-flurouracil. More interesting, however, is the observation that some drugs, such as cyclophosphamide and vincristine, are neither small nor lipid-soluble but still have activity against PCNSL. This probably relates to the fact that in areas of significant tumor burden, the BBB is variably disrupted, thus allowing access to certain drugs not normally capable of crossing an intact BBB. There are two important points, however, about this breakdown of the BBB by PCNSL. First, the disruption is not absolute, but rather variable, and thus even in the middle of a large tumor, drug delivery is unlikely to be as effective as it would be to a systemic tumor. Furthermore, since some components of the BBB still exist, certain very large, polar molecules (like the anthracyclines) are probably still excluded from the CNS. The second important aspect about the disrupted BBB is that it can be repaired after effective tumor treatment. PET scan data have demonstrated that a water-soluble drug like cyclophosphamide, which normally has only minimal BBB penetration, passes into a PCNSL very well when used before other treatments. As the tumor regresses, however, the BBB repairs itself,

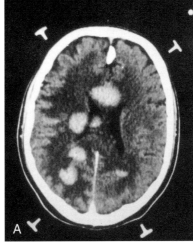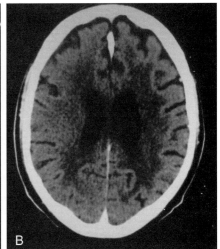

Figure 26–3. *A,* Before therapy. This CT scan is quite suggestive of the diagnosis of primary central nervous system lymphoma because of the brightly enhancing, multifocal, periventricular appearance of these lesions, with less mass effect than might otherwise be expected from other primary brain tumors or metastases. *B,* After chemotherapy. This CT scan of the same patient, obtained after just three cycles of systemic chemotherapy (cyclophosphamide, vincristine, and high-dose methotrexate), demonstrates a complete radiographic response. Of note, the patient no longer required glucocorticoids to control cerebral edema and was neurologically asymptomatic at the time of this scan.

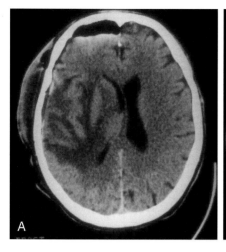 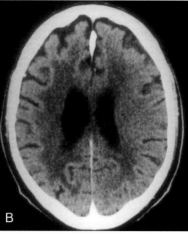

Figure 26–4. *A,* Before therapy. This CT scan reveals a large, heterogeneous mass with a significant amount of edema and mass effect. The radiographic characteristics are most suggestive of a high-grade astrocytoma, although the biopsy revealed a large cell lymphoma. The patient had significant cognitive and behavioral changes at this point and was hemiparetic. *B,* After chemotherapy. This CT scan of the same patient, obtained after just three cycles of systemic chemotherapy (cyclophosphamide, vincristine, and high-dose methotrexate), demonstrates a complete radiographic response. The patient no longer required glucocorticoids after the second cycle of chemotherapy, and he regained full neurologic function.

making subsequent delivery of cyclophosphamide much less efficient. This is a very important consideration when designing treatment strategies.

The other unique challenge to the use of chemotherapy in the treatment of PCNSL is the potential for serious neurotoxicity. Historical data from the experience with childhood leukemia suggests that methotrexate (possibly the most active agent for PCNSL) is synergistic with cranial radiation for predisposing to long-term neurotoxicity, particulary leukoencephalopathy. It has been suggested that the timing of drug administration relative to cranial radiation is an important factor for the likelihood that the patient will develop this treatment complication. In general it appears that chemotherapy given before cranial radiation is safer than chemotherapy given after radiation. This appears to be the case from the childhood leukemia experience with methotrexate, and data from Children's Hospital of Boston indicate that children treated with cisplatin before radiation have less sensorineural hearing loss than children treated in the reverse order.[119, 120] Thus, for reasons of both improved drug delivery and decreased chances of neurotoxicity, preradiation chemotherapy is probably the optimal way to incorporate drugs into the initial treatment regimen of PCNSL.

The first series of patients treated prospectively with preradiation chemotherapy was reported by Gabbai and coworkers, who used methotrexate 3.5 g/m², followed by leucovorin rescue, for three cycles before cranial radiation (Table 26–4).[121] Of the 13 initially reported patients, there were 9 complete and 4 partial responses to the chemotherapy alone. With longer followup and an additional 9 patients, the current median survival is more than 27 months. Neuwelt and associates reported the results of a technically difficult protocol whereby patients were treated with the combination of cyclophosphamide 15 to 30 mg/kg intravenously and methotrexate 1.5 g given by intracarotid injection along with mannitol-induced hyperosmotic BBB disruption.[62] In addition, patients were treated with procarbazine 100 to 150 mg/day and dexamethasone (Decadron) 24 mg/day for a total of 14 days. Patients were treated with 5000 cGy whole-brain radiation only at the time of tumor progression. With this regimen, 13 of 16 patients experienced a complete response to chemotherapy. Eventually 6 of the 13 patients relapsed and required radiation therapy. The median survival of the group as a whole was 44.5 months. Treatment was associated with a moderate degree of acute neurologic toxicity, although the authors claim that long-term neurologic toxicity was minimal. A major unresolved question is the need for BBB disruption. Clearly, methotrexate can cross an intact BBB, and some animal data suggest that BBB disruption increases the entry of the drug into normal brain to a much greater extent than into the area of the brain involved by tumor. Thus it is possible that BBB disruption, with its associated risks and difficulties, may not

Table 26–4. Results of Three Preradiation Chemotherapy Trials

Study	No. of Patients	Median Age (yr)	Chemotherapy	Response	Radiation (cGy)	Median Survival (mo)
Gabbai et al[121]	13	62	Methotrexate (3.5 g/m² × 3)	Complete response: 9/13 (69%) Partial response: 4/13 (31%)	3000 (12/13 patients)	9+ (27+)*
Neuwelt et al[62]	16	53.7	Blood-brain barrier disruption; cyclophosphamide/methotrexate + procarbazine	Complete response: 13/16 (81%) Partial response: 3/16 (19%)	5000 (9/16 patients)	44.5
DeAngelis[21]	31	58	Methotrexate (IV + via Ommaya shunt) + cytarabine	Complete response: 0 Partial response: 17/22 (77%) Stable disease: 5/22	4000 + 1440 boost	42.5

*Nine patients added to the original report with longer followup.

be necessary if the proper drugs are administered correctly. Certainly, one important point demonstrated by the study of Neuwelt and colleagues is the fact that when effective chemotherapy is administered to patients with PCNSL, it may be possible to withhold radiation therapy.

In another prospective series of PCNSL patients, DeAngelis treated 22 newly diagnosed patients with two doses of intravenous methotrexate (1 g/m^2) along with six doses of intrathecal methotrexate (12 mg).[21] After radiation therapy given as 4000 cGy to the whole brain plus a 1440-cGy boost to the tumor, patients were treated with high-dose cytarabine. With this regimen, 17 of 22 patients experienced partial responses to the chemotherapy. The median survival was 42.5 months. It is of interest that DeAngelis observed no complete responses, in contrast to the findings of Gabbai and colleagues. It is likely that the significantly lower doses of methotrexate in the regimen of DeAngelis (a total of 2 versus 10.5 g/m^2 in the study of Gabbai and colleagues) at least partially accounted for this difference. Observing these patients for long-term neurotoxicity will be important given that they were treated with both intravenous and intrathecal methotrexate and cytarabine (the latter a known neurotoxic agent) in combination with cranial irradiation.

The RTOG has recently completed a less encouraging study (protocol 88-06) in which 51 patients were treated with preradiation chemotherapy consisting of cyclophosphamide, doxorubicin, vincristine, and dexamethasone followed by 41.4-Gy whole-brain radiation with an 18-Gy boost to the tumor.[122] Overall the median survival was a disappointing 12.8 months. When patients were separated by age, it was found that those older than 60 years of age had much poorer outcomes than those younger than 60 years (2-year survival 30% versus 62%, respectively). In fact, the survival of patients younger than 60 years of age treated on this protocol was statistically superior to that of a similar group of patients treated on RTOG protocol 83-15, which used the same radiation therapy but no chemotherapy. This trial can be criticized for the choice of the chemotherapy regimen, for although CHOP (cyclophosphamide, hydroxydaunomycin, Oncovin, prednisone) chemotherapy is clearly an effective regimen for systemic high-grade lymphomas, it does not have an optimal pharmacokinetic profile for the treatment of PCNSL. In particular, the use of doxorubicin must be considered suspect given that the anthracyclines are large water-soluble, polar molecules that probably do not penetrate even a disrupted BBB. The toxicity of the regimen is increased and the dose intensity of the effective drugs (i.e., cyclophosphamide) are diminished by the addition of the anthracycline with its associated additional myelosuppression.

In conclusion, growing data suggest that preradiation chemotherapy may improve the outcome of some immunocompetent patients with PCNSL. Many questions still remain, however, including identification of the specific patient population that benefits from chemotherapy, the correct regimen, the need for intrathecal drug administration, and the optimal radiation therapy dose, fractionation, and volume. Indeed, with optimization of the chemotherapy regimen, it remains to be seen whether some patients can be spared cranial radiation altogether, thus lessening the chances of long-term neurotoxicity.

IMMUNOCOMPROMISED PATIENTS

Unfortunately, the recent advances made in the treatment of PCNSL in immunocompetent patients have not carried over to immunosuppressed patients. In our retrospective review of all cases of PCNSL, the overall survival of AIDS patients was significantly lower than that seen in immunocompetent patients regardless of treatment (2.6 versus 18.8 months, respectively) (Table 26–5). Even when matched for similar treatment approaches, such as radiation therapy alone, survival was much worse in the AIDS population (3 versus 16.6 months). There are several possible explanations for this difference, including the fact that AIDS patients may have intrinsically more radioresistant tumors as reflected by the fact that complete response rates are lower in the AIDS patients than in immunocompetent patients. Certainly, the differences in the biology of these tumors (i.e., EBV-positive, high-grade morphology) are consistent with a possible difference in sensitivity to cytotoxic stimuli. Another possible explanation for decreased responsiveness to radiation therapy and lower overall survival may be the tendency for AIDS patients to be treated with lower doses of radiation than their immunocompetent counterparts (12% of immunocompetent patients treated over the last 15 years were treated with less than 35 Gy, whereas nearly 56% of AIDS patients were.[29]

Although factors such as differences in the biology of the tumor and treatment approaches may partially account for differences in the poorer survival of AIDS patients with PCNSL, clearly the most important reason is their underlying HIV disease. Levine[30] was the first to point out that the average CD4 lymphocyte count in AIDS patients who develop PCNSL is less than 50 cells/mm^3. Thus, most of these patients are in the terminal phase of their HIV disease. Baumgartner and colleagues reported autopsy results on 21 AIDS patients with PCNSL.[83] Of 13 patients not treated, all had disease disseminated throughout the CNS, with 10 deaths directly attributable to tumor progression. However, an additional eight patients were treated with radiation, and two of them had residual tumor at autopsy. Only one of these patients died from tumor progression, with the remaining patients dying from opportunistic infections. The survival of both groups of patients was similar regardless of treatment.

Table 26–5. Type of Treatment and Survival

Treatment and Survival	Immunocompetent Group	AIDS Group
Treatment		
None	66 (9.6%)	45 (25.9%)
Radiation	450 (65.8%)	115 (66.1%)
Chemotherapy	168 (24.6%)	14 (8.0%)
Total	**684**°	**174**†
Survival (mo)		
No therapy	2.69	0.93
Radiation	16.61	2.96
Chemotherapy	29.07	No data
Overall average (mo)	**18.85**	**2.61**

°Treatment data available for 86% of all patients.
†Treatment data available for 55% of all patients.
AIDS, acquired immunodeficiency syndrome.

Thus, it does not appear that eradication of PCNSL in the majority of patients with AIDS is likely to significantly prolong survival. Ultimately, prolonging survival in this patient population will require improvements in the treatment of their HIV disease.

The generally poor outcome seen in the AIDS population should not be automatically interpreted to mean that a nihilistic treatment approach is appropriate. On the contrary, there is a subgroup of AIDS patients (10%) who present with PCNSL as their AIDS-defining illness. These patients are generally less advanced in the natural history of their HIV disease and can be expected to have a more prolonged survival than other PCNSL AIDS patients. Certainly this group of patients should be treated with aggressive radiation therapy. The role of chemotherapy in these patients remains unclear. It is also important to note that most AIDS patients with PCNSL can experience significant neurologic palliation by radiation. Thus, for quality-of-life reasons, most AIDS patients should be offered at least an accelerated course of treatment (i.e., 30 Gy over 10 fractions to the whole brain).

CONCLUSION

PCNSL is a disease distinct from other extranodal systemic lymphomas in its biology, clinical presentation, and treatment. Both in immunocompetent patients and in the AIDS population, the incidence of this tumor appears to be dramatically rising. PCNSL in the AIDS and immunocompetent host appears to be a different disease entity with respect to clinical and radiographic presentation, histologic type, and response to treatment. Although radiation therapy has historically been the standard of treatment, early data suggest that the addition of preradiation chemotherapy may significantly improve outcomes in some immunocompetent hosts. The optimal chemotherapy regimen and the actual need for radiation therapy have yet to be determined. Treatment for AIDS patients with PCNSL has not been as successful and is generally considered palliative. Substantial improvement in the prognosis of these patients awaits advances in the treatment of their underlying HIV and opportunistic infections.

REFERENCES

1. Bleyer W, Byrne T: Leptomeningeal cancer in leukemia and solid tumors. Curr Probl Cancer 1988; 12:181.
2. Hanbery JW, Dugger GS: Perithelial sarcoma of the brain. A clinicopathologic study of thirteen cases. Arch Neurol Psychiatry 1964;74:732.
3. Barnett LB, Schwartz E: Cerebral reticulum cell sarcoma after multiple renal transplants. J Neurol Neurosurg Psychiatry 1974; 37:966.
4. Benedek L, Juba A: Uber das Microgliom. Dtsch Z Nervehnheilk 1941; 152:159.
5. Schaumburg HH, Plank CR, Adams RD: The reticulum cell sarcoma-microglioma group of brain tumors. Brain 1972; 95:199.
6. Freeman C, Berg JW, Cutler SJ: Occurrence and prognosis of extranodal lymphomas. Cancer 1972; 29:252.
7. Jellinger K, Radaskiewics TH, Slowik F: Primary malignant lymphomas of the central nervous system in man. Acta Neuropathol (Berl) 1975; 6(suppl):95.
8. Zimmerman HM: Malignant lymphomas of the nervous system. Acta Neuropathol (Berl) 1975; 6(suppl):69.
9. Brand MM, Marinkovich VA: Primary malignant reticulosis of the brain in Wiskott-Aldrich syndrome. Report of a case. Arch Dis Child 196 44:536.
10. Model LM: Primary reticulum cell sarcoma of the brain in Wiskott-Aldrich syndrome. Report of a case. Arch Neurol 1977; 34:633.
11. Littman P, Wang CC: Reticulum cell sarcoma of the brain: A review of the literature and a study of 19 cases. Cancer 1975; 35:1412.
12. DeWeese TL, Hazuka MB, Hommel DJ, et al: AIDS-related non-Hodgkin's lymphoma: The outcome and efficacy of radiation therapy. Int J Radiat Oncol Biol Phys 1991; 20:803.
13. Penn I: Development of cancer as a complication of clinical transplantation. Transplant Proc 1977; 9:1121.
14. Weintraub J, Warnke RA: Lymphoma in cardiac allotransplant recipients. Clinical and histological features and immunologic phenotypes. Transplantation 1982; 33:347.
15. Diette KM, Caro WA, Roenigk HH Jr: Malignant lymphoma presenting with cutaneous granulomas. J Am Acad Dermatol 1984; 10:896.
16. Good AE, Russo HR, Schnitzer B, et al: Intracranial histiocytic lymphoma with rheumatoid arthritis. J Rheumatol 1978; 5:75.
17. Lipsmeyer EA: Development of malignant cerebral lymphoma in a patient with systemic lupus erythematosus treated with immunosuppression. Arthritis Rheum 1972; 15:183.
18. Snider WD, Simpson DM, Nielsen S, et al: Neurological complications of acquired immune deficiency syndrome: Analysis of 50 patients. Ann Neurol 1983; 14:403.
19. Pluda M, Yarchoan R, Jaffe ES, Feuerstein IM, et al: Development of non-Hodgkin lymphoma in a cohort of patients with severe human immunodeficiency virus (HIV) infection on long-term antiretroviral therapy. Ann Intern Med 1990; 113:276.
20. Eby NL, Grufferman S, Flannelly CM, et al: Increasing incidence of primary brain lymphoma in the U.S. Cancer 1988; 62:2461.
21. DeAngelis LM: Primary central nervous system lymphoma. PPO Update 1992; 6:1.
22. Bashir R, Freedman A, Harris N, et al: Immunophenotypic profile of CNS lymphoma: A review of eighteen cases. J Neurooncol 1989; 7:249.
23. Reese TS, Karnovsky MJ: Fine structural localization of a blood-brain barrier to exogenous peroxidase. J Cell Biol 1967; 37:207.
24. Rall DP, Zubrand CG: Mechanisms of drug absorption and excretion: Passage of drugs in and out of the central nervous system. Ann Rev Pharmacol 1962; 2:109.
25. Murphy JB, Sturm E: Conditions determining the transplantability of tissues in the brain. J Exp Med 1923; 38:183.
26. Medawar PB: Immunity to homologous grafted skin. The fate of skin homografts transplanted to the brain, to subcutaneous tissue and to the anterior chamber of the eye. Br J Exp Pathol 1948; 29:58.
27. Greene HSN: Heterotransplantation of tumours. Ann NY Acad Sci 1957; 69:818.
28. Weiner HL, Hauser SL: Neuroimmunology: I. Immunoregulation in neurological disease. Ann Neurol 1982; 11:437.
29. Fine HA, Mayer RJ: Primary central nervous system lymphoma. Ann Intern Med 1993; 119:1093.
30. Levine AM: Acquired immunodeficiency syndrome–related lymphoma. Blood 1992; 80:8.
31. Hochberg FH, Miller G, Schooley RT: Central-nervous-system lymphoma related to Epstein-Barr virus. N Engl J Med 1983; 309:745.
32. Bashir RM, Haris NL, Hochberg FH, Singer, RM: Detection of Epstein-Barr virus in CNS lymphomas by in-situ hybridization. N Engl J Med 1989; 39:813.
33. Ho M, Miller G, Atchison RW, et al: Epstein-Barr virus infections and DNA hybridization studies in posttransplant lymphoma and lymphoproliferative lesions: The role of primary infection. J Infect Dis 1985; 152:876.
34. Ho M, Jaffe R, Miller G, et al: The frequency of Epstein-Barr virus infection and associative lymphoproliferative syndrome after transplantation and its manifestations in children. Transplantion 1988; 45:719.
35. Magrath I: Clinical and pathological features of Burkitt's lymphoma and their relevance to treatment. *In* Levine PH, Ablash DV, Pearson GR, et al (eds): Epstein-Barr and Associated Diseases. Boston, Martinus Nijhoff, 1985, pp 631–643.
36. Klein G: Lymphoma development in mice and human: Diversity of inhibition is followed by convergent cytogenetic evaluation. Proc Natl Acad Sci USA 1979; 76:2442.

37. Hochberg FH, Miller DC: Primary central nervous system lymphoma. J Neurosurg 1988; 68:835.

38. O'Neil BP, Illig JJ: Primary central nervous system lymphoma. Mayo Clin Proc 1989; 64:1005.

39. DeAngelis LM, Yahalom J, Thaler HT, Kher U: Combined modality therapy for primary CNS lymphoma. J Clin Oncol 1992; 10:635.

40. Neuwelt EA, Frenkel EP, Gumerlock MK, et al: Developments in the diagnosis and treatment of primary CNS lymphoma: A prospective series. Cancer 1986; 58:1609.

41. Kawakami Y, Tabuchi K, Ohnishi R, et al: Primary central nervous system lymphoma. J Neurosurg 1985; 62:522.

42. Freeman CR, Shustik C, Brisson ML, et al: I. Primary malignant lymphoma of the central nervous system. Cancer 1986; 58:1106.

43. Mendenhall NP, Thar TL, Agee OF, et al. Primary lymphoma of the central nervous system: Computerized tomography scan characteristics and treatment results for 12 cases. Cancer 1983; 52:1993.

44. Gonzalez DG, Schuster-Uitterhoeve AL: Primary non-Hodgkin's lymphoma of the central nervous system. Cancer 1983; 51:2048.

45. Grant JW, Gallagher PJ, Jones DB: Primary cerebral lymphoma. Arch Pathol Lab Med 1986; 110:897.

46. Murray K, Kun L, Cox J: Primary malignant lymphoma of the central nervous system. J Neurosurg 1986; 65:600.

47. Di Marco A, Rosta L, Campostrini F, et al: The role of radiation therapy in the management of primary non-Hodgkin's lymphomas of the central nervous system: Clinical study of 10 cases. Tumori 1986; 72:565.

48. Hobson DE, Anderson BA, Carr I, et al: Primary lymphoma of the central nervous system: Manitoba experience and literature review. Can J Neurol Sci 1986; 13:55.

49. Bertoncelli C, Zigrossi P, Campanini M, et al: Primary lymphoma of the central nervous system. A clinical and immunohistological study of 8 patients. Haematologica 1987; 72:137.

50. Pollack IF, Lunsford LD, Flickinger JC, Dameshek HL: Prognostic factors in the diagnosis and treatment of primary central nervous system lymphoma. Cancer 1989; 63:939.

51. McLaughlin P, Velasquez WS, Redman JR, et al: Chemotherapy with dexamethasone, high-dose cytarabine, and cisplatin for parenchymal brain lymphomas. J Natl Cancer Inst 1988; 80:1408.

52. Allegranza A, Mariani C, Giardini R, et al: Primary malignant lymphomas of the central nervous system: A histological and immunohistological study of 12 cases. Histopathology 1984; 8:781.

53. Stewart DJ, Russell N, Atack EA, et al: Cyclophosphamide, doxorubicin, vincristine, and dexamethasone in primary lymphoma of the brain: A case report. Cancer Treat Rep 1983; 67:287.

54. Cohen IJ, Vogel R, Matz S, et al: Successful non-neurotoxic therapy [without radiation] of a multifocal primary brain lymphoma with a methotrexate, vincristine, and BCNU protocol [DEMOB]. Cancer 1986; 57:6.

55. Vakili ST, Muller J, Shidnia, H, Campbell, RL: Primary lymphoma of the central nervous system: A clinico-pathologic analysis of 26 cases. J Surg Oncol 1986; 33:95.

56. Schiffer D, Chio A, Giordana MT, et al: Primary lymphomas of the brain: A clinicopathologic review of 37 cases. Tumori 1987; 73:585.

57. Loeffler JS, Ervin TJ, Mauch P, et al: Primary lymphomas of the central nervous system: Patterns of failure and factors that influence survival. J Clin Oncol 1985; 3:490.

58. Yasunaga T, Takahashi M, Uozumi H, et al: Radiation therapy of primary malignant lymphoma of the brain. Acta Radiol Oncol 1986; 25:23.

59. Woodman R, Shin, K, Pineo G: Primary non-Hodgkin's lymphoma of the brain. Medicine (Baltimore) 1985; 64:425.

60. Michalski JM, Garcia DM, Kase E, et al: Primary central nervous system lymphoma: Analysis of prognostic variables and patterns of treatment failure. Radiology 1990; 176:855.

61. Pittman K, Olweny CL, North JB, Blumbergs, PC: Primary central nervous system lymphoma. Oncology 1991; 48:184.

62. Neuwelt EA, Goldman DL, Dahlborg SA, et al: Primary CNS lymphoma treated with osmotic blood brain barrier disruption: Prolonged survival and presentation of cognitive function. J Clin Oncol 1991; 9:1580.

63. Rampen FH, van Andel JG, Sizoo W, van Unnik AM: Radiation therapy in primary non-Hodgkin's lymphomas of the CSN. Eur J Cancer 1980; 16:177.

64. Berry MP, Simpson, WJ: Radiation therapy in the management of primary malignant lymphoma of the brain. Int J Radiat Oncol Biol Phys 1981; 7:55.

65. Spilane JA, Kendall BE, Moseley, IF: Cerebral lymphoma: Clinical radiological correlation. J Neurol Neurosurg Psychiatry 1982; 45:199.

66. Merkel KH, Hansmann ML: Primary non-Hodgkin's lymphomas of the central nervous system. Pathol Res Pract 1986; 181:430.

67. Watanabe M, Tanaka R, Takeda N, et al: Correlation of computed tomography with the histopathology of the primary malignant lymphoma of the brain. Neuroradiology 1992; 34:36.

68. Bogdahn U, Bogdahn S, Mertens HG, et al: Primary non-Hodgkin's lymphomas of the CNS. Acta Neurol Scand 1986; 73:602.

69. Sagerman RH, Collier CH, King GA: Radiation therapy of microgliomas. Radiology 1983; 149:567.

70. Helle TL, Britt RH, Colby TV: Primary lymphoma of the central nervous system. Clinicopathological study of experience at Stanford. J Neurosurg 1984; 60:94.

71. Frank G, Ferracini R, Spagnolli F, et al: Primary intracranial lymphomas. Surg Neurol 1985; 23:3.

72. Spaun E, Midholm S, Pederson NT, Ringsted J: Primary malignant lymphoma of the central nervous system. Surg Neurol 1985; 24:646.

73. Remick SC, Diamond C, Migliozzi JA, et al: Primary central nervous system lymphoma in patients with and without the acquired immune deficiency syndrome. Medicine (Baltimore) 1990; 69:345.

74. Casadei GP, Gambacorta M: A clinicopathological study of seven cases of primary high-grade malignant non-Hodgkin's lymphoma of the central nervous system. Tumori 1985; 71:501.

75. So YT, Beckstead JH, Davis RL: Primary central nervous system lymphoma in acquired immune deficiency syndrome: A clinical and pathological study. Ann Neurol 1986; 20:566.

76. Poon T, Matoso I, Tchertkoff V, et al: CT features of primary cerebral lymphoma in AIDS and non-AIDS patients. J Comput Assist Tomogr 1989; 13:6.

77. Formenti SC, Gill PS, Lean E, et al: Primary central nervous system lymphoma in AIDS. Cancer 1989; 63:1101.

78. Loureiro C, Gill PS, Meyer PR, et al: Autopsy findings in AIDS-related lymphoma. Cancer 1988; 62:735.

79. Levine AM, Sullivan-Halley J, Pike MC, et al: Human immunodeficiency virus–related lymphoma. Cancer 1991; 68:2466.

80. MacMahon EM, Glass JD, Hayward SD, et al: Epstein-Barr virus in AIDS-related primary central nervous system lymphoma. Lancet 1991; 338:969.

81. Goldstein JD, Zeifer B, Chao C, et al: CT appearance of primary CNS lymphoma in patients with acquired immunodeficiency syndrome. J Comput Assist Tomogr 1991; 15:39.

82. Dina TS: Primary central nervous system lymphoma versus toxoplasmosis in AIDS. Radiology 1991; 179:823.

83. Baumgartner JE, Rachlin JR, Beckstead JH, et al: Primary central nervous system lymphomas: Natural history and response to radiation therapy in 55 patients with acquired immune deficiency syndrome. Cancer 1990; 67:2756.

84. Chappell ET, Guthrie BL, Orenstein J: The role of stereotactic biopsy in the management of HIV-related focal brain lesions. Neurosurgery 1992; 30:825.

85. Goldstein JD, Dickson DW, Moser FG, et al: Primary central nervous system lymphoma in acquired immune deficiency syndrome. Cancer 1991; 67:2756.

86. Ziegler JL, Beckstead JA, Volberding PA, et al: Non-Hodgkin's lymphoma in 90 homosexual men. N Engl J Med 1984; 311:565.

87. DiCarlo EF, Amberson JB, Metroka CE, et al: Malignant lymphomas and the acquired immunodeficiency syndrome. Arch Pathol Lab Med 110:1986.

88. Nakleh RE, Manivel JC, Hurd D, Sung JH: Central nervous system lymphomas. Arch Pathol Lab Med 1989; 113:1050.

89. Pitlick SD, Fainstein V, Bolivar R, et al: Spectrum of central nervous system complications in homosexual men with acquired immune deficiency syndrome [Letter]. J Infect Dis 1983; 148:771.

90. Italian, CG f. A.-R. T. Malignant lymphomas in patients with or at risk for AIDS in Italy. J Natl Cancer Inst 1988; 80:855.

91. McArthur JC: Neurologic manifestations of AIDS. Medicine (Baltimore) 1987; 66:407.

92. Capanna AH, LaMancusa JJ, Erculei F, et al: Primary cerebral lymphoma in two consortial partners afflicted with acquired immune deficiency syndrome. Neurosurgery 1987; 21:920.

93. Mernick MH, Malamud SC, Haubenstock A, et al: Non-Hodgkin's lymphoma in AIDS: Report of 11 cases and literature review. Mt Sinai J Med 1986; 53:664.

94. Snow RB, Lavyne MH: Intracranial space-occupying lesions in acquired immune deficiency syndrome patients. Neurosurgery 1985; 16:148.

95. Koppel BS, Wormser GP, Tuchman AJ, et al: Central nervous system involvement in patients with acquired immune deficiency syndrome (AIDS). Acta Neurol Scand 1985; 71:337.

96. Gill PS, Levine AM, Meyer PR, et al: Primary central nervous system lymphoma in homosexual men. Clinical, immunologic, and pathologic features. Am J Med 1985; 78:742.

97. Anders KH, Latta H, Chang BS, et al: Lymphomatoid granulomatosis and malignant lymphoma of the central nervous system in the acquired immunodeficiency syndrome. Hum Pathol 1989; 20:326.

98. Kaplan MH, Susin B, Pahwa G, et al: Neoplastic complications of HTLV-III infection. Am J Med 82:1987.

99. Kalter SP, Riggs SA, Cabanillas F, et al: Aggressive non-Hodgkin's lymphoma in immunocompromised homosexual males. Blood 1985; 66:655.

100. Lowenthal DA, Straus DJ, Campbell SW, et al: AIDS-related lymphoid neoplasia: The Memorial Hospital experience. Cancer 1988; 61:2325.

101. Ahmed T, Wormser GP, Stahl RE, et al: Malignant lymphomas in a population at risk for acquired immune deficiency syndrome. Cancer 1987; 60:719.

102. Knowles DM, Chamulak GA, Subar M, et al: Lymphoid neoplasia associated with the acquired immunodeficiency syndrome (AIDS). Ann Intern Med 1988; 108:744.

103. Kaplan LD, Abrams DI, Feiget AL, et al: AIDS-associated non-Hodgkin's lymphoma in San Francisco. JAMA 1989; 261:719.

104. Song SK, Schwartz IS, Breakstone BA: Lymphoproliferative disorder of the central nervous system in AIDS. Mt Sinai J Med 1986; 53:686.

105. Gabuzda DH, Hirsch MS: Neurologic manifestations of infection with human immunodeficiency virus. Clinical features and pathogenesis. Ann Intern Med 1987; 107:383.

106. Appen RE: Posterior uveitis and primary cerebral reticulum cell sarcoma. Arch Ophthalmol 93:123, 1975.

107. Char DH, Ljung B-M, Miller T, et al: Primary intraocular lymphoma (ocular reticulum cell sarcoma) diagnosis and management. Ophthalmology 95:625, 1988.

108. Rockwood EJ, Zakov ZN, Bay JW: Combined malignant lymphoma of the eye and CNS (reticulum-cell sarcoma). J Neurosurg 61:369, 1984.

109. Duggan DB, Ehrlich GD, Davey FP, et al: HTLV-I-induced lymphoma mimicking Hodgkin's disease: Diagnosis by polymerase chain reaction amplification of specific HTLV-1 sequences in tumor DNA. Blood 1988; 71:1027.

110. Ezrin-Waters C, Klein M, Deck J, Lang AE: Diagnostic importance of immunological markers in lymphoma involving the central nervous system. Ann Neurol 1984; 16:668.

111. Jones GR, Mason WH, Fishman LS, DeClerek YA: Primary central nervous system lymphoma without intracranial mass in a child. Diagnosis by documentation of monoclonality. Cancer 1985; 56:2804.

112. Anders KH, Guerra WF, Tomiyasu U, et al: The neuropathology of AIDS. Am J Pathol 1986; 124:537.

113. Luft BJ, Hafner R, Korzun AH, et al: Toxoplasmic encephalitis in patients with the acquired immunodeficiency syndrome: Members of the ACTG 077p/ANRS 009 Study Team. N Engl J Med 1993; 329:995.

114. Hoffman JM, Waskin HA, Schifter T, et al: FDG-PET in determining lymphoma from nonmalignant central nervous system lesions in patients with AIDS. J Nucl Med 1993; 34:567.

115. Henry JM, Heffner RRJ, Dillard SH, et al: Primary malignant lymphomas of the central nervous system. Cancer 1974; 34:1293.

116. Sagerman RH, Cassady JR, Chang CH: Radiation therapy for intracranial lymphoma. Radiology 1967; 88:552.

117. Nelson DF, Martz KL, Bonner H, et al: Non-Hodgkin's lymphoma of the brain: Can high dose, large volume radiation therapy improve survival? Report on a prospective trial by the Radiation Therapy Oncology Group (RTOG): RTOG 83-15. Int J Radiat Oncol Biol Phys 1992; 23:9.

118. Tatsuta T, Naito M, Oh HT, et al: Functional involvement of P-glycoprotein in blood-brain barrier. J Biol Chem 1992; 267:20383.

119. Shapiro WR, Young DF: Neurologic complications of antineoplastic therapy. Acta Neurol Scand 1984; 70:125.

120. Kretschmar CS, Warren MP, Levally BL, et al: Ototoxicity of pre-radiation cisplatin for children with central nervous system tumors. J Clin Oncol 1990; 8:1191.

121. Gabbai AA, Hochberg FH, Linggood RM, et al: High-dose methotrexate for non-AIDS primary central system lymphoma. J Neurosurg 1989; 70:190.

122. Schultz C, Scott CTW, Fisher B, et al: Pre-irradiation chemotherapy (CTX) with cytoxan, Adriamycin, vincristine, and Decadron (CHOD) for primary central nervous system lymphoma (PCNSL): Initial report of Radiation Therapy Oncology Group (RTOG) protocol 88-06. Proc ASCO 485:174, 1994.

Twenty-Seven

——Mycosis Fungoides and Other —— Cutaneous Lymphomas

Richard T. Hoppe

The cutaneous lymphomas are a group of lymphomas that involve primarily the skin and affect other sites only secondarily. They include mycosis fungoides and Sézary syndrome, as well as other T-cell or B-cell non-Hodgkin's lymphomas. The major part of this chapter deals with mycosis fungoides and Sézary syndrome. The final section deals with the other cutaneous lymphomas.

MYCOSIS FUNGOIDES AND SÉZARY SYNDROME

Mycosis fungoides is a cutaneous lymphoma that was first described by the French dermatologist Alibert in 1806. The name was intended to describe the characteristic mushroom-like appearance of the tumorous lesions, and no relationship to a fungal etiology was implied. Mycosis fungoides may be included in the spectrum of diseases referred to as "cutaneous T-cell lymphomas." This group of diseases also includes Sézary syndrome, which may be considered to be an erythrodermic, leukemic variant of mycosis fungoides.[1]

EPIDEMIOLOGY

Mycosis fungoides is a rare disease, accounting for only 2% to 3% of cases of non-Hodgkin's lymphoma. The estimated annual incidence rate in the United States is 0.29 per 100,000, which is nearly twice that reported in western European nations.[2] The apparent incidence rate may be even higher in areas where dermatologists and pathologists are especially alert to the diagnosis.[3] There are 500 to 600 new cases and 100 to 200 deaths attributable to mycosis fungoides in the United States each year. It commonly affects older adults (median age 55 to 60 years) and the male-to-female ratio is 2:1.

ETIOLOGY

The cause of mycosis fungoides remains unknown. Some retrospective studies have implicated environmental chemical exposure in its etiology,[4] and there have been reports that identify an increased risk for developing the disease among people in the cotton, manufacturing, trolley and bus transportation, or construction industries.[4, 5] Other studies have suggested that the etiology may be related to chronic antigenic stimulation secondary to exposure to chemicals or pesticides.[6] However, a case-controlled study of patients in the western United States failed to reveal any relationship between occupational or recreational exposures to chemicals and the development of mycosis fungoides and refutes the hypothesis that the disease may develop as a result of chronic antigenic stimulation by contact allergens.[7] Another study, based on data from the Surveillance, Epidemiology, and End Results (SEER) program, also failed to confirm a relationship to any of these proposed etiologic factors.[2]

A viral cause for mycosis fungoides has been suggested. In fact, a retrovirus with type C morphology, later named the "human T-cell lymphotrophic virus, type I (HTLV-I)," was first isolated from two lymphoblastoid cell lines and the peripheral blood lymphocytes of a patient with presumed mycosis fungoides.[8] Actually, the patient had another peripheral T-cell lymphoma involving the skin, which simply resembled mycosis fungoides. The clinical characteristics of HTLV-I–associated T-cell lymphoma are now well described and are quite different from typical mycosis fungoides.[9] Nearly all patients with mycosis fungoides are HTLV-I seronegative. Nevertheless, using polymerase chain reaction techniques, HTLV-I–related DNA sequences have been identified in the peripheral blood mononuclear cells and cutaneous lesions of some patients with mycosis fungoides, despite their seronegativity, lending continued support to a viral etiology for the disease.[10, 11] In addition, HTLV-like particles have been identified in cultures of peripheral blood lymphocytes from a group of 18 patients with mycosis fungoides.[12] However, other studies have failed to demonstrate HTLV-I DNA fragments in either peripheral blood lymphocytes[13] or cutaneous lesions[14] of patients with mycosis fungoides.

Another virus, named HTLV-V, was grown from a continuous cell line derived from the peripheral blood lymphocytes of a patient with documented mycosis fungoides.[15] Closely related DNA sequences to those of the cloned provirus were identified in the cell lines and tumor cells from seven other patients with mycosis fungoides. The existence of this virus has not been confirmed, but it contributes to the suspicion that a viral link exists.

PATHOLOGY

The essential criteria for a diagnosis of mycosis fungoides vary among pathologists, and there may even be disagreement in individual cases among pathologists using the same criteria.[16] Individual pathologists also may disagree with themselves as often as 30% of the time reviewing the same biopsy specimen from a patient with suspected mycosis fungoides.[16]

Based on the severity of the epidermal and dermal involvement, the categories of "diagnostic of," "consistent with," and "suggestive of" mycosis fungoides have been recommended.[1, 17] Treatment programs specific for mycosis fungoides should be considered only in patients who have a biopsy "diagnostic of" or "consistent with," not merely "suggestive of," mycosis fungoides. Recently, some pathologists have required that monoclonal antibody–stained biopsy sections also be consistent with the immunophenotype of mycosis fungoides, before a firm diagnosis is made.

The characteristic histopathology of mycosis fungoides includes an epidermal infiltrate of mononuclear cells that may be present in clusters, called "Pautrier's microabscesses." Although Pautrier's microabscesses are not essential, abnormal cells must be present in the epidermis to make a firm diagnosis of mycosis fungoides. Typically, there is also an upper dermal infiltrate of similar cells, in addition to variable numbers of histiocytes, eosinophils, and plasma cells. The dermal infiltrate usually is intimate with the epidermis, obscuring the dermoepidermal junction, or Grenz zone. The extent of the mononuclear cell infiltrate does not correlate with clinical stage or prognosis.[16]

The density of the dermal infiltrate and extent of involvement of the epidermis may be minimal in skin biopsies from patients with Sézary syndrome, making this diagnosis more difficult to establish. The proximal use of topical corticosteroids, especially in patch stage disease, may ablate the epidermal component of the infiltrate and make a diagnosis more challenging to establish.

Under oil immersion light microscopy, the nuclei of the neoplastic mononuclear cells of mycosis fungoides have a hyperconvoluted surface. Electron microscopic studies demonstrate marked infolding of the nuclear membrane and on three-dimensional reconstruction there is a cerebriform appearance.[18] The degree of nuclear irregularity may be quantitated as a "nuclear contour index," which has proved useful to some in the differential diagnosis between mycosis fungoides and benign dermatoses.[19] Similar criteria may be used to distinguish peripheral blood lymphocytes of Sézary syndrome from reactive lymphocytosis or other leukemias.[20]

Mycosis fungoides was among the first lymphomas to be well characterized immunologically.[21] Functional studies and monoclonal antibody staining demonstrate that most cases are associated with the helper T-cell phenotype (CD4+).[22] Monoclonal antibody staining studies reveal a retention of the CD4 antigen on the cell surface of the mononuclear cells but loss of other mature T-cell antigens such as Leu-8 or Leu-9.[23] The loss of mature T-cell antigens may help in the differential diagnosis of mycosis fungoides.

Rare cases of mycosis fungoides have been demonstrated to be CD8+ (cytotoxic/suppressor T-cell phenotype).

Southern blot analysis has demonstrated monoclonal rearrangements of the T-cell receptors in the skin, lymph nodes, and peripheral blood of patients with mycosis fungoides.[24] These rearrangements are concordant about 80% of the time in multiple lesions from a single patient.[24, 25] Genotyping, the evaluation of skin biopsies to detect T-cell receptor gene rearrangements, is sometimes helpful in the differential diagnosis of early lesions of mycosis fungoides.

The pathology of extracutaneous disease poses special problems. Often, enlarged lymph nodes demonstrate only the changes of dermatopathic lymphadenitis, with paracortical expansion, sinus histiocytosis, an abundance of pigment-laden macrophages, and a small number of atypical lymphocytes with cerebriform nuclei. The potential prognostic relevance of different degrees of infiltration by these abnormal cells led to the development of a "lymph node classification system."[26] In this system, lymph nodes are classified as LN-0 to LN-4 corresponding to lymph node involvement ranging from "no atypical lymphocytes" (LN-0) to "partial or complete replacement of nodal architecture by atypical lymphocytes or frankly neoplastic cells" (LN-4). This descriptive system for grading lymph node involvement has been shown to have prognostic relevance.[27]

The detection of abnormal cells in lymph nodes and other extracutaneous sites may be facilitated by the use of special studies, including T-cell cytology, electron microscopy, cytogenetic studies[28] and Southern blot analysis to detect rearrangements of the T-cell receptor.[29, 30] With these special studies, the likelihood of detecting rearrangements of the T-cell receptor correlates with the lymph node classification system cited earlier and the majority of lymph nodes that show only dermatopathic lymphadenitis on routine evaluation demonstrate neoplastic involvement with these special studies. Although the clinical implication of lymph node involvement that is detectable only at the molecular level is not clear, one study shows a somewhat worse prognosis for patients with LN-3 disease when T-cell antigen receptor gene rearrangements are present,[30] and another shows a significantly worse prognosis for patients with dermatopathic lymphadenitis when β T-cell receptor gene rearrangements are present.[31]

NATURAL HISTORY

Mycosis fungoides often has a long natural history. A "premycotic" phase is characterized by nonspecific, slightly scaling skin lesions and nondiagnostic biopsies. These lesions may wax and wane over a period of years, and a diagnosis of parapsoriasis en plaque is often made. During this phase of disease, patients may respond to treatment with topical corticosteroids. Some experience an evolution of the disease and develop more typical patches or infiltrated plaques with characteristic biopsy changes of mycosis fungoides. It is not uncommon for a history of skin lesions to precede the diagnosis of mycosis fungoides by 5 years or longer.[1] Continued careful followup and repeat biopsies are indicated in patients suspected of having mycosis fungoides.

The typical patches of mycosis fungoides are erythematous and slightly scaling. Many patients present with involvement in the "bathing trunk" distribution, although any part of the body may be involved. Sometimes the sites of disease are curiously symmetric. The palms or soles may be heavily involved, or they may be spared. Scalp involvement may cause alopecia. Pruritus is the most common symptom, even in early phases of disease, and is often the problem that prompts the patient's initial visit to the dermatologist.

More infiltrated lesions are present as palpable plaques that are erythematous, slightly scaling, and have variable shape and well-defined borders. The distribution of lesions may vary substantially among patients.

The evolution of plaques into nodules or ulcerated or exophytic tumors was first described by Alibert. Ulcerated tumors may become infected, and sepsis secondary to infection is the most common immediate cause of death in mycosis fungoides. Generalized dermal thickening from infiltrative disease may cause the classic but highly unusual "leonine facies" of mycosis fungoides.

Some patients may demonstrate only the premycotic or patch phase of skin involvement throughout the course of their disease. However, many others demonstrate progression from patches to plaques and finally to tumorous involvement. The rapidity of this progression is unpredictable. The likelihood of developing clinical evidence of extracutaneous disease correlates with the extent of skin involvement. It is exceedingly rare among patients with limited plaque disease, relatively uncommon among those with generalized plaque (8%), and most likely among patients who develop cutaneous tumors (30%).[1] The development of extracutaneous disease may be accompanied by cytologic transformation, with the appearance of large cells similar to those seen in large cell lymphoma.[32] In this setting, the phenotypic characteristics of the tumor may also change.[33]

Another manifestation of skin involvement in mycosis fungoides is generalized erythroderma, with or without superimposed plaques or tumors. The skin may be either atrophic or lichenified. The erythroderma is accompanied by cold intolerance and intense pruritus. These patients may also have lymphadenopathy and circulating abnormal cells in the peripheral blood. These cells have the same microscopic appearance, immunophenotyping, and genotyping characteristics as the cells that infiltrate the epidermis.[24] Patients with this complex of findings have Sézary syndrome.[34] Although patients with erythroderma usually present in that phase of skin involvement, occasional patients develop erythroderma superimposed over preexisting plaque or tumorous disease.

Although mycosis fungoides may be a systemic disease from the outset, its clinical behavior suggests that progressive skin disease precedes lymph node and visceral involvement. The likelihood of developing symptomatic extracutaneous disease is related to the extent of skin disease. Only 15% to 20% of patients with mycosis fungoides develop clinical problems related to extracutaneous disease during their lifetimes. The first manifestations of extracutaneous disease are often in peripheral nodes, draining the sites of the most extensive skin involvement. Generally, lymph node involvement tends to be peripheral, with central nodal areas such as the mediastinum and paraaortic nodes involved only late in the course of disease.[35] Visceral disease often follows documented lymph node involvement. The involved visceral sites most commonly identified include the lungs, upper aerodigestive tract, central nervous system, spleen, and liver, but virtually any organ may be involved at autopsy.[36]

STAGING

The most useful staging classification system for mycosis fungoides is the Tumor, Node, Metastasis, Blood (TNMB) system first proposed at the Workshop on Mycosis Fungoides held at the National Cancer Institute (NCI) in 1978.[37] Tables 27–1 and 27–2 summarize the TNMB categories and staging classification.

The T stage represents the extent of skin involvement and it correlates closely with survival.[38] The N stage indicates the presence or absence of lymph node involvement. A biopsy specimen of enlarged lymph nodes should always be obtained, since palpable enlargement may be associated only with dermatopathic lymphadenitis, which has only minor prognostic significance.[27, 39] It is only when frank lymph node involvement is detected (LN-3 or LN-4) that the prognosis is substantially worse. The biopsy status of nodes should be designated by the appropriate subscripts.

The M category defines visceral disease. Suspected sites of visceral involvement should be confirmed by biopsy. Other neoplasms, as well as benign diseases, may be confused with mycosis fungoides if a diagnosis is based solely on imaging studies. This is important, since the presence of visceral disease has important prognostic implications. Treatment programs for visceral disease should be considered only if definite proof of extracutaneous disease exists.

The B category signifies the absence or presence of a significant proportion (≥10%) of abnormal cells in the peripheral blood. This is not an independent prognostic

Table 27–1. TNMB Classification for Mycosis Fungoides

Classification	Description
T (skin)	
T1	Limited plaques, papules, or eczematous lesions covering <10% of the skin surface
T2	Generalized plaques, papules, or eczematous lesions covering ≥10% of the skin surface
T3	Tumors
T4	Generalized erythroderma
N (nodes)	
N0	No clinically abnormal peripheral lymph nodes; biopsies (if performed) are negative
N1	Clinically abnormal peripheral lymph nodes
N2	No clinically abnormal peripheral lymph nodes, but biopsy specimens show involvement by mycosis fungoides
N3	Clinically abnormal peripheral lymph nodes; pathologic findings positive for mycosis fungoides
M (viscera)	
M0	No visceral involvement
M1	Visceral involvement (biopsy documented)
B (blood)	
B0	Atypical circulating cells not present in peripheral blood (<5%)
B1	Atypical circulating cells present (≥5%)

TNMB, tumor, node, metastasis, blood.

Table 27–2. Staging Classification for Mycosis Fungoides

	Classification		
Stage	**T**	**N**	**M**
IA	1	0	0
IB	2	0	0
IIA	1–2	1	0
IIB	3	0–1	0
IIIA	4	0	0
IIIB	4	1	0
IVA	1–4	2–3	0
IVB	1–4	0–3	1

See Table 27–1 for abbreviations.

factor but is closely linked with the extent of skin involvement and presence of extracutaneous disease.[27] The B designation does not alter the stage classification.

All patients with mycosis fungoides should undergo at least a limited staging evaluation, including a careful examination of the skin and lymph nodes, complete blood count, Sézary count, screening chemistries, and a chest radiograph. Further staging studies are dictated by the results of those screening evaluations.[1] Any blood or radiographic abnormalities should be evaluated further, as appropriate. If enlarged lymph nodes are detected on physical examination, a biopsy specimen should be obtained. If nodes are involved by mycosis fungoides, then additional staging studies, such as computed tomographic (CT) scans, should be performed to evaluate for the possibility of visceral disease.[1]

However, there is little value in completing radiographic imaging studies beyond a routine chest radiograph, unless indicated by the circumstances cited earlier. Screening CT scans of the chest/abdomen/pelvis, gallium scans, liver-spleen scans, and lymphangiograms are inevitably unrevealing unless there is known lymph node involvement.[40] Historically, series that have examined the usefulness of a staging bone marrow biopsy have concluded that the examination is not worth doing because of the low frequency of marrow involvement.[39] However, one recent analysis identified marrow involvement in 41% of patients, including diffuse lymphomatous infiltrates, and cytologically typical or atypical nodules, some of which included large transformed cells.[41] The likelihood of bone marrow infiltration correlates with the extent of skin involvement and prognosis. The prognosis of patients whose marrow shows cytologically normal lymphoid aggregates is similar to that of patients with an uninvolved marrow.

THERAPY

For the treatment of minor manifestations of mycosis fungoides, topical corticosteroids may achieve good responses and provide short-term palliation. However, complete responses are uncommon, and this treatment does not alter the long-term course of the disease. More definitive treatment of mycosis fungoides may be quite challenging but rewarding because of the good response rates to standard therapies. Only occasional patients are asymptomatic at the time of diagnosis, and the nature of the disease is such that prompt initiation of treatment is almost always indicated.

Control of disease is most likely achieved by treatment directed at the skin, by means of phototherapy, topical chemotherapy, or irradiation. A few patients (10% to 20%) require treatment for systemic involvement.

Phototherapy

Psoralen plus ultraviolet A (PUVA) therapy consists of treatment with 8-methoxypsoralen, an oral photosensitizing drug, followed by controlled exposure to long-wave ultraviolet light (UVA) in a specially designed box.[42] Psoralen intercalates with DNA in the presence of UVA in the 320- to 400-nm range, forming monofunctional and bifunctional adducts with DNA base pairs, which inhibit DNA synthesis. The effective depth of penetration of the UVA is into the epidermis and upper dermis, making it ideally suited for the treatment of mycosis fungoides, especially patch or minimally infiltrated plaque disease.

During the induction (clearing) phase, which may require as long as 6 months, patients are treated two or three times weekly with a dose (in joules) that varies with the patient's skin type, severity of skin reaction, and degree of response.[43] After the clearing phase has been completed, patients continue on a maintenance program with decreased frequency of treatment, as infrequently as once per month. If the disease begins to recur during the maintenance phase, then the intensity of treatment is increased to achieve better control.

The most common acute complications of PUVA therapy include erythema and blistering. These risks are highest among patients with erythroderma, who must be treated with very low exposures to UVA. Patients shield their skin from sunlight with sunscreens and protective clothing for at least 24 hours following psoralen ingestion. Cataract formation and secondary cutaneous malignancies are the most important potential long-term complications of PUVA.[44] To reduce the risk of cataracts, patients wear specially designed ultraviolet goggles while outdoors.

The results of PUVA therapy have been reported from several centers.[43, 45, 46] The clearance rate is about 50% and varies with the initial extent of skin involvement. The response of patients with highly infiltrated plaques or tumors may be accelerated by the addition of localized irradiation. Indications for PUVA treatment include the primary therapy of patients with limited or generalized plaque phase of skin involvement or as a secondary therapy following the failure of other topical modalities. Patients with erythroderma are also suitable candidates for PUVA, provided that very low daily exposures are used to avoid phototoxic reactions.[43] PUVA, combined with systemic therapy such as chlorambucil and prednisone, is one approach to the management of patients with Sézary syndrome.

Home phototherapy is another form of phototherapy.[47] Home phototherapy units with light sources that emit ultraviolet light in the UVA and UVB range (280 to 350 nm) are available for general use. Patients expose themselves to the ultraviolet treatment without using psoralen. Exposures are timed carefully to minimize adverse skin reactions. This treatment approach is most useful in patients who are fair skinned and have minimally infiltrative disease. Some of these patients may remain disease free, even after discontinuation of therapy.

Topical Chemotherapy

Topical nitrogen mustard (HN2) is an effective and convenient treatment for mycosis fungoides. The activity of intravenous HN2 as an alkylating agent for the management of systemic malignancy is well documented. The mechanism of action when HN2 is applied topically for the management of mycosis fungoides is less certain and may not be related simply to its alkylating agent properties.[48] Its activity may be mediated by immune mechanisms or by interaction with the epidermal cell/Langerhans' cell/T-cell axis. There is no detectable systemic absorption of topical HN2, so hematologic monitoring during therapy is unecessary.[49]

The technique of topical HN2 treatment for patients with mycosis fungoides was first developed by Van Scott and Kalmanson.[50] The chemical is mixed in water or in an ointment base (Aquaphor), generally in a concentration of 10 to 20 mg/dL. It is applied at least once daily during the clearing phase.[17, 51] If involvement is particularly limited, local treatment alone may be employed; however, for most patients with more generalized disease, total skin application is recommended. The concentration of the drug and frequency of application may be changed, depending on tolerance and response. It is important to be certain that coverage of involved skin regions is adequate, since certain surfaces, such as the back, neck, and portions of the arms and legs may not be covered adequately when the medication is self-applied.[52] The average time to skin clearance is about 6 months, and subsequent maintenance treatment is continued for at least 6 months.

The most common complication of topical nitrogen mustard is a cutaneous hypersensitivity reaction, which occurs in as many as 30% of patients treated with the aqueous solution and about 5% of patients treated with the ointment base.[17] Hypersensitivity reactions may be overcome by a variety of topical or systemic desensitization programs.[17, 51] The primary long-term hazard of long-term nitrogen mustard use is the potential development of secondary squamous and basal cell cancers.[17, 51] This risk is the greatest among patients who have had long-term sequential therapy with nitrogen mustard, PUVA, and irradiation.[44]

Nearly all patients treated with topical HN2 respond to treatment and complete response rates range from 32% to 61%. The likelihood of a complete response is dependent on the initial extent of skin involvement.[17] Because of its efficacy and ease of application, topical HN2 is employed widely in the management of patients with mycosis fungoides, especially those who have limited or generalized plaque phase of skin involvement, as either primary or secondary therapy.[17, 51, 53] As with PUVA, the response of patients with a limited number of refractory plaques or tumors may be accelerated by the addition of localized irradiation. Although the overall response rate to topical nitrogen mustard is high, only 10% to 15% maintain a long-term continuous complete response after treatment is discontinued.

Another type of topical chemotherapy used occasionally for mycosis fungoides is carmustine (BCNU).[54] Treatment is generally limited to the specific lesions. Clearance rates with BCNU are similar to those with HN2; however, the toxicity may be greater, with cutaneous telangiectasia observed quite commonly after its use. In addition, there is systemic absorption of topical BCNU, requiring hematologic monitoring and limiting the duration of therapy.

Radiation Therapy

Mycosis fungoides is an exquisitely radiosensitive neoplasm and ionizing irradiation is the most effective single agent in the treatment of the disease. Irradiation may be exploited in several ways. Individual plaques or tumors may be treated with small-field irradiation for palliation, with fractionated total doses of 15 to 25 Gy. Complete response of individual lesions is generally achieved with doses greater than 20 Gy, although higher doses may be necessary to ensure long-term local control.[55] Since the response to treatment is prompt, the total dose may be titrated to response. Small daily doses (1.25 to 1.5 Gy) may be used, especially in areas such as the eyelids and face, to minimize normal tissue reactions. Larger individual fractions may be used on other surfaces, but the use of fractions in excess of 2 Gy may result in the administration of a larger total dose than is really needed to achieve regression. Individual lesions can be treated most effectively with electrons (≤6 MeV), although orthovoltage x-rays (≤100 KV) may also be used. Electrons have an intrinsic advantage over photons since the depth of penetration of electrons can be controlled by appropriate selection of electron energy, whereas the depth dose contribution to the subcutaneous tissues is even greater with low-energy photons.

Some patients present with disease that extends into the deep soft tissues, girdles an extremity, or involves large portions of a hand or foot. In these instances, megavoltage photons (4 to 10 MV) are used most easily to provide an adequate depth of penetration and a homogeneous dose to the treatment volume; however, tissue-equivalent surface bolus is necessary to avoid the "skin-sparing" effects of high-energy x-rays.

Megavoltage photon therapy is also an effective palliative treatment for patients with extracutaneous mycosis fungoides, especially involving lymph nodes. Extensive or symptomatic nodal involvement may be treated with total doses similar to those used for cutaneous disease (≤30 Gy). Other extracutaneous sites that may be palliated effectively with irradiation include the brain, upper aerodigestive tract, and gastrointestinal tract.

In the late 1950s techniques were developed to permit the treatment of large skin surfaces by means of electrons.[56, 57] Commercially available linear accelerators may be modified to treat patients in the standing position at an extended distance to achieve the large field size. By standing in multiple positions (or on a rotational platform), the entire skin surface may be irradiated. The treatment technique employed at Stanford University Medical Center (and adopted at many other specialized centers) uses a six-field technique (anterior, posterior, and four opposed oblique fields). Treatment is administered four times a week, 4 Gy per week, to a total dose of 30 to 36 Gy. Electron energies of 4 to 9 MeV are used, providing an 80% depth dose at 0.35 to 0.8 cm.[58] Only the eyes are shielded routinely during treatment. Lead external shields are taped on the closed eyelids, or paraffin-coated, specially shaped lead shields may be placed under the lids (with the use of topical anesthesia).

Internal eye shields are preferable if there is disease involving the lids or in close proximity on the face. Other areas, such as the hands, elbows, and heels, may be shielded throughout or during a part of the course of treatment to help control localized cutaneous reactions.[56, 57] The scalp may be shielded after a dose of 24 Gy has been administered (provided there is no involvement of the scalp) to reduce the likelihood of permanent alopecia. Supplementary boost treatment with small-field electron therapy is required for the soles of the feet, the perineum, under the breasts, or any other areas of the body that are shadowed from the electron beam and do not receive an adequate dose of irradiation. A variety of fractionation schemes may be employed in these areas, such as 1 Gy fractions to a total of 20 Gy.

The acute complications of total skin electron beam therapy include acute erythema, desquamation, and temporary epilation. Patients experience temporary loss of their fingernails and toenails (usually after the completion of therapy), as well as an inability to sweat for at least 6 to 12 months. There is probably an increased risk of secondary squamous and basal cell cancers of the skin in long-term followup, but this is most evident in patients who have received protracted therapy with a variety of topical agents, including PUVA and topical HN_2.[44] Of special concern are the few patients who develop metastatic squamous cell cancers of the skin or lesions of the scrotum. In most patients, a few scattered telangiectasia and tendency to dry skin are the only long-term effects of treatment. However, there may be significant sequelae of treatment if the technique was administered improperly.

A number of centers have developed expertise in the use of total-skin electron beam therapy for mycosis fungoides.[1, 57, 59–61] Nearly all patients respond to treatment, with complete response rates dependent on the extent of skin involvement. At Stanford, the reported complete response rates are 98%, 64%, 34%, and 36% for patients with T1, T2, T3, and T4 disease, respectively. Just over one half of patients with limited plaque disease (T1) and about 20% of patients with generalized plaque disease (T2) remain free of disease more than 5 years after completion of a single course of therapy.[1, 56, 57] Although the curative potential of this treatment is questioned, it definitely provides an important palliative benefit, especially for patients with extensive disease. In addition, when disease recurs after electron beam therapy, it is often in a limited distribution and may be controlled readily with local topical therapy.

Electron beam therapy is often indicated in the primary or secondary management of patients with generalized plaque or tumorous involvement of the skin. Topical treatment with nitrogen mustard is often employed as an adjuvant after completion of electron beam therapy to prolong the response duration.[62] Maintenance PUVA treatment may be used in a similar fashion.

Occasional patients who have had an initial good response to electron beam therapy and later develop progressive disease may be candidates for a repeat course of treatment. In addition to an initial good response, these patients should have exhausted other topical therapies and have generalized progressive or refractory disease. Ideally, they should also have had a good duration of initial response. Second courses of treatment to total doses of 20 to 35 Gy with standard fractionation are tolerated well.[63]

Chemotherapy

The efficacy of systemic chemotherapy in mycosis fungoides has been disappointing.[1, 64] Virtually all drugs that are effective as single agents or in combination therapy in the treatment of patients with the non-Hodgkin's lymphomas have been tested in mycosis fungoides.[64] The largest experience is with combinations that include cyclophosphamide, vincristine, and prednisone, with or without doxorubicin (Adriamycin).[65–68] Complete response rates are only about 25% (range 11% to 57%) and response durations range from 3 to 20 months.[1, 64] Fortunately, only a few patients with mycosis fungoides (10% to 20%) require systemic management; however, an effective systemic treatment would potentially be beneficial in managing cutaneous disease, as well.

Systemic management provides an important palliative therapy for patients with Sézary syndrome.[1, 34] One common approach combines oral chlorambucil and prednisone.[69] Chlorambucil is administered daily, initially in 2-mg doses, titrating the dose according to response and toxicity (leukopenia and thrombocytopenia). Prednisone may be given initially at a dose of 20 mg per day, decreasing the dose as palliation is achieved. If a systemic response is achieved, but cutaneous symptoms persist, topical therapy such as low potency corticosteroids, low-dose PUVA, or low concentrations of nitrogen mustard may be added.[1]

Some newer drugs show promise in early clinical trials. Fludarabine, a purine antimetabolite that causes profound decreases in peripheral T-cell counts, has demonstrated clinical activity against mycosis fungoides, chronic lymphocytic leukemia, and the low-grade lymphomas.[70] Another drug of some usefulness is 2′-deoxycoformycin (pentostatin), which inhibits adenosine deaminase, an enzyme with a high level of activity in T cells. Adenosine deaminase inhibition leads to inhibition of DNA synthesis. This drug has demonstrated activity in mycosis fungoides and in a variety of other non-Hodgkin's lymphomas, as well as hairy cell leukemia. The response rate in mycosis fungoides may be as high as 50%.[71]

Combined-Modality Therapy

Combined-modality therapy plays an important role in the management of patients with mycosis fungoides. This may take the form of sequential topical therapies or combined topical and systemic treatment. Following electron beam therapy, response may be prolonged by use of a topical adjuvant, such as nitrogen mustard and PUVA.[62] Combined topical therapies may be helpful in the palliative management of patients with persistent skin disease. For example, a program emphasizing topical nitrogen mustard therapy may be supplemented by the judicious use of irradiation to tumors or symptomatic plaques. Occasionally, PUVA or photopheresis may be combined with topical nitrogen mustard. The main risk to consider in these cases is the potential for developing squamoproliferative lesions of the skin after prolonged therapy.[44]

Systemic chemotherapy has been combined with topical treatment and the wide range of responses reported (23% to 88%) is likely reflective of differences in patient selection.[1, 72–74] Responses are often attributable to the topical therapy. The ultimate test of the combined-modality approach was in the context of a prospective, randomized clinical trial reported from the NCI.[73] Patients were randomized to be treated aggressively with electron beam therapy plus chemotherapy with cyclophosphamide, doxorubicin, VP-16, and vincristine, or conservatively with sequential topical and then systemic therapies. There were no differences in outcome (survival) for conservative versus aggressive therapy for patients with either limited or advanced disease.

Another aggressive form of combined modality therapy is autologous bone marrow transplantation. However, although the concept is attractive and it has been shown that patients can tolerate the procedure, the limited experience reported thus far has been disappointing.[75]

Interferon

Although the outcome of management of mycosis fungoides with traditional systemic therapy has been disappointing, there is now a substantial experience supporting the use of interferon. The interferons have antiproliferative, cytotoxic, and immunoregulatory functions. Interferon-α was the first biologic tested in mycosis fungoides.[76–78] Response rates are reported to be about 50%, with a duration of about 6 months. The likelihood of response correlates with stage of disease, intensity of prior therapy, and dose of interferon. The greatest likelihood of response is in patients with limited disease, little prior therapy, and interferon doses as high as 50×10^6 U/day for 5 days, every 3 weeks. Patients experience mild to moderate systemic reactions to interferon, including fatigue, anorexia, decreased performance status, and leukopenia.

Interferon may play an even more important role in the context of combined-modality therapy. In a series combining interferon-alfa with PUVA, 80% of patients (primarily with stage I-II disease) achieved a complete response, often maintained as long as maintenance PUVA and interferon were continued.[79] Likewise, interferon appears to enhance the activity of deoxycoformycin, where a response rate of 41% has been reported.[80] There is also experience combining interferon with etretinate, with apparently enhanced activity over either treatment used alone.[81]

Novel Therapies

The frustration of dealing with patients who have refractory mycosis fungoides has led to the use of a variety of novel therapies. Treatments employed for other skin diseases, for extracutaneous lymphomas, or those with an immunologic basis of action have all been used with occasional success.

Photopheresis is also known as "extracorporeal PUVA."[82] It is a variation of PUVA in which the psoralen drug is administered orally, followed within 2 hours by pheresis of the peripheral white blood cells. The lymphocyte enriched fraction of the blood, combined with the psoralen-rich plasma, is passed through an extracorporeal circuit, exposed to a UVA irradiator, and then reinfused into the patient. Patients are generally treated on 2 consecutive days once a month. A response should be seen within 6 months. The mechanism of action of photopheresis has not been elucidated. It may be by a direct lymphotoxic effect, although an immune-mediated mechanism also has been proposed. The overall response rate to this treatment is 83%, with half of those patients demonstrating at least a 50% improvement.[83] Patients with erythroderma, especially those with low CD4+:CD8+ ratios in the peripheral blood, are the most likely to respond. Responses are less likely in patients who present with a large number of circulating Sézary cells. Unfortunately, this treatment approach has little usefulness among patients with more classic infiltrative disease.

Vitamin A regulates the growth and differentiation of epithelial tissues and is used in the prevention or treatment of many skin diseases. Retinoids are natural or synthetic vitamin A analogues. Patients with mycosis fungoides may achieve responses to treatment with retinoids.[84] The mechanisms of action are not known but may include decrease in cell proliferation, enhanced differentiation, or immunomodulation. Retinoids also are used in combination with other modalities, including PUVA (retinoids plus PUVA [RePUVA]) and interferon.[81]

Anti-T-cell monoclonal antibodies have also been used for the management of patients with mycosis fungoides. There have been trials with a pan-T-cell murine monoclonal antibody (anti-Leu-1),[85] an ^{131}I radiolabeled version of a similar antibody (T101),[86] and a pan-T-cell anti-CD5 antibody linked to ricin.[87] Responses to antibody therapy are generally brief and the duration of treatment is commonly limited by the development of human antimouse antibodies (HAMAs). In a more recent trial, a chimeric antihelper T-cell (anti-CD4) antibody has been used to minimize the development of HAMA and provide a more specific treatment against the mycosis fungoides subset of T cells.[88] The responses to this antibody were also modest and short-lived. Despite the minimal responses to antibody therapy that have been observed thus far, further studies are appropriate with different antibodies or with radiolabeled versions of existing antibodies. It is possible that antibody therapy will have a role to play in the management of minimal disease, perhaps as an adjuvant after electron beam therapy.

Another novel approach to treatment has been with a cytotoxic fusion protein.[89] With this technique, a fusion protein is genetically engineered and manufactured in which diphtheria toxin is linked to interleukin-2 (IL-2). The protein is administered intravenously and binds to cells that express high-affinity IL-2 receptors. It is internalized, and the toxin causes cell death. In a phase 1 trial, three of five patients with mycosis fungoides achieved significant tumor responses.

Cyclosporine, a potent anti-T-cell drug used as an immunosuppressive agent in organ transplantation, has achieved occasional responses in mycosis fungoides. In vitro, it inhibits the growth of mycosis fungoides cells by suppressing IL-2 production.[90]

THERAPEUTIC APPROACHES AND PROGNOSIS

The median survival of patients with mycosis fungoides is nearly 10 years.[1] The long-term survival of a cohort of more than 500 patients with all stages of mycosis fungoides seen at Stanford since 1960 is displayed in Figure 27–1. Treatment selection and prognosis are both linked closely to the extent of skin involvement and the presence of extracutaneous disease. Patients who present with extracu-

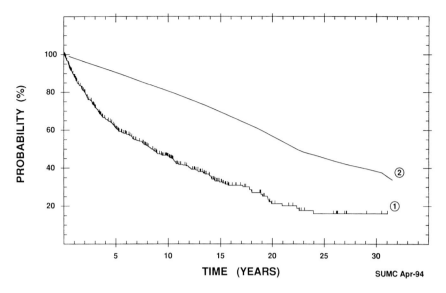

Figure 27–1. Actuarial survival of 502 patients with a confirmed diagnosis of mycosis fungoides or Sézary syndrome seen and treated at Stanford University Medical Center from 1960 to 1993 (curve 1) compared with the expected survival for an age- and sex-matched population (curve 2).

taneous disease have a median survival a little longer than 1 year (Fig. 27–2). Among patients who have disease apparently limited to the skin, the prognosis is linked closely to the extent of skin involvement (Fig. 27–3).

Patients with limited plaque (T1) disease are usually treated effectively with either topical nitrogen mustard or PUVA. When nitrogen mustard is used, treatment with a 10 to 20 mg/dL solution is initiated to the entire skin, since other areas of disease activity may thereby become evident. After several weeks, treatment is then restricted to the affected region. Treatment is continued daily until complete skin clearance is achieved and for as long as 1 year thereafter. If response is particularly slow, the concentration of the nitrogen mustard may be increased to 30 to 40 mg/dL, especially to small areas, or the frequency of application may be increased to twice a day.

PUVA may also be employed for limited plaque disease. Treatment is initiated on a three-times-weekly basis until skin clearance is achieved. Thereafter, the frequency of treatment is gradually decreased to as infrequently as once every 2 weeks. Maintenance therapy should be discontinued within 1 year.

The prognosis for patients with limited plaque (T1) disease is quite good. In our experience at Stanford, only 15% of patients treated in the limited plaque phase later progress to a more generalized extent of skin involvement.[1] Nearly all deaths are due to causes other than mycosis fungoides, such as cardiopulmonary disease and other cancers.

Patients with generalized plaque disease (T2) may be treated with nitrogen mustard, PUVA, or total-skin electron beam therapy. Irradiation should be considered for patients with very thickened plaques (since its depth of penetration is better than that of either nitrogen mustard or PUVA) and for patients with a recent history of rapid progression of disease (because of its more prompt effect). Patients treated with either nitrogen mustard or PUVA should be followed closely, and treatment with electron beam therapy should be initiated if disease progresses despite treatment intensification. Generally, following completion of electron beam therapy, adjuvant treatment with topical nitrogen mustard is appropriate and may be continued for a year or longer. Patients with limited or generalized plaque disease who fail to respond to one therapy, or who begin to progress after an

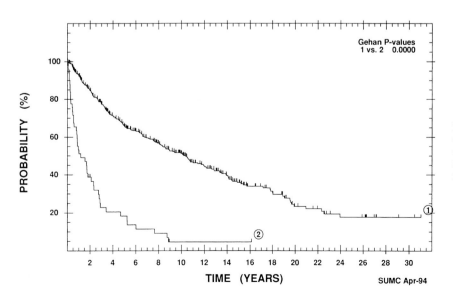

Figure 27–2. Actuarial survival of 451 patients (treated at Stanford University Medical Center) with mycosis fungoides apparently limited to the skin (curve 1) and 51 patients with extracutaneous manifestations at the time of diagnosis (curve 2).

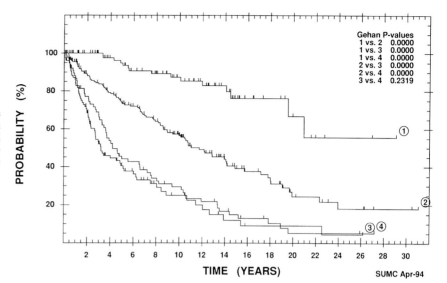

Figure 27–3. Actuarial survival of 451 patients (treated at Stanford University Medical Center) with mycosis fungoides limited to the skin, categorized according to the extent of skin involvement. Curve 1 = T1; curve 2 = T2; curve 3 = T3; and curve 4 = T4 (see Table 27–1 for stage classification).

initial response, may be treated with an alternative topical therapy. There is no evidence that the development of resistance to one modality affects subsequent response to an alternative modality.

Patients with more generalized disease (T2) at diagnosis are at greater risk for disease progression (30%) than patients with limited plaque. Nearly one third of deaths among patients with T2 disease are from causes related to mycosis fungoides, such as infection.[1]

Most patients with tumorous involvement (T3) have generalized cutaneous involvement, and the greatest likelihood of a response is with electron beam therapy, generally followed by adjuvant topical nitrogen mustard. Some patients, with a discrete number of tumors, may be treated with either topical nitrogen mustard or PUVA, combined with localized irradiation to individual tumors. Most patients who present with tumorous involvement ultimately die of mycosis fungoides. There is no evidence that treatment has any curative potential in this stage, but it does have tremendous palliative benefit.

Patients with erythroderma (T4) are challenging to manage. If there is no peripheral blood involvement, treatment may be initiated cautiously with low-dose PUVA. Photopheresis may also be effective treatment for these patients. If Sézary syndrome is present, systemic management such as management with chlorambucil and prednisone may have an important palliative role.[69] If there is a systemic response, but cutaneous symptoms persist, topical therapy such as low-potency corticosteroids, low-dose PUVA, or low concentrations of HN2 may be added. Patients who are young and have no peripheral blood involvement or extracutaneous disease may live quite long with palliative therapy only (median survival of 10 years).[91] However, once a patient develops Sézary syndrome, with circulating peripheral cells, the median survival is only about 3 years.

Patients with extracutaneous disease may be treated with megavoltage photon irradiation for palliation, especially for disease involving lymph nodes. Systemic chemotherapy or biologic therapies are appropriate to consider in these patients, as well. Because of the inadequacy of standard therapy, all patients with extracutaneous disease should be considered candidates for investigational therapies. Patients with extracutaneous disease and any extent of skin involvement have a median survival of only 1 year, and nearly all die of causes directly related to mycosis fungoides.

OTHER CUTANEOUS LYMPHOMAS

Non-mycosis fungoides cutaneous lymphomas represent only 5% to 7% of extranodal non-Hodgkin's lymphoma.[92] Among these patients there is a male predominance, and the median age is about 60 years.

Most are intermediate- or high-grade lymphomas according to modified criteria of the Working Formulation.[93] Immunoperoxidase studies demonstrate that they may be of either B-cell or T-cell phenotype. The proportion of B-cell lymphomas in different series ranges from 50%[94] to 75%.[95] They may be further categorized according to the expression of specific cell surface antigens, such as CD30 (Ki-1). In contrast with mycosis fungoides, the T-cell types often lack one or more of the mature T-cell antigens and do not exhibit either a helper or suppressor T-cell phenotype.

The pathologic aspects of the cutaneous non-Hodgkin's lymphomas differ from mycosis fungoides in that they are nonepidermatropic. That is, the neoplastic cells are usually absent from the epidermis and are limited to the dermis and subcutaneous tissues. The region between the dermis and epidermis (the Grenz zone) is spared; however, relatively advanced lesions may ulcerate secondarily into the epidermis.

The low-grade cutaneous lymphomas must be differentiated from benign lymphocytic proliferations such as lymphocytoma cutis.[96] This is done best by immunophenotyping, since lymphocytoma cutis is a polyclonal proliferation, in contrast with the monoclonal B-cell nature of the cutaneous lymphomas.

The most common histologic subtypes of cutaneous lymphoma are diffuse large cell or immunoblastic, which account for one half to two thirds of cases.[94, 97] The clinical presentation of cutaneous lymphomas is that of nodules rather than plaques or patches. The predominant site of primary involvement is the head and neck region.[98] The draining lymphatics are not commonly involved.

The staging evaluation for these patients should include those studies employed for evaluating patients with non-Hodgkin's lymphomas in other sites. These include a thorough physical examination with detailed examination of the skin, complete blood counts, screening chemistries, chest radiograph, CT scan of the chest and abdomen, and bone marrow biopsy.

For patients with localized involvement of the skin only (stage IE), treatment may be restricted to local irradiation. A dose of 30 to 36 Gy for low-grade and 40 to 44 Gy for intermediate- or high-grade lymphomas generally suffices. At least half of these patients are cured with local treatment.[97, 98] Systemic treatment may be restricted to those patients who have disease progression after localized radiation treatment, or those rare patients who present with lymphoblastic or undifferentiated lymphoma. After local treatment, the most common site of failure is in skin sites distant from the primary site of involvement. The 10-year survival of patients who present with stage IE disease ranges from 60% to 70%.[95, 97, 98]

Patients with stage IIE disease (regional lymph nodes involved) are treated most effectively with combined-modality therapy, as are other patients with stage II intermediate- or high-grade lymphoma.[99] In patients with stage III or IV disease, the cutaneous involvement is merely incidental unless it is particularly bulky and poses a problem for local control, in which case adjuvant irradiation may be added to the primary chemotherapy program.

A distinct subtype of lymphoma, anaplastic large cell lymphoma of the skin, has been described recently.[100] These lymphomas are generally Ki-1 (CD30) positive. They may arise de novo (primary) or develop in the face of preexisting cutaneous T-cell lymphoproliferative diseases such as mycosis fungoides and lymphomatoid papulosis (secondary).[101] The behavior of primary anaplastic large cell lymphoma is usually indolent, and treatment may be similar to other cutaneous non-Hodgkin's lymphomas.[102] The behavior of secondary cutaneous anaplastic large cell lymphoma may be more aggressive and require more intensive local therapy.[100]

REFERENCES

1. Hoppe RT, Wood GS, Abel EA: Mycosis fungoides and the Sézary syndrome: Pathology, staging, and treatment. Curr Probl Cancer 1990; 14:295.
2. Weinstock MA, Horm JW: Mycosis fungoides in the United States: Increasing incidence and descriptive epidemiology. JAMA 1988; 260:42.
3. Chuang TY, Su WPD, Muller SA: Incidence of cutaneous T-cell lymphoma and other rare skin cancers in a defined population. J Am Acad Dermatol 1990; 23:254.
4. Cohen SR, Stenn KS, Braverman IM, et al: Mycosis fungoides: Clinicopathologic relationships between survival and therapy in 59 patients with observations on occupation as a new prognostic factor. Cancer 1980; 46:2654.
5. Linet MS, McLaughlin JK, Fraumeni JF, et al: Mycosis fungoides and occupation in Sweden. J Natl Cancer Inst 1989; 81:1842.
6. Greene MH, Dalager NA, Lamberg SI, et al: Mycosis fungoides: Epidemiologic observations. Cancer Treat Rep 1979; 63:597.
7. Whittemore AS, Holly EA, Lee IM, et al: Mycosis fungoides in relation to environmental exposures and immune response: A case control study. J Natl Cancer Inst 1989; 81:1560.
8. Poiesz BJ, Ruscetti FW, Gazdar AF, et al: Detection and isolation of type C retrovirus particles from fresh and cultured lymphocytes of a patient with cutaneous T-cell lymphoma. Proc Natl Acad Sci U S A 1980; 77:7415.
9. Bunn PA, Schechter GP, Blayney D, et al: Clinical course of retrovirus-associated adult T-cell lymphoma in the United States. N Engl J Med 1983; 309:257.
10. Ranki A, Niemi K, Nieminen P, et al: Antibodies against retroviral core proteins in relation to disease outcome in patients with mycosis fungoides. Arch Dermatol Res 1990; 282:532.
11. Hall WW, Liu C, Schneewind O, et al: Deleted HTLV-1 provirus in blood and cutaneous lesions of patients with mycosis fungoides. Science 1991; 253:317.
12. Zucker-Franklin D, Coutavas EE, Rush MG, et al: Detection of human T-lymphotropic virus–like particles in cultures of peripheral blood lymphocytes from patients with mycosis fungoides. Proc Natl Acad Sci U S A' 1991; 88:7630.
13. Capesius C, Saal F, Maero E, et al: No evidence for HTLV-I infection in 24 cases of French and Portuguese mycosis fungoides and Sézary syndrome (as seen in France). Leukemia 1991; 5:416.
14. Lisby G, Reitz MS, Vejlsgaard GL: No detection of HTLV-1 DNA in punch skin biopsies from patients with cutaneous T-cell lymphoma by the polymerase chain reaction. J Invest Dermatol 1992; 98:417.
15. Manzari V, Gismondi A, Barillari G, et al: HTLV-V: A new human retrovirus isolated in a Tac-negative T-cell lymphoma/leukemia. Science 1987; 238:1581.
16. Olerud JE, Kulin PA, Chew DE, et al: Cutaneous T-cell lymphoma: Evaluation of pretreatment skin biopsy specimens by a panel of pathologists. Arch Dermatol 1992; 128:501.
17. Hoppe RT, Abel EA, Deneau DG, et al: Mycosis fungoides: Management with topical nitrogen mustard. J Clin Oncol 1987; 5:1796.
18. Lutzner MA, Edelson RL, Schein P, et al: Cutaneous T cell lymphomas: The Sézary syndrome, mycosis fungoides, and related disorders. Ann Intern Med 1975; 83:534.
19. Meijer CJLM, van der Loo EM, van Vloten WA, et al: Early diagnosis of mycosis fungoides and Sézary syndrome by morphometric analysis of lymphoid cells in the skin. Cancer 1980; 45:2864.
20. Payne CM, Glasser L: Ultrastructural morphometry in the diagnosis of Sézary syndrome. Arch Pathol Lab Med 1990; 114:661.
21. Brouet JC, Flandrin G, Seligmann M: Indications of the thymus-derived nature of the proliferating cells in six patients with Sézary's syndrome. N Engl J Med 1973; 289:341.
22. Wood GS, Weiss LM, Warnke RA, et al: The immunopathology of cutaneous lymphomas: Immunophenotypic and immunogenotypic characteristics. Semin Dermatol 1986; 5:334.
23. Michie SA, Abel EA, Hoppe RT, et al: Expression of T-cell receptor antigens in mycosis fungoides and inflammatory skin lesions. J Invest Dermatol 1989; 93:116.
24. Weiss LM, Wood GS, Hu E, et al: Detection of clonal T-cell receptor gene rearrangements in the peripheral blood of patients with mycosis fungoides/Sézary syndrome. J Invest Dermatol 1989; 92:601.
25. Bignon Y-J, Souteyrand P, Roger H, et al: Clonotypic heterogeneity in cutaneous T-cell lymphomas. Cancer Res 1990; 50:6620.
26. Sausville EA, Worsham GF, Matthews MJ, et al: Histologic assessment of lymph nodes in mycosis fungoides/Sézary syndrome: Clinical correlation and prognostic import of a new classification system. Hum Pathol 1985; 16:1098.
27. Sausville EA, Eddy JL, Makuch RW, et al: Histopathologic staging at initial diagnosis of mycosis fungoides and the Sézary syndrome: Definition of three distinctive prognostic groups. Ann Intern Med 1988; 109:372.
28. Bunn PA, Huberman MS, Whang-Peng J, et al: Prospective staging evaluation of patients with cutaneous T-cell lymphomas: Demonstration of a high frequency of extracutaneous dissemination. Ann Intern Med 1980; 93:223.
29. Weiss LM, Hu E, Wood GS, et al: Clonal rearrangements of the T-cell receptor gene in mycosis fungoides and dermatopathic lymphadenopathy. N Engl J Med 1985; 313:539.
30. Lynch JW, Linoilla I, Sausville EA, et al: Prognostic implications of evaluation for lymph node involvement by T-cell antigen receptor gene rearrangement in mycosis fungoides. Blood 1992; 79:3293.
31. Bakels V, Van Oostveen JW, Geerts ML, et al: Diagnostic and prognostic significance of clonal T-cell receptor beta gene rearrangements in lymph nodes of patients with mycosis fungoides. J Pathol 1993; 170:249.
32. Dmitrovsky E, Matthews MJ, Bunn PA, et al: Cytologic transformation

in cutaneous T cell lymphoma: A clinicopathologic entity associated with poor prognosis. J Clin Oncol 1987; 5:208.

33. Salhany KE, Cousar JB, Greer JP, et al: Transformation of cutaneous T-cell lymphoma to large cell lymphoma: A clinicopathologic and immunologic study. Am J Pathol 1988; 132:265.

34. Wieselthier JS, Koh HK: Sézary syndrome: Diagnosis, prognosis, and critical review of treatment options. J Am Acad Dermatol 1990; 22:381.

35. Miketic LM, Chambers TP, Lembersky BC: Cutaneous T-cell lymphoma: Value of CT in staging and determining prognosis. AJR 1993; 160:1129.

36. Epstein EH, Devin DL, Croft JD, et al: Mycosis fungoides: Survival, prognostic features, response to therapy, and autopsy findings. Medicine 1972; 15:61.

37. Bunn PA, Lamberg SI: Report of the Committee on Staging and Classification of Cutaneous T-Cell Lymphomas. Cancer Treat Rep 1979; 63:725.

38. Fuks ZY, Bagshaw MA, Farber EM: Prognostic signs in the management of the mycosis fungoides. Cancer 1973; 32:1385.

39. Hoppe RT, Cox RS, Fuks Z, et al: Electron beam therapy for mycosis fungoides: The Stanford University experience. Cancer Treat Rep 1979; 63:691.

40. Kulin PA, Marglin SI, Shuman WP, et al: Diagnostic imaging in the initial staging of mycosis fungoides and Sézary syndrome. Arch Dermatol 1990; 126:914.

41. Graham SJ, Sharpe RW, Steinberg SM, et al: Prognostic implications of a bone marrow histopathologic classification system in mycosis fungoides and the Sézary syndrome. Cancer 1993; 72:726.

42. Gilchrest BA, Parrish JA, Tanenbaum L, et al: Oral methoxsalen photochemotherapy of mycosis fungoides. Cancer 1976; 38:683.

43. Abel EA, Sendagorta E, Hoppe RT, et al: PUVA treatment of erythrodermic and plaque-type mycosis fungoides: Ten-year follow-up study. Arch Dermatol 1987;123:897.

44. Abel EA, Sendagorta E, Hoppe RT: Cutaneous malignancies and metastatic squamous cell carcinoma following topical therapy for mycosis fungoides. J Am Acad Dermatol 1986; 14:1029.

45. Honigsmann H, Brenner W, Rauschmeier W, et al: Photochemotherapy for cutaneous T cell lymphoma. J Am Acad Dermatol 1984; 10:238.

46. Rosenbaum MM, Roenigk HH, Caro WA, et al: Photochemotherapy in cutaneous T-cell lymphoma and parapsoriasis en plaques: Long-term follow-up in forty-three patients. J Am Acad Dermatol 1985; 13:613.

47. Resnik KS, Vonderheid EC: Home UV phototherapy of early mycosis fungoides: Long-term follow-up observations in thirty-one patients. J Am Acad Dermatol 1993; 29:73.

48. Vonderheid EC: Topical mechlorethamine chemotherapy: Considerations on its use in mycosis fungoides. Int J Dermatol 1984; 23:180.

49. Studstrup L, Beck HI, Bjerring P, et al: No detectable increase in sister chromatid exchanges in lymphocytes from mycosis fungoides patients after topical treatment with nitrogen mustard. Br J Dermatol 1988; 119:711.

50. Van Scott EJ, Kalmanson JD: Complete remissions of mycosis fungoides lymphoma induced by topical nitrogen mustard (HN_2): Control of delayed hypersensitivity to HN_2 by desensitization and by induction of specific immunologic tolerance. Cancer 1973; 32:18.

51. Vonderheid EC, Tan ET, Kantor AF, et al: Long-term efficacy, curative potential, and carcinogenicity of topical mechlorethamine chemotherapy in cutaneous T-cell lymphoma. J Am Acad Dermatol 1989; 20:416.

52. Breneman DL, Nartker AL, Ballman EA, et al: Topical mechlorethamine in the treatment of mycosis fungoides: Uniformity of application and potential for environmental contamination. J Am Acad Dermatol 1991; 25:1059.

53. Ramsay DL, Halperin PS, Zeleniuch-Jacquotte A: Topical mechlorethamine therapy for early-stage mycosis fungoides. J Am Acad Dermatol 1988; 9:684.

54. Zackheim HS, Epstein EH, Crain WR: Topical carmustine (BCNU) for cutaneous T cell lymphoma: A 15-year experience in 143 patients. J Am Acad Dermatol 1990; 22:802.

55. Cotter GW, Baglan RJ, Wasserman TH, et al: Palliative radiation treatment of cutaneous mycosis fungoides—a dose response. Int J Radiat Oncol Biol Phys 1983; 9:1477.

56. Hoppe RT, Fuks Z, Bagshaw MA: Radiation therapy in the management of cutaneous T-cell lymphomas. Cancer Treat Rep 1979; 63:625.

57. Hoppe RT: Total skin electron beam therapy in the management of mycosis fungoides. *In* Vaeth J, Meyer J (eds): Frontiers of Radiation Therapy and Oncology, Vol 25. Basel, Karger, 1990.

58. Cox RS, Heck RJ, Fessenden P, et al: Development of total-skin electron therapy at two energies. Int J Radiat Oncol Biol Phys 1990; 18:659.

59. Lo TCM, Salzman FA, Moschella SL, et al: Whole-body surface electron irradiation in the treatment of mycosis fungoides: An evaluation of 200 patients. Radiology 1979; 130:453.

60. Nisce LZ, Safai B, Kim JH: Effectiveness of once-weekly total skin electron beam therapy in mycosis fungoides and Sézary syndrome. Cancer 1981; 47:870.

61. Jones GW, Tadros A, Hodson DI, et al: Prognosis with newly diagnosed mycosis fungoides after total skin electron radiation of 30 or 35 Gy. Int J Radiat Oncol Biol Phys 1994; 28:839.

62. Price NM, Hoppe RT, Constantine VS, et al: The treatment of mycosis fungoides: Adjuvant topical mechlorethamine after electron beam therapy. Cancer 1977; 40:2851.

63. Becker M, Hoppe RT, Knox SJ: Multiple courses of high-dose total skin electron beam therapy in the management of mycosis fungoides. Int J Radiat Oncol Biol Phys 1995; 32:1239.

64. Broder S, Bunn PA: Cutaneous T-cell lymphomas. Semin Oncol 1980; 7:310.

65. Case DC: Combination chemotherapy for mycosis fungoides with cyclophosphamide vincristine, methotrexate, and prednisone. Am J Clin Oncol 1984; 7:453.

66. Molin L, Thomsen K, Volden G, et al: Combination chemotherapy in the tumour stage of mycosis fungoides with cyclophosphamide, vincristine, VP-16, Adriamycin, and prednisolone (COP, CHOP, CAVOP): A report from the Scandinavian Mycosis Fungoides Study Group. Acta Derm Venereol (Stockh) 1980; 60:542.

67. Raafat J, Oster MW, LoGerfo P, et al: Combination chemotherapy for advanced cutaneous T-cell lymphomas. Cancer Treat Rep 1980; 64:1371.

68. Tirelli U, Carbone A, Veronesi A, et al: Combination chemotherapy with cyclophosphamide, vincristine and prednisone (CVP) in TNM-classified stage IV mycosis fungoides. Cancer Treat Rep 1982; 66:167.

69. Winkelmann RK, Diaz-Perez JL, Buechner SA: The treatment of Sézary syndrome. J Am Acad Dermatol 1984; 10:1000.

70. Von Hoff D, Dahlberg S, Hartstock R, et al: Activity of fludarabine monophosphate in patients with advanced mycosis fungoides: A Southwest Oncology Group Study. J Natl Cancer Inst 1990; 82:1353.

71. Cummings FJ, Kim K, Neiman RS, et al: Phase II trial of pentostatin in refractory lymphomas and cutaneous T-cell lymphomas. J Clin Oncol 1991; 9:565.

72. Braverman IM, Yager NB, Chen M, et al: Combined total body electron beam irradiation and chemotherapy for mycosis fungoides. J Am Acad Dermatol 1987; 16:45.

73. Kaye FJ, Bunn PA, Steinberg SM, et al: A randomized trial comparing combination electron-beam radiation and chemotherapy with topical therapy in the initial treatment of mycosis fungoides. N Engl J Med 1989; 321:1784.

74. Zakem MH, Davis BR, Adelstein DJ, et al: Treatment of advanced-stage mycosis fungoides with bleomycin, doxorubicin, and methotrexate with topical nitrogen mustard (BAM-M). Cancer 1986; 58: 2611.

75. Bigler RD, Crilley P, Micaily B, et al: Autologous bone marrow transplantation for advanced-stage mycosis fungoides. Bone Marrow Transplant 1991; 7:133.

76. Kohn EC, Steis RG, Sausville EA, et al: Phase II trial of intermittent high-dose recombinant interferon alfa-2a in mycosis fungoides and the Sézary syndrome. J Clin Oncol 1990; 8:155.

77. Olsen EA, Rosen ST, Vollmer RT, et al: Interferon alfa-2a in the treatment of cutaneous T cell lymphoma. J Am Acad Dermatol 1989; 20:395.

78. Vegna MI, Papa G, Defazio D, et al: Interferon alpha-2a in cutaneous T-cell lymphoma. Eur J Haematol 1990; 45:32.

79. Kuzel TM, Gilyon K, Springer E, et al: Interferon alfa-2a combined with phototherapy in the treatment of cutaneous T-cell lymphoma. J Natl Cancer Inst 1990; 82:203.

80. Foss FM, Ihde DC, Breneman DL, et al: Phase II study of pentostatin and intermittent high-dose recombinant interferon alfa-2a in advanced mycosis fungoides/Sézary syndrome. J Clin Oncol 1992; 10:1907.

81. Dreno B, Claudy A, Meynadier J, et al: The treatment of 45 patients

with cutaneous T-cell lymphoma with low doses of interferon-2α and eretinate. Br J Dermatol 1991; 125:456.

82. Edelson R, Berger C, Gasparro F, et al: Treatment of cutaneous T-cell lymphoma by extracorporeal photochemotherapy: Preliminary results. N Engl J Med 1987; 316:297.

83. Heald P, Rook A, Perez M, et al: Treatment of erythrodermic cutaneous T-cell lymphoma with extracorporeal photochemotherapy. J Am Acad Dermatol 1992; 27:427.

84. Molin L, Thomsen K, Volden G, et al: Oral retinoids in mycosis fungoides and Sézary syndrome: A comparison of isotretinoin and etretinate—a study from the Scandinavian Mycosis Fungoides Group. Acta Derm Venereol 1987; 67:232.

85. Miller RA, Oseroff AR, Stratte PT, et al: Monoclonal antibody therapeutic trials in seven patients with T-cell lymphoma. Blood 1983; 62:988.

86. Dillman RO, Beauregard J, Shawler DL, et al: Continuous infusion of T101 monoclonal antibody in chronic lymphocytic leukemia and cutaneous T-cell lymphoma. J Biol Response Mod 1986; 5:394.

87. LeMaistre CF, Rosen S, Frankel A, et al: Phase I trial of H65-RTA immunoconjugate in patients with cutaneous T-cell lymphoma. Blood 1991; 78:1173.

88. Knox SJ, Levy R, Hodgkinson S, et al: Observations on the effect of chimeric anti-CD4 monoclonal antibody in patients with mycosis fungoides. Blood 1991; 77:20.

89. Hesketh P, Caguioa P, Koh H, et al: Clinical activity of a cytotoxic fusion protein in the treatment of cutaneous T-cell lymphoma. J Clin Oncol 1993; 11:1682.

90. Jensen JR, Thestrup-Pedersen K, Zachariae H, et al: Cyclosporin A therapy for mycosis fungoides. Arch Dermatol 1987; 123:161.

91. Kim YH, Bishop K, Vanghese A, et al: Prognostic factors in erythrodermic mycosis fungoides and the Sézary syndrome. Arch Dermatol 1995; 131:1003.

92. Paryani S, Hoppe RT, Burke JS, et al: Extralymphatic involvement in diffuse non-Hodgkin's lymphomas. J Clin Oncol 1983; 1:682.

93. The Non-Hodgkin's Lymphoma Pathology Classification Project: National Cancer Institute–sponsored study of classifications of non-Hodgkin's lymphomas: Summary and description of a working formulation for clinical usage. Cancer 1982; 49:2112.

94. Wood GS, Burke JS, Horning S, et al: The immunologic and clinicopathologic heterogeneity of cutaneous lymphomas other than mycosis fungoides. Blood 1983; 62:464.

95. Joly P, Charlotte F, Leibowitch M, et al: Cutaneous lymphomas other than mycosis fungoides: Follow-up study of 52 patients. J Clin Oncol 1991; 9:1994.

96. Garcia CF, Weiss LM, Warnke RA, et al: Cutaneous follicular lymphoma. Am J Surg Pathol 1986; 10:454.

97. Esche BA, Fitzpatrick PJ: Cutaneous malignant lymphoma. Int J Radiat Oncol Biol Phys 1986; 12:2111.

98. Burke JS, Hoppe RT, Cibull ML, et al: Cutaneous malignant lymphoma: A pathologic study of 50 cases with clinical analysis of 37. Cancer 1981; 47:300.

99. Prestidge BR, Horning SJ, Hoppe RT: Combined-modality therapy for stage I-II large cell lymphoma. Int J Radiat Oncol Biol Phys 1988; 15:633.

100. Kaudewitz P, Stein H, Dallenbach F, et al: Primary and secondary Ki-1+ (CD30+) anaplastic large cell lymphomas: Morphologic, immunohistologic, and clinical characteristics. Am J Pathol 1989; 135:359.

101. Willemze R, Beljaard R: Spectrum of primary cutaneous CD30 (Ki-1)-positive lymphoproliferative disorders. J Am Acad Dermatol 1993; 28:973.

102. Beljaards RC, Kaudewitz P, Berti E, et al: Primary cutaneous large cell lymphomas: Definition of a new type of cutaneous lymphoma with a favorable prognosis—an European multicenter study on 47 patients. Cancer 1993; 71:2097.

Twenty-Eight

——Lymphoma in the Setting of —— Human Immunodeficiency Virus Infection

Alexandra M. Levine

BACKGROUND

Lymphoma is known to occur in patients with underlying immunodeficiency, dysregulation, or both, and its incidence is statistically increased in these settings. Thus, patients with congenital immunodeficiency diseases, such as Wiskott-Aldrich syndrome,[1] ataxia telangectasia,[2] and X-linked lymphoproliferative disorder,[3] all are at increased risk for lymphoma. Patients with autoimmune disorders such as Sjögren's syndrome[4, 5] and Hashimoto's thyroiditis[6] are diagnosed with lymphoma more frequently than expected; the lymphomas that ensue may occur at the specific sites of prior autoimmune disease.[7]

Monoclonal B-cell lymphomas or polyclonal lymphoproliferative disorders are also seen with increased frequency in patients who have undergone organ transplantation,[8] occurring 25 to 50 times more commonly than expected in the general population, with a latent period of approximately 33 months from transplantation. The association between profound immunodeficiency and the subsequent development of transplant-related lymphoma may be also surmised by the data from Swinnen and colleagues, who demonstrated that the use of more intensive regimens of immunosuppression, such as monoclonal antibody–induced T-cell depletion, was associated with a greater likelihood of subsequent lymphoma, occurring at shorter latent periods.[9] Patients who have undergone cardiac transplantation appear most at risk. This may be related to the fact that episodes of incipient cardiac rejection are more likely to be treated with increasing immunosuppressive regimens in an attempt to preserve the transplant, in contrast with renal allografts, which can more easily be removed, with return to long-term dialysis.

In 1982, approximately 1 year after the first descriptions of *Pneumocystis carinii* pneumonia (PCP) and Kaposi's sarcoma, the Centers for Disease Control and Prevention (CDC) first reported a small group of homosexual men with Burkitt's-like (diffuse undifferentiated) lymphomas.[10] Lymphoma primary to the brain, occurring in patients younger than 60 years of age, was included as an acquired immuno-

deficiency syndrome (AIDS)–defining diagnosis in the same year,[11] and systemic lymphoma, high-grade or intermediate-grade large cell type occurring in human immunodeficiency virus (HIV)–seropositive patients, became AIDS defining in 1985.[12] Although lymphoma occurred in only 2.9% of patients diagnosed with AIDS in the United States between 1981 and 1989,[13] recent estimates suggest that the incidence has increased to the range of 4% to 10%.

The known relationship between underlying immune dysfunction and the subsequent development of lymphoma would be fully consistent with the occurrence of lymphomas in the setting of HIV-induced immune dysregulation. Indeed, certain similarities exist among all these immunodeficiency-related lymphomas, including the B-lymphoid origin of the disease; the development of high-grade pathologic types; the frequent presence of extranodal disease at initial presentation; and short survival times, despite therapy.[14]

EPIDEMIOLOGY

INCIDENCE

The incidence of lymphoma doubled in the United States between 1940 and 1980,[15] for reasons that are not well understood. The AIDS epidemic has had an additional impact, associated with a risk of lymphoma between 60 and 100 times that expected in the usual population.[13, 16, 17]

Lymphoma is the second most common malignancy occurring in patients with AIDS, serving as the initial AIDS-defining diagnosis in approximately 3% of HIV-infected persons in the United States and Europe.[13, 18] Data regarding the true incidence of AIDS-related lymphoma in the United States are problematic, however, since the CDC collects inclusive information only on initial AIDS-defining conditions.[13] Thus, lymphoma developing in a person initially diagnosed with PCP will remain unknown to the CDC in statistical terms. The impact of this reporting structure on the true incidence of AIDS-related lymphoma may be seen from the data of Levine and colleagues,[19] who noted that 73% of patients with AIDS-related primary central nervous system lymphoma (PCNSL) and 37% of those with systemic lymphoma had been diagnosed with an AIDS-defining illness before the development of lymphoma. None of these cases would have been reported to the CDC or accounted for in the analyses of AIDS occurring in the United States. In several areas in Europe, where all AIDS diagnoses are reportable, lymphoma has accounted for as many as 12% to 16% of all deaths occurring in patients with AIDS, as reported from one large hospital.[20]

AIDS-LYMPHOMA IN VARIOUS GROUPS AT RISK FOR HIV

In sharp distinction to Kaposi's sarcoma, which occurs primarily in homosexual or bisexual men,[21] lymphoma appears to occur with relatively equal frequency in persons in all categories of risk for the acquisition of HIV infection. Thus, as shown in data on 53,042 AIDS cases in 21 European countries,[18] the frequency of lymphoma ranged from 1.1% in children infected perinatally to 2.6% in injection drug users; 2.6% in heterosexuals; 3.2% in blood transfusion recipients; 3.4% in homosexual men; and 3.9% in hemophiliacs. After controlling for the effects of age, sex, and year of AIDS diagnosis, an excess of borderline statistical significance was found among homosexual or bisexual patients (odds ratio = 1.2; confidence interval 95%: 1.0–1.3).[18] Similarly, although the incidence of lymphoma among homosexual or bisexual men in the United States (3.4% as an initial AIDS diagnosis) is identical to that described in Europe, the incidence in injection drug users also appears somewhat less (1.6%).[13]

The demographic features of patients with AIDS-related lymphoma may differ among HIV risk groups. Thus, as described by Monfardini and colleagues in a study of 150 cases from the Italian Cooperative Group,[22] the median age of homosexual men diagnosed with AIDS-related lymphoma was 38 years, whereas that of injection drug users was 26 years. No differences were seen in pathologic type or sites of lymphomatous disease. Likewise, median survival after diagnosis of lymphoma was similar in both groups.[22]

In a recent prospective study of 1295 HIV-infected men with hemophilia, 5.5% developed lymphoma, at a median interval of 59 months from the initial HIV infection.[23] The relative risk of lymphoma was 36.5 times higher than that observed in a group of HIV-negative hemophiliacs, followed prospectively in the same study, and 29 times higher than expected in the general population. The mean CD4 cell count at diagnosis of AIDS-related lymphoma was 64 × 10^9/L. All pathologic and clinical characteristics of lymphomatous disease appeared similar to those described in patients with history of homosexuality or injection drug use.

DEMOGRAPHIC FEATURES

The usual age of patients with AIDS-related lymphoma seems to vary in a bimodal distribution pattern.[13, 18] Thus, the first peak of disease appears in adolescence (10 to 19 years of age), with the second peak in middle age (50 to 59 years). In data from the United States, where the relationship between age and pathologic type was also studied, the younger patients tended to present with Burkitt's lymphoma, whereas immunoblastic lymphoma was seen with increasing age.[13]

In the United States, AIDS-related lymphoma is more common in men than in women and is diagnosed in whites more often than in African Americans.[13] These data are fully consistent with the demographic pattern of "de novo" lymphoma in the United States, occurring in patients without underlying HIV infection.[17]

ROLE OF ANTIRETROVIRAL THERAPY

The role of specific antiretroviral therapy in the development of HIV-associated lymphoma remains somewhat controversial. Moore and associates[24] reported on 1030 patients with symptomatic HIV disease, all of whom were taking zidovudine and were followed over a 2-year period. The incidence of lymphoma was 2.3% overall, ranging from 1.6 per 100 person years of followup after beginning zidovudine therapy to 3.2% by 24 months of therapy. The relative hazard of developing lymphoma was stable throughout the period of followup, with a risk of 0.8% for each additional 6 months of antiretroviral therapy. Since the relative risk of developing lymphoma was constant over time, zidovudine per se was not believed to be etiologic. Consistent with this hypothesis, Baselga and associates[25] have reported a patient with AIDS-related lymphoma primary to the lung whose tumor underwent significant regression after the use of zidovudine therapy alone.

In contrast with these data, d'Arminio Monforte and associates[26] reported an association between higher cumulative doses of zidovudine and the development of PCNSL in an autopsy series of 637 AIDS cases. It is possible, however, that higher cumulative zidovudine dosages may have served as a surrogate marker for longer overall survival, thus permitting time for the development of these lymphomas.

Pluda and colleagues[27] also studied the development of lymphoma among a cohort of 116 patients with symptomatic HIV disease, noting an incidence of 19% within 36 months of institution of antiretroviral therapy. Although most patients had received zidovudine, others had received either didanosine (ddI), or zalcitabine (ddC). The characteristics of lymphomatous disease were identical in all groups and also identical to those described in patients who had never received antiretroviral therapy. The authors concluded that the antiretroviral agents per se had not contributed to the pathogenesis of lymphomatous disease.

Thus, although the use of antiretroviral agents is not believed to have directly contributed to the development of AIDS-related lymphoma, a recent report has documented the unexpected occurrence of thymic lymphoma among laboratory mice receiving ddC.[28] To clarify the precise role of zidovudine in the subsequent development of AIDS-related lymphoma, Levine and associates performed a population-based case control study of patients with AIDS-related lymphoma within the County of Los Angeles.[29] A total of 112 HIV-infected homosexual/bisexual men with lymphoma were matched to 112 homosexual/bisexual men with asymptomatic HIV infection; 49 of the lymphoma cases were also matched to 49 control subjects with AIDS, as defined by conditions other than lymphoma. In comparing the lymphoma cases with controls, the unmatched relative odds of lymphoma associated with zidovudine use was 0.93 (95% confidence interval = 0.47–1.83). It is thus apparent from these data that zidovudine is not associated with an increased risk of development of lymphoma among HIV-infected homosexual or bisexual men.

PROJECTIONS: INCIDENCE OF AIDS-LYMPHOMA IN FUTURE YEARS

Lymphoma is a relatively late manifestation of HIV infection, first noted to have increased statistically in occurrence in 1985,[30] a full 4 years after the initial descriptions of opportunistic infections and Kaposi's sarcoma. The expected increase in AIDS-lymphoma may also be seen from the data of Pluda and colleagues, who documented an increasing incidence of lymphoma over time in a group of 116 patients with symptomatic HIV infection (AIDS, or significant AIDS-related complex). At 36 months of followup, 19% of the cohort were projected to develop lymphoma[27, 31]; these projections have already been fulfilled.

ETIOLOGY AND PATHOGENESIS

The development of lymphoma in patients with underlying HIV infection represents the accumulation of multiple factors occurring over a relatively short period in a given person. The full description of those factors that are necessary and sufficient for the development of lymphoma is not yet available. However, multiple insights have already been made, and this allows the beginning of an understanding of those factors that may lead to the development of lymphoma in persons infected by HIV.

UNDERLYING IMMUNODEFICIENCY

Immunodeficient states per se may be associated with the development of lymphoma, as evidenced by its increased incidence in patients with congenital immunodeficiency diseases[1, 3]; in those with acquired autoimmune disorders; and in the setting of organ transplantation with iatrogenic immunosuppression.[8] The latter example is of particular interest, in that lymphoma has been shown to increase in patients who have received more profound immunosuppressive agents, including the use of monoclonal antibodies to deplete T lymphocytes.[9]

The importance of significant immunosuppression in the development of AIDS-lymphoma may be surmised by the fact that lymphoma is a relatively late manifestation of HIV infection, occurring in approximately 3% of patients as the first AIDS-defining diagnosis but in as many as 20% of patients with symptomatic HIV disease who are alive 2 or 3 years after an earlier AIDS diagnosis.[27] Likewise, lymphoma is most likely to occur in patients with more profound degrees of CD4 lymphocytopenia. Thus, the median CD4 cell count at diagnosis of systemic AIDS-lymphoma was 189×10^9/L in one study, whereas the median CD4 count in patients with AIDS-related PCNSL was only 30×10^9/L.[19] In Pluda and associates' study of lymphoma arising in patients with symptomatic HIV disease, the median CD4 count at the time of institution of zidovudine therapy was 74×10^9/L, whereas that at the onset of didanosine therapy

was 62×10^9/L. The median CD4 cell count at the time of lymphoma diagnosis was 6×10^9/L and 9×10^9/L, respectively[27]; most of these patients actually developed lymphoma primary to the central nervous system (CNS).[27] Thus, although AIDS-lymphoma can develop at higher CD4 cell counts, it is more often the rule that affected persons have lower CD4 cells, often less than 200×10^9/L, especially in those with PCNSL, in whom severe CD4 depletion is expected.

ONGOING B-CELL EXPANSION AND ACTIVATION

Aside from the myriad of qualitative and quantitative abnormalities of T lymphocytes in HIV-infected persons,[32] B-lymphocytic function is also deranged, with polyclonal activation induced by HIV, as well as by other antigens, mitogens, and additional infecting organisms.[33] This polyclonal expansion results in the florid follicular hyperplasia seen in enlarged reactive lymph nodes ("persistent generalized lymphadenopathy"), and in the polyclonal hypergammaglobulinemia that often accompanies HIV infection.[32, 33] The recent description of an HIV-infected patient with multiple myeloma, in whom the abnormal paraprotein was found to have activity against the p24 antigen of HIV, lends further credence to the concept that HIV per se may lead to ongoing B-cell expansion, with eventual clonal selection.[34]

Although associated with polyclonal expansion of B lymphocytes, HIV infection may also be associated with an intrinsic impairment in B-cell maturation, as described by Berberian and colleagues,[35] who noted a clonal defect in rearrangement of the VH3L genes that encode the variable region of the immunoglobulin heavy chain. This clonal defect, occurring in B cells within the germinal centers of lymph nodes, leads to a maturational arrest, with subsequent deficit in memory B cells. Thus, the ongoing B-cell expansion in HIV infection, with subsequent intrinsic impairment in B-cell maturation, may mimic the usual setting in lymphoproliferative malignancies, characterized by clonal expansion of cells that have been arrested at a specific stage of maturation or activation.[36]

CYTOKINE NETWORKS

Ongoing activation of various cytokines or growth factors may contribute to the chronic B-cell proliferation that characterizes HIV infection. Numerous cytokines are responsible for B-cell proliferation and differentiation, including interleukin-1 (IL-1); IL-2; IL-4; IL-6; IL-7; IL-10; and tumor necrosis factor-α (TNF-α).[37–42] B cells from HIV-infected patients with polyclonal hypergammaglobulinemia constitutively express TNF-α and IL-6.[43]

IL-6 may play a critical role in the development of AIDS-related lymphoma, as is the case in other lymphoproliferative malignancies. Thus, IL-6 functions as an autocrine growth factor in multiple myeloma[44] and is constitutively expressed in chronic lymphocytic leukemia[45] and in Castleman's disease.[46] High levels of IL-6 expression have been demonstrated in both HIV-positive and HIV-negative cases of B-cell large cell lymphoma, independent of Epstein-Barr virus (EBV) status, but dependent on the presence of immunoblasts within the lymphoma tissue.[47] Thus, although not unique to AIDS lymphoma, IL-6 may play an important role in the pathogenesis of diverse types of B-cell neoplasia, in which terminally differentiated cells predominate. Elevations levels of serum IL-6 levels at study entry, with subsequent further elevations in time, were documented before the development of large cell lymphoma in the group of patients with symptomatic HIV infection followed by Pluda and associates[27]; elevated serum IL-6 levels and depressed CD4 cells were the only predictors of lymphoma in this cohort. Emilie and associates[48] recently tested the use of a monoclonal antibody against IL-6 in a small group of patients with AIDS-lymphoma. Although no objective antitumor responses were observed, stabilization of disease was documented in several persons, and systemic B symptoms seemed to regress.[48]

IL-10 may also play an important role in the development of AIDS-related lymphoma. Human IL-10 shares significant homology with the EBV-associated protein BCRF-1.[49] IL-10 and BCRF-1 specifically impair the ability of the activated Th-1 subset of CD4 cells to synthesize interferon-γ and IL-2, serving to suppress T-helper cell antiviral and antitumor surveillance activities.[50] These functions alone could have an impact in terms of lymphomagenesis. In addition, however, constitutive expression of large amounts of IL-10 has been demonstrated in EBV-positive B-cell lines derived from patients with AIDS-related lymphoma.[51] Further, human IL-10 has been shown to function as an autocrine growth factor in similar cell lines.[52]

It is thus apparent that several cytokines may be operative in the full pathogenesis of AIDS-related lymphoma. HIV itself may induce the production of a cascade of such cytokines from infected monocytes, T cells, and bone marrow stromal cells, serving to upregulate HIV. These cytokines may also effect the proliferation, differentiation, and expression of both B cells and cytotoxic T cells, creating the milieu in which polyclonal B-cell expansion may occur, with eventual clonal selection and continued paracrine- and autocrine-induced B-cell growth.

EPSTEIN-BARR VIRUS

In addition to links to cytokine pathways, EBV may be implicated in the pathogenesis of HIV-associated lymphoma, per-haps related to the impaired immunosurveillance of EBV-infected cells in patients with AIDS.[53] EBV has consistently been implicated in the etiology of Burkitt's lymphoma in Africa, in which the EBV genome is uniformly present within tumor cells,[54] and EBV infection has been shown to precede the development of lymphoma.[55] Additional relationships between EBV infection and subsequent lymphoma may be seen in the model of X-linked lymphoproliferative disorder, in which affected boys may develop high-grade B-cell lymphomas after primary infection with EBV.[56]

Theoretically, EBV could lead to malignant transformation via multiple diverse mechanisms. First, activation of various EBV latent genes, encoding Epstein-Barr nuclear antigens (EBNAs), and latent membrane proteins (LMPs) may prolong the survival of EBV-infected host cells by blocking apoptosis.[57] LMP has also been shown to have direct transforming and oncogenic properties in the rodent model.[58] Expression of the *EBNA2* gene has been shown to induce the expression of CD21 and CD23 B-cell surface

antigens, which in turn induce B-cell proliferation. In this regard, CD21 is a receptor for EBV, possibly allowing EBV-induced autostimulation.[59]

In addition, EBV could participate in an eventual malignant phenotype by its downregulation of lymphocyte function–associated antigens (LFA-1 and LFA-3), leading to a "non-adhesive" phenotype that could then allow cells to escape immune surveillance by cytotoxic T cells.[60]

Another mechanism whereby EBV could cause malignant transformation relates to its ability to form complexes with the p53 protein so as to inactivate the protein's tumor suppressor function.[61] A similar interaction has been described for the E6 oncoprotein of human papillomavirus (types 16 and 18), which binds to the *p53* tumor suppressor gene, abrogating its suppressor activity.[62]

Furthermore, EBV could lead to ongoing B-cell activation and polyclonal expansion by means of its BCRF-1 protein, which is similar in its functional and structural characteristics to human IL-10.[49] BCRF-1 leads to a decrease in interferon-γ and IL-2 production from T cells, resulting in decreased T-cell-induced antiviral activity, enhanced viral survival, and resultant ongoing B-cell activation and expansion.[50] This ongoing B-cell proliferation may generate increased numbers of B cells that are susceptible to genetic errors, such as chromosome breaks and translocations.

Although EBV may thus induce malignant transformation through multiple pathways, its precise relationship to the etiology of AIDS-lymphomas remains somewhat controversial. Shibata and associates[63] studied the reactive lymphadenopathy tissues from 35 HIV-infected patients, employing polymerase chain reaction (PCR) and in situ hybridization. EBV DNA was detected in 13 (35%) of the 35 patients; the presence of detectable amounts of EBV DNA in these 13 reactive biopsies was associated with an increased incidence of concurrent lymphoma at another site, or development of lymphoma.

Primary CNS AIDS-related lymphoma has been uniformly associated with the presence of EBV DNA within tumor cells, with identification of the EBV early region (EBER) protein in 21 of 21 cases described by MacMahon and colleagues,[64] and LMP expressed in 45%. These PCNSLs were all of large cell or immunoblastic pathologic subtype.

Although AIDS-related PCNSLs are thus associated with EBV, the relationship between EBV and systemic HIV-associated lymphoma is less clear. Thus, MacMahon and colleagues[64] detected EBV genome in only 3 (43%) of 7 such cases, whereas Subar and associates[65] found EBV sequences or protein in only 6 (36%) of 16 systemic lymphoma cases. The differences in EBV expression may be a function of the site of disease or may be related to differing histologic types. Thus, Hamilton-Dutoit and associates detected the EBV genome by in situ hybridization in 11 (65%) of 17 cases of systemic immunoblastic lymphoma, versus only 1 of 5 cases of Burkitt's lymphoma, similar to the findings of others.[66–68] In a subsequent study of 101 cases of systemic AIDS-related lymphoma, Hamilton-Dutoit and associates[69] demonstrated EBER-1 expression in 46 (77%) of 60 immunoblast-rich, large cell lymphomas, but in only 12 (34%) of 35 small noncleaved cases, and in 1 (17%) of 6 cases of diffuse large noncleaved cell lymphoma.

In contrast, employing Southern blot analysis, PCR, and

in situ hybridization in 59 cases of systemic AIDS lymphoma, Shibata and colleagues[70] have demonstrated the presence of EBV in almost all cases, including 85% of immunoblastic, 55% of large cell, and 57% of small noncleaved lymphomas. These discrepancies may be related to differing assessments of histologic type, differing geographic patterns of disease, or other unidentified factors. However, clonal EBV infection has been demonstrated in all systemic EBV-positive cases yet reported, thus indicating that EBV integration occurred before clonal B-cell expansion and lymphomagenesis.[70, 71] Although not proving that EBV caused these lymphomas, the finding of clonal EBV would be consistent with the hypothesis that this virus was critically involved in the process of lymphomagenesis.

ABNORMAL B-CELL GENE REARRANGEMENTS

As discussed previously, ongoing B-cell expansion and activation is expected during the long asymptomatic course of HIV infection, induced by HIV itself, by multiple cytokines, and potentially by EBV as well. This continual B-cell proliferation may allow the milieu in which genetic "errors" may occur, simply because of the increased numbers of cells that may be susceptible to chromosome translocations and abnormal rearrangements. Thus, as hypothesized by Ames and Gold,[72] high proliferative activity alone may predispose cells to genomic mutations, leading eventually to neoplastic transformation.

In the adult, lymphocytes normally undergo DNA rearrangement during B-cell differentiation. These normal DNA rearrangements may provide vulnerable, abnormal recombination-prone sites, leading to chromosome translocations involving the immunoglobulin heavy-chain or light-chain genes. These recombinase errors could lead to the specific chromosome translocations that have been described in AIDS-lymphoma, as well as in Burkitt's lymphoma, including t(8;14), t(8;22), and t(8;2).[73–78] Consistent with this hypothesis, Pelicci and colleagues[79] described the presence of one or more faint or low-intensity immunoglobulin gene rearrangement bands within reactive persistent generalized lymphadenopathy tissues in 4 of 11 HIV-infected persons. The rearrangement bands were occasionally accompanied by a hybridization smear, suggesting the presence of additional oligoclonal B-cell expansions. These B-cell clones did not carry c-*myc* rearrangements, suggesting that they were immortalized but not fully transformed. These results suggest that within reactive lymphoid tissues there are one or several occult clonal B-cell populations that are not identifiable by morphologic or immunophenotypic analysis. The subsequent selection and growth advantage of one such clone, perhaps by abnormal activation of c-*myc* or other oncogenes, could explain the eventual development of monoclonal B-cell malignancy from an ongoing polyclonal B-cell response. The oligoclonal B-cell expansions would thus represent a premalignant condition, from which true lymphoma could develop. In this regard, chromosome abnormalities have been described in such reactive lymph nodes.[78] Furthermore, the development of lymphoma in patients with persistent generalized lymphadenopathy has been shown to occur 850 times more frequently than expected in the usual population.[80]

C-*MYC* DYSREGULATION

One mechanism that may lead to malignant transformation of B lymphocytes is the translocation of a normal growth-promoting gene ("protooncogene") to one of the immunoglobulin genes of the B cell in question. The juxtaposition of this protooncogene with the transcriptionally active enhancer sequences of the immunoglobulin molecule would result in overexpression of the translocated gene, now functioning as a true oncogene. The classic example of such a translocation is the t(8;14) rearrangement, which occurs uniformly in Burkitt's lymphoma.[73] This translocation leads to abnormal activation of the c-*myc* oncogene on chromosome 8 (8q24), which has been translocated to the immunoglobulin gene heavy-chain locus on chromosome 14 (q32). In this setting, transcriptional activation of c-*myc* can occur from direct juxtaposition to the immunoglobulin gene enhancer sequences or from the action of long-range enhancers on chromosome 14, without the need for proximity to c-*myc*.

Although both endemic and sporadic Burkitt's lymphoma are associated with t(8;14) or its variants—t(8;22); t(8;2)—the specific mechanisms of c-*myc* dysregulation differ in the two forms. Thus, in endemic (African) Burkitt's lymphoma, the c-*myc* gene is translocated in its intact form to the joining J$_H$ segment of the immunoglobulin gene. In this type, inactivation of the regulatory sequences of c-*myc* occurs primarily through point mutations within its first exon.[81] In contrast, in sporadic (American) Burkitt's lymphoma, the c-*myc* gene is disrupted within its 5′ region and is separated from its regulatory or "repressor" region. The first *myc* exon is then translocated, in truncated form to the J$_H$ region, or to the switch region of the heavy-chain gene of 14q32.[81–84] The consequence of either type of translocation is the constitutive expression of *myc*, under the control of genes that actively transcribe immunoglobulin determinants, thus resulting in the clonal proliferation of a neoplastic B-cell population.

Although c-*myc* dysregulation has been documented in many cases of AIDS-related lymphoma, this abnormality has not uniformly been observed. Thus, activation of c-*myc* has been detected in approximately 60% to 80% of AIDS-associated systemic lymphomas.[65, 79, 85, 86] Differences in c-*myc* dysregulation have been observed in different pathologic types of lymphoma. Thus, as shown by at least two groups of investigators, the AIDS-related small noncleaved lymphomas (Burkitt's or Burkitt's-like) are uniformly associated with c-*myc* dysregulation, whereas only one third or fewer of the immunoblastic or large cell lymphomas demonstrate this abnormality.[85, 86] The molecular mechanisms leading to c-*myc* dysregulation may also differ in the AIDS-related lymphomas. Thus, c-*myc* translocation, similar at the molecular level to sporadic Burkitt's lymphoma, has been observed in several series.[68, 79] In contrast, point mutation within c-*myc*, similar to that seen in endemic Burkitt's lymphoma, has been documented in another well-studied patient.[87]

Dysregulation of c-*myc* has been associated with transformation of human B cells in vitro and may cause B-cell lymphoma in transgenic animals carrying immunoglobulin-*myc* chimeric constructs.[88, 89] The important role of c-*myc* dysregulation in the pathogenesis of AIDS-lymphoma may also be seen from the work of Laurence and Astrin,[90] who demonstrated that HIV type I infection of immortalized B cell lines can itself result in upregulation of c-*myc* transcripts. Additionally, Pauza and associates[91] have demonstrated that HIV may directly affect cellular c-*myc* gene expression.

In summary, myc protein is a potent regulator of cell proliferation. Its abnormal expression may provide an important mechanism for the development of lymphoma in the setting of HIV infection. However, it is also clear that c-*myc* dysregulation is not present in all cases of AIDS-related lymphoma, indicating that alternative mechanisms of lymphomagenesis must also be operative.

ROLE OF OTHER PROTOONCOGENES

A putative new protooncogene was recently described on chromosome 3, consistent with chromosome breakpoints that have been described in cases of diffuse large cell lymphoma at chromosome 3q27. This protooncogene has been termed *BCL6*. Rearrangements of the *BCL6* gene have been found in 30% to 40% of de novo diffuse large cell lymphoma.[92, 93] Gaidano and colleagues[94] recently studied 24 cases of AIDS-associated diffuse large cell lymphoma, demonstrating rearrangements of *BCL6* in 20%, including 2 of 8 cases of large noncleaved lymphoma, and 3 of 16 cases of immunoblastic lymphoma. *BCL6* rearrangement was found in none of the 13 cases of small noncleaved lymphoma that were evaluated. *BCL6* rearrangements were found in both the presence and the absence of EBV infection of the tumor clone. The discovery of *BCL6* rearrangements exclusive to diffuse large cell lymphoma serves to broaden the understanding of the multiple molecular pathways that are operative in the eventual development of AIDS-related lymphoma.

The *ras* family of protooncogenes has also been evaluated in cases of lymphoma. Although mutations involving the H-, K-, or N-*ras* genes were not detected in any of 143 lymphomas in patients uninfected by HIV, a recent study has confirmed the presence of point mutations involving *ras* genes in 4 (15%) of 27 cases of AIDS-related lymphoma.[85] Further work is awaited in this regard.

There are no data to indicate involvement of additional protooncogenes in the pathogenesis of AIDS-related lymphoma. For example, there has been no evidence of rearrangement or abnormalities of the *BCL2* or *BCL1* oncogenes.[65, 70, 95]

ROLE OF TUMOR SUPPRESSOR GENES (*p53*)

Tumor suppressor genes such as the *p53* or retinoblastoma (*Rb*) genes are believed to play a significant role in the development and progression of various human malignancies when their loss or dysregulation removes the normal negative regulatory signals from affected cells. In this regard, *p53* gene mutations have been described in de novo lymphomas, specifically of the small noncleaved type, or its leukemic counterpart, French-American-British L3 acute lymphoblastic leukemia.[96, 97] In addition, *p53* gene mutations have been demonstrated in approximately 37% of AIDS-related lymphomas.[85] The presence of *p53* abnormalities was shown to vary between pathologic subtypes of disease, with approximately 60% of small noncleaved

lymphomas demonstrating *p53* abnormalities, whereas no case of immunoblastic or large cell lymphoma did so. A relationship was seen between the occurrence of *p53* suppressor gene inactivation and c-*myc* protooncogene dysregulation in the same tumor in vivo,[85] and in a lymphoma cell line in vitro,[94] suggesting that cells carrying the overexpressed c-*myc* are under additional pressure to delete a *p53* pathway. The c-*myc* protein may be involved in the regulation of *p53* gene expression.[98]

Aside from the tumor suppressor *p53* abnormalities in AIDS-related small noncleaved lymphoma, there is no current evidence to indicate inactivation of other such suppressor genes. Thus, abnormalities of the *Rb* gene have been demonstrated in none of 27 cases of AIDS-related lymphoma so far reported.[85]

PATHOLOGIC CHARACTERISTICS OF AIDS-LYMPHOMA

The AIDS-associated lymphomas are classically of B-lymphoid derivation and high-grade pathologic type,[99] described in approximately 70% to 90% of reported cases.[100–104] The more common subtypes of disease include B-immunoblastic or small noncleaved lymphomas,[105] the latter of which may be further subclassified into Burkitt's on non-Burkitt's types. Intermediate-grade, diffuse large cell lymphomas have also been included in the expanded case definition of AIDS published in 1987[106]; these intermediate-grade large cell lymphomas constitute approximately 30% of all cases.[107] The preponderance of high-grade disease is one of the characteristic features of AIDS-associated lymphomas, expected in only 10% to 15% of patients with de novo lymphoma, unassociated with HIV infection.[105]

Although unusual, HIV-infected patients with low-grade, B-cell lymphomas have also been described, including persons diagnosed with plasmacytomas, chronic lymphocytic leukemia, and multiple myeloma.[108–111] Such patients appear to fare reasonably well with standard approaches to management, similar to the expected course of disease in patients with de novo low-grade lymphoma.[112] A recent such case of multiple myeloma was reported, in which the monoclonal paraprotein was shown to have activity against the p24 core protein of HIV,[34] consistent with the hypothesis that the myeloma arose from the setting of chronic, specific antigenic stimulation by HIV.

IMMUNOPHENOTYPIC AND GENOTYPIC CHARACTERISTICS

Most AIDS-related lymphomas exhibit immunophenotypic evidence of B-cell lineage, including expression of CD19, CD20, and CD22 antigens, usually with monoclonal surface immunoglobulin and lack of T-cell-associated antigens.[113] Knowles and group[113] have reported that most small noncleaved lymphomas are monoclonal by surface immunophenotype, expressing immunoglobulin M (IgM), κ most commonly, whereas approximately 75% express CD10, and only 10% express CD21, the C3d EBV receptor. In contrast, a more variable isotype is expressed on the large cell and immunoblastic lymphomas, with 30% expressing CD10 and approximately two thirds expressing CD21.

Most cases demonstrate one or two immunoglobulin heavy-chain gene rearrangement bands, demonstrating the genotypic monoclonality expected in the AIDS-related lymphomas.[70, 79] One or more faint rearrangement bands may also be found, representing additional minor B-cell clones, as have been described in approximately 20% of reactive lymph nodes from HIV-infected persons.[78]

Polyclonal lymphomas have also been described at the molecular level by Shiramizu and associates,[114] who noted that approximately 40% of 40 cases of AIDS-lymphomas were polyclonal in genotype. Although multiple oligoclonal expansions have been documented before the development of monoclonal lymphoma,[79] the finding of such a high proportion of polyclonal lymphomas is most unusual, and its interpretation and significance await further confirmation.

T-CELL LYMPHOMAS

Although HIV-infected patients with various T-cell lymphomas have been reported, these cases are unusual and such conditions are not considered among the criteria for the diagnosis of AIDS. Thus, T-lymphoblastic lymphomas[115, 116]; cutaneous T-cell lymphomas[117–119]; and peripheral T-cell lymphomas[120] have been reported in HIV-infected patients. Further, human T-cell lymphotropic virus, type I (HTLV-I) associated lymphoma/leukemia has been diagnosed in several patients who were dually infected with HIV and HTLV-I.[121, 122] An HIV-infected patient with EBV-associated T-cell lymphoma confined to the oral cavity was recently reported.[123]

Ki-1–POSITIVE ANAPLASTIC LARGE CELL LYMPHOMA

Occasional cases of Ki-1–positive anaplastic lymphoma have been described in HIV-infected persons,[124] including a series of 12 cases recently reported from Italy.[125] One of these was found to be of both T-cell and B-cell origin, whereas the others were of B-lymphoid derivation. The presence of EBV DNA was detected in 10 of 12, whereas LMP-1 was found in 9 of 12. The expression of specific types of latent EBV proteins differed among the various types of AIDS-lymphoma, with similar patterns documented in patients with Ki-1–positive anaplastic lymphoma and in those with Hodgkin's disease.[125]

An additional eight cases of HIV-associated Ki-1 anaplastic lymphoma were recently reported from New York.[126] All the patients had extranodal disease, with skin involvement in four. Similar to what has been described in de novo anaplastic Ki-1–positive large cell lymphoma, four of the HIV-associated cases were of T-cell origin, one was of B-cell origin, and the remainder were indeterminate in origin. The molecular biologic characteristics of the HIV-associated cases were also similar to those described in de novo patients.[127, 128] Thus, EBV genome was found clonally expressed in two of the three cases studied, whereas c-*myc* mutations, or abnormalities of *p53* gene or p53 protein expression, were absent in all three cases so studied.[126] Likewise, both HIV and HTLV-I genomes were absent from tumor cell DNA.

The clinical, pathologic, and molecular characteristics of anaplastic large cell lymphoma thus appear identical in patients with or without underlying HIV infection. It is possible that these cases simply represent the chance occurrence of two unrelated events. However, further information is required to determine the true relationship between HIV infection and the subsequent development of Ki-1–positive anaplastic large cell lymphoma.

CLINICOPATHOLOGIC CORRELATIONS

Employing data from the CDC, which include only initial AIDS-defining diagnoses, Beral and colleagues[13] noted that small noncleaved lymphomas (Burkitt's or non-Burkitt's subtypes) were more likely to occur in younger persons (10 to 19 years of age), remaining relatively constant in incidence after the age of 30 years. In contrast, immunoblastic lymphoma became more common with increasing age.

There is some discrepancy in the data regarding the likelihood of one pathologic type of lymphoma versus another being more commonly associated with the initial AIDS-defining event. In persons with transfusion-associated HIV disease, when data from the United States were used, the mean incubation period for those with Burkitt's lymphoma was found to be 56 months, versus 49 months for those with immunoblastic lymphoma.[13] In contrast, in a series from France, where all cases of AIDS-lymphoma were available for review, Burkitt's lymphoma accounted for 46% of lymphomas occurring as the first manifestation of AIDS and for only 13% of lymphomas that developed after an earlier AIDS-defining illness.[129] These data would be consistent with the hypothesis that Burkitt's lymphoma is an earlier manifestation of the immunodeficient state induced by HIV, and that the incubation period from HIV infection to the development of lymphoma may be somewhat longer for immunoblastic lymphomas than for the small noncleaved Burkitt's type.

As suggested by these data from France, the degree of immunodeficiency at diagnosis of HIV-associated lymphoma may also vary with the pathologic type. Thus, as demonstrated in a series of 136 patients from France (including both initial AIDS-defining and subsequent AIDS-related lymphomas), the median CD4 cell count was 270 cells × 10^9/L in patients with Burkitt's lymphoma and only 99 × 10^9/L in those with immunoblastic or large cell lymphoma ($P<.01$).[129]

Aside from the degree of underlying immunodeficiency, the specific site of disease may also vary among the different pathologic types of AIDS-related lymphoma. Thus, PCNSLs are almost exclusively of the immunoblastic or large cell types[19, 64, 129] and are uniformly associated with EBV, expressing various EBV-related latent proteins.[64] In a series of 113 cases from France, in which all cases were reviewed by one group of pathologists, large cell or immunoblastic lymphomas were more likely to occur in the CNS, as well as in the gastrointestinal tract and oral cavity, whereas small noncleaved lymphomas were more likely to occur in lymph nodes, bone marrow, and muscles ($P<.0001$).[107]

The relationship between the response to therapy, survival, and pathologic type of AIDS-lymphoma is unclear at the present time. Knowles and colleagues[101] reported a survival advantage in patients with large cell lymphoma, although uniform therapy was not given in this series, and other prognostic factors for survival were not taken into account by multivariate analysis. In other prospective, multi-institutional trials, no differences in response or survival were seen among the various pathologic types of systemic AIDS-lymphoma.[111, 130] Patients with PCNSL do particularly poorly, with a median survival in the range of only 2 to 3 months; these patients are usually diagnosed with immunoblastic lymphomas. Whether the poor survival is related to the specific site of disease within the CNS or to the pathologic type of disease per se remains to be clarified. Nonetheless, patients with systemic immunoblastic lymphoma seem to fare the same as those with the other pathologic types.

CLINICAL FEATURES AT PRESENTATION

Significant systemic B symptoms are expected in most patients at the time of the initial diagnosis, often leading the physician to first consider the possibility of an occult opportunistic infection. In fact, these symptoms, including fever, drenching night sweats, and/or weight loss, may be seen in approximately 80% of patients with AIDS-related systemic lymphoma and 90% of those with disease primary to the CNS as a consequence of the lymphoma itself.[100–104] Emilie and associates[48] recently demonstrated resolution of these symptoms in a small group of patients after the administration of monoclonal antibody against IL-6.

Advanced-stage disease is expected in most patients, with extranodal involvement reported in 60% to 90% of all large series.[100–104] Once again, this would be distinct from de novo lymphoma, in which extranodal involvement has been reported in approximately 40% of newly diagnosed patients.[131] Indeed, the likelihood of disseminated disease is so great in patients with AIDS-related disease that for all practical purposes, such patients must be assumed to have extensive disease and receive treatment with multiagent chemotherapy, as opposed to local radiation.

Essentially any anatomic site may be involved with lymphoma in the setting of HIV infection. The more common sites of extranodal disease include the CNS, reported in approximately 30%; gastrointestinal tract, in approximately 25%; bone marrow, in 20% to 30%; and liver, in 9% to 26%.[100–104] Other, more unusual sites of involvement include the myocardium[132, 133]; testes[134]; rectum and anus[135–137]; oral cavity; gall bladder fossa; skeletal muscle; skin; soft tissues; earlobes; adrenals; and other organs.[100–104] Multiple sites of extranodal disease are frequently encountered.

STAGING EVALUATION

Routine staging evaluation is similar to that employed in patients with de novo lymphomas, including chest radiographs; computed tomographic (CT) scans of the chest, abdomen and pelvis; bone marrow biopsy, usually obtained from two sites; and gallium 67 scanning, expected to reveal intense uptake in the areas of lymphomatous involvement.[138] Serum lactate dehydrogenase (LDH) levels should also be determined, as elevated levels are expected in most

and may be used to monitor the response to therapy in time.[139]

In addition to these routine studies, lumbar puncture should also be obtained as part of the routine staging evaluation of patients with AIDS-related lymphoma, since asymptomatic leptomeningeal involvement has been reported in approximately 20% of newly diagnosed patients.[130] It is now common practice to administer the first dose of intrathecal chemotherapy at the time of this initial lumbar puncture, in an attempt to provide prophylactic therapy to this common site of lymphomatous relapse.

Radin and colleagues[140] recently reviewed the abdominal CT scan findings in 112 patients with newly diagnosed AIDS-related lymphoma. Evidence of intraabdominal lymphoma was seen in 64% of the group, and in 58 (98%) of 59 patients in whom the predominant symptoms of disease were related to the abdomen. Intraabdominal masses were documented in 14 (26%) of 53 patients who denied such abdominal symptoms. In patients with abdominal abnormalities on CT scan, the gastrointestinal tract was involved in 54%; liver in 29%; kidney in 11%; adrenal gland in 11%; lower genitourinary tract in 10%; spleen in 7%; peritoneum and omentum in 7%; pancreas in 5%; epidural space in 4%; bone in 3%; and muscle in 1%. Moderate or marked hepatomegaly (span >20 cm) or splenomegaly (span >15 cm) was seen only in the presence of focal hepatic lesions as well.[140]

The CT scan findings of the chest were reviewed by Sider and associates[141] in 35 patients with AIDS-related lymphoma, of whom 11 (31%) had biopsy-proven thoracic involvement. Pleural effusion, interstitial and alveolar lung disease, nodules, and/or hilar and mediastinal adenopathy were described. No predominant pattern of pulmonary parenchymal involvement was defined.[141]

PROGNOSTIC FACTORS FOR SURVIVAL

In de novo lymphoma, the prognosis is related to (1) tumor bulk, as defined by the stage, the serum LDH level, and the presence of more than one extranodal site; and (2) patient vigor, as defined by age and performance status.[142] In AIDS-related lymphoma, the prognosis appears to depend on certain of these "lymphoma-related" factors, as well as on other considerations related to the severity of underlying HIV-induced immunodeficiency.[19]

In a multivariate analysis of prognostic factors in 60 patients with newly diagnosed AIDS-lymphoma, four factors were independently associated with shorter survival: AIDS before the diagnosis of lymphoma; low CD4 cell counts as a continuous variable; a Karnofsky performance status less than 70%; and stage IV disease, as evidenced by bone marrow involvement.[19] In patients with systemic AIDS-lymphoma, the median survival was 11.3 months in those who lacked all such factors and 4.0 months in those who presented with one or more of these poor prognostic factors.[19] A similar study also defined that a history of AIDS, fewer than 200×10^9/L CD4 cells, a low performance status, and stage IV disease were associated with shorter survival in patients with AIDS-related lymphoma.[103]

Patients with PCNSL have the worst prognosis of all, with a median survival in the range of only 2 to 3 months, despite therapy.[19] These patients have evidence of profound HIV-related immunodeficiency, with a history of AIDS before the lymphoma in 73%, and median CD4 cell counts of only 30×10^9/L.[19]

In a prospective study of 116 patients with symptomatic HIV disease receiving various antiretroviral agents at the National Cancer Institute (NCI), 19% eventually developed lymphoma within a 3-year period. The only factors predictive of lymphoma were very low CD4 cell counts ($<50 \times 10^9$/L) and elevated levels of serum IL-6 at study entry, which then rose over time.[27]

Spontaneous regression of AIDS-related lymphoma has been reported, although rarely.[143, 144] In one such case, an 11×7 cm cervical mass spontaneously disappeared, with recurrence in the testes 14 months later.[143] An additional patient with isolated pulmonary involvement experienced significant regression of lymphoma after the use of zidovudine alone.[25]

TREATMENT

The optimal therapy for patients with AIDS-related lymphoma remains to be defined. However, certain progress has been made over the past decade, such that it is no longer appropriate to leave such patients untreated in the belief that no intervention is likely to be successful.

At the onset of the AIDS epidemic in the early 1980s, the use of dose-intensive regimens was common in patients with intermediate- or high-grade lymphoma, in the belief that multidrug resistance might be avoided, with greater likelihood of response.[145] Thus, building on the CHOP (cyclophosphamide, hydroxydaunomycin, Oncovin, prednisone) regimen,[146] additional combinations were designed, including M-BACOD (methotrexate, bleomycin, Adriamycin, cyclophosphamide, Oncovin, dexamethasone)[147]; ProMACE-cytaBOM (prednisone, methotrexate, Adriamycin, cyclophosphamide, etoposide; cytarabine, bleomycin, Oncovin),[148, 149]; MACOP-B[150] (methotrexate, Adriamycin, cyclophosphamide, Oncovin, prednisone, bleomycin) and others, which appeared to be associated with higher response rates, from 60% complete remission with CHOP to over 80% with MACOP-B. However, although initially promising, a large, prospective, randomized national trial subsequently demonstrated no real differences in complete remission rates, or rates of long-term disease-free survival, when the CHOP regimen was compared with MACOP-B, ProMACE-CytaBOM, or M-BACOD.[151]

With this background, it is not surprising that similar dose-intensive regimens were employed at the outset of the epidemic in patients with AIDS-related lymphoma, who were known to have extensive, bulky, high-grade disease. Unfortunately, these regimens were associated with low rates of response and high rates of complicating opportunistic infection. Thus, the COMP (CCNU, Oncovin, methotrexate, procarbazine) regimen was associated with a 28% complete remission (CR) rate in 19 patients with AIDS-related small noncleaved lymphoma,[152] whereas ProMACE-MOPP (ProMACE; mechlorethamine, Oncovin, procarbazine, prednisone) resulted in a 20% CR rate in 15 patients.[153]

A novel regimen containing high-dose cyclophosphamide and other agents resulted in a CR rate of only 33%, whereas 78% of patients developed opportunistic infections, from which they died.[154] A similar regimen, termed COMET-A (cyclophosphamide, vincristine, methotrexate, etoposide, cytosine arabinoside), yielded CR in 58% of a group of 38 patients, although the median duration of survival was only 5.2 months, which was statistically shorter than that achieved with other, less intensive "standard" regimens.[103]

In an attempt to consider the possibility that "less might be better," the national AIDS Clinical Treatment Group (ACTG) of the U.S. National Institutes of Allergy and Infectious Disease (NIAID) tested a low-dose modification of the M-BACOD regimen. In this regimen, the doses of doxorubicin (Adriamycin) and cyclophosphamide were halved, and methotrexate was given on day 15, at a dose of 500 mg/m². A total of only four cycles of therapy was administered, in contrast with the 10 cycles originally described in the M-BACOD regimen. A complete remission rate of approximately 50% was achieved in 35 evaluable patients, with durable remissions in 75%, and a median survival of 18 months in complete responders.[130] With the routine use of prophylactic intrathecal cytosine arabinoside (50 mg, given once per week × 4), no case of isolated CNS relapse was encountered. Opportunistic infections developed in 20%, consisting of PCP in all, despite the use of prophylactic therapy against *P. carinii*. No differences in the response rate or survival were documented in patients with various pathologic subtypes of disease, although those with prior AIDS, low CD4 counts, or bone marrow involvement fared less well.[130] Despite the relatively low dosages of chemotherapy employed and the shortened total treatment time, absolute granulocyte counts (AGCs) less than 1000×10^9/L developed in 60%, and 20% had AGC nadirs less than 500×10^9/L.

ADDITIONAL USE OF HEMATOPOIETIC GROWTH FACTORS

In an attempt to improve on response rates and hematologic toxicity, Walsh and associates[155] conducted a phase I/II trial of the low-dose M-BACOD regimen with the addition of granulocyte-macrophage colony-stimulating factor (GM-CSF). Sequential dose escalations of low-dose M-BACOD were found to be feasible, and full-dose M-BACOD could safely be administered under these conditions, with acceptable toxicity. Although this was not designed as an efficacy study, response rates and complicating infections appeared to be similar to those described with the low-dose M-BACOD regimen.[130, 155] Further, although in vitro data had suggested the possibility of upregulation of HIV by the GM-CSF, this finding was not observed in vivo, when measured by HIV p24 antigen levels over time.

Chemotherapy with CHOP, given with or without GM-CSF, was also evaluated by Kaplan and colleagues,[156] who began the GM-CSF either 24 hours after the completion of chemotherapy or later, given from days 4 to 13 after chemotherapy. The later institution of GM-CSF was associated with statistically higher mean nadir absolute neutrophil counts, as well as fewer days in the hospital and fewer chemotherapy cycles complicated by neutropenia and fever.[156] Serum HIV p24 antigen levels fell after the first week of chemotherapy in the GM-CSF–treated patients, with a transient increase in p24 antigen at week 3, which was not observed in the subjects treated with CHOP alone. The clinical significance of this finding could not be determined.

ADDITION OF ANTIRETROVIRAL AGENTS

With the continued development of opportunistic infections despite the use of hematopoietic growth factors, and with the understanding that HIV per se may be indirectly involved in the pathogenesis of AIDS-related lymphoma, the addition of antiretroviral agents to multiagent chemotherapy appeared reasonable. However, the addition of zidovudine, itself myelosuppressive, was found to be ineffective and associated with severe myelosuppression when tested in a group of 37 patients with poor-prognosis AIDS-lymphoma.[157] Thus, only 57% of patients actually received any zidovudine during the trial, and only 12 (32%) were actually able to complete a full course of combined chemotherapy and antiretroviral therapy. Opportunistic infections occurred in 43% of those receiving zidovudine and in 31% of those who did not. The complete remission rate was only 14%, and the median survival for the group was 3.5 months.

The addition of ddC to the low-dose M-BACOD regimen was tested by Levine and colleagues[158] in a phase I/II trial administered to 28 patients. Because of the known neurotoxicity of both ddC and vincristine, the latter was initially withheld and then added in escalating doses to successive cohorts of patients. Only minimal (grades 1 and 2) neurotoxicity was documented, occurring in two patients who had not received vincristine. Bone marrow toxicity was also relatively mild, with 15% of patients experiencing nadir granulocyte counts less than 500/mm^3, and with only four patients requiring the addition of hematopoietic growth factor support (granulocyte colony-stimulating factor [G-CSF]). Opportunistic infections occurred in 11%. The complete remission rate was 56%, with durable remissions in 75%. The median survival of complete responders was 18 months. CR rates were equivalent in patients with poor prognostic indicators of disease, including a history of AIDS (CR of 50%); CD4 cells less than 200/mm^3 (CR of 47%); and bone marrow involvement.[158] It is apparent, then, that additional study of the combined use of antiretroviral agents with combination chemotherapy is indicated, provided that less marrow toxic antiretroviral agents are employed.

USE OF CHEMOTHERAPY BY ALTERNATIVE ROUTES OF ADMINISTRATION

An oral regimen for the treatment of AIDS-related lymphoma was recently studied by Remick and associates[159] in 18 patients, of whom 27% had a history of AIDS-defining opportunistic infection, and the median CD4 cell count was 73 × 10^9/L. The regimen consisted of CCNU (100 mg/m^2 on day 1); etoposide (200 mg/m^2, days 1 to 3); cyclophosphamide (100 mg/m^2, days 22 to 31); and procarbazine (100 mg/m^2, days 22 to 31). A complete remission rate of 39% was achieved; the median duration of the CR was 7 months, and the median survival of complete responders was 15 months. Grade 3 or 4 neutropenia occurred in 64% of cycles, whereas opportunistic infections developed in 11%. Therapy-related

death occurred in 11%, and treatment was discontinued secondary to toxicity in 40%. Only one patient completed all five planned cycles of therapy.[159]

Infusional therapy has also been employed, with early evidence of efficacy. Thus, Sparano and associates[160] studied the use of a 4-day continuous infusion of cyclophosphamide (750 mg/m^2), doxorubicin (50 mg/m^2), and etoposide (240 mg/m^2). These doses represent the full amounts of drugs administered over the 4-day period. The regimen was repeated every 28 days, for a total of six cycles. Twelve patients were initially reported, with a recent update including a total of 21 patients.[160] Complete remission was achieved in 62%, with a median survival of 18 months. Severe neutropenia (<500/mm^3) occurred in 38% of the cycles. Dose reduction for toxicity was required in 47% of the cycles and for 79% of the patients who received at least two cycles of therapy. Fourteen episodes of opportunistic infection occurred, and death resulted in one patient with disseminated aspergillosis.[160]

USE OF DOSE-INTENSIVE REGIMENS

Various regimens of dose-intensive chemotherapy have been employed, primarily in patients with good-prognosis AIDS-lymphoma. Thus, Bermudez and associates[161] used the MACOP-B regimen in 12 patients, half of whom had intermediate-grade lymphoma. A complete remission rate of 67% was achieved, with a median survival of 7 months. Five of the eight complete responders had Karnofsky performance scores of 100%, without a history of prior AIDS.

Gisselbrecht and colleagues[162] employed the intensive LNH-84 regimen in 141 patients with good-prognosis AIDS-lymphoma, as evidenced by excellent performance status, no history of prior opportunistic infections, and relatively high CD4 cell counts (median of 227 × 10^9/L). A complete response rate of 63% was documented, with a median survival of 9 months. Drug dosages were given as planned in 80% of the patients, although 70% experienced treatment delays secondary to bone marrow suppression, which reduced the relative dose intensity actually administered. Factors that were independently associated with shorter survival included CD4 cell counts less than 100 × 10^9/L; a performance status of 3 or 4; an immunoblastic pathologic type; and a history of AIDS before the lymphoma, present in 9%. In the absence of all such factors, the median survival was 2 years.[162]

It is evident from these data that patients with good-prognosis AIDS-related lymphoma may be able to tolerate various dose-intensive regimens of combination chemotherapy. However, the real issue has been whether dose-intensive regimens actually confer an advantage in terms of response or survival. To address this issue, a large, prospective randomized trial has recently been completed through the ACTG of the National Institutes of Allergy and Infectious Disease.[163] A total of 192 patients were stratified by prognostic characteristics and then randomized to receive either low-dose M-BACOD[130] or standard-dose M-BACOD with GM-CSF.[155] CR rates were equivalent, at approximately 50%. Median time to recurrence following complete response was 106 weeks for the standard dose and in excess of 190 weeks for the low-dose group (*P* = .06). Median survival time was 35 weeks for patients receiving low-dose therapy and 31 weeks for patients who received standard-dose therapy (*P* = ns). Grade 3 or higher chemotherapy toxicity occurred in 66 (70%) of 94 patients assigned to standard-dose therapy and in 50 (51%) of 98 patients assigned to low-dose treatment (*P* = .008). These results were similar in patients with good-prognostic and poor-prognostic disease. It is thus apparent from this large, randomized trial that low-dose chemotherapy is associated with significantly less toxicity and similar response rates and survival time when compared with standard-dose therapy with adjunctive colony-stimulating factor (CSF) support.[163]

USE OF BIOLOGIC AGENTS

Various biologic agents have recently been employed in patients with AIDS-related lymphoma, and their use is expected to increase. One such approach involves an attempt to block the effects of IL-6, important in the pathogenesis of disease. In this regard, retinoic acid has been shown to downregulate IL-6 receptors and to inhibit IL-6–mediated autocrine growth stimulation in multiple myeloma.[164] IL-4 has also been shown capable of downregulating IL-6 production.[165] Such agents are currently under study in patients with refractory AIDS-lymphoma.

Monoclonal antibodies represent another avenue by which IL-6 binding or signaling may be blocked. In this regard, Emilie and colleagues[48] have employed a monoclonal antibody against IL-6 in 10 patients with AIDS-related lymphoma. Stabilization of disease was seen in four, with disappearance of systemic B symptoms in all. However, no patient experienced a tumor response. Conjugation of IL-6 to a mutant *Pseudomonas* exotoxin (IL-6–PE-4E) has been performed by Kreitman and colleagues,[166] producing an immunotoxin molecule that was shown to be cytotoxic to myeloma cells, while sparing normal hematopoietic cells. Such an approach would also appear warranted in patients with AIDS-related lymphoma.

A B4 (anti-CD19) blocked ricin has been generated by conjugating the potent toxin ricin to a mouse-derived IgG1 monoclonal antibody directed against the CD19 antigen on normal and malignant B lymphocytes.[167] This immunotoxin has been administered to nine patients with refractory or relapsed AIDS-lymphoma,[168] in a dose-escalating, phase I trial. No significant toxicity has been encountered at doses of 5, 10, and 20 µg/kg, given by continuous infusion over 28 days. Responses have been documented in 22%, including the complete remission of a large rectal mass in one and a partial remission of hepatic disease in a second individual. The development of human antimouse antibody (HAMA) and human antiricin antibody (HARA) occurred in three persons.[168]

With evidence of efficacy in patients with refractory disease, Scadden and colleagues[169] have employed B4-blocked ricin, given by continuous infusion over 7 days, together with the low-dose M-BACOD regimen, in a phase I/II study. The immunotoxin was administered during cycles 3 and 4 in those patients achieving complete or partial remission after two cycles of low-dose M-BACOD alone. The maximally tolerated dose of B4-blocked ricin appears to be 20 µg/kg in this setting. In 18 evaluable patients to date, a CR rate of 67% was achieved after the low-dose M-BACOD. The precise efficacy of B4-blocked ricin could

not yet be assessed, although toxicity appeared acceptable. Four patients developed either HAMA and/or HARA responses.

PRIMARY CENTRAL NERVOUS SYSTEM LYMPHOMA

Lymphoma primary to the CNS (PCNSL) was considered an AIDS-defining diagnosis from the outset of the epidemic. The precise number of such cases is unknown, since most affected patients have had another AIDS-defining diagnosis before the PCNSL and would thus be unknown in a statistical sense to the CDC.[13, 19] It is believed, however, that the incidence of AIDS-related PCNSL is increasing significantly, as patients with far-advanced HIV disease live long enough to develop this complication.

Patients with AIDS-related PCNSL tend to be quite frail, with a history of AIDS before the lymphoma in approximately 73%, and a median CD4 cell count of only 30/mm[3].[19] Indeed, in the large series of 116 patients with symptomatic HIV disease followed by Pluda and associates[27] at the NCI, the median CD4 cell count at diagnosis of lymphoma was only 6/mm[3].

Most patients with AIDS-related PCNSL are diagnosed with either immunoblastic or large cell lymphoma, similar to the situation in patients with de novo PCNSL.[19, 64, 107, 170] However, approximately 25% of AIDS-related cases have been diagnosed with small noncleaved lymphoma, which is distinctly unusual in patients without underlying HIV infection, occurring in less than 5% of cases.[170] Another characteristic of AIDS-related PCNSL is the almost universal association with EBV, with expression of EBV-related latent proteins in 21 of 21 such cases studied by MacMahon and colleagues.[64] In this study, the EBV EBER was found by in situ hybridization in 100% of cases, whereas the EBV LMP-1 was detected in 45%. Although 14 cases of de novo PCNSL were similar in terms of the pathologic type of lymphoma, EBV-related proteins were detected in only one such case (7%), indicating that the biology of AIDS-associated PCNSL is distinct. Meeker and associates[171] have also described the uniform presence of the EBV genome in five cases of AIDS-related PCNSL.

Patients with AIDS-related PCNSL usually present with mass lesions in the brain, as opposed to primary leptomeningeal involvement. The masses are usually relatively large (3 to 4 cm) and may be multifocal in approximately half.[172, 173] In the latter cases, approximately two to three mass lesions are expected. Ring enhancement may be seen, similar to the case with cerebral toxoplasmosis; of interest, ring enhancement is not expected in patients with de novo PCNSL.[170]

A patient with PCNSL may be evaluated by either CT scan or magnetic resonance imaging (MRI) techniques, although the MRI scan may be more sensitive and more helpful in distinguishing PCNSL from other pathologic processes.[173] Lumbar puncture may also be helpful in establishing a diagnosis of PCNSL, if the procedure is not clinically contraindicated. Malignant cells may be found in the cerebrospinal fluid in approximately 25% of patients with AIDS-related PCNSL and if present may obviate the need for brain biopsy. In the absence of diagnostic material from the CSF, definitive diagnosis may be made only by brain biopsy.[174] Unfortunately, many such patients never actually undergo biopsy, because of the unjustified fear of potential contagion to operating room personnel[175] or in the belief that treatment would be ineffective and precise diagnosis therefore not necessary.[174] It is currently common practice to begin empiric therapy for cerebral toxoplasmosis in HIV-infected patients with mass lesions within the brain; CT or MRI scans are repeated in 1 to 2 weeks. If definite improvement is documented, the patient is assumed to have toxoplasmosis and therapy is continued. With no improvement on repeat scans, brain biopsy should be performed for definitive diagnosis and treatment. PCNSL is often the underlying diagnosis in such cases.

Like de novo PCNSL, AIDS-related PCNSL may involve any site within the brain.[170, 176] In fact, autopsy series have demonstrated that such lymphomas are universally multicentric.[177] The more common sites of antemortem involvement include the cerebrum, cerebellum, and brain stem.[177] Approximately 75% are located adjacent to ventricular surfaces or cortical convexities, with subsequent propensity to spread along pathways of cerebrospinal fluid flow.[170]

Symptoms of PCNSL include focal neurologic deficits, dependent on the precise areas of anatomic involvement within the brain. Seizures occur in approximately 25%,[170, 178] and headaches are also fairly common. Although usually of dramatic onset, altered mental status may be the only presenting complaint and may be extremely subtle in degree, such as a change in personality or behavior. Confusion, lethargy, and/or memory loss have also been described.[177, 178] The incidence of these changes in mental status differs among patients with AIDS-related versus de novo disease, occurring in approximately 50% of the former and 35% of the latter group.[170]

The optimal therapy for patients with AIDS-related PCNSL remains to be defined. In de novo PCNSL, whole-brain radiation therapy is expected to result in complete remission in approximately 90%, although disease-free survival is usually in the range of 18 months.[170, 179] Recently, systemic chemotherapy has been used before radiation, in an attempt to improve this long-term outcome. Early results are quite promising, with a median survival of approximately 4 years.[180] Although potentially efficacious, the use of systemic chemotherapy in patients with AIDS-related disease may be quite problematic, owing to the inherent immunosuppression of chemotherapy per se in these frail patients with far-advanced HIV disease.

The use of cranial radiation in patients with AIDS-related PCNSL has resulted in complete remission in approximately 20% to 50%.[181–184] Unfortunately, the median survival has been only in the range of 2 to 3 months, with death often caused by opportunistic infections. If the disease is left untreated, the median survival is approximately the same, with death often due to lymphoma.[185] It is important to realize, however, that radiation therapy has been associated with significant improvement in the quality of survival in approximately 75% of treated persons, indicating a definite role for such therapy, even if used solely for palliation of symptoms.[183]

National protocols have recently been activated that seek to explore the role of short courses of systemic chemotherapy given before whole-brain radiation in patients with AIDS-related PCNSL. The results of these studies are awaited with interest and are of great importance since the incidence of PCNSL is expected to increase substantially as survival in HIV disease is prolonged.

SUMMARY

AIDS-related lymphoma represents a late manifestation of HIV infection, occurring in the setting of significant immunocompromise. All groups at risk for HIV infection appear to be at similar risk for the development of AIDS-lymphoma. The lymphomatous disease is usually widespread at initial diagnosis, involving one or more extranodal sites, including the CNS, bone marrow, gastrointestinal tract, and other areas. PCNSL may occur, presenting as space-occupying lesion(s) within the brain, which must be differentiated by biopsy from cerebral toxoplasmosis or other pathologic processes. Although radiation therapy may improve the quality of survival in patients with PCNSL, no intervention has yet been shown to improve the overall median survival, which has been in the range of approximately 2 to 3 months. In patients with systemic AIDS-related lymphoma, low-dose chemotherapy, or infusional chemotherapy with CNS prophylaxis, may result in complete remission in approximately 50% to 60% of persons; these remissions are durable in most patients. The pathogenesis of AIDS-related lymphoma is complex and still not fully understood. The HIV may be indirectly operative, by inducing chronic B-cell proliferation and stimulation itself, or via release of IL-6, IL-10, and other cytokines from infected mononuclear cells. EBV may also participate in this ongoing B-cell proliferation. In the setting of such B-cell activity, genetic errors may occur, leading to activation of the c-*myc* oncogene, with *p53* tumor suppressor gene abnormalities, as documented in the small noncleaved lymphomas. The monoclonal presence of EBV within immunoblastic and other large cell lymphomas may implicate this virus in the pathogenesis of these types of lymphoma, whereas activation of the *BCL6* oncogene may be operative in the pathogenesis of diffuse large cell lymphomas seen in the setting of AIDS.

REFERENCES

1. Frizzera G, Rosai J, Dehner LP, et al: Lymphoreticular disorders in primary immunodeficiency: New findings based on an updated histologic classification of 35 cases. Cancer 1980; 46:692.
2. Penn I: Tumors of the immunocompromised patient. Annu Rev Med 1988; 39:63.
3. Purtilo DT: Opportunistic non-Hodgkin's lymphoma in X-linked recessive immunodeficiency and lymphoproliferative syndromes. Semin Oncol 1977; 4:335.
4. Zulman J, Jaffe R, Talal N: Evidence that the malignant lymphoma of Sjögren's syndrome is a monoclonal B cell neoplasm. N Engl J Med 1978; 299:1215.
5. Anderson LG, Talal N: The spectrum of benign to malignant lymphoproliferation in Sjögren's syndrome. Clin Exp Immunol 1972; 10:199.
6. Burke JS, Butler JJ, Fuller LM: Malignant lymphomas of the thyroid: A clinical-pathologic study of 35 patients including ultrastructural observations. Cancer 1977; 39:1587.
7. Levine AM, Taylor CR, Schneider DR, et al: Immunoblastic sarcoma of T cell versus B cell origin: I. Clinical features. Blood 1981; 58:52.

8. Penn I: Cancers complicating organ transplantation. N Engl J Med 1990; 323:1767.

9. Swinnen LJ, Costanzo-Nordin MR, Fisher SG, et al: Increased incidence of lymphoproliferative disorder after immunosuppression with the monoclonal antibody OKT3 in cardiac transplant recipients. N Engl J Med 1990; 323:1723.

10. Centers for Disease Control: Diffuse, undifferentiated non-Hodgkin's lymphoma among homosexual males—United States. MMWR Morb Mortal Wkly Rep 1982; 31:277.

11. Centers for Disease Control: Update on acquired immune deficiency syndrome (AIDS)—United States. MMWR Morb Mortal Wkly Rep 1982; 31:507.

12. Centers for Disease Control: Revision of the case definition of acquired immunodeficiency syndrome for national reporting—United States. Ann Intern Med 1985; 103:402.

13. Beral V, Peterman T, Berkelman R, Jaffe H: AIDS-associated non-Hodgkin lymphoma. Lancet 1991; 337:805.

14. Levine AM: Lymphoma complicating immunodeficiency disorders. Ann Oncol 1994; 4(Suppl 2):S29.

15. DeVesa SS, Fears T: Non-Hodgkin's lymphoma time trends: U.S. and international data. Cancer Res 1992; 52:5432.

16. Rabkin CS, Biggar RJ, Horm JW: Increasing incidence of cancers associated with the human immunodeficiency virus epidemic. Int J Cancer 1991; 47:692.

17. Biggar RJ, Rabkin CS: The epidemiology of acquired immuno-deficiency syndrome–related lymphomas. Curr Opin Oncol 1992; 4:883.

18. Serraino D, Salamina G, Franceschi S, et al: The epidemiology of AIDS-associated non-Hodgkin's lymphoma in the World Health Organization European Region. Br J Cancer 1992; 66:912.

19. Levine AM, Sullivan-Halley J, Pike MC, et al: HIV-related lymphoma: Prognostic factors predictive of survival. Cancer 1991; 68:2466.

20. Peters BS, Beck EJ, Coleman DG, et al: Changing disease patterns in patients with AIDS in a referral center in the United Kingdom: The changing face of AIDS. Br Med J 1991; 302:203.

21. Jaffe HW, Choi K, Thomas PA, et al: National case-control study of Kaposi's sarcoma and *Pneumocystis carinii* pneumonia in homosexual men: I. Epidemiologic results. Ann Intern Med 1983; 99:145.

22. Monfardini S, Vaccher E, Tirelli U: AIDS associated non-Hodgkin's lymphoma in Italy: Intravenous drug users versus homosexual men. Ann Oncol 1990; 1:208.

23. Ragni MV, Belle SH, Jaffe RA, et al: Acquired immunodeficiency syndrome–associated non-Hodgkin's lymphomas and other malignan-cies in patients with hemophilia. Blood 1993; 81:1889.

24. Moore RD, Kessler H, Richman DD, et al: Non-Hodgkin's lymphoma in patients with advanced HIV infection treated with zidovudine. JAMA 1991; 265:2208.

25. Baselga J, Krown SE, Telzak EE, et al: AIDS-related pulmonary NHL regressing after zidovudine therapy. Cancer 1993; 71:2332.

26. D'Arminio Monforte A, Vago L, Mainini F: Primitive cerebral lymphoma and systemic lymphomas in 637 autopsies from AIDS cases. The Eighth International Conference on AIDS, Amsterdam, 1992.

27. Pluda JM, Venzon DJ, Tosato G, et al: Parameters affecting the development of non-Hodgkin's lymphoma in patients with severe human immunodeficiency virus infection receiving antiretroviral therapy. J Clin Oncol 1993; 11:1099.

28. National Toxicology Program: Subchronic toxicity study of 2′,3′-dideoxycytidine (ddC) in female B6C3F1 mice. Research Triangle Park, NC; National Institute of Health Sciences, National Toxicology Program, 1993.

29. Levine AM, Bernstein L, Sullivan-Halley J, et al: Role of zidovudine antiretroviral therapy in the pathogenesis of acquired immunodefi-ciency syndrome–related lymphoma. Blood 1995; 86:4612.

30. Ross R, Dworsky R, Paganini-Hill A, et al: Non-Hodgkin's lymphomas in never married men in Los Angeles. Br J Cancer 1985; 52:785.

31. Pluda JM, Yarchoan R, Jaffe ES, et al: Development of non-Hodgkin's lymphoma in a cohort of patients with severe human immunodefi-ciency virus (HIV) infection on long-term antiretroviral therapy. Ann Intern Med 1990; 113:276.

32. Pantaleo G, Graziosi C, Fauci AS: Mechanisms of disease: The immunopathogenesis of human immunodeficiency virus infection. N Engl J Med 1993; 328:327.

33. Schnittman SM, Lane HC, Higgins SE, et al: Direct polyclonal activation of human B lymphocytes by the AIDS virus. Science 1986; 233:1084.

34. Konrad RJ, Kricka LJ, Goodman DBP, et al: Myeloma-associated paraprotein directed against the HIV-1 p24 antigen in an HIV-1 seropositive patient. N Engl J Med 1993; 328:1817.

35. Berberian L, Valles-Ayoub Y, Sun N, et al: A V_H clonal deficit in human immunodeficiency virus–positive individuals reflects a B-cell matura-tional arrest. Blood 1991; 78:175.

36. Karp J: Overview of AIDS-related lymphomas: A paradigm of AIDS malignancies. *In* Broder S, Merigan TC Jr, Bolognesi D (eds): Textbook of AIDS Medicine. Baltimore, Williams & Wilkins, 1994, p 415.

37. Paul WE: Interleukin 4/B cell stimulatory factor 1: One lymphokine, many functions. FASEB J 1987; 1:456.

38. Jelinek DF, Lipsky PE: Enhancement of human B cell proliferation and differentiation by tumor necrosis factor-alpha and interleukin 1. J Immunol 1987; 139:2970.

39. Jelinek DF, Splawski JB, Lipsky PE: The roles of interleukin-2 and interferon-gamma in human B cell activation, growth, and differen-tiation. Eur J Immunol 1986; 16:925.

40. Hirano T, Yasukawa K, Harada H, et al: Complementary DNA for a novel human interleukin (BSF-2) that induces B lymphocytes to produce immunoglobulin. Nature 1986; 324:73.

41. Saeland S, Duvert V, Pandrau D, et al: Interleukin-7 induces the proliferation of normal human B cell precursors. Blood 1991; 78:2229.

42. Zlotnik A, Morre KW: Interleukin 10. Cytokine 1991; 3:366.

43. Fauci A, Schnittman SM, Poli G, et al: Immunopathogenetic mechanisms in human immunodeficiency virus (HIV) infection. Ann Intern Med 1991; 114:678.

44. Kawano M, Hirano T, Matsuda T, et al: Autocrine generation and requirement of BSF-2/IL-6 for human multiple myelomas. Nature 1988; 332:83.

45. Biondi A, Rossi V, Bassan R, et al: Constitutive expression of IL-6 gene in chronic lymphocytic leukemia. Blood 1989; 73:1279.

46. Yoshizaki K, Matsuda T, Nishimoto N, et al: Pathogenic significance of IL-6 (IL-6/BSF-2) in Castleman's disease. Blood 1989; 74:1360.

47. Emilie D, Coumbaras J, Raphael M, et al: Interleukin-6 production in high-grade B lymphomas: Correlation with the presence of malignant immunoblasts in acquired immunodeficiency syndrome and in human immunodeficiency virus–seronegative patients. Blood 1992; 80:498.

48. Emilie D, Marfaing A, Merrien D, et al: Treatment of AIDS-lymphomas with an anti-IL-6 monoclonal antibody. Blood 1993; 82:387a.

49. Moore KW, Vieria P, Fiorentino DF, et al: Homology of cytokine synthesis inhibitory factor (IL-10) to the Epstein-Barr virus gene (BCRF). Science 1990; 248:1230.

50. Fiorentino DF, Bond MW, Mossmann TR: Two types of mouse helper T cells: IV. Th2 clones secrete a factor that inhibits cytokine production by Th1 clones. J Exp Med 1989; 170:2081.

51. Benjamin D, Knobloch TJ, Dayton MA: Human B cell interleukin-10: B cell lines derived from patients with acquired immunodeficiency syndrome and Burkitt's lymphoma constitutively secrete large quan-tities of interleukin-10. Blood 1992; 80:1289.

52. Masood R, Bond M, Scadden D, et al: Interleukin-10: An autocrine B cell growth for human B-cell lymphoma and their progenitors [Abstract]. Blood 1992; 80:115.

53. Birx DI, Redfield RR, Tosato G: Defective regulation of Epstein-Barr virus infection in patients with acquired immunodeficiency syndrome (AIDS) or AIDS-related disorders. N Engl J Med 1986; 314:874.

54. Lindahl T, Klein G, Reedman BM, et al: Relationship between Epstein-Barr virus DNA and the EBV determines nuclear antigen (EBNA) in Burkitt lymphoma biopsies and other lymphoproliferative malignancies. Int J Cancer 1974; 13:764.

55. Geser A, DeThe G, Lenoir G, et al: Final case reporting from the Uganda prospective study of the relationship between EBV and lymphoma. Int J Cancer 1982; 29:397.

56. Purtilo DT: Opportunistic non-Hodgkin's lymphoma in X-linked recessive immunodeficiency and lymphoproliferative syndromes. Semin Oncol 1977; 4:335.

57. Gregory CD, Dive C, Henderson S, et al: Activation of Epstein-Barr virus latent genes protects human B cells from death by apoptosis. Nature 1991; 349:612.

58. Wang D, Liebowitz D, Kieff E: An EBV membrane protein expressed in immortalized lymphocytes transforms established rodent cells. Cell 1985; 43:831.

59. Calender A, Cordier M, Billaud M, Lenoir GM: Modulation of cellular gene expression in B lymphoma cells following in vitro infection by Epstein-Barr virus (EBV). Int J Cancer 1990; 46:658.

60. Gregory CD, Murray RJ, Edwards CF, Rickinson AB: Downregulation of cell adhesion molecules LFA-3 and ICAM-1 in Epstein-Barr virus–positive Burkitt's lymphoma underlies tumor cell escape from virus-specific T cell surveillance. J Exp Med 1988; 167:1811.

61. Luka J, Jornvall H, Klein G: Purification and biochemical characterization of the Epstein-Barr virus–determined nuclear antigen and an associated protein with a 53,000-dalton subunit. J Virol 1980; 35:2.

62. Werness BA, Levine AJ, Howley PM: Association of human papillomavirus types 16 and 18 E6 proteins with p53. Science 1990; 248:76.

63. Shibata D, Weiss LM, Nathwani BN, et al: Epstein-Barr virus in benign lymph node biopsies from individuals infected with the human immunodeficiency virus is associated with concurrent or subsequent development of non-Hodgkin's lymphoma. Blood 1991; 77:1527.

64. MacMahon EME, Glass JD, Hayward SD, et al: Epstein-Barr virus in AIDS-related primary central nervous system lymphoma. Lancet 1991; 338:969.

65. Subar M, Neri A, Inghirami G, et al: Frequent c-myc oncogene activation and infrequent presence of Epstein-Barr virus genome in AIDS-associated lymphoma. Blood 1988; 72:667.

66. Hamilton-Dutoit SJ, Pallesen G, Franzmann MB, et al: AIDS-related lymphoma: Histopathology, immunophenotype, and association with Epstein-Barr virus as demonstrated by in situ nucleic acid hybridization. Am J Pathol 1991; 138:149.

67. Pederson C, Gerstoft J, Luundgren JD, et al: HIV-associated lymphoma: Histopathology and association with Epstein-Barr virus genome related to clinical, immunological, and prognostic features. Eur J Cancer 1991; 27:1416.

68. Ballerini P, Gaidano G, Gong JZ, et al: Molecular pathogenesis of HIV-associated lymphomas. AIDS Res Hum Retroviruses 1992; 8:731.

69. Hamilton-Dutoit SJ, Raphael M, Audouin J, et al: In situ demonstration of Epstein-Barr virus small RNAs (EBER 1) in acquired immunodeficiency syndrome–related lymphomas: Correlation with tumor morphology and primary site. Blood 1993; 82:619.

70. Shibata D, Weiss LM, Hernandez AM, et al: Epstein-Barr virus–associated non-Hodgkin's lymphoma in patients infected with the human immunodeficiency virus. Blood 1993; 81:2102.

71. Neri A, Barriga F, Inghirami G, et al: Epstein-Barr virus infection precedes clonal expansion in Burkitt's and acquired immunodeficiency–associated lymphoma. Blood 1991; 77:1092.

72. Ames BN, Gold LS: Too many rodent carcinogens: Mitogenesis increases mutagenesis. Science 1990; 249:970.

73. Zech I, Haglund U, Nilsson K, Klein G: Characteristic chromosomal abnormalities in biopsies and lymphoid cell lines from patients with Burkitt and non-Burkitt lymphomas. Int J Cancer 1976; 17:47.

74. Berger R, Bernheim A, Bertrand S, et al: Variant chromosomal t(8;22) translocation in four French cases with Burkitt lymphoma-leukemia. Nouv Rev Fr Hematol 1981; 23:39.

75. Chaganti RSK, Jhanwar SC, Koziner B, et al: Specific translocations characterize Burkitt's-like lymphoma of homosexual men with the acquired immunodeficiency syndrome. Blood 1983; 61:1269.

76. Peterson JM, Tubbs RR, Savage RA, et al: Small noncleaved B cell Burkitt-like lymphoma with chromosome t(8;14) translocation and Epstein Barr virus nuclear associated antigen in a homosexual man with acquired immunodeficiency syndrome. Am J Med 1985; 78:141.

77. Groopman JE, Sullivan JL, Mulder C, et al: Pathogenesis of B-cell lymphoma in a patient with AIDS. Blood 1986; 67:612.

78. Alonso ML, Richardson ME, Metroka CE, et al: Chromosome abnormalities in AIDS-associated lymphadenopathy. Blood 1987; 69:855.

79. Pelicci PG, Knowles DM II, Arlin ZA, et al: Multiple monoclonal B cell expansions and c-myc oncogene rearrangements in acquired immune deficiency syndrome–related lymphoproliferative disorders: Implications for lymphomagenesis. J Exp Med 1986; 164:2049.

80. Levine AM, Gill PS, Krailo M, et al: Natural history of persistent generalized lymphadenopathy (PGL) in gay men: Risk of lymphoma and factors associated with development of lymphoma. Blood 1986; 68:130a.

81. Shiramizu B, Barriga F, Neequaye I, et al: Patterns of chromosomal breakpoint locations in Burkitt's lymphoma: Relevance to geography and Epstein-Barr virus association. Blood 1991; 77:1516.

82. Ladanyi M, Offitt K, Jhanwar SC, et al: MYC rearrangement and translocations involving band 8q24 in diffuse large cell lymphomas. Blood 1991; 7:1057.

83. Klein G: Multiple phenotypic consequences of the Ig/Myc translocation in B-cell-derived tumors. Genes Chromosomes Cancer 1989; 1:3.

84. Gauwerky CE, Croce CM: Molecular biology of leukemias and lymphomas. In Broder S (ed): Molecular Foundations of Oncology. Baltimore, Williams & Wilkins, 1991, pp 295–310.

85. Ballerini P, Gaidano G, Gong JZ, et al: Multiple genetic lesions in AIDS-related non-Hodgkin's lymphoma. Blood 1993; 81:166.

86. Delecluse HJ, Raphael M, Magaud JP, Felman P: Variable morphology of human immunodeficiency virus–associated lymphomas with c-myc rearrangements. Blood 1993; 82:552.

87. Haluska FG, Russo G, Kant J, et al: Molecular resemblance of an AIDS-associated lymphoma and endemic Burkitt lymphomas: Implications for their pathogenesis. Proc Natl Acad Sci U S A 1989; 86:8907.

88. Lombardi L, Newcomb EW, Dalla-Favera R: Pathogenesis of Burkitt lymphoma: Expression of an activated c-myc oncogene causes the tumorigenic conversion of EBV infected human B lymphoblasts. Cell 1987; 46:161.

89. Adams JM, Harris AW, Pinkert CA, et al: The c-myc oncogene driven by immunoglobulin enhancers induces lymphoid malignancy in transgenic mice. Nature 1985; 318:553.

90. Laurence J, Astrin SM: Human immunodeficiency virus induction of malignant transformation in human B lymphocytes. Proc Natl Acad Sci U S A 1991; 88:7635.

91. Pauza CD, Galindo J, Richman DD: Human immunodeficiency virus infection of monoblastoid cells: Cellular differentiation determines the pattern of virus replication. J Virol 1988; 62:3558.

92. Ye BH, Lista F, Lo Coco F, Knowles DM, et al: Alterations of a zinc finger–encoding gene, BCL-6, in diffuse large cell lymphoma. Science 1993; 262:747.

93. Lo Coco F, Ye BH, Lista F, et al: Rearrangements of the BCL-6 gene in diffuse large cell non-Hodgkin's lymphoma. Blood 1994; 83:1757.

94. Gaidano G, LoCoco F, Ye BH, et al: Rearrangement of the Bcl-6 gene in AIDS-associated non-Hodgkin's lymphoma: Association with diffuse large cell type. Blood 1994; 84:397.

95. Athan E, Foitl DR, Knowles DM: Bcl-1 gene rearrangement: Frequency and clinical significance among B cell chronic lymphocytic leukemias and non-Hodgkin's lymphomas. Am J Pathol 1991; 138:591.

96. Gaidano G, Ballerini P, Gong JZ, et al: p53 mutations in human lymphoid malignancies: Association with Burkitt lymphoma and chronic lymphocytic leukemia. Proc Natl Acad Sci U S A 1991; 88:5413.

97. Cesarman E, Chadburn A, Inghirami G, et al: Structural and functional analysis of oncogenes and tumor suppressor genes in adult T cell leukemia/lymphoma (ATLL) reveals frequent p53 mutations. Blood 1992; 80:3205.

98. Dryja TP, Rapaport JM, Joyce JM, Peterson RA: Molecular detection of deletions involving band q14 of chromosome 13 in retinoblastoma. Proc Natl Acad Sci U S A 1986; 83:7391.

99. NCI Non-Hodgkin's Lymphoma Classification Project Writing Committee: Classification of non-Hodgkin's lymphomas: Reproducibility of major classification systems. Cancer 1985; 55:91.

100. Levine AM, Gill PS, Meyer PR, et al: Retrovirus and malignant lymphoma in homosexual men. JAMA 1985; 254:1921.

101. Knowles DM, Chamulak GA, Subar M, et al: Lymphoid neoplasia associated with the acquired immunodeficiency syndrome (AIDS): The New York University experience. Ann Intern Med 1988; 108:744.

102. Lowenthal DA, Straus DJ, Campbell SW, et al: AIDS-related lymphoid neoplasia: The Memorial Hospital experience. Cancer 1988; 61:2325.

103. Kaplan LD, Abrams DI, Feigal E, et al: AIDS-associated non-Hodgkin's lymphoma in San Francisco. JAMA 1989; 261:719.

104. Ziegler JL, Beckstead JA, Volberding PA, et al: Non-Hodgkin's lymphoma in 90 homosexual men: Relation to generalized lymphadenopathy and the acquired immunodeficiency syndrome. N Engl J Med 1984; 311:565.

105. Lukes RJ, Parker JW, Taylor CR, et al: Immunologic approach to non-Hodgkin's lymphomas and related leukemias: Analysis of the results of multiparameter studies of 425 cases. Semin Hematol 1978; 15:322.

106. Centers for Disease Control: Revision of the CDC surveillance case definition for acquired immunodeficiency syndrome. MMWR Morb Mortal Wkly Rep 1987; 36(Suppl):1S.

107. Raphael J, Gentihomme O, Tulliez M, et al: Histopathologic features of high-grade non-Hodgkin's lymphomas in acquired immunodeficiency syndrome. Arch Pathol Lab Med 1991; 115:15.

108. Carbone A, Tirelli U, Vaccher E, et al: A clinicopathologic study of lymphoid neoplasms associated with human immunodeficiency virus infection in Italy. Cancer 1991; 68:842.

109. Ioachim HL, Dorsett B, Cronin W, et al: Acquired immunodeficiency syndrome–associated lymphomas: Clinical, pathological, immunologic and viral characteristics of 111 cases. Hum Pathol 1991; 22:659.

110. Levine AM, Burkes RL, Walker M, et al: Development of B cell lymphoma in two monogamous homosexual men. Arch Intern Med 1985; 145:479.

111. Levine AM: Acquired immunodeficiency syndrome–related lymphoma [Review]. Blood 1992; 80:8.

112. Horning SJ, Rosenberg SA: The natural history of initially untreated low-grade non-Hodgkin's lymphomas. N Engl J Med 1984; 311:1471.

113. Knowles DM, Chamulak GA, Subar M, et al: Clinicopathologic, immunophenotypic, and molecular genetic analysis of AIDS-associated lymphoid neoplasia: Clinical and biologic implications. Pathol Annu 1988; 23:33.

114. Shiramizu B, Herndier B, Meeker T, et al: Molecular and immunophenotypic characterization of AIDS-associated EBV-negative polyclonal lymphoma. J Clin Oncol 1992; 10:383.

115. Ciobanu N, Andreef M, Safai B, et al: Lymphoblastic neoplasia in a homosexual patient with Kaposi's sarcoma. Ann Intern Med 1983; 98:151.

116. Presant CA, Gala K, Wiseman C, et al: Human immunodeficiency virus–associated T-cell lymphoblastic lymphoma in AIDS. Cancer 1987; 60:1459.

117. Janier M, Katlama C, Flageul B, et al: The pseudo-Sézary syndrome with CD8 phenotype in a patient with the acquired immunodeficiency syndrome (AIDS). Ann Intern Med 1989; 110:738.

118. Goldstein J, Becker N, DelRowe J, Davis L: Cutaneous T-cell lymphoma in a patient infected with HIV, type 1. Cancer 1990; 66:1130.

119. Crane GA, Variakojis D, Rosen ST, et al: Cutenaous T-cell lymphoma in patients with human immunodeficiency virus infection. Arch Dermatol 1991; 127:989.

120. Sternlieb J, Mintzer D, Kwa D, Gluckman S: Peripheral T-cell lymphoma in a patient with the acquired immunodeficiency syndrome. Am J Med 1988; 85:445.

121. Baurmann H, Miclea JM, Ferchal F, et al: Adult T-cell leukemia associated with HTLV-I and simultaneous infection by HIV type 2 and human herpesvirus 6 in an African woman: A clinical, virologic, and familial serologic study. Am J Med 1988; 85:853.

122. Shibata D, Brynes R, Rabinowitz A, et al: HTLV-I associated adult T cell leukemia lymphoma in a patient infected with HIV-1. Ann Intern Med 1989; 111:871.

123. Thomas JA, Cotter F, Hanby AM, et al: Epstein-Barr virus–related oral T-cell lymphoma associated with human immunodeficiency virus immunosuppression. Blood 1993; 81:3350.

124. Gonzalez-Clemente JM, Ribera JM, Campo E, et al: Ki-1 positive anaplastic large cell lymphoma of T cell origin in an HIV-infected patient. AIDS 1991; 5:751.

125. Carbone A, Tirelli U, Gloghini A, et al: Human immunodeficiency virus–associated systemic lymphomas may be subdivided into two main groups according to Epstein-Barr viral latent gene expression. J Clin Oncol 1993; 11:1674.

126. Chadburn A, Cesarman E, Jagirdar J, et al: CD30 (Ki-1) positive anaplastic large cell lymphomas in individuals infected with the HIV. Cancer 1993; 72:3078.

127. Anagnostopoulos I, Herbst H, Niedobitek G, Stein H: Demonstration of monoclonal EBV genomes in Hodgkin's disease and Ki-1-positive anaplastic large cell lymphoma by combined Southern blot and in situ hybridization. Blood 1989; 74:810.

128. Herbst H, Dallenbach F, Hummel M, et al: Epstein-Barr virus DNA and latent gene products in Ki-1 (CD30)-positive anaplastic large cell lymphomas. Blood 1991; 78:2666.

129. Roithmann S, Tourani JM, Andrieu JM: AIDS-associated non-Hodgkin's lymphoma. Lancet 1991; 338:884.

130. Levine AM, Wernz JC, Kaplan L et al: Low-dose chemotherapy with central nervous system prophylaxis and azidothymidine maintenance in AIDS-related lymphoma: A prospective multi-institutional trial. JAMA 1991; 266:84.

131. Jones SE, Fuks Z, Bellm M, et al: Non-Hodgkin's lymphoma: IV. Clinicopathologic correlation of 405 cases. Cancer 1973; 31:806.

132. Holladay AO, Siegel RJ, Schwartz DA: Cardiac malignant lymphoma in acquired immune deficiency syndrome. Cancer 1992; 70:2203.

133. Gill PS, Chandraratna P, Meyer PR, Levine AM: Malignant lymphoma: Cardiac involvement at initial presentation. J Clin Oncol 1987; 5:216.

134. Armenakas NA, Schevchuk MM, Brodherson M, Fracchia JA: AIDS presenting as primary testicular lymphoma. Urology 1992; 40:162.

135. Burkes RL, Meyer RP, Gill PS, et al: Rectal lymphoma in homosexual men. Arch Intern Med 1986; 146:913.

136. Ioachim HL, Weinstein MA, Robbins RD, et al: Primary anorectal lymphoma: A new manifestation of the acquired immune deficiency syndrome (AIDS). Cancer 1987; 60:1449.

137. Lee MH, Waxman M, Gillooley JF: Primary malignant lymphoma - of the anorectum in homosexual men. Dis Colon Rectum 1986; 29:413.

138. Podzamczer D, Ricat I, Bolao F, et al: Gallium 67 scan for distinguishing follicular hyperplasia from other AIDS associated diseases in lymph nodes. AIDS 1990; 4:683.

139. Silverman BA, Rubinstein A: Serum lactate dehydrogenase levels in adults and children with acquired immunodeficiency syndrome (AIDS) and AIDS-related complex: Possible indicator of B-cell lymphoproliferation and disease activity. Am J Med 1985; 78:728.

140. Radin DR, Esplin J, Levine AM, Ralls PW: AIDS-related non-Hodgkin's lymphoma: Abdominal CT findings in 112 patients. AJR Am J Roentgenol 1993; 160:1133.

141. Sider L, Weiss AJ, Smith MD, et al: Varied appearance of AIDS-related lymphoma in the chest. Radiology 1989; 171:629.

142. Shipp MA, et al (The International Non-Hodgkin's Lymphoma Prognostic Factors Project): A predictive model for aggressive non-Hodgkin's lymphoma. N Engl J Med 1993; 329:987.

143. Daniels D, Lowdell CP, Glaser MG: The spontaneous regression of lymphoma in AIDS. Clin Oncol (R Coll Radiol) 1992; 4:196.

144. Karnad AB, Jaffar A, Lands RH: Spontaneous regression of acquired immune deficiency syndrome–related high-grade, extranodal non-Hodgkin's lymphoma. Cancer 1992; 69:1856.

145. Goldie JH, Coldman AJ, Gudauskas GA: Rationale for the use of alternating non-cross resistant chemotherapy. Cancer Treat Rep 1982; 66:439.

146. McKelvey EM, Gottlieb JA, Wilson HE, et al: Hydroxydaunomycin (Adriamycin) combination chemotherapy in malignant lymphoma. Cancer 1976; 38:1484.

147. Skarin AT, Canellos GP, Rosenthal DS, et al: Improved prognosis of diffuse histiocytic and undifferentiated lymphoma by use of high-dose methotrexate alternating with standard agents (M-BACOD). J Clin Oncol 1983; 1:91.

148. Fisher RI, DeVita VT Jr, Hubbard SM, et al: Diffuse aggressive lymphomas: Increased survival after alternating flexible sequence of ProMACE and MOPP chemotherapy. Ann Intern Med 1983; 98:304.

149. Fisher RI, DeVita VT, Hubbard SM, et al: Randomized trial of ProMACE-MOPP versus ProMACE-CytaBOM in previously untreated, advanced stage, diffuse aggressive lymphomas. Proc Am Soc Clin Oncol 1984; 3:242.

150. Klimo P, Connors JM: MACOP-B chemotherapy for the treatment of diffuse large cell lymphoma. Ann Intern Med 1985; 102:596.

151. Fisher RI, Gaynor E, Dahlberg S, et al: Comparison of a standard regimen (CHOP) with three intensive chemotherapy regimens for advanced non-Hodgkin's lymphoma. N Engl J Med 1993; 328:1002.

152. Odajnyk C, Subar M, Dugan M, et al: Clinical features and correlates with immunopathology and molecular biology of a large group of patients with AIDS associated small noncleaved lymphoma (SNCL) [Abstract]. Blood 1986; 68:1331a.

153. Dugan M, Subar M, Odajnyk C, et al: Intensive multiagent chemotherapy for AIDS-related diffuse large cell lymphoma [Abstract]. Blood 1986; 68:124a.

154. Gill PS, Levine AM, Krailo M, et al: AIDS-related malignant lymphoma: Results of prospective treatment trials. J Clin Oncol 1987; 5:1322.

155. Walsh C, Wernz J, Levine AM, et al: Phase I study of M-BACOD and granulocyte-macrophage colony-stimulating factor (GM-CSF) in HIV-associated non-Hodgkin's lymphoma. J AIDS 1993; 6:265.

156. Kaplan LD, Kahn JO, Crowe S, et al: Clinical and virologic effects of recombinant human granulocyte-macrophage colony-stimulating factor in patients receiving chemotherapy for human immunodeficiency virus–associated non-Hodgkin's lymphoma: Results of a randomized trial. J Clin Oncol 1991; 9:929.

157. Tirelli U, Errante D, Okssenhendler E, et al: Prospective study with combined low-dose chemotherapy and zidovudine in 37 patients with

poor-prognosis AIDS-related non-Hodgkin's lymphoma. Ann Oncol 1992; 3:843.

158. Levine AM, Tulpule A, Espina B, et al: Low-dose methotrexate, bleomycin, doxorubicin, cyclophosphamide, vincristine, and dexamethasone with zalcitabine in patients with acquired immunodeficiency syndrome–related lymphoma: Effect on HIV and serum interleukin-6 levels over time. Cancer 1996; 78:517.

159. Remick SC, McSharry JJ, Walt BC, et al: Novel oral combination chemotherapy in the treatment of intermediate-grade and high-grade AIDS-related non-Hodgkin's lymphoma. J Clin Oncol 1993; 11:1691.

160. Sparano JA, Wiernik PH, Dutcher JP, et al: Infusion cyclophosphamide, doxorubicin, and etoposide in HIV-related non-Hodgkin's lymphoma: A followup report of a highly active regimen [Abstract]. Blood 1993; 82:386a.

161. Bermudez M, Grant KM, Rodvien R, Mendes F: Non-Hodgkin's lymphoma in a population with or at risk for acquired immunodeficiency syndrome: Indications for intensive chemotherapy. Am J Med 1989; 86:71.

162. Gisselbrecht C, Oksenhendler E, Tirelli U, et al, for the French Italian Cooperative Group: Human immunodeficiency virus–related lymphoma treatment with intensive combination chemotherapy. Am J Med 1993; 95:188.

163. Kaplan L, Straus D, Testa M, Levine AM: Randomized trial of standard-dose mBACOD with GM-CSF versus reduced-dose mBACOD for systemic HIV-associated lymphoma: ACTG 142. Proc Am Soc Clin Oncol 1995; 14:288.

164. Sidell N, Taga T, Hirano T, et al: Retinoic acid–induced growth inhibition of a human myeloma cell line via downregulation of IL-6 receptors. J Immunol 1991; 146:3809.

165. Tepper RI, Pattengale PK, Leder P: Murine interleukin-4 displays potent antitumor activity in vivo. Cell 1989; 57:503.

166. Kreitman RJ, Siegall CB, FitzGerald DJP, et al: Interleukin-6 fused to a mutant form of *Pseudomonas* exotoxin kills malignant cells from patients with multiple myeloma. Blood 1992; 79:1775.

167. Anti-B4 Blocked Ricin [Investigator's Brochure]. Boston, Immuno-Gen, 1990.

168. Tulpule A, Anderson LJJ, Levine AM, et al: Anti-B4 (CD19) monoclonal antibody, conjugated with ricin (B4-blocked ricin) in refractory AIDS-lymphoma. Proc Am Soc Clin Oncol 1994; 13:52.

169. Scadden DT, Doweiko J, Schenkein D, et al: A phase I/II trial of combined immunoconjugate and chemotherapy for AIDS-related lymphoma [Abstract]. Blood 1993; 82:386a.

170. Fine HA, Mayer RJ: Primary central nervous system lymphoma [Review]. Ann Intern Med 1993; 119:1093.

171. Meeker TC, Shiramizu B, Kaplan L, et al: Evidence for molecular subtypes of HIV-associated lymphoma: Division into peripheral monoclonal, polyclonal, and central nervous system lymphoma. AIDS 1991; 5:669.

172. Gill PS, Graham RA, Boswell W, et al: A comparison of imaging, clinical, and pathologic aspects of space-occupying lesions within the brain in patients with acquired immunodeficiency syndrome. Am J Physiol Imaging 1986; 1:134.

173. Ciricillo SF, Rosenblum ML: Use of CT and MR imaging to distinguish intracranial lesions and to define the need for biopsy in AIDS patients. J Neurosurg 1990; 73:720.

174. Galetto G, Levine AM: AIDS-related primary central nervous system lymphoma. JAMA 1993; 269:92.

175. Corn BW, Trock BD: Impact of medical specialty on the approach to AIDS patients with intracranial mass lesions. Proc Am Soc Clin Oncol 1992; 11:44.

176. Shibata S: Sites of origin of primary intracerebral malignant lymphoma. Neurosurgery 1989; 25:14.

177. So YT, Beckstead JH, Davis RL: Primary central nervous system lymphoma in acquired immune deficiency syndrome: A clinical and pathological study. Ann Neurol 1986; 20:566.

178. Gill PS, Levine AM, Meyer PR, et al: Primary central nervous system lymphoma in homosexual men: Clinical, immunologic, and pathologic features. Am J Med 1985; 78:742.

179. DeAngelis LM, Yahalom J, Rosenblum M, Posner JB: Primary CNS lymphoma: Managing patients with spontaneous and AIDS-related disease. Oncology 1987; 1:52.

180. DeAngelis LM, Yahalom J, Heinemann MH, et al: Primary CNS lymphoma: Combined treatment with chemotherapy and radiotherapy. Neurology 1990; 40:80.

181. Formenti SC, Gill PS, Lean E, et al: Primary central nervous system lymphoma in AIDS: Results of radiation therapy. Cancer 1989; 63:1101.

182. Goldstein JD, Dickson DW, Moser FG, et al: Primary central nervous system lymphoma in acquired immunodeficiency syndrome: A clinical and pathologic study with results of treatment with radiation. Cancer 1991; 67:2756.

183. Baumgartner JE, Rachlin JR, Beckstead JH, et al: Primary central nervous system lymphomas: Natural history and response to radiation therapy in 55 patients with acquired immunodeficiency syndrome. J Neurosurg 1990; 73:206.

184. Nisce LZ, Kaufmann T, Metroka C: Radiation therapy in patients with AIDS-related central nervous system lymphomas. JAMA 1992; 267:192.

185. Bishburg E, Eng RHK, Slim J, et al: Brain lesions in patients with acquired immunodeficiency syndrome. Arch Intern Med 1989; 149:941.

CLINICAL ASPECTS

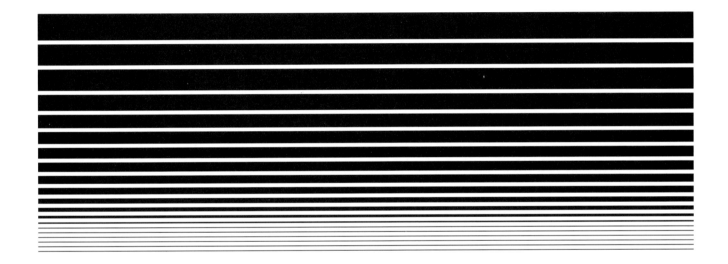

Twenty-Nine

Paraneoplastic Syndromes

Arthur T. Skarin

Paraneoplastic syndromes are signs and symptoms of a malignancy not directly related to the tumor itself. The "remote effects," or indirect manifestations, of an underlying malignancy have been long recognized, and there have been many extensive reviews of patients with a variety of cancers.[1, 2] The categories of remote effects include endocrinologic, neurologic, hematologic, renal, dermatologic, gastrointestinal, rheumatologic and connective tissue, and miscellaneous. In this chapter, paraneoplastic syndromes associated with lymphomas are emphasized.

Many of the paraneoplastic syndromes are due to secretion of cytokines, growth factors, or other biologically active proteins by tumor cells. Tumor cells, however, may also induce normal cells to produce polypeptides or antibodies that then result in specific tumor-related syndromes. The etiology and pathogenesis of paraneoplastic syndromes are summarized in Table 29–1.[2]

The clinical importance of paraneoplastic syndromes relates to several areas, which are summarized as follows:

1. The syndrome may predate the first sign of the underlying malignancy, thus allowing for an early diagnosis and greater chance for cure when minimal disease is present.
2. The syndrome may suggest advanced disease and thus prevent or delay curative treatment.
3. The syndrome may mask underlying disease complications (such as infection), resulting in withholding of appropriate therapy.
4. The syndrome may be used as a "tumor marker" for monitoring treatment or detecting early relapse.
5. The syndrome may be disabling, especially in patients with advanced (incurable) or refractory disease, and modern management of the paraneoplastic manifestations may offer reasonable palliation.
6. The syndrome resolves with successful therapy of the underlying neoplasm.
7. The syndrome, particularly if caused by hormone secretion involving an "autocrine loop," may be interrupted with specific antihormone therapy.[3] Although this mechanism may not be common, it offers an opportunity for further research into the elucidation of the pathogenesis of some paraneoplastic syndromes.

Since paraneoplastic syndromes are uncommon, other problems directly related to the underlying malignancy must always be considered in the differential diagnosis. These include direct tumor invasion; obstruction by the malignancy; vascular abnormalities; infections; fluid, electrolyte, and metabolic abnormalities; and toxicity of antineoplastic therapy, including cytotoxic chemotherapy, radiation therapy, antibiotics, and resultant (or inherent disease-related) immunosuppression.

ENDOCRINOLOGIC MANIFESTATIONS

Endocrinologic abnormalities in lymphoma due to paraneoplastic syndromes are relatively rare and include a number of clinicopathologic entities.[2] Most of the polypeptide hormones involved in these syndromes have been identified within the central nervous system (CNS) or gastrointestinal tract. The paraneoplastic features are usually independent of normal regulatory mechanisms.

The most common paraneoplastic endocrinopathy in patients with lymphoma is nonmetastatic hypercalcemia, occurring in 0.3% to 4% of patients.[4] Mechanisms for hypercalcemia include the following[5, 6]:

1. Production of parathyroid hormone-related peptide (PTH-RP) by tumor cells—a rare cause in lymphomas and leukemias but more commonly seen in solid tumors.
2. Production of cytokines—osteoclast-activating factors were originally isolated from lymphoma cells and are associated with a variety of transforming growth factors (TGFs) that act in an autocrine fashion. TGF-α, secreted by malignant cells, shares partial amino acid homology with epidermal growth factor (EGF) and induces bone resorption by binding to the EGF receptor. TGF-β, in contrast, is secreted by osteoblasts and may act as an autocrine regulator for growth and differentiation of osteoblasts. Imbalance in secretion and function of these factors may account for mixed lytic and blastic bone lesions.[5] Other cytokines involved in bone resorption include interleukin-1 (IL-1), platelet-derived growth factor (PDGF), tumor necrosis factor (TNF), and certain hematopoietic growth factors (colony-stimulating factors [CSFs]). It may be concluded that the cytokines cause hypercalcemia

Table 29–1. Mechanisms in the Pathogenesis of Paraneoplastic Syndromes

Tumor-produced or related biologically active products
  Peptide hormones
  Growth factors
  Interleukins
  Cytokines
  Prostaglandins
  Fetal proteins (carcinoembryonic antigen, α-fetoprotein, other)
  Immunoglobulins
  Enzymes
Autoimmune or immune complex disease
"Ectopic receptor" production or competitive blockade of normal hormone action by tumor produced biologically in active hormones
"Forbidden contact"—release of enzymes or other products that cause antigenic response, inappropriate physiologic functions, or other toxic manifestations
Unknown causes

Modified from Bunn PA Jr, Ridgway EC: Paraneoplastic syndromes. *In* DeVita VT Jr, Hellman S, Rosenberg SA (eds): Cancer: Principles and Practice of Oncology, 4th ed. Philadelphia, JB Lippincott, 1993, p 2026.

by local action within sites of bony involvement since few data are available regarding their role as circulating "hormonal" mediators.[5]

3. Vitamin D—elevated levels of 1,25-dihydroxyvitamin D_3 [1,25$(OH)_2D_3$] (calcitriol) have been reported in patients with non-Hodgkin's lymphoma (NHL) and Hodgkin's disease (HD).[7] The elevated levels are due to increased activity of 1α-vitamin D-hydroxylase, similar to that reported in patients with granulomatous disease such as sarcoidosis and berylliosis. The role of vitamin D in causing or sustaining hypercalcemia or merely acting as a marker of tumor burden is unclear.[5]

4. Prostaglandins—release of prostaglandins (especially of the E series) has been implicated in hypercalcemia for a number of solid tumors but has not been implicated in hypercalcemia associated with lymphoma.

The most common type of lymphoma associated with paraneoplastic hypercalcemia is adult T-cell leukemia/lymphoma caused by the type C retrovirus known as the human T-cell lymphotropic virus (HTLV), type I. In a large series from Japan, increased serum calcium levels were present at diagnosis in 16 (21%) of 77 patients.[8] In the National Cancer Institute (NCI) series, 5 of 11 patients presented with signs and symptoms of hypercalcemia, but eventually all patients developed hypercalcemia.[9] The paraneoplastic syndrome also includes increased bone turnover and abnormal bone scintigraphy (generalized and symmetric increase in tracer activity). Bone biopsies showed increased osteoblastic and osteoclastic activation with paratrabecular bone scalloping but often without the presence of malignant cells. Blood levels of PTH, cyclic adenosine monophosphate, and prostaglandins were normal. Studies of cultured lymphoma cells in two patients showed an osteolytic substance consistent with the presence of a circulating lymphokine as a cause for hypercalcemia. A subsequent study confirmed normal prostaglandin E and PTH levels but also showed low levels of 25-hydroxyvitamin D and 1,25-dihydroxyvitamin D.[10] An elevated serum level of PTH-RP,

however, was reported in two hypercalcemic patients and one normocalcemic patient, including detection of PTH-like activity in pleural and ascitic fluids.[11] Elevated serum TNF-β level was detected in seven of eight hypercalcemic patients with adult T-cell leukemia, suggesting a role for this tumor-secreted cytokine in the pathogenesis of paraneoplastic hypercalcemia.[12]

Hypercalcemia may also occur in other subtypes of lymphoma. In an NCI report, elevated serum calcium level was documented in 2 of 28 cases of large cell lymphoma, 1 of 20 cases of diffuse PDL lymphoma, but none of 21 cases of diffuse mixed or 39 patients with nodular PDL lymphoma.[13] Only 1 of 109 patients with HD had hypercalcemia. Of all 217 cases, 58 (27%) had bone lesions and 63 (29%) had bone marrow infiltration by malignant cells. All instances of hypercalcemia occurred in patients with bone involvement, suggesting the release of calcium by bone destruction. Effective chemotherapy resulted in reversal of hypercalcemia.

Humoral factors have been implicated in the hypercalcemia of some lymphomas. In a study of 22 hypercalcemic patients, most with large cell lymphoma, elevated levels of serum calcitriol—an active vitamin D metabolite—were found in 12 patients (55%) by radioreceptor assay.[14] Serum PTH levels were normal. An increase in calcium excretion was noted in hypercalcemic patients as well as in 71% of normocalcemic patients. One presumed mechanism of vitamin D–mediated hypercalcemia is enhanced absorption of calcium. In HD, tumor-related production of calcitriol is also implicated in patients with hypercalcemia and hypercalciuria. The paraneoplastic syndrome appears to predominantly affect middle-aged men with bulky intraabdominal disease.[15] A prompt response to steroids was noted in the latter study.[15] In two patients with NHL (one diffuse mixed and one Lennert's T-cell type) and hypercalcemia, increased activity of serum angiotensin-converting enzyme was found.[16] A mechanism similar to that in sarcoidosis may have caused the elevated calcium level, namely, cytokine elaboration by the lymphoma causing activated macrophages to produce calcitriol. Multiple mechanisms may be involved in some patients.[15]

An unusual endocrinopathy rarely occurring with lymphomas is hypoglycemia.[2] This paraneoplastic syndrome, although more common with mesotheliomas, hemangiopericytomas, and hepatomas, results from several mechanisms, including ectopic insulin production and nonsuppressible insulin-like activity (somatomedins), insulin-like growth factors I and II, or production of an inhibitor of hepatic glucose output. Autoimmunity to the insulin receptor with resultant hypoglycemia was reported in a patient with HD.[17] In this latter case, the hypoglycemia did not respond to azathioprine or plasmapheresis but remitted after the use of prednisolone, and the erythrocyte-receptor binding of insulin became normal.

Hypertension in a pediatric patient with HD is an unusual paraneoplastic phenomenon. An elevated serum renin level resulting in hypertension in a 14-year-old girl with stage IIIB disease declined with a successful response to combination chemotherapy.[18] On the other hand, paraneoplastic orthostatic hypotension has been rarely seen, mainly with thoracic malignancies. It appears to arise from interference in the transmission of impulses from intrathoracic baroreceptors causing abnormalities in the antidiuretic hormone level and sodium excretion[19]; however, it is more likely a toxic complication of the vinca alkaloids used in the treatment of lymphoma.

NEUROLOGIC MANIFESTATIONS

The differential diagnosis of neurologic syndromes in patients with malignancy is quite extensive, including direct effects of primary or distant spread of disease, syndromes due to endocrine or metabolic tumor products (e.g., antidiuretic hormone and calcium, glucose, and electrolyte disturbances), the effects of cerebral or spinal vascular disease, toxicity of specific treatment, neurologic manifestation of CNS infections, and paraneoplastic syndromes.[2]

The neurologic paraneoplastic syndromes are uncommon, occurring in about 7% of cancer patients; they are most common in lung cancer,[20] with an estimated 2.5% incidence in HD.[21] Many of the paraneoplastic syndromes are caused by "autoimmune" reactions wherein the malignant cells have antigens that are shared with the normal neural tissue. The immune response results in nervous system damage with a variety of manifestations. Antineuronal antibodies have been reported in 38% of patients with paraneoplastic syndromes with a high specificity of 98.6%.[22]

Numerous neurologic syndromes have been described in a variety of cancers.[2] The following is a discussion of the more commonly reported paraneoplastic syndromes reported in lymphomas, grouped together by area within the nervous system.

CENTRAL NERVOUS SYSTEM

Subacute cerebellar degeneration has been reported in HD. It is characterized by ataxia, dysarthria, hypotonia, and pendular reflexes. Dementia may occur. In a series of 21 patients, HD preceded neurologic symptoms by 1 to 54 months in 17 of 21 patients.[23] The stage of HD did not correlate with severity of neurologic disease. The median age was 44 years. Six patients developed paraneoplastic cerebellar degeneration (PCD) while in HD remission. Serum antibodies that reacted specifically with Purkinje's cells were present in six cases. The pattern of reaction was distinct from that of PCD with gynecologic cancer (anti-Yo) or small cell cancer (anti-Hu). Two patients improved spontaneously, but corticosteroids, other immunosuppressive therapy, and plasmapheresis did not affect the PCD.

Limbic encephalitis, characterized by dementia and memory loss (Ophelia's syndrome), occurs rarely in HD. It may be reversible with successful therapy of HD.[24] Other paraneoplastic causes of dementia include angioendotheliosis, with magnetic resonance imaging findings consistent with multiple strokes.[25] It may be related to tumor secretion of angiogenic peptides.[26]

Progressive multifocal leukoencephalopathy (PML), most often occurring in malignancies associated with impaired or altered immunity, is characterized by demyelination of white matter throughout the brain. Patients develop dementia, paralysis, aphasia, ataxia, dysarthria, and visual field defects.

PML is rapidly progressive, with death occurring usually within 6 months. Although this entity was previously considered to be a paraneoplastic syndrome, most of the evidence suggests a viral etiology.[27]

Paraneoplastic myelopathy has been reported rarely in HD.[28] Neurologic features include progressive paraparesis, numbness and paresthesias, urinary or fecal incontinence, hypertonia, and bilateral up-going Babinski reflexes. Extensive evaluation is required to rule out other causes. In one patient, the syndrome responded to intrathecal dexamethasone.[28]

PERIPHERAL NERVES

Paraneoplastic disorders reported in HD include subacute sensory neuropathy, subacute motor neuropathy, and acute and chronic inflammatory polyradiculoneuropathy.[29] An unusual brachial plexopathy, characterized by asymmetric weakness and paresthesias of both upper extremities responded to corticosteroids in one patient.[29] Ascending acute polyneuropathy (Guillain-Barré syndrome) has been seen in patients with both HD and NHLs.[2] The syndrome is similar to that without associated malignancy, and the association may be coincidental.

Peripheral polyneuropathy occurs in about 5% of patients with lymphoplasmacytic lymphoma (Waldenström's macroglobulinemia). The pathogenesis has been recently elucidated by the finding of antibody activity against myelin sheath mediated by the $F(ab')_2$ fragments of the immunoglobulin M (IgM) monoclonal protein in 40% of patients. The polyneuropathy was usually sensory in type and could precede the detection of monoclonal IgM by many years.[30]

AUTONOMIC NERVES

Disorders of the autonomic nervous system related to paraneoplastic phenomena include orthostatic hypotension, neurogenic bladder, and intestinal pseudo-obstruction (Ogilvie's syndrome). These conditions are rarely seen in lymphomas. However, a study of patients with advanced disease revealed one or more abnormal cardiovascular function tests in 16 of 20 patients.[31] The subclinical findings improved with treatment in most patients.

NEUROMUSCULAR FUNCTION

Rare patients with lymphoma may develop a myasthenic syndrome (Eaton-Lambert syndrome), characterized by weakness and fatigability of proximal muscles, mouth dryness, dysphagia, dysarthria, and peripheral paresthesias. Myasthenia gravis has also been reported.[32] In one patient with thymic lymphoblastic lymphoma, chemotherapy resulted in a complete remission of both conditions.[33] Of importance is the fact that both these neuromuscular entities may predate the clinical appearance of lymphoma.

HEMATOLOGIC MANIFESTATIONS

Paraneoplastic hematologic disorders often occur in the lymphoproliferative diseases. The abnormalities occur in all hematopoietic cell lines and in the clotting proteins and are related to autoimmune mechanisms or aberrant production of hematopoietic CSFs.[34]

Autoimmune hemolytic anemia (AIHA) due to warm-reacting antibodies occurs mainly in B-cell lymphoproliferative disorders, although it has been reported in HD.[35] Other autoimmune cytopenias include thrombocytopenia[36] and a combination of the latter conditions, called Evans's syndrome.[37] Mechanisms for the development of these syndromes include cross-reacting antibodies, tumor production of autoantibodies, or tumor production of product-altering erythrocytes and/or platelets, making them immunogenic.

AIHA due to cold-reacting autoantibodies (cold agglutinins) has been reported rarely in patients with NHL.[38] Histologic B-cell types include most commonly diffuse lymphocytic poorly or well differentiated, diffuse large cell, and occasionally nodular lymphocytic. One case report of a patient with low-grade mucosal-associated lymphoid tissue (MALT) lymphoma of the lung showed that the hemolytic anemia was due to production of an anti-I cold agglutinin present in the serum as a monoclonal IgM λ light chain–restricted protein.[39] The monoclonal gammopathy and AIHA responded to steroid therapy, suggesting that the autoantibodies were released from the B-cell maltomas.

Microangiopathic hemolytic anemia (MAHA), related to various causes of erythrocyte shearing, occurs mainly in patients with metastatic mucin-producing adenocarcinoma.[40] MAHA is exceedingly rare in lymphomas.[2]

Severe anemia due to selective marrow red blood cell aplasia has been reported in thymomas and other neoplasms but also in T-cell lymphoproliferative disorders. In the latter patients, T-cell–mediated suppression of erythropoiesis has been demonstrated, with improvement in the anemia after cyclophosphamide therapy.[41]

A paraneoplastic leukemoid reaction has been noted in many patients with malignancy, including HD and NHL. Monocytosis and granulocytosis with elevation of peripheral cells to more than 20,000/μL without infection or leukemia is usually asymptomatic.[42] The mechanism of leukemoid reactions relates to tumor production of a CSF, including granulocyte-CSF, granulocyte-macrophage-CSF, macrophage-CSF/CSF-1, IL-3, or IL-1.[34, 43, 44]

Eosinophilia occurs in about 20% of patients with HD.[2] Studies in lymphoproliferative disorders show eosinophilia (>570/μL) in 21% of patients with acute T-cell leukemia/lymphoma, 11% of patients with T-cell lymphoma, and 10% of patients with B-cell lymphoma.[45] The mechanism relates to secretion of lymphokines by lymphoma cells. In a study of lymphocytes from three patients with T-cell lymphoma extensively infiltrated by eosinophils, IL-5 mRNA was detected by polymerase chain reaction.[46] It was concluded that IL-5, a cytokine that promotes eosinophil differentiation, growth, and migration, was responsible for the hypereosinophilia in certain T-cell lymphomas. Enhanced expression of the IL-5 gene has also been reported in HD.[47]

Thrombocytosis (platelet counts >400,000/μL) occurs in 30% to 40% of patients with malignancy.[2] The mechanism undoubtedly involves release of a thrombopoietin.[48] Other causes of thrombocytosis should be ruled out, including underlying myeloproliferative disorder, gastrointestinal bleeding, hemolytic anemia, acute and chronic inflammatory disorders, and after splenectomy and other surgical procedures. Thrombosis and hemorrhage rarely occur with paraneoplastic thrombocytosis. Platelet counts decrease to normal with successful therapy of the underlying neoplasm.

Various clotting abnormalities, migratory thrombophlebitis (Trousseau's syndrome), and disseminated intravascular coagulation (DIC) occur in patients mainly with solid tumors. Lymphomas accounted for less than 1% of cases in a large review.[2] The mechanism for these disorders relates to many factors, including a hypercoagulable state induced by the underlying malignancy, local tissue disruption from tumor or therapy, infection, vitamin deficiency, liver disease, and circulating anticoagulants. Nonbacterial thrombotic endocarditis (NBTE), another cause of thrombosis or hemorrhagic complications, may be seen with or without DIC. NBTE ordinarily occurs late in the clinical course and is characterized by sterile verrucous, bland, fibrin-platelet lesions usually on the left-sided heart valves.[49] Clinical features include arterial emboli causing focal neurologic deficits or diffuse abnormalities such as confusion, generalized seizures, and coma. Bleeding into the skin, genitourinary tract, and ear, nose, and throat sites also occurs. The autopsy incidence of NBTE is most common in lung cancer (7.5%), twice that of pancreatic and prostatic cancer (3% to 4%), and more than seven times that of other tumors, lymphomas, or leukemias.[49] Of note, symptoms of NBTE may predate diagnosis of the underlying malignancy.[50]

RENAL MANIFESTATIONS

Renal abnormalities are common in lymphomas, usually directly related to the disease process but also to electrolyte and fluid imbalances and infection. Paraneoplastic manifestations usually relate to glomerular lesions and the resultant nephrotic syndrome. The nephrotic syndrome, however, can also result from neoplastic infiltration of the kidneys, renal vein thrombosis, or amyloid infiltration.

Fewer than 50 cases of paraneoplastic nephrotic syndrome in HD have been reported.[51] The most common glomerular lesion (80% of cases) is lipoid nephrosis, or minimal change disease. The remaining 20% of cases reveal typical membranous glomerulopathy, focal sclerosis, or membranoproliferative glomerulonephritis.[2] Of note, patients with nephrotic syndrome related to an underlying carcinoma most often have membranous glomerulonephritis. Also, patients may present with paraneoplastic nephrotic syndrome long before a diagnosis of malignancy has been established.

The pathogenesis of lipoid nephrosis in HD appears related to abnormal T-cell function, although other factors such as viral and tumor antigens, fetal antigen expression, and immune complex disease may also play a role.

The nephrotic syndrome is less common in NHL, usually seen in Burkitt's lymphoma or diffuse large cell lymphoma. In 35 cases of paraneoplastic nephrotic syndrome, 5 had minimal change lesions, 7 had membranous lesions, and 7 had membranoproliferative lesions.[51] Immunoglobulin deposits have also been detected, suggesting an immune complex cause of the syndrome.[52]

DERMATOLOGIC MANIFESTATIONS

Malignancies have been associated with a great number of paraneoplastic skin lesions.[2] Some of the more typical syndromes are reviewed by pattern of cutaneous reaction in this section.

Numerous *pigmented lesions* and keratoses may occur. *Acanthosis nigricans*, characterized by symmetric brown areas of hyperpigmentation and hyperkeratosis especially in the axillae, neck flexures, and anogenital area, is usually associated with abdominal adenocarcinomas, but occasional patients with lymphoma have been reported.[53] Tumor secretion of TGF-α may be involved in the pathogenesis. *Sweet's syndrome* consists of fever, neutrophilia, and multiple cutaneous plaques with intense infiltration of the dermis by neutrophils. It is seen in various hematologic malignancies and some carcinomas.[54] The syndrome may be related to secretion of a lymphokine such as IL-1. Rapid response occurs with steroids. A large area of distinctive inflammatory plaques was reported in a 12-year-old girl with an adjacent diffuse large cell lymphoma.[55] Biopsied tissue showed infiltration of the epidermal spongiosis with neutrophils. The lymphoma and dermatosis responded dramatically to chemotherapy.

Erythematous skin lesions may be related to a paraneoplastic syndrome. Exfoliative dermatitis has been reported in HD and NHL including cutaneous T-cell lymphoma (CTCL).[56]

Bullous and urticarial lesions have been reported in patients with HD and NHL. Paraneoplastic pemphigus is a distinct and rare autoimmune disease characterized by extensive and painful mucosal ulcerations and polymorphic skin lesions. The mucocutaneous eruption resembles both erythema multiforme major (Stevens-Johnson syndrome) and pemphigus vulgaris. Autoantibodies against epidermal proteins desmoplakin I and II have been detected by direct immunofluorescent studies on skin biopsy and immunoprecipitation studies on serum.[57] Although the clinical course is usually rapid and fatal despite immunosuppressive therapy, rare patients have prolonged survival.[57–59] One patient with previous diffuse large cell lymphoma in remission after chemotherapy and subsequent bone marrow transplantation developed paraneoplastic pemphigus within 6 months of the transplant.[60] In addition to very tense skin blisters suggestive of bullous pemphigoid, tracheal, pulmonary, and esophageal involvement occurred. IgG autoantibody deposits were demonstrated within the bronchial epithelium.

Lichen planus, a unique inflammatory reaction pattern in the skin, was reported in three patients with low-grade lymphomas.[61] Observations regarding pathogenesis suggested a cell-mediated immune response compared with paraneoplastic pemphigus, which is caused primarily by a humoral response to tumor-related antigens.

Miscellaneous paraneoplastic cutaneous lesions include fasciitis panniculitis syndrome (FPS), eosinophilic fasciitis, and progressive atrophying chronic dermohypodermitis (PACGD). FPS has a female predominance and predilection for hematologic malignancies.[54] It is characterized by swelling and patchy induration of the skin of the upper or lower extremities and occasionally the trunk or neck.

Biopsied tissue shows chronic inflammation and fibrous thickening of the subcutaneous septa, fascia, and perimysium. The pathogenesis is unknown but may be related to activated T lymphocytes producing chemotactic and growth factors and other mediators of inflammation.[62] Eosinophilic fasciitis has been reported with leukemias, HD, and CTCL.[63] It is characterized by painful, sclerodermatous lesions on the extremities and trunk without acrosclerosis. Histologic features include edema and lymphocytic inflammation in the superficial fascia and dermis along with deposition of immune reactants. Peripheral eosinophilia and circulating immune complexes were noted in one patient with CTCL.[63] These conditions are not related to L-tryptophan-induced eosinophilia myalgia syndrome, except for a similar distribution of lesions in the fascia and muscles.[64]

PACGD has been associated with HD and often predates the clinical onset of HD.[65] The granulomatous skin disease partially responds to corticosteroids as well as azathioprine. The abundance of macrophages in PACGD may result in the characteristic skin looseness since elastase and other macrophage surface proteolytic enzymes could destroy the connective tissue responsible for normal skin elastic properties.[65] The pathogenesis of PACGD is unknown.

GASTROINTESTINAL MANIFESTATIONS

Patients with malignancy often present with anorexia, loss of taste, weight loss, and cachexia. These symptoms may predate the diagnosis of a tumor. With proper anticancer therapy, the anorexia syndrome is reversible. These paraneoplastic manifestations are related to many factors, including elaboration of cytokines such as TNF-α (cachectin) and IL-1β by tumor cells.[66] TNF-α inhibits lipoprotein lipase activity in peripheral tissues and may facilitate metabolic abnormalities resulting in anorexia-cachexia.[66]

Protein-losing enteropathy (PLE) has been associated with many neoplasms, unusually carcinomas, but occasionally lymphomas.[67] Unexplained edema and hypoproteinemia may be the presenting clinical features. Many mechanisms for low albumin levels other than protein loss through the bowel may be involved, including decreased albumin synthesis and abnormal distribution of albumin in effusions. Thus, the true paraneoplastic nature of PLE has been debated.[2] In rare patients, treatment of the underlying malignancy results in improvement in the PLE.

Malabsorption rarely occurs as a paraneoplastic syndrome in malignancies, including lymphomas.[2] It may be associated with direct involvement of bowel wall and mesenteric nodes. Rarely, lymphoma complicates the natural history of celiac disease.[68] Histologic features include flat mucosa with simple or partial villous atrophy.[69]

Unexplained abdominal symptoms suggestive of intestinal obstruction may be the presenting features of patients with occult lymphoma who have acquired angioedema.[70] In this disorder, which may also be hereditary, there is a deficiency of complement component (C1) inhibitor. The resultant angioedema can occur in the face, throat, mouth, larynx, neck, and scrotum and result in peripheral edema and episodes of pseudointestinal obstruction with nausea, emesis, and abdominal pain. Acquired angioedema occurs most often in low-grade B-cell lymphomas, often with associated circulating paraproteins.[71] C1 inhibitor deficiency is a consequence of increased consumption or destruction by one or several mechanisms.[71] Use of danazol reverses angioedema by increasing the synthesis of the C1 inhibitor.

RHEUMATOLOGIC AND CONNECTIVE TISSUE MANIFESTATIONS

Rheumatoid arthritis and asymmetric polyarthritis have been associated with a variety of neoplasms, including lymphomas, but this relationship may be the result of chance alone.[2] Polymyalgia rheumatica may herald an underlying neoplasm in a high percentage of patients, possibly related to arterial emboli to muscle from NBTE.[2] The interrelationship of polymyalgia rheumatica, giant cell arteritis, and tissue cytokine patterns has been recently reviewed.[72] The shoulder-hand syndrome, a variant of reflex sympathetic dystrophy, has also been reported with malignancies.[73] Palmar fasciitis and arthritis are characterized by complete loss of upper extremity function and contracture. It has been seen typically with ovarian cancer but also rarely in HD.[74] Immunoglobulin deposits have been seen in the fascial tissue, suggesting an immunologic cause.

Systemic lupus erythematosus (SLE) has been associated with increased frequency in NHL as well as HD.[75] Of note, SLE usually precedes the diagnosis of lymphoma, and often hypergammaglobulinemia is present. The pathogenesis relates to several autoimmune mechanisms, including an antinuclear antibody recognizing a novel antigen.[76] Successful treatment of the underlying lymphoma usually results in resolution of SLE.

Polymyositis (PM) and dermatomyositis (DM) are inflammatory myopathies that can occur in all age groups.[77] They have been categorized as paraneoplastic syndromes with a fivefold to sevenfold increase in the incidence of malignancies.[78] PM is characterized by the subacute onset of weakness in proximal muscles. About one third of patients have dysphagia, with rare patients developing cardiac arrhythmias and interstitial lung disease. Muscle-derived serum enzyme levels are increased, typical electromyographic findings are noted, and muscle biopsy specimens show necrosis and inflammation. DM includes the just-delineated features plus a characteristic skin rash (erythematous, pruritic, and scaly lesions over sun-exposed areas). PM has been reported in a child with an occult immunoblastic lymphoma.[79] Both regressed with systemic chemotherapy. DM is more frequently associated with malignancy but not commonly with a lymphoma. A review of 12 patients with HD and DM showed a more advanced stage and older age of HD patients without DM.[78] Also, the myopathy either preceded or presented simultaneously with the lymphoma in all patients. Pathogenesis of the paraneoplastic syndrome remains obscure.

The first case of orbital myositis identified as a paraneoplastic syndrome in a patient with a large cell lymphoma was recently reported.[80] The patient had presented with multiple cranial neuropathies, a sensory polyneuropathy, and serum and spinal fluid paraproteins. Although the paraneoplastic features responded to immunosuppressive therapy, the lymphoma progressed despite intensive chemotherapy. The paraneoplastic orbital myositis and other symptoms were explained by an immunologic mechanism involving antibodies directed against antigens shared by the lymphoma and neuromuscular tissues.[81]

MISCELLANEOUS MANIFESTATIONS

Fever is a relatively common paraneoplastic feature of malignancy, occurring in an estimated 5% of cases.[2] Underlying occult infection, drug fever, and adrenal insufficiency must always be ruled out. Fever occurs mainly in patients with lymphomas but also with myxomas, renal cell carcinoma, and osteogenic sarcoma. The mechanism of fever relates to release of pyrogens from malignant cells or normal adjacent cells. IL-6 has been reported as the pyrogen in some cases and has been shown to be released by tumor cells.[82]

Hypertrophic pulmonary osteoarthropathy (HPO) is a well-recognized paraneoplastic syndrome consisting of digital clubbing, periostitis of the long bones, and sometimes polyarthritis, suggestive of rheumatoid arthritis. Although most frequently seen in lung cancer patients (about 12% of patients with adenocarcinoma), it has been reported in intrathoracic HD. Successful chemotherapy of HD has resulted in complete reversal of HPO.[83] The pathogenesis of HPO is complex, with estrogens, growth factors (such as PDGF and TGF-β), neurogenic factors, and growth hormones postulated to play a role.[2, 84]

Amyloidosis, although most often related to multiple myeloma (6% to 15% of cases), occurs in 4% of patients with HD and 10% of those with B-cell lymphomas.[2] Deposition of amyloid (i.e., paraneoplastic β-fibrils) is a pathologic process involving the formation of a specific unique protein conformation—the twisted β-pleated sheet fibril.[85] The fibrils are resistant to normal proteolytic digestion and accumulate in tissues, causing a variety of clinical features such as peripheral neuropathy, gastrointestinal motility disturbances, restrictive cardiomyopathy, purpura, and macroglossia.

Unusual paraneoplastic features have been noted in some patients with T-cell lymphomas. Four patients with isolated bone marrow lymphoma (three T-cell mixed and large cell types and one B large cell type) presented with unexplained fever, abnormal liver function tests, polyserositis, and neurologic symptoms.[86] The features were attributed to release of humoral factors. Multiple paraneoplastic manifestations simulating collagen vascular disorders, infections, or liver disease were also reported in patients with extranodal peripheral T-cell lymphomas.[87] Clinically, the unusual multiple signs and symptoms in these lymphomas without peripheral adenopathy may be ascribed to other disease processes; therefore, early diagnosis of the lymphoma may be difficult. The pathogenesis of paraneoplastic processes relates in part to circulating cytokines and soluble cytokine receptors, often seen in T-cell lymphomas.[88]

Two rare paraneoplastic syndromes reported in patients with lymphoma are digital ischemia and high cardiac output. In the former, a pediatric patient presented with acrocyanosis, and workup revealed underlying Burkitt's lymphoma.[89] Serologic studies showed the presence of antinuclear antibodies, antineutrophil cytoplasmic antibodies, antiendothelial antibodies, and elevated serum IgG. In the latter paraneoplastic syndrome, high cardiac output with failure developed in a young woman with lymphoplasmacytic lymphoma.[90] The condition regressed with therapy but recurred with lymphoma relapse. Anemia, sepsis, and hyperthyroidism were not present. The hyperkinetic circulation (high cardiac output with low vascular resistance) has been reported in other hematologic malignancies and may be related to vasoactive substances secreted by tumor cells, causing vasodilation and hypotension.[90]

REFERENCES

1. Hall TC (ed): Paraneoplastic syndromes. Ann NY Acad Sci 1974; 230:1.
2. Bunn PA Jr, Ridgway EC: Paraneoplastic syndromes. *In* DeVita VT Jr, Hellmann S, Rosenberg SA (eds): Cancer: Principles and Practice of Oncology, 4th ed. Philadelphia, JB Lippincott, 1993, p 2026.
3. De Larco JE, Todaro GJ: Growth factors from murine sarcoma virus–transformed cells. Proc Natl Acad Sci U S A 1978; 75:4001.
4. Muggia FM: Overview of cancer-related hypercalcemia: Epidemiology and etiology. Semin Oncol 1990; 17(Suppl 5):3.
5. Singer FR: Pathogenesis of hypercalcemia of malignancy. Semin Oncol 1991; 18:4.
6. Mundy GR: Pathophysiology of cancer-associated hypercalcemia. Semin Oncol 1990; 17(Suppl 5):10.
7. Seymour JF, Gagel RF: Calcitriol: The major humoral mediator of hypercalcemia in Hodgkin's disease and non-Hodgkin's lymphomas. Blood 1993; 82:1383.
8. Shimoyama M, Ota K, Kikuchi M, et al: Major prognostic factors of adult patients with advanced T-cell lymphoma/leukemia. J Clin Oncol 1988; 6:1088.
9. Bunn PA Jr, Schechter GP, Jaffe E, et al: Clinical course of retrovirus-associated adult T-cell lymphoma in the United States. N Engl J Med 1983; 309:257.
10. Kiyokasw T, Yamaguchi K, Motohiro T, et al: Hypercalcemia and osteoclast proliferation in adult T-cell leukemia. Cancer 1987; 59:1187.
11. Motokura T, Fukumoto S, Matsumoto T, et al: Parathyroid hormone–related protein in adult T-cell leukemia-lymphoma. Ann Intern Med 1989; 111:484.
12. Ishibashi K, Ishitsuka K, Chuman Y, et al: Tumor necrosis factor-β in the serum of adult T-cell leukemia with hypercalcemia. Blood 1991; 77:2451.
13. Canellos GP: Hypercalcemia in malignant lymphoma and leukemia. Ann NY Acad Sci 1974; 230:240.
14. Seymour J, Gagel RF, Hagemeister FR, et al: Calcitriol production in hypercalcemic and normocalcemic patients with non-Hodgkin's lymphoma. Ann Intern Med 1994; 121:633.
15. Jacobson JO, Bringhurst RF, Harris NL, et al: Humoral hypercalcemia in Hodgkin's disease. Cancer 1989; 63:917.
16. DeRemee RA, Banks PM: Non-Hodgkin's lymphoma associated with hypercalcemia and increased activity of serum angiotensin-converting enzyme. Mayo Clin Proc 1986; 61:714.
17. Braund WJ, Williamson DH, Clark A, et al: Autoimmunity to insulin receptor and hypoglycaemia in patient with Hodgkin's disease. Lancet 1987; 1:237.
18. Singh AP, Charan VD, Desai N, et al: Hypertension as a paraneoplastic phenomenon in childhood Hodgkin's disease. Leuk Lymphoma 1993; 11:315.
19. Boasberg PD, Henry JP, Rosenbloom AA, et al: Case reports and studies of paraneoplastic hypotension: Abnormal low-pressure baroreceptor responses. Med Pediatr Oncol 1977; 3:59.
20. Croft P, Wilkinson M: The incidence of carcinomatous neuromyopathy in patients with various types of carcinoma. Brain 1965; 88:427.
21. Currie S, Henson RA, Morgan HG, Poole AJ: The incidence of the nonmetastatic neurological syndromes of obscure origin in the reticuloses. Brain 1970; 93:629.
22. Moll JWB, Henzen-Logmans SC, Splinter TAW, et al: Disystem. J Neurol Neurosurg Psychiatry 1990; 53:940.
23. Hammack J, Kotanides H, Rosenblum MK, Posner JB: Paraneoplastic cerebellar degeneration. Neurology 1992; 42:1938.
24. Carr I: The Ophelia syndrome: Memory loss in Hodgkin's disease. Lancet 1982; 1:844.
25. Petito CK, Gottlieb GJ, Dougherty JH, Petito FH: Neoplastic angioendotheliosis: Ultrastructural study and review of the literature. Ann Neurol 1978; 3:393.
26. Folkman J: A family of angiogenic peptides. Nature 1987; 329:671.
27. Wiener LP, Henden RM, Narayan O, et al: Virus-related TSV40 in patients with progressive multifocal leukoencephalopathy. N Engl J Med 1972; 286:385.
28. Hughes M, Ahern V, Kefford R, Boyages J: Paraneoplastic myelopathy at diagnosis in a patient with pathologic stage IA Hodgkin disease. Cancer 1992; 70:1598.
29. Lachance DH, O'Neill BP, Harper CM Jr, et al: Paraneoplastic brachial plexopathy in a patient with Hodgkin's disease. Mayo Clin Proc 1991; 66:97.
30. Dellagi K, Dupouey P, Billecoq A, et al: Waldenström's macroglobulinemia and peripheral neuropathy: A clinical and immunologic study of 25 patients. Blood 1983; 62:280.
31. Turner ML, Boland OM, Parker AC, Ewing DJ: Subclinical autonomic dysfunction in patients with Hodgkin's disease and non-Hodgkin's lymphoma. Br J Haematol 1993; 84:623.
32. Tyler HR: Paraneoplastic syndromes of nerve, muscle, and neuromuscular junction. Ann NY Acad Sci 1974; 230:348.
33. Liu KL, Herbrecht R, Tranchant C, et al: Malignant thymic lymphoblastic lymphoma and myasthenia gravis: An exceptional association. Nouv Rev Fr Hematol 1992; 34:221.
34. Clark SC, Kamen R: The human hematopoietic colony-stimulating factors. Science 1987; 236:1229.
35. Kedar A, Khan AB, Mattern JQA II, et al: Autoimmune disorders complicating adolescent Hodgkin's disease. Cancer 1979; 44:112.
36. Berkman AW, Kickler T, Braine H: Platelet-associated IgG in patients with lymphoma. Blood 1984; 63:944.
37. Evans RS, Takahasi K, Duane RT, et al: Primary thrombocytopenic purpura and acquired hemolytic anemia: Evidence for a common etiology. Arch Intern Med 1957; 87:48.
38. Crisp D, Pruzanski W: B-cell neoplasms with homogenous cold-reacting antibodies (cold agglutinins). Am J Med 1982; 72:915.
39. Liaw Y, Yang P, Su I, et al: Mucosa-associated lymphoid tissue lymphoma of the lung with cold-reacting autoantibody-mediated hemolytic anemia. Chest 1994; 105:288.
40. Antman KH, Skarin AT, Mayer RJ, et al: Microangiopatic hemolytic anemia and cancer: A review. Medicine (Baltimore) 1979; 58:377.
41. Akard LP, Brandt J, Lee L, et al: Chronic T-cell lymphoproliferative disorder and pure red cell aplasia. Am J Med 1987; 83:1069.
42. Waterbury L: Hematologic problems. *In* Abeloff MD (ed): Complications of Cancer: Diagnosis and Management. Baltimore, Johns Hopkins Press, 1979, pp 121–145.
43. Hocking W, Goodman J, Goolde D: Granulocytosis associated with tumor production of colony-stimulating factor. Blood 1983; 61:600.
44. Okabe T, Sato N, Knodo Y, et al: Establishment and characterization of a human cancer cell line that produces human colony-stimulating factor. Cancer Res 1978; 38:3910.
45. Murata K, Yamada Y, Kamihira S, et al: Frequency of eosinophilia in adult T-cell leukemia/lymphoma. Cancer 1992; 69:966.
46. Samoszuk M, Ramzi E, Cooper DL: Interleukin-5 mRNA in three T-cell lymphomas with eosinophilia. Am J Hematol 1993; 42:402.
47. Samoszuk M, Nansen L: Detection of interleukin-5 messenger RNA in Reed-Sternberg cells of Hodgkin's disease with eosinophilia. Am Soc Hematol 1990; 75:13.
48. Paulus JM, Aster RH: Production, distribution, life span, and fate of platelets. *In* Williams WJ, Beutler E, Erslev AJ, Lichtman MA (eds): Hematology, 4th ed. New York, McGraw-Hill, 1990, p 1251.
49. Rosen P, Armstrong D: Nonbacterial thrombotic endocarditis in patients with malignant neoplastic disease. Am J Med 1973; 54:23.
50. Chad DA, Recht LD: Neurological paraneoplastic syndromes. Cancer Invest 1988; 6:67.
51. Dabbs DJ, Striker L, Mignon F, et al: Glomerular lesions in lymphomas and leukemias. Am J Med 1986; 80:63.
52. Hyman LR, Burkholder PM, Joo PA, Segar WE: Malignant lymphoma and the nephrotic syndrome: A clinicopathologic analysis with light

immunofluorescence and electron microscopy of the renal lesions. J Pediatr 1973; 82:207.

53. Curth HO: Classification of acanthosis nigricans. Int J Dermatol 1976; 15:592.

54. Cohen PR, Kurzrock R: Sweet's syndrome and malignancy. Am J Med 1987; 82:1220.

55. Tope WT, Fishbein JD, White PF, et al: Large cell lymphoma presenting with a distinctive inflammatory dermatosis. J Am Acad Dermatol 1991; 25:912.

56. Nicolis GD, Helwig EB: Exfoliative dermatitis: A clinicopathologic study of 135 cases. Arch Dermatol 1973; 108:788.

57. Perniciaro C, Kuechle MK, Colon-Otero G, et al: Paraneoplastic pemphigus: A case of prolonged survival. Mayo Clin Proc 1994; 69:851.

58. Rybojad M, Leblanc T, Flageul B, et al: Paraneoplastic pemphigus in a child with a T-cell lymphoblastic lymphoma. Br J Dermatol 1993; 128:418.

59. Tankel M, Tannenbaum S, Parekh S: Paraneoplastic pemphigus presenting as an unusual bullous eruption. J Am Acad Dermatol 1993; 29:825.

60. Fullerton SH, Woodley DT, Smoller RS, Anhalt GJ: Paraneoplastic pemphigus with autoantibody deposition in bronchial epithelium after autologous bone marrow transplantation. JAMA 1992; 267:1500.

61. Helm TN, Camisa C, Liu AY, et al: Lichen planus associated with neoplasia: A cell-mediated immune response to tumor antigens? J Am Acad Dermatol 1994; 30:219.

62. Naschitz JE, Yeshurun D, Zuckerman E, et al: Cancer-associated fasciitis panniculitis. Cancer 1994; 73:231.

63. Chan LS, Hanson CA, Cooper KD: Concurrent eosinophilic fasciitis and cutaneous T-cell lymphoma. Arch Dermatol 1991; 127:862.

64. Alonzo-Ruiz A, Zea-Mendoza AC, Salazar-Valinas JM, et al: Toxic oil syndrome: A syndrome with features overlapping those of various forms of scleroderma. Semin Arthritis Rheum 1986; 15:200.

65. Benisovich V, Papadopoulos E, Amorosi EL, et al: The association of progressive, atrophying, chronic granulomatous dermohypodermitis with Hodgkin's disease. Cancer 1988; 62:2425.

66. Yoneda T, Alsina MA, Chavez JB, et al: Evidence that tumor necrosis factor plays a role in the paraneoplastic syndromes of cachexia and leukocytosis in a human tumor in nude mice. J Clin Invest 1991; 87:977.

67. Waldman TA, Broder S, Strober W: Protein-losing enteropathies in malignancy. Ann NY Acad Sci 1974; 230:306.

68. Mathus-Vliegen EMH, Van Halteren H, Tutgat GNJ: Malignant lymphoma in coeliac disease: Various manifestations with distinct symptomatology and prognosis. J Intern Med 1994; 236:43.

69. Gilat T, Fischel B, Danon J, Lowenthal M: Morphology of small bowel mucosa and malignancy. Digestion 1972; 12:147.

70. Eck SL, Morse JH, Janssen DA, et al: Angioedema presenting as chronic gastrointestinal symptoms. Am J Gastroenterol 1993; 88:436.

71. Bain BJ, Catovsky D, Ewan PW: Acquired angioedema as the presenting feature of lymphoproliferative disorders of mature B lymphocytes. Cancer 1993; 72:3318.

72. Weyand CM, Hicok KC, Hunder GG, Goronzy JJ: Tissue cytokine patterns in patients with polymyalgia rheumatica and giant cell arthritis. Ann Intern Med 1994; 121:484.

73. Michaels RM, Sorber JA: Reflex sympathetic dystrophy as a probable paraneoplastic syndrome: Case report and literature review. Arthritis Rheum 1984; 27:1183.

74. Pfinsgraff J, Buckingham RB, Killian PJ, et al: Palmar fasciitis and arthritis with malignant neoplasms: A paraneoplastic syndrome. Semin Arthritis Rheum 1986; 16:118.

75. Efremidis A, Eiser AR, Grishman E, Rosenberg V: Hodgkin's lymphoma in an adolescent with systemic lupus erythematosus. Cancer 1984; 53:142.

76. Freundlich B, Makover D, Maul GG: A novel antinuclear antibody associated with a lupuslike paraneoplastic syndrome. Ann Intern Med 1988; 109:295.

77. Bohan A, Peter JB, Bowman RL, et al: A computer-assisted analysis of 153 patients with polymyositis and dermatomyositis. Medicine 1977; 56:255.

78. Dowsett RJ, Wong RL, Robert N, Abeles M: Dermatomyositis and Hodgkin's disease. Am J Med 1986; 80:719.

79. Sherry DD, Haas JE, Milstein JM: Childhood polymyositis as a paraneoplastic phenomenon. Pediatr Neurol 1993; 9:155.

80. Harris GJ, Murphy ML, Schmidt EW, et al: Orbital myositis as a paraneoplastic syndrome. Arch Ophthalmol 1994; 112:380.

81. Posner JB: Paraneoplastic syndromes. Neurol Clin 1991; 9:919.

82. Fukumoto S, Matsumoto T, Harada S, et al: Pheochromocytoma with pyrexia and marked inflammatory signs: A paraneoplastic syndrome with possible relation to interleukin-6 production. J Clin Endocrinol Metab 1991; 73:877.

83. Atkinson MK, McElwain TJ, Peckham MJ, et al: Hypertrophic pulmonary osteoarthropathy in Hodgkin's disease. Cancer 1976; 38:1729.

84. Martinez-Lavin M: Hypertrophic osteoarthropathy may occur as a primary condition. More often it is a clue to another underlying disease. Provocative new data may explain its pathogenesis. Contemp Intern Med 1992:75.

85. Glenner GC: Amyloid deposits and amyloidosis: The β-fibriloses. N Engl J Med 1966; 19:539.

86. Ponzoni M, Chin-Yang L: Isolated bone marrow non-Hodgkin's lymphoma: A clinicopathologic study. Mayo Clin Proc 1994; 69:37.

87. Diez-Martin JL, Lust JA, Witzig TE, et al: Unusual presentation of extranodal peripheral T-cell lymphomas with multiple paraneoplastic features. Cancer 1991; 68:834.

88. Raziuddin S, Sheikha A, Abu-eshy S, Al-Janadi M: Circulating levels of cytokines and soluble cytokine receptors in various T-cell malignancies. Cancer 1994; 73:2426.

89. Smith P, Ricci N, Toogood I, et al: A case of Burkitt's lymphoma presenting with digital ischaemia. Acta Paediatr 1993; 82:217.

90. Somerville JF, Lenaers AP, Abramowicz M, Neve PE: High cardiac output as a paraneoplastic syndrome. J Intern Med 1990; 229:89.

Chapter Thirty

Disorders that Mimic Lymphomas or May Predate Lymphoma

Arthur T. Skarin

EPSTEIN-BARR VIRUS AND BENIGN AND MALIGNANT LYMPHOPROLIFERATIVE DISORDERS

Years ago Dameshek and Gunz stated that infectious mononucleosis (IM) is a regulated neoplasm.[1] In the immunocompetent patient Epstein-Barr virus (EBV) infects B lymphocytes with induction of a set of nuclear proteins that presumably causes the well-known lymphoproliferative disorder (LPD) called IM. This polyclonal proliferative disorder, characterized mainly by lymphadenopathy, is then brought under control when T lymphocytes recognize the foreign peptides on the surface of the infected B lymphocytes by the major histocompatibility complex, resulting in eradication of the EBV-infected B cells. Clinical and laboratory manifestations of the illness resolve within a few weeks. In immunosuppressed patients, fatal IM can occur, as for example in the X-linked LPD described by Purtilo and Stevenson.[2] EBV may well be an important cofactor in the development of many LPDs in patients with primary and acquired immunodeficiencies.[3] Of great concern is the increasing number of posttransplant fatal LPDs implicating EBV (e.g., from a normal donor) as the etiologic agent.[4] The distinction between benign and malignant LPD may be difficult to clarify.[5] Furthermore, the significance of monoclonal and polyclonal proliferation remains poorly understood. EBV is detected in the chronic generalized adenopathy syndrome associated with acquired immunodeficiency syndrome. These histologically benign nodes are associated with an increased risk of subsequent high-grade B-cell lymphomas.[6] An understanding of the evolution from EBV infection of a benign polyclonal B-cell population to a malignant monoclonal population is critically important but as yet not worked out.[5]

AUTOIMMUNE LYMPHADENOPATHY

A number of autoimmune disorders are associated with lymphadenopathy and occasionally splenomegaly. These disorders are mainly rheumatoid arthritis, systemic lupus erythematosus (SLE), and Sjögren's syndrome, but also included are other less common entities such as dermatomyositis, Hashimoto's thyroiditis, Graves' disease, primary biliary cirrhosis, mixed connective tissue disease, and essential mixed cryoglobulinemia.[7] Most lymph node biopsy results show reactive lymphoid hyperplasia. Occasionally, the features may be confused with an early lymphoma. Since many patients have a risk of subsequent lymphoma, adequate tissue should be removed during the biopsy to permit optimal evaluation and diagnosis. Fresh, unfixed tissue should be available for special studies if necessary.

In rheumatoid arthritis, lymphadenopathy may occur in as many as 75% of patients at some time during the illness. The enlarged nodes may be regional (near inflamed joints), but generalized adenopathy can also occur.[8] Lymph node biopsy shows extensive reactive follicular hyperplasia and paracortical (interfollicular) plasmacytosis. Immunophenotyping reveals the presence of polyclonal B cells. The predominant T lymphocytes are CD4+ with CD4-to-CD8 ratios of 2:1 to 7:1, depending on the origin of the data or nodal location (paracortical versus follicular).[8, 9] Interleukin-6 (IL-6) has been found at high concentrations in a lymph node of one patient with rheumatoid arthritis.[10] Since IL-6 is a multifunctional cytokine that assists B-cell differentiation to plasma cells, it may play a role in the pathogenesis of rheumatoid arthritis–related adenopathy. Chronic immune stimulation has also been postulated.[7] Patients with rheumatoid arthritis appear to be at increased risk of malignant LPDs (usually large B-cell lymphoma), particularly with long-standing disease of at least 15 years.[11] Immunosuppressive therapy with azathioprine may also play a role in development of secondary lymphomas. Felty's syndrome, a rare complication of severe rheumatoid arthritis that occurs in 1% of patients, consists of splenomegaly, neutropenia, and recurrent infections.[12] In a retrospective review of 906 men from a Veterans Affairs Hospital, the risk for subsequent non-Hodgkin's lymphoma (NHL) was much greater that the twofold risk reported in rheumatoid arthritis and was similar to the risk of lymphoma in Sjögren's syndrome.[13]

Lymphadenopathy in patients with SLE is also common, occurring in 25% to 67% of patients.[14] Patients are generally younger than those with rheumatoid arthritis, and adenopathy and enlarged nodes may be the presenting complaint. Biopsy shows diffuse hyperplasia of small lymphocytes and plasma cells along with a conspicuous population of large immunoblasts.[7] The latter may contain two nuclei and simulate Reed-Sternberg cells. The most characteristic features, however, are coagulation necrosis, hematoxylin bodies (extracellular amorphous material composed of degenerated cellular contents, mostly DNA), and DNA deposition within vessel walls.[15] Detailed immunophenotypic and molecular biologic studies were not available in older studies, but evaluation of a recent case has been carried out[16]: The lymph node showed paracortical hyperplasia of T lymphocytes (CD4-to-CD8 ratio, 3:1) with scattered hyperplastic secondary follicles composed of polytypic B lymphocytes. Necrotic foci in the node were surrounded by histiocytes and small reactive T cells with a predominance of CD8+ lymphocytes (CD4-to-CD8 ratio, 1:5).[16] The pathogenesis of SLE adenopathy is unknown but apparently is not related to vasculitis. One theory is that lymphocytotoxic autoantibodies mediate abortive lymphocyte transformation, resulting in multifocal karyorrhexis, debris, and necrosis. A related reaction occurs in the animal model for SLE, the New Zealand B-mouse.[17] Cancers and lymphomas occur in patients with SLE at variable rates, suggesting an association perhaps related to therapy or other unknown factors. An early report described and reviewed lymphoma in 18 cases of SLE, with simultaneous diagnoses in 4, lymphoma predating SLE in 2, and occurring after SLE in 16.[18] More recently, 5 cases of lymphoma were reported in patients with autoimmune disorders, including 2 with SLE.[19] The lymphomas in these reports included Hodgkin's disease, NHL (usually large cell type), and chronic lymphocytic leukemia.[19] An overexpression of oncogenes was postulated as partly responsible for the malignancy, particularly since oncogene activation (c-*myc*, c-*myb*, and c-*ras*) has been detected in peripheral blood of patients with SLE.[20]

Sjögren's syndrome is an autoimmune disorder characterized by dryness of the eyes and mouth along with serum autoantibodies and abnormal lymphoid infiltrates on lower lip or minor salivary gland biopsy.[21] The disease may be primary or associated with other connective tissue diseases such as rheumatoid arthritis. Clinical features appear to be a consequence of CD4+ T-cell-mediated attack on autoantigenic epitopes of glandular and ductal elements.[21] Lymphadenopathy occasionally occurs in patients with Sjögren's syndrome and may be localized or generalized. The initial biopsy usually shows reactive follicular hyperplasia and interfollicular plasmacytosis, which is characteristic of rheumatoid arthritis. Atypical features may also be present similar to features of angioimmunoblastic lymphadenopathy (AILD; see later); this condition is often called "pseudolymphoma." Patients are at increased risk of LPD, which has been reported in excised enlarged lymph nodes of 18 of 138 patients.[22] Types of LPD vary from low-grade small lymphocytic to large cell B-immunoblastic. Salivary gland enlargement in patients with Sjögren's syndrome indicates development of an LPD, as does hepatosplenomegaly, pulmonary infiltrates, renal insufficiency, cytopenias, and increased or even decreased serum immunoglobulin M (IgM) levels. Mikulicz's disease (myoepithelial sialadenitis) refers to classic histopathologic features seen in enlarged salivary glands of patients with Sjögren's syndrome. Although the features appear to be benign, modern immunohistologic and molecular genetic studies have revealed monoclonal B-cell populations that undoubtedly evolve into malignant LPD.[23] The development of Sjögren's syndrome–associated LPD appears to be related to several factors, including chronic immune stimulation, EBV-driven B-cell expansion, genetic alterations, and defective immune surveillance.[7, 21]

HYPERSENSITIVITY LYMPHADENOPATHY

DRUG HYPERSENSITIVITY

Patients may develop lymphadenopathy as a hypersensitivity reaction to medications (Table 30–1). Other features such as fever, rash, arthralgias, and eosinophilia are usually present but rarely may be absent.[7] In either case, an underlying lymphoma may be considered, and lymph node biopsies are often carried out, with findings suggesting a lymphoma. An existing or subsequent malignant LPD may develop, particularly in patients taking anticonvulsant drugs.

The adenopathy in patients receiving phenytoin and related hydantoin derivatives has been described most extensively with a classic report in 1959 that detailed the clinical and laboratory features.[24] Most patients with this adenopathy have been on the drug for less than 4 months, although some have had drug exposure for years. Adenopathy is particularly prominent in the cervical lymph nodes. Biopsy most often shows features similar to viral-induced lymphadenopathy, with partial or complete effacement of nodal architecture by a polymorphous infiltrate of immunoblasts, small lymphocytes, eosinophils, and plasma cells. Areas of necrosis may be present along with large binucleated immunoblasts suggestive of Reed-Sternberg cells.[25]

Terms such as "pseudolymphoma" and "pseudo-pseudolymphoma" have been used to describe drug-induced adenopathy, but these only cause confusion and should be abandoned. A diagnosis of atypical LPD is most often used. In a recent review, a wide range of histologic features, varying from reactive to malignant, was reported by the Armed Forces Institute of Pathology.[26] Among 25 patients with phenytoin exposure for 6 weeks to 30 years who developed adenopathy, 15 had benign LPD and 10 had malignant LPD. The former included typical and atypical follicular and mixed hyperplasias, paracortical immunoblas-

Table 30–1. Medications Associated with Lymphadenopathy

Phenytoin (Dilantin; Parke-Davis, Morris Plains, NJ)	Carbamazepine (Tegretol; Basel, Summit, NJ)
Para-amino salicylic acid	Phenylbutazone
Indomethacin	Aspirin
Sulphonamides	Iron dextran
Penicillins	Erythromycin
Gentamicin	Tetracycline
Thiouracil compounds	Sulfasalazine
Griseofulvin	Antithymocyte globulin
OKT-3	Gold
Halothane	Bacillus Calmette-Guérin
Allopurinol	Insulin
Primidone	Methyldopa, levodopa

From Segal G, Clough JD, Tubbs RR: Autoimmune and iatrogenic causes of lymphadenopathy. Semin Oncol 1993; 20:611.

tic proliferations, and LPD resembling AILD (see later). The malignant LPDs were composed of seven cases of NHL and three cases of Hodgkin's disease. Serial study of two cases showed progression of atypical hyperplasia to NHL. Unfortunately, immunophenotyping, T- and B-cell gene rearrangement studies, and use of molecular probes have not been carried out in most studies.

An unusual but reversible hypersensitivity reaction consists of adenopathy, hepatosplenomegaly, eosinophilia, and generalized pruritic exfoliative erythroderma suggesting mycosis fungoides that developed in three patients receiving phenytoin.[27] The patients also had circulating Sézary-like cells. Studies showed a "hyperimmune" status with an increase in peripheral blood T lymphocytes, significant stimulation of lymphocyte-blastic transformation by phenytoin and low response to pokeweed mitogen stimulation, and the impaired ability of T-suppressor lymphocytes to suppress B-cell differentiation and immunoglobulin production.[27] The clinical and laboratory abnormalities in all patients regressed after discontinuation of phenytoin.

More than 30 cases of adenopathy related to carbamazepine, a newer anticonvulsant than phenytoin, have been reported.[7] Histologically, features suggestive of AILD or NHL have been observed in a small number of patients. Some patients have been studied by use of immunophenotypic markers. Abnormalities vary and include a CD4+ T-cell immunoblastic proliferation with loss of CD7 antigen,[28] a mixture of CD4+ and CD8+ T cells,[29] and a B-cell IgM, κ-restricted large cell lymphoma.[30] When carbamazepine (as well as phenytoin) is discontinued, adenopathy regresses in most patients. However, long-term followup is important, particularly when adenopathy persists or progresses owing to the risk of an evolving malignant LPD. When a lymph node biopsy is performed, multiple diagnostic studies should be carried out (as outlined earlier) for optimal definition of a clonal (malignant) disorder.

Multiple factors have been suggested for the association of phenytoin and related drugs with subsequent benign and malignant LPDs. Chronic immunosuppression from the drugs was implied in an epidemiologic study.[31] It was found that 8 (1.6%) of 516 patients with Hodgkin's disease or NHL had a history of phenytoin therapy compared with 3 (0.6%) of 516 patients with other cancers and 2 (0.4%) of 516 tumor-free subjects. Abnormalities of the immune system occur in as many as 70% of patients receiving phenytoin and carbamazepine[7, 32, 33] and include (1) suppressor T-cell abnormalities, both decreased and increased function; (2) depressed cellular and humoral responses; (3) serum sickness–like (immune complex) disease; (4) abnormal lymphocyte metabolism; (5) autoimmune phenomenon; and (6) severe immune dysregulation.[29]

It has been estimated that the incidence of hypersensitivity to phenytoin is about 1 in 10^3 to 10^5 people.[34] There appears to be a genetic predisposition to anticonvulsant hypersensitivity reactions that is an autosomal recessive inheritance of an enzyme defect.[34] The abnormality prevents detoxification of electrophilic metabolites (arene oxides) of aromatic anticonvulsants. As a result, the metabolites combine with cellular macromolecules, creating haptenlike neoantigenic epitopes that may result in abnormal immune responses.[34, 35] Of clinical relevance, in vitro tests are available to determine individual susceptibility, which is especially useful in patients with a family history of

anticonvulsant drug hypersensitivity reactions.[34] Although most patients with anticonvulsant-related LPD have benign lesions that regress after discontinuation of drug, others develop malignant LPD (as reviewed earlier). The latter process is undoubtedly multifactorial, including many immune disturbances owing to the drugs, familial or genetic predispositions, and other unknown factors affecting DNA that all result in the emergence of a malignant clone.

SILICONE-ASSOCIATED LYMPHADENOPATHY (IATROGENIC)

Adenopathy related to silicone has become increasingly recognized since silicone-elastomer prostheses became available for joint replacement surgery 25 years ago.[36] Most cases occur in patients with rheumatoid arthritis who have had replacement surgery for hand deformities resulting in subsequent axillary adenopathy.[37] Inguinal adenopathy has rarely been reported, usually related to insertion of a silicone prosthesis in the lower extremities.[37]

Lymph node biopsy shows reactive lymphoid hyperplasia with many multinucleated giant cells, most containing refractile, nonbirefringent material that proves to be silicone.[38] Confluent noncaseating granulomas may also be present.[39] It has been estimated that as many as 15% of patients undergoing silicone implant arthroplasty may develop regional adenopathy.[38] Over many years, particulate silicone generated by small fractures of the prosthesis is trapped in draining lymph nodes, resulting in slowly progressive asymptomatic enlargement. A lymphoma may be suspected, particularly in patients with underlying rheumatoid arthritis, and biopsy can be justified. Nonsilicone large joint implants using polyester or polyethylene may also result in regional lymphadenopathy by a similar mechanism.[40] Lymph node biopsy shows characteristic sinus histiocytosis with polarizing, birefringent material in the cytoplasm of histiocytes.

Liquid silicone used in breast augmentation procedures may eventually result in regional adenopathy. Although axillary nodes are mainly asymptomatic, occasional tender nodes have occurred.[38] Breast prostheses may rupture or particulate silicone may slowly leak from an intact prosthesis, eventually resulting in lymph node enlargement.[41, 42] Histologic findings are less reactive than those related to solid silicone joint prostheses and include only occasional multinucleated giant cells and clear silicone-containing vacuoles.[41]

Recently, the association of silicone breast implants with certain autoimmune disorders, including scleroderma, has been suggested.[43] The data appear to be controversial, and the disorders ordinarily would not suggest an LPD.

ATYPICAL LYMPHOPROLIFERATIVE DISORDERS (POTENTIALLY MALIGNANT)

A variety of entities have been described that can be termed "atypical" LPDs.[44] These disorders are characterized by indolent lymphadenopathy, organomegaly, and occasionally systemic symptoms. They represent lymphoid proliferation in response to unknown stimuli but poor regulation by a defective immune system that is prone to clonal evolution resulting in malignancy.[45] The morphologic features of these atypical LPDs include (1) extensive alteration of nodal architecture, but without loss of the normal anatomic compartments; (2) expansion of the interfollicular areas by an intense immunoblastic proliferation and an increase in endothelial venules; and (3) alterations of the germinal centers (including regressive transformation, follicle lysis, and proteinaceous deposits).[46] Several well-defined clinicopathologic entities of atypical LPD exist and are reviewed in the following sections.

ANGIOFOLLICULAR (GIANT) LYMPH NODE HYPERPLASIA (CASTLEMAN'S DISEASE)

In 1956 Castleman and coworkers described a patient with a localized mediastinal mass that on biopsy showed hyperplasia resembling a thymoma.[47] Various confusing terms were subsequently employed, including "localized hamartoma," "angiomatous lymphoid hamartoma," "benign giant lymphoma," and, more recently, "angiofollicular or giant lymph node hyperplasia."[46] Detailed studies have described two forms of the same disease, referred to as the plasma cell type (10% of cases) and the hyaline vascular type (90% of cases).[48] Patients may present with the same histologic features with either unicentric-localized or more generalized and extensive lymphadenopathy called "multicentric angiofollicular lymphoid hyperplasia"[49] or systemic LPD with morphologic features of Castleman's disease.[50]

The diagnosis of systemic or multicentric Castleman's disease is based on the following clinicopathologic criteria: (1) histologic features, of plasma cell type (see later); (2) generalized peripheral lymphadenopathy; (3) multisystem involvement; and (4) idiopathic etiology.[46] Clinical features include weakness, fever, night sweats, weight loss, anorexia, enlargement of multiple lymph node sites, hepatosplenomegaly, edema and effusions, skin rash, and neurologic abnormalities. Laboratory findings show anemia in most cases but also thrombocytopenia and leukopenia, proteinuria, abnormal liver tests, hypoalbuminemia, and elevated gamma globulin levels. Of considerable importance is that subsequent NHL occurs in 18% of patients and Kaposi's sarcoma in 13% of patients.[46]

The histopathologic features of multicentric Castleman's disease in enlarged lymph nodes include recognizable architecture, germinal center abnormalities, and plasmacytosis. A nodular architectural pattern predominates. The interfollicular areas are expanded with a florid plasmacytosis. The germinal centers are also expanded, hypervascularized, and often ill defined. A predominant component of endothelial cells and large pale eosinophilic cells (follicular dendritic reticulum cells) are present. The partially hyalinized and atrophic germinal centers and prominent mantle cells often present a characteristic "onion skin" appearance. In some patients depletion of germinal center lymphoid cells and the resulting collapse of the stromal vascular component may result in hyaline vascular structures, as initially described by Castleman and coworkers.[47] Plasma cells may also be sparse. When the latter features are prominent, the condition has been classified as the hyaline vascular form of Castleman's disease.

As noted earlier, the histopathologic findings are not specific for multicentric Castleman's disease but may be seen in other autoimmune disorders, primary immunodeficiencies, human immunodeficiency virus (HIV) infection, and in association with Kaposi's sarcoma.[46] Immunophenotypic studies in a small number of cases of multicentric Castleman's disease have revealed the presence of polyclonal as well as monoclonal plasma cells.[51] The mantle zones are composed of IgM+ D+ polyclonal B lymphocytes (CD19+, CD20+, CD22+), which also express HLA-DR and the pan-T antigen CD5.[52] Within the follicles, both CD4+ and CD8+ T cells as well as CD57 (Leu 7)-positive cells are found. Large amounts of IL-6 have been detected in the germinal centers, with the IL-6 gene expressed by follicular dendritic reticulum cells as well as by other reactive cells in the interfollicular areas.[53, 54] Elevation of blood IL-6 levels has also been reported in patients having POEMS syndrome (*p*olyneuropathy, *o*rganomegaly, *e*ndocrinopathy, *M*-component, and *s*kin changes) with enlarged lymph nodes and spleen compatible with Castleman's disease.[55, 56] These patients also have a clonal plasma cell component occurring either diffusely throughout the node or forming several nodular areas.[52]

The pathogenesis of Castleman's disease appears to be related to several factors, including antigenic-driven lymphoproliferation, autoimmunity, and defective immune regulation.[46] It has been proposed that the stimulus for B-cell proliferation is dysregulated IL-6 production, a B-cell growth factor, by the germinal centers.[53] As noted earlier, excessive expression of the IL-6 gene has been detected in lymph node biopsies; furthermore, retroviral transduction of IL-6 coding sequences in bone marrow cells has reproduced the clinical and laboratory features of Castleman's disease in mice.[57] Additional findings of interest include the presence of CD5+ lymphocytes in lymph node follicles (contrary to normal nodes), which are an autoantibody-producing lymphocyte subset.[52] It has been suggested that the pathogenesis of multicentric Castleman's disease is related to lymphoproliferation of a specific autoantibody-producing B-cell subset, driven toward plasma cell differentiation by abnormal IL-6 production and unregulated by a defective immune system.[46]

Limited data are available concerning therapy for multicentric Castleman's disease. Spontaneous remission may occur. In symptomatic patients, relatively high doses of corticosteroids have resulted in prolonged remissions. Systemic manifestations of Castleman's disease in a patient with elevated serum IL-6 levels were alleviated by monoclonal anti-IL-6 antibody.[58] Standard-dose chemotherapeutic regimens used in NHL have often been used with some success. Radiation therapy, used in localized disease, may also result in responses.[46]

ANGIOIMMUNOBLASTIC LYMPHADENOPATHY WITH DYSPROTEINEMIA

The atypical LPD called AILD, an entity with clinical features of lymphoma, was described more than 20 years ago by several investigators.[59–61] Characteristically, patients present with systemic symptoms, generalized adenopathy, hepatosplenomegaly, fever, skin rash, arthralgias, Coombs'-

positive hemolytic anemia, and, frequently, polyclonal hypergammaglobulinemia. The patients are at high risk for developing an NHL, usually of large cell histology and T-cell immunophenotype. AILD-like peripheral T-cell lymphomas are closely associated (see Chapter 24).

Lymph node biopsy shows a diffuse effacement of architecture with loss of reactive germinal centers, sinuses, and blurring of the distinction between the cortex and paracortex.[60, 61] A prominent arborizing vasculature is readily evident, and amorphous pink-staining proteinaceous material is present in the interstitium. Interspersed throughout the lymph node are large immunoblasts, along with a polymorphous infiltrate of plasma cells, lymphocytes, eosinophils, and epithelioid histiocytes. The overall picture is similar to other atypical and viral-related LPDs. In some instances, however, AILD and AILD-like lymphomas may be difficult to distinguish from each other.

Immunophenotyping shows that the predominant cells are CD4+ and CD8+ lymphocytes, with the former more frequent. Polyclonal B lymphocytes are also present, expressing both κ and λ light chains.[44]

Gene arrangement studies have not been helpful in distinguishing benign from malignant disease. Both T-cell-receptor β-chain gene rearrangements and immunoglobulin heavy chain rearrangements have been detected, occasionally in the same patient.[62] However, use of a polymerase chain reaction–based method for detecting clonal T-cell-receptor rearrangements in a patient with cutaneous T-cell lymphoma demonstrated T-cell clones in all skin nodules undergoing biopsy but not in the original lymph node involved by AILD.[63] It was postulated that in some patients with AILD, T-cell expansion may not be detectable until a later stage of the disease. It has been concluded that AILD is an oligoclonal LPD, involving either T or B lymphocytes, in which proliferating clones might spontaneously regress.[59] The pool of proliferating lymphocytes, however, might be at risk of secondary genetic damage (e.g., chromosome translocations and mutations) that may result in a subsequent malignant lymphoma.

Cytogenetic studies have not revealed any consistent chromosome markers that might distinguish AILD from AILD lymphoma. Chromosome translocations, however, have been reported involving breakpoints carrying assignments of antigen receptor genes (e.g., 7q35, the location of the T-cell-receptor β-chain gene) that are involved in other T-cell malignancies (e.g., peripheral T-cell lymphoma).[64] Further studies of the chromosome rearrangements involving antigen receptor genes may shed some light on their involvement in the pathogenesis of AILD and AILD-like lymphomas.

Molecular pathogenesis is currently under investigation.[59] The c-*myb* oncogene that is involved in lymphocyte cell division is expressed in AILD tissues.[65] In addition, DNA viruses (e.g., cytomegalovirus and EBV) have also been detected, but it is not known whether the latter are involved in inducing the clonal expansion of lymphoid cells or present only in the setting of an altered immune response.

The clinical course of AILD is rapidly progressive, with mortality rates of 48% to 72% and median survival ranging from 11 to 30 months.[59] Most patients die from infections, including opportunistic types. Encouraging results have been recently reported with the use of doxorubicin-con-taining regimens, including complete remission in 7 (58%) of 12 patients in one study.[66] Cisplatin-based chemotherapy has also been effective.[67] Other treatment programs include the use of prednisone, human interferon-α,[68] and cyclosporine.[69]

Between 5% and 20% of patients with AILD develop a lymphoma, most commonly large cell immunoblastic lymphoma but also peripheral T-cell lymphoma and Hodgkin's disease.[66] In a recent study of AILD-type peripheral T-cell lymphoma, 32 (78%) of 41 patients showed aberrant clones detected by combined interphase and metaphase cytogenetics.[70] The abnormalities included trisomy 3, trisomy 5, and an additional X chromosome. The lymphomas are usually advanced with extranodal sites of disease and respond poorly to therapy. In a recent German multicenter study, however, prednisone with or without COP-BLAM (cyclophosphamide, Oncovin, prednisone, bleomycin, Adriamycin, Matulane)/IMVP-16 chemotherapy was administered to 39 patients, with a complete remission in about half the patients and long-term disease-free survival in one third.[71] A large cell immunoblastic B-cell lymphoma developed in a patient with AILD.[72] Studies showed oligoclonal gene rearrangements associated with EBV in lymphoma cells but not in the AILD lymph nodes. It was postulated that the deficit in cellular immunity that accompanies AILD might permit primary EBV infection or reactivation of latent infection, eventually with a second genetic event in one or more clones of EBV-infected cells resulting in the malignant lymphoma.[71] Finally, patients with AILD have a 4% incidence of various carcinomas and HIV-negative Kaposi's sarcoma.[73, 74]

ANGIOCENTRIC IMMUNOPROLIFERATIVE DISORDERS

The term "angiocentric immunoproliferative disorder" refers to several conditions that have similar histologic features but quite variable clinical courses.[75, 76] The disorders include lymphomatoid granulomatosis, lymphomatoid papulosis, lethal midline granuloma (polymorphic reticulosis), and Wegener's granulomatosis. The diseases may be localized or generalized and may present with skin lesions, adenopathy, and pulmonary and other organ involvement. Histologic features include polymorphous lymphoid infiltrates surrounding a prominent vasculitis with necrosis owing to lymphocytic involvement of arteries and veins (angiocentric and angiodestructive). The focal necrosis within lymphoid nodules results in "granulomatosis," which should not be confused with granulomatous inflammation. A unifying concept proposes that these disorders are part of a spectrum of peripheral (postthymic) T-cell lymphomas, which vary from low grade, characteristically involving the upper aerodigestive tract, to high-grade disease, which involves the lower respiratory tract or causes multisystem disease.[75]

Lymphomatoid granulomatosis usually affects men more than women (2 to 3:1) in the fifth or sixth decade.[77, 78] Most patients present with respiratory symptoms and bilateral discrete, rounded pulmonary nodules, often with cavitation. Extrathoracic manifestations are common and include skin involvement in 37% and nervous system involvement in 30% of patients.[78] About 12% of cases develop a recognizable malignant lymphoma, usually a large T-cell type. Cytogenetic studies in one patient with lymphomatoid granulomatosis of 3 year's duration showed an abnormal clone supporting a neoplastic process.[79] Genotypic analysis, however, failed to reveal clonal T-cell proliferation. Another report showed rearranged DNA, indicating the presence of a clonal T-cell proliferative disorder.[80] The prognosis is generally poor, with a mortality rate higher than 50%. Chemotherapy substantially improves survival.[75]

Wegener's granulomatosis may occasionally simulate a lymphoma. Characteristically, patients present with pulmonary and renal lesions.[81] Other features include proptosis, musculoskeletal symptoms, skin infiltrates, and systemic complaints. Histologically, the inflammatory lesions are characterized by vasculitis, necrosis, and granulomatous changes. The clinical course varies from indolent to rapidly progressive. Benefit is achieved by the use of glucocorticoids and cyclophosphamide. Despite many years of research, the etiology remains unknown. Only 2.5% of patients die from a subsequent malignancy.[81]

UNUSUAL CAUSES OF LYMPHADENOPATHY

INFLAMMATORY PSEUDOTUMOR OF LYMPH NODES

Inflammatory pseudotumor of lymph nodes is an entity that occurs mainly in young adults who present with enlarged lymph nodes in single or multiple sites, with or without systemic complaints.[82, 83] The nodes may be quite large (>3 cm) and involve central as well as peripheral sites. Mild anemia and hypergammaglobulinemia are often present. Lymph node biopsy reveals expansion of the hilum and fibrous trabeculae with proliferation of spindle cells and vessels, admixed with lymphocytes and plasma cells. The uninvolved nodal parenchyma shows only nonspecific reactive changes. These features may at times be mistaken for Kaposi's sarcoma, Castleman's disease, Hodgkin's disease, or NHL.[84] The inflammatory pseudotumor of lymph nodes probably represents the end result of an inflammatory response to multiple etiologies, including *Pseudomonas psittici* or toxoplasmosis infection.[84] Spontaneous regression occurs in most patients.

HISTIOCYTIC NECROTIZING LYMPHADENITIS (KIKUCHI'S LYMPHADENITIS)

Histiocytic necrotizing lymphadenitis (Kikuchi's lymphadenitis) is a benign self-limiting disease that was first described in 1972.[85] It occurs worldwide; most patients are younger than 40 years of age and there is a female predominance. Solitary or multiple lymph nodes are enlarged, most often in the cervical area, usually nontender, and rarely larger than 2 cm in diameter.[84] Constitutional symptoms often occur including a recent flulike illness. Lymph node histopathology consists of histiocytic proliferation with karyorrhectic foci often exhibiting a "starry-sky" appearance. The center of the karyorrhectic foci shows coagulative necrosis surrounded by histiocytes, plasmacytoid monocytes, and immunoblasts (T-cell lineage). Characteristic "crescentic histiocytes" are phagocytic cells with eccentrically located crescentic nuclei.[84] The clinical course is usually self-limited, although corticosteroids may occasionally be indicated.[86] An infectious etiology has been postulated with a number of organisms implicated, including EBV, parainfluenza virus, and toxoplasmosis.[84]

SINUS HISTIOCYTOSIS WITH MASSIVE LYMPHADENOPATHY (ROSAI-DORFMAN DISEASE)

Sinus histiocytosis with massive lymphadenopathy (Rosai-Dorfman disease) is an unusual entity that was initially described in 1969.[87] It is characterized by greatly enlarged and matted lymph nodes in an otherwise healthy person. Subsequent studies, however, have shown that in about 40% of cases the disease can occur in extranodal sites.[88] These sites include the skin, nasal sinuses, soft tissues, orbit, bone, salivary gland, and central nervous system. Rosai-Dorfman disease usually occurs in young adults, with a mean age of about 20 years.[88] About 25% of patients have fever. The systemic features include fever, elevated sedimentation rate, low serum albumin level, polyclonal hypergammaglobulinemia, reversal of CD4-to-CD8 ratio in peripheral blood lymphocytes, and anemia. About 10% of cases have one or more immune disorders preceding or associated with onset of the disease.[88, 89]

Lymph node biopsy shows a thickened fibrous capsule with distention of the sinuses by large, benign histiocytes characterized by abundant cytoplasm and vesicular nuclei with prominent nucleoli. The latter cells apparently have no known morphologic counterpart; however, immunophenotypic and histochemical features suggest they are activated macrophages.[84] Plasma cells are also present in the sinuses and parenchyma. The differential diagnosis includes metastatic carcinoma, melanoma, and malignant lymphoma. The etiology of Rosai-Dorfman disease is unknown. It appears to represent an unusual histiocytic reaction possibly mediated by secretion of cytokines. It has rarely been noted as an incidental finding in lymph nodes involved by lymphoma, Langerhans' cell histiocytosis, or nonspecific reactive hyperplasia.[84]

Most patients have a self-limited clinical course with spontaneous remission in several weeks. Rarely, relapse or progressive disease may occur with life-threatening complications necessitating the use of corticosteroids, radiation therapy, or chemotherapy.[90]

VASCULAR TRANSFORMATION OF SINUSES

Vascular transformation of sinuses, also called "nodal angiomatosis" and "stasis lymphadenopathy," is an uncommon entity that is a reactive condition characterized by transformation of lymph node sinuses into complex endothelial-lined channels.[91–93] The entity represents an incidental finding in draining lymph nodes obtained at the time of surgery for cancer or lymphoma. Other causative factors that contribute to lymphatic or vascular obstruction include thrombosis, severe heart failure, and previous regional surgery or radiation therapy. Rarely, patients have no obvious predisposing factors.[84]

Microscopically, vascular transformation of the sinuses

shows expansion and sclerosis of nodal sinuses with sparing of the nodal capsule. The normal lymphoid parenchymal shows variable degrees of atrophy. Within the sinuses vessel proliferation is prominent, with irregular slits or rounded vascular spaces lined by flat endothelium along with solid vascular foci. Kaposi's sarcoma may be confused with these features, but it usually extends beyond a pure sinusoidal location.[84]

PROGRESSIVE TRANSFORMATION OF GERMINAL CENTERS

Progressive transformation of germinal centers (PTGC) was initially described in 1975 as a closely associated lesion in nodular lymphocyte predominance Hodgkin's disease (NLPHD).[94] Subsequent studies suggested that PTGC often predated NLPHD by months to years.[95, 96] A recent detailed evaluation of five patients concluded that florid PTGC and lymphoid hyperplasia represented a syndrome in young men and adolescent boys that did not always progress to NLPHD.[97]

Most patients with PTGC are young men who present with asymptomatic solitary lymphadenopathy. Generalized lymph node enlargement is more common in pediatric patients, although florid PTGC, defined as more than nine PTGCs per lymph node cross section (see later), was associated with generalized adenopathy as well as persistent or recurrent adenopathy.[97]

Histologically, PTGCs are large lymphoid follicles in which mantle zone lymphocytes accumulate and expand the germinal center. In most reported cases, one to several PTGCs are noted in a single cross section, and most of the lymph node shows reactive changes.[97] Immunohistochemical studies show that PTGCs comprise mainly polyclonal B cells with the immunophenotype of mantle zone lymphocytes. Also present are T cells (especially CD4+), natural killer cells, and a dense network of dendritic reticulum cells.[97] The etiology of PTGC is unknown. It might reflect an ineffective immune response to certain antigens since PTGCs contain relatively few transformed lymphocytes. The finding of PTGC in patients with previous or active Hodgkin's disease, as well as hypogammaglobulinemia—both disorders associated with T-cell defects—also supports an immunologic abnormality as causative.[97]

Patients with PTGC require no therapy. Adenopathy often regresses spontaneously. Most important, a diagnosis of NLPHD or follicular lymphoma must be excluded. Long-term followup is indicated owing to a risk for subsequent NLPHD, which may be minimal in cases showing the florid form of PTGC.[97]

MISCELLANEOUS BENIGN DISORDERS

A number of benign disorders may be associated with reactive lymphadenopathy (see Table 10–1 in Chapter 10). The histopathologic findings are described in standard pathology textbooks, and only certain conditions that may be confused with lymphoma are discussed here.

Sarcoidosis is a multisystem disease of unknown cause, characterized by noncaseating granulomas throughout vari-ous tissues and organs. Many clinical presentations occur, particularly bilateral hilar adenopathy or lung involvement, eye and skin lesions, and lymphadenopathy. Lymph node biopsy specimens show noncaseating granulomas composed of epithelioid cells, often with Langhans' or foreign body–type giant cells. Within the granulomas are found two characteristic features: (1) laminated concretions composed of calcium and proteins known as Schaumann's bodies and (2) stellate-shaped inclusions called asteroid bodies within giant cells. Their features are not pathognomonic of sarcoidosis, since they may also be seen in other granulomatous diseases such as berylliosis.[98]

Patients usually have deficient T-cell responses as well as reduction in peripheral blood T lymphocytes, particularly T-helper cells.[98] In contrast, T-helper cells are increased in the lung. Peripheral blood B-cells are normal in number but show an enhanced humoral immunity as evidenced by hypergammaglobulinemia with abnormally high levels of antibodies to commonly encountered antigens. There appears to be no excess risk of lymphomas in patients with sarcoidosis.[99]

Dermatopathic adenopathy (DA) refers to enlarged lymph nodes often found in patients with chronic skin diseases, particularly generalized exfoliative dermatitis and mycosis fungoides. In mycosis fungoides, about 25% of early cases have dermatopathic adenopathy, 70% to 75% of advanced cases, and 90% of patients with generalized erythroderma (Sézary syndrome).[100] Lymph node biopsy shows the normal follicular pattern and an intact capsule. The follicles, however, show slight enlargement of their germinal centers surrounded by a rim of lymphocytes. The paracortical areas stand out as pale patches, owing to an increase in large histiocytes or macrophages with abundant pale cytoplasm and large pale nucleoli. Interspersed are small lymphocytes with cerebriform nuclei, which are difficult to distinguish from mycosis fungoides cells. Special studies show that the large, pale cells are composed of dendritic cells, Langerhans' cells, and indeterminate cells.[100]

Most patients with *primary systemic amyloidosis* present with nephrotic syndrome, congestive heart failure, orthostatic hypotension, carpal tunnel syndrome, and peripheral neuropathy. Only occasionally is generalized adenopathy or splenomegaly the presenting feature.[101] Tissue biopsy shows deposition of the amorphous hyaline-like substance that stains pink with hematoxylin and eosin. Under polarized light, Congo red produces an apple-green birefringence. Electron microscopy reveals the diagnostic rigid, linear, nonbranching aggregated fibrils of indefinite length and with hollow cases.[101] Recent data suggest that amyloidosis is a generic term referring to a final common pathway for tissue protein deposition in a wide variety of diseases.[102] It is rarely associated with underlying lymphomas.[103]

REFERENCES

1. Dameshek W, Gunz F: Leukemia, 2nd ed. New York, Grune & Stratton, 1964, p 316.
2. Purtilo DT, Stevenson M: Lymphotropic viruses as etiologic agents of lymphoma. Hematol Oncol Clin North Am 1991; 5:901.
3. Filipovich AH, Mathur A, Kamat D, et al: Primary immunodeficiencies: Genetic risk factors for lymphoma. Cancer Res 1992; 52(Suppl 19):5465s.

4. Seiden MV, Sklar J: Molecular genetic analysis of post-transplant lymphoproliferative disorders. Hematol Oncol Clin North Am 1993; 7:447.

5. Yarbro JW: The Epstein-Barr virus and the distinction between benign and malignant lymphoproliferative processes. Semin Oncol 1993; 20:658.

6. Shibata D, Weiss LM, Nathwani BN, et al: Epstein-Barr virus in benign lymph node biopsies from individuals infected with the human immunodeficiency virus is associated with concurrent or subsequent development of non-Hodgkin's lymphoma. Blood 1991; 77:1527.

7. Segal G, Clough JD, Tubbs RR: Autoimmune and iatrogenic causes of lymphadenopathy. Semin Oncol 1993; 20:611.

8. Kojima M, Hosomura Y, Itoh H, et al: Reactive proliferative lesions in lymph nodes from rheumatoid arthritis patients: A clinicopathological and immunohistochemical study. Acta Pathol Jpn 1990; 40:249.

9. Kondratowicz GM, Symmons DPM, Bacon PA, et al: Rheumatoid lymphadenopathy: A morphological and immunohistochemical study. J Clin Pathol 1990; 143:106.

10. Numata Y, Matsuura Y, Onishi S, et al: Interleukin-6 positive follicular hyperplasia in lymph node of a patient with rheumatoid arthritis. Am J Hematol 1991; 36:282.

11. Symmons DPM: Neoplasms of the immune system in rheumatoid arthritis. Am J Med 1985; 78(Suppl 1A):22.

12. Rosenstein ED, Kramer N: Felty's and pseudo-Felty's syndrome. Semin Arthritis Rheum 1991; 21:129.

13. Gridley G, Klippel JH, Hoover RN, et al: Incidence of cancer among men with the Felty syndrome. Ann Intern Med 1994; 120:35.

14. Estes D, Christian CC: The natural history of systemic lupus erythematosus by prospective analysis. Medicine 1971; 50:85.

15. Schnitzer B: Reactive lymphoid hyperplasia. In Jaffe ES (ed): Surgical Pathology of the Lymph Nodes and Related Organs. Philadelphia, WB Saunders, 1985, pp 22–56.

16. Medeiros LJ, Kaynor B, Harris NL: Lupus lymphadenitis: Report of a case with immunohistologic studies on frozen sections. Hum Pathol 1989; 20:295.

17. Paradinas F: Primary and secondary immune disorders. In Stansfeld AG, d'Ardenne AJ (eds): Lymph Node Biopsy Interpretation, 2nd ed. London, Churchill Livingstone, 1992, pp 143–186.

18. Green JA, Dawson AA, Walker W: Systemic lupus erythematosus and lymphoma. Lancet 1978; 2:753.

19. Houssiau FA, Kirkove C, Asherson RA, et al: Malignant lymphoma in systemic rheumatic diseases: A report of five cases. Clin Exp Rheumatol 1991; 9:515.

20. Boumpas DT, Tsokos GC, Mann DL, et al: Increased proto-oncogene expression in peripheral blood lymphocytes from patients with systemic lupus erythematosus and other autoimmune diseases. Arthritis Rheum 1986; 29:755.

21. Fox RI, Luppi M, Kang HI, et al: Reactivation of Epstein-Barr virus in Sjögren's syndrome. Springer Semin Immunopathol 1991; 13:217.

22. McCurley TL, Collins RD, Ball E, et al: Nodal and extranodal lymphoproliferative disorders in Sjögren's syndrome: A clinical and immunopathologic study. Hum Pathol 1990; 21:482.

23. Segal GH, Wittwer CT, Fishleder AJ, et al: Identification of monoclonal B-cell populations by rapid-cycle PCR: A practical screening method for the detection of immunoglobulin gene rearrangements. Am J Pathol 1992; 141:1291.

24. Saltzstein SJ, Ackerman LV: Lymphadenopathy induced by anticonvulsant drugs and mimicking clinically and pathologically malignant lymphomas. Cancer 1959; 12:164.

25. Harris NL, Widder DJ: Phenytoin and generalized lymphadenopathy. Arch Pathol Lab Med 107:663, 1983.

26. Abbondanzo SL, Irey NS, Frizzera G: Dilantin-associated lymphadenopathy: Spectrum of histopathologic patterns [Abstract]. Lab Invest 1992; 66:73A.

27. Rosenthal CJ, Noguera CA, Coppola A, et al: Pseudolymphoma with mycosis fungoides manifestations, hyperresponsiveness to diphenylhydantoin, and lymphocyte disregulation. Cancer 1982; 49:2305.

28. Katzin WE, Julius CJ, Tubbs RR, et al: Lymphoproliferative disorders associated with carbamazepine. Arch Pathol Lab Med 1990; 114:1244.

29. Sinnige HAM, Boender CA, Kuypers EW, et al: Carbamazepine-induced pseudolymphoma and immune dysregulation. J Intern Med 1990; 227:355.

30. Schlaifer D, Arlet P, Ollier S, et al: Carbamazepine update. Lancet 1989; 2:980.

31. Li FP, Willard DR, Goodman R, et al: Malignant lymphoma after diphenylhydantoin (Dilantin) therapy. Cancer 1975; 36:1359.

32. Sorrell TC, Forbes IJ: Depression of immune competence by phenytoin and carbamazepine: Studies in vivo and in vitro. Clin Exp Immunol 1975; 20:273.

33. Dosch HM, Jason J, Gelfand EW: Transient antibody deficiency and abnormal T suppressor cells induced by phenytoin. N Engl J Med 1982; 306:406.

34. Gennis MA, Vemuri R, Burns EA, et al: Familial occurrence of hypersensitivity to phenytoin. Am J Med 1991; 91:631.

35. Gerson WT, Fine DG, Spielberg SP, et al: Anticonvulsant-induced aplastic anemia: Increased susceptibility to toxic drug metabolites in vitro. Blood 1983; 61:889.

36. Swanson AB: Finger joint replacement by silicone rubber implants and the concept of implant fixation by encapsulation. Ann Rheuma Dis 1969; 28(Suppl):47.

37. Endo LP, Edwards NL, Longley S, et al: Silicone and rheumatic diseases. Semin Arthritis Rheum 1987; 17:112.

38. Paplanus SH, Payne CM: Axillary lymphadenopathy 17 years after silicone implants: Study with x-ray microanalysis. J Hand Surg 1988; 13a:411.

39. Rogers LA, Longtine J, Garnick MB, et al: Silicone lymphadenopathy in a long distance runner: Complication of a Silastic prosthesis. Hum Pathol 1988; 19:1237.

40. Gray MH, Talbert ML, Talbert WM, et al: Changes seen in lymph nodes draining the sites of large joint prostheses. Am J Surg Pathol 1989; 13:1050.

41. Wintsch W, Smahel J, Clodius L, et al: Local and regional lymph node response to ruptured gel-filled mammary prostheses. Br J Plastic Surg 1978; 31:349.

42. Truong LD, Cartwright J, Goodman MD, et al: Silicone lymph adenopathy associated with augmentation mammoplasty: Morphologic features of nine cases. Am J Surg Pathol 1988; 12:484.

43. Bridges AJ, Conley C, Wang G, Burns PE, et al: A clinical and immunological evaluation of women with silicone breast implants and symptoms of rheumatic disease. Ann Intern Med 1993; 118:929.

44. Frizzera G: Atypical lymphoproliferative disorders. In Knowles DM (ed): Neoplastic Hematopathology. Baltimore, Williams & Wilkins, 1992, pp 459–495.

45. Lipford EH, Smith HR, Pittaluga S, et al: Clonality of angioimmunoblastic lymphadenopathy and implications for its evolution to malignant lymphoma. J Clin Invest 1987; 79:637.

46. Peterson BA, Frizzera G: Multicentric Castleman's disease. Semin Oncol 1993; 20:636.

47. Castleman B, Iverson L, Menendez VP: Localized mediastinal lymph node hyperplasia resembling thymoma. Cancer 1956; 9:822.

48. Keller AR, Hocholzer L, Castleman B: Hyaline-vascular and plasma-cell types of giant lymph node hyperplasia of the mediastinum and other locations. Cancer 1972; 29:670.

49. Gaba AR, Stein RS, Sweet DL, et al: Multicentric giant lymph node hyperplasia. Am J Clin Pathol 1978; 69:86.

50. Frizzera G, Peterson BA, Bayrd ED, et al: A systemic lymphoproliferative disorder with morphologic features of Castleman's disease: Clinical findings and clinicopathologic correlations in 15 patients. J Clin Oncol 1985; 3:1202.

51. Radaszkiewicz T, Hansmann M-L, Lennert K: Monoclonality and polyclonality of plasma cells in Castleman's disease of the plasma cell variant. Histopathology 1989; 14:11.

52. Hall PA, Donaghy M, Cotter FE, et al: An immunohistological and genotypic study of the plasma cell form of Castleman's disease. Histopathology 1989; 14:333.

53. Yoshizaki K, Matsuda T, Nishimoto H, et al: Pathogenic significance of interleukin-6 (IL-6/BSF-2) in Castleman's disease. Blood 1989; 74:1360.

54. Leger-Ravet MB, Peuchmaur M, Devergne O, et al: Interleukin-6 gene expression in Castleman's disease. Blood 1991; 78:2923.

55. Mandler RN, Kerrigan DP, Smart J: Castleman's disease in POEMS syndrome with elevated interleukin-6. Cancer 1992; 69:2697.

56. Soubrier M, Dubost J, Sauvezie, B, et al: POEMS Syndrome: A study of 25 cases and a review of the literature. Am J Med 1994; 97:543.

57. Brandt SJ, Bodine DM, Dunbar CE, Nienhuis AW: Dysregulated interleukin-6 expression produces a syndrome resembling Castleman's disease in mice. J Clin Invest 1990; 86:592.

58. Beck J, Hsu S, Wijdens J, et al: Alleviation of systemic manifestations

of Castleman's disease by monoclonal anti-interleukin-6 antibody. N Engl J Med 1994; 330:602.

59. Freter CE, Cossman J: Angioimmunoblastic lymphadenopathy with dysproteinemia. Semin Oncol 1993; 20:627.

60. Lukes RJ, Tindle BH: Immunoblastic lymphadenopathy. A hyperimmune entity resembling Hodgkin's disease. N Engl J Med 1975; 292:1.

61. Frizzera G, Moran EM, Rappaport H: Angioimmunoblastic lymphadenopathy with dysproteinaemia. Lancet 1974; 1:1070.

62. Lipford EH, Smith HR, Pittaluga S, et al: Clonality of angioimmunoblastic lymphadenopathy and implications for its evolution to malignant lymphoma. J Clin Invest 1987; 79:637.

63. Yu R, Schofiel J, Path MRC, et al: Angioimmunoblastic lymphadenopathy with dysproteinemia and dermal T-cell lymphoma. Cancer 1994; 74:1801.

64. Haluska TG, Finger KR, Kagan J, et al: Molecular genetics of chromosomal translocations in B- and T-lymphoid malignancies. *In* Cossman J (ed): Molecular Genetics in Cancer Diagnostics. New York, Elsevier, 1990, pp 73–104.

65. Mountz JD, Steinberg AD, Klinmann DM, et al: Autoimmunity and increased c-*myb* transcription. Science 1984; 266:1087.

66. Ohsaka A, Saito K, Sakai T, et al: Clinicopathologic and therapeutic aspects of angioimmunoblastic lymphadenopathy–related lesions. Cancer 1992; 69:1259.

67. Uphouse WJ, Woods JC: Angioimmunoblastic lymphadenopathy with dysproteinemia: Complete remission with cisplatin-based chemotherapy. Cancer 1987; 60:2161.

68. Seigert W, Neri C, Methuen I, et al: Recombinant human interferon-alpha in the treatment of angioimmunoblastic lymphadenopathy: Results in 12 patients. Leukemia 1991; 5:892.

69. Murayama T, Imoto S, Takahashi T, et al: Successful treatment of angioimmunoblastic lymphadenopathy with dysproteinemia with cyclosporin A. Cancer 1992; 69:2567.

70. Schlegelberger B, Zhang Y, Matthiesen K, et al: Detection of aberrant clones in nearly all cases of angioimmunoblastic lymphadenopathy with dysproteinemia-type T-cell lymphoma by combined interphase and metaphase cytogenetics. Blood 1994; 84:2640.

71. Siegert W, Agthe A, Griesser H, et al: Treatment of angioimmunoblastic lymphadenopathy (AILD)-type T-cell lymphoma using prednisone with or without the COP-BLAM/IMVP-16 regimen. Ann Intern Med 1992; 117:364.

72. Abruzzo LV, Schmidt K, Weiss LM, et al: B-cell lymphoma after angioimmunoblastic lymphadenopathy: A case with oligoclonal gene rearrangements associated with Epstein-Barr virus. Blood 1993; 82:241.

73. Knecht G, Schwarze EW, Lennert K, et al: Histological, immunohistochemical, and autopsy findings in lymphogranulomatosis X (including angioimmunoblastic lymphadenopathy). Virchows Arch A Pathol Anat Histopathol 1985; 406:105.

74. Steinberg AD, Seldin MF, Jaffee ES, et al: Angioimmunoblastic lymphadenopathy with dysproteinemia. Ann Intern Med 1988; 108:575.

75. Lipford EH Jr, Margolick JB, Longo DL, et al: Angiocentric immunoproliferative lesions: A clinicopathologic spectrum of post-thymic T-cell proliferations. Blood 1988; 72:1674.

76. Jaffe ES: Angiocentric immunoproliferative lesions. *In* Jaffe ES (ed): Surgical Pathology of the Lymph Nodes and Related Organs. Philadelphia, WB Saunders, 1985, pp 241–246.

77. Liebow AA, Carrington CRB, Friedman PJ: Lymphomatoid granulomatosis. Hum Pathol 1972; 3:457.

78. Myers JL: Lymphomatoid granulomatosis: Past, present, future? Mayo Clin Proc 1990; 65:274.

79. Donner LR, Dobin S, Harrington D: Angiocentric immunoproliferative lesion (lymphomatoid granulomatosis). Cancer 1990; 65:249.

80. Gaulard P, Henni T, Marolleau JP, et al: Lethal midline granuloma (polymorphic reticulosis) and lymphomatoid granulomatosis. Cancer 1988; 62:705.

81. Hoffman GS, Kerr GS, Leavitt RY, et al: Wegener granulomatosis: An analysis of 158 patients. Ann Intern Med 1992; 116:488.

82. Davis RE, Warnke RA, Dorfman RF: Inflammatory pseudotumor of lymph nodes: Additional observations and evidence for an inflammatory etiology. Am J Surg Pathol 1991; 15:744.

83. Perrone T, de Wolf-Peeters C, Frizzera G: Inflammatory pseudotumor of lymph nodes: A distinctive pattern of nodal reaction. Am J Surg Pathol 1988; 12:351.

84. Chan JKC, Tsang WYW: Uncommon syndromes of reactive lymphadenopathy. Semin Oncol 1993; 20:648.

85. Dorfman RF: Histiocytic necrotizing lymphadenitis of Kikuchi and Fujimoto. Arch Pathol Lab Med 1987; 111:1026.

86. Sumiyoshi Y, Kikuchi M, Ohshima K, et al: A case of histiocytic necrotizing lymphadenitis with bone marrow and skin involvement. Virchows Arch A Pathol Anat Histopathol 1992; 420:275.

87. Rosai J, Dorfman RF: Sinus histiocytosis with massive lymphadenopathy: A newly recognized benign clinicopathologic entity. Arch Pathol 1969; 87:63.

88. Foucar E, Rosai J, Dorfman R: Sinus histiocytosis with massive lymphadenopathy (Rosai-Dorfman disease): Review of the entity. Semin Diagn Pathol 1990; 7:19.

89. Foucar E, Rosai J, Dorfman RF, et al: Immunological abnormalities and their significance in sinus histiocytosis with massive lymphadenopathy. Am J Clin Pathol 1984; 82:515.

90. Komp DM: The treatment of sinus histiocytosis with massive lymphadenopathy (Rosai-Dorfman disease). Semin Diagn Pathol 1990; 7:83.

91. Fayemi AO, Toker C: Nodal angiomatosis. Arch Pathol Lab Med 1975; 99:170.

92. Michal M, Koza V: Vascular transformation of lymph node sinuses—a diagnostic pitfall, histopathologic, and immunohistochemical study. Pathol Res Pract 1989; 185:441.

93. Haferkamp O, Rosenau W, Lennert K: Vascular transformation of lymph node sinuses due to venous congestion. Arch Pathol 1971; 92:81.

94. Lennert K, Hansmann ML: Progressive transformation of germinal centers: Clinical significance and lymphocytic predominance Hodgkin's disease—the Kiel experience. Am J Surg Pathol 1987; 11:149.

95. Burns BF, Colby TV, Dorfman RF: Differential diagnostic features of nodular L&H Hodgkin's disease, including progressive transformation of germinal centers. Am J Surg Pathol 1984; 8:253.

96. Osborne BM, Butler JJ: Clinical implications of progressive transformation of germinal centers. Am J Surg Pathol 1984; 8:725.

97. Ferry JA, Zukerberg LR, Harris NL: Florid progressive transformation of germinal centers. Am J Surg Pathol 1987; 11:149.

98. Robbins SL, Cotran RS, Kumar V: Infectious disease. *In* Robbins SL, Cotran RS, Kumar V (eds): Pathologic Basis of Disease, 3rd ed. Philadelphia, WB Saunders, 1984, pp 390–392.

99. Reich JM, Mullooly JP, Johnson RE: Linkage analysis of malignancy-associated sarcoidosis. Chest 1995; 107:605.

100. Lever WF, Schaumburg-Lever G: Dermatopathic lymphadenopathy. *In* Histopathology of the Skin, 7th ed. Philadelphia, JB Lippincott, 1990, pp 113–114.

101. Kyle RA, Greipp PR: Amyloidosis (AL): Clinical and laboratory features in 229 cases. Mayo Clin Proc 1983; 58:665.

102. Stone MJ: Amyloidosis: A final common pathway for protein deposition in tissues. Blood 75:531.

103. Kaplan HS: Hodgkin's Disease, 2nd ed. Cambridge, Harvard University Press, 1980, p 220.

Thirty-One

―――――Lymphoma in the Elderly ―――――
and in Pregnancy

Non-Hodgkin's Lymphoma in Elderly Patients

Bertrand Coiffier

The median age for lymphoma patients is approximately 65 years, and the incidence of non-Hodgkin's lymphoma (NHL) in patients older than 65 years of age increases regularly in developed countries with the increasing age of the population. However, the data presented during the last 10 years on characteristics and outcome of these patients are surprisingly inadequate and difficult to interpret. This chapter reviews the characteristics, prognostic factors, and treatment of elderly patients with NHL.

In cancer registries, the median age of lymphoma patients is somewhere between 60 and 65 years but often only the younger patients are referred to university centers, and in these centers median age is generally near 50 years. In our center we have treated 1425 lymphoma patients with a median age of 55 years, and if 39% of these patients were older than 59 years, only 16% were older than 69 years.

"Elderly" was defined in most recent reviews as age older than 60 years. This definition must probably be revised according to the new standard of life in Europe and North America. In Table 31–1, several definitions of elderly patients are presented. The ideal definition would be the age above which the treatment should be modified in comparison with younger patients. In this review, we have chosen to use 65 to 70 years as the threshold to elderly status because we believe that patients aged between 60 and 65 may and have to receive a curative treatment not different from that for younger patients. The international consensus on the definition of aged patients should probably be redefined.

Data concerning NHL incidence in European countries or North America are available through different registries. In the United States, these data are collected by the Surveillance, Epidemiology, and End Results (SEER) program of the National Cancer Institute. In recent SEER data, NHL represents 3.6% of all cancers and its incidence increases exponentially with age between 20 and 79 years (Fig. 31–1). The increased incidence of NHL in recent years was more marked in the elderly patient group.[1] If lymphoma rates stayed relatively stable in patients younger than 45, they increased at least 100% in each 10-year age group between 45 and 75 during the last 40 years and they increased nearly 400% in patients older than 75 years. The

same increase was observed in European cancer registries.[2] This increase in incidence is specific to NHL and was not observed for other hematologic neoplasias such as acute leukemia, myeloma, and Hodgkin's disease.[3]

CHARACTERISTICS OF LYMPHOMA IN ELDERLY PATIENTS

Few studies have compared on a population-based analysis the characteristics of aged with young adult lymphoma patients. In such an analysis, d'Amore and associates[2] found that elderly patients (defined as >70 years) had a significantly higher number of female cases (P = .0002) (in fact, proportional to the female predominance seen in the general population for that age group), of localized disease (46% versus 36% in younger patients, $P<.0001$), and of extranodal manifestations (41% versus 33% in younger patients, $P<.01$). No difference was found between aged and young patients as to the presence of B symptoms or the distribution of main histologic subgroups. As in other series, the most frequent extranodal localizations were the gastrointestinal tract, bone marrow, and skin.

We have recently performed an analysis of all lymphoma patients seen in 2 years in two European centers (Lyon, France, and Aviano, Italy) and in two North American centers (Omaha, Nebraska, and Vancouver, Canada)[4] (J. R. Anderson, personal communication, 1995). Four hundred one patients had an aggressive lymphoma and 225 (56%) were older than 60 years, 26% aged 60 to 69 years, 21% aged 70 to 79 years, and 8% older than 80 years. In terms of presenting features, the older patients differed significantly from the younger patients by performance status and by the presence of massive tumor bulk: older patients were more likely to have poor performance status ($P<.05$) but less likely to have massive tumor bulk ($P<.05$) (Table 31–2). The most frequent extranodal localizations were bone marrow, gastrointestinal tract, and liver.

According to the two studies previously mentioned and to smaller studies not comparing young and elderly patients, the initial picture of NHL in elderly patients shows nothing specific. Follicular lymphomas are less frequent than in patients younger than 70 years and nonfollicular small cell lymphomas (small lymphocytic, immunocytoma, and mantle cell) are more frequent.[2, 5] However, diffuse large cell lymphomas represent the main category of lymphoma in

Table 31–1. Definition of "Elderly" Patients According to Different Standards

Standard	Definition	Elderly (yr)
Age	Median age of lymphoma patients	>60–65
Work	Age of retiring	>65–70
Daily work	Capacity to do day-to-day work	>75
Diseases	Alteration of different organ diseases	>65
Renal function	Decline of glomerular filtration and tubular secretion rates <50%	>70
Hormonal status	Menopause in women	>50–55
Treatment	Capacity to tolerate allogeneic marrow transplantation	>50
Treatment	Capacity to tolerate autologous stem cell transplantation	>60 (65?)
Prognosis	Modification of survival curves in International Prognostic Index	>60–65

these patients in all analyses.[4, 6, 7] True lymphoblastic subtype is nearly absent in these patients but some patients with a small noncleaved cell lymphoma, Burkitt's or non-Burkitt's type, are seen in all series. The percentage of patients with a peripheral T-cell lymphoma does not seem different from what is seen in younger patients. In a study of 70 lymphoma cases in patients older than 80 years, Hoerni and colleagues[8] did not find any difference for histologic repartition in comparison with younger patients or to younger aged patients.

In small therapeutic series, the clinical picture of elderly patients is not different from that of younger patients: no difference was observed in comparing the percentage of patients with B symptoms, advanced stage, poor performance status, anemia, increased lactate dehydrogenase (LDH) level, high tumoral mass, number of extranodal sites of disease, or different extranodal sites involved.[9–11] Elderly patients have a concomitant disease more often and are less often included in a prospective therapy protocol.[9, 11]

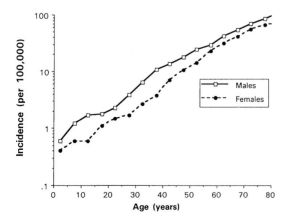

Figure 31–1. SEER data showing the incidence of non-Hodgkin's lymphoma that increased exponentially with age between 20 and 79 years. (From Rabkin CS, Devesa SS, Zahm SH, Gail MH: Increasing incidence of non-Hodgkin's lymphoma. Semin Hematol 1993; 30:286.)

Table 31–2. Initial Presentation of Aggressive Lymphoma Patients According to Age Groups[4]

	No. of Patients	Age Groups (yr)		
		<60 (%)	60–69 (%)	≥70 (%)
Sex				
Male	206	54	52	47
Female	195	46	48	53
Stage				
I	50	14	9	15
II	94	31	21	18
III	45	10	10	15
IV	196	45	60	51
B symptoms present	124	30	40	31
Performance status*				
0–1	287	84	72	58
≥2	106	16	28	42
Tumor size ≥ 10 cm*	111	34	26	19
No. of extranodal sites				
0–1	299	77	75	72
≥2	100	23	25	28
Extranodal sites involved				
Bone marrow	104	21	34	26
Gastrointestinal tract	70	20	17	14
Pleura	30	7	8	8
Skin	29	6	7	9
Liver	28	6	11	5
Lung	28	9	5	6
LDH level above normal	151	42	46	43

*Log-rank test *P* <.05.
LDH, lactate dehydrogenase.

SURVIVAL AND PROGNOSTIC FACTORS

In the analysis by d'Amore and associates,[2] the 7-year survival of NHL patients older than 70 was 35% (median 1.7 years) compared with 57% (median not reached) for younger patients (*P*<.0001). This expected difference persisted after correction of survival data for causes of death that did not appear to be related to the lymphoma. The corrected 7-year survival for patients older than 70 years was 52% versus 66% for those younger than 70 (*P*<.0001). In the recent comparative analysis we have conducted in four centers (J. R. Anderson, personal communication, 1995), median survival was not reached for patients aged between 60 and 69 years but was 1.3 years for those older than 70 (*P*<.01) (Fig. 31–2*A*). Median failure-free survival (from time of treatment onset to first progression or death from any cause) was 1.6 years for patients aged 60 to 69 years, 0.6 year for those between 70 and 79 years, and 0.46 years for those older than 80 years of age (*P* = .01; Fig. 31–2*B*).

AGE AS A SPECIFIC PROGNOSTIC FACTOR

The effect of age on treatment results has been analyzed differently in several published studies, and the importance of age as a prognostic indicator of survival has been controversial. In a Southwest Oncology Group study, older patients (>60 years of age) had a worse outcome because they responded less to treatment and they relapsed more often. This poorer outcome was related to a decrease in chemotherapy dose intensity given to these patients because

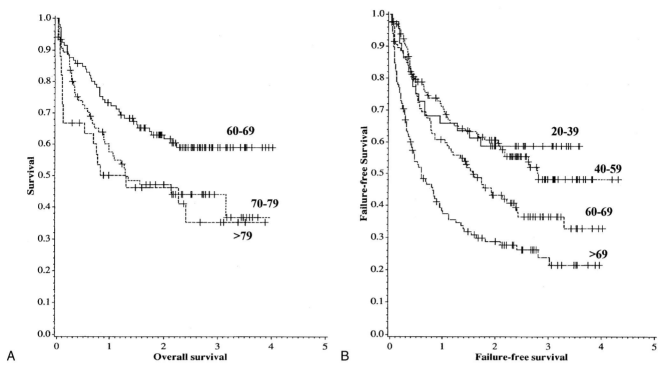

Figure 31–2. Overall survival (*A*) and failure-free survival (*B*) of 401 patients included in a comparative analysis of lymphoma patients treated in four centers in Europe and North America[4] according to age.

aged patients should receive only 50% of the drug dosage.[10] However, aged patients who received the full-dose chemotherapy regimen also had a shorter survival. In other analyses, aged patients were observed to die more often during the first courses of treatment, but those who responded to this treatment did well after response was achieved.[11, 12] It was then concluded that aged patients are more likely to present complications after chemotherapy because of their age and the possible disabilities that are often observed in aged patients. Whatever the reason, age was isolated as an adverse prognostic factor in nearly all studies.[4, 9, 13–19] However, Grogan and coworkers, in a study of a group of patients treated with CHOP (cyclophosphamide, hydroxydaunomycin, Oncovin, prednisone) or M-BACOD (methotrexate, bleomycin, Adriamycin, cyclophosphamide, Oncovin, dexamethasone), found that elderly patients have a comparable survival with that of younger patients.[20]

As an example, Figure 31–3 shows the survival of patients treated for an aggressive lymphoma in the Groupe d'Etudes des Lymphomes de l'Adulte showing three subgroups of patients: those younger than 55 years with the best outcome, those aged between 55 and 65 years with an intermediate outcome, and those older than 65 years with the worst outcome. The adverse effects of aging have to be considered when evaluating the presence or absence of other adverse prognostic factors such those described in the following section.

PROGNOSTIC FACTORS IN ELDERLY PATIENTS

In their analysis of a large group of elderly patients, d'Amore and associates[2] found the same prognostic parameters associated with shorter survival times as those in other

prognostic analyses done in younger groups of patients: presence of B symptoms, liver involvement, elevated LDH level, high-grade histology, more than one extranodal site of disease, hypercalcemia, splenic involvement, and stage IV disease. The variables were entered in a multiparametric Cox regression analysis, and those associated with short survival were, in order of relative risk magnitude: hepatic involvement, presence of B symptoms, high-grade histology, and elevated LDH level.

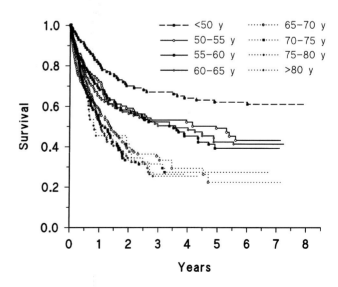

Figure 31–3. Survival of 1800 patients included in the LNH-80, LNH-84, and LNH-87 protocols according to age. Patients were divided into classes of 5 years. Three subgroups of patients are clearly defined: younger than 55 years, between 55 and 65 years, and older than 65 years of age.

In our recent analysis of four centers,[4] the factors most associated with failure-free survival or overall survival were age younger or older than 70 years (P = .002), localized or advanced stage (P = .005), performance status (P<.001), presence or absence of B symptoms (P<.001), normal or elevated LDH level (P<.001), number of extranodal sites of disease (P<.058), and presence or absence of a bulky tumor (P <.05). In a multivariate analysis, performance status (0 to 1 versus ≥2), stage (localized or disseminated), LDH level (normal or increased), and B symptoms (present or not) were demonstrated to be independent predictors. Figure 31–4 shows the survival of young and old patients included in this analysis according to the number of adverse prognostic factors. Elderly patients without adverse factors had a survival that is nearly comparable with that of patients younger than 60 years (3-year survival of 67% versus 87%, P = .05). However, elderly patients with adverse prognostic factors had a shorter survival than younger patients with the same adverse prognostic factors (3-year survival of 6%, 30%, and 36% for patients older than 70, 60 to 69, and <60 years, respectively, P<.001).

When prognostic parameters were analyzed separately for patients younger or older than 60 years, few differences could be found between the groups.[4, 7, 9, 20] Older patients often have a poorer performance status or a stage IV disease, but these differences are rarely statistically significant. Finally, the predictive capacity of chronologic age and the tolerance to the therapy are related to the poor performance status, the presence of concomitant diseases, the patients' physiologic resources, and the dose intensity of chemotherapy regimen. In elderly patients with a good performance status and few or no debilitating concomitant dis-

eases, no reason exists not to give them treatment with a curative intent.

TREATMENT OF ELDERLY PATIENTS

As in younger patients, the treatment of elderly patients with lymphoma has to be designed according to the histologic subtype of the lymphoma and the presence or absence of adverse prognostic factors.[14, 21]

Follicular Lymphomas. No specific study exists for elderly patients with follicular lymphoma. Some rules appear in the literature and seem to be followed.[22–25] Patients with localized disease have to be treated with localized radiation therapy. Patients with disseminated disease but without adverse prognostic factors are the best candidates to be included in a "watch-and-wait" strategy. Those patients with adverse prognostic factors must be treated at diagnosis and intermittent courses of chlorambucil (16 mg/m² daily × 5 days a month) habitually allow good results. Multidrug chemotherapy regimens may be reserved for patients progressing after the earlier mentioned treatments.

Nonfollicular Small Cell Lymphomas. These lymphoma subtypes appear more frequently in elderly patients and are difficult to treat even in young patients.[5] No specific treatment has to be considered for elderly patients. Patients with a small lymphocytic lymphoma or an immunocytoma may be treated with chlorambucil or fludarabine.[26, 27] Those patients with a mucosal-associated lymphoid tissue lymphoma may be treated with surgery, local radiation therapy,

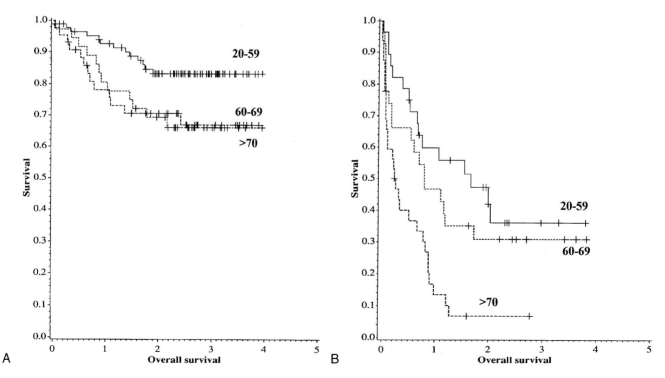

Figure 31–4. Overall survival of the patients presented in Figure 31–2 according to age and the number of adverse prognostic factors at diagnosis: (A) no adverse prognostic factors; (B) three or more adverse prognostic factors.

Table 31–3. Standard Chemotherapy Regimens Used in Elderly Patients with Aggressive Lymphoma

Regimen°	No. of Patients	Median Age	Percentage of Patients >70 Yr	Toxic Deaths (%)	Complete Remission (%)	Median Survival (mo)	3-Year Survival (%)	3-Year Disease-Free Survival (%)
CHOP[12]	20	75	100	30	45	13	25	NA
CHOP[10]	81	NA	—	17†	37	14†	32	48
CHOP[49]	42	75	60	7	44	38†	50†	NA
CTVP[36]	43	73	74	0†	30	18†	NA	NA
COPA[32]	141	NA	—	1	NA	37	48†	NA
CAP/BOP[11]	112	NA	—	7	61	15†	36†	70†
M-BACOD[20]	60	71	—	0	65	NA	58	48
VNCOP-B[38]	29	66	—	0	76	NA	NA	NA
CHOP/CNOP[34]	100	70	50	10	54	18	35†	NA
CEMP[50]	31	72	68	19	58	18+	NA	NA

°COPA = Cytoxin, Oncovin, prednisone, Adriamycin; CEMP = cyclophosphamide, etoposide, mitoxantrone, prednisone. See text for other regimens.
†Value calculated from the original article by the author (B. C.).
NA, not available in the article.

or chlorambucil. For patients with mantle cell lymphoma, no good recipe exists to prolong survival. We propose to our patients intermittent courses of chlorambucil if they do not have adverse prognostic features or six courses of CHOP if they have adverse prognostic parameters and may tolerate this treatment. Otherwise, an association of ifosfamide plus VP-16 may be a good alternative.[28]

Aggressive Lymphomas. The specific problems of treating elderly patients come from those patients with a diffuse large cell lymphoma, a disease that is curable,[21] because these patients may not receive full high-dose chemotherapy regimens owing to their age and concomitant diseases. Two approaches appear in the literature for these patients. The first one favors standard treatment whatever the age if the patient does not have severe concomitant disease. The second one designs specific chemotherapy regimens "adapted" for elderly patients.

STANDARD CHEMOTHERAPY REGIMENS (Table 31–3)

The gold standard chemotherapy regimen for patients with diffuse large cell lymphoma is CHOP.[29] In some trials, when CHOP doses were decreased because of the older age of the patients, the complete remission (CR) rate decreased and the survival shortened.[10, 30] With standard doses, the CHOP regimen allowed longer survival for responding elderly patients but the percentage of toxic death increased dramatically, sometimes to 15% to 30%.[12, 31, 32] Identical experiences were observed with CHOP-like regimens: CNOP (cyclophosphamide, Novantrone, Oncovin, prednisone) with mitoxantrone in place of doxorubicin,[33, 34] CAP/BOP (cyclophosphamide, Adriamycin, procarbazine, bleomycin, Oncovin, prednisone),[11] COP-BLAM (cyclophosphamide, Oncovin, prednisone, bleomycin, Adriamycin, Matulane),[35] M-BACOD,[20] CTVP (cyclophosphamide, THP=Adriamycin [pirarubicin], VM-26, prednisone) with pirarubicin in place of doxorubicin,[36, 37] or VNCOP-B (VP-16, Novantrone, cyclophosphamide, Oncovin, prednisone, bleomycin).[38]

The conclusion of these different prospective trials was that for patients not too old (<75 years), without severe concomitant disease, and with a good performance status, CHOP or CHOP-like regimens may allow a long survi-val probably not different from that observed in patients younger than 65 years. Some preliminary reports have showed that hematopoietic growth factors may allow a better tolerance of standard-dose chemotherapy regimens in these elderly patients.[39]

CHEMOTHERAPY REGIMENS SPECIFICALLY DESIGNED FOR ELDERLY PATIENTS (Table 31–4)

Recently, some centers have devised specific chemotherapy regimens for elderly patients presenting an aggressive lymphoma. Most of them included mitoxantrone in place of doxorubicin, as in the CNOP (cyclophosphamide, Novantrone, Oncovin, prednisone).[33] The Aviano group and the European Organization for the Research and Treatment of Cancer have proposed a VMP regimen based on etoposide (VP-16), mitoxantrone, and prednimustine.[40–42] The Padua group proposed an MVP regimen with mitoxantrone, etoposide, and prednisone.[43] The Vancouver group described a series of weekly regimens based on their MACOP-B regimen: low-dose ACOP-B (Adriamycin, cyclophosphamide, Oncovin, prednisone, bleomycin)[44]; VABE (vincristine, Adriamycin, bleomycin, etoposide, and prednisone)[44]; and P/DOCE (epirubicin/doxorubicin, Oncovin, cyclophosphamide, etoposide, and prednisone).[45] No difference was observed between these regimens (Fig. 31–5). McMaster and coworkers have reported the results obtained in 26 patients with BECLAM (bleomycin, etoposide, cyclophosphamide, leucovorin, Adriamycin, methotrexate),[46] but the percentage of toxic death rose to 15% without a longer median survival. Goss and associates did not observe toxic death with the PEN (prednisone, etoposide, Novantrone) regimen,[47] but median survival was only 6 months. We obtained identical results with an association of ifosfamide plus etoposide over 3 days.[28] The longer survival observed with elderly-device chemotherapy regimen was obtained by Martelli and colleagues with P-VABEC regimen (prednisone, vincristine, Adriamycin, bleomycin, etoposide, cyclophosphamide)[48] but their patients were much younger than in other series (only 28% were >70 years).

No comparative trials have been realized between all the regimens described earlier. Results obtained in terms of percentage of CR or survival rates are presented in Table

Table 31–4. Specifically Designed Chemotherapy Regimens for Elderly Patients with Aggressive Lymphoma

Regimen*	No. of Patients	Median Age (yr)	Percentage of Patients >70 Years	Toxic Deaths (%)	Complete Remission (%)	Median Survival (mo)	3-yr Survival (%)	3-yr Disease-Free Survival (%)
E + P[51]	21	76	100	0	48	NA	21†	12†
Ifm VP[28]	21	NA	100	0	75	NA	NA	NA
CNOP[33]	30	70	50	0	60	12	NA	NA
VMP[40]	52	76	100	6	48	12	30†	37
MVP[43]	55	75	65	2	55	16	45†	30†
ld-ACOP-B[44]	40	72	—	5	65	22†	48†	52†
VABE[44]	32	73	—	6	63	20†	40†	45†
P/DOCE[45]	63	75	77	8	62	48	45	41
BECALM[46]	26	75	88	15	42	9	38	50†
PEN[47]	40	74	70†	0	59	6	NA	NA
P-VABEC[48]	60	67	28	2	75	25	55†	45†

E + P = etoposide + prednisone; Ifm VP = ifosfamide, etoposide; ld-ACOP-B = low-dose Adriamycin, cyclophosphamide, Oncovin, prednisone, bleomycin; BECALM = bleomycin, etoposide, cyclophosphamide, Adriamycin, leucovorin, methotrexate. See text for other regimens.
†Value calculated from the original article by the author (B. C.).
NA, not available in the article.

31–4. However, to interpret these results, one should note the low number of patients included in these trials and their extreme heterogeneity. The standard deviation of these results is probably large even if not presented in most of the studies, and all these results must be considered as nearly equivalent. The main characteristics of these specifically designed regimens for elderly lymphoma patients are a lower CR rate but a lower mortality rate during treatment and thus an equivalent 3- or 4-year survival rate compared with CHOP or CHOP-like regimens.

Two recent studies have specifically addressed the therapeutic efficiency of CHOP compared with less intensive CHOP-like regimens in elderly patients with aggressive lymphoma. Sonneveld and associates demonstrated that the CHOP regimen was well tolerated in 72 patients older than

60 years of age (half of them >70 years) and that toxicity was not different from a regimen containing less toxic drugs (mitoxantrone).[52] Moreover, CHOP treatment resulted in a higher CR rate and a longer survival than CNOP (mitoxantrone). This study was supported by another one in which standard CHOP was compared with weekly CHOP in an attempt to decrease the adverse events.[53] In this trial, patients treated with standard CHOP had a longer 2-year survival and progression-free survival compared with those treated with weekly CHOP. These data confirm that the response rate that can be achieved in elderly patients is comparable with that achieved in younger patients and that patients with a complete response have a good probability of long survival.

WHICH REGIMEN TO CHOOSE

Except for the two most recent studies,[52, 53] there are no good indications in the literature review about how to treat elderly patients with aggressive lymphoma. We urgently need comparative prospective trials, particularly comparing a standard-dose chemotherapy regimen with hematopoietic growth factor support and a low-dose regimen containing a doxorubicin analogue less cardiotoxic and less toxic for hematopoietic cells. For patients without concomitant disease we need a regimen that is curative because the chances are high that this patient will die from the lymphoma before any other disease appears. CHOP or CHOP-like regimens are the best candidates. For patients with poor performance status or concomitant diseases, a curative treatment may be too toxic and thus increase the chance of fatal direct or indirect toxicity of the treatment. In this latter case, regimens incorporating ifosfamide and etoposide with or without mitoxantrone may be sufficient to stop the lymphoma progression for 1 or 2 years.

CONCLUSION

Aggressive lymphoma in elderly patients increases in frequency as a function of age. There is a huge gap between

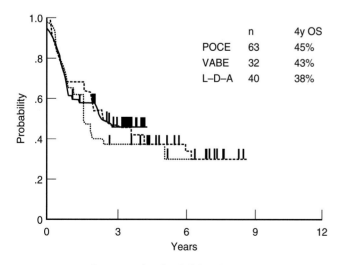

	n	4y OS
POCE	63	45%
VABE	32	43%
L–D–A	40	38%

Figure 31–5. Kaplan-Meier plot of probability of overall survival according to the three specifically designed chemotherapy regimens for elderly patients as described by O'Reilly and associates[45]: P/DOCE (POCE), VABE, and low-dose ACOP-B (L-D-A). (From O'Reilly SE, Connors JM, Howdle S, et al: In search of an optimal regimen for elderly patients with advanced-stage diffuse large cell lymphoma: Results of a phase II study of P/DOCE chemotherapy. J Clin Oncol 1993; 11:2250.)

the high number of elderly lymphoma patients and the paucity of prospective clinical trials in these patients. There are no differences in clinical presentation and prognostic factors in elderly lymphoma patients in comparison with lymphoma in younger patients. The difficulty in treating this disease comes from the concomitant diseases that occur in patients older than 70 years of age and the poor tolerance of visceral organs to the toxic effects of treatment. Patients with diffuse large cell lymphoma should be treated with a curative intent whenever possible.

(See Reference List at the end of the chapter.)

Lymphoma and Pregnancy

N. Dhedin
Bertrand Coiffier

The occurrence of a lymphoma during pregnancy is rare for non-Hodgkin's lymphoma (NHL) (131 cases reported), but it is more frequent for Hodgkin's disease (HD): 1 in 1500 deliveries in one hospital[1] to 1 in 140,000 deliveries in Germany in 10 years (1970 to 1979).[2] The association of pregnancy and lymphoma raises some important questions about either the influence of lymphoma and its treatment on fetal development and on pregnancy outcome or the effect of pregnancy on lymphoma course. To protect the fetus, staging procedures require noninvasive radiologic examinations, but the treatment comprises chemotherapy and/or radiation therapy, both of which may have teratogenic effects. Moreover, waiting until after delivery with an aggressive lymphoma to begin the treatment may be fatal for both mother and child. Thus, the management of a lymphoma in a pregnant woman presents difficult therapeutic decisions for the physician, in particular, when treatment should start and whether an early termination of the pregnancy is needed.

INCIDENCE OF LYMPHOMAS DURING PREGNANCY

The incidence of lymphomas in pregnant women has not been definitively determined. Overall, HD and NHLs are the fourth most frequent malignancies among pregnant women, after breast, cervix, and ovarian neoplasms.[2, 3] HD is a disease of young adults, with a median age at diagnosis around 30 years, thus representing the most common type of lymphoma during the reproductive years. Its association with pregnancy is estimated to be 1 in 1000 to 6000 deliveries.[1, 2] NHLs occur among older adults with a median age at diagnosis older than 60 years[4] and are rarer during the pregnancy period. In a review of the literature, we found 131 cases of NHL associated with pregnancy and 6 cases that occurred during the immediate postpartum period (Table 31–5).[5–21] In one case, the NHL was associated with maternal human immunodeficiency virus infection and placental involvement[12] and in another case of T-cell lymphoma with a maternal human T-cell lymphotropic virus, type I infection.[22] The prevalence of NHL during pregnancy has been described as being significantly higher in women having their first pregnancy after 30 years of age.[23]

HOW TO STAGE LYMPHOMA IN WOMEN DURING PREGNANCY

Usually lymphoma patients are staged through physical examination, bone marrow biopsy, radiographic imaging, and biologic tests. This staging process and the interpretation of biologic parameters may present some problems during pregnancy. Because of potential risk of abortion, teratogenicity, and mutagenicity after use of radiologic imaging, computed tomographic scans, lymphangiography, and other radioisotopic examinations are contraindicated.[24] However, the milligray doses associated with chest radiographs apparently are safe during pregnancy. Because of the absence of any adverse effect on the fetus, ultrasonography is used for abdominal and pelvic examinations. Although there is no evidence that magnetic and electric fields associated with magnetic resonance imaging (MRI) may interfere with the fetal development, the toxicity of MRI in staging lymphoma patients remains undefined, and MRI should be used only during the first trimester when ultrasonographic examinations have not provided valuable results.[25] However, staging with chest radiographs and abdominal ultrasonography is rarely optimal, and MRI may have to be used, particularly for patients with mediastinal or abdominal localizations. LDH and β_2-microglobulin levels have prognostic implication for NHL and HD patients and should always be measured. Acute-phase protein levels are associated with outcome in HD patients, but most of these protein levels increase during pregnancy and lose their significance.

EFFECTS OF PREGNANCY ON LYMPHOMA

In a series of 84 women with HD during pregnancy reported by Barry and associates, there was no evidence that pregnancy may have any influence on the lymphoma outcome; specifically, response rate and median duration of survival seemed identical to what is expected for nonpregnant patients with the same lymphoma.[26] Similar conclusions were presented by Gobbi and colleagues in a series of 21 patients[27] and by Thomas and Peckham in a series of 15 patients.[24] On the other hand, a study of Jouet and coworkers on 25 patients suggested that HD in late pregnancy or after delivery might be more active with a 55% treatment failure and relapse rates.[28]

The effect of pregnancy on NHL outcome is more difficult to assess because of the lower NHL incidence. In a review of 42 cases where maternal survival was known, outcome was poor, with only 13 women alive, 11 in complete remission and 2 with active disease. Only 6 of these 42 women received a multidrug regimen during their pregnancy; 14 were treated whether with a single agent, radiation therapy, or steroids or with surgery; and 22 patients received no treatment at all.[29] In some series it was suggested that NHL during pregnancy is more commonly of an aggressive subtype[5, 29–31] but this has to be correlated with the predominance of aggressive subtypes in young patients (>50% of all lymphoma cases). In our review of literature (see Table

Table 31–5. Stage, Histologic Subtype, Treatment, and Maternal and Fetal Outcome of 73 Pregnant Women with Lymphoma

Year and Reference	Trimester	Stage at Diagnosis	Histologic Subtype[*]	Treatment During Pregnancy (1) and After Delivery (2)	Maternal Outcome		Fetal Outcome	
					Status	Date (mo)	Status	Date (mo)
1960[39]	1	I	—	2: RT	CR	30	Alive	—
1963[62]	2	—	—	1: Surgery	Death	—	Death	—
1963[35]	PP	IV	J	—	Death	<1	—	—
1965[35]	2	IV	J	1: SA	Death	<1	Alive at delivery	—
1965[35]	3	IV	J	2: SA	Death	9	Death	<1
1965[35]	PP	IV	J	—	Death	<1	—	—
1964[36]	2	IV	—	1: Surgery; 2: RT	Death	6	Death	<1
1966[63]	PP	IV	J	—	Death	<1	—	—
1966[64]	2	—	—	1: SA	Death	—	Alive	—
1966[65]	PP	—	I	—	Death	—	—	—
1968[33]	1	III	—	2: SA	Death	20	Therapeutic abortion	—
1969[34]	3	IV	G	1: Surgery	Death	1	Alive	30
1970[66]	3	I	J	1: RT + SA	Death	6	Alive	12
1971[37]	2	IV	G	1: RT	Death	<1	Alive, prematurate	—
1972[67]	3	I	—	1: RT	CR	2	Alive	—
1974[38]	2	IV	J	2: RT + SA	Death	4	Therapeutic abortion	—
1974[50]	2	IV	F	1: COP	CR	19	Alive	—
1974[33]	2	III	I	1: RT; 2: COP	Death	35	Alive	36
1976[40]	PP	—	J	—	Death	—	—	—
1976[40]	PP	—	J	—	Death	—	—	—
1976[68]	2	—	J	1: Surgery	Death	—	Therapeutic abortion	—
1977[32]	2	IV	J	1: SA	Death	5	Therapeutic abortion	—
1977[69]	2	IV	I	—	Death	<1	Spontaneous abortion	—
1977[70]	2	IV	I	1: COP	CR	17	Alive	24
1978[71]	3	—	G	1: Surgery	CR	—	Alive	—
1979[40]	3	I	J	1: SA	Death	2	Alive	1
1979[41]	1	I	—	2: RT + SA	CR	12	Alive, premature	—
1979[42]	2	IV	J	—	Death	<1	Spontaneous abortion	—
1980[72]	2	IV	J	2: SA	Death	3	Spontaneous abortion	—
1980[73]	3	IV	H	2: CHOP	CR	6	Alive, premature	6
1980[61]	1	IV	E	1: SA	Death	—	Alive, premature	—
1981[20]	3	IV	—	1: CHOP	CR	40	Alive	26
1981[33]	3	I	I	2: CHOP	Death	36	Alive	42
1982[74]	2	IV	J	1: CHOP-like	Death	6	Alive	2
1982[30]	3	I	I	2: CHOP-like	Death	12	Alive	—
1982[30]	3	IV	I	2: RT + CHOP	CR	24	Alive	—
1983[30]	3	IV	E	2: CHOP-like	CR	9	Alive	—
1983[30]	3	IV	G	2: CHOP-like	Death	6	Alive	—
1983[75]	3	—	J	2: COP	Death	—	Alive	—
1983[56]	2	I	I	1: RT; 2: CHOP-like	CR	6	Development failure	72
1984[56]	3	I	G	2: CHOP-like	CR	12	Alive	12
1984[56]	2	IV	J	—	Death	<1	Death	<1
1985[8]	3	IV	G	2: CHOP-like	CR	60	Alive	60
1987[79]	2	III	G	1: CHOP	CR	36	Alive	36
1990[7]	2	IV	G	1: CHOP-like	—	—	Alive	—
1990[7]	1	II	J	1: CHOP-like	—	—	Alive	—
1990[7]	2	IV	G	1: CHOP-like	—	—	Alive	—
1990[7]	1	III	G	1: CHOP-like	—	—	Alive	—
1990[7]	3	IV	H	1: CHOP-like	—	—	Alive	—
1990[7]	1	IV	J	1: CHOP-like	—	—	Alive	—
1990[7]	1	IV	I	1: CHOP-like	—	—	Alive	—
1990[7]	3	III	I	1: CHOP	—	—	Alive	—
1990[7]	1	IV	G	1: CHOP	—	—	Alive	—
1990[7]	2	IV	F	1: CHOP-like	—	—	Alive	—
1990[7]	1	III	G	1: CHOP-like	—	—	Alive	—
1990[7]	2	IV	J	1: CHOP-like	—	—	Alive	—
1990[7]	3	III	G	1: CHOP-like	—	—	Alive	—
1990[7]	1	IV	G	1: CHOP-like	—	—	Alive	—
1990[7]	3	II	F	1: CHOP	—	—	Alive	—
1990[7]	1	IV	G	1: CHOP-like	—	—	Alive	—

[*]Working Formulation subtypes: E, diffuse small cell; F, diffuse mixed; G, diffuse large cell; H, immunoblastic; L, lymphoblastic; J, small noncleaved cell.
PP, postpartum; RT, radiation therapy; CR, complete remission; SA, single-agent chemotherapy; MR, multidrug regimen; COP, cyclophosphamide, Oncovin, prednisone; CHOP = COP + doxorubicin.

Table 31–5. Stage, Histologic Subtype, Treatment, and Maternal and Fetal Outcome of 73 Pregnant Women with Lymphoma (*Continued*)

Year and Reference	Trimester	Stage at Diagnosis	Histologic Subtype°	Treatment During Pregnancy (1) and After Delivery (2)	Maternal Outcome Status	Date (mo)	Fetal Outcome Status	Date (mo)
1990[12]	3	IV	H	2: CHOP-like	CR	—	Alive	—
1990[19]	2	—	H	1: CHOP-like	CR	—	Alive, prematurate	—
1990[10]	2	IV	—	1: MR	—	—	Alive	—
1990[13]	1	—	—	1: RT + SA	CR	—	Alive	5
1990[14]	2	II	G	1: CHOP-like	CR	—	Alive	—
1991[6]	2	—	—	1: CHOP	—	—	Alive	—
1991[6]	1	—	—	1: COP	—	—	Therapeutic abortion	—
1991[6]	1	—	—	1: SA	—	—	Alive	20
1991[6]	1	—	—	1: COP	—	—	Spontaneous abortion	—
1991[5]	3	IV	H	2: MR	CR	24	Alive	24
1992[11]	3	IV	G	2: MR	CR	—	Death	<1
1993[17]	2	IV	G	2: MR	Death	10	Death before term	<1
1993[18]	—	—	—	No treatment	Death	<1	Death in utero	—

°Working Formulation subtypes: E, diffuse small cell; F, diffuse mixed; G, diffuse large cell; H, immunoblast; L, lymphoblastic; J, small noncleaved cell.
PP, postpartum; RT, radiation therapy; CR, complete remission; SA, single-agent chemotherapy; MR, multidrug regimen; COP, cyclophosphamide, Oncovin, prednisone; CHOP = COP + doxorubicin.

31–5), we found 27% of Burkitt's lymphoma, 8% of lymphoblastic lymphoma, and 60% of diffuse large cell lymphoma. None of these women had a low-grade lymphoma. This high percentage of Burkitt's lymphoma is not the proportion usually observed in young patients.

Breast, uterine, and ovarian involvement are often reported during pregnancy, although these localizations are rare in nonpregnant women.[8, 32–45] In our review, among the 45 patients who had correctly described localizations, 13 (28%) had breast involvement, 5 (11%) uterus involvement, and 5 (11%) ovarian involvement. Patients with breast localization usually had a Burkitt's lymphoma subtype, and they typically had a short survival. These organs are obviously stimulated during pregnancy, and their involvement may suggest a hormonal influence on the progress of the lymphoma. Only 3 cases of placenta involvement were reported.[5, 12, 17] Two cases of fetal involvement were reported: in 1 case by an NHL and another case by an HD.[46] Thus, the risk of metastatic involvement of the fetus by the lymphoma appears negligible.

Most NHL occurring during pregnancy had a disseminated stage: 67% were stage IV, 12% stage III, 5% stage II, and 16% stage I (see Table 31–5). One explanation for this pattern may be that diagnosis of the lymphoma is often delayed during pregnancy. Indeed, some of the symptoms that a lymphoma patient may have are often observed during a normal pregnancy, and this may have contributed to an initial misdiagnosis or a delayed diagnosis. In the 37 pregnant NHL women reported by Moore and Taslimi, the correct diagnosis was delayed for more than 3 weeks in 40% of the cases and by more than 3 months in 20%.[11]

It is unclear if pregnancy affects the clinical course of NHL patients. However, in most of the reported cases, there was a relative quiescence of the lymphoma during pregnancy and a rapid clinical progression in the immediate postpartum period.[30, 33] It has been suggested that hormonal and immunologic changes occurring during pregnancy may stabilize the lymphoma cell proliferation until delivery.[29] Ioachim and Moroson verified this clinical observation and demonstrated in animals a maternal and fetal antilymphoma

effect during pregnancy.[31] In pregnant rats inoculated with NHL, cells had a slower growth than in nonpregnant animals and 30% of the pregnant rats remained free of tumor compared with 0% in the nonpregnant group. However, other investigators have suggested that pregnancy has no influence on the NHL course and that response to treatment, failure, and progression rates were similar to those of patients without pregnancy.[47, 48]

EFFECT OF LYMPHOMA ON PREGNANCY

In 1976 Sweet presented a review of pregnant women with HD in which he found no deleterious effect on gestation, delivery, incidence of spontaneous abortions and prematurity, and fetal outcome.[49]

It is more difficult to evaluate the NHL effect on the course of pregnancy because fewer cases were reported and because most of the reported patients died from progressive disease before delivery or after abortion. In 1977, Ortega reported the first successful pregnancy associated with advanced NHL after treatment with a multidrug chemotherapy regimen including cyclophosphamide, vincristine, bleomycin, and prednisone.[50] In a series of 56 pregnant women with associated hematologic malignancies, the incidence of spontaneous abortion, prematurity, and malformations was not different than that observed in a healthy population.[6]

CHEMOTHERAPY AGENTS AND RADIATION TREATMENT DURING PREGNANCY

Treatment choices during pregnancy raise difficult problems because of the putative immediate and delayed adverse effects of chemotherapy and radiation on the fetus.

Immediate adverse effects of antineoplastic agents comprise spontaneous abortion, teratogenicity, organ toxicity, prematurity, and low birth weight. Potential adverse effects include carcinogenesis, sterility, retarded physical and/or mental growth and development, and mutation and teratogenicity in the second generation.

CHEMOTHERAPY AGENTS AND PREGNANCY

Pharmacology of Antineoplastic Agents During Pregnancy. Drug pharmacokinetics may be altered by physiologic changes that occur during pregnancy: the increase in plasma volume results in a dilution of chemotherapy agents; the binding of antineoplastic drugs is modified because of a decreased serum albumin concentration. In addition, the hepatic metabolism is more rapid and there is an increased renal plasma flow, glomerular filtration rate, and creatinine clearance.[51] The transplacental crossing of antineoplastic drugs is conditioned by their physicochemical characteristics: passive diffusion increases with decreasing molecular weight, increasing liposolubility, and decreasing protein-binding capacity.[52] Most of the antineoplastic drugs have a high placental diffusion.

Adverse Effects of Antineoplastic Agents on the Fetus.. The timing of exposure to antineoplastic agents is critical for potential adverse effects. Drug administration during the first weeks after conception produces an all-or-nothing phenomenon that is either a spontaneous abortion or a normal fetus.[53] During the first trimester, when organogenesis occurs, antineoplastic drugs can produce congenital malformations or abortion and should be avoided if possible.[53] However, the incidence of malformations depends on the drug used. Doll and colleagues reported 20% fetal malformations with antimetabolites.[51] Alkylating agents and plant alkaloids were less frequently associated with fetal abnormalities: 1 in 25 cases after an alkylating agent and 1 in 14 after a vinca alkaloid.[51] The prevalence of fetal abnormalities after a multidrug regimen chemotherapy was 16%, and in more than 50% of these cases the regimen included procarbazine. Thus, procarbazine should be avoided whenever possible.[51]

During the second and third trimesters, the use of these drugs is not associated with significant malformations but it may impair fetal growth and functional development. Brain growth continues during this period, and exposure to anticancer drugs after the first trimester may be followed by microcephaly, mental retardation, and impaired learning behavior.[51] No specific adverse event has been related to the use of corticosteroids during pregnancy, and they may be included in any multidrug regimen.

Little is known about possible delayed effects of exposure to antineoplastic agents in utero.

RADIATION TREATMENT AND PREGNANCY

The effects of x-rays on fetal development are estimated from extrapolation of experimental animal irradiation or from accidental and therapeutic human exposure. The classic effects of radiation on the fetal development are congenital malformations, intrauterine growth retardation, and embryonic death. Growth retardation and central nervous system side effects, such as microcephaly and eye malformations, are the cardinal manifestations of intrauterine irradiation.[53, 54] Radiation exposure of 200 or 300 cGy before the 20th week of gestation caused mental retardation, microcephaly, cataracts, retinal degeneration, low birth weight, and skeletal and genital abnormalities.[55] Between 20 and 25 weeks, no organ abnormality occurred, and children were apparently normal except for radiation skin changes similar to those expected in postnatal radiation exposure.[55] The long-term sequelae of fetal radiation exposure are unknown, but they may include an increasing incidence of childhood leukemias or other cancers, chromosome aberrations, or impaired future fertility.[51] There is no safe dose of radiation during pregnancy, and radiation damage follows a dose-response curve. However, most authorities agree that a delivered dose of less than 10 cGy leads to a negligible risk for the fetus.[56]

Therapeutic irradiation in a pregnant women with lymphoma usually involves only supradiaphragmatic fields. Wong and associates have estimated the doses received by the fetus during a mantle field irradiation with 10-MV x-rays. When a dose of 4400 cGy was delivered to the mother on midline of the central axis, doses to the fetus in early, mid, and late pregnancy were estimated to be 63, 88, and 220 cGy, respectively.[57] Therapeutic abortion is recommended for fetal exposure of greater than 10 cGy in the first trimester.[58]

TREATMENT

HODGKIN'S DISEASE

The literature offers a limited consensus for the treatment of pregnant patients with HD. The three largest series concern no more than 15 cases each,[24, 59, 60] and HD treatment has changed these last 10 years with a larger use of chemotherapy even in localized stage patients. Many women have been treated successfully while pregnant without adverse effects for the fetus. Thus, some recommendations may be given regarding timing of the pregnancy, disease stage, and patient's desire of pregnancy.

HD in the first trimester is not an indication for a therapeutic abortion, but it may be proposed when a delay in treatment is unacceptable, or in case of bulky disease, B symptoms, visceral involvement, subdiaphragmatic disease, or rapid disease progression. If continuation of pregnancy is elected despite an urgent need to treat the patient, the experience to date suggests that vinblastine may be used with minimal risk.

Many patients presenting in the second half of pregnancy with a localized disease may be treated only after delivery. If a significant progression occurs and delivery is not possible, a multidrug chemotherapy regimen is the best treatment choice because of the high radiation delivered to the fetus even with abdominal shielding. The multidrug regimen may be modified ABVD (Adriamycin, bleomycin, vinblastine, dacarbazine) without dacarbazine, or a modified CHOP; these regimens are known to be associated with the smallest risk for the fetus.

NON-HODGKIN'S LYMPHOMA

Fetal and Maternal Outcome After Therapy. One hundred thirty-one NHL cases associated with pregnancy were reported in literature. Table 31–5 summarizes the reported 73 women in whom sufficient data were available concerning the date of diagnosis according to the duration of pregnancy, the histologic NHL subtype, the maternal and fetal outcomes, and treatments during and after pregnancy. Maternal outcome was known in 58 of these cases and in only 38 of them the date of followup was known. Among the 73 cases reported in Table 31–5, diagnosis of lymphoma occurred during pregnancy in 66 cases (16 during the first trimester, 27 during the second trimester, and 23 during the third trimester), and it occurred in postpartum in 6 cases. Among the 66 cases where maternal treatment and fetal outcome were known, 13 received chemotherapy or radiation therapy during the first trimester of pregnancy. In 11 of these 13 cases, the infants were delivered alive, in 1 case there was a spontaneous abortion, and in the last one a therapeutic abortion was done. One of the newborns was premature, but none of them showed apparent malformations, although cyclophosphamide was used in 10 cases and methotrexate in 2 cases.[7, 12, 13, 61] Among the 33 women treated with a multidrug regimen or with radiation therapy during the second and the third trimester, 4 gave birth to premature infants and 29 to normal infants. One premature infant died, but all the others were alive in good health. A transitory decrease of leukocyte and platelet counts after birth was reported in 4 of these infants, secondary to maternal treatment with cyclophosphamide during breast-feeding in 1 case.[7, 40]

Among the 58 cases where maternal outcome was reported, 28 patients were alive with a 17-month median followup (range of 6 to 60 months), 26 were in complete remission, and 2 had an active disease. Among the 26 patients who reached a complete remission, 13 were treated with a multidrug chemotherapy regimen during pregnancy and 9 were treated only after delivery. Thirty patients died from the lymphoma: 14 of these patients received a multidrug chemotherapy regimen, 9 during pregnancy and 5 after delivery or abortion. Five of the 6 women who presented NHL during postpartum died with rapidly progressive disease (see Table 31–5). The overall survival of the 38 patients with a known followup is presented in Figure 31–6. These results concern a heterogeneous period longer than 30 years and represent only a fraction of the reported NHL cases in pregnant women, but they show the poor outcome clearly associated with lymphoma during pregnancy. Median duration of survival is only 6 months, and nearly all untreated or incorrectly treated patients died rapidly (Fig. 31–7). In this analysis optimal treatment was defined as the use of single-agent chemotherapy or irradiation in localized stage and as multidrug regimen in disseminated stage.

Recommendations. Lymphomas associated with pregnancy usually have an aggressive histology, and maternal prognosis is poor without an efficient treatment administered as soon as possible, that is, during pregnancy. Treatment with a multidrug regimen may allow patients to reach high complete remission rates and long survival. Multidrug regimens have been used in the second and third trimester without apparent deleterious effect to the fetus.

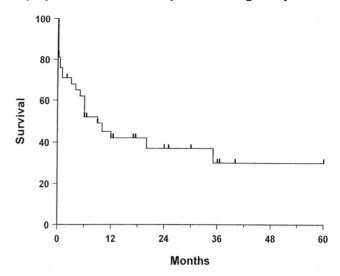

Figure 31–6. Overall survival of 38 pregnant women with lymphoma. To be included in these data a patient should have relevant information described in the original article reporting her case. Only 38 of the 73 women descibed in Table 31–5 have a followup identified. These data must be considered as a good estimate of the survival of pregnant women with lymphoma.

No case of low-grade nodular lymphoma during pregnancy has been reported. However, in a pregnant woman with a low-grade lymphoma treatment may be delayed until delivery when staging can be completed and appropriate therapy instituted.

Women with an aggressive lymphoma during the first trimester should be considered for a therapeutic abortion and immediate multidrug regimen treatment. In a small fraction of these patients with stage I lymphoma, localized irradiation or no treatment may be realized till the second trimester of pregnancy, when a multidrug regimen may be

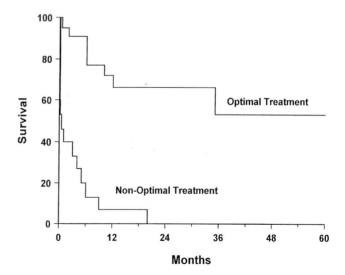

Figure 31–7. Overall survival of the 38 pregnant women with lymphoma included in Figure 31–6 according to the type of treatment they have received for the lymphoma. "Optimal treatment" was defined as the use of single-agent chemotherapy or local radiation therapy for localized-stage patients and as the use of a multidrug regimen for disseminated-stage patients.

proposed without adverse effect for the fetus. In patients with disseminated disease, supradiaphragmatic radiation therapy or single-drug chemotherapy to stabilize the disease until the second trimester is not a valid option for the mother. However, when the patient and the family refuse therapeutic abortion, a decision regarding treatment must be made that balances the prognosis of the mother and the hazards to the fetus.

During the second and third trimester of pregnancy, patients must be treated with full doses of a multidrug regimen known to have efficacy in this lymphoma subtype because the risk of teratogenicity is absent, although the possibility that the child may develop a malignancy in early life has not been evaluated.

In a woman patient treated for HD or NHL and free from disease for 2 years, is there any risk to envisage a pregnancy? This is a crucial problem for these young patients, but no good evidence may be found in the literature. The absence of reported studies demonstrating an adverse effect of pregnancy on the course of a cure regimen for HD may be acknowledged as the absence of effect and, in fact, it is the opinion of the authors that pregnancy is not associated with an increased risk of progression in a patient in stable response after correct treatment. This may be true for NHL patients, but no more evidence has been presented in the literature. In our experience we have seen 22 women who became pregnant after being successfully treated for an NHL and none of them had an NHL recurrence.

REFERENCES

Non-Hodgkin's Lymphoma in Elderly Patients

1. Rabkin CS, Devesa SS, Zahm SH, Gail MH: Increasing incidence of non-Hodgkin's lymphoma. Semin Hematol 1993; 30:286.
2. d'Amore F, Brincker H, Christensen BE: Non-Hodgkin's lymphoma in the elderly: A study of 602 patients aged 70 or older from a Danish population-based registry. Ann Oncol 1992; 3:379.
3. Moller Jensen O, Estève J, Moller H, Renard H: Cancer in the European Community and its member states. Eur J Cancer 1990; 12:1167.
4. Dumontet C, Anderson JR, Sebban C, et al: Elderly non-Hodgkin's lymphoma patients have comparable prognostic factors but a poorer outcome than younger patients [Abstract 1118]. *In* 11th American Society of Clinical Oncology Meeting, 1992, San Diego, p 328.
5. Berger F, Felman P, Sonet A, et al: Nonfollicular small B-cell lymphomas: A heterogenous group of patients with distinct clinical features and outcome. Blood 1994; 83:2829.
6. Carbone A, Tirelli U, Volpe R, et al: Non-Hodgkin's lymphoma in the elderly: A retrospective clinicopathologic study of 50 patients. Cancer 1986; 57:2185.
7. Carbone A, Volpe R, Gloghini A, et al: Non-Hodgkin's lymphoma in the elderly: I. Pathologic features at presentation. Cancer 1990; 66:1991.
8. Hoerni B, Sotto JJ, Eghbali H, et al: Non-Hodgkin's malignant lymphomas in patients older than 80: 70 cases. Cancer 1988; 61:2057.
9. Ansell SM, Falkson G, van der Merwe R, Uys A: Chronological age is a multifactorial prognostic variable in patients with non-Hodgkin's lymphoma. Ann Oncol 1992; 3:45.
10. Dixon DO, Neilan B, Jones SE, et al: Effect of age on therapeutic outcome in advanced diffuse histiocytic lymphoma: The Southwest Oncology Group experience. J Clin Oncol 1986; 4:295.
11. Vose JM, Armitage JO, Weisenburger DD, et al: The importance of age in survival of patients treated with chemotherapy for aggressive non-Hodgkin's lymphoma. J Clin Oncol 1988; 6:1838.
12. Armitage JO, Potter JF: Aggressive chemotherapy for diffuse histiocytic lymphoma in the elderly: Increased complications with advancing age. J Am Geriatr Soc 1984; 32:269.
13. Solal-Celigny P, Chastang C, Herrera A, et al: Age as the main prognostic factor in adult aggressive non-Hodgkin's lymphoma. Am J Med 1987; 83:1075.
14. International Non-Hodgkin's Lymphoma Prognostic Factors Project: A predictive model for aggressive non-Hodgkin's lymphoma. N Engl J Med 1993; 329:987.
15. Stein RS, Greer JP, Flexner JM, et al: Large cell lymphomas: Clinical and prognostic features. J Clin Oncol 1990; 8:1370.
16. Coiffier B, Gisselbrecht C, Vose JM, et al: Prognostic factors in aggressive malignant lymphomas: Description and validation of a prognostic index that could identify patients requiring a more intensive therapy. J Clin Oncol 1991; 9:211.
17. Velasquez WS, Jagannath S, Tucker SL, et al: Risk classification as the basis for clinical staging of diffuse large cell lymphoma derived from 10-year survival data. Blood 1989; 74:551.
18. Hayward RL, Leonard RCF, Prescott RJ: A critical analysis of prognostic factors for survival in intermediate- and high-grade non-Hodgkin's lymphoma. Br J Cancer 1991; 63:945.
19. Coiffier B, Bryon PA, French M, et al: Intensive chemotherapy in aggressive lymphomas: Updated results of LNH-80 protocol and prognostic factors affecting response and survival. Blood 1987; 70:1394.
20. Grogan L, Corbally N, Dervan PA, et al: Comparable prognostic factors and survival in elderly patients with aggressive non-Hodgkin's lymphoma treated with standard-dose Adriamycin-based regimens. Ann Oncol 1994; 5:47s.
21. Salles G, Shipp MA, Coiffier B: Chemotherapy of non-Hodgkin's aggressive lymphomas. Semin Hematol 1994; 31:46.
22. Coiffier B: How should prognostic factors influence therapy in follicular lymphomas? Ann Oncol 1991; 2:619.
23. Coiffier B, Bastion Y, Berger F, et al: Prognostic factors in follicular lymphomas. Semin Oncol 1993; 20:89.
24. Horning SJ: Low-grade lymphoma, 1993: State of the art. Ann Oncol 1994; 5:23s.
25. Horning SJ: Treatment approaches to the low-grade lymphomas. Blood 1994; 83:881.
26. Richards M, Hall P, Gregory W, et al: Lymphoplasmocytoid and small cell centrocytic non-Hodgkin's lymphoma: A retrospective analysis from St. Bartholomew's Hospital. Hematol Oncol 1989; 7:29.
27. Whelan JS, Davis CL, Rule S, et al: Fludarabine phosphate for the treatment of low-grade lymphoid malignancy. Br J Cancer 1991; 64:120.
28. Tigaud JD, Demolombe S, Bastion Y, et al: Ifosfamide continuous infusion plus etoposide in the treatment of elderly patients with aggressive lymphoma: A phase II study. Hematol Oncol 1991; 9:225.
29. Fisher RI, Gaynor ER, Dahlberg S, et al: Comparison of a standard regimen (CHOP) with three intensive chemotherapy regimens for advanced non-Hodgkin's lymphoma. N Engl J Med 1993; 328:1002.
30. Orlandi E, Lazzarino M, Brusamolino E, et al: Non-Hodgkin's lymphoma in the elderly: The impact of advanced age on therapeutic options and clinical results. Haematologica 1991; 76:204.
31. Armitage JO, Dick FR, Corder MP, et al: Predicting therapeutic outcome in patients with diffuse histiocytic lymphoma treated with cyclophosphamide, Adriamycin, vincristine, and prednisone (CHOP). Cancer 1982; 50:1695.
32. O'Connell MJ, Earle JD, Harrington DP, et al: Initial chemotherapy doses for elderly patients with malignant lymphoma. J Clin Oncol 1986; 4:1418.
33. Sonneveld P, Michiels JJ: Full-dose chemotherapy in elderly patients with non-Hodgkin's lymphoma: A feasibility study using a mitoxantrone-containing regimen. Br J Cancer 1990; 62:105.
34. Sonneveld P, Hop W, Mulder AH, et al: Full-dose chemotherapy for non-Hodgkin's lymphoma in the elderly. Semin Hematol 1994; 31:s9.
35. Arai N, Hara A, Kaneko H, Shirai T: The COP/BLAM therapy for non-Hodgkin's lymphoma in elderly patients. Nippon Ronen Igakkai Zasshi 1990; 27:357.
36. Kitamura K, Tabaru F: Pirarubicin, a novel derivative of doxorubicin: THP-COP therapy for non-Hodgkin's lymphoma in the elderly. Am J Clin Oncol 1990; 13:s15.
37. Coiffier B, Gisselbrecht C, Bosly A, et al: Treatment of Aggressive Lymphomas in Patients Older than 69 Years: First Interim Report of a Randomized Study from the GELA. Fourth International Conference on Malignant Lymphoma, Lugano, Switzerland, June 1990.
38. Zinzani PL, Bendandi M, Gherlinzoni F, et al: VNCOP-B regimen in the treatment of high-grade non-Hodgkin's lymphoma in the elderly. Haematologica 1993; 78:378.
39. Zagonel V, Babare R, Merola MC, et al: Cost-benefit of granulocyte colony-stimulating factor administration in older patients with non-

Hodgkin's lymphoma treated with combination chemotherapy. Ann Oncol 1994; 5:s127.

40. Tirelli U, Zagonel V, Errante D: A prospective study of a new combination chemotherapy regimen in patients older than 70 years with unfavorable non-Hodgkin's lymphoma. J Clin Oncol 1992; 10:228.

41. Tirelli U, Zagonel V, Serraino D, et al: Non-Hodgkin's lymphomas in 137 patients aged 70 years or older: A retrospective European Organization for Research and Treatment of Cancer Lymphoma Group study. J Clin Oncol 1988; 6:1708.

42. Tirelli U, Zagonel V, Sorio R, et al: Mitoxantrone in combination with etoposide and prednimustine in patients older than 70 years with unfavorable non-Hodgkin's lymphoma: A prospective study in 52 patients. Semin Hematol 1994; 31:s13.

43. Salvagno L, Contu A, Bianco A: A combination of mitoxantrone, etoposide, and prednisone in elderly patients with non-Hodgkin's lymphoma. Ann Oncol 1992; 3:833.

44. O'Reilly SE, Klimo P, Connors JM: Low-dose ACOP-B and VABE: Weekly chemotherapy for elderly patients with advanced stage diffuse large cell lymphoma. J Clin Oncol 1991; 9:741.

45. O'Reilly SE, Connors JM, Howdle S, et al: In search of an optimal regimen for elderly patients with advanced-stage diffuse large cell lymphoma: Results of a phase II study of P/DOCE chemotherapy. J Clin Oncol 1993; 11:2250.

46. McMaster ML, Johnson DH, Greer JP, et al: A brief-duration combination chemotherapy for elderly patients with poor-prognosis non-Hodgkin's lymphoma. Cancer 1991; 67:1487.

47. Goss PE, Burkes R, Rudinskas L, et al: Prednisone, oral etoposide, and Novantrone for treatment of non-Hodgkin's lymphoma: A preliminary report. Semin Hematol 1994; 31:s23.

48. Martelli M, Guglielmi C, Coluzzi S, et al: P-VABEC: A prospective study of a new weekly chemotherapy regimen for elderly aggressive non-Hodgkin's lymphoma. J Clin Oncol 1993; 11:2362.

49. Brice P, Lepage E, Gisselbrecht C, et al: Aggressive non-Hodgkin lymphoma in the elderly: A retrospective study of 72 patients with clinical features and treatment. Nouv Rev Fr Hematol 1990; 32:153.

50. Ansell SM, Falkson G: A phase II trial of chemotherapy combination in elderly patients with aggressive lymphoma. Ann Oncol 1993; 4:172.

51. Tirelli U, Carbone A, Zagonel V, et al: Non-Hodgkin's lymphomas in the elderly: Prospective studies with specifically devised chemotherapy regimens in 66 patients. Eur J Cancer Clin Oncol 1987; 23:535.

52. Sonneveld P, Deridder M, Vanderlelie H, et al: Comparison of doxorubicin and mitoxantrone in the treatment of elderly patients with advanced diffuse non-Hodgkin's lymphoma using CHOP versus CNOP chemotherapy. J Clin Oncol 1995; 13:2530.

53. Meyer RM, Browman GP, Samosh ML, et al: Randomized phase II comparison of standard CHOP with weekly CHOP in elderly patients with non-Hodgkin's lymphoma. J Clin Oncol 1995; 13:2386.

Lymphoma and Pregnancy

1. Riva HL, Andreson PS, O'Grady JW: Pregnancy and Hodgkin's disease: A report of eight cases. Am J Obstet Gynecol 1953; 66:866.

2. Haas JF: Pregnancy in association with a newly diagnosed cancer: A population-based epidemiologic assessment. Int J Cancer 1984; 34:229.

3. du Bois A, Meerpohl HG, Gerner K, et al: Einfluss einer Schwangerschaft auf Inzidenz und Verlauf von Malignomerkrankungen. Geburtshilfe Frauenheilkd 1993; 53:619.

4. d'Amore F, Brincker H, Christensen BE, et al: Non-Hodgkin's lymphoma in the elderly: A study of 602 patients aged 70 or older from a Danish population-based registry. Ann Oncol 1992; 3:379.

5. Kurtin PJ, Gaffey TA, Habermann TM: Peripheral T-cell lymphoma involving the placenta. Cancer 1992; 70:2963.

6. Zuazu J, Julia A, Sierra J, et al: Pregnancy outcome in hematologic malignancies. Cancer 1991; 67:703.

7. Aviles A, Diaz-Maqueo JC, Torras V, et al: Non-Hodgkin's lymphomas and pregnancy: Presentation of 16 cases. Gynecol Oncol 1990; 37:335.

8. Roumen FJ, de Leeuw JW, van der Linden PJ, Pannebakker MA: Non-Hodgkin's lymphoma of the puerperal uterus. Obstet Gynecol 1990; 75:527.

9. Toki H, Okabe K, Kamei H, et al: Successful chemotherapy on a pregnant non-Hodgkin's lymphoma patient. Acta Med Okayama 1990; 44:321.

10. du Bois A, Runge M, Schmid J, Hillemanns HG: Disseminiertes, hochmalignes Non-Hodgkin-Lymphom und Schwangerschaft: Poly-chemothrapie im 2. und 3. Trimester. Geburtshilfe Frauenheilkd 1990; 50:405.

11. Moore DT, Taslimi MM: Non-Hodgkin's lymphoma in pregnancy: A diagnostic dilemma: Case report and review of the literature. J Tenn Med Assoc 1992; 85:467.

12. Pollack RN, Sklarin NT, Rao S, Divon MY: Metastatic placental lymphoma associated with maternal human immunodeficiency virus infection. Obstet Gynecol 1993; 81:856.

13. Ba-Thike K, Oo N: Non-Hodgkin's lymphoma in pregnancy. Asia Oceania J Obstet Gynaecol 1990; 16:229.

14. Lambert J, Wijermans PW, Dekker GA, Ossenkoppele GJ: Chemotherapy in non-Hodgkin's lymphoma during pregnancy. Neth J Med 1991; 38:80.

15. Valenzuela PL, Montalban C, Matorras R, et al: Pregnancy and relapse of peripheral T-cell lymphoma: A case report. Gynecol Obstet Invest 1991; 32:59.

16. Engert A, Lathan B, Cremer R, et al: Non-Hodgkin-Lymphom und Schwangerschaft. Med Klin 1990; 85:734.

17. Tsujimura T, Matsumoto K, Aozasa K: Placental involvement by maternal non-Hodgkin's lymphoma. Arch Pathol Lab Med 1993; 117:325.

18. Morice P, Cristalli B, Heid M, Briere J, Levardon M: Grossesse et lymphome non-hodgkinien: Un cas. J Gynecol Obstet Biol Reprod 1993; 22:68.

19. Nantel S, Parboosingh J, Poon MC: Treatment of an aggressive non-Hodgkin's lymphoma during pregnancy with MACOP-B chemotherapy. Med Pediatr Oncol 1990; 18:143.

20. Garg A, Kochupillai V: Non-Hodgkin's lymphoma in pregnancy. South Med J 1985; 78:1263.

21. Lishner M, Zelickis D, Sutcliffe SB, Koren G: Non-Hodgkin's lymphoma and pregnancy. Leuk Lymphoma 1994; 14:411.

22. Ohba T, Matsuo I, Katabuchi H, et al: Adult T-cell leukemia/lymphoma in pregnancy. Obstet Gynecol 1988; 72:445.

23. Olsson H, Olsson ML, Ranstam J: Late age at first full-term pregnancy as a risk factor for women with malignant lymphoma. Neoplasma 1990; 37:185.

24. Thomas PRM, Peckham MJ: The investigation and management of Hodgkin's disease in the pregnant patient. Cancer 1976; 38:1443.

25. Consensus Conference: Magnetic resonance imaging. JAMA 1988; 259:2132.

26. Barry RM, Diamond HD, Graver LF: Influence of pregnancy on the course of Hodgkin's disease. Am J Obstet Gynecol 1962; 84:445.

27. Gobbi PG, Attardo-Parrinello G, Danesino M, et al: Hodgkin's disease and pregnancy. Haematologica 1984; 69:336.

28. Jouet JP, Buchet-Bouverne B, Fenaux P, et al: Influence de la grossesse sur lévolutivité de la maladie de Hodgkin? Presse Méd 1988; 17:423.

29. Ward FT, Weiss RB: Lymphoma and pregnancy. Semin Oncol 1989; 16:397.

30. Steiner-Salz D, Yahalom J, Samuelov A, Polliack A: Non-Hodgkin's lymphoma associated with pregnancy: A report of six cases, with a review of the literature. Cancer 1985; 56:2087.

31. Ioachim HL, Moroson H: Lymphoma and pregnancy: Clinical observations and experimental investigations. Leukemia 1994; 8:s198.

32. Armitage JO, Feagler JR, Skoog DP: Burkitt lymphoma during pregnancy with bilateral breast involvement. JAMA 1977; 237:151.

33. Ioachim HL: Non-Hodgkin's lymphoma in pregnancy: Three cases and review of the literature. Arch Pathol Lab Med 1985; 109:803.

34. Ludanyi VI, Donko A: Retikulosarkom in der Gravidität. Zentralbl Gynäkol 1969; 49:1609.

35. Shepherd JJ, Wright DH: Burkitt's tumour presenting as bilateral swelling of the breast in women of child-bearing age. Br J Surg 1967; 54:776.

36. Henderson M, Paterson WG: Perforation of jejunum by reticulum cell sarcoma in pregnancy. Am J Surg 1968; 115:385.

37. Bergamaschi P, Magni M, Ricevuti G: Reticulosarcoma in gravidanza: Studio anatomoclinico. Ann Obstet Gin Med Perin 1973; 94:255.

38. Finkle HI, Goldman RL: Burkitt's lymphoma: Gynecologic considerations. Obstet Gynecol 1974; 43:281.

39. Vieaux JW, McGuire DE: Reticulum cell sarcoma of the cervix. Am J Obstet Gynecol 1964; 89:134.

40. Durudola JI: Administration of cyclophosphamide during late pregnancy and early lactation: A case report. J Natl Med Assoc 1979; 71:165.

41. Tunca JC, Reddi PR, Shah SH, Slack ST: Malignant non-Hodgkin's–type lymphoma of the cervix uteri occurring during pregnancy. Gynecol Oncol 1979; 7:385.
42. Jones DED, d'Avignon MB, Lawrence R, Latshaw RF: Burkitt's lymphoma: Obstetric and gynecologic aspects. Obstet Gynecol 1980; 56:533.
43. Arber DA, Simpson JF, Weiss LM, Rappaport H: Non-Hodgkin's lymphoma involving the breast. Am J Surg Pathol 1994; 18:288.
44. Azouri J, Afif N, Ghosn M, et al: Lymphome primitif du sein: A propos d'un cas. J Med Liban 1992; 40:202.
45. Bobrow LG, Richards MA, Happerfield LC, et al: Breast lymphomas: A clinicopathologic review. Hum Pathol 1993; 24:274.
46. Rothman LA, Cohen CJ, Astarlova J: Placental and fetal involvement by maternal malignancy: A report of rectal carcinoma and review of literature. Am J Obstet Gynecol 1973; 116:1023.
47. Aviles A: Peripheral T-cell lymphoma involving the placenta. Cancer 1993; 72:300.
48. du Bois A, Meerpohl HG, Gerner K, et al: Schwangerschaftsverlauf bei Patientinnen mit Malignomen. Geburtshilfe Frauenheilkd 1993; 53:547.
49. Sweet DL: Malignant lymphoma: Implications during the reproductive years and pregnancy. J Reprod Med 1976; 17:198.
50. Ortega J: Multiple agent chemotherapy including bleomycin of non-Hodgkin's lymphoma during pregnancy. Cancer 1977; 40:2829.
51. Doll DC, Ringenberg S, Yarbo JW: Antineoplastic agents and pregnancy. Semin Oncol 1989; 16:337.
52. Delmer A, Bauduer F, Ajchenbaum-Cymbalista F, et al: Grossesse et hémopathies malignes: Approche thérapeutique. Bull Cancer 1994; 81:277.
53. Miller RW, Mulvihill JJ: Small head size after atomic irradiation: Teratogen update. Teratology 1976; 14:355.
54. Dekaban AS: Abnormalities in children exposed to X irradiation during various stages of gestation: Tentative timetable of radiation injury to the human fetus. J Nucl Med 1968; 9:471.
55. Orr JW, Shingleton HM: Cancer in pregnancy. Curr Probl Cancer 1983; 8:1.
56. Spitzer M, Citron M, Ilardi CF, Saxe B: Non-Hodgkin's lymphoma during pregnancy. Gynecol Oncol 1991; 43:309.
57. Wong PS, Rosemark PJ, Wexler MC, et al: Doses to organs at risk from mantle-field radiation therapy using 10 MV x-rays. Mt Sinai J Med 1985; 52:216.
58. Hammer-Jacobsen E: Therapeutic abortion on account of x-ray examination during pregnancy. Dan Med Bull 1959; 6:122.
59. Niesce LZ, Tome MA, He S, et al: Management of coexisting Hodgkin's disease and pregnancy. Am J Clin Oncol 1986; 9:146.
60. Jacobs C, Donaldson SS, Rosenberg SA, Kaplan HS: Management of the pregnant patient with Hodgkin's disease. Ann Intern Med 1981; 95:669.
61. Schapira DV, Chudley AE: Successful pregnancy following continuous treatment with combination chemotherapy before conception and throughout pregnancy. Cancer 1984; 54:800.
62. Lysyj A, Bergquist JR: Pregnancy complicated by sarcoma: Report of two cases. Obstet Gynecol 1963; 21:506.
63. Bannerman RHO: Burkitt's tumour in pregnancy. Br Med J 1966; 2:1136.
64. Mehta A, Vakil RM: Use of Endoxan in case of lymphosarcoma with pregnancy during the third trimester. Indian J Cancer 1966; 3:198.
65. Leeks SR: Lymphosarcoma complicating pregnancy. NZ J Med 1966; 65:465.
66. Hardin JA: Cyclophosphamide treatment of lymphoma during third trimester of pregnancy. Obstet Gynecol 1972; 39:850.
67. Inoue Y, Masuda H, Shiojima Y: Pregnancy complicated by sarcoma. Acta Obstet Gynaecol Jpn 1972; 19:222.
68. Armon PJ: Burkitt's lymphoma of the ovary in association with pregnancy: Two case reports. Br J Obstet Gynaecol 1976; 83:169.
69. Case BW, Benaroya S: Dyspnea in a pregnant young woman. Can Med Assoc J 1980; 122:890.
70. Falkson HC, Simson IW, Falkson G: Non-Hodgkin's lymphoma in pregnancy. Cancer 1980; 45:1679.
71. Villasanta U, Attar S, Jiji R: Malignant histiocytic lymphoma (reticulum cell sarcoma) in pregnancy. Gynecol Oncol 1978; 6:383.
72. Bornkamm GW, Kaduk B, Kachel G, et al: Epstein-Barr virus–positive Burkitt's lymphoma in a German woman during pregnancy. Blut 1980; 40:167.
73. Cheson BD, Johnston JL, Junco DD, Kjeldsberg CR: Cytologic evidence for disseminated immunoblastic lymphoma. Am J Clin Pathol 1981; 75:621.
74. Lowenthal RM, Funnell CF, Hope DM, et al: Normal infant after combination chemotherapy including teniposide for Burkitt's lymphoma in pregnancy. Med Pediatr Oncol 1982; 10:165.
75. Berrebi A, Schattner A, Mogilner BM: Disseminated Burkitt's lymphoma during pregnancy. Acta Haematol 1983; 70:139.

Index

Note: Page numbers in *italics* indicate illustrations; those followed by t indicate tables.

ISBN 0-7216-5030-9

9 780721 650302

DATE DUE

SEP 1 4 1998			